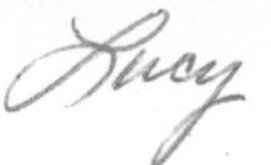

Formulas for drug calculations

Surface area rule:

$$\text{Child dose} = \frac{\text{Surface area (m}^2\text{)}}{1.73\text{m}^2} \times \text{Adult dose}$$

Calculating strength of a solution:

Solution Strength: *Desired Solution:*

$$\frac{x}{100} = \frac{\text{Amount of drug desired}}{\text{Amount of finished solution}}$$

Calculating flow rate for IV:

$$\text{Rate of Flow} = \frac{\text{Amount of fluid} \times \text{Administration set calibration}}{\text{Running time}}$$

$$\frac{x}{1} = \frac{\text{(ml) (gtt/min)}}{\text{min}}$$

Calculation of medication dosages:

Formula method:

$$\frac{\text{Amount ordered}}{\text{Amount on hand}} \times \text{Vehicle}$$

$$= \text{Number of tablets, capsules, or amount of liquid}$$

Vehicle is the drug form or amount of liquid containing the dosage. Amounts used in calculation by formula must be in the same system.

Ratio—proportion method:

1 tablet: tablet in mg on hand:: x tablet order in mg
Know or have:: Want to know or order

Multiply means and extremes, divide both sides by known amount to get X. Amounts used in equation must be in same system.

Dimensional analysis method:

$$\text{Order in mg} \times \frac{\text{1 tablet or capsule}}{\text{What 1 tablet or capsule is in mg}}$$

$$= \text{Tablets or capsules to be given}$$

If amounts are in different systems:

$$\text{Order in mg} \times \frac{\text{1 tablet or capsule}}{\text{What 1 tablet or capsule is in g}} \times \frac{1}{\text{1000 mg}}$$

$$= \text{Tablets or capsules to be given}$$

Mosby's

1993 Nursing Drug Reference

Linda Skidmore-Roth, R.N., M.S.N., N.P.

Formerly, New Mexico State University,
Nursing Faculty, Las Cruces, New Mexico;
El Paso Community College, El Paso, Texas

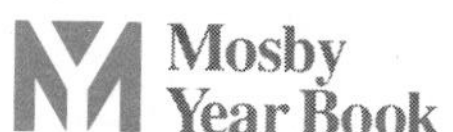

St. Louis Baltimore Boston Chicago London Philadelphia Sydney Toronto

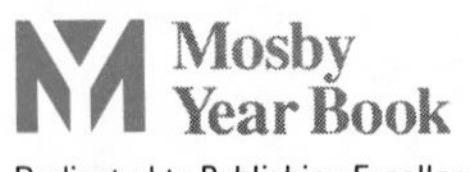

Dedicated to Publishing Excellence

Executive Editor: Don Ladig
Managing Editor: Robin Carter
Editorial Assistant: Chris Kuehne
Project Manager: Gayle May Morris
Production Editor: Mary Cusick Drone
Design: Elizabeth Fett

A NOTE TO THE READER

The authors and publisher have made every attempt to check dosages and nursing content for accuracy. Because the science of pharmacology is continually advancing, our knowledge base continues to expand. Therefore, we recommend that the reader always check product information for changes in dosage or administration before administering any medication. This is particularly important with new or rarely used drugs.

Printed in the United States of America

Mosby–Year Book, Inc.
11830 Westline Industrial Drive
St. Louis, Missouri 63146

ISSN 1044-8470
ISBN 0-8016-6662-7

GW/D 9 8 7 6 5 4 3 2 1

Clinical nursing consultants

Marie B. Andrews, R.N., Ph.D.
Lecturer, Texas Woman's University, Houston, Texas

Janet T. Barrett, R.N., Ph.D.
Director, BSN Program, Deaconess College of Nursing, St. Louis, Missouri

Alice Bledig, R.N., Ph.D.
Professor, Southeastern Illinois Community College, Harrisburg, Illinois

Donnie F. Booth, R.N., Ph.D.
Director, School of Nursing, Southeastern Louisiana University, Hammond, Louisiana

Ruth Bowen, R.N., M.S.
Lecturer, Texas Woman's University, Denton, Texas

June Chandler, R.N., Ed.D.
Instructor, Florida Community College, Jacksonville, Florida

Rosemary Chappell, R.N., M.S.
Coordinator, Undergraduate Curriculum, South Dakota State University, College of Nursing, Brookings, South Dakota

Mary Lou Cheatham, R.N., M.S.N.
Associate Professor, Ball State University, Muncie, Indiana

Leah M. Cleveland, R.N., Ed.D.
Professor, Saddleback College, Mission Viejo, California

Mary B. Gardner, R.N., M.S.
Lecturer, Assumption College, Worcester, Massachusetts

Barbara H. Goodkin, R.N., M.S.
Instructor, Washtenaw Community College, Ann Arbor, Michigan

Brenda Goodner, R.N., M.S.N., C.S.
Assistant Professor, Abilene Intercollegiate School of Nursing, Abilene, Texas

Jyneal Linton Greer, R.N., M.S.N.
Instructor, Nursing, Normandale Community College, Bloomington, Minnesota

Kathy Gutierrez, R.N., M.S.N.
Assistant Professor, Loretto Heights College, Denver, Colorado

Milly Gutkoski, R.N.C., M.N.
Assistant Professor, Montana State University, Bozeman, Montana

Mark Hamelink, R.N., M.S.N., C.R.N.A.
Lakeshore Anesthesia, P.C., South Haven, Michigan

Jane Hartsock, R.N., M.A.
Instructor, Nursing, Minneapolis Community College, Minneapolis, Minnesota

Patricia Hong, R.N., M.A.
Instructor, Anchorage Community College, Anchorage, Alaska

Joan M. Jenks, R.N., M.S.N.
Assistant Professor, Thomas Jefferson University, Philadelphia, Pennsylvania

Barbara Johnst
Assistant Profess
College, Rockvil
York

Linda L. Lilley, R.N., M.S.
Assistant Professor, Old Dominion University, Norfolk, Virginia

Edwina McConnell, R.N., Ph.D.
Independent Nurse Consultant, Madison, Wisconsin

Bernadette Maucher McKay, R.N.C., M.S.
Nurse Practitioner and Assistant Professor, School of Nursing, The University of Texas, Galveston, Texas

Cheryl Macejkovik, R.N., M.S.
Adult Health Instructor, University of North Dakota, Grand Forks, North Dakota

Suzanne E. Malloy, R.N., M.S.N.
Assistant Professor, San Jose State University, San Jose, California

Marylou Medlin, R.N., B.S.N., M.N.
Instructor, Charity Hospital School of Nursing, New Orleans, Louisiana

Michaelene P. Mirr, R.N., Ph.D., C.C.R.N.
Assistant Professor, School of Nursing, University of Wisconsin-Eau Claire, Eau Claire, Wisconsin

Shirley Moore, R.N., M.S.N., M.S.
Faculty, Barnes College, St. Louis, Missouri

M. Joan Owen, R.N., M.A.
Instructor, Mesa College, Mesa, Arizona

Judy A. Peterson, R.N., M.S.N., C.S.
Associate Professor, University of Alaska, Anchorage, Alaska

Celeste Phillips, R.N., Ed.D.
Principal, Phillips & Fenwick, [illegible]cotts Valley, California

[illegible]ele Poradzisz, R.N., M.S.
[illegible]r, De Paul University, [illegible]linois

Joyce Powers, R.N., M.S.N., C.S.
Clinical Nurse Specialist, Cardiology Consultants, Albuquerque, New Mexico

Camille Rabitoy, R.N., M.A.Ed.
Nursing Educator, Bay de Noc Community College, Escanaba, Michigan

Tracy Riley, R.N., B.S.N.
Instructor, Aultman Hospital School of Nursing, Canton, Ohio

Carol Ruscin, R.N., B.S.
Level I Faculty, Baptist Medical System School of Nursing, Little Rock, Arkansas

Robert E. St. John, R.N., R.R.T., B.S.N., B.A.
Cardiopulmonary Nurse Clinician, Jewish Hospital, St. Louis, Missouri

Jean Schneewind, R.N., M.S.N.
Assistant Professor, Imperial Valley College, Imperial, California

Brenda K. Shelton, R.N., B.S., C.C.R.N., O.C.N.
Critical Care Instructor, The Johns Hopkins Oncology Center, Baltimore, Maryland

Cynthia Mills Spiro, R.N., M.S.N.
Faculty, Barnes College, St. Louis, Missouri

Carol A. Stephenson, R.N., Ed.D.
Associate Professor, Texas Christian University, Fort Worth, Texas

Ruth Stieglitz-Hooley, R.N., Ph.D.
Associate Professor, University of Wyoming, Laramie, Wyoming

Regina Stroud, R.N., M.S.
Instructor, Rancho Santiago College, Santa Ana, California

Janice A. Traylor, R.N., M.Ed., M.S.
Instructor, Nursing, Casper College, Casper, Wyoming

Richard E. Watters, R.N., M.Ed.
Nursing Consultant, Wembley, Western Australia

Pamela Becker Weilitz, R.N., M.S.N. (R)
Clinical Nurse Specialist, Barnes Hospital at Washington University Medical Center, St. Louis, Missouri

Judith M. Wilkinson, R.N.C., M.A., M.S.N.
Instructor, Johnson County Community College, Overland Park, Kansas

Rita Yaeger, R.N., M.S.N., M.A.
Associate Professor of Nursing, West Virginia Northern Community College, Wheeling, West Virginia

---

Clinical pharmacology consultants

Carmen Aceves-Blumenthal, M.S., R.Ph.
Assistant Professor, Southeastern College of Pharmaceutical Sciences, North Miami Beach, Florida

Richard H. Alper, Ph.D.
Assistant Professor, University of Kansas Medical Center, Kansas City, Kansas

Danial E. Baker, Pharm.D.
Assistant Professor, Washington State University, Pullman, Washington

R. Keith Campbell, Pharm.D.
Professor, Washington State University, Pullman, Washington

Catherine Celestin, Pharm.D.
Assistant Professor, Southeastern College of Pharmaceutical Sciences, North Miami Beach, Florida

Bruce D. Clayton, Pharm.D.
Professor, University of Arkansas, Little Rock, Arkansas

Edward H. Clouse, Ph.D.
Associate Professor, Southeastern College of Pharmaceutical Sciences, North Miami Beach, Florida

Jackson Como, Pharm.D.
Supervisor, Drug Information Service, University of Alabama, Birmingham, Alabama

David E. Domann, M.S., F.A.S.C.P.
Professional Services Manager, E.R. Squibb and Sons, Princeton, New Jersey

Mark W. Garrison, Pharm.D.
Assistant Professor of Pharmacy, Washington State University at Spokane, Spokane, Washington

William Gerthoffer, Ph.D.
Associate Professor, University of Nevada School of Medicine, Reno, Nevada

Patricia A. Howard, B.S., R.Ph.
Clinical Instructor, University of Kansas Medical Center, Kansas City, Kansas

Norman Keltner, R.N., Ed.D.
Associate Professor, California State University, Bakersfield, California

James Lipp, Ph.D.
Associate Professor, Grand Valley State University, Allendale, Michigan

Lori A. Mangels, B.S.
Pharmacologist, The University of Michigan Medical School, Ann Arbor, Michigan

Judith K. Marquis, Ph.D.
Assistant Professor, Boston University School of Medicine, Boston, Massachusetts

Bozena B. Michniak, Ph.D., M.P.S.
Assistant Professor, University of South Carolina, Columbia, South Carolina

Keith M. Olsen, Pharm.D.
Assistant Professor, University of Arkansas, Little Rock, Arkansas

Robert T. Reilly, Pharm.D.
Assistant Director of Pharmacy, Clinical Services, Thomason Hospital, El Paso, Texas

Roberta J. Secrest, Ph.D., Pharm.D., R.Ph.
Senior Research Pharmacologist, Marion Merrell Dow Research Institute, Indianapolis, Indiana

Kay See-Lasley, M.S.
Pharmacology Consultant, Lawrence, Kansas

Roberta J. Secrest, Ph.D., R.Ph.
Associate Scientist, Marion Merrell Dow Research Institute, Indianapolis, Indiana

Donald J. Sefcik, D.O., R.Ph.
Adjunct Assistant Professor, Butler University, Indianapolis, Indiana

Katherine Stefos, Ph.D., R.Ph.
Staff Development Coordinator, The University of Texas M.D. Anderson Cancer Center, Houston, Texas

Carol Walsh, Ph.D.
Associate Professor, Boston University School of Medicine, Boston, Massachusetts

John R. White, Jr., Pharm.D.
Assistant Professor, Washington State University, Spokane, Washington

Lynn Roger Willis, Ph.D.
Professor, Indianapolis University School of Medicine, Indianapolis, Indiana

Canadian consultants

Linda Albert, R.N., B.N.
Instructor, Prince Edward Island School of Nursing, Charlottetown, Prince Edward Island

Susanne Guy Alcolado, R.N., B.N., M.Ed.
Assistant Director, Halifax Infirmary Hospital School of Nursing, Halifax, Nova Scotia

Linda M. Cameron, R.N., B.N.
Instructor, Foothills Hospital School of Nursing, Calgary, Alberta

Margaret Chad, B.S.N.
Instructor, Diploma Nursing Program, Saskatchewan Institute of Applied Science and Technology, Saskatoon, Saskatchewan

Tim Engelhardt, B.Sc., Pharm.D.
Manager, Pharmacy Services, Calgary District Hospital Group, Calgary, Alberta, Canada

Edythe Ann Fleming, B.Sc.N.
Professor, Fanshawe College, London, Ontario

Jacqueline Murphy, R.N., M.Sc.
Instructor and Staff Nurse, Foothills Hospital School of Nursing, Calgary, Alberta

Maureen J. Osis, R.N., M.N.
Clinical Nurse Specialist, Calgary, Alberta

Kenneth W. Renton, Ph.D.
Professor and Head, Dalhousie University Department of Pharmacology, Halifax, Nova Scotia

Roberta Ronayne, R.N., B.Sc.N., M.Sc.
Assistant Professor, University of Ottawa, Ottawa, Ontario

Shiela M. Stanton, R.N., M.S.N.
Associate Professor Emerita Nursing, University of British Columbia,
Vancouver, British Columbia

Linda Strand, Ph.D.
Executive Director, Saskatchewan Health, Regina, Saskatchewan

Sheila Rankin Zerr, R.N., M.Ed.
Assistant Professor, University of Victoria, Victoria, British Columbia

Preface

Mosby's 1993 Nursing Drug Reference has been completely revised and updated with the addition of over 1800 new drug facts, 30 new drugs recently approved by the FDA, and—completely new to this edition—over 85 geriatric considerations. Nursing considerations have been extensively revised to include over 800 new nursing guidelines. In addition, over 400 therapeutic responses and 200 newly researched side effects have been added. Another major revision is a complete updating of the combination products appendix. New drugs include biologics such as sargramostim (Leukine), used for myeloid recovery in non-Hodgkin's lymphoma and Hodgkin's disease; and filgrastin (Neupogen), used to reduce infection in patients with nonmyeloid malignancy. Other important drugs approved this year include didanosine (Videx), used for treatment of adult and pediatric patients with advanced HIV infection who are unable to use zidovudrine; pamidronate sodium (Aredia), used to treat hypercalcemia associated with malignancy; and fludarubine phosphate (Fludaor), used for palliative treatment of chronic lymphocytic leukemia.

Although drug references abound, few are available that are truly portable and geared specifically for clinical use by the practicing nurse or student. The guiding principle of this reference remains to provide the user with a book that allows easy access to drug information and nursing considerations that specifically tell the nurse what to do in terms consistent with the nursing process. Every detail—down to the choice of paper, typeface, cover, binding, use of color, and appendixes—has been carefully chosen with the user in mind.

Over 1000 generic and 4000 trade medications, alphabetized by generic name, are included. Trade names are given for all medications commonly used in the United States and Canada. Drugs available only in Canada are identified by an asterisk. The following information is provided, whenever possible, for safe and effective administration of each drug:

Pronunciations: Pronunciations are provided to help the nursing student master the more complex generic names.

Functional and chemical classifications: All known broad functional and chemical classifications are given. These classifications allow the nurse to see similarities and dissimilarities among drugs in the same functional but different chemical classes.

Controlled-substance schedule: Schedules are included for the United States (I, II, III, IV, V) and Canada (F, G).

Action: Pharmacologic properties are described in concise terms. Action is discussed to the cellular level when known.

Side effects/adverse reactions: Grouped by body system, common side effects are *italicized,* and life-threatening reactions are in ***bold italic***

type, allowing the nurse to quickly identify common and life-threatening reactions.

Dosages and routes: All available and approved dosages and routes are given for adult, pediatric, and geriatric patients.

Available forms: All available forms—including tablets, capsules, extended-release, injectables (IV, IM, SC), solutions, creams, ointments, lotions, gels, shampoos, elixirs, suspensions, suppositories, sprays, aerosols, and lozenges—are provided.

Contraindications: Contraindications are instances in which a medication should absolutely not be given. When the FDA has assigned pregnancy safety category D or X, it appears here.

Precautions: Special precautionary steps are given here, including FDA pregnancy safety categories A, B, and C.

Pharmacokinetics: Metabolism, distribution, and elimination are provided for all dosage forms, if known.

Interactions/incompatibilities: This section includes confirmed drug, food, and smoking interactions. The reaction is listed first, followed by the drug or nutrient causing that interaction, when applicable.

Nursing considerations: Highlighted nursing considerations are organized to foster use of the nursing process: Assess, Administer, Perform/provide, Evaluate, and Teach patient/family. Nursing considerations are consistently grouped under these headings to help the nurse group interventions that can be used for planning nursing care.

Lab test interferences: When known, lab test interferences are provided.

Treatment of overdose: Drugs and treatment for overdoses are provided for appropriate drugs.

The following appendixes are included to further enhance the usability of this reference: abbreviations, commonly used antibiotics in adults and children, nomogram, how to prepare a medication card, controlled substances, FDA pregnancy categories, bibliography, and combination products. A compatibility chart has been printed on the inside front cover for quick access, and weights and measurements and formulas for drug calculations have been printed on the inside back cover.

I am indebted to the nursing and pharmacology consultants who reviewed the manuscript and galley pages and thank them for their criticism and encouragement. I would also like to thank Don Ladig and Robin Carter, my editors, whose active encouragement and enthusiasm have made this book better than it might otherwise have been. I am likewise grateful to Gayle May Morris, Mary Drone, and Elizabeth Fett. I also wish to thank the many users who have offered comments and suggestions concerning previous editions. I, along with the publisher, welcome comments from users of *Mosby's Nursing Drug Reference* so that we may continue to provide current and useful information in future editions.

Linda Skidmore-Roth

Contents

ALPHA-ADRENERGIC BLOCKERS

Action: Acts by binding to α-adrenergic receptors, causing dilation of peripheral blood vessels. Lowers peripheral resistance, resulting in decreased blood pressure.

Uses: Used for pheochromocytoma.

Side effects/adverse reactions: The most common side effects are: hypotension, tachycardia, nasal stuffiness, nausea, vomiting, and diarrhea.

Contraindications: Hypersensitive reactions may occur, and allergies should be identified before these products are given. Patients with myocardial infarction, coronary insufficiency, angina, or other evidence of coronary artery disease should not use these products.

Pharmacokinetics: Onset, peak, and duration vary among products.

Interactions/incompatibilities: Vasoconstrictive and hypertensive effects of epinephrine are antagonized by α-adrenergic blockers.

Possible nursing diagnoses:

- Altered tissue perfusion *[uses]*
- High risk for injury *[adverse reactions]*
- Sleep pattern disturbance *[adverse reactions]*

NURSING CONSIDERATIONS

Assess:

- Electrolytes: K, Na, Cl, CO_2
- Weight daily, I&O
- B/P lying, standing before starting treatment, q4h thereafter

Administer:

- Starting with low dose, gradually increasing to prevent side effects
- With food or milk for GI symptoms

Evaluate:

- Therapeutic response: decreased B/P, increased peripheral pulses
- Nausea, vomiting, diarrhea
- Skin turgor, dryness of mucous membranes for hydration status

Teach patient/family:

- To avoid alcoholic beverages
- To report dizziness, palpitations, fainting
- To change position slowly or fainting may occur
- To take drug exactly as prescribed
- To avoid all OTC products (cough, cold, allergy) unless directed by physician

Generic names:

phenoxybenzamine (p. 766) phentolamine (p. 769)

ANTACIDS

Action: Antacids are basic compounds that neutralize gastric acidity and decrease the rate of gastric emptying. Products are divided into those containing aluminum, magnesium, calcium, or a combination of these.

Uses: Hyperacidity is decreased by antacids in conditions such as peptic ulcer disease, reflux esophagitis, gastritis, or hiatal hernia.

Side effects/adverse reactions: The most common side effect caused by aluminum-containing antacids is constipation, which may lead to fecal impaction and bowel obstruction. Diarrhea occurs often when magnesium products are given. Alkalosis may occur when systemic products are used. Constipation occurs more frequently than laxation with calcium carbonate. The release of CO_2 from carbonate-containing antacids causes belching, abdominal distention, and flatulence. Sodium bicarbonate may act as a systemic antacid and produce systemic electrolyte disturbances and alkalosis. Calcium carbonate and sodium bicarbonate may cause rebound hyperacidity and milk-alkali syndrome. Alkaluria may occur when products are used on a long-term basis, particularly in persons with abnormal renal function.

Contraindications: Sensitivity to aluminum or magnesium products may cause hypersensitive reactions. Aluminum products should not be used by persons sensitive to aluminum; magnesium products should not be used by persons sensitive to magnesium. Check for sensitivity before administering.

Precautions: Magnesium products should be given cautiously to patients with renal insufficiency and during pregnancy and lactation. Sodium content of antacids may be significant; use with caution for patients with hypertension, CHF, or those on a low-sodium diet.

Pharmacokinetics: Duration is 20-40 min. If ingested 1 hr after meals, acidity is reduced for at least 3 hr.

Interactions/incompatibilities: Drugs whose effects may be increased by some antacids: quinidine, amphetamines, pseudoephedrine, levodopa, valproic acid, dicumarol. Drugs whose effects may be decreased by some antacids: cimetadine, corticosteroids, ranitidine, iron salts, phenothiazines, phenytoin, digoxin, tetracyclines, ketoconazole, salicylates, isoniazid.

Possible nursing diagnoses:

- Pain *[uses]*
- Constipation *[adverse reactions]*
- Diarrhea *[adverse reactions]*

NURSING CONSIDERATIONS

Assess:

• Aggravating and alleviating factors of epigastric pain or hyperacidity; identify the location, duration, and characteristics of epigastric pain
• GI symptoms, including constipation, diarrhea, abdominal pain; if severe abdominal pain with fever occurs, these drugs should not be given
• Renal symptoms, including increasing urinary pH, electrolytes

Administer:

• All products with an 8-oz glass of water to ensure absorption in the stomach
• Another antacid if constipation occurs with aluminum products

Evaluate:

• The therapeutic effectiveness of the drug; absence of epigastric pain and decreased acidity should occur

Teach patient/family:

• Not to take other drugs within 1-2 hr of antacid administration, since antacids may impair absorption of other drugs

---

Generic names:

aluminum carbonate gel (p. 61)
aluminum hydroxide (p. 62)
aluminum phosphate (p. 63)
bismuth subsalicylate (p. 141)
calcium carbonate (p. 162)
dihydroxyaluminum (p. 335)
magaldrate (p. 575)
magnesium carbonate (p. 576)
magnesium oxide (p. 576)
magnesium trisilicate (p. 580)
sodium bicarbonate (p. 868)

ANTICONVULSANTS

Action: Anticonvulsants are divided into the barbiturates (p. 18), benzodiazepines (p. 20), hydantoins, succinimides, and miscellaneous products. Barbiturates and benzodiazepines are discussed in separate sections. Hydantoins act by inhibiting the spread of seizure activity in the motor cortex. Succinimides act by inhibiting spike and wave formation; they also decrease amplitude, frequency, duration, and spread of discharge in seizures.

Uses: Hydantoins are used in generalized tonic-clonic seizures, status epilepticus, and psychomotor seizures. Succinimides are used for absence (petit mal) seizures. Barbiturates are used in generalized tonic-clonic and cortical focal seizures.

Side effects/adverse reactions: Bone marrow depression is the most life-threatening adverse reaction associated with hydantoins or succinimides. The most common side effects are GI symptoms. Other common side effects for hydantoins are gingival hyperplasia and CNS effects such as nystagmus, ataxia, slurred speech, and mental confusion.

Contraindications: Hypersensitive reactions may occur, and allergies should be identified before these products are given.

Precautions: Persons with renal or hepatic disease should be watched closely.

Pharmacokinetics: Onset, peak, and duration vary widely among products. Most products are metabolized in the liver and excreted in urine, bile, and feces.

Interactions/incompatibilities: Decreased effects of estrogens, oral contraceptives (hydantoins).

Possible nursing diagnoses:

- High risk for injury *[uses]*
- Noncompliance
- Sleep pattern disturbance *[adverse reactions]*

NURSING CONSIDERATIONS

Assess:

- Renal function studies, including BUN, creatinine, serum uric acid, urine creatinine clearance before and during therapy
- Blood studies: RBC, Hct, Hgb, reticulocyte counts qwk for 4 wk then qmo
- Hepatic studies: AST, ALT, bilirubin, creatinine

Administer:

- With food, milk to decrease GI symptoms

Perform/provide:

- Good oral hygiene is important for hydantoins

Evaluate:

- Therapeutic response, including decreased seizure activity; document on patient's chart
- Mental status, including mood, sensorium, affect, behavorial changes; if mental status changes, notify physician
- Eye problems, including need for ophthalmic examinations before, during, and after treatment (slit lamp, funduscopy, tonometry)
- Allergic reaction, including red raised rash; if this occurs, drug should be discontinued
- Blood dyscrasia, including fever, sore throat, bruising, rash, jaundice
- Toxicity, including bone marrow depression, nausea, vomiting, ataxia, diplopia, cardiovascular collapse, Stevens-Johnson syndrome

Teach patient/family:

- To carry ID card or Medic-Alert bracelet stating drugs taken, condition, physician's name, phone number
- To avoid driving, other activities that require alertness

Generic names:

Hydantoins: ethotoin (p. 398)
mephenytoin (p. 602)
phensuximide (p. 767)
phenytoin (p. 774)

Succinimides: ethosuximide (p. 396)
methsuximide (p. 627)
phensuximide (p. 767)

Miscellaneous: acetazolamide (p. 42)
carbamazepine (p. 168)
clonazepam (p. 254)
diazepam (p. 314)
magnesium sulfate (p. 579)
paraldehyde (p. 733)
paramethadione (p. 734)
phenacemide (p. 758)
primidone (p. 807)
trimethadione (p. 963)
valproate acid (p. 979)

ANTIDIABETICS

Action: Antidiabetics are divided into the insulins that decrease blood sugar, phosphate, and potassium and increase blood pyruvate and lactate; and oral antidiabetics that cause functioning beta cells in the pancreas to release insulin, improves the effect of endogenous and exogenous insulin.
Uses: Insulins are used for ketoacidosis and diabetes mellitus types I (IDDM) and II (NIDDM); oral antidiabetics are used for stable adult-onset diabetes mellitus type II (NIDDM).
Side effects/adverse reactions: The most common side effect of insulin and oral antidiabetics is hypoglycemia. Other adverse reactions for oral antidiabetics include blood dyscrasias, hepatotoxicity, and, rarely, cholestatic jaundice. Adverse reactions for insulin products include allergic responses and, more rarely, anaphylaxis.
Contraindications: Hypersensitive reactions may occur, and allergies should be identified before these products are given. Oral antidiabetics should not be used in juvenile or brittle diabetes, diabetic ketoacidosis, severe renal disease, or severe hepatic disease.
Precautions: Oral antidiabetics should be used with caution in the elderly, in cardiac disease, pregnancy, lactation, and in the presence of alcohol.
Pharmacokinetics: Onset, peak, and duration vary widely among products. Oral antidiabetics are metabolized in the liver, with metabolites excreted in urine, bile, and feces.

Interactions/incompatibilities: Interactions vary widely among products. Check individual monograph for specific information.

Possible nursing diagnosis:

• Altered nutrition: more than body requirements *[uses]*

NURSING CONSIDERATIONS

Assess:

• Blood, urine glucose levels during treatment to determine diabetes control (oral products)

• Fasting blood glucose, 2 hr PP (60-100 mg/dl normal fasting level) (70-130 mg/dl—normal 2-hr level)

Administer:

• Insulin, after warming to room temperature by rotating in palms to prevent lipodystrophy from injecting cold insulin

• Human insulin to those allergic to beef or pork

• Oral antidiabetic 30 min before meals

Perform/provide:

• Rotation of injection sites when giving insulin; use abdomen, upper back, thighs, upper arm, buttocks; rotate sites within one of these regions; keep a record of sites

Evaluate:

• Therapeutic response, including decrease in polyuria, polydipsia, polyphagia, clear sensorium, absence of dizziness, stable gait

• Hypoglycemic reaction that can occur during peak time

Teach patient/family:

• To avoid alcohol and salicylates except on advice of physician

• Symptoms of ketoacidosis: nausea, thirst, polyuria, dry mouth, decreased B/P, dry, flushed skin, acetone breath, drowsiness, Kussmaul respiration

• Symptoms of hypoglycemia: headache, tremors, fatigue, weakness; and that candy or sugar should be carried to treat hypoglycemia

• To test urine for glucose/ketones tid if this drug is replacing insulin

• To continue weight control, dietary restrictions, exercise, hygiene

---

Generic names:

Oral antidiabetics: acetohexamide (p. 44)
chlorpropamide (p. 229)
insulin, regular (p. 513)
insulin, regular concentrated (p. 514)
insulin, zinc suspension (extended) (p. 517)
insulin, zinc suspension (intermediate) (p. 516)
insulin, zinc suspension (prompt) (p. 518)

ANTIDYSRHYTHMICS

Action: Antidysrhythmics are divided into four classes and miscellaneous antidysrhythmics:

• Class I increases the action potential duration and the effective refractory period and reduces disparity in the refractory period between a normal and infarcted myocardium; further subclasses include Ia, Ib, Ic

• Class II decreases the rate of SA node discharge, increases recovery time, slows conduction through the AV node, and decreases heart rate, which decreases O_2 consumption in the myocardium

• Class III increases the action potential duration and the effective refractory period

• Class IV inhibits calcium ion influx across the cell membrane during cardiac depolarization; decreases SA node discharge, decreases conduction velocity through the AV node

• Miscellaneous antidysrhythmics include those such as adenosine, which slows conduction through the AV node, and digoxin, which decreases conduction velocity and prolongs the effective refractory period in the AV node

Uses: These products are used for PVCs, tachycardia, hypertension, atrial fibrillation, angina pectoris.

Side effects/adverse reactions: Side effects and adverse reactions vary widely among products.

Contraindications: Contraindications vary widely among products.

Precautions: Precautions vary widely among products.

Pharmacokinetics: Onset, peak, and duration vary widely among products.

Interactions/incompatibilities: Interactions vary widely among products; check individual monograph for specific information.

Possible nursing diagnoses:

• Altered tissue perfusion: cardiopulmonary *[uses]*

• Decreased cardiac output *[uses]*

• Diarrhea *[adverse reactions]*

• Impaired gas exchange *[adverse reactions]*

NURSING CONSIDERATIONS

Assess:

• ECG continuously to determine drug effectiveness, PVCs or other dysrhythmias

• IV infusion rate to avoid causing nausea, vomiting

• For dehydration or hypovolemia

• B/P continuously for hypotension, hypertension

• I&O ratio

Evaluate:

- Therapeutic response, including decrease in B/P in hypertension, decreased B/P, edema moist rales in CHF
- Edema in feet and legs daily

Teach patient/family:

- To comply with dosage schedule, even if patient is feeling better
- To report bradycardia, dizziness, confusion, depression, fever

---

Generic names:

Class I: moricizine (p. 663)

Class Ia: disopyramide (p. 344)
procainamide (p. 810)
quinidine (p. 843)

Class Ib: lidocaine (p. 555)
mexiletine (p. 647)
phenytoin (p. 774)
tocainide (p. 939)

Class Ic: indecainide (p. 507)
flecainide (p. 419)
propafenone (p. 821)

Class II: acebutolol (p. 39)
esmolol (p. 381)
propranolol (p. 825)

Class III: amiodarone HCl (p. 75)
bretylium (p. 144)

Class IV: verapamil HCl (p. 984)

Miscellaneous: adenosine (p. 51)
digoxin (p. 331)

ANTIHISTAMINES

Action: Antihistamines compete with histamines for H_1 receptor sites. They antagonize in varying degrees most of the pharmacologic effects of histamines.

Uses: Products are used to control the symptoms of allergies, rhinitis, and pruritus.

Side effects/adverse reactions: Most products cause drowsiness; however, two of the newer products, astemizole and terfenadine, produce little, if any, drowsiness. Other common side effects are headache and thickening of bronchial secretions. Serious blood dyscrasias may occur, but are rare. Urinary retention occurs with many of these products.

Contraindications: Hypersensitivity to H_1-receptor antagonists occurs rarely. Patients with acute asthma and lower respiratory tract disease should not use these products, since thick secretions may result. Other contraindications include narrow-angle glaucoma, bladder neck obstruction, stenosing peptic ulcer, symptomatic prostatic hypertrophy, newborn, lactation.

Precautions: These products must be used cautiously in conjunction with intraocular pressure, since they increase intraocular pressure. Caution should also be used in patients with renal and cardiac disease, hypertension, and seizure disorders and in the elderly.

Pharmacokinetics: Onset varies from 20-60 min, with duration lasting 4-12 hr. In general pharmacokinetics vary widely among products.

Drug interactions/incompatibilities: Barbiturates, narcotics, hypnotics, tricyclic antidepressants, or alcohol can increase CNS depression when taken with antihistamines.

Possible nursing diagnoses:

- Ineffective airway clearance *[uses]*

NURSING CONSIDERATIONS

Assess:

- I&O ratio; be alert for urinary retention, frequency, dysuria; drug should be discontinued if these occur
- CBC during long-term therapy, since hemolytic anemia, although rare, may occur

Administer:

- With food or milk to decrease GI symptoms; absorption may be decreased slightly

Perform/provide:

- Hard candy, gum, frequent rinsing of mouth for dryness

Evaluate:

- Therapeutic response, including absence of allergy symptoms, itching
- Blood dyscrasias: thrombocytopenia, agranulocytosis (rare)
- Respiratory status, including rate rhythm, increase in bronchial secretions, wheezing, chest tightness
- Cardiac status, including palpitations, increased pulse, hypotension

Teach patient/family:

- To notify physician if confusion, sedation, hypotension occur
- To avoid driving or other hazardous activity if drowsiness occurs
- To avoid concurrent use of alcohol or other CNS depressants

---

Generic names:

astemizole (p. 105)
azatadine maleate (p. 113)
brompheniramine maleate (p. 146)
chlorpheniramine maleate (p. 225)
diphenhydramine HCl (p. 339)
promethazine HCl (p. 819)
terfenadine (p. 903)
trimeprazine tartrate (p. 962)
tripelennamine HCl (p. 969)

ANTIHYPERTENSIVES

Action: Antihypertensives are divided into angiotensin-converting enzyme (ACE) inhibitors, β-adrenergic blockers, calcium channel blockers, centrally acting adrenergics, diuretics, peripherally acting antiadrenergics, and vasodilators. Beta blockers, calcium channel blockers, and diuretics are discussed in separate sections. Angiotensin-converting enzyme inhibitors act by selectively suppressing renin-angiotensin I to angiotensin II; dilation of arterial and venous vessels occurs. Centrally acting adrenergics act by inhibiting the sympathetic vasomotor center in the CNS that reduces impulses in the sympathetic nervous system; blood pressure, pulse rate, and cardiac output decrease. Peripherally acting antiadrenergics inhibit sympathetic vasoconstriction by inhibiting release of norepinephrine and/or depleting norepinephrine stores in adrenergic nerve endings. Vasodilators act on arteriolar smooth muscle by producing direct relaxation or vasodilation; a reduction in blood pressure, with concomitant increases in heart rate and cardiac output, occurs.

Uses: Used for hypertension and for heart failure not responsive to conventional therapy. Some products are used in hypertensive crisis, angina, and for some cardiac dysrhythmias.

Side effects/adverse reactions: The most common side effects are marked hypotension, bradycardia, tachycardia, headache, nausea, and vomiting. Side effects and adverse reactions may vary widely between classes and specific products.

Contraindications: Hypersensitive reactions may occur, and allergies should be identified before these products are given. Antihypertensives should not be used in patients with heart block or children.

Precautions: Antihypertensives should be used with caution in the elderly, in dialysis patients, and in the presence of hypovolemia, leukemia, and electrolyte imbalances.

Pharmacokinetics: Onset, peak, and duration vary widely among products. Most products are metabolized in the liver, with metabolites excreted in urine, bile, and feces.

Interactions/incompatibilities: Interactions vary widely among products; check individual monograph for specific information.

Possible nursing diagnoses:

- Altered tissue perfusion *[uses]*
- Decreased cardiac output *[uses]*
- Diarrhea *[adverse reactions]*
- Impaired gas exchange *[adverse reactions]*

NURSING CONSIDERATIONS

Assess:

- Blood studies: neutrophil; decreased platelets occur with many of the products
- Renal studies: protein, BUN, creatinine; watch for increased levels that may indicate nephrotic syndrome; obtain baselines in renal and liver function studies before beginning treatment

Perform/provide:

- Supine or Trendelenburg position for severe hypotension

Evaluate:

- Therapeutic response, including decrease in B/P in hypotension; decreased B/P, edema, moist rales in CHF
- Edema in feet and legs daily
- Allergic reaction, including rash, fever, pruritus, urticaria: drug should be discontinued if antihistamines fail to help
- Symptoms of CHF: edema, dyspnea, wet rales, B/P
- Renal symptoms: polyuria, oliguria, frequency

Teach patient/family:

- To comply with dosage schedule, even if feeling better
- To rise slowly to sitting or standing position to minimize orthostatic hypotension

---

Generic names:

Angiotensin-converting enzyme inhibitors: benazepril HCl (p. 126)
enalapril (p. 367)
fosinopril sodium (p. 444)
quinapril HCl (p. 840)
ramipril (p. 847)

Centrally acting adrenergics:
clonidine HCl (p. 255)
guanabenz (p. 464)
guanfacine (p. 467)
methyldopa (p. 629)

Peripherally acting antiadrenergics: guanadrel (p. 465)
guanethidine (p. 466)
prazosin (p. 801)
reserpine (p. 849)
terazosin (p. 900)

Vasodilators: diazoside (p. 315)
hydralazine (p. 481)
minoxidil (p. 655)
nitroprusside (p. 696)

Antiadrenergic: combined alpha/beta blocker—labetalol (p. 543)

ANTIINFECTIVES

Action: Antiinfectives are divided into several groups, which include but are not limited to penicillins, cephalosporins, aminoglycosides, sulfonamides, tetracyclines, monobactam, erythromycins, and quinolones. These drugs act by inhibiting the growth and replication of susceptible bacterial organisms.

Uses: Used for infections of susceptible organisms. These products are effective against bacterial, rickettsial, and spirochete infections.

Side effects/adverse reactions: The most common side effects are nausea, vomiting, and diarrhea. Adverse reactions include bone marrow depression and anaphylaxis.

Contraindications: Hypersensitive reactions may occur, and allergies should be identified before these products are given. Cross-sensitivity can occur between products of different classes (penicillins or cephalosporins). Often persons allergic to penicillins will also be allergic to cephalosporins.

Precautions: Antiinfectives should be used with caution in persons with renal and liver disease.

Pharmacokinetics: Onset, peak, and duration vary widely among products. Most products are metabolized in the liver, and metabolites are excreted in urine, bile, and feces.

Interactions/incompatibilities: Interactions vary widely among products; check individual monograph for specific information.

Possible nursing diagnoses:

- High risk for infection *[uses]*
- Diarrhea *[adverse reactions]*

NURSING CONSIDERATIONS

Assess:

- Nephrotoxicity, including increased BUN, creatinine
- Blood studies: AST, ALT, CBC, Hct, bilirubin; test monthly if patient is on long-term therapy
- Bowel pattern qd; if severe diarrhea occurs, drug should be discontinued

Administer:

- For 10-14 days to ensure organism death, prevention of superimposed infection
- After C&S completed, drug may be taken as soon as culture is taken

Evaluate:

- Therapeutic response, including absence of fever, fatigue, malaise, draining wounds
- Urine output; if decreasing, notify physician; may indicate nephrotoxicity

• Allergic reaction, including rash, fever, pruritus, urticaria; drug should be discontinued
• Bleeding: ecchymosis, bleeding gums, hematuria, stool guaiac daily
• Overgrowth of infection: perineal itching, fever, malaise, redness, pain, swelling, drainage, rash, diarrhea, change in cough, sputum

Teach patient/family:

• To comply with dosage schedule, even if feeling better
• To report sore throat, bruising, bleeding, joint pain; may indicate blood dyscrasias (rare)

Generic names:

ANTINEOPLASTICS

Action: Antineoplastics are divided into alkylating agents, antimetabolites, antibiotic agents, hormonal agents, and miscellaneous agents. Alkylating agents act by cross-linking strands of DNA. Antimetabolites act by inhibiting DNA synthesis. Antibiotic agents act by inhibiting RNA synthesis and by delaying or inhibiting mitosis. Hormones alter the effect of androgens, luteinizing hormone, follicle-stimulating hormone, or estrogen by changing the hormonal environment.

Uses: Uses vary widely among products and classes of drugs. They are used to treat leukemia, Hodgkin's disease, lymphomas, and other tumors throughout the body.

Side effects/adverse reactions: Most products cause thrombocytopenia, leukopenia, and anemia, and, if these reactions occur, the drug may need to be stopped until the problem is corrected. Other side effects include nausea, vomiting, glossitis, and hair loss. Some products also cause hepatotoxicity, nephrotoxicity, and cardiotoxicity.

Contraindications: Hypersensitive reactions may occur, and allergies should be identified before these products are given. Also, persons with severe liver and kidney disease should not use these products unless the benefits outweigh the risks.

Precautions: Persons with bleeding, severe bone marrow depression, or renal or hepatic disease should be watched closely.

Pharmacokinetics: Onset, peak, and duration vary widely among products. Most products cross the placenta and are excreted in breast milk and in urine.

Interactions/incompatibilities: Toxicity may occur when used with other antineoplastics or radiation.

Possible nursing diagnoses:

- High risk for infection *[adverse reactions]*
- Altered nutrition: less than body requirements *[adverse reactions]*
- Altered oral mucous membrane *[adverse reactions]*

NURSING CONSIDERATIONS

Assess:

- CBC, differential, platelet count weekly; withhold drug if WBC is <4000 or platelet count is <75,000; notify physician of results
- Renal function studies, including BUN, creatinine, serum uric acid, and urine creatinine clearance before and during therapy
- I&O ratio; report fall in urine output of 30 ml/hr
- Monitor temperature q4h (may indicate beginning infection)
- Liver function tests before and during therapy (bilirubin, AST, ALT, LDH) as needed or monthly

Administer:
- Checking IV site for irritation; phlebitis
- Epinephrine for hypersensitivity reaction
- Antibiotics for prophylaxis of infection

Perform/provide:
- Strict medical asepsis, protective isolation if WBC levels are low
- Comprehensive oral hygiene, using careful technique and soft-bristle brush

Evaluate:
- Therapeutic response, including decreased tumor size
- Bleeding, including hematuria, guaiac, bruising or petechiae, mucosa, or orifices q8h; obtain prescription for viscous xylocaine
- Yellowing of skin, sclera, dark urine, clay-colored stools, itchy skin, abdominal pain, fever, diarrhea
- Edema in feet, joint pain, stomach pain, shaking
- Inflammation of mucosa, breaks in skin

Teach patient/family:
- To report signs of infection, including increased temperature, sore throat, malaise
- To report signs of anemia, including fatigue, headache, faintness, shortness of breath, irritability
- To report bleeding and avoid use of razors or commercial mouthwash

---

Generic names:

Alkylating agents: busulfan
p. 154)
carboplatin (p. 171)
carmustine (p. 174)
chlorambucil (p. 213)
cisplatin (p. 241)
cyclophosphamide (p. 279)
dacarbazine (p. 286)
lomustine (p. 566)
mechlorethamine (p. 588)
melphalan (p. 596)
streptozocin (p. 881)
thiotepa (p. 922)
uracil mustard (p. 974)

Antimetabolites: cytarabine
(p. 284)
fludarabine phosphate (p. 424)
fluorouracil (p. 431)
doxorubicin (p. 354)
mitomycin (p. 656)
mitoxantrone (p. 659)
plicamycin (p. 788)

Hormonal agents:
aminoglutethimide (p. 73)
estramustine (p. 387)
flutamide (p. 441)
goserelin acetate (p. 462)
leuprolide (p. 546)
megestrol (p. 595)
mitotane (p. 658)
tamoxifen (p. 897)
testolactone (p. 904)
trilostane (p. 961)

Miscellaneous agents:
altretamine (p. 60)

mercaptopurine (p. 606)
methotrexate (p. 622)
thioguanine (p. 918)

Antibiotic agents: bleomycin (p. 142)
dactinomycin (p. 287)
daunorubicin HCl (p. 293)
asparaginase (p. 101)
etoposide (p. 404)
interferon alfa-2A (p. 520)
interferon alfa-2B (p. 520)
pentostatin (p. 753)
procarbazine (p. 812)
vinblastine (p. 986)
vincristine (p. 988)

ANTIPSYCHOTICS

Action: Antipsychotics/neuroleptics are divided into several subgroups: phenothiazines, thioxanthenes, butyrophenones, dibenzoxazepines, dibenzodiazepines, and indolones and other heterocyclic compounds. Although chemically different, these subgroups share many pharmacologic and clinical properties. All antipsychotics work to block postsynaptic dopamine receptors in the brain that are responsible for psychotic behavior, including hallucinations, delusions, and paranoia.

Uses: Antipsychotic behavior is decreased in conditions such as schizophrenia, paranoia, and mania. These agents are also effective for severe anxiety, intractable hiccups, nausea, vomiting, behavioral problems in children, and before surgery for relaxation.

Side effects/adverse reactions: The most common side effects include extrapyramidal symptoms such as pseudoparkinsonism, akathisia, dystonia, and tardive dyskinesia, which may be controlled by use of antiparkinsonian agents. Serious adverse reactions such as hypotension, agranulocytosis, cardiac arrest, and laryngospasm have occurred. Other common side effects include dry mouth and photosensitivity.

Contraindications: Persons with liver damage, severe hypertension or coronary disease, cerebral arteriosclerosis, blood dyscrasias, bone marrow depression, parkinsonism, severely depressed persons, narrow-angle glaucoma, children <12 yr, or persons withdrawing from alcohol or barbiturates should not use antipsychotics until these conditions are corrected.

Precautions: Caution must be used when antipsychotics are given to the elderly, since metabolism is slowed and adverse reactions can occur rapidly. Hepatic and renal disease may cause poor metabolism and excretion of the drug. Seizure threshold is decreased with these products; increases in the dose of anticonvulsants may be required. Persons with diabetes mellitus, prostatic hypertrophy, chronic respiratory disease, and peptic ulcer disease should be monitored closely.

Pharmacokinetics: Onset, peak, and duration vary widely with different products and routes. Products are metabolized by the liver, are excreted in urine as metabolites, are highly bound to plasma proteins, cross the placenta, and enter breast milk. Half-life can be extended over 3 days.
Interactions/incompatibilities: Because other CNS depressants can cause oversedation, these combinations should be used carefully. Anticholinergics may decrease the therapeutic actions of phenothiazines and also cause increased anticholinergic effects.
Possible nursing diagnoses:
• Altered thought processes *[uses]*
• Sensory-perceptual alterations *[uses]*

NURSING CONSIDERATIONS

Assess:
• Bilirubin, CBC, liver function studies monthly, since these drugs are metabolized in the liver and excreted in urine
• I&O ratio: palpate bladder if low urinary output occurs, since urinary retention occurs with many of these products
• Affect, orientation, LOC, reflexes, gait, coordination, sleep pattern disturbances
• Dizziness, faintness, palpitations, tachycardia on rising
Administer:
• Antiparkinsonian agent if extrapyramidal symptoms occur
• Liquid concentrates mixed in glass of juice or cola, since taste is unpleasant; avoid contact with skin when preparing liquid concentrate or parental medications
Perform/provide:
• Supervised ambulation until stabilized on medication; do not involve in strenuous exercise program because fainting is possible; patient should not stand still for long periods of time
• Increased fluids to prevent constipation
• Sips of water, candy, gum for dry mouth
Evaluate:
• Therapeutic response: decrease in excitement, hallucinations, delusions, paranoia, reorganization of thought patterns, speech
• B/P lying and standing; wide fluctuations between lying and standing B/P may require dosage or product change since orthostatic hypotension is occurring
• Extrapyramidal symptoms, including akathisia, tardive dyskinesia, pseudoparkinsonism
Teach patient/family:
• To rise from sitting or lying position gradually, since fainting may occur

- To remain lying down for at least 30 min after IM injections
- To avoid hot tubs, hot showers, or tub baths, since hypotension may occur
- To wear a sunscreen or protective clothing to prevent burns
- To take extra precautions during hot weather to stay cool; heat stroke can occur
- To avoid driving or other activities requiring alertness until response to medication is known
- That drowsiness or impaired mental/motor activity is evident the first 2 wk, but tends to decrease over time

---

Generic names:

Phenothiazines: chlorpromazine HCl (p. 226)
fluphenazine (p. 436)
mesoridazine (p. 608)
perphenazine (p. 756)
prochlorperazine (p. 813)
promazine (p. 817)
thioridazine (p. 920)
thiothixene (p. 924)
trifluoperazine (p. 955)

Butyrophenone: haloperidol (p. 471)

Miscellaneous: loxapine (p. 572)
molindone (p. 661)

BARBITURATES

Action: Barbiturates act by decreasing impulse transmission to the cerebral cortex.

Uses: All forms of epilepsy can be controlled, since the seizure threshold is increased. Uses also include febrile seizures in children, sedation, insomnia, hyperbilirubinemia, chronic cholestasis with some of these products. Ultra-short acting barbiturates are used as anesthetics.

Side effects/adverse reactions: The most common side effects are drowsiness and nausea. Serious adverse reactions such as Stevens-Johnson syndrome and blood dyscrasias may occur with high doses and long-term treatment.

Contraindications: Hypersensitivity may occur, and allergies should be identified before administering. Barbiturates are identified as pregnancy category (D) and should not be used in pregnancy. Other contraindications include porphyria and marked impairment of liver function.

Precautions: Caution must be used when these products are given to the elderly or debilitated; usually smaller doses are needed, since metabolism is slowed. Persons with renal and hepatic disease may show delayed excretion. Barbiturates may produce excitability in children.

Pharmacokinetics: Onset of action can be slow, up to 1 hr, with a peak of 8 hr and a duration of 3-10 hr. These drugs are metabolized by the liver, excreted by the kidneys, cross the placenta, and enter breast milk.
Drug interactions/incompatibilities: Increased CNS depressant effect may occur with alcohol, MAOIs, sedatives, or narcotics. These products should be used together cautiously. Oral anticoagulants, corticosteroids, griseofulvin, quinidine, oral contraceptives, and theophylline may show a decreased effect when used with barbiturates.
Possible nursing diagnoses:
• Sleep pattern disturbance *[uses]*
• High risk for injury *[adverse reactions]*

NURSING CONSIDERATIONS

Assess:
• Hepatic and renal studies: AST, ALT, bilirubin, creatinine, LDH, alkaline phosphatase, BUN if patient is on long-term therapy, since these products are metabolized and excreted by the liver and kidney
• Blood studies: CBC, hematocrit, hemoglobin, and prothrombin time if patient is on long-term therapy, since these products increase the possibility of bleeding and blood dyscrasias
Evaluate:
• Therapeutic response, including appropriate sedation or seizure control
• Barbiturate toxicity: hypotension, pulmonary constriction; cold, clammy skin; cyanosis of lips; insomnia; nausea; vomiting, hallucinations, delirium, weakness
Teach patient/family:
• That physical dependency may result when used for extended periods of time (45-90 days, depending on dose)
• To avoid driving and activities that require alertness, since drowsiness and dizziness may occur
• To abstain from alcohol or other psychotropic medications unless prescribed by physician
• Not to discontinue medication abruptly after long-term use; withdrawal symptoms will occur

---

Generic names:

amobarbital (p. 80)
mephobarbital (p. 603)
pentobarbital (p. 751)
phenobarbital (p. 764)
secobarbital (p. 860)
talbutal (p. 895)
thiopental (p. 919)

BENZODIAZEPINES

Action: Benzodiazepines potentiate the effects of γ-aminobutyrate (GABA), including any other inhibitory transmitters in the CNS, resulting in decreased anxiety.

Uses: Anxiety is relieved in conditions such as phobic disorders. Benzodiazepines are also used for acute alcohol withdrawal to relieve the possibility of delirium tremens, and some products are used before surgery for relaxation.

Side effects/adverse reactions: The most common side effects are dizziness, drowsiness, blurred vision, and orthostatic hypotension. Most adverse effects are mediated through the CNs. There is a risk for physicial dependence and abuse.

Contraindications: Hypersensitivity, acute narrow-angle glaucoma, children <6 months, liver disease (clonazepam), lactation (diazepam).

Precautions: Caution must be used when these products are given to the elderly or debilitated; usually smaller doses are needed, since metabolism is slowed. Persons with renal and hepatic disease may show delayed excretion. Clonazepam may increase incidence of seizures.

Pharmacokinetics: Onset of action is ½-1 hr, with a peak of 1-2 hr and a duration of 4-6 hr. These drugs are metabolized by the liver, excreted by the kidneys, cross the placenta, and enter breast milk.

Drug interactions/incompatibilities: Increased CNS depressant effect may occur with other CNS depressants. These products should be used together cautiously. Alcohol should not be used; fatal reactions can occur. The serum concentration and toxicity of digoxin may be increased.

Possible nursing diagnoses:
- Anxiety *[uses]*
- High risk for injury *[adverse reactions]*

NURSING CONSIDERATIONS

Assess:
- B/P (lying, standing), pulse; if systolic B/P drops 20 mm Hg, hold drug, notify physician; orthostatic hypotension is severe
- Hepatic and renal studies: AST, ALT, bilirubin, creatinine, LDH, alkaline phosphatase

Administer:
- With food or milk for GI symptoms; may give crushed if patient is unable to swallow medication whole

Evaluate:
- Therapeutic response, including relaxation or decreased anxiety
- Physical dependency, withdrawal symptoms, including headache, nausea, vomiting, muscle pain, weakness after long-term use

Teach patient/family:

• That drug should not be used for everyday stress or long-term; not to take more than prescribed amount, since drug is habit forming

• To avoid driving and activities that require alertness, since drowsiness and dizziness occur

• To abstain from alcohol or other psychotropic medications unless prescribed by physician

• Not to discontinue medication abruptly after long-term use; withdrawal symptoms will occur

---

Generic names:

alprazolam (p. 57)
chlordiazepoxide HCl (p. 217)
clonazepam (p. 254)
diazepam (p. 314)
flurazepam (p. 439)
halazepam (p. 469)
lorazepam (p. 570)
midazolam (p. 652)
oxazepam (p. 717)
prazepam (p. 799)
quazepam (p. 837)
temazepam (p. 899)
triazolam (p. 953)

BETA-ADRENERGIC BLOCKERS

Action: Beta blockers are divided into selective and nonselective blockers. Nonselective blockers produce a fall in blood pressure without reflex tachycardia or reduction in heart rate through a mixture of beta blocking effects; elevated plasma renins are reduced. Selective beta blockers competitively block stimulation of β-1 receptors in cardiac smooth muscle; these drugs produce chronotropic and inotropic effects.

Uses: Beta blockers are used for hypertension, ventricular dysrhythmias, and prophylaxis of angina pectoris.

Side effects/adverse reactions: The most common side effects are orthostatic hypotension, bradycardia, diarrhea, nausea, vomiting. Serious adverse reactions include blood dyscrasias, bronchospasm, and CHF.

Contraindications: Hypersensitive reactions may occur, and allergies should be identified before these products are given. β-adrenergic blockers should not be used in heart block, CHF, or cardiogenic shock.

Precautions: Beta blockers should be used with caution in the elderly or in renal and thyroid disease, COPD, CAD, diabetes mellitus, or pregnancy.

Pharmacokinetics: Onset, peak, and duration vary widely among products. Most products are metabolized in the liver, with metabolites excreted in urine, bile, and feces.

Interactions/incompatibilities: Interactions vary widely among products; check individual monograph for specific information.

Possible nursing diagnoses:

- Altered tissue perfusion *[uses]*
- Decreased cardiac output *[uses]*
- Diarrhea *[adverse reactions]*
- Impaired gas exchange *[adverse reactions]*

NURSING CONSIDERATIONS

Assess:

- Renal studies, including protein, BUN, creatinine; watch for increased levels that may indicate nephrotic syndrome; obtain baselines in renal and liver function studies before beginning treatment
- I&O, weight daily
- B/P during beginning treatment and periodically thereafter, pulse q4h, note rate, rhythm, quality
- Apical/radial pulse before administration; notify physician of significant changes

Administer:

- PO ac, hs, tablets may be crushed or swallowed whole
- Reduced dosage in renal dysfunction

Evaluate:

- Therapeutic response, including decrease in B/P in hypertension, decreased B/P, edema, moist rales in CHF
- Edema in feet and legs daily

Teach patient/family:

- To comply with dosage schedule, even if feeling better
- To rise slowly to sitting or standing position to minimize orthostatic hypotension
- To report bradycardia, dizziness, confusion, depression, fever
- To take pulse at home; advise when to notify physician
- To comply with weight control, dietary adjustment, modified exercise program
- To wear support hose to minimize effects of orthostatic hypotension
- Not to discontinue drug abruptly; taper over 2 wk; may precipitate angina

---

Generic names:

Selective β-1 receptor blockers:
acebutolol (p. 39)
atenolol (p. 106)
esmolol (p. 381)
metoprolol (p. 642)
nadolol (p. 670)
pindolol (p. 780)
propranolol (p. 825)
timolol (p. 933)

Nonselective β-1 and β-2 blockers: carteolol (p. 175)

Combined α-1, β-1, and β-2 receptor blocker: labetalol (p. 543)

CALCIUM-CHANNEL BLOCKERS

Action: These products act by inhibiting calcium ion influx across the cell membrane in cardiac and vascular smooth muscle. This action produces relaxation of coronary vascular smooth muscle, dilates coronary arteries, slows SA/AV node conduction, and dilates peripheral arteries.
Uses: These products are used for chronic stable angina pectoris, vasospastic angina, dysrhythmias, hypertension, and unstable angina.
Side effects/adverse reactions: The most common side effects are dysrhythmias and edema. Also common are headache, fatigue, drowsiness, and flushing.
Contraindications: Persons with 2nd or 3rd degree heart block, sick sinus syndrome, hypotension of <90 mm Hg systolic, Wolff-Parkinson-White syndrome or cardiogenic shock should not use these products, since worsening of those conditions may occur.
Precautions: CHF may worsen, since edema may be increased. Hypotension may worsen, since B/P is decreased. Patients with renal and liver disease should use these products cautiously, since they are metabolized in the liver and excreted by the kidneys.
Pharmacokinetics: Onset, peak, and duration vary widely with route of administration. Drugs are metabolized by the liver and excreted in the urine primarily as metabolites.
Interactions/incompatibilities: Increased levels of digoxin and theophylline may occur when used with these products. Increased effects of beta blockers and antihypertensives may occur with calcium channel blockers.
Possible nursing diagnoses:
- Altered tissue perfusion: cardiopulmonary *[uses]*
- Decreased cardiac output *[adverse reactions]*

NURSING CONSIDERATIONS

Assess:
- Cardiac system, including B/P, pulse, respirations, ECG intervals (PR, QRS, QT)

Administer:
- PO before meals and hs

Evaluate:
- Therapeutic response, including decreased anginal pain, decreased B/P, dysrhythmias

Teach patient/family:

• How to take pulse before taking drug; patient should record or graph pulses to identify changes

• To avoid hazardous activities until stabilized on this drug, since dizziness occurs frequently

• Need for compliance to all areas of medical regimen, including diet, exercise, stress reduction, drug therapy

---

Generic names:

diltiazem (p. 336)
felodipine (p. 410)
nicardipine (p. 689)
nifedipine (p. 692)
verapamil HCl (p. 984)

CARDIAC GLYCOSIDES

Action: Products act by inhibiting sodium and potassium ATPase and then making more calcium available to activate contracted proteins. Cardiac contractility and cardiac output are increased.

Uses: These products are used for CHF, atrial fibrillation, atrial flutter, atrial tachycardia, and rapid digitalization in these disorders.

Side effects/adverse reactions: The most common side effects are cardiac disturbances, headache, hypotension, GI symptoms. Also common are blurred vision and yellow-green halos.

Contraindications: Hypersensitive reactions may occur, and allergies should be identified before these products are given. Also, persons with ventricular tachycardia, ventricular fibrillation, and carotid sinus syndrome should not use these products.

Precautions: Persons with acute MI and those who have or may develop serum potassium, calcium, or magnesium imbalances should use these products cautiously. Also, persons with AV block, severe respiratory disease, hypothyroidism, renal and liver disease, and the elderly should exercise caution when these drugs are prescribed.

Pharmacokinetics: Onset, peak, and duration vary widely with the route of administration. Digitoxin is inactivated by the liver, and inactive metabolites are excreted in urine. Digoxin is excreted in urine mainly as the parent drug and metabolites.

Interactions/incompatibilities: Toxicity may occur when used with diuretics, succinylcholine, quinidine, and thioamines. Increased blood levels may occur with propantheline bromide, spironolactone, quinidine, verapamil, aminoglycosides (PO), amiodarone, anticholinergics, and quinine. Diuretics may increase toxicity.

Possible nursing diagnoses:
- Altered tissue perfusion: cardiopulmonary *[uses]*
- Decreased cardiac output *[adverse reactions]*

NURSING CONSIDERATIONS

Assess:
- Cardiac system, including B/P, pulse, respirations, and increased urine output
- Apical pulse for 1 min before giving drug; if pulse <60, take again in 1 hr; if <60 notify physician
- Electrolytes, including potassium, sodium, chloride, calcium, magnesium; renal function studies, including BUN and creatinine; and blood studies, including AST, ALT, bilirubin
- I&O ratio, daily weights
- Monitor therapeutic drug levels

Administer:
- Potassium supplements if ordered for potassium levels <3.0

Evaluate:
- Therapeutic response, including decreased weight, edema, pulse, respiration, and increased urine output

Teach patient/family:
- How to take pulse before taking drug; patient should record or graph pulse to identify changes
- To avoid hazardous activities until stabilized on this drug, since dizziness occurs frequently
- Need for compliance to all areas of medical regimen, including diet, exercise, stress reduction, drug therapy

Generic names:

digitoxin (p. 330) digoxin (p. 331)

CHOLINERGIC BLOCKERS

Action: Cholinergic blockers inhibit or block acetylcholine at receptor sites in the autonomic nervous system.

Uses: Many products are used to decrease secretions before surgery, to reverse neuromuscular blockade, and to decrease motility of GI, biliary, urinary tracts. Other products are used for parkinsonian symptoms, including dystonia associated with neuroleptic drugs.

Side effects/adverse reactions: The most common side effects are dry-

ness of the mouth and constipation, which can be prevented by frequent rinsing of the mouth and increasing water and bulk in the diet.
Contraindications: Hypersensitivity can occur, and allergies should be identified before administering these products. Persons with GI and GU obstruction should not use these products, since constipation and urinary retention may occur. They are also contraindicated in angle-closure glaucoma and myasthenia gravis.
Precautions: Caution must be used when these products are given to the elderly, since metabolism is slowed. Also, persons with tachycardia or prostatic hypertrophy should use these products with caution.
Pharmacokinetics: Onset, peak, and duration vary with route.
Drug interactions/incompatibilities: Increase in anticholinergic effect occurs when used with narcotics, barbiturates, antihistamines, MAOIs, phenothiazines, amantadine.
Possible nursing diagnoses:
• Impaired physical mobility *[uses]*
• Pain *[uses]*

NURSING CONSIDERATIONS

Assess:
• I&O ratio; be alert for urinary retention, frequency, dysuria; drug should be discontinued if these occur
Administer:
• With food or milk to decrease GI symptoms
• Parenteral dose with patient recumbent to prevent postural hypotension; give parenteral dose slowly, monitoring vital signs
Perform/provide:
• Hard candy, gum, frequent rinsing of mouth for dryness
Evaluate:
• Therapeutic response, including absence of cramps, absence of extrapyramidal symptoms
• Urinary hesitancy, retention; palpate bladder if retention occurs
• Constipation; increase fluids, bulk, exercise
• For tolerance over long-term therapy, dose may need to be increased or changed
• Mental status: affect, mood, CNS depression, worsening of mental symptoms during early therapy
Teach patient/family:
• To avoid driving or other hazardous activity if drowsiness occurs
• To avoid concurrent use of cough, cold preparations with alcohol, antihistamines unless directed by physician
• To use with caution in hot weather, since medication may increase susceptibility to heat stroke

Generic names:

atropine sulfate (p. 108)
benztropine mesylate (p. 131)
biperiden HCl (p. 139)
glycopyrrolate (p. 459)
procyclidine HCl (p. 814)
scopolamine hydrobromide (p. 858)
trihexyphenidyl HCl (p. 960)

CORTICOSTEROIDS

Action: Corticosteroids are divided into glucocorticoids and mineralocorticoids. Glucocorticoids decrease inflammation by the suppression of migration of polymorphonuclear leukocytes, fibroblasts, increased capillary permeability, and lysosomal stabilization. They also have varied metabolic effects and modify the body's immune responses to many different stimuli. Mineralocorticoids act by increasing resorption of sodium by increasing hydrogen and potassium excretion in the distal tubule.
Uses: Glucocorticoids are used to decrease inflammation and for immunosuppression. In addition, some products may be given for allergy, adrenal insufficiency, or cerebral edema. Mineralocorticoids are given for adrenal insufficiency or adrenogenital syndrome.
Side effects/adverse reactions: The most common side effects include change in behavior, including insomnia and euphoria; GI irritation, including peptic ulcer; metabolic reactions, including hypokalemia, hyperglycemia, and carbohydrate intolerance; and sodium and fluid retention. Most adverse reactions are dose dependent.
Contraindications: Hypersensitivity may occur and should be identified before administering. Since these products mask infection, they should not be used in systemic fungal infections or amebiasis. Mothers taking pharmacologic doses of corticosteroids should not nurse.
Precautions: Caution must be used when these products are prescribed for diabetic patients, since hyperglycemia may occur. Also, patients with glaucoma, seizure disorders, peptic ulcer, impaired renal function, CHF, hypertension, ulcerative colitis, or myasthenia gravis should be monitored closely if corticosteroids are given. Use with caution in children and the elderly and during pregnancy.
Pharmacokinetics: For oral preparations the onset of action occurs between 1-2 hr, and duration can be up to 2 days, with a half-life of 2-4 days. Pharmacokinetics vary widely among products. These products cross the placenta and appear in breast milk.
Drug interactions/incompatibilities: Decreased corticosteroid effect may occur with barbiturates, rifampin, phenytoin; corticosteroid dose may

need to be increased. There is a possibility of GI bleeding when used with salicylates, indomethacin. Steroids may reduce salicylate levels. When using with digitalis glycosides, potassium-depleting diuretics, and amphotericin, serum potassium levels should be monitored.

Possible nursing diagnoses:

- High risk for infection *[adverse reactions]*
- Body-image disturbance *[adverse reactions]*
- High risk for violence: self-directed (suicide) *[adverse reactions]*

NURSING CONSIDERATIONS

Assess:

- Potassium, blood sugar, urine glucose while on long-term therapy; hypokalemia and hyperglycemia are common
- Weight daily; notify physician if weekly gain of >5 lb, since these products alter fluid and electrolyte balance
- I&O ratio; be alert for decreasing urinary output and increasing edema
- Plasma cortisol levels during long-term therapy (normal level is 138-635 nmol/L SI U when drawn at 8 AM
- Infection, including increased temperature, WBC, even after withdrawal of medication; drug masks symptoms of infection
- Adrenal insufficiency: nausea, anorexia, fatigue, dizziness, dyspnea, weakness, joint pain

Administer:

- With food or milk to decrease GI symptoms

Evaluate:

- Therapeutic response, including decreased inflammation
- Potassium depletion, including paresthesias, fatigue, nausea, vomiting, depression, polyuria, dysrhythmias, weakness
- Mental status, including affect, mood, behavioral changes, aggression; if severe personality changes occur, including depression, drug may need to be tapered and then discontinued

Teach patient/family:

- That ID as steroid user should be carried
- Not to discontinue this medication abruptly or adrenal crisis can result
- Teach patient all aspects of drug use, including cushingoid symptoms
- That single daily or alternate-day doses should be taken in the morning before 9 AM
- To take with meals or a snack

Generic names:

Glucocorticoids: beclomethasone dipropionate (p. 123)

methylprednisolone acetate (p. 634)

betamethasone (p. 134)
betamethasone benzoate (p. 136)
betamethasone disodium phosphate (p. 134)
betamethasone sodium phosphate (p. 134)
cortisone acetate (p. 268)
dexamethasone (p. 301)
dexamethasone acetate (p. 302)
dexamethasone sodium phosphate (p. 304)
flunisolide (p. 428)
hydrocortisone (p. 484)
hydrocortisone acetate (p. 485)
hydrocortisone sodium phosphate (p. 486)
hydrocortisone sodium succinate (p. 486)
methylprednisolone (p. 634)
methylprednisolone sodium succinate (p. 634)
paramethasone acetate (p. 735)
prednisolone (p. 802)
prednisolone acetate (p. 802)
prednisolone phosphate (p. 802)
prednisolone sodium phosphate (p. 804)
prednisolone tebutate (p. 802)
prednisone (p. 805)
triamcinolone (p. 949)
triamcinolone acetonide (p. 949)
triamcinolone diacetate (p. 949)
triamcinolone hexacetonide (p. 949)

Mineralocorticoid: fludrocortisone acetate (p. 426)

DIURETICS

Action: Diuretics are divided into subgroups: thiazides and thiazide-like diuretics, loop diuretics, carbonic anhydrase inhibitors, osmotic diuretics, and potassium-sparing diuretics. Each one of these subgroups differs in its mechanism of action. Thiazides and thiazide-like diuretics increase excretion of water and sodium by inhibiting resorption in the early distal tubule. Loop diuretics inhibit resorption of sodium and chloride in the thick ascending limb of the loop of Henle. Carbonic anhydrase inhibitors increase sodium excretion by decreasing sodium–hydrogen ion exchange throughout the renal tubule. Carbonic anhydrase inhibitors also decrease secretion of aqueous humor in the eye and thus decrease intraocular pressure. Osmotic diuretics increase the osmotic pressure of glomerular filtrate, thus decreasing net absorption of sodium. The potassium-sparing diuretics interfere with sodium resorption at the distal tubule, thus decreasing potassium excretion.

Uses: Blood pressure is reduced in hypertension; edema is reduced in CHF; intraocular pressure is decreased in glaucoma.

Side effects/adverse reactions: Hypokalemia, hyperuricemia, and hyperglycemia occur most frequently with thiazide diuretics. Aplastic anemia, blood dyscrasias, volume depletion, and dehydration may occur when thiazide-like diuretics, loop diuretics, or carbonic anhydrase inhibitors are given. Side effects and adverse reactions vary widely for the miscellaneous products.

Contraindications: Persons with electrolyte imbalances (sodium, chloride, potassium), dehydration, or anuria should not be given these products until the problem is corrected.

Precautions: Caution must be used when diuretics are given to the elderly, since electrolyte disturbances and dehydration can occur rapidly. Hepatic and renal disease may cause poor metabolism and excretion of the drug.

Pharmacokinetics: Onset, peak, and duration vary widely among the different subgroups of these drugs.

Interactions/incompatibilities: Cholestyramine and colestipol will decrease the absorption of thiazide diuretics. Concurrent use of thiazides with diazoxide may increase hyperuricemia, hyperglycemia, and antihypertensive effects of thiazides. Ototoxicity may occur when loop diuretics are used with aminoglycosides. Thiazide and loop diuretics may increase therapeutic and toxic effects of lithium.

Possible nursing diagnoses:

- Fluid volume excess *[uses]*
- Decreased cardiac output *[adverse reactions]*

NURSING CONSIDERATIONS

Assess:

- Weight, I&O daily to determine fluid loss; check skin turgor for dehydration
- Electrolytes: potassium, sodium, chloride: include BUN, blood sugar, CBC, serum creatinine, blood pH, ABGs, uric acid, calcium; electrolyte imbalances may occur quickly
- B/P lying, standing; postural hypotension may occur, since fluid loss occurs from intravascular spaces first

Administer:

- In AM to avoid interference with sleep if using drug as a diuretic
- Potassium replacement if potassium is less than 3.0

Evaluate:

- Therapeutic response: improvement in edema of feet, legs, sacral area daily if medication is being used in CHF; improvement in B/P if medication is being used as a diuretic; improvement in intraocular pressure if medication is being used to decrease aqueous humor in the eye
- Signs of metabolic alkalosis, including drowsiness and restlessness
- Signs of hypokalemia with some products, including postural hypotension, malaise, fatigue, tachycardia, leg cramps, weakness

Teach patient/family:

- To take drug early in the day (diuretic) to prevent nocturia

Generic names:

Thiazides: chlorothiazide (p. 221)
hydrochlorothiazide (p. 482)

Thiazide-like: chlorthalidone (p. 231)
indapamide (p. 506)
metolazone (p. 641)

Loop: bumetanide (p. 148)
ethacrynate acid (p. 391)
ethacrynate sodium (p. 391)
furosemide (p. 446)

Carbonic anhydrase inhibitors:
acetazolamide (p. 42)
acetazolamide sodium (p. 42)
methazolamide (p. 615)

Potassium-sparing: amiloride (p. 69)
spironolactone (p. 876)
triamterene (p. 952)

Osmotic: mannitol (p. 581)
urea (p. 975)

NARCOTICS

Action: Narcotics act by depressing pain impulse transmission at the spinal cord level by interacting with opioid receptors. Products are divided into opiates and nonopiates.

Uses: Most products are used to control moderate-to-severe pain and are used before and after surgery.

Side effects/adverse reactions: GI symptoms, including nausea, vomiting, anorexia, constipation, and cramps are the most common side effects. Other common side effects include lightheadedness, dizziness, sedation. Serious adverse reactions such as respiratory depression, respiratory arrest, circulatory depression, and increased intracranial pressure may result, but are less common and usually dose dependent.

Contraindications: Hypersensitive reactions occur frequently. Check for sensitivity before administering. These drugs should not be used if narcotic addiction is suspected, and they are also contraindicated in acute bronchial asthma and upper airway obstruction.

Precautions: Caution must be used when these products are given to persons with an addictive personality, since the possibility of addiction is so great. Also, persons with increased intracranial pressure may experience an even greater increase in intracranial pressure. Persons with severe heart disease, hepatic or renal disease, respiratory conditions, and seizure disorders should be monitored closely for worsening condition.

Pharmacokinetics: Onset of action is immediate by IV route and rapid by IM and PO routes. Peak occurs from 1-2 hr, depending on route, with a duration of 2-8 hr. These agents cross the placenta and appear in breast milk.

Drug interactions/incompatibilities: Barbiturates, other narcotics, hypnotics, antipsychotics, or alcohol can increase CNS depression when taken with narcotics.

Possible nursing diagnoses:
- Pain *[uses]*
- Impaired gas exchange *[adverse reactions]*

NURSING CONSIDERATIONS

Assess:
- I&O ratio; be alert for urinary retention, frequency, dysuria; drug should be discontinued if these occur

Administer:
- With antiemetic if nausea or vomiting occurs
- When pain is beginning to return; determine dosage interval by patient response

Perform/provide:
- Assistance with ambulation; patient should not be ambulating during drug peak

Evaluate:
- Therapeutic response, including decrease in pain
- Respiratory dysfunction, including respiratory depression, rate, rhythm, character; notify physician if respirations are <12/min
- CNS changes: dizziness, drowsiness, hallucinations, euphoria, LOC, pupil reaction
- Allergic reactions: rash, urticaria
- Need for pain medication, physical dependence

Teach patient/family:
- To report any symptoms of CNS changes, allergic reactions, or shortness of breath
- That physical dependency may result when used for extended periods of time
- That withdrawal symptoms may occur, including nausea, vomiting, cramps, fever, faintness, anorexia
- To avoid alcohol and other CNS depressants

Generic names:

alfentanil HCl (p. 54)
buprenorphine HCl (p. 150)
butorphanol tartrate (p. 156)
codeine phosphate (p. 263)
codeine sulfate (p. 263)
dezocine (p. 313)
meperidine HCl (p. 600)
methadone HCl (p. 611)
morphine sulfate (p. 664)
nalbuphine HCl (p. 673)
oxycodone HCl (p. 720)
oxymorphone HCl (p. 724)

NONSTEROIDAL ANTIINFLAMMATORIES

Action: These products act by inhibition of prostaglandin synthesis. Products have analgesic, antiinflammatory, antipyretic properties.

Uses: Products are used to control pain, inflammation associated with acute, chronic rheumatoid arthritis, osteoarthritis, and ankylosing spondylitis. Some products may be used for relief of mild-to-moderate pain, tendinitis, bursitis, fever, sunburn, migraine, dysmenorrhea.

Side effects/adverse reactions: GI symptoms, including nausea, vomiting, anorexia, are the most common side effects. May cause dizziness, drowsiness, or blurred vision. Serious adverse reactions include nephrotoxicity and blood dyscrasias.

Contraindications: Hypersensitive reactions occur frequently. Check for sensitivity before administering. Patients sensitive to aspirin or iodides should not use these agents.

Precautions: Patients with bleeding disorders should use cautiously, since bleeding tendencies may increase. GI disorders may be intensified, since these products are irritating to the GI system. Use with caution in lactation and in impaired renal or hepatic function.

Pharmacokinetics: Peak occurs from 0.5-4 hr after oral ingestion, and elimination half-life may be as long as 5 hr. They are highly bound to plasma proteins and metabolized in the liver, with metabolites excreted in the urine.

Interactions/incompatibilities: Increased anticoagulant effect may occur with coumarin. Increased toxicity may occur when used with phenytoin, sulfonamide, or sulfonylureas. Aspirin may decrease activity of nonsteroidals.

Possible nursing diagnoses:

- Pain *[uses]*
- Impaired physical mobility *[uses]*
- Activity intolerance *[uses]*
- Sensory/perceptual alteration: auditory *[adverse reactions]*

NURSING CONSIDERATIONS

Assess:

- Hepatic and renal studies: AST, ALT, bilirubin, creatinine, LDH, al-

kaline phosphatase, BUN if patient is on long-term therapy, since these products are metabolized and excreted by the liver and kidney
• Blood studies: CBC, hematocrit, hemoglobin, and prothrombin time if patient is on long-term therapy, since these products increase the possibility of bleeding and blood dyscrasias

Administer:
• With food or milk to decrease gastric irritation; give 30 min before or 1 hr after meals with a full glass of water

Evaluate:
• Therapeutic response, including decreased pain, inflammation
• Hepatotoxicity: dark urine, clay-colored stools, yellowing of skin, sclera, itching, abdominal pain, fever, diarrhea, which may occur with long-term use

Teach patient/family:
• Not to exceed recommended dosage; acute poisoning may result
• That therapeutic response takes 2 wk in arthritis
• To avoid use of alcohol, since GI bleeding may result
• To avoid taking with aspirin while on nonsteroidal therapy
• Signs and symptoms of hepatotoxicity and when to notify physician

Generic names:

diclofenac (p. 318)
etodolac (p. 403)
fenoprofen calcium (p. 412)
ibuprofen (p. 498)
indomethacin (p. 508)
ketoprofen (p. 541)
ketorolac tromethamine (p. 542)
meclofenamate (p. 590)
mefenamic acid (p. 593)
nabumetone (p. 669)
naproxen (p. 680)
naproxen sodium (p. 680)
piroxicam (p. 786)
sulindac (p. 894)
tolmetin sodium (p. 943)

SALICYLATES

Action: Salicylates have analgesic, antipyretic, and antiinflammatory effects. The antiinflammatory and analgesic activities may be mediated through the inhibition of prostaglandin synthesis. Antipyretic action results from inhibition of the hypothalamic heat-regulating center.

Uses: The primary uses of salicylates are relief of mild-to-moderate pain and fever and in inflammatory conditions such as arthritis, thromboembolic disorders, and rheumatic fever.

Side effects/adverse reactions: The most common side effects are GI symptoms and rash. Serious blood dyscrasias and hepatotoxicity may result when used for long periods of time at high doses. Tinnitus or impaired hearing may indicate that blood salicylate levels are reaching or exceeding the upper limit of the therapeutic range.

Contraindications: Hypersensitivity to salicylates is common. Check for sensitivity before administering. Persons with bleeding disorders, GI bleeding, and vitamin K deficiency should not use these products, since salicylates increase prothrombin time. Children should not use these products, since salicylates have been associated with Reye's syndrome.

Precautions: Caution is needed when salicylates are given to patients with anemia, hepatic or renal disease, or Hodgkin's disease. Caution should also be exercised in pregnancy and lactation.

Pharmacokinetics: Onset of action occurs in 15-30 min, with a peak of 1-2 hr and a duration up to 6 hr. These drugs are metabolized by the liver and excreted by the kidneys.

Drug interactions/imcompatibilities: Increased effects of anticoagulants, insulin, methotrexate, heparin, valproic acid, and oral sulfonylureas may occur when used with salicylates. Aspirin may decrease serum concentrations of nonsteroidal antiinflammatory agents.

Possible nursing diagnoses:

- Pain *[uses]*
- Impaired physical mobility *[uses]*
- Activity intolerance *[uses]*
- Sensory/perceptual alteration: auditory *[adverse reactions]*
- Thermoregulation *[uses]*

NURSING CONSIDERATIONS

Assess:

- Hepatic and renal studies: AST, ALT, bilirubin, creatinine, LDH, alkaline phosphatase, BUN if patient is on long-term therapy, since these products are metabolized and excreted by the liver and kidney
- Blood studies: CBC, hematocrit, hemoglobin, and prothrombin time if patient is on long-term therapy, since these products increase the possibility of bleeding and blood dyscrasias

Administer:

- With food or milk to decrease gastric irritation; give 30 min before or 1 hr after meals with a full glass of water

Evaluate:

- Therapeutic response/including decreased pain, fever
- Hepatotoxicity: dark urine, clay-colored stools, yellowing of skin, sclera, itching, abdominal pain, fever, diarrhea, which may occur with long-term use

• Ototoxicity: tinnitus, ringing, roaring in ears; audiometric testing is needed before and after long-term therapy

Teach patient/family:

• That blood sugar levels should be monitored closely, if patient is diabetic
• Not to exceed recommended dosage; acute poisoning may result
• That therapeutic response takes 2 wk in arthritis
• To avoid use of alcohol, since GI bleeding may result
• To notify physician if ringing in the ears or persistent GI pain occurs
• To take with full glass of H_2O to reduce risk of lodging in esophagus

---

Generic names:

aspirin (p. 103)
choline salicylate (p. 234)
magnesium salicylate (p. 577)
salsalate (p. 855)
sodium thiosalicylate (p. 873)

THYROID HORMONES

Action: Acts by increasing metabolic rates, resulting in increased cardiac output, O_2 consumption, body temperature, blood volume, growth, development at cellular level, respiratory rate, enzyme system activity.

Uses: Products are used for thyroid replacement.

Side effects/adverse reactions: The most common side effects include insomnia, tremors, tachycardia, palpitations, angina, dysrhythmias, weight loss, and changes in appetite. Serious adverse reactions include thyroid storm.

Contraindications: Persons with adrenal insufficiency, myocardial infarction, or thyrotoxicosis should not use these products.

Precautions: The elderly and patients with angina pectoris, hypertension, ischemia, cardiac disease, or diabetes mellitus or insipidus should be watched closely when using these products. Caution should be used in pregnancy (A) and lactation.

Pharmacokinetics: Pharmacokinetics vary widely among products; check specific monographs.

Interactions/incompatibilities:

• Impaired absorption of thyroid products may occur when administered with cholestyramine (separate by 4-5 hr)
• Increased effects of anticoagulants, sympathomimetics, tricyclic antidepressants, catecholamines may occur
• Decreased effects of digitalis, glycosides, insulin, hypoglycemics may occur
• Decreased effects of thyroid products may occur with estrogens

Possible nursing diagnoses:
- Knowledge deficit
- Noncompliance
- Body image disturbance [adverse reactions]

NURSING CONSIDERATIONS

Assess:
- B/P, pulse before each dose
- I&O ratio
- Weight qd in same clothing, using same scale, at same time of day
- Height, growth rate if given to a child
- T3, T4, which are decreased; radioimmunoassay of TSH, which is increased; ratio uptake, which is decreased if patient is on too low a dosage of medication

Administer:
- At same time each day to maintain drug level
- Only for hormone imbalances, not to be used for obesity, male infertility, menstrual conditions, lethargy

Perform/provide:
- Removal of medication 4 wk before RAIU test

Evaluate:
- Therapeutic response: absence of depression; increased weight loss; diuresis; pulse; appetite; absence of constipation; peripheral edema; cold intolerance; pale, cool, dry skin; brittle nails; alopecia; coarse hair; menorrhagia; night blindness; paresthesias; syncope; stupor; coma; rosy cheeks
- Increased nervousness, excitability, irritability; may indicate too high doses of medication usually after 1-3 wk of treatment
- Cardiac status: angina, palpitation, chest pain, change in VS

Teach patient/family:
- That hair loss will occur in child and is temporary
- To report excitability, irritability, anxiety; indicates overdose
- Not to switch brands unless directed by physician
- That hypothyroid child will show almost immediate behavior/personality change
- That treatment drug is not to be taken to reduce weight
- To avoid OTC preparations with iodine; read labels
- To avoid iodine food, salt-iodinized, soy beans, tofu, turnips, some seafood, some bread

---

Generic names:

levothyroxine sodium (T_4) (p. 553)
thyroglobulin (p. 926)
thyroid USP (p. 928)

liothyronine sodium (T_3) (p. 559)
liotrix (p. 561)
thyrotropin (TSH) (p. 929)

VITAMINS

Action: Action varies widely among products and classes; check specific monographs.

Uses: Vitamins are used to correct and prevent vitamin deficiencies.

Side effects/adverse reactions: There is an absence of side effects or adverse reactions with the water-soluble vitamins (C, B). However, fat-soluble vitamins (A, D, E, K) may accumulate in the body and cause adverse reactions (refer to specific monographs).

Contraindications: Hypersensitive reactions may occur, and allergies should be identified before these products are given.

Pharmacokinetics: Onset, peak, and duration vary widely among products; check individual monograph for specific information.

Possible nursing diagnosis:

- Nutrition, less than body requirements *[uses]*

NURSING CONSIDERATIONS

Administer:

- PO with food for better absorption

Perform/provide:

- Storage in tight, light-resistant container

Evaluate:

- Therapeutic response

Teach patient/family:

- Not to take more than prescribed amount

Generic names:

Fat-soluble: phytonadione (p. 777)
vitamin A (p. 989)
vitamin D (p. 990)
vitamin E (p. 991)
vitamin K-menadiol (p. 597)

Water-soluble: ascorbic acid (C) (p. 100)
cyanocobalamin hydroxocobalimin (B_{12}) (p. 274)
pyridoxine (B_6) (p. 835)
riboflavin (B_2) (p. 851)
thiamine (B_1) (p. 916)

Miscellaneous: multi vitamins (p. 667)

A

absorbable gelatin

Gelfoam

Func. class.: Hemostatic
Chem. class.: Purified gelatin solution

Action: Absorbs blood, provides area for clot formation, healthy tissue growth
Uses: Hemostasis during surgery, decubitus ulcers
Dosage and routes:
• *Adult:* TOP hold in place for 15 sec after saturating with isotonic NaCl injection
Decubitus ulcer
• *Adult:* TOP place into ulcer, may add more as needed, not to be removed
Available forms include: Sponge, pack, cone, powder
Side effects/adverse reactions: None reported
Contraindications: Hypersensitivity, frank infection, abnormal bleeding, postpartum bleeding
Pharmacokinetics:
IMPLANT: Absorbed in 4-6 wk
NURSING CONSIDERATIONS
Administer:
• By lightly packing, do not overpack foam
• Dry, hold for 10-15 sec, remove
• Moist, place in sterile saline or thrombin solution, squeeze after removing, blot before applying
• After debridement of decubiti unless dressing change qd; do not remove sponge, may add more sponges over top of old ones
Perform/provide:
• Discard unused portion; do not resterilize
Evaluate:
• Therapeutic response: Control of bleeding during surgery or healing of decubitus ulcer
• Infection: fever, redness, inflammation
Teach patient/family:
• That foam is absorbed in 4-6 wk, does not need to be removed

acebutolol

(ase-bute'-oh-lole)
Monitan,* Sectral

Func. class.: Antihypertensive
Chem. class.: Nonselective β-blocker

Action: Competitively blocks stimulation of β-adrenergic receptor within vascular smooth muscle; produces chronotropic, inotropic activity (decreases rate of SA node discharge, increases recovery time), slows conduction of AV node, decreases heart rate, which decreases O_2 consumption in myocardium; also, decreases renin-aldosterone-angiotensin system at high doses, inhibits β-2 receptors in bronchial system (high doses)
Uses: Mild to moderate hypertension, sinus tachycardia, persistent atrial extrasystoles, tachydysrhythmias, prophylaxis of angina pectoris
Dosage and routes:
Hypertension
• *Adult:* PO 400 mg qd or in 2 divided doses, may be increased to desired response
Ventricular dysrhythmia
• *Adult:* PO until dose 200 mg bid, may increase gradually, usual range 600-1200 mg daily
Available forms include: Caps 200, 400 mg, tabs 100, 200, 400 mg (Canada only)
Side effects/adverse reactions:
CV: ***Profound hypotension, bradycardia, CHF,*** *cold extremities,*

postural hypotension, ***2nd or 3rd degree heart block***
CNS: Insomnia, fatigue, dizziness, mental changes, memory loss, hallucinations, depression, lethargy, drowsiness, strange dreams, catatonia
GI: Nausea, diarrhea, vomiting, ***mesenteric arterial thrombosis, ischemic colitis***
INTEG: Rash, fever, alopecia
HEMA: Agranulocytosis, thrombocytopenia, purpura
EENT: Sore throat, dry burning eyes
GU: Impotence
ENDO: Increased hypoglycemic response to insulin
RESP: ***Bronchospasm,*** dyspnea, wheezing

Contraindications: Hypersensitivity to β-blockers, cardiogenic shock, heart block (2nd, 3rd degree), sinus bradycardia, CHF, cardiac failure

Precautions: Major surgery, pregnancy (B), lactation, diabetes mellitus, renal disease, thyroid disease, COPD, asthma, well compensated heart failure, aortic, mitral valve disease

Pharmacokinetics:
PO: Peak 2-4 hr; half-life 6-7 hr, excreted unchanged in urine, protein binding 5%-15%

Interactions/incompatibilities:
- Increased hypotension, bradycardia: reserpine, hydralazine, methyldopa, prazosin, anticholinergics
- Decreased antihypertensive effects: indomethacin
- Increased hypoglycemic effect: insulin
- Decreased bronchodilation: theophyllines

NURSING CONSIDERATIONS

Assess:
- B/P during beginning treatment, periodically thereafter; pulse q4h; note rate, rhythm, quality
- Apical/radial pulse before administration; notify physician of any significant changes (pulse <60 bpm)
- Baselines in renal, liver function tests before therapy begins

Administer:
- PO ac, hs, tablet may be crushed or swallowed whole
- Reduced dosage in renal dysfunction

Perform/provide:
- Storage protected from light, moisture; placed in cool environment

Evaluate:
- Therapeutic response: decreased B/P after 1-2 wk
- Edema in feet, legs daily
- Skin turgor, dryness of mucous membranes for hydration status, especially elderly

Teach patient/family:
- Not to discontinue drug abruptly, taper over 2 wk, may cause precipitate angina
- Not to use OTC products containing α-adrenergic stimulants (such as nasal decongestants, OTC cold preparations) unless directed by physician
- To report bradycardia, dizziness, confusion, depression, fever
- To take pulse at home, advise when to notify physician
- To avoid alcohol, smoking, sodium intake
- To comply with weight control, dietary adjustments, modified exercise program
- To carry Medic Alert ID to identify drug that you are taking, allergies
- To avoid hazardous activities if dizziness is present
- To report symptoms of CHF: dif-

ficult breathing, especially on exertion or when lying down, night cough, swelling of extremities

Lab test interferences:

Interference: Glucose/insulin tolerance tests

Treatment of overdose: Lavage, IV atropine for bradycardia, IV theophylline for bronchospasm, digitalis, O_2, diuretic for cardiac failure, hemodialysis, IV glucose for hyperglycemia, IV diazepam (or phenytoin) for seizures

acetaminophen

(a-seat-a-mee'noe-fen)

Anapap, Atasol,* Campain,* Dapa, Datril, Liquiprin, Panadol, Parten, Pedric, Robigesic,* Rounax,* Tempra, Tylenol, Valadol, Valcrin

Func. class.: Nonnarcotic analgesic

Chem. class.: Nonsalicylate, para aminophenol derivative

Action: Blocks pain impulses in CNS that occur in response to inhibition of prostaglandin synthesis; antipyretic action results from inhibition of hypothalamic heat-regulating center.

Uses: Mild to moderate pain or fever

Dosage and routes:

- *Adult and child >10 yr:* PO 325-650 mg q4h prn, not to exceed 4 g/day; REC: 325-650 mg q4h prn, not to exceed 4 g/day
- *Child 0-3 mo:* 40 mg/dose
- *Child 4-11 mo:* 80 mg/dose
- *Child <1 yr:* PO/REC 15-60 mg/dose q4-6h, not to exceed 65 mg/kg/day
- *Child 1-2 yr:* PO/REC 60 mg/dose
- *Child 2-3 yr:* PO/REC 120 mg/dose
- *Child 3-4 yr:* PO/REC 180 mg/dose
- *Child 4-5 yr:* PO/REC 240 mg/dose
- *Child 5-10 yr:* PO/REC 325 mg/dose

Available forms include: Rectal supp 120, 125, 325, 600, 650 mg; chewable tab 80 mg; caps 325, 500, 650 mg; elix 120, 160, 325 mg/5 ml; liq 160 mg/5 ml, 500mg/15ml; sol 100 mg/1 ml, 120 mg/2.5 ml

Side effects/adverse reactions:

SYST: ***Anaphylaxis***

HEMA: ***Leukopenia, neutropenia, hemolytic anemia*** (long-term use), ***thrombocytopenia, pancytopenia***

CNS: Stimulation, drowsiness

GI: Nausea, vomiting, abdominal pain, ***hepatotoxicity***

INTEG: Rash, urticaria, ***angioedema***

TOXICITY: ***Cyanosis, anemia, neutropenia, jaundice, pancytopenia, CNS stimulation, delirium then vascular collapse, convulsions, coma, death***

Contraindications: Hypersensitivity

Precautions: Anemia, hepatic disease, renal disease, chronic alcoholism, pregnancy (B)

Pharmacokinetics:

PO: Onset 10-30 min, peak ½-2 hr, duration 4-6 hr

REC: Onset slow, duration 4-6 hr

Metabolized by liver, excreted by kidneys, crosses placenta, excreted in breast milk, half-life 1-4 hr

Interactions/incompatibilities:

- Increased effects of: chloramphenicol
- Decreased effects of acetaminophen: cholestyramine, oral contraceptives, anticholinergics

• Increased effect of acetaminophen: diflunisal, caffeine

NURSING CONSIDERATIONS

Assess:

• Liver function studies: AST, ALT, bilirubin, creatinine if patient is on long-term therapy
• Renal function studies: BUN, urine creatinine if patient is on long-term therapy
• Blood studies: CBC, pro-time if patient is on long-term therapy
• I&O ratio; decreasing output may indicate renal failure (long-term therapy)

Administer:

• To patient crushed or whole; chewable tablets may be chewed
• With food or milk to decrease gastric symptoms

Evaluate:

• Therapeutic response: absence of pain, fever
• Hepatotoxicity: dark urine, clay-colored stools, yellowing of skin, sclera, itching, abdominal pain, fever, diarrhea if patient is on long-term therapy
• Allergic reactions: rash, urticaria; if these occur, drug may need to be discontinued
• Renal dysfunction: decreased urine output

Teach patient/family:

• Not to exceed recommend dosage; acute poisoning may result
• To read label on other OTC drugs; many contain acetaminophen

Treatment of overdose: Drug level q4h, gastric lavage, administer acetylcysteine

---

acetazolamide/ acetazolamide sodium

(a-set-a-zole'a-mide)

Cetazol, Diamox, Hydrazol/Diamox Parenteral

Func. class.: Diuretic; carbonic anhydrase inhibitor

Chem. class.: Sulfonamide derivative

Action: Inhibits carbonic anhydrase activity in proximal renal tubules to decrease reabsorption of water, sodium, potassium, bicarbonate; decreases carbonic anhydrase in CNS, increasing seizure threshold; able to decrease aqueous humor in eye, which lowers intraocular pressure

Uses: Open-angle glaucoma, narrow-angle glaucoma (preoperatively, if surgery delayed), epilepsy (petit mal, grand mal, mixed), edema in CHF, drug-induced edema, acute mountain sickness

Dosage and routes:

Closed-angle glaucoma

• *Adult:* PO/IM/IV 250 mg q4h, or 250 mg bid, to be used for short-term therapy

Open-angle glaucoma

• *Adult:* PO/IM/IV 250 mg-1g/day in divided doses for amounts over 250 mg

Edema

• *Adult:* IM/IV 250-375 mg/day in AM
• *Child:* IM/IV 5 mg/kg/day in AM

Seizures

• *Adult:* PO/IM/IV 8-30 mg/kg/day, usual range 375-1000 mg/day
• *Child:* PO/IM/IV 8-30 mg/kg/day in divided doses tid or qid, or 300-900 mg/m^2/day, not to exceed 1.5 g/day

*Available in Canada only

Mountain sickness
• *Adult:* PO 250 mg q8-12h
Available forms include: Tabs 125, 250 mg; caps sust rel 500 mg; inj IM/IV 500 mg

Side effects/adverse reactions:
GU: Frequency, hypokalemia, polyuria, ***uremia,*** glucosuria, hematuria, dysuria
CNS: Drowsiness, paresthesia, anxiety, depression, headache, dizziness, confusion, stimulation, fatigue, ***convulsions,*** sedation, nervousness
GI: Nausea, vomiting, anorexia, constipation, diarrhea, melena, weight loss, ***hepatic insufficiency***
EENT: Myopia, tinnitus
INTEG: Rash, pruritus, urticaria, fever, ***Stevens-Johnson syndrome,*** photosensitivity
ENDO: Hyperglycemia
HEMA: ***Aplastic anemia, hemolytic anemia, leukopenia, agranulocytosis, thrombocytopenia, purpura, pancytopenia***

Contraindications: Hypersensitivity to sulfonamides, severe renal disease, severe hepatic disease, electrolyte imbalances (hyponatremia, hypokalemia), hyperchloremic acidosis, Addison's disease, long-term use in narrow-angle glaucoma, COPD

Precautions: Hypercalciuria, pregnancy (C)

Pharmacokinetics:
PO: Onset 1-1½ hr, peak 2-4 hr, duration 6-12 hr
PO—SUS REL: Onset 2 hr, peak 8-12 hr, duration 18-24 hr
IV: Onset 2 min, peak 15 min, duration 4-5 hr
65% absorbed if fasting (oral), 75% absorbed if given with food; half-life 2½-5½ hr; excreted unchanged by kidneys (80% within 24 hr), crosses placenta

Interactions/incompatibilities:
• Increased action of: amphetamines, procainamide, quinidine, tricyclics, flecainide, ephedrine, pseudoephedrine
• Toxicity: salicylates
• Hypokalemia: with other diuretics, corticosteroids, amphotericin B
• IV compatibility: cimetidine, D_5W, $D_{10}W$, NaCl, LR

NURSING CONSIDERATIONS

Assess:
• Weight daily, I&O daily to determine fluid loss; effect of drug may be decreased if used qd
• Rate, depth, rhythm of respiration, effect of exertion
• B/P lying, standing; postural hypotension may occur
• Electrolytes: potassium, sodium, chloride; include BUN, blood sugar, CBC, serum creatinine, blood pH, ABGs, liver function tests

Administer:
• PO or IV if possible, IM administration is painful
• In AM to avoid interference with sleep if using drug as diuretic
• Potassium replacement if potassium level is less than 3.0
• With food if nausea occurs; absorption may be decreased slightly

Perform/provide:
• Storage in dark, cool area; use reconstituted solution within 24 hr
• Dilute 500 mg in >5 ml sterile H_2O for injection; direct IV—give at 100-500 mg/min; may be diluted further in compatible IV solutions and infused over 4-8 hr

Evaluate:
• Therapeutic response: improvement in edema of feet, legs, sacral area daily if medication is being used in CHF; or decrease in

aqueous humor if medication is being used in glaucoma
• Improvement in CVP q8h
• Signs of metabolic acidosis: drowsiness, restlessness
• Signs of hypokalemia: postural hypotension, malaise, fatigue, tachycardia, leg cramps, weakness
• Rashes, temperature elevation qd
• Confusion, especially in elderly; take safety precautions if needed

Teach patient/family:
• To increase fluid intake 2-3 L/day unless contraindicated; to rise slowly from lying or sitting position
• To notify physician if sore throat, unusual bleeding, bruising, paresthesias, tremors, flank pain, or skin rash occurs
• To avoid hazardous activities if drowsiness occurs

Lab test interferences:
False positive: Urinary protein

Treatment of overdose: Lavage if taken orally, monitor electrolytes, administer dextrose in saline, monitor hydration, CV, renal status

---

acetohexamide

(a-seat-oh-hex'a-mide)
Dimelor,* Dymelor

Func. class.: Antidiabetic
Chem. class.: Sulfonylurea (1st generation)

Action: Causes functioning β-cells in pancreas to release insulin, leading to drop in blood glucose levels; may improve binding between insulin and insulin receptors or increase number of insulin receptors; not effective if patient lacks functioning β-cells

Uses: Stable adult-onset diabetes mellitus (type II), NIDDM

Dosage and routes:
• *Adult:* PO 250 mg-1.5 g/day; usually given before breakfast, unless large dose is required, then dose is divided in two

Available forms include: Tabs 250, 500 mg scored

Side effects/adverse reactions:
CNS: Headache, weakness, tinnitus, fatigue, dizziness, vertigo
GI: Nausea, vomiting, diarrhea, ***hepatotoxicity, jaundice,*** heartburn
HEMA: ***Leukopenia, thrombocytopenia, agranulocytosis, aplastic anemia,*** increased AST, ALT, alk phosphatase
INTEG: Rash, allergic reactions, pruritus, urticaria, eczema, photosensitivity, erythema
ENDO: ***Hypoglycemia***

Contraindications: Hypersensitivity to sulfonylureas, juvenile or brittle diabetes

Precautions: Pregnancy (C), elderly, cardiac disease, renal disease, hepatic disease, thyroid disease, severe hypoglycemic reactions

Pharmacokinetics:
PO: Completely absorbed by GI route, onset 1 hr, peak 2-4 hr, duration 12-24 hr, half-life 6-8 hr, metabolized in liver, excreted in urine (active metabolites, unchanged drug)

Interactions/incompatibilities:
• Increased hypoglycemic effects: oral anticoagulants, salicylates, sulfonamides, nonsteroidal antiinflammatories, guanethidine, methyldopa, MAOIs, chloramphenicol, insulin, cimetidine
• Decreased action of acetohexamide: calcium channel blockers, corticosteroids, oral contraceptives, thiazide diuretics, thyroid preparations, estrogens, phenobarbital, phenothiazines, phenytoin, rifampin, sympathomimetics

---

* Available in Canada only

• Decreased effect of both drugs: diazoxide

NURSING CONSIDERATIONS

Administer:

• Drug 30 min before meals

Perform/provide:

• Storage in tight container in cool environment

Evaluate:

• Therapeutic response: decrease in polyuria, polydipsia, polyphagia, clear sensorium, absence of dizziness, stable gait

• Hypoglycemic/hyperglycemic reaction that can occur soon after meals

Teach patient/family:

• To check for symptoms of cholestatic jaundice: dark urine, pruritus, yellow sclera; if these occur physician should be notified

• To use capillary blood glucose test or Chemstrip 3 ×/day

• Symptoms of hypo/hyperglycemia, what to do about each

• That drug must be continued on daily basis; explain consequence of discontinuing drug abruptly

• To take drug in morning to prevent hypoglycemic reactions at night

• Not to drink alcohol

• To avoid OTC medications unless prescribed by physician

• That diabetes is life-long illness; that this drug is not a cure

• That all food included in diet plan must be eaten in order to prevent hypoglycemia

• To carry Medic-Alert ID for emergency purposes

Treatment of overdose: 10%-50% glucose solution or 1 mg glucagon

acetohydroxamic acid

(a-set-oh-hye-drox-am'ic)

Lithostat

Func. class.: Ammonia detoxicant, reversible urease inhibitor

Chem. class.: Hydroxylamine, ethyl acetate compound

Action: Inhibits bacterial enzyme urease, which decreases conversion of urea to ammonia; the reduced ammonia levels and decreased pH increase the effectiveness of antimicrobial agents

Uses: Adjunctive treatment in chronic urea-splitting urinary infection

Dosage and routes:

• *Adult:* PO 250 mg tid-qid q6-8h when stomach is empty, not to exceed 1.5 g/day

• *Child:* PO 10 mg/kg/day in 2-3 divided doses

Available forms include: Tabs 250 mg

Side effects/adverse reactions:

HEMA: ***Hemolytic anemia, reticulocytosis***

CNS: Headache, depression, restlessness, anxiety, nervousness

GI: Nausea, vomiting, anorexia, malaise

INTEG: Rash on face, arms, alopecia

CV: Phlebitis, ***deep vein thrombosis, pulmonary embolism,*** palpitation

Contraindications: Hypersensitivity, severe renal disease, nonurease-producing organisms, pregnancy (X)

Precautions: Deep vein thrombosis, hepatic disease, renal disease, lactation

Pharmacokinetics:

PO: Peak 15-60 min, half-life 3½-

10 hr, metabolized, excreted in urine as unchanged drug (15%-60%)

Interactions/incompatibilities:

• Decreased absorption of both drugs: iron preparations

• Rash: alcohol

NURSING CONSIDERATIONS

Assess:

• I&O ratio; observe for decrease in urinary output

• CBC, platelets, reticulocytes before, during therapy (q3 mo)

Administer:

• On empty stomach only, to facilitate absorption

Perform/provide:

• Storage in tight container at room temperature

Evaluate:

• Therapeutic response: decrease in stone formation on x-ray, decreased pain in kidney region, absence of hematuria, signs of anemia

Teach patient/family:

• To avoid alcohol, OTC preparations that contain alcohol; skin rashes have occurred

• To report any pain, redness, or hard area, usually in legs, may indicate phlebitis

• The importance of patient compliance with medical regimen; bone marrow depression may occur

• To increase fluids to 3-4 L/day

• To use contraception during treatment

---

acetylcholine chloride

(a-se-teel-koe'leen)

Miochol direct-acting

Func. class.: Miotic, cholinergic

Chem. class.: Quaternary ammonium compound

Action: Intense, immediate miosis (pupil constriction) by causing contraction of sphincter muscle of iris

Uses: Miosis during anterior segment surgery; cataract removal keratoplasty, peripheral iridectomy or cyclodialysis

Dosage and routes:

• *Adult and child:* INSTILL 0.5-2 ml of a 1% sol in anterior chamber of eye (instillation by physician)

Available forms include: Sol 1:100

Side effects/adverse reactions:

CV: Hypotension, bradycardia

EENT: Blurred vision, lens opacities

Contraindications: Hypersensitivity, when miosis is undesirable

Precautions: Acute cardiac failure, bronchial asthma

Pharmacokinetics:

INSTILL: Miosis occurs immediately, duration 10 min

NURSING CONSIDERATIONS

Administer:

• Check vial for percentage of solution

• Check label for expiration date

• After shaking vial to mix drug to clear solution, push stopper to mix solvent with powder; do not use if stopper cannot be forced down

• After cleaning stopper with alcohol or other germicidal

• IV atropine 0.6-0.8 mg for systemic reactions

Perform/provide:

• Used reconstituted solution immediately; discard unused portion

Evaluate:

• Therapeutic response: miosis during surgery

Teach patient/family:

• To report change in vision, blurring or loss of sight, trouble breathing, sweating, flushing

A

acetylcysteine

(a-se-til-sis'tay-een)
Airbron,* Mucomyst, Parvolex
Func. class.: Mucolytic
Chem. class.: Amino acid L-cysteine

Action: Decreases viscosity of secretions by breaking disulfide links of mucoproteins; increases hepatic glutathione, which is necessary to inactivate toxic metabolites in acetaminophen overdose
Uses: Acetaminophen toxicity, bronchitis, pneumonia, cystic fibrosis, emphysema, atelectasis, tuberculosis, complications of thoracic, cardiovascular surgery, diagnosis in bronchial lab tests
Dosage and routes:
• *Adult and child:* INSTILL 1-2 ml (10%-20% sol) q1-4h prn or 3-5 ml (20% sol) or 6-10 ml (10% sol) tid or qid
Acetaminophen toxicity
• *Adult and child:* PO 140 mg/kg, then 70 mg/kg q4h × 17 doses to total of 1330 mg/kg
Available forms include: Sol 10%, 20%
Side effects/adverse reactions:
CNS: Dizziness, drowsiness, headache, fever, chills
GI: Nausea, stomatitis, constipation, vomiting, anorexia, ***hepatotoxicity***
EENT: Rhinorrhea, tooth damage
CV: Hypotension
INTEG: Urticaria, rash, fever, clamminess
RESP: ***Bronchospasm,*** burning, hemoptysis, chest tightness
Contraindications: Hypersensitivity, increased intracranial pressure, status asthmaticus
Precautions: Hypothyroidism, Addison's disease, CNS depression, brain tumor, asthma, hepatic disease, renal disease, COPD, psychosis, alcoholism, convulsive disorders, lactation, pregnancy (B)
Pharmacokinetics:
INH/INSTILL: Onset 1 min, duration 5-10 min, metabolized by liver, excreted in urine
Interactions/incompatibilities:
• Do not use with iron, copper, rubber
• Do not mix with antibiotics: tetracycline, chlortetracycline, oxytetracycline, erythromycin, lactobionate, amphotericin-B, sodium ampicillin; iodized oil, chymotrypsin, trypsin, hydrogen peroxide

NURSING CONSIDERATIONS

Assess:
• VS, cardiac status including checking for dysrhythmias, increased rate, palpitations
• ABGs for increased CO_2 retention in asthma patients
• Antidotal use: liver function tests, acetaminophen levels; inform physician if dose is vomited or vomiting is persistent
Administer:
• Store in refrigerator: use within 96 hr of opening
• Before meals ½-1 hr for better absorption, to decrease nausea
• 20% solutions diluted with NS over water for injection; may give 10% solution undiluted
• Only after patient clears airway by deep breathing, coughing
• Antidotal use: give within 24 hr; give with cola or soft drink to disguise taste; can be given with H_2O through tubes; use within 1 hr
• By syringe 2-3 doses of 1-2 ml of 20% or 2-4 ml of 10% solution
• Decreased dose to elderly patients; their metabolism may be slowed

• Gum, hard candy, frequent rinsing of mouth for dryness of oral cavity
• Only if suction machine is available

Perform/provide:
• Storage in refrigerator after opening
• Assistance with inhaled dose: bronchodilator if bronchospasm occurs
• Mechanical suction if cough insufficient to remove excess bronchial secretions

Evaluate:
• Therapeutic response: absence of purulent secretions when coughing
• Cough: type, frequency, character including sputum
• Rate, rhythm of respirations, increased dyspnea; discontinue if bronchospasm occurs
• Antidotal use: decrease in hepatic encephalopathy

Teach patient/family:
• To avoid driving or other hazardous activities until patient is stabilized on this medication
• To avoid alcohol, other CNS depressants; will enhance sedating properties of this drug
• That unpleasant odor will decrease after repeated use
• That discoloration of solution after bottle is opened does not impair its effectiveness
• To avoid smoking, smoke-filled rooms, perfume, dust, environmental pollutants, cleaners

---

activated charcoal

Arm-a-char, Actidose-Aqua, Liqu-Char, Superchar, Charcoaide, Charcocaps, Charcodote, Charcotabs, Digestalin

Func. class.: Antiflatulent/antidote

Action: Binds poisons, toxins, irritants; increases adsorption in GI tract; inactivates toxins and binds until excreted

Uses: Flatulence, poisoning, dyspepsia, distention, deodorant in wounds, diarrhea

Dosage and routes:

Poisoning
• *Adult and child:* PO 5-10 × weight of substance ingested, minimum dose 30 g/250 ml of water, may give 20-40g q6h for 1-2 days in severe poisoning

Flatulence/dyspepsia
• *Adult:* PO 520-975 mg p.c. up to 4.16 g/day

Available forms include: Powder; liq 12.5, 25, 30,50 g; caps 260 mg; tabs 325 mg

Side effects/adverse reactions:
GI: Nausea, black stools, vomiting, constipation, diarrhea

Contraindications: Hypersensitivity to this drug, unconsciousness/semiconsciousness, poisoning of cyanide, mineral acids, alkalies

Pharmacokinetics:
PO: Not metabolized, excreted in feces

Interactions/incompatibilities:
• Decreased effectiveness of both drugs: ipecac, laxatives
• Do not mix with dairy products

NURSING CONSIDERATIONS

Assess:
• Respiration, pulse, B/P to determine charcoal effectiveness if taken for barbiturate/narcotic poisoning

Administer:
• After inducing vomiting first unless contraindicated (i.e., cyanide or alkalies)
• After mixing with water or fruit juice to form thick syrup; do not use dairy products to mix charcoal
• Repeat dose if vomiting occurs soon after dose
• After spacing at least 1 hr before

---

* Available in Canada only

or after other drugs, or absorption will be decreased
• With a laxative to promote elimination
• Alone; do not administer with ipecac
• Through a nasogastric tube if patient unable to swallow
• Keeping container tightly closed to prevent absorption of gases
Evaluate:
• Therapeutic response: LOC-alert (poisoning)
Teach patient/family:
• That stools will be black

acyclovir (topical)

(ay-sye'kloe-ver)
Zovirax

Func. class.: Local antiinfective
Chem. class.: Antiviral

Action: Interferes with viral DNA replication
Uses: Simple mucocutaneous herpes simplex, in immunocompromised clients with initial herpes genitalis
Dosage and routes:
• *Adult and child:* TOP apply to all lesions q3h while awake, 6 times/day × 1 wk
Available forms include: TOP oint 5% (50 mg/g)
Side effects/adverse reactions:
INTEG: Rash, urticaria, stinging, burning, pruritus, vulvitis
Contraindications: Hypersensitivity
Precautions: Pregnancy (C), lactation
NURSING CONSIDERATIONS
Administer:
• Using finger cot or rubber glove to prevent further infection
• Enough medication to completely cover lesions
• After cleansing with soap, water before each application, dry well
Perform/provide:
• Storage at room temperature in dry place
Evaluate:
• Allergic reaction: burning, stinging, swelling, redness, rash, vulvitis, pruritus
• Therapeutic response: decrease in size, number of lesions
Teach patient/family:
• Not to use in eyes, or use when there is not evidence of infection
• To apply with glove to prevent further infection
• To avoid use of OTC creams, ointments, lotions unless directed by physician
• To use medical asepsis (hand washing) before, after each application and avoid contact with eyes
• Strict adherence to prescribed regimen to maximize successful treatment outcome
• To begin taking drug when symptoms arise

acyclovir sodium

(ay-sye-kloe-ver)
Zovirax

Func. class.: Antiviral
Chem. class.: Acylic purine nucleoside analog

Action: Interferes with DNA synthesis needed for viral replication
Uses: Mucocutaneous herpes simplex virus, herpes genitalis (HSV-1, HSV-2)
Dosage and routes:
Herpes simplex
• *Adult and child >12 yr:* IV INF 5 mg/kg over 1 hr q8h × 5 days
• *Child <12 yr:* IV INF 250 mg/m² over 1 hr q8h × 5 days
Genital herpes

• *Adult:* PO 200 mg q4h 5 × /day while awake for 5 days to 6 mo depending whether initial, recurrent, or chronic

Available forms include: Caps 200 mg; inj IV 500 mg, oint (see topical listings)

Side effects/adverse reactions:

CNS: Tremors, confusion, lethargy, hallucinations, ***convulsions,*** dizziness, *headache*

HEMA: Anemia, increased bleeding time, ***bone marrow depression, granulocytopenia, thrombocytopenia, leukopenia, megaloblastic anemia***

GI: Nausea, vomiting, diarrhea, increased ALT, AST, abdominal pain, glossitis, colitis

GU: Oliguria, proteinuria, hematuria, *vaginitis, moniliasis,* ***glomerulonephritis, acute renal failure***, changes in menses

INTEG: Rash, urticaria, pruritus, phlebitis at IV site

Contraindications: Hypersensitivity, herpes zoster in immunosuppressed individual

Precautions: Lactation, hepatic disease, renal disease, electrolyte imbalance, dehydration, pregnancy (C)

Pharmacokinetics:

IV: Peak 1 hr, half-life 20 min-3 hr, (terminal), metabolized by liver, excreted by kidneys as unchanged drug (95%), crosses placenta

Interactions/incompatibilities:

• Increased neurotoxicity, nephrotoxicity: aminoglycosides, amphotericin, interferon, probenecid, methotrexate

• IV incompatibility: dobutamine, dopamine, all protein products

• IV-compatible solutions: D_5W, LR, or NaCl solutions

NURSING CONSIDERATIONS

Assess:

• Signs of infection, anemia

• I&O ratio; report hematuria, oliguria, fatigue, weakness; may indicate nephrotoxicity; check for protein in urine during treatment

• Any patient with compromised renal system, since drug is excreted slowly in poor renal system function; toxicity may occur rapidly

• Liver studies: AST, ALT

• Blood studies: WBC, RBC, Hct, Hgb, bleeding time; blood dyscrasias may occur; drug should be discontinued

• Renal studies: urinalysis, protein, BUN, creatinine, CrCl

• C&S before drug therapy; drug may be taken as soon as culture is taken; repeat C&S after treatment

Administer:

• Increased fluids to 3 L/day to decrease crystalluria when given IV

• After reconstituting with 10 ml compatible solution/500 mg of drug, concentration of 50 mg/ml, shake, use within 12 hr; give over at least 1 hr by infusion pump to prevent nephrotoxicity

Perform/provide:

• Storage at room temperature for up to 12 hr after reconstitution

• Adequate intake of fluids (2000 ml) to prevent deposit in kidneys

Evaluate:

• Therapeutic response: absence of itching, painful lesions

• Bowel pattern before, during treatment; if severe abdominal pain with bleeding occurs, drug should be discontinued

• Skin eruptions: rash, urticaria, itching

• Allergies before treatment, reaction of each medication; place allergies on chart, Kardex in bright red letters

Teach patient/family:

• That drug may be taken orally before infection occurs; drug should

---

* Available in Canada only

be taken when itching or pain occurs, usually before eruptions
• That partners need to be told that patient has herpes; they could become infected
• That drug does not cure infection, just controls symptoms
• To report sore throat, fever, fatigue; could indicate superimposed infection
• That drug must be taken in equal intervals around the clock to maintain blood levels for duration of therapy
• To notify physician of side effects of bruising, bleeding, fatigue, malaise; may indicate blood dyscrasias

adenosine

(ah-den'oh-seen)
Adenocard

Func. class.: Antidysrhythmic
Chem. class.: Endogenous nucleoside

Action: Slows conduction through AV node, can interrupt reentry pathways through AV node, and can restore normal sinus rhythm in patients with paroxysmal supraventricular tachycardia (PSVT)
Uses: PSVT
Dosage and routes:
• *Adult:* IV BOL 6 mg; if conversion to normal sinus rhythm does not occur within 1-2 min, give 12 mg by rapid IV BOL; may repeat 12 mg dose again
Available forms include: Inj 3 mg/ml
Side effects/adverse reactions:
GI: Nausea, metallic taste, throat tightness, groin pressure
RESP: Dyspnea, chest pressure, hyperventilation
CNS: Lightheadedness, dizziness, arm tingling, numbness, apprehension, blurred vision, headache
CV: Chest pain, ***atrial tachydysrhythmias,*** sweating, palpitations, hypotension, *facial flushing*
Contraindications: Hypersensitivity, 2nd or 3rd degree heart block, AV block, sick sinus syndrome, atrial flutter, atrial fibrillation, ventricular tachycardia
Precautions: Pregnancy (C), lactation, children, asthma, elderly
Pharmacokinetics: Cleared from plasma in <30 sec, half-life 10 sec
Interactions/incompatibilities:
• Increased effects of adenosine: dipyridamole
• Decreased activity of adenosine; theophylline or other methylxanthines (caffeine)
• Higher degree of heart block: car-

NURSING CONSIDERATIONS

Assess:
• Cardiac status continually
• B/P continuously for fluctuations
• I&O ratio, electrolytes (K, Na, Cl)
Administer:
• IV bolus undiluted; give 6 mg or less over 1 min
Perform/provide
• Storage at room temperature, sol should be clear
Evaluate:
• Therapeutic response: decreased anginal pain, decreased B/P, dysrhythmias
• Cardiac status: B/P, pulse, respiration, ECG intervals (PR, QRS, QT)
• Respiratory status: rate, rhythm, lung fields for rales, watch for respiratory depression
• CNS effects: dizziness, confusion, psychosis, paresthesias, convulsions; drug should be discontinued

• Lung fields, bilateral rales may occur in CHF patient
• Increased respiration, increased pulse; drug should be discontinued
Lab test interferences:
Increase: Liver function tests
Treatment of overdose: Defibrillation, vasopressor for hypotension

albumin, normal serum 5%/25%

(al-byoo'min)
Albuminar 5%, Albutein 5%, Buminate 5%, Plasbumin 5%, Albuminar 25%, Albumisol 25%, Buminate 25%, Plasbumin 25%
Func. class.: Blood derivative
Chem. class.: Placental human plasma

Action: Exerts oncotic pressure, which expands volume of circulating blood
Uses: Restores plasma volume in burns, hyperbilirubinemia, shock, hypoproteinemia, varicella zoster infections (supportive treatment)
Dosage and routes:
Burns
• *Adult:* IV dose to maintain plasma albumin at 30-50 g/L, use 5% sol initially, then 25% sol after 24 hr
Shock
• *Adult:* IV 500 ml of 5% sol q30 min, as needed
• *Child:* ¼-½ adult dose in nonemergencies
Hypoproteinemia
• *Adult:* IV 1000-2000 ml of 5% sol qd, not to exceed 5-10 ml/min or 25-100 g of 25% sol qd, not to exceed 3 ml/min, titrated to patient response
Hyperbilirubinemia/erythroblastosis fetalis
• *Infant:* IV 1 g of 25% sol/kg before transfusion
Available forms include: Inj IV 50, 250 mg/ml
Side effects/adverse reactions:
GI: Nausea, vomiting, increased salivation
INTEG: Rash, urticaria
CNS: Fever, chills, flushing, headache
RESP: Altered respirations, pulmonary edema
CV: Fluid overload, hypotension, erratic pulse, tachycardia
Contraindications: Hypersensitivity, congestive heart failure, severe anemia
Precautions: Decreased salt intake, decreased cardiac reserve, lack of albumin deficiency, hepatic disease, renal disease, pregnancy (C)
Pharmacokinetics: In hyponutrition states metabolized as protein/energy source.

NURSING CONSIDERATIONS

Assess:
• Blood studies Hct, Hgb; if serum protein declines, dyspnea, hypoxemia can result
• Decreased B/P, erratic pulse, respiration
• I&O ratio: urinary output may decrease
• CVP, pulmonary wedge pressure will increase if overload occurs
Administer:
• IV slowly, to prevent fluid overload; dilute with NS for injection or D_5W; may be given undiluted; use infusion pump
• Within 4 hr of opening
Perform/provide:
• Adequate hydration before, during administration
• Check type of albumin, some stored at room temperature, some need to be refrigerated

* Available in Canada only

Evaluate:
• Therapeutic response: increased B/P, decreased edema, increased serum albumin
• Allergy: fever, rash, itching, chills, flushing, urticaria, nausea, vomiting, hypotension, requires discontinuation of infusion, use of new lot if therapy reinstituted
• CVP reading: distended neck veins indicate circulatory overload; shortness of breath, anxiety, insomnia, expiratory rales, frothy blood-tinged cough, cyanosis indicate pulmonary overload

Lab test interferences:
False increase: Alk phosphatase

---

albuterol

(al-byoo'ter-ole)
Proventil, Salbutamol,* Ventolin
Func. class.: Adrenergic β-2 agonist

Action: Causes bronchodilation by action on β_2 receptors by increasing levels of cAMP, which relaxes smooth muscle with very little effect on heart rate

Uses: Prevention of exercise-induced asthma, bronchospasm

Dosage and routes:
Asthma
• *Adult:* INH 2 puffs 15 min before exercising, Neb/LPPB 5 mg tid-qid
Bronchospasm
• *Adult:* INH 1-2 puffs q4-6h PO 2-4 mg tid-qid, not to exceed 8 mg
Available forms include: Aerosol 90 μg/actuation; tabs 2, 4 mg; syr 2 mg/5 ml

Side effects/adverse reactions:
CNS: Tremors, anxiety, insomnia, headache, dizziness, stimulation, restlessness, hallucinations, flushing, irritability
EENT: Dry nose, irritation of nose and throat
CV: Palpitations, tachycardia, hypertension, angina, hypotension, dysrhythmias
GI: Heartburn, nausea, vomiting
MS: Muscle cramps
RESP: ***Bronchospasm***
GU: Difficulty in urination

Contraindications: Hypersensitivity to sympathomimetics, tachydysrhythmias, severe cardiac disease

Precautions: Lactation, pregnancy (C), cardiac disorders, hyperthyroidism, diabetes mellitus, hypertension, prostatic hypertrophy, narrow angle glaucoma, seizures

Pharmacokinetics:
PO: Onset ½ hr, peak 2½ hr, duration 4-6 hr, half-life 2½ hr
INH: Onset 5-15 min, peak ½-2 hr, duration 3-6 hr, half-life 4 hr
Metabolized in the liver, excreted in urine, crosses placenta, breast milk, blood-brain barrier

Interactions/incompatibilities:
• Increased action of: aerosol bronchodilators
• Increased action of albuterol: tricyclic antidepressants, MAOIs
• May inhibit action of albuterol: other β-blockers

NURSING CONSIDERATIONS

Assess:
• Respiratory function: vital capacity, forced expiratory volume, ABGs, lung sounds, heart rate and rhythm

Administer:
• After shaking, exhale, place mouthpiece in mouth, inhale slowly, hold breath, remove, exhale slowly
• Gum, sips of water for dry mouth
• PO with meals to decrease gastric irritation

Perform/provide:
• Storage in light-resistant container, do not expose to temperatures over 86° F
Evaluate:
• Therapeutic response: absence of dyspnea, wheezing after 1 hr
Teach patient/family:
• Not to use OTC medications, extra stimulation may occur
• Use of inhaler, review package insert with patient
• To avoid getting aerosol in eyes
• To wash inhaler in warm water qd and dry
• To avoid smoking, smoke-filled rooms, persons with respiratory infections
Treatment of overdose: Administer a β_2-adrenergic blocker

alfentanil HCl

(al-fen'ta-nil)
Alfenta

Func. class.: Narcotic analgesic
Chem. class.: Opiate, synthetic

Action: Inhibits ascending pain pathways in limbic system, thalamus, midbrain, hypothalamus
Uses: In combination with other drugs in general anesthesia, as a primary anesthetic in general surgery
Dosage and routes:
Combination
• *Adult:* IV 8-50 μg/kg, may increase by 3-15 μg/kg
Anesthetic induction
• *Adult:* IV 130-245 μg/kg, then 0.5-1.5 μg/kg/min
Available forms include: Inj 500 μg/ml
Side effects/adverse reactions:
CNS: Drowsiness, dizziness, confusion, headache, sedation, euphoria, delirium, agitation, anxiety
GI: Nausea, vomiting, anorexia, constipation, cramps, dry mouth
GU: Urinary retention, dysuria
INTEG: Rash, urticaria, bruising, flushing, diaphoresis, pruritus
EENT: Tinnitus, blurred vision, miosis, diplopia
CV: Palpitation, bradycardia, change in B/P, facial flushing, syncope, asystole
RESP: ***Respiratory depression, apnea***
MS: Rigidity
Contraindications: Child <12 yr, hypersensitivity
Precautions: Pregnancy (C), lactation, increased intracranial pressure, acute MI, severe heart disease, renal disease, hepatic disease, asthma, respiratory conditions, convulsive disorders, elderly
Pharmacokinetics: Half-life 1-2 hr, 90% bound to plasma proteins, duration 30 min
Interactions/incompatibilities:
• Respiratory depression, hypotension, profound sedation: alcohol, sedative hypnotics, or other CNS depressants, antihistamines, phenothiazines
• Compatible IV solution: LR, 0.9% NaCl, D_5W, D_5/0.9% NaCl

NURSING CONSIDERATIONS

Assess:
• I&O ratio, check for decreasing output; may indicate urinary retention, especially elderly
• CNS changes: dizziness, drowsiness, hallucinations, euphoria, LOC, pupil reaction
Administer:
• Direct IV over 1½-3 min
• Cont. IV by diluting 20 ml of drug in 230 ml of diluent (40 μg/ml)
Perform/provide:
• Storage in light-resistant area at room temperature

Evaluate:
• Therapeutic response: maintenance of anesthesia
• Allergic reactions: rash, urticaria
• Respiratory dysfunction: respiratory depression, character, rate, rhythm: notify physician if respirations are <12/min

Lab test interferences:
Increase: Amylase

Treatment of overdose: Narcan 0.2-0.8 IV, O_2, IV fluids, vasopressors

alglucerase

Ceredase

Func. class.: Enzyme

Action: Stimulates proliferation and differentiation of hematopoietic progenitor cells

Uses: Long-term enzyme replacement for a confirmed diagnosis of type I Gaucher's disease

Dosage and routes:
• *Adult and child:* IV 60 U/kg diluted in up to 100 ml of 0.9% NaCl given over 1-2 hr; dose is repeated q2wk, but may be given QOD or as infrequently as q4wk; dose should be adjusted downward at intervals of 3-6 mo

Available forms include: Inj 80 IU/ml

Side effects/adverse reactions:
CNS: Fever, malaise, chills
GI: Nausea, vomiting, diarrhea, abdominal discomfort
INTEG: Pain on injection, burning and swelling at site of injection

Contraindications: Hypersensitivity

Precautions: Pregnancy (C), lactation

Pharmacokinetics: Steady-state enzymatic activity occurs within 60 min after a single injection, elimination half-life 4-20 min

NURSING CONSIDERATIONS

Assess:
• GI status: transient nausea, vomiting, abdominal discomfort
• Hypersensitive reactions; rashes and local injection site reactions may occur
• For increased fluid retention in cardiac disease

Administer:
• By IV infusion over 1-2 hr
• Dilute 60 U/kg in up to 10 ml of 0.9% NaCl

Perform/provide:
• Storage in refrigerator; do not freeze, do not shake as this may inactivate the drug

Evaluate:
• Therapeutic response: Reduction of splenomegaly and hepatomegaly; improvement of hematologic deficiencies, reduced cachexia and wasting in children

Teach patient/family:
• To use medication only as directed by physician
• To report unusual side effects and avoid all other medications unless prescribed by physician

allopurinol

(al-oh-pure'i-nole)

Apoallopurinol,* Novapurol,* Lopurin, Purimol,* Zyloprim, Zurinol

Func. class.: Antigout drug
Chem. class.: Enzyme inhibitor

Action: Inhibits the enzyme xanthine oxidase, reducing uric acid synthesis

Uses: Chronic gout, hyperuricemia associated with malignancies, recurrent calcium oxalate calculi

Dosage and routes:
Gout/hyperuricemia

• *Adult:* PO 200-600 mg qd depending on severity, not to exceed 800 mg/day
• *Child 6-10 yr:* 300 mg qd
• *Child <6 yr:* 150 mg qd

Impaired renal function
• *Adult:* PO 200 mg qd when CrCl is 20 to 10 ml/min

Recurrent calculi
• *Adult:* PO 200-300 mg qd

Uric acid nephropathy prevention
• *Adult:* PO 600-800 mg qd × 2-3 days

Available forms include: Tabs 100, 300 mg

Side effects/adverse reactions:
HEMA: ***Agranulocytosis, thrombocytopenia, aplastic anemia, pancytopenia, leukopenia, bone marrow depression, eosinophilia***
CNS: Headache, drowsiness, neuritis, paresthesia
GI: Nausea, vomiting, anorexia, malaise, metallic taste, cramps, peptic ulcer, diarrhea, stomatitis
MISC: Myopathy, arthralgia, hepatomegaly, cholestatic jaundice, renal failure
EENT: Retinopathy, cataracts, epistaxis
INTEG: Fever, chills, dermatitis, pruritus, purpura, erythema, ecchymosis, alopecia

Contraindications: Hypersensitivity

Precautions: Pregnancy (B), lactation, renal disease, hepatic disease, children

Pharmacokinetics:
PO: Peak 2-4 hr; excreted in feces, urine, half-life 2-3 hr, terminal half-life 18-30 hr

Interactions/incompatibilities:
• Increased action of: oral anticoagulants, chlorpropamide, cyclophosphamide, hydantoin, theophylline, vidarabine, ACE inhibitors
• Decreased effects of: probenecid
• Rash: ampicillin, amoxicillin
• Increased hypersensitivity: thiazide diuretics
• Decreased effects of allopurinol: aluminum salts

NURSING CONSIDERATIONS

Assess:
• Uric acid levels q2 wk; uric acid levels should be 6 mg/dl
• CBC, AST, BUN, creatinine before starting treatment, monthly
• I&O ratio; increase fluids to prevent stone formation

Administer:
• With meals, to prevent GI symptoms
• A few days before antineoplastic therapy

Evaluate:
• Therapeutic response: decreased pain in joints, decreased stone formation in kidney
• Nutritional status: discourage organ meat, sardines, salmon, legumes, gravies (high purine foods)

Teach patient/family:
• To increase fluid intake to 3-4 L/day
• To report skin rash, stomatitis, malaise, fever, aching; drug should be discontinued
• To avoid hazardous activities if drowsiness or dizziness occurs
• To avoid alcohol, caffeine; will increase uric acid levels
• Avoid large doses of vitamin C; kidney stone formation may occur

Lab test interferences:
Increase: AST/ALT, alk phosphatase
Decrease: Hct/Hgb, leukocytes, serum glucose

A

alprazolam

(al-pray'zoe-lam)

Xanax

Func. class.: Antianxiety
Chem. class.: Benzodiazepine

Controlled Substance Schedule IV

Action: Depresses subcortical levels of CNS, including limbic system, reticular formation

Uses: Anxiety, panic disorders, anxiety with depressive symptoms

Dosage and routes:

• *Adult:* PO 0.25-0.5 mg tid, not to exceed 4 mg in divided doses/day

• *Geriatric:* PO 0.25 mg bid-tid

Available forms include: Tab 0.25, 0.5, 1 mg

Side effects/adverse reactions:

CNS: Dizziness, drowsiness, confusion, headache, anxiety, tremors, stimulation, fatigue, depression, insomnia, hallucinations

GI: Constipation, dry mouth, nausea, vomiting, anorexia, diarrhea

INTEG: Rash, dermatitis, itching

CV: Orthostatic hypotension, ***ECG changes, tachycardia,*** hypotension

EENT: Blurred vision, tinnitus, mydriasis

Contraindications: Hypersensitivity to benzodiazepines, narrow-angle glaucoma, psychosis, pregnancy (D), child <18 yr

Precautions: Elderly, debilitated, hepatic disease, renal disease

Pharmacokinetics:

PO: Onset 30 min, peak 1-2 hr, duration 4-6 hr, therapeutic response 2-3 days, metabolized by liver, excreted by kidneys, crosses placenta, breast milk, half-life 12-15 hr

Interactions/incompatibilities:

• Increased CNS depression: anticonvulsants, alcohol, antihistamines, sedative/hypnotics

• Decreased action of alprazolam: disulfiram, cimetidine

• Decreased action of: levodopa

NURSING CONSIDERATIONS

Assess:

• B/P (lying, standing), pulse; if systolic B/P drops 20 mm Hg, hold drug, notify physician

• Blood studies: CBC during long-term therapy; blood dyscrasias have occurred rarely

• Hepatic studies: AST, ALT, bilirubin, creatinine, LDH, alk phosphatase

• I&O; may indicate renal dysfunction

• For indications of increasing tolerance and abuse

Administer:

• With food or milk for GI symptoms

• Crushed if patient is unable to swallow medication whole

• Sugarless gum, hard candy, frequent sips of water for dry mouth

Perform/provide:

• Assistance with ambulation during beginning therapy; drowsiness/dizziness occurs

• Safety measures, including siderails

• Check that PO medication has been swallowed

Evaluate:

• Therapeutic response: decreased anxiety, restlessness, sleeplessness

• Mental status: mood, sensorium, affect, sleeping pattern, drowsiness, dizziness, especially elderly

• Physical dependency, withdrawal symptoms: anxiety, panic attacks, agitation, convulsions, headache, nausea, vomiting, muscle pain, weakness

• Suicidal tendencies

Teach patient/family:
• That drug may be taken with food
• Not to use for everyday stress or longer than 3 mo, unless directed by physician; not to take more than prescribed amount, may be habit forming
• To avoid OTC preparations unless approved by physician
• To avoid driving, activities that require alertness, since drowsiness may occur
• To avoid alcohol ingestion or other psychotropic medications, unless prescribed by physician
• Not to discontinue medication abruptly after long-term use
• To rise slowly or fainting may occur, especially elderly
• That drowsiness might worsen at beginning of treatment

Lab test interferences:
Increase: AST/ALT, serum bilirubin
False increase: 17-OHCS
Decrease: RAIU

Treatment of overdose: Lavage, VS, supportive care

---

alprostadil

(al-pros'ta-dil)
Prostin VR Pediatric
Func. class.: Hormone
Chem. class.: Prostaglandin E_1

Action: Relaxes smooth muscles of ductus arteriosus; results in increased O_2 content throughout body

Uses: Patent ductus arteriosus (temporary treatment)

Dosage and routes:
• *Infants:* IV INF 0.1 μg/kg/min, until desired response, then reduce to lowest effective amount, not to exceed 0.4 μg/kg/min

Available forms include: Inj IV 500 μg/ml

Side effects/adverse reactions:
MISC: Sepsis, hypokalemia, peritonitis, hypoglycemia, hyperkalemia
RESP: ***Apnea, bradypnea, wheezing, respiratory depression***
HEMA: ***DIC*** (disseminated intravascular coagulation), ***thrombocytopenia,*** anemia, ***bleeding***
CNS: Fever, ***convulsions,*** lethargy, hypothermia, stiffness
GI: Diarrhea, regurgitation
GU: Oliguria, hematuria, ***anuria***
CV: ***Bradycardia, tachycardia,*** *hypotension,* ***CHF, ventricular fibrillation, shock,*** flushing, ***cardiac arrest***

Contraindications: ***Hypersensitivity,*** respiratory distress syndrome (RDS)

Precautions: Bleeding disorders

Pharmacokinetics: Metabolized in lungs, up to 80%, excreted in urine (metabolites)

NURSING CONSIDERATIONS

Assess:
• ABGs, arterial pH, arterial pressure, continuous ECG; if arterial pressure decreases, reduce or stop drug

Administer:
• Only with emergency equipment available by trained clinicians
• After diluting with NS or D_5W injection to a concentration of 500 μg/ml, dilute further with 0.9% NaCl, D_5W; 500 μg of drug/250 mg of dilute = 2 μg/ml

Perform/provide:
• Arterial pressure measurement during infusion
• Refrigeration for drug; discard all mixed unused portion

Evaluate:
• Therapeutic response: increased PO_2 (cyanotic heart disease)
• Apnea and bradycardia; if these occur, discontinue drug

• Increased pH, B/P, output, decreased ratio of PA to AP (restricted systemic blood flow)
Teach patient/family:
• About diagnosis, prognosis, treatment

alteplase

(al-teep'lase)
Activase

Func. class.: Antithrombotic
Chem. class.: Tissue plasminogen activator (TPA)

Action: Produces fibrin conversion of plasminogen to plasmin; able to bind to fibrin, convert plasminogen in thrombus to plasmin, which leads to local fibrinolysis, limited systemic proteolysis
Uses: Lysis of obstructing thrombi associated with acute MI
Dosage and routes:
• *Adult:* IV a total of 100 mg; 6-10 mg given IV Bol over 1-2 min, 60 mg given over first hour, 20 mg given over second hour, 20 mg given over third hour; or 1.25 mg/kg given over 3 hr for smaller patients
Available forms include: Powder for inj 20 mg (11.6 million IU)/vial, 50 mg (29 million IU)/vial
Side effects/adverse reactions:
SYST: ***GI, GU, intracranial, retroperitoneal bleeding,*** *surface bleeding*
CV: ***Sinus bradycardia, ventricular tachycardia, accelerated idioventricular rhythm***
INTEG: Urticaria, rash
Contraindications: Hypersensitivity, active internal bleeding, recent CVA, severe uncontrolled hypertension, intracranial/intraspinal surgery/trauma, aneurysm
Precautions: Pregnancy (C), lactation, children
Pharmacokinetics: Cleared by liver, 80% cleared within 10 min of drug termination
Interactions/incompatibilities:
• Increased bleeding: heparin, acetylsalicylic acid, dipyridamole
• Do not add other drugs to IV solution

NURSING CONSIDERATIONS

Assess:
• VS, B/P, pulse, respirations, neurologic signs, temperature at least q4h; temperature >104° F is indicator of internal bleeding; monitor rhythm closely; ventricular dysrhythmias may occur with hyperfusion; monitor heart, breath sounds, neuro status, peripheral pulses
• For bleeding during first hr of treatment: hematuria, hematemesis, bleeding from mucous membranes, epistaxis, ecchymosis; guaiac all body fluids, stools
Administer:
• After reconstituting with provided diluent, add appropriate amount of sterile water for injection (no preservatives) to 1 mg/ml, mix by slow inversion or dilute with NaCl, D_5W to a concentration of 0.5 mg/ml; flush line with NaCl after administration
• Heparin therapy after thrombolytic therapy is discontinued, TT, ACT, or APTT less than 2 × control (about 3-4 hr)
• Reconstituted IV solution within 8 hr
• Within 6 hr of coronary occlusion for best results
Perform/provide:
• Avoidance of invasive procedures, injection, rectal temperature
• Pressure for 30 sec to minor bleeding sites; inform physician if

this does not attain hemostasis, apply pressure dressing

• Storage of powder at room temperature or refrigerate, protect from excessive light

Evaluate:

• Therapeutic response: lysis of thrombi

• Allergy: fever, rash, itching, chills; mild reaction may be treated with antihistamines

• Blood studies (Hct, platelets, PTT, PT, TT, APTT) before starting therapy; PT or APTT must be less than 2 × control before starting therapy TT or PT q3-4h during treatment

Lab test interferences:

Increase: PT, APTT, TT

altretamine

(al-tray'ta-meen)

Hexalen

Func. class.: Misc. antineoplastic

Chem. class.: s-triazine derivative (formerly known as hexamethylmelamine)

Action: Products of metabolism form covalent adducts with tissue macromolecules including DNA, which may be responsible for cytotoxicity

Uses: Palliative treatment of recurrent, persistent ovarian cancer following first line treatment with cisplatin or alkylating agent–based combination

Dosage and routes:

• *Adult:* PO 260 mg/m^2 day for 14 or 21 days in a 28-day cycle; give in 4 divided doses after meals and at hs

Available forms include: Caps 50 mg

Side effects/adverse reactions:

GI: Nausea, anorexia, vomiting, increased alk phosphatase, ***hepatic toxicity***

CNS: Peripheral sensory neuropathy, fatigue, ***seizures,*** mood disorders, disorders of consciousness, ataxia, dizziness, vertigo

HEMA: ***Leukopenia, thrombocytopenia, anemia***

GU: Increased BUN, serum creatinine

INTEG: Rash, pruritus, alopecia

Contraindications: Hypersensitivity, severe bone marrow depression, severe neurologic toxicity

Precautions: Pregnancy (D), lactation, children

Pharmacokinetics:

PO: Well absorbed orally, rapidly metabolized in liver, metabolites excreted in urine; peak ½-3 hr

Interactions/incompatibilities:

• Possible increased toxicity of altretamine: cimetidine

• Severe orthostatic hypotension: MAOI

NURSING CONSIDERATIONS

Assess:

• CBC, differential, platelet count weekly, withhold drug if WBC is <2000 or platelet count is <75,000 or granulocyte count is <1000/mm^3; notify physician of results

• Renal function studies: BUN, serum uric acid, urine CrCl before, during therapy

• I&O ratio; report fall in urine output of 30 ml/hr

• Temperature q4h, may indicate beginning infection

• Liver function tests before, during therapy (bilirubin, AST, ALT, LDH) as needed or monthly

Administer:

• Antacid before oral agent, give drug after meals, at hs

• Antiemetic 30-60 min before giving drug to prevent vomiting

• Antibiotics for prophylaxis of infection

Perform/provide:

• Strict medical asepsis, protective isolation if WBC levels are low

Evaluate:

• Therapeutic response: decreased tumor size, spread of malignancy

Teach patient/family:

• To report signs of infection: increased temperature, sore throat, flu symptoms

• To report signs of anemia: fatigue, headache, faintness, shortness of breath, irritability

• To report bleeding; avoid use of razors or commercial mouthwash

• To avoid use of aspirin products or ibuprofen

• That hair may be lost during therapy; a wig or hairpiece may make patient feel better; new hair may be different in color, texture (rare)

aluminum acetate

Acid Mantle, Burow's solution, Buro-Sol, modified Burow's solution, Bluboro, Domeboro

Func. class.: Astringent
Chem. class.: Aluminum product

Action: Maintains skin acidity, which is protective to skin surface

Uses: Skin irritation, inflammation, athlete's foot, insect bites, poison ivy, eczema, acne, rash, bruises, pruritus (anal)

Dosage and routes:

• *Adult and child:* TOP apply for 15-30 min, q4-8h (1 : 10-40); gargle use 1 : 10 sol prn

Available forms include: Solution, cream (Canada only)

Side effects/adverse reactions:

INTEG: Irritation, increasing inflammation

Contraindications: Tight, occlusive dressing

Interactions/incompatibilities:

• Inhibits action of: topical collagenase ointment

• Decreased action of aluminum acetate: soap

NURSING CONSIDERATIONS

Administer:

• 1 pk/1 pt water (1 : 10-40 water)

Perform/provide:

• Wet dressings using only loose fitting dressing

Evaluate:

• Therapeutic response: decreased skin irritation

• Area of body to receive topical application, irritation, rash, breaks, dryness

Teach patient/family:

• To discontinue use if irritation occurs

• To avoid using near eye area

• To retain otic preparation for 2-3 min

aluminum carbonate gel

Basaljel

Func. class.: Antacid
Chem. class.: Aluminum product

Action: Neutralizes gastric acidity, binds phosphates in GI tract, these phosphates are excreted

Uses: Antacid, phosphate stones (prevention), phosphate binder in chronic renal failure

Dosage and routes:

Urinary phosphate stones

• *Adult:* SUSP 5-10 ml as needed; EXTRA STREN SUSP 2.5-5 ml as needed; PO 1-2 as needed

Antacid

• *Adult:* SUSP 15-45 ml in water or juice 1 hr pc, hs; EXTRA STREN SUSP 5-15 ml in water or juice 1 hr pc, hs; PO 2-6 1 hr pc, hs

Available forms include: Caps 500, 608 mg; tabs 500, 608 mg; susp 400 mg/5 ml; extra stren susp 1000 mg/ml

Side effects/adverse reactions:

GI: Constipation, anorexia, obstruction, fecal impaction

META: Hypophosphatemia, hypercalciuria

Contraindications: Hypersensitivity to this drug or aluminum products, appendicitis

Precautions: Elderly, fluid restriction, decreased GI motility, GI obstruction, dehydration, renal disease, sodium-restricted diets, pregnancy (C)

Pharmacokinetics:

PO: Excreted in feces

Interactions/incompatibilities:

• Decreased effectiveness of: tetracyclines, ketoconazole

• Decreased absorption of: anticholinergics, chlordiazepoxide, cimetidine, corticosteroids, iron salts, phenothiazines, phenytoin, digitalis

• Enteric-coated drugs: separate by 1 hr

NURSING CONSIDERATIONS

Administer:

• Laxatives, or stool softeners if constipation occurs, especially elderly

• After shaking

Perform/provide:

• I&O, strain urine if using for urinary calculi

Evaluate:

• Therapeutic response: absence of pain, decreased acidity

• Hypophosphatemia: anorexia, weakness, fatigue, bone pain, hyporeflexia

• Constipation, if product is being used as an antacid, may need to switch to magnesium antacid

• Phosphate levels, urinary pH, Ca^{++}, electrolytes

Teach patient/family:

• Increase fluids to 2000 ml/day unless contraindicated

• Avoid phosphate foods (most dairy products, eggs, fruits, carbonated beverages) during drug therapy

• Add cheese, corn, pasta, plums, prunes, lentils after drug is discontinued

• Limit sodium intake

---

aluminum hydroxide

AlternaGEL, Alu-Cap, Al-U-Creme, Aluminett, Amphojel, Basaljel,* Dialume, Hydroxal, Nephrox, No-Co-Gel, Nutrajel

Func. class.: Antacid

Chem. class.: Aluminum product

Action: Neutralizes gastric acidity, binds phosphates in GI tract; these phosphates are excreted

Uses: Antacid, hyperphosphatemia in chronic renal failure

Dosage and routes:

• *Adult:* SUSP 5-10 ml 1 hr pc, hs; PO 600 mg 1 hr pc, hs, chewed with milk or water

Hyperphosphatemia in renal failure

• *Adult:* SUSP 500 mg-2 g bid-qid

Available forms include: Caps 475, 500 mg; tabs 300, 500 mg; chewable tabs 600 mg; susp (4%) 600 mg/5 ml; liq 320 mg/5ml, 600 mg/5 ml

Side effects/adverse reactions:

GI: Constipation, anorexia, ***obstruction,*** fecal impaction

META: Hypophosphatemia, hypercalciuria

Contraindications: Hypersensitiv-

*Available in Canada only

ity to this drug or aluminum products

Precautions: Elderly, fluid restriction, decreased GI motility, GI obstruction, dehydration, renal disease, sodium-restricted diets, pregnancy (C)

Pharmacokinetics:

PO: Onset 20-40 min, excreted in feces

Interactions/incompatibilities:

- Decreased effectiveness of: tetracyclines, anticholinergics, phenothiazines, isoniazid, quinidine, phenytoin, digitalis, iron salts, warfarin, ketoconazole; separate by at least 2 hr

NURSING CONSIDERATIONS

Assess:

- Phosphate levels since drug is bound in GI system

Administer:

- Laxatives, or stool softeners if constipation occurs, especially elderly
- After shaking liquid
- By nasogastric tube if patient unable to swallow
- With small amount of water or milk

Evaluate:

- Therapeutic response: absence of pain, decreased acidity
- Hypophosphatemia: anorexia, weakness, fatigue, bone pain, hyporeflexia
- Constipation, increase bulk in diet if needed
- Phosphate levels, urinary pH, Ca^{++}, electrolytes

Teach patient/family:

- Increase fluids to 2000 ml/day unless contraindicated
- Avoid phosphate foods (most dairy products, eggs, fruits, carbonated beverages) during drug therapy
- Add cheese, corn, pasta, plums, prunes, lentils after drug is discontinued
- Stools may appear white or speckled
- To check with physician after 2 wk of self-prescribed antacid use

---

aluminum phosphate

Phosphaljel

Func. class.: Antacid
Chem. class.: Aluminum products

Action: Neutralizes gastric acidity, binds phosphates in GI tract, these phosphates are excreted

Uses: Antacid

Dosage and routes:

- *Adult:* SUSP 15-30 ml 1 hr pc, hs
- *Adult:* Intragastric dilute 1:3 or 1:4

Available forms include: Susp 233 mg/5 ml

Side effects/adverse reactions:

GI: Constipation, anorexia, ***obstruction,*** fecal impaction

META: Hyperphosphatemia

Contraindications: Hypersensitivity to this drug or aluminum products

Precautions: Elderly, fluid restriction, decreased GI motility, GI obstruction, dehydration, renal disease, sodium-restricted diets, pregnancy (C)

Pharmacokinetics:

PO: Onset 20-40 min, excreted in feces

Interactions/incompatibilities:

- Decreased effectiveness of: tetracyclines, ketoconazole, isoniazid, phenothiazines, iron salts, digitalis

NURSING CONSIDERATIONS

Administer:

- Laxatives, or stool softeners if

constipation occurs, especially elderly
• After shaking solution

Evaluate:
• Therapeutic response: absence of pain, decreased acidity
• Constipation, increase bulk in diet if needed or alternate with magnesium antacids
• Phosphate levels, urinary pH, Ca^{++}, electrolytes

Teach patient/family:
• To increase fluids to 2000 ml unless contraindicated
• Not to switch antacids unless directed by physician
• To use PO meds 1-2 hrs after antacid
• That antacid may cause premature dissolution of enteric-coated tablets

amantadine HCl

(a-man'ta-deen)
Symmetrel
Func. class.: Antiviral, antiparkinsonian agent
Chem. class.: Tricyclic amine

Action: Prevents uncoating of nucleic acid in viral cell, preventing penetration of virus to host; causes release of dopamine from neurons

Uses: Prophylaxis or treatment of influenza type A, extrapyramidal reactions, parkinsonism, respiratory tract infections

Dosage and routes:
Influenza type A
• *Adult and child >9 yr:* PO 200 mg/day in single dose or divided bid
• *Child 1-9 yr:* PO 4.4-8.8 mg/kg/day divided bid-tid, not to exceed 200 mg/day

Extrapyramidal reaction/parkinsonism
• *Adult:* PO 100 mg bid, up to 400 mg/day in EPS; give for 1 wk then 100 mg as needed in parkinsonism

Available forms include: Caps 100 mg; syr 50 mg/5 ml

Side effects/adverse reactions:
CNS: Headache, dizziness, drowsiness, fatigue, anxiety, psychosis, depression, hallucinations, tremors, ***convulsions***
CV: Orthostatic hypotension, ***CHF***
INTEG: Photosensitivity, dermatitis
EENT: Blurred vision
HEMA: **Leukopenia**
GI: Nausea, vomiting, constipation, dry mouth
GU: Frequency, retention

Contraindications: Hypersensitivity, lactation, child <1 yr, pregnancy (C)

Precautions: Epilepsy, CHF, orthostatic hypotension, psychiatric disorders, hepatic disease, renal disease

Pharmacokinetics:
PO: Onset 48 hr, half-life 24 hr, not metabolized, excreted in urine (90%) unchanged, crosses placenta, excreted in breast milk

Interactions/incompatibilities:
• Increased anticholingeric response: atropine, other anticholinergics
• Increased CNS stimulation: CNS stimulants

NURSING CONSIDERATIONS

Assess:
• I&O ratio; report frequency, hesitancy
• CHF, confusion, mottling of skin

Administer:
• Before exposure to influenza; continue for 10 days after contact
• At least 4 hr before hs to prevent insomnia
• After meals for better absorption, to decrease GI symptoms
• In divided doses to prevent CNS

disturbances: headache, dizziness, fatigue, drowsiness

Perform/provide:

• Storage in tight, dry container

Evaluate:

• Therapeutic response: absence of temperature, malaise, cough, dyspnea in infection; tremors, shuffling gait in Parkinson's disease

• Bowel pattern before, during treatment

• Skin eruptions, photosensitivity after administration of drug

• Respiratory status: rate, character, wheezing, tightness in chest

• Allergies before initiation of treatment, reaction of each medication; place allergies on chart, Kardex in bright red letters

• Signs of infection

Teach patient/family:

• To change body position slowly to prevent orthostatic hypotension

• About aspects of drug therapy: need to report dyspnea, weight gain, dizziness, poor concentration, dysuria, behavioral changes

• To avoid hazardous activities if dizziness occurs

• To take drug exactly as prescribed; parkinsonian crisis may occur if drug is discontinued abruptly

• To avoid alcohol

Treatment of overdose: Withdraw drug, maintain airway, administer epinephrine, aminophylline, O_2, IV corticosteroids, physostigmine

ambenonium chloride

(am-be-noe'nee-um)

Mytelase caplets

Func. class.: Cholinergics

Chem. class.: Synthetic quaternary ammonium compound

Action: Inhibits destruction of acetylcholine, which increases concentration at sites where acetylcholine is released; this facilitates transmission of impulses across myoneural junction

Uses: Myasthenia gravis when other drugs cannot be used

Dosage and routes:

• *Adult:* PO 5 mg q3-4h, then gradually increased q1-2 days, usually 5-40 mg is sufficient

Available forms include: Tabs 10 mg

Side effects/adverse reactions:

INTEG: Rash, urticaria

CNS: Dizziness, headache, sweating, confusion, weakness, ***convulsions,*** incoordination, ***paralysis***

GI: Nausea, diarrhea, vomiting, cramps, increased salivary, gastric secretions, dysphagia

CV: Tachycardia, dysrhythmias, bradycardia, hypotension, AV block, ECG changes, cardiac arrest

GU: Frequency, incontinence

RESP: ***Respiratory depression, bronchospasm, constriction, laryngospasm, respiratory arrest***

EENT: Miosis, blurred vision, lacrimation

Contraindications: Obstruction of intestine, renal system, hypersensitivity

Precautions: Seizure disorders, bronchial asthma, coronary occlusion, hyperthyroidism, dysrhythmias, peptic ulcer, megacolon, poor GI motility, pregnancy (C), bradycardia, hypotension, lactation, children

Pharmacokinetics:

PO: Onset 2-30 min, duration 3-8 hr

Interactions/incompatibilities:

• Decreased action of ambenonium: aminoglycosides, anesthetics, antidysrhythmics, mecamyl-

amine, polymyxin, quinidine, magnesium, corticosteroids
• Increased action of: neuromuscular blockers

NURSING CONSIDERATIONS

Assess:
• VS, respiration q2h
• I&O ratio; check for urinary retention or incontinence

Administer:
• Only with atropine sulfate available for cholinergic crisis
• Only after all other cholinergics have been discontinued
• Increased doses if tolerance occurs
• With food or milk to decrease GI symptoms; may decrease action of this drug
• Larger doses after exercise or fatigue
• On empty stomach for better absorption

Perform/provide:
• Storage at room temperature

Evaluate:
• Therapeutic response: increased muscle strength, improved gait, absence of labored breathing (if severe)
• Bradycardia, hypotension, bronchospasm, headache, dizziness, convulsions, respiratory depression; drug should be discontinued if toxicity occurs
• Muscle strength: hand grasp

Teach patient/family:
• To take drug exactly as prescribed
• That drug is not a cure; it only relieves symptoms
• To wear Medic Alert ID specifying myasthenia gravis, drugs taken

Treatment of overdose: Discontinue med, respiratory support, atropine 1-4 mg

amcinonide

(am-sin'oh-nide)

Cyclocort

Func. class.: Topical corticosteroid
Chem. class.: Synthetic fluorinated agent, group II potency

Action: Possesses antipruritic, antiinflammatory actions

Uses: Psoriasis, eczema, contact dermatitis, pruritus

Dosage and routes:
• *Adult and child:* Apply to affected area bid-tid, rub completely into skin

Available forms include: Cream 0.1%; oint 0.1%

Side effects/adverse reactions:
INTEG: Burning, dryness, itching, irritation, acne, folliculitis, hypertrichosis, perioral dermatitis, hypopigmentation, atrophy, striae, miliaria, allergic contact dermatitis, secondary infection

Contraindications: Hypersensitivity to corticosteroids, fungal infections

Precautions: Pregnancy (C), lactation, viral infections, bacterial infections

NURSING CONSIDERATIONS

Assess:
• Temperature, worsening of rash; if fever develops drug should be discontinued

Administer:
• Only to affected areas; do not get in eyes
• Medication, then cover with occlusive dressing (only if prescribed), seal to normal skin, change q12h; systemic absorption may occur
• Only to dermatoses; do not use on weeping, denuded, or infected area

Perform/provide:
• Cleansing before application of drug
• Treatment for a few days after area has cleared
• Storage at room temperature
Evaluate:
• Therapeutic response: absence of severe itching, patches on skin, flaking
• For systemic absorption: increased temperature, inflammation, irritation
Teach patient/family:
• To avoid sunlight on affected area; burns may occur
• To discontinue drug, notify physician if local irritation or fever develops

---

amikacin sulfate

(am-i-kay'sin)
Amikin

Func. class.: Antibiotic
Chem. class.: Aminoglycoside

Action: Interferes with protein synthesis in bacterial cell by binding to ribosomal subunit, which causes misreading of genetic code; inaccurate peptide sequence forms in protein chain, causing bacterial death
Uses: Severe systemic infections of CNS, respiratory, GI, urinary tract, bone, skin, soft tissues caused by *P. aeruginosa, E. coli, Enterobacter, Acinetobacter, Providencia, Citrobacter, Staphylococcus, Serratia, Proteus*
Dosage and routes:
Severe systemic infections
• *Adult and child:* IV INF 15 mg/kg/day in 2-3 divided doses q8-12h in 100-200 ml D_5W over 30-60 min, not to exceed 1.5 g; decreased doses are needed in poor renal function as determined by blood levels, renal function studies; IM 15 mg/kg/day in divided doses q8-12h
• *Neonates:* IV INF 10 mg/kg initially, then 7.5 mg/kg q12h in D_5W over 1-2 hr
Severe urinary tract infections
• *Adults:* IM 250 mg bid
• *Adults with poor renal function:* 7.5 mg/kg initially, then increased as determined by blood levels, renal function studies
Available forms include: Inj IM, IV 50, 250 mg/ml
Side effects/adverse reactions:
GU: ***Oliguria, hematuria, renal damage, azotemia, failure, nephrotoxicity***
CNS: Confusion, depression, numbness, tremors, ***convulsions,*** muscle twitching, ***neurotoxicity,*** dizziness, vertigo, tinnitus
EENT: ***Ototoxicity,*** deafness, visual disturbances
HEMA: ***Agranulocytosis, thrombocytopenia, leukopenia, eosinophilia, anemia***
GI: Nausea, vomiting, anorexia, increased ALT, AST, bilirubin, hepatomegaly, ***hepatic necrosis,*** splenomegaly
CV: Hypotension or hypertension, palpitations
INTEG: Rash, burning, urticaria, dermatitis, alopecia
Contraindications: Mild to moderate infections, severe renal disease, hypersensitivity to aminoglycosides
Precautions: Neonates, mild renal disease, pregnancy (D), myasthenia gravis, lactation, hearing deficits, Parkinson's disease, elderly
Pharmacokinetics:
IM: Onset rapid, peak 1-2 hr
IV: Onset immediate, peak 1-2 hr
Plasma half-life 2-3 hr; not metab-

olized, excreted unchanged in urine, crosses placental barrier

Interactions/incompatibilities:

• Increased ototoxicity, neurotoxicity, nephrotoxicity: other aminoglycosides, amphotericin B, polymyxin, vancomycin, ethacrynic acid, furosemide, mannitol, methoxyflurane, cisplatin, cephalosporins

• Increased neuromuscular blockade, respiratory depression: anesthetics, nondepolarizing neuromuscular blockers, succinylcholine

• Do not mix in solution or syringe: carbenicillin, ticarcillin, amphotericin B, cephalothin, erythromycin, heparin

NURSING CONSIDERATIONS

Assess:

• Weight before treatment; calculation of dosage is usually based on ideal body weight, but may be calculated on actual body weight

• I&O ratio; urinalysis daily for proteinuria, cells, casts; report sudden change in urine output

• VS during infusion, watch for hypotension, change in pulse

• IV site for thrombophlebitis including pain, redness, swelling q30 min, change site if needed; apply warm compresses to discontinued site

• Serum peak, drawn at 30-60 min after IV infusion or 60 min after IM injection, trough level drawn just before next dose; blood level should be 2-4 times bacteriostatic level

• Urine pH if drug is used for UTI; urine should be kept alkaline

Administer:

• IV, dilute 500 mg of drug/100-200 ml of compatible solutions and give over ½-1hr; flush after administration with D_5W or 0.9% NaCl

• IM injection in large muscle mass, rotate injection sites

• In evenly spaced doses to maintain blood level

• Bicarbonate to alkalinize urine if ordered for UTI, as drug is most active in alkaline environment

Perform/provide:

• Adequate fluids of 2-3 L/day unless contraindicated to prevent irritation of tubules

• Flush of IV line with NS or D_5W after infusion

• Supervised ambulation, other safety measures with vestibular dysfunction

Evaluate:

• Therapeutic response: absence of fever, draining wounds, negative C&S after treatment

• Renal impairment by securing urine for CrCl testing, BUN, serum creatinine; lower dosage should be given in renal impairment (CrCl <80 ml/min)

• Deafness by audiometric testing, ringing, roaring in ears, vertigo; assess hearing before, during, after treatment

• Dehydration: high sp gr, decrease in skin turgor, dry mucous membranes, dark urine

• Overgrowth of infection including increased temperature, malaise, redness, pain, swelling, perineal itching, diarrhea, stomatitis, change in cough, sputum

• C&S before starting treatment to identify organism

• Vestibular dysfunction: nausea, vomiting, dizziness, headache; drug should be discontinued if severe

• Injection sites for redness, swelling, abscesses; use warm compresses at site

Teach patient/family:

• To report headache, dizziness,

* Available in Canada only

symptoms for overgrowth of infection, renal impairment
• To report loss of hearing, ringing, roaring in ears or feeling of fullness in head
Treatment of overdose: Hemodialysis, monitor serum levels of drug

amiloride HCl

(a-mill'oh-ride)
Midamor
Func. class.: Potassium-sparing diuretic
Chem. class.: Pyrazine

Action: Acts primarily on distal tubule, secondarily by inhibiting reabsorption of sodium, and increasing potassium retention
Uses: Edema in CHF in combination with other diuretics, for hypertension, adjunct with other diuretics to maintain potassium
Dosage and routes:
• *Adult:* PO 5 mg qd, may be increased to 10-20 mg qd if needed
Available forms include: Tab 5 mg
Side effects/adverse reactions:
GU: Polyuria, dysuria, frequency, impotence
ELECT: Acidosis, hyponatremia, ***hyperkalemia,*** hypochloremia
CNS: Headache, dizziness, fatigue, weakness, paresthesias, tremor, depression, anxiety
GI: Nausea, diarrhea, dry mouth, vomiting, anorexia, cramps, constipation, dry mouth, abdominal pain, jaundice, bleeding
EENT: Loss of hearing, tinnitus, blurred vision, nasal congestion, increased intraocular pressure
INTEG: Rash, pruritus, alopecia, urticaria
MS: Cramps, joint pain
CV: Orthostatic hypotension
HEMA: ***Agranulocytopenia, leukopenia, thrombocytopenia*** (rare)
Contraindications: Anuria, hypersensitivity, hyperkalemia, impaired renal function
Precautions: Dehydration, pregnancy (B), diabetes, acidosis, lactation
Pharmacokinetics:
PO: Onset 2 hr, peak 6-10 hr, duration 24 hr; excreted in urine, feces, half-life 6-9 hr
Interactions/incompatibilities:
• Enhanced action of: antihypertensives, lithium toxicity may be provoked
• Hyperkalemia: other potassium-sparing diuretics, potassium products, ACE inhibitors, salt substitutes

NURSING CONSIDERATIONS

Assess:
• Weight, I&O daily to determine fluid loss; effect of drug may be decreased if used qd
• Rate, depth, rhythm of respiration, effect of exertion
• B/P lying, standing; postural hypotension may occur
• Electrolytes: potassium, sodium, chloride; include BUN, CBC, serum creatinine, blood pH, ABGs
Administer:
• In AM to avoid interference with sleep if using drug as a diuretic
• With food, if nausea occurs, absorption may be decreased slightly
Evaluate:
• Therapeutic response: improvement in edema of feet, legs, sacral area daily if medication is being used in CHF
• Improvement in CVP q8h
• Signs of drowsiness, restlessness
• Rashes, temperature elevation qd
• Confusion especially in elderly; take safety precautions if needed
Teach patient/family:
• About adverse reactions:

muscle cramps, weakness, nausea, dizziness, blurred vision
• To take with food or milk for GI symptoms
• To take early in day to prevent nocturia
• To avoid potassium-rich foods: oranges, bananas; salt substitutes
Lab test interferences:
Interfere: GTT
Treatment of overdose: Lavage if taken orally, monitor electrolytes, administer sodium bicarbonate for K^+ >6.5 mEq/L, monitor hydration, CV, renal status

---

amino acid injection

(a-mee'noe)
FreAmine HBC, HepatAmine
Func. class.: Nitrogen product

Action: Needed for anabolism to maintain structure, decrease catabolism, promote healing
Uses: Hepatic encephalopathy, cirrhosis, hepatitis, nutritional support in cancer
Dosage and routes:
• *Adult:* IV 80-120 g/day; 500 ml of amino acids/500 ml D_{50} given over 24 hr
Available forms include: Inj IV many strengths, types
Side effects/adverse reactions:
CNS: Dizziness, headache, confusion, ***loss of consciousness***
CV: Hypertension, ***CHF, pulmonary edema***
GI: Nausea, vomiting, liver fat deposits, abdominal pain
GU: Glycosuria, osmotic diuresis
ENDO: Hyperglycemia, rebound hypoglycemia, electrolyte imbalances, hyperosmolar syndrome, hyperosmolar hyperglycemic nonketotic syndrome, alkalosis, acidosis, hypophosphatemia, hyperammonemia, dehydration, hypocalcemia
INTEG: Chills, flushing, warm feeling, rash, urticaria, extravasation necrosis, phlebitis at injection site
Contraindications: Hypersensitivity, severe electrolyte imbalances, anuria, severe liver damage, maple syrup urine disease, PKU
Precautions: Renal disease, pregnancy (C), children, diabetes mellitus, CHF

NURSING CONSIDERATIONS

Assess:
• Electrolytes (K, Na, Ca, Cl, Mg), blood glucose, ammonia, phosphate
• Renal, liver function studies: BUN, creatinine, ALT, AST, bilirubin
• Injection site for extravasation: redness along vein, edema at site, necrosis, pain, hard tender area; site should be changed immediately
• Monitor respiratory function q4h: auscultate lung fields bilaterally for crackles, respirations, quality, rate, rhythm
• Monitor temperature q4h for increased fever, indicating infection; if infection suspected, infusion is discontinued, tubing bottle cultured
• Monitor for impending hepatic coma: asterixis, confusion, fetor, lethargy
• Urine glucose q6h using Chemstrips, which are not affected by infusion substances
Administer:
• TPN only mixed with dextrose to promote protein synthesis
• Immediately after mixing in pharmacy under strict aseptic technique using laminar flowhood, use infusion pump, in-line filter
• Using careful monitoring technique; do not speed up infusion;

---

* Available in Canada only

pulmonary edema, glucose overload will result

Perform/provide:

- Storage depends on type of solution; consult manufacturer
- Changing dressing and IV tubing to prevent infection q24-48h or q5-7 days if transparent dressing is used

Evaluate:

- Therapeutic response: weight gain, decrease in jaundice in liver disorders, increased LOC
- Hyperammonemia: nausea, vomiting, malaise, tremors, anorexia, convulsions

Teach patient/family:

- Reason for use of TPN
- If chills, sweating are experienced, report at once

amino acid solution

Aminosyn, FreAmine III, Novamine, Travasol

Func. class.: Nitrogen product

Action: Needed for anabolism to maintain structure, decrease catabolism, promote healing

Uses: Nutritional support in cancer, trauma, intestinal obstruction, short bowel syndrome, severe malabsorption

Dosage and routes:

- *Adult:* IV 1-1.5 g/kg/day titrated to patient's needs
- *Child:* IV 2-3 g/kg/day titrated to patient's needs

Available forms include: Inj IV many types, strengths

Side effects/adverse reactions:

CNS: Dizziness, headache, confusion, ***loss of consciousness***

CV: Hypertension, ***CHF, pulmonary edema***

GI: Nausea, vomiting, liver fat deposits, abdominal pain, jaundice

GU: Glycosuria, osmotic diuresis

ENDO: Hyperglycemia, rebound hypoglycemia, electrolyte imbalances, hyperosmolar syndrome, hyperosmolar hyperglycemic nonketotic syndrome, alkalosis, acidosis, hypophosphatemia, hyperammonemia, dehydration, hypocalcemia

INTEG: Chills, flushing, warm feeling, rash, urticaria, extravasation necrosis, phlebitis at injection site

Contraindications: Hypersensitivity, severe electrolyte imbalances, anuria, severe liver damage, maple syrup urine disease, PKU

Precautions: Renal disease, pregnancy (C), children, diabetes mellitus, CHF

NURSING CONSIDERATIONS

Assess:

- Electrolytes (K, Na, Ca, Cl, Mg), blood glucose, ammonia, phosphate
- Renal, liver function studies: BUN, creatinine, ALT, AST, bilirubin
- Injection site for extravasation: redness along vein, edema at site, necrosis, pain, hard tender area; site should be changed immediately
- Monitor respiratory function q4h: auscultate lung fields bilaterally for crackles, respirations, quality, rate, rhythm
- Monitor temperature q4h for increased fever, indicating infection; if infection suspected, infusion is discontinued, tubing, bottle cultured
- Urine glucose q6h using Tes-Tape, Clinistix, Keto-Diastix, which are not affected by infusion substances; blood glucose is preferred testing method

Administer:

- TPN only mixed with dextrose to promote protein synthesis

• Immediately after mixing in pharmacy under strict aseptic technique using laminar flowhood, use infusion pump, in-line filter
• Using careful monitoring technique; do not speed up infusion; pulmonary edema, glucose overload will result

Perform/provide:
• Storage depends on type of solution; consult manufacturer
• Changing dressing and IV tubing to prevent infection q24-48h

Evaluate:
• Therapeutic response: weight gain, decrease in jaundice in liver disorders, increased serum albumin
• Hyperammonemia: nausea, vomiting, malaise, tremors, anorexia, convulsions

Teach patient/family:
• Reason for use of TPN
• If chills, sweating are experienced, they should be reported at once

---

aminocaproic acid

(a-mee-noe-ka-proe'ik)
Amicar, (EACA)
Func. class.: Hemostatic
Chem. class.: Synthetic monoaminocarboxylic acid

Action: Inhibits fibrinolysis by inhibiting plasminogen activator substances
Uses: Hemorrhage from hyperfibrinolysis, adjunctive therapy in hemophilia
Dosage and routes:
• *Adult:* PO/IV 5 g loading dose, then 1-1.25 g q1h if needed, not to exceed 30 g/day
Available forms include: Inj IV 250 mg/ml; tab 500 mg; syr 250 mg/ml
Side effects/adverse reactions:
GU: Dysuria, frequency, oliguria, ***renal failure,*** ejaculatory failure, menstrual irregularities
GI: Nausea, vomiting, abdominal cramps, diarrhea
INTEG: Rash
CNS: Headache, dizziness, malaise, fatigue, hallucinations, delirium, psychosis, ***convulsions,*** weakness
HEMA: ***Thrombosis***
CV: ***Dysrhythmias,*** orthostatic hypotension, bradycardia
EENT: Tinnitus, nasal congestion, conjunctival suffusion
Contraindications: Hypersensitivity, abnormal bleeding, postpartum bleeding, DIC, upper urinary tract bleeding, new burns
Precautions: Neonates/infants, mild or moderate renal disease, hepatic disease, thrombosis, cardiac disease, pregnancy (C)
Pharmacokinetics:
PO/IV: Peak 2 hr, excreted by kidneys as unmetabolized drug rapidly absorbed
Interactions/incompatibilities:
Increased coagulation: estrogens, oral contraceptives
• Do not mix with other drugs in solution

NURSING CONSIDERATIONS

Assess:
• I&O; if urinary output decreases, notify physician and stop drug
• Blood studies: coagulation factors, platelets, protamine coagulation test for extravascular clotting, thrombophlebitis
• B/P, pulse for increase
• Drug level: 0.13 mg/ml is required to decrease fibrinolysis
• Creatine phosphokinase, urinalysis

Administer:
• Give IV loading dose over 30 min to avoid hypotension

---

* Available in Canada only

• IV push slowly, with plastic syringe only; check for extravasation
• IV after dilution with 4-5 g/250 ml NS, D_5W, LR, give over 1 hr; may give by continuous infusion after loading dose(s) of 1 g/hr diluted in 50-100 ml of compatible solutions; use infusion pump

Perform/provide:
• Storage in tight container in cool environment, do not freeze

Evaluate:
• Therapeutic response: decreased bleeding
• Allergy: fever, rash, itching, jaundice
• Myopathy: if weakness, fever, myoglobinemia, or oliguria; discontinue drug
• Bleeding: mucous membrane, epistaxis, ecchymosis, petechiae, hematuria, hematemesis

Teach patient/family:
• To report any signs of bleeding (gums, under skin, urine, stools, emesis) or myopathy
• To change position slowly to decrease orthostatic hypotension
• Proper administration for 8-10 days following dental procedure in hemophilia
• To inform physicians that drug is being taken
• To change position slowly

Lab test interferences:
Increased: K^+, CPK

---

aminoglutethimide

(a-meen-noe-gloo-te-th'i-mide)
Cytadren

Func. class.: Antineoplastic, adrenal steroid inhibitor
Chem. class.: Hormone

Action: Acts by inhibiting DNA, RNA, protein synthesis; is derived from *Streptomyces verticillus;* replication is decreased by binding to DNA, which causes strand splitting; phase specific in G_2 and M phases; blocks biosynthesis of all steroid hormones (cortisol, androgens, progestins)

Uses: Suppression of adrenal function in Cushing's syndrome, metastatic breast cancer, adrenal cancer

Dosage and routes:
• *Adult:* PO 250 mg qid at 6 hr intervals, may increase by 250 mg/day q1-2 wk, not to exceed 2 g/day

Available forms include: Tabs 250 mg

Side effects/adverse reactions:
GI: Nausea, vomiting, anorexia, ***hepatotoxicity***
INTEG: Rash, pruritus, hirsutism
CV: ***Hypotension,*** *tachycardia*
CNS: Drowsiness, morbilliform skin rash, dizziness, headache, lethargy

Contraindications: Hypersensitivity, hypothyroidism, pregnancy (D)

Precautions: Renal disease, hepatic disease, respiratory disease

Pharmacokinetics: Half-life 13 hr, metabolized in liver, excreted in urine, crosses placenta

Interactions/incompatibilities:
• Accelerated metabolism of: dexamethasone

NURSING CONSIDERATIONS

Assess:
• Renal function studies: BUN, serum uric acid, urine CrCl, electrolytes before, during therapy
• I&O ratio; report fall in urine output of 30 ml/hr
• Monitor temperature q4h; may indicate beginning infection
• Liver function tests before, during therapy (bilirubin, AST, ALT, LDH) as needed or monthly
• RBC, Hct, Hgb, since these may be decreased

Administer:
- Antacid before oral agent; give last dose of the day after evening meal before bedtime
- Local or systemic drugs for infection if indicated

Perform/provide:
- Special skin care
- Liquid diet, including cola, Jell-O; dry toast or crackers as ordered may be added if patient is not nauseated or vomiting
- Nutritious diet with iron and vitamin supplements as ordered

Evaluate:
- Therapeutic response: decrease in size of tumor or decrease in Cushing's syndrome
- Food preferences; list likes, dislikes
- Inflammation of mucosa, breaks in skin
- Yellowing of skin, sclera, dark urine, clay-colored stools, itchy skin, abdominal pain, fever, diarrhea
- Symptoms indicating severe allergic reaction: rash, pruritus, urticaria, purpuric skin lesions, itching, flushing

Teach patient/family:
- To report any complaints, side effects to nurse or physician
- That masculinization can occur, is reversible after discontinuing treatment
- Correct self-administration of adjuvant corticosteroids

aminophylline (theophylline ethylenediamine)

(am-in-off'i-lin)

Amoline, Corophyllin,* Lixaminol, Phyllocontin, Somophyllin-DF, Truphylline

Func. class.: Spasmolytic
Chem. class.: Xanthine, ethylenediamide

Action: Relaxes smooth muscle of respiratory system by blocking phosphodiesterase, which increases cyclic AMP

Uses: Bronchial asthma, bronchospasm, Cheyne-Stokes respirations

Dosage and routes:
- *Adult:* PO 500 mg, then 250-500 mg q6-8h; CONT IV 0.3-0.9 mg/kg/hr (maintenance); RECT 500 mg q6-8h
- *Child:* PO 7.5 mg/kg, then 3-6 mg/kg q6-8h; IV 7.5 mg/kg, then 3-6 mg/kg q6-8h injected over 5 min, do not exceed 25 mg/min; may give loading dose of 5.6 mg/kg over ½ hr; CONT IV 1 mg/kg/hr (maintenance)
- *Neonates:* IV/PO 1 mg/kg initially for plasma increases of each 2 μg/ml, then 1 mg/kg q6h

Available forms include: Inj IV, IM, rectal supp 250, 500 mg; rectal sol 300 mg/5 ml; elix 250 mg/5 ml; oral liq 105 mg/5 ml; tabs 100, 200 mg, tabs con-rel 225 mg; tabs sust-rel 300 mg

Side effects/adverse reactions:

CNS: Anxiety, restlessness, insomnia, dizziness, ***convulsions,*** headache, light-headedness, muscle twitching

CV: Palpitations, sinus tachycardia, hypotension, flushing, dysrhythmias

GI: Nausea, vomiting, anorexia,

*Available in Canada only

diarrhea, bitter taste, dyspepsia, anal irritation (suppositories), epigastric pain
RESP: Increased rate
INTEG: Flushing, urticaria
GU: Urinary frequency
Contraindications: Hypersensitivity to xanthines, tachydysrhythmias
Precautions: Elderly, CHF, cor pulmonale, hepatic disease, active peptic ulcer disease, diabetes mellitus, hyperthyroidism, hypertension, children, pregnancy (C), glaucoma, prostatic hypertrophy
Pharmacokinetics:
IV: Peak 30 min
Interactions/incompatibilities:
- Do not mix in syringe with other drugs
- Increased action of aminophylline: cimetidine, propranolol, erythromycin, troleandomycin
- May increase effects of: anticoagulants
- Cardiotoxicity: β-blockade
- Increased elimination: smoking
- Decreased effects of: lithium

NURSING CONSIDERATIONS

Assess:
- Theophylline blood levels (therapeutic level is 10-20 μg/ml); toxicity may occur with small increase above 20 μg/ml, especially elderly
- Monitor I&O; diuresis occurs, dehydration may result in elderly or children
- Whether theophylline was given recently

Administer:
- PO after meals to decrease GI symptoms; absorption may be affected
- IV after diluting in 5% dextrose to decrease burning sensation at injection site; only clear solutions
- May be diluted for IV INF in 100-200 ml compatible solution
- Avoid IM injection; pain occurs
- Rectal dose if patient is unable to take PO

Perform/provide:
- Storage of diluted solution for 24 hr if refrigerated

Evaluate:
- Therapeutic response: decreased dyspnea, respiratory rate, rhythm
- Respiratory rate, rhythm, depth; auscultate lung fields bilaterally; notify physician of abnormalities
- Allergic reactions: rash, urticaria; if these occur, drug should be discontinued

Teach patient/family:
- To check OTC medications, current prescription medications for ephedrine; will increase CNS stimulation
- To avoid hazardous activities; dizziness may occur
- If GI upset occurs, to take drug with 8 oz water; avoid food, since absorption may be decreased
- To remain in bed 15-20 min after rectal suppository is inserted to avoid removal
- To notify physician of toxicity: insomnia, anxiety, nausea, vomiting, rapid pulse, convulsions
- To notify physician of change in smoking habit; a change in dose may be required

---

amiodarone HCl

(a-mee'-oh-da-rone)
Cordarone
Func. class.: Antidysrhythmic (Class III)
Chem. class.: Iodinated benzofuran derivative

Action: Prolongs action potential duration and effective refractory period, noncompetitive α- and β-adrenergic inhibition
Uses: Severe ventricular tachycar-

dia, ventricular fibrillation not controlled by first-line agents

Dosage and routes:

• *Adult:* Loading dose 800-1600 mg/day 1-3 wk; then 600-800 mg/day 1 mo; maintenance 200-600 mg/day

Available forms include: Tabs 200 mg

Side effects/adverse reactions:

CNS: Headache, dizziness, involuntary movement, tremors, peripheral neuropathy, malaise, fatigue, ataxia, paresthesias, insomnia

GI: Nausea, vomiting, diarrhea, abdominal pain, anorexia, constipation, ***hepatotoxicity***

CV: Hypotension, bradycardia, ***sinus arrest, CHF,*** *dysrhythmias,* ***SA node dysfunction***

INTEG: Rash, photosensitivity, blue-gray skin discoloration, rash, alopecia, spontaneous ecchymosis

EENT: Blurred vision, halos, photophobia, ***corneal microdeposits,*** dry eyes

ENDO: Hyperthyroidism or hypothyroidism

MS: Weakness, pain in extremities

RESP: ***Pulmonary fibrosis***, pulmonary inflammation

MISC: Flushing, abnormal taste or smell, edema, abnormal salivation, coagulation abnormalities

Precautions: Goiter, Hashimoto's thyroiditis, SN dysfunction, 2nd or 3rd degree AV block, electrolyte imbalances, pregnancy (C), bradycardia, lactation

Pharmacokinetics:

PO: Onset 1-3 wk, peak 2-10 hr; half-life 15-100 days; metabolized by liver, excreted by kidneys

Interactions/incompatibilities:

• Bradycardia: β-blockers, calcium channel blockers

• Increased levels of: digitalis, quinidine, procainamide, flecainide, disopyramide, phenytoin

• Increased anticoagulant effects: warfarin

• Bradycardia, arrest: lidocaine

NURSING CONSIDERATIONS

Assess:

• I&O ratio; electrolytes: K, Na, Cl

• Liver function studies: AST, ALT, bilirubin, alk phosphatase

• ECG continuously to determine drug effectiveness, measure PR, QRS, QT intervals, check for PVCs, other dysrhythmias

• For dehydration or hypovolemia

• B/P continuously for hypotension, hypertension

Administer:

• Reduced dosage slowly with ECG monitoring

Evaluate:

• Therapeutic response: decrease in ventricular tachycardia or fibrillation

• For rebound hypertension after 1-2 hr

• CNS symptoms: confusion, psychosis, numbness, depression, involuntary movements; if these occur drug should be discontinued

• Hypothyroidism: lethargy, dizziness, constipation, enlarged thyroid gland, edema of extremities, cool, pale skin

• Hyperthyroidism: restlessness, tachycardia, eyelid puffiness, weight loss, frequent urination, menstrual irregularities, dyspnea, warm, moist skin

• Pulmonary toxicity: dyspnea, fatigue, cough, fever, chest pain; drug should be discontinued

• Cardiac rate, respiration: rate, rhythm, character, chest pain

Teach patient/family:

• To use sunscreen or stay out of sun to prevent burns

• To report side effects immediately
• That skin discoloration is usually reversible
• That dark glasses may be needed for photophobia

Treatment of overdose: O_2, artificial ventilation, ECG, administer dopamine for circulatory depression, administer diazepam or thiopental for convulsions, isoproterenol

---

amitriptyline HCl

(a-mee-trip'ti-leen)

Amitril, Apo-Amitriptyline,* Elavil, Emitrip, Endep, Enovil, Levate,* Meravil,* Novotriptyn,* Rolavil*

Func. class.: Antidepressant—tricyclic

Chem. class.: Tertiary amine

Action: Blocks reuptake of norepinephrine, serotonin into nerve endings, increasing action of norepinephrine, serotonin in nerve cells

Uses: Major depression

Dosage and routes:

• *Adult:* PO 50-100 mg hs, may increase to 200 mg qd, not to exceed 300 mg/day; IM 20-30 mg qid, or 80-120 mg hs
• *Adolescent/geriatric:* PO 30 mg/day in divided doses, may be increased to 150 mg/day

Available forms include: Tabs 10, 25, 50, 75, 100, 150 mg; inj IM 10 mg/ml

Side effects/adverse reactions:

HEMA: ***Agranulocytosis, thrombocytopenia, eosinophilia, leukopenia***

CNS: Dizziness, drowsiness, confusion, headache, anxiety, tremors, stimulation, weakness, insomnia, nightmares, EPS (elderly), increased psychiatric symptoms

GI: Diarrhea, dry mouth, nausea, vomiting, ***paralytic ileus,*** increased appetite, cramps, epigastric distress, jaundice, ***hepatitis,*** stomatitis

GU: Retention

INTEG: Rash, urticaria, sweating, pruritus, photosensitivity

CV: Orthostatic hypotension, ***ECG changes, tachycardia, hypertension,*** palpations

EENT: Blurred vision, tinnitus, mydriasis, ophthalmoplegia

Contraindications: Hypersensitivity to tricyclic antidepressants, recovery phase of myocardial infarction

Precautions: Suicidal patients, convulsive disorders, prostatic hypertrophy, schizophrenia, psychotic, severe depression, increased intraocular pressure, narrow-angle glaucoma, urinary retention, cardiac disease, hepatic disease/renal disease, hyperthyroidism, electroshock therapy, elective surgery, child <12 yr, pregnancy (C), elderly

Pharmacokinetics:

PO/IM: Onset 45 min, peak 2-12 hr, therapeutic response 2-3 wk; metabolized by liver, excreted in urine/feces, crosses placenta, excreted in breast milk, half-life 10-50 hr

Interactions/incompatibilities:

• Decreased effects of: guanethidine, clonidine, indirect acting sympathomimetics (ephedrine)
• Increased effects of: direct acting sympathomimetics (epinephrine), alcohol, barbiturates, benzodiazepines, CNS depressants
• Hyperpyretic crisis, convulsions, hypertensive episode: MAOI (pargyline [Eutonyl])

NURSING CONSIDERATIONS

Assess:

- B/P (lying, standing), pulse q4h; if systolic B/P drops 20 mm Hg hold drug, notify physician; take vital signs q4h in patients with cardiovascular disease
- Blood studies: CBC, leukocytes, differential, cardiac enzymes if patient is receiving long-term therapy
- Hepatic studies: AST, ALT, bilirubin, creatinine
- Weight qwk, appetite may increase with drug
- ECG for flattening of T wave, bundle branch block, AV block, dysrhythmias in cardiac patients

Administer:

- Increased fluids, bulk in diet if constipation, urinary retention occur, especially elderly
- With food or milk for GI symptoms
- Crushed if patient is unable to swallow medication whole
- Dosage hs if over-sedation occurs during day; may take entire dose hs; elderly may not tolerate once/day dosing
- Gum, hard sugarless candy, or frequent sips of water for dry mouth

Perform/provide:

- Storage at room temperature, do not freeze
- Assistance with ambulation during beginning therapy since drowsiness/dizziness occurs
- Safety measure including siderails primarily in elderly
- Checking to see PO medication swallowed

Evaluate:

- Therapeutic response: decrease in depression, absence of suicidal thoughts
- EPS primarily in elderly: rigidity, dystonia, akathisia
- Mental status: mood, sensorium, affect, suicidal tendencies; increase in psychiatric symptoms: depression, panic
- Urinary retention, constipation; constipation is more likely to occur in children or elderly
- Withdrawal symptoms: headache, nausea, vomiting, muscle pain, weakness; do not usually occur unless drug was discontinued abruptly
- Alcohol consumption; if alcohol is consumed, hold dose until morning

Teach patient/family:

- That therapeutic effects may take 2-3 wk
- Use caution in driving or other activities requiring alertness because of drowsiness, dizziness, blurred vision, avoid rising quickly from sitting to standing, especially elderly
- To avoid alcohol ingestion, other CNS depressants
- Not to discontinue medication quickly after long-term use, may cause nausea, headache, malaise
- To wear sunscreen or large hat since photosensitivity occurs

Lab test interferences:

Increase: Serum bilirubin, blood glucose, alk phosphatase

Decrease: VMA, 5-HIAA

False increase: Urinary catecholamines

Treatment of overdose: ECG monitoring, induce emesis, lavage, activated charcoal, administer anticonvulsant

---

ammonia, aromatic spirit

Func. class.: Respiratory stimulants

Chem. class.: Aromatic hydroalcoholic solution of ammonia

Action: Stimulates medulla (res-

*Available in Canada only

piratory, vasomotor areas) by irritation of sensory receptors in mucosa of nasal passages, esophagus, stomach

Uses: To treat, prevent fainting

Dosage and routes:

- *Adult and child:* INH prn; PO 2-4 ml diluted in water

Available forms include: Inh 0.33, 0.4 ml; sol

Side effects/adverse reactions: None known

NURSING CONSIDERATIONS

Assess:

- Vital signs, B/P after administration of inhalant

Administer:

- By inhalation, do not place packets in pockets, may open, cause caustic burns
- Orally by diluting 2-4 ml in >30 ml of water

Perform/provide:

- Storage protected from light at room temperature

Evaluate:

- Therapeutic response: revival after fainting
- Cause of fainting

---

ammonium chloride

Func. class.: Acidifier
Chem. class.: Ammonium

Action: Lowers urinary pH, liberates hydrogen and chloride ions in blood and extracellular fluid with decreased pH and correction of alkalosis

Uses: Alkalosis (metabolic), systemic and urinary acidifer, expectorant, diuretic

Dosage and routes:

Alkalosis

- *Adult and child:* IV INF 0.9-1.3 ml/min of a 2.14% sol, not to exceed 2 ml/min

Acidifier

- *Adult:* PO 4-12 g/day in divided doses
- *Child:* PO 75 mg/kg/day in divided doses

Expectorant

- *Adult:* PO 250-500 mg q2-4h as needed

Available forms include: Tabs 500 mg, 1 g; inj IV 0.4, 5 mEq/ml

Side effects/adverse reactions:

CNS: Drowsiness, headache, confusion, stimulation, tremors, *twitching, hyperreflexia,* ***tetany,*** *EEG changes*

CV: Bradycardia, dysrhythmias, bounding pulse

GU: Glycosuria, thirst

GI: Gastric irritation, nausea, vomiting, anorexia, diarrhea

INTEG: Rash, pain at infusion site

META: Acidosis, hypokalemia, hyperchloremia, hyperglycemia

RESP: ***Apnea,*** irregular respirations, hyperventilation

Contraindications: Hypersensitivity, severe hepatic disease, severe renal disease

Precautions: Severe respiratory disease, cardiac edema, infants, pregnancy (C), children, elderly

Pharmacokinetics:

PO: Absorbed in 3-6 hr; metabolized in liver, excreted in urine and feces

Interactions/incompatibilities:

- Increased toxicity: PAS
- Decreased effects of: amphetamines, tricyclic antidepressants, salicylates, sulfonylureas
- Increased risk of systemic acidosis: spironolactone

NURSING CONSIDERATIONS

Assess:

- Respiratory rate, rhythm, depth, notify physician of abnormalities that may indicate acidosis

• Electrolytes and CO_2, chloride before and during treatment
• Urine pH, urinary output, urine glucose, specific gravity during beginning treatment
• I&O ratio, report large increases or decreases

Administer:
• PO with meals if GI symptoms occur
• IV slowly to avoid pain at infusion site and toxicity
• After diluting solutions to 2.14% (IV), each 20-ml vial must be further diluted by adding 1-2 vials/500-1000 ml of compatible solution given at a rate of 5 ml/min or less
• With water for expectorant not compatible with milk or other alkaline solutions

Evaluate:
• Therapeutic response: decreasing metabolic alkalosis or increasing urinary acidity or diuresis
• For CNS symptoms: confusion, twitching, hyperreflexia, stimulation, headache that may indicate ammonia toxicity
• For cardiac dysrhythmias
• For respiratory symptoms: hyperventilation

Teach patient/family:
• To increase potassium in diet: bananas, oranges, cantaloupe, honeydew, spinach, potatoes, dry fruit

Lab test interferences:
Increase: Blood ammonia, AST/ALT
Decrease: Serum magnesium, urine urobilinogen

amobarbital/amobarbital sodium

(am-oh-bar'bi-tal)
Amytal, Isobec/Amytal sodium
Func. class.: Sedative/hypnotic-barbiturate (intermediate acting)
Chem. class.: Amylobarbitone

Controlled Substance Schedule II (USA), Schedule G (Canada)

Action: Depresses activity in brain cells primarily in reticular activating system in brain stem, also selectively depresses neurons in posterior hypothalamus, limbic structures; able to decrease seizure activity by inhibition of impulses in CNS

Uses: Sedation, preanesthetic sedation, insomnia, anticonvulsant, adjunct in psychiatry, hypnotic

Dosage and routes:
Preanesthetic sedation
• *Adult and child:* PO/IM 200 mg 1-2 hr preoperatively
Sedation
• *Adult:* PO 30-50 mg bid or tid, may be from 15-120 mg bid-qid
• *Child:* PO 2 mg/kg/day in 4 divided doses
Anticonvulsant/psychiatry
• *Adult:* IV 65-500 mg given over several min, not to exceed 100 mg/min; not to exceed 1 g
• *Child* <6 yr: IV/IM 3-5 mg/kg over several min
Insomnia
• *Adult:* PO/IM 65-200 mg hs, not to exceed 5 ml in one site
• *Child:* IM 3-5 mg/kg at hs, not to exceed 5 ml in one site

Available forms include: Tabs 30, 50, 100 mg; caps 65, 200 mg; powder for inj IM, IV 250, 500 mg/vial

Side effects/adverse reactions:
CNS: Lethargy, drowsiness, hang-

over, dizziness, stimulation in the elderly and children, lightheadedness, physical dependence, CNS depression, mental depression, slurred speech
GI: Nausea, vomiting, diarrhea, constipation
INTEG: Rash, urticaria, pain, abscesses at injection site, ***angioedema,*** thrombophlebitis, ***Stevens-Johnson syndrome***
CV: Hypotension, bradycardia
RESP: ***Depression, apnea, laryngospasm, bronchospasm***
HEMA: ***Agranulocytosis, thrombocytopenia, megaloblastic anemia*** (long-term treatment)
Contraindications: Hypersensitivity to barbiturates, respiratory depression, addiction to barbiturates, severe liver impairment, porphyria
Precautions: Anemia, pregnancy (B), lactation, hepatic disease, renal disease, hypertension, elderly, acute/chronic pain
Pharmacokinetics:
PO: Onset 45-60 min, duration 6-8 hr
IV: Onset 5 min, duration 3-6 hr
Metabolized by liver, excreted by kidneys (inactive metabolites), crosses placenta, highly protein bound, excreted in breast milk, half-life 16-40 hr
Interactions/incompatibilities:
• Increased CNS depression: alcohol, MAOIs, sedative, narcotics
• Decreased effect of: oral anticoagulants, corticosteroids, griseofulvin, quinidine, oral contraceptives, estrogens
• Increased half-life of: doxycycline

NURSING CONSIDERATIONS

Assess:
• VS q30min after parenteral route for 2 hr
• Blood studies: Hct, Hgb, RBCs, serum folate, vitamin D (if on long-term therapy); pro-time in patients receiving anticoagulants
• Hepatic studies: AST, ALT, bilirubin; if increased, drug is usually discontinued
Administer:
• After removal of cigarettes, to prevent fires
• Deep IM injection in large muscle mass to prevent tissue sloughing, abscesses, no more than 5 ml/site
• After trying conservative measures for insomnia
• After mixing with sterile water for injection to a concentration of 100 mg/ml, may dilute further with compatible solution: inject within 30 min of preparation; don't shake solution or use cloudy solution
• IV only with resuscitative equipment available, administer at <100 mg/min (only by qualified personnel)
• ½-1 hr before hs for expected sleeplessness
• On empty stomach for best absorption
Perform/provide:
• Assistance with ambulation after receiving dose
• Safety measures: siderails, nightlight, call bell within easy reach
• Checking to see PO medication swallowed
Evaluate:
• Therapeutic response: ability to sleep at night, decreased amount of early morning awakening if taking drug for insomnia, or decrease in number, severity of seizures if taking drug for seizure disorder
• Mental status: mood, sensorium, affect, memory (long, short), especially elderly
• Physical dependency: more fre-

quent requests for medication, shakes, anxiety

- Barbiturate toxicity: hypotension; pulmonary constriction; cold, clammy skin; cyanosis of lips; insomnia; nausea; vomiting; hallucinations; delirium; weakness; coma, pupillary constriction, mild symptoms may occur in 8-12 hr without drug
- Respiratory dysfunction: respiratory depression, character, rate, rhythm; hold drug if respirations are <10/min or if pupils are dilated
- Blood dyscrasias: fever, sore throat, bruising, rash, jaundice, epistaxis

Teach patient/family:

- That hangover is common
- That drug is indicated only for short-term treatment of insomnia and is probably ineffective after 2 wk
- That physical dependency may result when used for extended time (45-90 days depending on dose)
- To avoid driving or other activities requiring alertness
- To avoid alcohol ingestion or CNS depressants; serious CNS depression may result
- Not to discontinue medication quickly after long-term use; drug should be tapered over 1 wk
- To tell all prescribers that a barbiturate is being taken
- That withdrawal insomnia may occur after short-term use; do not start using drug again, insomnia will improve in 1-3 nights, may experience increased dreaming
- That effects may take 2 nights for benefits to be noticed
- Alternate measures to improve sleep: reading, exercise several hours before hs, warm bath, warm milk, TV, self-hypnosis, deep breathing

Lab test interferences:
False increase: Sulfobromophthalein

Treatment of overdose: Lavage, activated charcoal, warming blanket, vital signs, hemodialysis, alkalinize urine

---

amoxapine

(a-mox'a-peen)

Asendin

Func. class.: Antidepressant—tricyclic

Chem. class.: Dibenzoxazepine derivative—secondary amine

Action: Blocks reuptake of norepinephrine, serotonin into nerve endings, increasing action of norepinephrine, serotonin in nerve cells

Uses: Depression

Dosage and routes:

- *Adult:* PO 50 mg tid, may increase to 100 mg tid on 3rd day of therapy; not to exceed 300 mg/day unless lower doses have been given for at least 2 wk, may be given daily dose hs, not to exceed 600 mg/day in hospitalized patients

Available forms include: Tabs 10, 25, 50, 75, 100, 150 mg

Side effects/adverse reactions:

HEMA: ***Agranulocytosis, thrombocytopenia, eosinophilia, leukopenia***

CNS: Dizziness, drowsiness, confusion, headache, anxiety, tremors, stimulation, weakness, insomnia, nightmares, EPS (elderly), increased psychiatric symptoms, paresthesia

GI: Diarrhea, dry mouth, constipation, nausea, vomiting, ***paralytic ileus,*** increased appetite, cramps,

---

* Available in Canada only

epigastric distress, jaundice, ***hepatitis,*** stomatitis
GU: Retention, ***acute renal failure***
INTEG: Rash, urticaria, sweating, pruritus, photosensitivity
CV: Orthostatic hypotension, ECG changes, tachycardia, ***hypertension,*** palpitations
EENT: Blurred vision, tinnitus, mydriasis, ophthalmoplegia
Contraindications: Hypersensitivity to tricyclic antidepressants, recovery phase of myocardial infarction, convulsive disorders, prostatic hypertrophy
Precautions: Suicidal patients, severe depression, increased intraocular pressure, narrow-angle glaucoma, urinary retention, cardiac disease, hepatic disease, hyperthyroidism, electroshock therapy, elective surgery, elderly, pregnancy (C)
Pharmacokinetics:
PO: Steady state 7 days; metabolized by liver, excreted by kidneys, crosses placenta, half-life 8 hr
Interactions/incompatibilities:
- Decreased effects of: guanethidine, clonidine, indirect-acting sympathomimetics (ephedrine)
- Increased effects of: direct-acting sympathomimetics (epinephrine), alcohol, barbiturates, benzodiazepines, CNS depressants
- Hyperpyretic crisis, convulsions, hypertensive episode: MAOI (pargyline [Eutonyl])

NURSING CONSIDERATIONS

Assess:
- B/P (lying, standing), pulse q4h; if systolic B/P drops 20 mm Hg hold drug, notify physician; take vital signs q4h in patients with cardiovascular disease
- Blood studies: CBC, leukocytes, differential, cardiac enzymes if patient is receiving long-term therapy
- Hepatic studies: AST, ALT, bilirubin, creatinine
- Weight qwk, appetite may increase with drug
- ECG for flattening of T wave, bundle branch block, AV block, dysrhythmias in cardiac patients

Administer:
- Increased fluids, bulk in diet if constipation, urinary retention occur, especially in elderly
- With food or milk for GI symptoms
- Crushed if patient is unable to swallow medication whole
- Dosage hs if over-sedation occurs during day; may take entire dose hs; elderly may not tolerate once/day dosing
- Gum, hard candy, or frequent sips of water for dry mouth

Perform/provide:
- Storage at room temperature, do not freeze
- Assistance with ambulation during beginning therapy since drowsiness/dizziness occurs
- Safety measures including siderails primarily in elderly
- Checking to see PO medication swallowed

Evaluate:
- Therapeutic response: decreased depression, absence of suicidal thoughts
- EPS primarily in elderly: rigidity, dystonia, akathisia
- Mental status: mood, sensorium, affect, suicidal tendencies, increase in psychiatric symptoms: depression, panic
- Urinary retention, constipation; constipation is more likely to occur in children, elderly
- Withdrawal symptoms: headache, nausea, vomiting, muscle pain, weakness; do not usually oc-

cur unless drug was discontinued abruptly
• Alcohol consumption; if alcohol is consumed, hold dose until morning

Teach patient/family:
• That therapeutic effects may take 2-3 wk
• To use caution in driving or other activities requiring alertness because of drowsiness, dizziness, blurred vision
• To avoid alcohol ingestion, other CNS depressants
• Not to discontinue medication quickly after long-term use, may cause nausea, headache, malaise
• To wear sunscreen or large hat since photosensitivity occurs

Lab test interferences:
Increase: Serum bilirubin, blood glucose, alk phosphatase
False increase: Urinary catecholamines
Decrease: VMA, 5-HIAA

Treatment of overdose: ECG monitoring, induce emesis, lavage, activated charcoal, administer anticonvulsant

---

amoxicillin/clavulanate potassium

(a-mox-i-sill'in)
Augmentin, Clavulin*

Func. class.: Broad spectrum antibiotic
Chem. class.: Aminopenicillin-B lactamase inhibitor

Action: Interferes with cell wall replication of susceptible organisms; the cell wall, rendered osmotically unstable, swells, and bursts from osmotic pressure

Uses: Sinus infections, pneumonia, otitis media, skin, urinary tract infections; effective for strains of *E. coli, P. mirabilis, H. influenzae, S. faecalis, S. pneumoniae,* and β-lactamase-producing organisms

Dosage and routes:
• *Adult:* PO 250-500 mg q8h depending on severity of infection
• *Child:* PO 20-40 mg/kg/day in divided doses q8h

Available forms include: Tabs 250, 500 mg; chew tabs 125, 250 mg; powder for oral susp 125, 250 mg/5 ml

Side effects/adverse reactions:
HEMA: Anemia, ***bone marrow depression, granulocytopenia, leukopenia, eosinophilia,*** thrombocytopenic purpura
GI: Nausea, diarrhea, vomiting, increased AST, ALT, abdominal pain, glossitis, colitis, black tongue
GU: Oliguria, proteinuria, hematuria, *vaginitis, moniliasis,* ***glomerulonephritis***
CNS: Headache
META: Hyperkalemia, hypokalemia, alkalosis, hypernatremia

Contraindications: Hypersensitivity to penicillins; neonates

Precautions: Pregnancy (B), hypersensitivity to cephalosporins

Interactions/incompatibilities:
• Decreased antimicrobial effectiveness of amoxicillin: tetracyclines, erythromycins
• Increased amoxicillin concentrations: aspirin, probenecid

Pharmacokinetics:
PO: Peak 2 hr, duration 6-8 hr; half-life 1-1⅓ hr, metabolized in liver, excreted in urine, crosses placenta, enters breast milk

NURSING CONSIDERATIONS

Assess:
• I&O ratio; report hematuria, oliguria since penicillin in high doses is nephrotoxic
• Any patient with a compromised renal system, since drug is excreted

* Available in Canada only

slowly in poor renal system function; toxicity may occur rapidly
- Liver studies: AST, ALT
- Blood studies: WBC, RBC, H&H, bleeding time
- Renal studies: urinalysis, protein, blood
- Culture, sensitivity before drug therapy; drug may be taken as soon as culture is taken

Administer:
- After C&S completed

Perform/provide:
- Adrenaline, suction, tracheostomy set, endotracheal intubation equipment on unit
- Adequate intake of fluids (2000 ml) during diarrhea episodes
- Scratch test to assess allergy after securing order from physician; usually done when penicillin is only drug of choice
- Storage refrigerated for 2 wk, or room temperature for 1 wk

Evaluate:
- Therapeutic response: absence of temperature, draining wounds
- Bowel pattern before, during treatment
- Skin eruptions after administration of penicillin to 1 wk after discontinuing drug
- Respiratory status: rate, character, wheezing, tightness in chest
- Allergies before initiation of treatment, reaction of each medication; place allergies on chart, Kardex in bright red

Teach patient/family:
- Aspects of drug therapy: need to complete entire course of medication to ensure organism death (10-14 days); culture may be taken after completed course of medication
- To report sore throat, fever, fatigue (could indicate a superimposed infection)
- That drug must be taken in equal intervals around the clock to maintain blood levels, take on empty stomach with full glass of water
- To wear or carry a Medic Alert ID if allergic to penicillins
- To notify nurse of diarrhea

Lab test interferences:
False positive: Urine glucose, urine protein

Treatment of overdose: Withdraw drug, maintain airway, administer epinephrine, aminophylline, O_2, IV corticosteroids for anaphylaxis

amoxicillin trihydrate

(a-mox-i-sill'in)

Amoxican,* Amoxil, Apo-Amoxi,* Larotid, Novamoxin,* Polymox, Robamox, Sumox, Trimox, Utimox, Wymox

Func. class.: Broad-spectrum antibiotic

Chem. class.: Aminopenicillin

Action: Interferes with cell wall replication of susceptible organisms; the cell wall, rendered osmotically unstable, swells, and bursts from osmotic pressure

Uses: Effective for gram-positive cocci *(S. aureus, S. pyogenes, S. faecalis, S. pneumoniae)*, gram-negative cocci *(N. gonorrhoeae, N. meningitidis, E. coli)*, gram-positive bacilli *(C. diphtheriae, L. monocytogenes)*, gram-negative bacilli *(H. influenzae, P. mirabilis, Salmonella)*

Dosage and routes:

Systemic infections
- *Adult:* PO 750 mg-1.5 g qd in divided doses q8h
- *Child:* PO 20-40 mg/kg/day in divided doses q8h

Gonorrhea/urinary tract infections

• *Adult:* PO 3 g given with 1 g probenecid as a single dose

Available forms include: Caps 250, 500 mg; chew tabs 125, 250 mg; powder for oral susp 50, 125, 250 mg/5 ml

Side effects/adverse reactions:

HEMA: Anemia, increased bleeding time, ***bone marrow depression, granulocytopenia***

GI: Nausea, vomiting, diarrhea, increased AST, ALT, abdominal pain, glossitis, colitis

CNS: Headache

SYST: ***Anaphylaxis, respiratory distress***

Contraindications: Hypersensitivity to penicillins; neonates

Precautions: Pregnancy (B), hypersensitivity to cephalosporins

Interactions/incompatibilities:

• Decreased antimicrobial effectiveness of amoxicillin: tetracyclines, erythromycins

• Increased amoxicillin concentrations: aspirin, probenecid

Pharmacokinetics:

PO: Peak 2 hr, duration 6-8 hr; half-life 1-1⅓ hr, metabolized in liver, excreted in urine, crosses placenta, enters breast milk

NURSING CONSIDERATIONS

Assess:

• I&O ratio; report hematuria, oliguria since penicillin in high doses is nephrotoxic

• Any patient with a compromised renal system, since drug is excreted slowly in poor renal system function; toxicity may occur rapidly

• Liver studies: AST, ALT

• Blood studies: WBC, RBC, H&H, bleeding time

• Renal studies: urinalysis, protein, blood

• Culture, sensitivity before drug therapy; drug may be taken as soon as culture is taken

Administer:

• After C&S completed

Perform/provide:

• Adrenaline, suction, tracheostomy set, endotracheal intubation equipment on unit

• Adequate intake of fluids (2000 ml) during diarrhea episodes

• Scratch test to assess allergy after securing order from physician; usually done when penicillin is only drug of choice

• Storage in tight container; after reconstituting, oral suspension refrigerated for 2 wk or stored at room temperature for 1 wk

Evaluate:

• Therapeutic response: absence of temperature, draining wounds

• Bowel pattern before, during treatment

• Skin eruptions after administration of penicillin to 1 wk after discontinuing drug

• Respiratory status: rate, character, wheezing, tightness in the chest

• Allergies before initiation of treatment, reaction of each medication; place allergies on chart, Kardex in bright red

Teach patient/family:

• Aspects of drug therapy: need to complete entire course of medication to ensure organism death (10-14 days); culture may be taken after completed course of medication

• To report sore throat, fever, fatigue, diarrhea (could indicate a superimposed infection)

• That drug must be taken in equal intervals around the clock to maintain blood levels, take on empty stomach with a full glass of water

• To wear or carry a Medic Alert ID if allergic to penicillins

Lab test interferences:

False positive: Urine glucose, urine protein

---

* Available in Canada only

Treatment of overdose: Withdraw drug, maintain airway, administer epinephrine, aminophylline, O_2, IV corticosteroids for anaphylaxis

---

amphetamine sulfate

(am-fet'a-meen)

Racemic Amphetamine Sulfate

Func. class.: Cerebral stimulant
Chem. class.: Amphetamine

Controlled Substance Schedule II
Action: Increases release of norepinephrine, dopamine in cerebral cortex to reticular activating system
Uses: Narcolepsy, exogenous obesity, attention deficit disorder
Dosage and routes:
Narcolepsy
• *Adult:* PO 5-60 mg qd in divided doses
• *Child >12 yr:* PO 10 mg qd increasing by 10 mg/day at weekly intervals
• *Child 6-12 yr:* PO 5 mg qd increasing by 5 mg/wk, max 60 mg/day
Attention deficit disorder
• *Child >6 yr:* PO 5 mg qd-bid increasing by 5 mg/day at weekly intervals
• *Child 3-6 yr:* PO 2.5 mg qd increasing by 2.5 mg/day at weekly intervals
Obesity
• *Adult:* PO 5-30 mg in divided doses 30-60 min before meals
Available forms include: Tabs 5, 10 mg; sus rel caps 15 mg
Side effects/adverse reactions:
CNS: Hyperactivity, insomnia, restlessness, talkativeness, dizziness, headache, chills, stimulation, dysphoria, irritability, aggressiveness, tremor, dependence, addiction
GI: Nausea, vomiting, anorexia, dry mouth, diarrhea, constipation, weight loss, metallic taste, cramps
GU: Impotence, change in libido
CV: Palpitations, tachycardia, hypertension, dysrhythmias, decreased heart rate
INTEG: Urticaria
Contraindications: Hypersensitivity to sympathomimetic amines, hyperthyroidism, hypertension, glaucoma hypertrophy, severe arteriosclerosis, drug abuse, cardiovascular disease, anxiety
Precautions: Gilles de la Tourette's disorder, pregnancy (X), lactation, child <3 yr
Pharmacokinetics:
PO: Onset 30 min, peak 1-3 hr, duration 4-20 hr, metabolized by liver, excreted by kidneys, crosses placenta, breast milk, half-life 10-30 hr
Interactions/incompatibilities:
• Hypertensive crisis: MAOIs or within 14 days of MAOIs
• Increased effect of amphetamine: acetazolamide, antacids, sodium bicarbonate
• Decreased effect of amphetamine: barbiturates, tricyclics
• Decreased effect of: guanethidine

NURSING CONSIDERATIONS

Assess:
• VS, B/P since this drug may reverse antihypertensives; check patients with cardiac disease more often
• CBC, urinalysis, in diabetes: blood sugar, urine sugar; insulin changes may need to be made since eating will decrease
• Height, growth rate in children, growth rate may be decreased
Administer:
• At least 6 hr before hs to avoid sleeplessness
• For obesity only if patient is on weight reduction program that includes dietary changes, exercise;

patient will develop tolerance, and weight loss won't occur without additional methods; give 30-60 min before meals
• Gum, hard candy, frequent sips of water for dry mouth

Evaluate:
• Therapeutic response: decreased activity in attention deficit disorder; absence of sleeping during day in narcolepsy; decrease in weight
• Mental status: mood, sensorium, affect, stimulation, insomnia; aggressiveness may occur
• Physical dependency; should not be used for extended time; dose should be discontinued gradually
• Withdrawal symptoms: headache, nausea, vomiting, muscle pain, weakness
• Drug tolerance will develop after long-term use
• Dosage should not be increased if tolerance develops

Teach patient/family:
• To decrease caffeine consumption (coffee, tea, cola, chocolate), which may increase irritability, stimulation
• To avoid OTC preparations unless approved by physician
• To taper off drug over several weeks, or depression, increased sleeping, lethargy may occur
• To avoid alcohol ingestion
• To avoid hazardous activities until patient is stabilized on medication
• To get needed rest; patients will feel more tired at end of day

Treatment of overdose: Administer fluids, hemodialysis, peritoneal dialysis, antihypertensives for increased B/P; ammonium Cl for increased excretion

amphotericin B

(am-foe-ter'i-sin)
Fungizone
Func. class.: Antifungal
Chem. class.: Amphoteric polyene

Action: Increases cell membrane permeability in susceptible organisms by binding sterols; decreases K, Na, and nutrients in cell

Uses: Histoplasmosis, blastomycosis, coccidioidomycosis, cryptococcosis, aspergillosis, phycomycosis, candidiasis, sporotrichosis causing severe meningitis, septicemia, skin infections

Dosage and routes:
• *Adult and child:* IV INF 1 mg/250 ml D_5W (0.1 mg/ml) over 2-4 hr or 0.25 mg/kg/day over 6 hr; may be increased gradually up to 1 mg/kg/day, not to exceed 1.5 mg/kg; INTRATHECAL 0.1 mg, gradually increased to 0.5 mg q48-72 hr

Available forms include: Powder for inj 50 mg

Side effects/adverse reactions:
EENT: Tinnitus, deafness, diplopia, blurred vision
INTEG: Burning, irritation, necrosis at injection site, flushing, dermatitis, skin rash (topical route)
CNS: Headache, fever, chills, peripheral nerve pain, paresthesias, peripheral neuropathy, ***convulsions,*** dizziness
GU: Hypokalemia, axotemia, hyposthenuria, ***renal tubular acidosis,*** nephrocalcinosis, ***permanent renal impairment, anuria, oliguria***
GI: Nausea, vomiting, anorexia, diarrhea, cramps, ***hemorrhagic gastroenteritis, acute liver failure***
MS: ***Arthralgia, myalgia,*** generalized pain, weakness

* Available in Canada only

HEMA: Normochromic, normocytic anemia, ***thrombocytopenia, agranulocytosis, leukopenia, eosinophilia,*** hypokalemia, hyponatremia, hypomagnesemia

Contraindications: Hypersensitivity, severe bone marrow depression

Precautions: Renal disease, pregnancy (B)

Pharmacokinetics:

IV: Peak 1-2 hr, initial half-life 24 hr, metabolized in liver, excreted in urine (metabolites), breast milk, highly bound to plasma proteins; penetrates poorly CSF, bronchial secretions, aqueous humor, muscle, bone

Interactions/incompatibilities:

- Increased nephrotoxicity: other nephrotoxic antibiotics (aminoglycosides, cisplatin, vancomycin, cyclosporine, polymixin B)
- Increased hypokalemia: corticosteroids, digitalis, skeletal muscle relaxants
- Antagonism: miconazole
- Do not mix in sodium solutions or diluent with preservatives

NURSING CONSIDERATIONS

Assess:

- VS q15-30 min during first infusion; note changes in pulse, B/P
- I&O ratio; watch for decreasing urinary output, change in sp gr; discontinue drug to prevent permanent damage to renal tubules
- Blood studies: CBC, K, Na, Ca, Mg q2 wk
- Weight weekly; if weight increases over 2 lb/wk, edema is present, renal damage should be considered

Administer:

- After diluting with 10 ml sterile water (no preservatives) or NS, then dilute with 500 ml of solution to concentration of 0.1 mg/ml
- Test dose of 1 mg/20 ml D_5W; give over 10-30 min
- IV using in-line filter (mean pore diameter >1 μm) using distal veins, check for extravasation, necrosis q8h
- Drug only after C&S confirms organism, drug needed to treat condition; make sure drug is used in life-threatening infections

Perform/provide:

- Protection from light during infusion, cover with foil
- Symptomatic treatment as ordered for adverse reactions: aspirin, antihistamines, antiemetics, antispasmodics
- Storage, protected from moisture and light; diluted solution is stable for 24 hr

Evaluate:

- Therapeutic response: decreased fever, malaise, rash, negative C&S for infecting organism
- For renal toxicity: increasing BUN, serum creatinine; if BUN is >40 mg/dl or if serum creatinine >3 mg/dl, drug may be discontinued or dosage reduced
- For hepatotoxicity: increasing AST, ALT, alk phosphatase, bilirubin
- For allergic reaction: dermatitis, rash; drug should be discontinued, antihistamines (mild reaction) or epinephrine (severe reaction) administered
- For hypokalemia: anorexia, drowsiness, weakness, decreased reflexes, dizziness, increased urinary output, increased thirst, paresthesias
- For ototoxicity: tinnitus (ringing, roaring in ears) vertigo, loss of hearing (rare)

Teach patient/family:

- That long-term therapy may be

needed to clear infection (2 wk-3 mo depending on type of infection)

amphotericin B (topical)

(am-foe-ter'i-sin)

Fungizone

Func. class.: Local antiinfective
Chem. class.: Antifungal (polyene)

Action: Increases cell membrane permeability in susceptible organisms by binding sterols

Uses: Cutaneous, mucocutaneous infections caused by *Candida*

Dosage and routes:

• *Adult and child:* TOP bid-qid for 7-21 days or longer if needed

Available forms include: Cream, lotion, oint 3%

Side effects/adverse reactions:

INTEG: Urticaria, stinging, burning, dry skin, pruritus, contact dermatitis, erythema, staining of nail lesions

Contraindications: Hypersensitivity

Precautions: Pregnancy (B), lactation

NURSING CONSIDERATIONS

Administer:

• Enough medication to completely cover lesions, apply liberally and rub thoroughly into affected area

• After cleansing with soap, water before each application, dry well (as ordered)

Perform/provide:

• Storage at room temperature in dry place

Evaluate:

• Therapeutic response: decrease in size, number of lesions

• Allergic reaction: burning, stinging, swelling, redness

Teach patient/family:

• That skin and clothing may become discolored

• To apply with glove to prevent further infection; not to cover with occlusive dressing

• To avoid use of OTC creams, ointments, lotions unless directed by physician

• To use medical asepsis (hand washing) before, after each application to prevent further infection

• To continue even if condition improves

• To report increased itching, burning, rash, redness

ampicillin/ampicillin sodium/ampicillin trihydrate

(am-pi-sill'in)

Amcap, Amcill, Ampicin, Ampilean,* Ampicin-PRB,* Apo-Ampi,* D-Amp, NovoAmpicillin,* Omnipen, Penbritin,* Pfizerpen A, Principen, Roampicillin, Supen, Omnipen-N, Pen A/N, Polycillin-N, Totacillin-N

Func. class.: Broad-spectrum antibiotic
Chem. class.: Aminopenicillin

Action: Interferes with cell wall replication of susceptible organisms; the cell wall, rendered osmotically unstable, swells, bursts from osmotic pressure

Uses: Effective for gram-positive cocci *(S. aureus, S. pyogenes, S. faecalis, S. pneumoniae)*, gram-negative cocci *(N. gonorrhoeae, N. meningitidis)*, gram-negative bacilli *(H. influenzae, P. mirabilis, Salmonella, Shigella, L. monocytogenes)*, gram-positive bacilli

Dosage and routes:

Systemic infections

• *Adult:* PO 1-2 g qd in divided

*Available in Canada only

doses q6h; IV/IM 2-8 g qd in divided doses q4-6h
- *Child:* PO 50-100 mg/kg/day in divided doses q6h; IV/IM 100-200 mg/kg/day in divided doses q6h

Meningitis
- *Adult:* IV 8-14 g/day in divided doses q3-4h × 3 days
- *Child:* IV 200-300 mg/kg/day in divided doses q3-4h × 3 days

Gonorrhea
- *Adult:* PO 3.5 g given with 1 g probenecid as a single dose

Available forms include: Powder for inj IV, IM 125, 250, 500 mg, 1, 2, 10 g; IV inf 500 mg, 1, 2 g; caps 250, 500 mg; powder for oral susp 100, 125, 250, 500 mg/5 ml

Side effects/adverse reactions:
INTEG: Rash, urticaria
HEMA: Anemia, increased bleeding time, ***bone marrow depression, granulocytopenia***
GI: Nausea, vomiting, diarrhea
GU: Oliguria, proteinuria, hematuria, *vaginitis, moniliasis,* ***glomerulonephritis***
CNS: Lethargy, hallucinations, anxiety, depression, twitching, ***coma, convulsions***

Contraindications: Hypersensitivity to penicillins

Precautions: Pregnancy (B); hypersensitivity to cephalosporins; neonates

Pharmacokinetics:
PO: Peak 2 hr
IV: Peak 5 min
IM: Peak 1 hr
Half-life 50-110 min; metabolized in liver, excreted in urine, bile, breast milk, crosses placenta

Interactions/incompatibilities:
- Possible increased bleeding: oral anticoagulants
- Decreased antimicrobial effectiveness of ampicillin: tetracyclines, erythromycins
- Increased ampicillin concentrations: aspirin, probenecid
- Decreased effectiveness of: oral contraceptives
- Increased ampicillin-induced skin rash: allopurinol

NURSING CONSIDERATIONS

Assess:
- I&O ratio; report hematuria, oliguria since penicillin in high doses is nephrotoxic
- Any patient with compromised renal system, since drug is excreted slowly in poor renal system function; toxicity may occur rapidly
- Liver studies: AST, ALT
- Blood studies: WBC, RBC, H&H, bleeding time
- Renal studies: urinalysis, protein, blood
- Culture, sensitivity before drug therapy; drug may be taken as soon as culture is taken
- Sodium levels when high doses of injectables are given to cardiac patients

Administer:
- After diluting with sterile H_2O 0.9-1.2 ml/125 mg drug, administer over 3-5 min (up to 500 mg), 10-15 min, (>500 mg) by direct IV; may be diluted in 50 ml or more of compatible solutions to a concentration of 30 mg/ml or less
- After C&S completed
- On empty stomach for best absorption

Perform/provide:
- Adrenaline, suction, tracheostomy set, endotracheal intubation equipment on unit
- Adequate intake of fluids (2000 ml) during diarrhea episodes
- Scratch test to assess allergy after securing order from physician; usually done when penicillin is only drug of choice
- Storage in tight container; after

reconstituting oral suspension refrigerated for 2 wk or stored at room temperature for 1 wk

Evaluate:

• Therapeutic response: absence of temperature, draining wounds

• Bowel pattern before, during treatment

• Skin eruptions after administration of penicillin to 1 wk after discontinuing drug

• Respiratory status: rate, character, wheezing, tightness in chest

• Allergies before initiation of treatment; reaction of each medication; place allergies on chart, Kardex in bright red

Teach patient/family:

• To take oral penicillin on empty stomach with full glass of water

• Aspects of drug therapy: need to complete entire course of medication to ensure organism death (10-14 days); culture may be taken after completed course of medication

• To report sore throat, fever, fatigue, diarrhea (could indicate superimposed infection)

• That drug must be taken in equal intervals around the clock to maintain blood levels

• To wear or carry a Medic Alert ID if allergic to penicillins

Lab test interferences:

False positive: Urine glucose, urine protein

Treatment of overdose: Withdraw drug, maintain airway, administer epinephrine, aminophylline, O_2, IV corticosteroids for anaphylaxis

ampicillin sodium, sulbactam sodium

Unasyn

Func. class.: Broad-spectrum antibiotic

Chem. class.: Aminopenicillin

Action: Interferes with cell wall replication of susceptible organisms; the cell wall, rendered osmotically unstable, swells, bursts from osmotic pressure

Uses: Skin infections (*S. aureus, E. coli, Klebsiella, P. mirabilis, B. fragilis, Enterobacter, A. calcoaceticus*), intraabdominal infections (*Enterobacter, Klebsiella, Bacteroides, E. coli*) gynecologic infections (*E. coli, Bacteroides.*)

Dosage and routes:

• *Adult:* IV 1 g ampicillin, 0.5 g sulbactam to 2 g ampicillin and 1 g sulbactam q6h, not to exceed 4 g/day sulbactam

Available forms include: Powder for inj 1.5 g (1 g ampicillin, 0.5 g sulbactam), 3.0 g (2 g ampicillin, 1 g sulbactam)

Side effects/adverse reactions:

HEMA: Anemia, increased bleeding time, ***bone marrow depression, granulocytopenia***

GI: Nausea, vomiting, diarrhea, increased AST, ALT, abdominal pain, glossitis, colitis

GU: Oliguria, proteinuria, hematuria, *vaginitis, moniliasis,* ***glomerulonephritis***

CNS: Lethargy, hallucinations, anxiety, depression, twitching, ***coma, convulsions***

Contraindications: Hypersensitivity to penicillins

Precautions: Pregnancy, hypersensitivity to cephalosporins, neonates

Pharmacokinetics:
IV: Peak 5 min; half-life 50-110 min; little metabolized in liver, 75% to 85% of both drugs excreted in urine, diffuses to breast milk, crosses placenta

Interactions/incompatibilities:
- Decreased antimicrobial effectiveness of ampicillin: tetracyclines, erythromycins
- Increased ampicillin concentration: aspirin, probenecid

NURSING CONSIDERATIONS

Assess:
- Bowel pattern before, during treatment
- Respiratory status: rate, character, wheezing, tightness in chest
- I&O ratio; report hematuria, oliguria, since penicillin in high doses is nephrotoxic
- Any patient with compromised renal system, since drug is excreted slowly in poor renal system function; toxicity may occur rapidly
- Liver studies: AST, ALT
- Blood studies: WBC, RBC, Hct/Hgb, bleeding time
- Renal studies: urinalysis, protein, blood
- C&S before drug therapy; drug may be taken as soon as culture is taken

Administer:
- IV after diluting 1.5 g/4 ml or more sterile H_2O for inj; may be given over 15 min directly or diluted in 50 ml or more of compatible solution
- After C&S completed; on empty stomach

Perform/provide:
- Adrenaline, suction, tracheostomy set, endotracheal intubation equipment on unit for possible anaphylaxis
- Adequate intake of fluids (2000 ml) during diarrhea episode
- Scratch test to assess allergy after securing order from physician; usually done when penicillin is only drug choice
- Storage in tight container, out of light

Evaluate:
- Therapeutic response: absence of temperature, draining wounds, negative C&S
- Skin eruptions after administration of ampicillin 1 wk after discontinuing drug
- Allergies before initiation of treatment; reaction of each medication; place allergies on chart

Teach patient/family:
- To report sore throat, fever, fatigue (could indicate superimposed infection)
- To wear or carry Medic Alert ID if allergic to penicillin products

Lab test interferences:
False positive: Urine glucose, urine protein

Treatment of overdose: Withdraw drug, maintain airway, administer epinephrine, aminophylline, O_2, IV corticosteroids for anaphylaxis

---

amrinone lactate

(am'ri-none)

Inocor

Func. class.: Cardiac inotropic agent

Chem. class.: Bipyrimidine derivative

Action: Positive inotropic agent with vasodilator properties; reduces preload and afterload by direct relaxation on vascular smooth muscle

Uses: Short-term management of CHF that has not responded to other medication; can be used with digitalis

Dosage and routes:
• *Adult:* IV BOL 0.75 mg/kg given over 2-3 min; start infusion of 5-10 μg/kg/min; may give another bolus ½ hr after start of therapy, not to exceed 10 mg/kg total daily dose
Available forms include: Inj 5 mg/ml
Side effects/adverse reactions:
HEMA: ***Thrombocytopenia***
CV: Dysrhythmias, hypotension, headache, chest pain
GI: Nausea, vomiting, anorexia, abdominal pain, ***hepatotoxicity, ascites,*** jaundice, hiccups
INTEG: Allergic reactions, burning at injection site
RESP: Pleuritis, ***pulmonary densities, hypoxemia***
Contraindications: Hypersensitivity to this drug or bisulfites, severe aortic disease, severe pulmonic valvular disease, acute myocardial infarction
Precautions: Lactation, pregnancy (C), children, renal disease, hepatic disease, atrial flutter/fibrillation, elderly
Pharmacokinetics:
IV: Onset 2-5 min, peak 10 min, duration variable; half-life 4-6 hr, metabolized in liver, excreted in urine as drug and metabolites 60%-90%
Interactions/incompatibilities:
• Excessive hypotension: antihypertensives

NURSING CONSIDERATIONS

Assess:
• B/P and pulse q5 min during infusion; if B/P drops 30 mm Hg, stop infusion and call physician
• Electrolytes: potassium, sodium, chloride, calcium; renal function studies: BUN, creatinine; blood studies: platelet count
• ALT, AST, bilirubin daily
• I&O ratio and weight qd, diuresis should increase with continuing therapy
• If platelets are <150,000/mm^3 drug is usually discontinued and another drug started
Administer:
• Do not mix with glucose solutions directly, chemical reaction occurs over 24 hr; precipitate forms if amrinone and furosemide come in contact
• Into running dextrose infusion through Y-connector or directly into tubing; dilute with normal saline to concentration of 1-3 mg/ml, do not mix with glucose for long-term infusion
• By infusion pump for doses other than bolus
• Potassium supplements if ordered for potassium levels <3.0
Evaluate:
• Therapeutic response: increased cardiac output, decreased PCWP, adequate CVP, decreased dyspnea, fatigue, edema, ECG
• Extravasation, change site q48h
Treatment of overdose: Discontinue drug, support circulation

---

amyl nitrite

(am'il)

Amyl Nitrite Aspirols, Amyl Nitrite Vaporole

Func. class.: Coronary vasodilator
Chem. class.: Nitrite

Action: Relaxes vascular smooth muscle, may dilate coronary blood vessels, resulting in reduced venous return, decreased cardiac output; reduces preload, afterload, which decreases left ventricular end diastolic pressure, systemic vascular resistance
Uses: Acute angina pectoris

A

Dosage and routes:
Angina
• ***Adult:*** INH 0.18-0.3 ml as needed, 1-6 inhalations from 1 cap, may repeat in 3-5 min
Cyanide poisoning
• ***Adult:*** INH 0.3 ml ampule inhaled 15 sec until preparation of sodium nitrite infusion is ready
Available forms include: Inh pearls 0.18, 0.3 ml
Side effects/adverse reactions:
CV: Postural hypotension, ***tachycardia, cardiovascular collapse,*** palpitations
CNS: Headache, dizziness, weakness, syncope
GI: Nausea, vomiting, abdominal pain
INTEG: Flushing, pallor, sweating
MISC: Muscle twitching, ***hemolytic anemia, methemoglobinemia***
Contraindications: Hypersensitivity to nitrites, severe anemia, acute myocardial infarction, increased intracranial pressure, hypertension, pregnancy (X)
Precautions: Lactation, children, drug abuse, head injury, cerebral hemorrhage, hypotension
Pharmacokinetics:
INH: Onset 30 sec, duration 3-5 min; metabolized by liver, ⅓ excreted in urine, half-life 1-4 min
Interactions/incompatibilities:
• Increased hypotension: alcohol, β-blockers, antihypertensive
NURSING CONSIDERATIONS
Assess:
• B/P, supine and sitting, pulse during treatment until stable
Administer:
• After wrapping, crushing ampule to avoid cuts
• Ordered analgesic if headache develops
• To patient who is sitting or lying down during treatment; keep head low, use deep breaths, which will decrease dizziness
• Drug, and have patient rest for 15 min
Perform/provide:
• Storage in light-resistant area in cool environment
Evaluate:
• Therapeutic response: relief of chest pain (angina)
• For drug tolerance: the need for more medication for each attack
• For postural hypotension, headache during treatment, which are common side effects because of vasodilation
Teach patient/family:
• To keep a record of angina attacks, and what aggravates condition; prolonged chest pain may indicate MI, seek emergency treatment
• That medication may explode in presence of flame
• To take several deep breaths despite foul odor
• To make position changes slowly to prevent orthostatic hypotension
• To keep drug out of reach of children and in secure place, as there is high abuse potential

---

anistreplase (APSAC)

(an-ih-strep'layz)
Eminase

Func. class.: Thrombolytic enzyme
Chem. class.: Anisolated plasminogen streptokinase activator complex

Action: Promotes thrombolysis by promoting conversion of plasminogen to plasmin
Uses: Management of acute myocardial infarction

Dosage and routes:

• *Adult:* IV 30 U over 4-5 min as soon as possible after onset of symptoms

Available forms include: Powder, lyophilized 30 U/vial

Side effects/adverse reactions:

HEMA: Decreased Hct, ***GI, GU, intracranial, retroperitoneal,*** surface bleeding, ***thrombocytopenia***

INTEG: Rash, urticaria, phlebitis at site, itching, flushing

CNS: Headache, fever, sweating, agitation, dizziness, paresthesia, tremor, vertigo

GI: Nausea, vomiting

RESP: Altered respirations, dyspnea, ***bronchospasm,*** lung edema

MS: Low back pain, arthralgia

CV: Hypotension, dysrhythmias, conduction disorders

SYST: ***Anaphylaxis***

Contraindications: Hypersensitivity, active internal bleeding, intraspinal or intracranial surgery, neoplasms of CNS, severe hypertension, cerebral embolism/thrombosis/hemorrhage

Precautions: Arterial emboli from left side of heart, pregnancy (B), ulcerative colitis/enteritis, renal disease, hepatic disease, hypocoagulation, COPD, subacute bacterial endocarditis, rheumatic valvular disease, intraarterial diagnostic procedure or surgery (10 days), recent major surgery

Pharmacokinetics: Half-life 105 min

Interactions/incompatibilities:

• Increased bleeding potential: aspirin, indomethacin, phenylbutazone, anticoagulants

NURSING CONSIDERATIONS

Assess:

• VS, B/P, pulse, respirations, neurologic signs, temperature at least q4h, temp >104° F or indicators of internal bleeding, cardiac rhythm after intracoronary administration

Administer:

• Reconstitute only with sterile water for injection (not bacteriostatic water), and roll (not shake) to enhance reconstitution

• As soon as thrombi are identified; not useful for thrombi more than 1 wk old

• Cryoprecipitate or fresh, frozen plasma if bleeding occurs

• Heparin therapy after thrombolytic therapy is discontinued, TT or APTT less than 2 times control (about 3-4 hr)

• About 10% of patients have high streptococcal antibody titers, requiring increased loading doses

Perform/provide:

• Bed rest during entire course of treatment; handle patient as little as possible during therapy

• Storage of powder in refrigerator; use within 30 min after reconstitution

• Avoid invasive procedures: inj, rectal temperature

• Treat fever with acetaminophen

• Pressure of 30 sec to minor bleeding sites; inform physician if hemostasis not attained, apply pressure dressing

Evaluate:

• Therapeutic response: absence of thrombi formation in MI, improved ventricular function

• Allergy: fever, rash, itching, chills; mild reaction may be treated with antihistamines

• Bleeding during 1st hr of treatment (hematuria, hematemesis, bleeding from mucous membranes, epistaxis, ecchymosis)

• Blood studies (Hct, platelets, PTT, PT, TT, APTT) before starting therapy; PT or APTT must be

less than 2 times control before starting therapy; TT or PT q3-4h during treatment
Lab test interferences:
Increase: PT, APTT, TT
Decrease: Fibrinogen, plasminogen

---

antihemophilic factor (AHF)

(an-tee-hee-moe-fill'ik)
Hemofil M, Koate H.P., Koate H.S., Kryobulin VH,* Monoclate
Func. class.: Hemostatic
Chem. class.: Factor VIII

Action: Necessary for clotting, activates factor X in conjunction with activated factor IX, transformation of prothrombin to thrombin
Uses: Hemophilia A, patients with acquired circulating factor VIII inhibitors, factor VIII deficiency
Dosage and routes: Depends on severity of deficiency
• *Adult and child:* IV 10-20 U/kg q8-24 h; INF 10-20 ml/3 min
Available forms include: Inj IV (number of units noted on label)
Side effects/adverse reactions:
GI: Nausea, vomiting, abdominal cramps, jaundice, ***viral hepatitis***
INTEG: Rash, flushing, *urticaria,* stinging at injection site
CNS: Headache, *lethargy, chills, fever, flushing*
HEMA: ***Thrombosis, hemolysis, AIDS***
CV: Hypotension, tachycardia
RESP: ***Bronchospasm***
Contraindications: Hypersensitivity, monoclonal antibody-derived factor VIII
Precautions: Neonates/infants, hepatic disease, blood types A, B, AB, pregnancy (C), factor VIII inhibitor
Pharmacokinetics:
IV: Half-life 4 hr, terminal 15 hr

NURSING CONSIDERATIONS

Assess:
• Blood studies (coagulation factors assay by % normal: 5% prevents spontaneous hemorrhage, 30%-50% for surgery, 80%-100% for severe hemorrhage)
• I&O, urine color; notify physician if urine becomes orange, red
• Pulse: discontinue infusion if significant increase
• Hct, Coombs' with blood types A, B, AB
• Test for factor VIII inhibitors before starting treatment, may require concomitant antiinhibitor coagulant complex therapy
Administer:
• After rotating gently to mix
• IV slowly, plastic syringe to reconstitute, administer; adheres to glass; use another needle as a vent when reconstituting
• After dilution with warm NS, D_5W, LR, give within 3 hr
• IV INF: give at ≤2 ml/min if concentration exceeds 34 U/ml or over 3 min if concentration is less than 34 U/ml
Perform/provide:
• Storage in refrigerator, do not freeze, after reconstitution, do not refrigerate
Evaluate:
• Therapeutic response: absence of bleeding
• Allergy: fever, rash, itching, jaundice; give Benadryl, continue therapy if reaction is mild
• Blood group of patient, donors (if applicable; most factor VIII not from specific blood group donors)
• Bleeding: ankles, knees, elbows, other joints
Teach patient/family:
• To report any signs of bleeding:

gums, under skin, urine, stools, emesis; review methods to prevent bleeding
• To avoid salicylates (increase bleeding tendencies)
• To prepare, administer factor VIII concentrates at first sign of danger
• To advise health professionals of treatment for hemophilia
• Signs of viral hepatitis, AIDS
• That immunization for hepatitis B may be given first
• To report hives, urticaria, chest tightness, hypotension; may be monoclonal antibody-derived factor VIII
• To be checked q2-3 mo for HIV screen
• To carry ID describing disease process

antithrombin III, human

ATnativ

Func. class.: Antithrombin
Chem. class.: Pooled human plasma

Action: Inactivates thrombin and the activated forms of factors IX, X, XI, XII, resulting in inhibition of coagulation
Uses: Hereditary antithrombin III deficiency in connection with surgical or obstetric procedures or for thromboembolism
Dosage and routes: Dosage is individualized. After first dose, antithrombin III level should increase to about 120% of normal; thereafter maintain at levels >80%; this is usually achieved by administering maintenance doses once every 24 hr
Available forms include: Lyophilized powder, 50 ml infusion bottles containing 500 IU antithrombin III with 10 ml sterile water for injection
Side effects/adverse reactions:
SYST: Bleeding, surface bleeding, ***anaphylaxis,*** vasodilatory effects
Precautions: Pregnancy (C), children
Pharmacokinetics: Unknown

NURSING CONSIDERATIONS

Assess:
• VS, B/P, pulse, respirations, neurologic signs, temperature at least q4h, temperature 104° F or indicators of internal bleeding, cardiac rhythm
• For neurologic changes that may indicate intracranial bleeding
• Retroperitoneal bleeding: back pain, leg weakness, diminished pulses
• Heparin after fibrinogen level is over 100 mg/dl; heparin infusion to increase PTT to 1.5-2 × baseline for 3-7 days
• After reconstituting with 10 ml of NS or D_5W; do not shake
• IV therapy using 0.22 or 0.45 micro filter
Perform/provide:
• Bed rest during entire course of treatment
• Avoidance of venous or arterial puncture, inj, rectal temperature
• Treatment of fever with acetaminophen or aspirin
Evaluate:
• Therapeutic response: absence of thrombi formation

apomorphine HCl

(a-poe-mor'feen)

Func. class.: Emetic, dopamine agonist
Chem. class.: Morphine, hydrochloric acid

Controlled Substance Schedule II

Action: Acts centrally by stimulating chemoreceptor trigger zone, which in turn acts on vomiting center

Uses: In poisoning/drug overdose to induce vomiting promptly (10-15 min); is almost 100% effective

Dosage and routes:

• *Adult:* IM/SC 2-10 mg then 7-10 oz evaporated milk or water, do not repeat

• *Child >1 yr:* IM/SC 0.07 mg/kg then 16 oz evaporated milk or water, do not repeat

• *Child <1 yr:* IM/SC 0.07 mg/kg then 8 oz evaporated milk or water, do not repeat

Available forms include: Soluble tabs (parenteral) 6 mg

Side effects/adverse reactions:

CNS: Euphoria, depression, restlessness, tremor, muscle weakness

GI: Nausea, anorexia, dry mouth, diarrhea, constipation, weight loss, metallic taste, cramps, salivation

CV: ***Circulatory failure, tachycardia,*** irregular rapid pulse, decreased B/P

RESP: ***Respiratory depression***

Contraindications: Hypersensitivity to narcotics, respiratory depression, corrosive poisoning, coma, shock, narcosis from CNS depressants

Precautions: Children, cardiac decompensation, elderly, pregnancy (C)

Pharmacokinetics:

PO: Onset 10-15 min

SC: Onset 1-2 min, metabolized by liver, excreted by kidneys

Interactions/incompatibilities:

• Incompatible with iodides, iron preparations, tannins, oxidizing agents

NURSING CONSIDERATIONS

Assess:

• Vital signs, B/P; check patients with cardiac disease more often, administer to conscious patients only

Administer:

• Dopamine antagonists to reverse emetic effect of this drug

• Activated charcoal if this drug doesn't work; may begin lavage after 10-15 min

• Only clear solutions; do not expose to light or air

Evaluate:

• Therapeutic response: vomiting rapidly

• Type of poisoning; do not administer if petroleum products or caustic substances have been ingested: kerosene, gasoline, lye, Drano

• Respiratory status before, during, after administration of emetic, check rate, rhythm, character; respiratory depression can occur rapidly with elderly or debilitated patients; record B/P, pulse; check for odor of alcohol on breath, clothes

---

apraclonidine HCl

(ap-raa-kloe'ni-deen)

Iopidine

Func. class.: Topical ophthalmic agent

Chem. class.: Selective α-adrenergic agonist

Action: Reduces intraocular pressure by reducing aqueous formation; exact mechanism of action unknown

Uses: Control elevations of intraocular pressure after laser iridotomy or trabeculoplasty

Dosage and routes

• *Adult:* Instill 1 gtt 1 hr before laser surgery, second gtt at completion of surgery

Available forms include: Sol 1%

apraclonidine HCl, 0.01% benzalkonium chloride

Side effects/adverse reactions:
EENT: Upper lid elevation, conjunctival blanching, mydriasis, burning, dryness, itching, blurred vision, conjunctival microhemorrhage, foreign body sensation, dry mouth, taste abnormalities, nasal dryness/burning
GI: Abdominal pain, diarrhea, cramps, emesis
CV: Bradycardia, palpitations, vasovagal attack, orthostatic episode
CNS: Insomnia, irritability, restlessness, headache, dream disturbances
OTHER: Shortness of breath, head cold sensation, sweaty palms, fatigue, paresthesia, pruritus

Contraindications: Hypersensitivity to this drug or clonidine, severe cardiovascular disease

Precautions: Pregnancy (C), lactation, children

NURSING CONSIDERATIONS

Assess:
- Cardiac status; watch for bradycardia, palpitations, especially in cardiac disease (including hypertension)
- Vasovagal attack during laser surgery primarily in individuals with history of such episodes

Perform/provide:
- Storage at room temperature, away from light

Evaluate:
Therapeutic response: absence of increased intraocular pressure

Teach patient/family
- Drug may cause burning, itching, blurring, dryness of eye area

ascorbic acid (vitamin C)

(a-skor'bic)

Ascorbicap, Ascorbineed, Best-C, Cecon, Cemill, C-Long, C-Syrup 500, Cenolate, Cetane, Cevalin, Cevi-Bid, Ce-Vi-Sol, Cevita, Redoxon,* Solucap C, Vitacee, Viterra C

Func. class.: Vitamin C, water-soluble vitamin

Action: Needed for wound healing, collagen synthesis, antioxidant, carbohydrate metabolism

Uses: Vitamin C deficiency, scurvy, delayed wound and bone healing, chronic disease, urine acidification, before gastrectomy

Dosage and routes:

Scurvy
- *Adult:* PO/SC/IM/IV 100 mg-500 mg qd, then 50 mg or more qd
- *Child:* PO/SC/IM/IV 100-300 mg qd, then 35 mg or more qd

Wound healing/chronic disease/fracture
- *Adult:* SC/IM/IV/PO 200-500 mg qd
- *Child:* SC/IM/IV/PO 100-200 mg added doses

Urine acidification
- *Adult:* 4-12 g qd in divided doses

Available forms include: Tabs 25, 50, 100, 250, 500, 1000, 1500 mg; tabs effervescent 1000 mg; tabs chewable 100, 250, 500 mg; tabs timed release 500, 750, 1000, 1500 mg; caps timed release 500 mg; crys 4 g/tsp; powd 4 g/tsp; liq 35 mg/0.6 ml; sol 100 mg/ml; syr 20 mg/ml, 500 mg/5 ml; inj SC, IM, IV 100, 250, 500 mg/ml

Side effects/adverse reactions:
CNS: Headache, insomnia, dizziness, fatigue, flushing
GI: Nausea, vomiting, diarrhea, anorexia, heartburn, cramps

* Available in Canada only

GU: Polyuria, urine acidification, oxalate or urate renal stones
HEMA: ***Hemolytic anemia in patients with G-6-PD***
Contraindications: None significant
Precautions: Gout, pregnancy (A)
Pharmacokinetics:
PO, INJ: Metabolized in liver, unused amounts excreted in urine (unchanged) and metabolites, crosses placenta, breast milk
Interactions/incompatibilities:
- Increased effects of: salicylates, oral contraceptives
- Increased side effects of: PAS, digitalis, sulfonamides
- Decreased effects of: phenothiazines, disulfiram, amphetamines, heparin, coumarin (massive doses)

NURSING CONSIDERATIONS
Assess:
- I&O ratio
- Ascorbic acid levels throughout treatment if continued deficiency is suspected

Administer:
- By direct IV 100 mg over at least 1 min
- By IV INF diluted with compatible solutions and given over 15 min

Evaluate:
- Therapeutic response: absence of anorexia, irritability, pallor, joint pain, hyperkeratosis, petechiae, poor wound healing
- Nutritional status: citrus fruits, vegetables
- Injection sites for inflammation

Teach patient/family:
- Necessary foods to be included in diet
- That if oral contraceptives are taken, increased levels of vitamin C are needed
- That smoking decreases vitamin C levels, not to exceed prescribed dose; increases will be excreted in urine, except time release

Lab test interferences:
- *False positive:* negatives in glucose tests
- *False negative:* occult blood

---

asparaginase (L-asparaginase)

(a-spar'a-gin-ase)
Elspar, Kidrolase

Func. class.: Antineoplastic
Chem. class.: *E. coli* enzyme

Action: Indirectly inhibits protein synthesis in tumor cells; without amino acid, DNA, RNA synthesis is halted; a nonvesicant
Uses: Acute lymphocytic leukemia in combination with other antineoplastics
Dosage and routes:
In combination
- *Adult:* IV 1000 IU/kg/day × 10 days given over 30 min; IM 6000 IU/m^2/day

Sole induction
- *Adult:* IV 200 IU/kg/day × 28 days

Available forms include: Inj 10,000 IU
Side effects/adverse reactions:
SYST: ***Anaphylaxis, hypersensitivity***
HEMA: ***Thrombocytopenia, leukopenia, myelosuppression, anemia, decreased clotting factors***
GI: Nausea, vomiting, anorexia, cramps, stomatitis, ***hepatotoxicity, pancreatitis***
GU: Urinary retention, ***renal failure,*** glycosuria, polyuria, azotemia, uric acid neuropathy
INTEG: Rash, urticaria, chills, fever
ENDO: Hyperglycemia

RESP: ***Fibrosis, pulmonary infiltrate***
CV: Chest pain
CNS: Neuritis, dizziness, headache, ***coma,*** depression, fatigue, confusion, hallucinations

Contraindications: Hypersensitivity, infants, pregnancy (D), lactation, pancreatitis

Precautions: Renal disease, hepatic disease

Pharmacokinetics: Half-life 4-9 hr, terminal 1.4-1.8 hr

Interactions/incompatibilities:

- Decreased action of: methotrexate
- Do not use with radiation
- Increased toxicity: vincristine, prednisone
- Synergism: in combination with cytarabine, 6-azauridine

NURSING CONSIDERATIONS

Assess:

- For signs and symptoms of pancreatitis (nausea, vomiting, severe abdominal pain), anaphylaxis (bronchospasm, dyspnea), cyanosis
- CBC, differential, platelet count weekly; withhold drug if WBC is <4000 or platelet count is <75,000; notify physician of these results
- Pulmonary function tests, chest x-ray studies before, during therapy; chest x-ray film should be obtained q2 wk during treatment
- Renal function studies: BUN, serum uric acid, ammonia urine CrCl, electrolytes before, during therapy
- I&O ratio; report fall in urine output of 30/ml/hr
- Monitor temperature q4h; may indicate beginning infection
- Liver function tests before, during therapy (bilirubin, AST, ALT, LDH) as needed or monthly
- RBC, Hct, Hgb since these may be decreased
- Serum, urine glucose levels

Administer:

- Allopurinol or sodium bicarbonate to reduce uric acid levels, alkalinization of urine
- IV infusion using 21-, 23-, 25-gauge needle; administer by slow IV infusion after diluting 10,000 IU/5 ml of sterile H_20 or 0.9% NaCl (no preservatives); use of filter may be necessary if fibers are present
- After intradermal skin testing and desensitization, give 0.1 ml (2 IU) intradermally after reconstituting with 5 ml sterile H_20 or 0.9% NaCl for injection; then add 0.1 ml of reconstituted drug to 9.9 ml diluent (20 IU/ml); observe for 1 hr, check for wheal
- Transfusion for anemia
- Antispasmodic

Perform/provide:

- Deep-breathing exercises with patient 3-4 × day; place in semi-Fowler's position
- Increase fluid intake to 2-3 L/day to prevent urate deposits, calculi formation
- Diet low in purines: absence of organ meats (kidney, liver), dried beans, peas to maintain alkaline urine
- Rinsing of mouth 3-4 × day with water, club soda
- Brushing of teeth 2-3 × day with soft brush or cotton-tipped applicators for stomatitis; use unwaxed dental floss
- Warm compresses at injection site for inflammation
- Nutritious diet with iron, vitamin supplements
- HOB raised to facilitate breathing

Evaluate:

- Therapeutic response: decreased exacerbations in A.L.L.

• Bleeding: hematuria, guaiac, bruising or petechiae, mucosa or orifices q8h
• Dyspnea, rales, nonproductive cough, chest pain, tachypnea fatigue, increased pulse, pallor, lethargy, or swelling around eyes or lips, anaphylaxis may occur
• Food preferences; list likes, dislikes
• Yellowing of skin and sclera, dark urine, clay-colored stools, itchy skin, abdominal pain, fever, diarrhea
• Local irritation, pain, burning, discoloration at injection site
• Symptoms indicating severe allergic reaction: rash, pruritus, urticaria, purpuric skin lesions, itching, flushing, dyspnea
• Frequency of stools, characteristics: cramping, acidosis; signs of dehydration: rapid respirations, poor skin turgor, decreased urine output, dry skin, restlessness, weakness

Teach patient/family:
• To report any complaints or side effects to nurse or physician
• To report any changes in breathing or coughing

Lab test interferences:
Decrease: Thyroid function tests

Treatment of anaphylaxis:
Administer epinephrine, diphenhydramine, IV corticosteroids

---

aspirin

(as'pir-in)

Ancasal,* ASA, Aspirin,* Ecotrin, Empirin, Entrophen,* Novasen,* Sal-Adult,* Sal-Infant,* Supasa*

Func. class.: Nonnarcotic analgesic
Chem. class.: Salicylate

Action: Acts by blocking pain impulses in CNS that occur in response to inhibition of prostaglandin synthesis; antipyretic action results from inhibition of hypothalamic heat-regulating center

Uses: Mild to moderate pain or fever including arthritis, thromboembolic disorders, transient ischemic attacks in men, rheumatic fever, postmyocardial infarction

Dosage and routes:

Arthritis
• *Adult:* PO 2.6-5.2 g/day in divided doses q4-6h
• *Child:* PO 90-130 mg/kg/day in divided doses q4-6h

Pain/fever
• *Adult:* PO/REC 325-650 mg q4h prn, not to exceed 4 g/day
• *Child:* PO/REC 40-100 mg/kg/day in divided doses q4-6h prn

Thromboembolic disorders
• *Adult:* PO 325-650 mg/day or bid

Transient ischemic attacks in men
• *Adult:* PO 650 mg bid or 325 mg qid

Available forms include: Tabs 65, 81, 325, 500, 650, 975 mg; chewable tabs 81 mg; caps 325, 500 mg; tabs controlled-release 800 mg; tabs time-release 650 mg; supp 60, 120, 125, 130, 195, 200, 300, 325, 600, 650 mg, 1.2 g; cream; gum 227.5 mg

Side effects/adverse reactions:
HEMA: ***Thrombocytopenia, agranulocytosis, leukopenia, neutropenia, hemolytic anemia,*** increased pro-time, PT, bleeding time
CNS: Stimulation, drowsiness, dizziness, confusion, ***convulsion,*** headache, flushing, hallucinations, ***coma***
GI: Nausea, vomiting, ***GI bleeding,*** diarrhea, heartburn, anorexia, ***hepatitis***
INTEG: Rash, urticaria, bruising

EENT: Tinnitus, hearing loss
CV: Rapid pulse, pulmonary edema
RESP: Wheezing, hyperpnea
ENDO: Hypoglycemia, hyponatremia, hypokalemia

Contraindications: Hypersensitivity to salicylates, GI bleeding, bleeding disorders, children < 3 yr, children with flulike symptoms, pregnancy (C), lactation, vitamin K deficiency, peptic ulcer

Precautions: Anemia, hepatic disease, renal disease, Hodgkin's disease, pre/postoperatively

Pharmacokinetics:
PO: Onset 15-30 min, peak 1-2 hr, duration 4-6 hr
REC: Onset slow, duration 4-6 hr; metabolized by liver, excreted by kidneys, crosses placenta, excreted in breast milk, half-life 1-3½ hr

Interactions/incompatibilities:
- Decreased effects of aspirin: antacids, steroids, urinary alkalizers
- Increased blood loss: alcohol, heparin
- Increased effects of: anticoagulants, insulin, methotrexate
- Decreased effects of: probenecid, spironolactone, sulfinpyrazone, sulfonylamides
- Toxic effects: PABA, furosemide, carbonic anhydrase inhibitors
- Decreased blood sugar levels: salicylates
- Gastric ulcer: steroids, antiinflammatories

NURSING CONSIDERATIONS

Assess:
- Liver function studies: AST, ALT, bilirubin, creatinine if patient is on long-term therapy
- Renal function studies: BUN, urine creatinine if patient is on long-term therapy
- Blood studies: CBC, Hct, Hgb, pro-time if patient is on long-term therapy
- I&O ratio; decreasing output may indicate renal failure (long-term therapy)

Administer:
- To patient crushed or whole; chewable tablets may be chewed
- With food or milk to decrease gastric symptoms; give 30 min before or 2 hr after meals

Evaluate:
- Therapeutic response: decreased pain, inflammation, fever
- Hepatotoxicity: dark urine, clay-colored stools, yellowing of skin, sclera, itching, abdominal pain, fever, diarrhea if patient is on long-term therapy
- Allergic reactions: rash, urticaria; if these occur, drug may need to be discontinued
- Renal dysfunction: decreased urine output
- Ototoxicity: tinnitus, ringing, roaring in ears; audiometric testing needed before, after long-term therapy
- Visual changes: blurring, halos, corneal, retinal damage
- Edema in feet, ankles, legs
- Prior drug history; there are many drug interactions

Teach patient/family:
- To report any symptoms of hepatotoxicity, renal toxicity, visual changes, ototoxicity, allergic reactions, bleeding (long-term therapy)
- Not to exceed recommended dosage; acute poisoning may result
- To read label on other OTC drugs; many contain aspirin
- That the therapeutic response takes 2 wk (arthritis)
- To avoid alcohol ingestion; GI bleeding may occur

Lab test interferences:
Increase: Coagulation studies, liver function studies, serum uric acid, amylase, CO_2, urinary protein
Decrease: Serum potassium, PBI, cholesterol
Interfere: Urine catecholamines, pregnancy test
Treatment of overdose: Lavage, activated charcoal, monitor electrolytes, VS

---

astemizole

(a-stem´mi-zole)
Hismanal

Func. class.: Antihistamine
Chem. class.: H_1-histamine antagonist

Action: Acts on blood vessels, GI, respiratory system by competing with histamine for H_1-receptor site; decreases allergic response by blocking pharmacologic effects of histamine
Uses: Rhinitis, allergy symptoms
Dosage and routes:
• *Adult and child > 12 yr:* PO 10 mg qd, to reduce time to steady state may take 30 mg day 1, 20 mg day 2, followed by 10 mg daily
Available forms include: Tabs 10 mg
Side effects/adverse reactions:
GU: Frequency, dysuria, urinary retention, impotence
HEMA: ***Hemolytic anemia, thrombocytopenia, leukopenia, agranulocytosis, pancytopenia***
RESP: Thickening of bronchial secretions, dry nose, throat
GI: Nausea, diarrhea, abdominal pain, vomiting, constipation
CNS: Headache, stimulation, drowsiness, sedation, fatigue, confusion, blurred vision, tinnitus, restlessness, tremors, paradoxical excitation in children or elderly
INTEG: Rash, eczema, photosensitivity, urticaria
CV: Hypotension, palpitations, bradycardia, tachycardia
Contraindications: Hypersensitivity, newborn or premature infants, lactation
Precautions: Pregnancy (C), elderly, children, respiratory disease, narrow-angle glaucoma, prostatic hypertrophy, bladder neck obstruction, asthma, elderly
Pharmacokinetics:
PO: Peak 1-2 hr, 97% bound to plasma proteins; half-life is biphasic 3½ hr, 16-23 hr
Interactions/incompatibilities:
• Increased CNS depression: alcohol, other CNS depressants, procarbazine
• Increased anticholinergic effects: MAOIs
• Decreased action of: oral anticoagulants

NURSING CONSIDERATIONS

Assess:
• I&O ratio: be alert for urinary retention, frequency, dysuria, especially elderly; drug should be discontinued if these occur
• CBC during long-term therapy
Administer:
• On empty stomach, 1 hr before or 2 hr after meals
Perform/provide:
• Hard candy, gum, frequent rinsing of mouth for dryness
• Storage in tight, light-resistant container
Evaluate:
• Therapeutic reponse: absence of running or congested nose or rashes
• Respiratory status: rate, rhythm, increase in bronchial secretions, wheezing, chest tightness
Teach patient/family:
• All aspects of drug use; to notify

physician if confusion, sedation, hypotension occurs
• To avoid driving or other hazardous activity if drowsiness occurs
• To avoid alcohol or other CNS depressants

Lab test interferences:
False negative: Skin allergy tests

Treatment of overdose: Administer ipecac syrup or lavage, diazepam, vasopressors, barbiturates (short-acting)

---

atenolol

(a-ten'oh-lole)
Apo-Atenol* Tenormin

Func. class.: Antihypertensive
Chem. class.: β-Blocker, β-1, 2 blocker (high doses)

Action: Competitively blocks stimulation of β-adrenergic receptor within vascular smooth muscle; produces negative chronotropic activity, positive inotropic activity (decreases rate of SA node discharge, increases recovery time), slows conduction of AV node, decreases heart rate, decreases O_2 consumption in myocardium; also, decreases renin-aldosterone-angiotensin system at high doses, inhibits β-2 receptors in bronchial system

Uses: Mild to moderate hypertension, prophylaxis of angina pectoris

Dosage and routes:
• *Adult:* PO 50 mg qd, increasing q1-2 wk to 100 mg qd; may increase to 200 mg qd for angina

Available forms include: Tabs 50, 100 mg

Side effects/adverse reactions:
CV: ***Profound hypotension, bradycardia, CHF,*** *cold extremities, postural hypotension, 2nd or 3rd degree heart block*
CNS: Insomnia, fatigue, dizziness, mental changes, memory loss, hallucinations, depression, lethargy, drowsiness, strange dreams, catatonia
GI: Nausea, diarrhea, vomiting, ***mesenteric arterial thrombosis, ischemic colitis***
INTEG: Rash, fever, alopecia
HEMA: ***Agranulocytosis, thrombocytopenia, purpura***
EENT: Sore throat, dry burning eyes
GU: Impotence
ENDO: Increased hypoglycemic response to insulin
RESP: ***Bronchospasm,*** dyspnea, wheezing

Contraindications: Hypersensitivity to β-blockers, cardiogenic shock, 2nd or 3rd degree heart block, sinus bradycardia, CHF, cardiac failure

Precautions: Major surgery, pregnancy (C), lactation, diabetes mellitus, renal disease, thyroid disease, COPD, asthma, well compensated heart failure

Pharmacokinetics:
PO: Peak 2-4 hr; half-life 6-7 hr, excreted unchanged in urine, protein binding 5%-15%

Interactions/incompatibilities:
• Increased hypotension, bradycardia: reserpine, hydralazine, methyldopa, prazosin, anticholinergics, digoxin
• Decreased antihypertensive effects: indomethacin
• Increased hypoglycemic effect: insulin
• Mutual inhibition: sympathomimetics (cough, cold preparations)
• Decreased bronchodilation: theophyllines
• Paradoxical hypertension: clonidine

NURSING CONSIDERATIONS

Assess:
• I&O, weight daily

---

*Available in Canada only

- B/P, pulse q4h; note rate, rhythm, quality
- Apical/radial pulse before administration; notify physician of any significant changes
- Baselines in renal, liver function tests before therapy begins

Administer:

- PO ac, hs, tablet may be crushed or swallowed whole
- Reduced dosage in renal dysfunction

Perform/provide:

- Storage protected from light, moisture; placed in cool environment

Evaluate:

- Therapeutic response: decreased B/P after 1-2 wk
- Edema in feet, legs daily
- Skin turgor, dryness of mucous membranes for hydration status

Teach patient/family:

- Not to discontinue drug abruptly, taper over 2 wk
- Not to use OTC products unless directed by physician
- To report bradycardia, dizziness, confusion, depression, fever
- To take pulse at home, advise when to notify physician
- To avoid alcohol, smoking, sodium intake
- To comply with weight control, dietary adjustments, modified exercise program
- To carry Medic Alert ID to identify drug that you are taking, allergies
- To avoid hazardous activities if dizziness is present

Lab test interferences:

Interference: Glucose/insulin tolerance tests

Treatment of overdose: Lavage, IV atropine for bradycardia, IV theophylline for bronchospasm, digitalis, O_2, diuretic for cardiac failure, hemodialysis

atracurium besylate

(a-tra-cyoor'ee-um)

Tracrium

Func. class.: Neuromuscular blocker (nondepolarizing)

Chem. class.: Biquaternary ammonium ester

Action: Inhibits transmission of nerve impulses by binding with cholinergic receptor sites, antagonizing action of acetylcholine

Uses: Facilitation of endotracheal intubation, skeletal muscle relaxation during mechanical ventilation, surgery, or general anesthesia

Dosage and routes:

- *Adult:* IV BOL 0.4-0.5 mg/kg, then 0.08-0.10 mg/kg 20-45 min after 1st dose if needed for prolonged procedures

Available forms include: Inj IV 10 mg/ml

Side effects/adverse reactions:

CV: Bradycardia, tachycardia, increase, decrease B/P

RESP: ***Prolonged apnea, bronchospasm, cyanosis, respiratory depression***

EENT: Increased secretions

INTEG: Rash, flushing, pruritus, urticaria

Contraindications: Hypersensitivity

Precautions: Pregnancy (C), cardiac disease, lactation, children <2 yr, electrolyte imbalances, dehydration, neuromuscular disease, respiratory disease

Pharmacokinetics:

IV: Onset 2 min, duration 20-60 min; half-life 2 min, 29 min (terminal), excreted in urine, feces (metabolites), crosses placenta

Interactions/incompatibilities:
• Increased neuromuscular blockade: aminoglycosides, clindamycin, lincomycin, quinidine, local anesthetics, polymyxin antibiotics, lithium, narcotic analgesics, thiazides, enflurane, isoflurane
• Dysrhythmias: theophylline
• Do not mix with barbiturates in solution or syringe

NURSING CONSIDERATIONS

Assess:
• For electrolyte imbalances (K, Mg), may lead to increased action of this drug
• Vital signs (B/P, pulse, respirations, airway) until fully recovered; rate, depth, pattern of respirations, strength of hand grip
• I&O ratio; check for urinary retention, frequency, hesitancy

Administer:
• Using nerve stimulator by anesthesiologist to determine neuromuscular blockade
• Anticholinesterase to reverse neuromuscular blockade
• By slow IV over 1-2 min (only by qualified person, usually an anesthesiologist), do not administer IM
• Only slightly discolored solution

Perform/provide:
• Storage in light-resistant area
• Reassurance if communication is difficult during recovery from neuromuscular blockade

Evaluate:
• Therapeutic response: paralysis of jaw, eyelid, head, neck, rest of body
• Recovery: decreased paralysis of face, diaphragm, leg, arm, rest of body
• Allergic reactions: rash, fever, respiratory distress, pruritus; drug should be discontinued

Treatment of overdose: Edrophonium or neostigmine, atropine, monitor VS; may require mechanical ventilation

atropine sulfate

(a'troe-peen)

Func. class.: Anticholinergic-parasympatholytic
Chem. class.: Belladonna alkaloid

Action: Blocks acetylcholine at parasympathetic neuroeffector sites; increases cardiac output, heart rate by blocking vagal stimulation in heart; dries secretions by blocking vagus

Uses: Bradycardia, bradydysrhythmia, anticholinesterase insecticide poisoning, blocking cardiac vagal reflexes, decreasing secretions before surgery, antispasmodic with GU, biliary surgery, bronchodilator

Dosage and routes:

Bradycardia/bradydysrhythmias
• *Adult:* IV BOL 0.5-1 mg given q1-2 hr, not to exceed 2 mg
• *Child:* IV BOL 0.01-0.03 mg/kg up to 0.4 mg or 0.3 mg/m^2, may repeat q4-6h

Insecticide poisoning
• *Adult and child:* IM/IV 2 mg qh until muscarinic symptoms disappear, may need 6 mg qh

Presurgery
• *Adult:* SC/IM/IV 0.4-0.5 mg before anesthesia
• *Child:* SC 0.1-0.3 mg 30 min before surgery

Available forms include: Inj 0.05, 0.1, 0.3, 0.4, 0.5, 0.8, 1 mg/ml, tabs 0.4 mg; tabs sol 0.4, 0.6 mg

Side effects/adverse reactions:
GU: Retention, hesitancy, impotence, dysuria
CNS: Headache, dizziness, involuntary movement, confusion, psy-

* Available in Canada only

chosis, anxiety, ***coma***, flushing, drowsiness, insomnia
GI: Dry mouth, nausea, vomiting, abdominal pain, anorexia, constipation, ***paralytic ileus,*** abdominal distention
CV: Hypotension, paradoxical bradycardia, angina, PVCs, hypertension, tachycardia, ectopic ventricular beats
INTEG: Rash, urticaria, contact dermatitis, dry skin, flushing
EENT: Blurred vision, photophobia, glaucoma, eye pain, pupil dilation, nasal congestion
MISC: Suppression of lactation, decreased sweating
Contraindications: Hypersensitivity to belladonna alkaloids, angle-closure glaucoma, GI obstructions, myasthenia gravis, thyrotoxicosis, ulcerative colitis, prostatic hypertrophy, tachycardia/tachydysrhythmias, asthma
Precautions: Pregnancy (C), renal disease, lactation, CHF, tachydysrhythmias, hyperthyroidism, COPD, hepatic disease, child <6 yr, hypertension
Pharmacokinetics:
IV: Peak 2-4 min
IM: Peak 30 min
Half-life 2-3 hr, excreted by kidneys (70%-90% in 24 hr); metabolized in liver, crosses placenta, excreted in breast milk
Interactions/incompatibilities:
• Decreased effects of: phenothiazines
• Increased anticholinergic effects of: anticholinergics, antidepressants, amantadine, MAOIs
• Incompatible with all drugs in solution or syringe (except analgesics)

NURSING CONSIDERATIONS
Assess:
• I&O ratio; check for urinary retention, daily output
• ECG for hypertension, ectopic ventricular beats, PVC, tachycardia
• For bowel sounds, check for constipation
Administer:
• IV undiluted or diluted with 10 ml sterile H_2O, give at a rate of 0.6 mg/min
• Increased bulk, water in diet if constipation occurs
Perform/provide:
• Sugarless hard candy, gum, frequent rinsing of mouth for dryness
Evaluate:
• Therapeutic response: decreased dysrhythmias, secretions, GI, GU spasms
• Respiratory status: rate, rhythm, cyanosis, wheezing, dyspnea, engorged neck veins
• Increased intraocular pressure: eye pain, nausea, vomiting, blurred vision, increased tearing
• Cardiac rate: rhythm, character, B/P continuously
• Allergic reaction: rash, urticaria
Teach patient/family:
• To report blurred vision, chest pain, allergic reactions
Treatment of overdose: O_2, artificial ventilation, ECG, administer dopamine for circulatory depression, administer diazepam or thiopental for convulsions; assess need for antidysrhythmics

---

atropine sulfate (optic)

(a'troe-peen)
Atropisol, BufOpto Atropine, Isopto Atropine
Func. class.: Mydriatic
Chem. class.: Belladonna alkaloid

Action: Blocks response of iris sphincter muscle, muscle of accommodation of ciliary body to cholinergic stimulation, resulting in dilation, paralysis of accommodation

Uses: Iritis, cycloplegic refraction

Dosage and routes:

• *Adult:* INSTILL SOL 1-2 gtt of a 1% sol qd-tid for iritis or 1 hr before refracting (cycloplegic refraction); INSTILL OINT 2-3 ×/day

• *Child:* INSTILL SOL 1-2 gtts of a 0.5% sol qd-tid for iritis or bid × 1-3 days before exam (cycloplegic refraction); INSTILL OINT qd-bid 2-3 days before exam

Available forms include: Oint 0.5%, 1%; sol 0.5%, 1%, 2%, 3%

Side effects/adverse reactions:

SYST: Tachycardia, confusion, fever, flushing, dry skin, dry mouth, abdominal discomfort (infants: bladder distention, irregular pulse, respiratory depression)

Contraindications: Hypersensitivity, infants <3 mo, open or narrow angle glaucoma, conjunctivitis, Down syndrome

Pharmacokinetics:

INSTILL: Peak 30-40 min (mydriasis), 60-180 min (cycloplegia), duration 6-12 days

NURSING CONSIDERATIONS

Evaluate:

• Therapeutic response: decrease in inflammation (iritis) or cycloplegic refraction

• Eye pain, discontinue use if pain occurs

Teach patient/family:

• To report change in vision, blurring or loss of sight, trouble breathing, sweating, flushing

• Method of instillation: pressure on lacrimal sac for 1 min, do not touch dropper to eye

• That blurred vision will decrease with repeated use of drug

• Not to do hazardous things until able to see

• To omit next instillation if side effects are present

• To wait 5 min to use other drops

• Not to blink more than usual

---

auranofin

(aur-an-oo-fin)

Ridaura

Func. class.: Gold salt

Chem. class.: Active gold compound (2%)

Action: Antiinflammatory action unknown, may decrease phagocytosis, lysosomal activity or decrease prostaglandin synthesis; decreases concentration of rheumatoid factor, immunoglobulins

Uses: Rheumatoid arthritis

Dosage and routes:

• *Adult:* PO 6 mg qd or 3 mg bid, may increase to 9 mg/day after 3 mo

Available forms include: Caps 3 mg

Side effects/adverse reactions:

HEMA: ***Thrombocytopenia, agranulocytosis, aplastic anemia, leukopenia, eosinophilia***

INTEG: Rash, pruritus, dermatitis, ***exfoliative dermatitis***, urticaria, alopecia, photosensitivity

CNS: Dizziness, syncope

GI: Diarrhea, abdominal cramping, stomatitis, nausea, vomiting, enterocolitis, anorexia, flatulence, metallic taste, dyspepsia, jaundice, increased AST, ALT, glossitis, gingivitis, melena, constipation

GU: ***Proteinuria, hematuria,*** increased BUN, creatinine, vaginitis

RESP: ***Interstitial pneumonitis, fibrosis,*** cough, dyspnea

Contraindications: Hypersensitivity to gold, necrotizing enterocoli-

---

* Available in Canada only

tis, bone marrow aplasia, child <6 yr, lactation, pulmonary fibrosis, exfoliative dermatitis, blood dyscrasias, recent radiation therapy
Precautions: Elderly, CHF, diabetes mellitus, allergic conditions, ulcerative colitis, renal disease, liver disease, pregnancy (C)
Pharmacokinetics:
PO: Absorbed by GI tract, peak 2 hr, steady state 8-16 wk, excreted in urine, feces

NURSING CONSIDERATIONS

Assess:
- Respiratory status: dyspnea, wheezing; if respiratory problems occur, drug should be discontinued
- I&O ratio
- Urine: hematuria, proteinuria, increased BUN, creatinine, may require decrease in dosage
- Platelet counts qmo, drug should be discontinued if <100,000/mm^3
- Hepatic test: ALT, AST, alk phosphatase

Administer:
- bid or may give as single dose qAM with food or drink

Evaluate:
- Therapeutic response: ability to move joints with less pain
- Diarrhea stools; if severe, drug should be discontinued
- Allergy: rash, dermatitis, pruritus; drug should be discontinued if any of these occur
- Gold toxicity: decreased Hgb, WBC <4000/mm^3, granulocytes <1500/mm^3, platelets <150,000/mm^3, severe diarrhea, stomatitis, hematuria, rash, itching, proteinuria

Teach patient/family
- That drug must be taken as prescribed to be useful, to obtain lab work monthly
- That diarrhea is common, but if blood appears in stools or urine notify physician at once, that patient should check for bruising, petechiae, bleeding gums
- To report skin conditions, stomatitis, fatigue, jaundice; may indicate blood dyscrasias
- To avoid exposure to sunlight or ultraviolet light; to use sunscreen to prevent burns
- That therapeutic effect may take 3-4 mo
- To use dilute hydrogen peroxide for mild stomatitis, avoid hot spicy foods, food with high acidic content; use soft toothbrush, rinse more frequently, floss daily
- That contraception should be used during treatment

Lab test interferences:
False positive: TB test

---

aurothioglucose/gold sodium thiomalate

(aur-oh-thye-oh-gloo'kose)
Solganal/Myochrysine
Func. class.: Gold salts
Chem. class.: Active gold compound

Action: Antiinflammatory action unknown; may decrease phagocytosis, lysosomal activity, prostaglandin synthesis
Uses: Rheumatoid arthritis, psoriatic arthritis
Dosage and routes:
- *Adult:* IM 10 mg, then 25 mg q wk × 2-3 wk, then 50 mg/wk until total of 1 g is administered, then 25-50 mg q3-4 wk if there is improvement without toxicity (aurothioglucose) total of 800 mg-1 g
- *Adult:* IM 10 mg, then 25 mg after 1 wk, then 50 mg q wk for total of 14-20 doses, then 50 mg q2 wk × 4, then 50 mg q3 wk × 4,

then 50 mg q mo for maintenance (gold sodium thiomalate)

• *Child 6-12 yr:* IM 1 mg/kg/wk × 20 wk, or ¼ of adult dose (aurothioglucose)

• *Child:* IM 1 mg/kg/wk × 20 wk, then q3-4 wk if improvement without toxicity (gold sodium thiomalate) not to exceed 2.5 mg

Available forms include: IM inj 50 mg/ml

Side effects/adverse reactions:

EENT: Iritis, corneal ulcers

HEMA: ***Thrombocytopenia, agranulocytosis, aplastic anemia, leukopenia, eosinophilia***

INTEG: Rash, pruritus, dermatitis, urticaria, alopecia, photosensitivity, ***exfoliative dermatitis, angioedema***

GI: Stomatitis, nausea, vomiting, metallic taste, jaundice, ***hepatitis,*** diarrhea

GU: Proteinuria, hematuria, ***nephrosis, tubular necrosis***

RESP: Interstitial pneumonitis, pharyngitis, ***pulmonary fibrosis***

CNS: Dizziness, syncope, EEG abnormalities, ***encephalitis***

CV: Bradycardia, rapid pulse

SYST: ***Anaphylaxis***

Contraindications: Hypersensitivity to gold, systemic lupus erythematosus, uncontrolled diabetes mellitus, marked hypertension, recent radiation therapy, CHF, lactation, renal disease, liver disease

Precautions: Decrease tolerance in elderly, children, blood dyscrasias, pregnancy (C)

Pharmacokinetics:

IM: Peak 4-6 hr; half-life 3-27 days, excreted in urine, feces

Interactions/incompatibilities:

• Increased blood dyscrasias: antimalarials, cytotoxic agents, immunosuppressants, oxyphenbutazone, phenylbutazone, penicillamine

NURSING CONSIDERATIONS

Assess:

• Respiratory status: dyspnea, wheezing; if respiratory problems occur, drug should be discontinued

• I&O ratio

• For pregnancy before administration; do not give in pregnancy

• Urine: hematuria, proteinuria, increased BUN, creatinine, may require decrease in dosage

• Platelet counts qmo, drug should be discontinued if $<100,000/mm^3$

• Hepatic test: ALT, AST, alk phosphatase

Administer:

• bid or may give as single dose qAM

• Deep IM, never IV

• Slowly, keep recumbent for 10 min after injection, monitor for transient reaction

Evaluate:

• Therapeutic response: ability to move joints with less pain

• Diarrhea stools; if severe, drug should be discontinued

• Allergy: rash, dermatitis, pruritus; drug should be discontinued if any of these occur

• Gold toxicity: decreased Hgb, WBC $<4000/mm^3$, granulocytes $<1500/mm^3$, platelets $<150,000/mm^3$, severe diarrhea, stomatitis, hematuria, rash, itching, proteinuria

Teach patient/family

• That drug must be taken as prescribed to be useful

• To obtain lab work monthly

• That diarrhea is common, but if blood appears in stools or urine, notify physician at once, that patient should check for bruising, petechiae, bleeding gums

• To report skin conditions, sto-

matitis, fatigue, jaundice, which may indicate blood dyscrasias; report fever, chills, which may indicate infection
• That therapeutic effect may take 3-4 months
• To use dilute hydrogen peroxide for mild stomatitis, avoid hot spicy foods or food with high acidic content; use soft toothbrush, rinse more frequently
• That contraception should be used during treatment
• To use sunscreen to prevent burns
Lab test interferences:
False positive: TB test

azatadine maleate

(a-za'ta-deen)
Optimine
Func. class.: Antihistamine
Chem. class.: Piperidine H_1-receptor antagonist

Action: Acts on blood vessels, GI, respiratory system by competing with histamine for H_1-receptor site; decreases allergic response by blocking histamine
Uses: Allergy symptoms, rhinitis, chronic urticaria
Dosage and routes:
• *Adult:* PO 1-2 mg bid, not to exceed 4 mg/day
Available forms include: Tabs 1 mg
Side effects/adverse reactions:
CNS: Dizziness, drowsiness, poor coordination, fatigue, anxiety, euphoria, confusion, paresthesia, neuritis, sweating, chills
CV: Hypotension, palpitations, tachycardia
RESP: Increased thick secretions, wheezing, chest tightness
HEMA: ***Thrombocytopenia, agranulocytosis, hemolytic anemia***
GI: Constipation, dry mouth, nausea, vomiting, anorexia, diarrhea
INTEG: Rash, urticaria, photosensitivity
GU: Retention, dysuria, frequency, impotence
EENT: Blurred vision, dilated pupils, tinnitus, nasal stuffiness, dry nose, throat, mouth
Contraindications: Hypersensitivity to H_1-receptor antagonist, acute asthma attack, lower respiratory tract disease, child <12 yr
Precautions: Increased intraocular pressure, renal disease, cardiac disease, bronchial asthma, seizure disorder, stenosed peptic ulcers, hyperthyroidism, prostatic hypertrophy, bladder neck obstruction, pregnancy (B), elderly
Pharmacokinetics:
PO: Peak 4 hr; metabolized in liver, excreted by kidneys, crosses placenta, crosses blood-brain barrier, minimally bound to plasma proteins, half-life 9-12 hr
Interactions/incompatibilities:
• Increased CNS depression: barbiturates, narcotics, hypnotics, tricyclic antidepressants, alcohol
• Decreased effect of: oral anticoagulants, heparin
• Increased effect of azatadine: MAOIs

NURSING CONSIDERATIONS

Assess:
• I&O ratio; be alert for urinary retention, frequency, dysuria, especially elderly; drug should be discontinued if these occur
• CBC during long-term therapy
Administer:
• With meals if GI symptoms occur; absorption may slightly decrease
Perform/provide:
• Hard candy, gum, frequent rinsing of mouth for dryness

• Storage in tight container at room temperature

Evaluate:

• Therapeutic response: absence of running or congested nose, or rashes

• Blood dyscrasias: thrombocytopenia, agranulocytosis; these occur rarely

• Respiratory status: rate, rhythm, increase in bronchial secretions, wheezing, chest tightness

Teach patient/family:

• All aspects of drug use; to notify physician if confusion, sedation, or hypotension occurs

• To avoid driving or other hazardous activities if drowsiness occurs

• To avoid concurrent use of alcohol or other CNS depressants

Lab test interferences:

False negative: Skin allergy tests

Treatment of overdose: Administer ipecac syrup or lavage, diazepam, vasopressors, barbiturates (short-acting)

---

azathioprine

(ay-za-thye'oh-preen)

Imuran

Func. class.: Immunosuppressant
Chem. class.: Purine analog

Action: Produces immunosuppression by inhibiting purine synthesis in cells

Uses: Renal transplants to prevent graft rejection, refractory rheumatoid arthritis, refractory ITP, glomerulonephritis, nephrotic syndrome, bone marrow transplant

Dosage and routes:

Prevention of rejection

• *Adult and child:* PO 3-5 mg/kg/day, then maintenance of at least 1-2 mg/kg/day

Refractory rheumatoid arthritis

• *Adult:* PO 1/mg/kg/day, may increase dose after 2 mo by 0.5 mg/kg/day, not to exceed 2.5 mg/kg/day

Available forms include: Tabs 50 mg; inj IV 100 mg

Side effects/adverse reactions:

GI: Nausea, vomiting, stomatitis, esophagitis, ***pancreatitis, hepatotoxicity, jaundice***

HEMA: ***Leukopenia, thrombocytopenia, anemia, pancytopenia***

INTEG: Rash

MS: Arthralgia, muscle wasting

Contraindications: Hypersensitivity, pregnancy (D)

Precautions: Severe renal disease, severe hepatic disease

Pharmacokinetics: Metabolized in liver, excreted in urine (active metabolite), crosses placenta

Interactions/incompatibilities:

• Increased action of azathioprine: allopurinol

NURSING CONSIDERATIONS

Assess:

• Blood studies: Hgb, WBC, platelets during treatment monthly; if leukocytes are $<3000/mm^3$ drug should be discontinued

• Liver function studies: alk phosphatase, AST, ALT, bilirubin

Administer:

• For several days before transplant surgery

• All medications PO if possible, avoiding IM injections since bleeding may occur

• With meals to reduce GI upset

Evaluate:

• Therapeutic response: absence of graft rejection, immunosuppression in autoimmune disorders

• Hepatotoxicity: dark urine, jaundice, itching, light-colored stools; drug should be discontinued

Teach patient/family:

• That therapeutic response may

---

* Available in Canada only

take 3-4 mo in rheumatoid arthritis
- To report fever, rash, severe diarrhea, chills, sore throat, fatigue since serious infections may occur
- To use contraceptive measures during treatment, for 12 wk after ending therapy
- To avoid crowds to reduce risk of infection

azithromycin

(ay-zi-thro-mye'sin)
Zithromax

Func. class.: Antibacterial
Chem. class.: Macrolide (azalide) antibiotic

Action: Binds to 50S ribosomal subunits of susceptible bacteria and suppresses protein synthesis; much greater spectrum of activity than erythromycin

Uses: Mild to moderate infections of the upper respiratory tract, lower respiratory tract, uncomplicated skin and skin structure infections caused by *M. catarrhalis, S. pneumoniae, S. pyogenes, S. aureus, S. agalactiae, H. influenzae, Clostridium, L. pneumophila,* nongonococcal urethritis or cervicitis due to *C. trachomatis*

Dosage and routes:
- *Adult:* PO 500 mg on day 1, then 250 mg qd on days 2-5 for a total dose of 1.5 g; may give a one time dose of 1 g of chlamydial infections

Available forms include: Caps 250

Side effects/adverse reactions:
INTEG: Rash, urticaria, pruritus, photosensitivity
CV: Palpitations, chest pain
CNS: Dizziness, headache, vertigo, somnolence
GI: Nausea, vomiting, diarrhea, ***hepatotoxicity,*** abdominal pain, stomatitis, heartburn, dyspepsia, flatulence, melena
GU: Vaginitis, moniliasis, nephritis

Contraindications: Hypersensitivity to azithromycin or erythromycin

Precautions: Pregnancy (C), lactation, hepatic, renal, cardiac disease, elderly, children <16 yrs

Pharmacokinetics: Peak 12 hr, duration 24 hr, half-life 11-57 hr, excreted in bile, feces, urine primarily as unchanged drug

Interactions/incompatibilities:
- Increased effects of: oral anticoagulants, digoxin, theophylline, methylprednisolone, cyclosporine, bromocriptine, disopyramide
- Decreased action of: clindamycin
- Toxicity: carbamazepine
- Decreased absorption of azithromycin: food, aluminium, magnesium antacids

NURSING CONSIDERATIONS

Assess:
- I&O ratio; report hematuria, oliguria in renal disease
- Liver studies: AST, ALT
- Renal studies: urinalysis, protein, blood
- C&S before drug therapy; drug may be taken as soon as culture is taken; C&S may be repeated after treatment

Administer:
- Adequate intake of fluids (2000 ml) during diarrhea episodes

Perform/provide:
- Storage at room temperature

Evaluate:
- Therapeutic response: C&S negative for infection
- Bowel pattern before, during treatment
- Skin eruptions, itching
- Respiratory status: rate, character, wheezing, tightness in chest; discontinue drug if these occur
- Allergies before treatment, reac-

tion of each medication; place allergies on chart, notify all people giving drugs

Teach patient/family:

• To take with a full glass of water; do not take with food, take 1 hr before or 2 hr after meals; do not take with fruit juices

• To report sore throat, fever, fatigue; could indicate superimposed infection

• Not to take aluminum, magnesium-containing antacids simultaneously with this drug

• To notify nurse of diarrhea stools, dark urine, pale stools, yellow discoloration of eyes or skin, severe abdominal pain

• To take at evenly spaced intervals; complete dosage regimen

Lab test interferences:

False increase: 17-OHCS/17-KS, AST, ALT

Decrease: Folate assay

Treatment of overdose: Withdraw drug, maintain airway, administer epinephrine, aminophylline, O_2, IV corticosteroids

---

azlocillin sodium

(az-loe-sill'in)

Azlin

Func. class.: Broad-spectrum antibiotic

Chem. class.: Extended-spectrum penicillin

Action: Interferes with cell wall replication of susceptible organisms; the cell wall, rendered osmotically unstable, swells, bursts from osmotic pressure

Uses: Lower respiratory infections, skin, bone, bacterial septicemia, urinary tract infections, yaws; effective for gram-positive cocci *(S. aureus, S. pyogenes, S. faecalis)*, gram-positive bacilli *(C. perfringens, C. tetani)*, gram-negative bacilli *(Bacteroides, P. aeruginosa, E. coli), H. influenzae, P. mirabilis*

Dosage and routes:

• *Adult:* IV 100-350 mg/kg/day in 4-6 divided doses, max 24 g

Cystic fibrosis

• *Child:* IV 75 mg/kg q4h max 24 g

Available forms include: Powder for inj 2, 3, 4 g

Side effects/adverse reactions:

HEMA: Anemia, increased bleeding time, ***bone marrow depression, granulocytopenia***

GI: Nausea, vomiting, diarrhea, increased AST, ALT, abdominal pain, glossitis, colitis

GU: Oliguria, proteinuria, hematuria, *vaginitis, moniliasis,* ***glomerulonephritis***

CNS: Lethargy, hallucinations, anxiety, depression, twitching, ***coma, convulsions***

META: Hypokalemia, alkalosis, hypernatremia

Contraindications: Hypersensitivity to penicillins

Precautions: Pregnancy (B), hypersensitivity to cephalosporins, neonates

Pharmacokinetics: Half-life 55-70 min, metabolized in liver, excreted in urine, bile, breast milk (small amount), crosses placenta

Interactions/incompatibilities:

• Decreased antimicrobial effectiveness of azlocillin: tetracyclines, erythromycins

• Increased azlocillin concentrations: aspirin, probenecid

NURSING CONSIDERATIONS

Assess:

• I&O ratio; report hematuria, oliguria since penicillin in high doses is nephrotoxic

---

* Available in Canada only

• Any patient with compromised renal system, since drug is excreted slowly in poor renal system function; toxicity may occur rapidly
• Liver studies: AST, ALT
• Blood studies: WBC, RBC, H&H, bleeding time
• Renal studies: urinalysis, protein, blood
• Culture, sensitivity before drug therapy; drug may be taken as soon as culture is taken

Administer:
• IV after reconstituting 1 g/10 ml of compatible solution, shake
• After C&S completed
• Slowly (direct IV) over 5 min to prevent chest discomfort
• After further dilution in 50-100 ml of compatible solution, give over 30 min; change IV site q48h

Perform/provide:
• Adrenaline, suction, tracheostomy set, endotracheal intubation equipment on unit
• Adequate intake of fluids (2000 ml) during diarrhea episodes
• Scratch test to assess allergy after securing order from physician; usually done when penicillin is only drug of choice
• Storage in cool environment; solution is stable for 24 hr at room temperature

Evaluate:
• Therapeutic response: absence of temperature, draining wounds
• Bowel pattern before, during treatment
• Skin eruptions after administration of penicillin to 1 wk after discontinuing drug
• Respiratory status: rate, character, wheezing, tightness in chest
• Allergies before initiation of treatment; reaction of each medication; place allergies on chart, Kardex in bright red

Teach patient/family:
• That culture may be taken after completed course of medication
• To report sore throat, fever, fatigue (could indicate superimposed infection)
• To wear or carry a Medic Alert ID if allergic to penicillins
• To notify nurse of diarrhea

Lab test interferences:
False positive: Urine glucose, urine protein
Decrease: Uric acid

Treatment of overdose: Withdraw drug, maintain airway, administer epinephrine, aminophylline, O_2, IV corticosteroids for anaphylaxis

---

aztreonam

(az-tree'oo nam)
Azactam

Func. class.: Misc antibiotic
Chem. class.: Monobactam

Action: Inhibits organisms by inhibiting bacterial cell wall synthesis, which causes death of organism (bactericidal)

Uses: Urinary tract infection; septicemia; skin, muscle, bone infection; and other infections caused by gram-negative organisms

Dosage and routes:
Urinary tract infections
• *Adult:* IV/IM 500 mg-1 g q8-12h
Systemic infections
Adult: IV/IM 1-2 g q8-12h
Severe systemic infections
Adult: IV/IM 2 g q6-8h, do not exceed 8 g/day
Continue treatment for 48 hr after negative culture or until patient is asymptomatic

Available forms include: Powder for inj 500 mg, 1, 2 g

Side effects/adverse reactions:
HEMA: Anemia, increased bleeding

time, ***bone marrow depression, granulocytopenia***
GI: Nausea, vomiting, diarrhea, increased AST, ALT, abdominal pain, glossitis, colitis
CNS: Lethargy, hallucinations, anxiety, depression, twitching, ***coma, convulsions,*** malaise
EENT: Tinnitus, diplopia, nasal congestion
GU: Vaginal candidiasis, vaginitis, breast tenderness
Contraindications: Hypersensitivity
Precautions: Pregnancy (B), lactation, children, impaired renal, hepatic function
Pharmacokinetics:
IV: Peak immediate, trough 8 hr
IM: Peak 1 hr
Half-life: 1.7 hr, half-life prolonged in renal disease; protein binding 56%; metabolized by liver, excreted in urine, small amounts appear in breast milk, placenta
Interactions/incompatibilities:
• Decreased effect of both drugs: β-lactamase antibiotics (cefoxitin, imipenem)
• Incompatible with nafcillin, metronidazole, cephradine

NURSING CONSIDERATIONS

Assess:
• Signs of bruising, bleeding, anemia
• Bowel pattern before, during treatment
• Respiratory status: rate, character, wheezing, tightness in chest
• I&O ratio; report hematuria, oliguria, since this drug in high doses is nephrotoxic
• Any patient with compromised renal system, since drug is excreted slowly in poor renal system function; toxicity may occur rapidly
• Liver studies: AST, ALT
• Blood studies: WBC, RBC, Hgb & Hct, bleeding time
• Renal studies: urinalysis, protein, blood
Administer:
• Direct IV after diluting with 6-10 ml sterile H_2O/15 ml drug; give over 3-5 min
• IV INF after diluting with 3 ml or more sterile H_2O/1 g drug; then dilute with 50-100 ml of compatible solution; give over ½-1 hr
• IM; dilute each g with at least 3 ml of 0.9% NaCl; give into large muscle
• Drug after C&S completed
Perform/provide:
• Adequate fluid intake (2000/ml) during diarrhea episodes
• Storage in refrigerator
Evaluate:
• Therapeutic response: absence of fever, purulent drainage, redness, inflammation
• Skin eruptions after administration of drug to 1 wk after discontinuing drug
• Allergies before initiation of treatment, reaction of medication; highlight allergies on chart
Teach patient/family:
• That culture may be taken after completed course of medication
• To report sore throat, fever, fatigue; could indicate superimposed infection

---

bacampicillin HCl

(ba-kam-pi-sill'in)
Penglobe,* Spectrobid
Func. class.: Broad-spectrum antibiotic
Chem. class.: Aminopenicillin

Action: Interferes with cell wall replication of susceptible organisms; the cell wall, rendered os-

*Available in Canada only

motically unstable, swells, bursts from osmotic pressure

Uses: Respiratory tract infections, skin urinary tract infections; effective for gram-positive cocci *(S. faecalis, S. pneumoniae)*, gram-negative cocci *(N. gonorrhoeae)*, gram-negative bacilli *(E. coli, H. influenzae, P. mirabilis)*

Dosage and routes:

• *Adult:* PO 400-800 mg q12h

• *Child:* PO 25-50 mg/kg/day in divided doses q12h

Available forms include: Tabs 400 mg; powder for oral susp 125 mg/5 ml

Side effects/adverse reactions:

HEMA: Anemia, increased bleeding time, ***bone marrow depression, granulocytopenia***

GI: Nausea, vomiting, diarrhea, increased AST, ALT, abdominal pain, glossitis, colitis

GU: Oliguria, proteinuria, hematuria, *vaginitis, moniliasis,* ***glomerulonephritis***

CNS: Lethargy, hallucinations, anxiety, depression, twitching, ***coma, convulsions***

Contraindications: Hypersensitivity to penicillins; neonates

Precautions: Pregnancy (B), hypersensitivity to cephalosporins

Pharmacokinetics:

PO: Peak 30-60 min, duration 5-6 hr, half-life ½-1 hr, metabolized in liver, excreted in urine

Interactions/incompatibilities:

• Decreased antimicrobial effectiveness of bacampicillin: tetracyclines, erythromycins

• Increased bacampicillin concentrations: aspirin, probenecid

• Do not give with disulfiram

NURSING CONSIDERATIONS

Assess:

• I&O ratio; report hematuria, oliguria since penicillin in high doses is nephrotoxic

• Any patient with compromised renal system, since drug is excreted slowly in poor renal system function; toxicity may occur rapidly

• Liver studies: AST, ALT

• Blood studies: WBC, RBC, H&H, bleeding time

• Renal studies: urinalysis, protein, blood

• Culture, sensitivity before drug therapy; drug may be taken as soon as culture is taken

Administer:

• After C&S completed

Perform/provide:

• Adrenaline, suction, tracheostomy set, endotracheal intubation equipment on unit

• Adequate intake of fluids (2000 ml) during diarrhea episodes

• Scratch test to assess allergy after securing order from physician; usually done when penicillin is only drug of choice

• Storage in dry tight container, oral suspension refrigerated for 2 wk or at room temperature for 1 wk

Evaluate:

• Therapeutic response: absence of temperature, draining wounds

• Bowel pattern before, during treatment

• Skin eruptions after administration of penicillin to 1 wk after discontinuing drug

• Respiratory status: rate, character, wheezing, tightness in chest

• Allergies before initiation of treatment; reaction of each medication; place allergies on chart, Kardex in bright red

Teach patient/family:

• Aspects of drug therapy: culture may be taken after completed course of medication

• To report sore throat, fever, fa-

tigue (could indicate superimposed infection)
• To wear or carry a Medic Alert ID if allergic to penicillins
• To notify nurse of diarrhea
• That drug should be taken on an empty stomach, with a full glass of water

Lab test interferences:
False positive: Urine glucose, urine protein
Decrease: Uric acid

Treatment of overdose: Withdraw drug, maintain airway, administer epinephrine, aminophylline, O_2, IV corticosteroids for anaphylaxis

bacitracin

(bass-i-tray'sin)
Baci-IM
Func. class.: Antibacterial
Chem. class.: Bacillus subtilis derivative

Action: Inhibits bacterial cell wall synthesis, thereby interfering with osmotic pressure within cell

Uses: Staphylococcal pneumonia, empyema, pseudomembranous colitis

Dosage and routes:
• *Infants >2.5 kg:* IM 1,000 U/kg/day in divided doses q8-12h
• *Infants <2.5 kg:* IM 900 U/kg/day in divided doses q8-12h
• *Adults:* 20,000-25,000 U q6h × 7-10 days

Available forms include: Inj IM 10,000, 50,000 U

Side effects/adverse reactions:
INTEG: Rash, pain at injection site
GI: Nausea, vomiting, diarrhea
GU: ***Proteinuria, casts, azotemia***

Contraindications: Hypersensitivity, severe renal disease

Precautions: Pregnancy (C)

Pharmacokinetics: Peak 1-2 hr, duration >12 hr, metabolized in liver, excreted in urine

Interactions/incompatibilities:
• Increased nephrotoxicity, neurotoxicity: aminoglycosides, polymyxin
• Increased neuromuscular blockage: nondepolarizing skeletal muscle relaxants, anesthetics

NURSING CONSIDERATIONS

Assess:
• I&O ratio; report oliguria, change in urinary output; high doses are nephrotoxic
• Any patient with compromised renal system; drug is excreted slowly in poor renal system function; toxicity may occur rapidly
• Renal studies: urinalysis, protein, blood, BUN, creatinine, urine pH (keep at 6.0)
• C&S before drug therapy; drug may be taken as soon as culture is taken; repeat C&S after treatment

Administer:
• After reconstituting with NS
• IM in deep muscle mass; rotate injection site; do not give IV/SC

Perform/provide:
• Storage in refrigerator; protect from direct sunlight
• Adrenalin, suction, tracheostomy set, endotracheal intubation equipment on unit
• Adequate intake of fluids (2000 ml) during diarrhea episodes

Evaluate:
• Therapeutic response: absence of fever, cough, dyspnea, malaise
• Bowel pattern before, during treatment; if severe diarrhea occurs, drug should be discontinued
• Skin eruptions, itching: rash, urticaria, erythema
• Respiratory status: rate, character, wheezing, tightness in chest, dyspnea on exertion
• Allergies before treatment, reac-

tion of each medication; place allergies on chart, Kardex in bright red; notify all people giving drugs

Teach patient/family:

- To report sore throat, fever, fatigue; could indicate superimposed infection

bacitracin (ophthalmic)

(bass-i-tray'sin)

Func. class.: Antiinfective

Action: Inhibits cell wall synthesis in bacteria

Uses: Infection of eye

Dosage and routes:

- *Adult and child:* Apply to conjunctival sac bid-qid until desired response

Available forms include: Oint 500 U/g

Side effects/adverse reactions:

EENT: Poor corneal wound healing, visual haze (temporary), overgrowth of nonsusceptible organisms

Contraindications: Hypersensitivity

Precautions: Antibiotic hypersensitivity, pregnancy (C)

NURSING CONSIDERATIONS

Administer:

- After washing hands, cleanse crusts or discharge from eye before application

Perform/provide:

- Storage at room temperature

Evaluate:

- Therapeutic response: absence of redness, inflammation, tearing
- Allergy: itching, lacrimation, redness, swelling

Teach patient/family:

- To use drug exactly as prescribed
- Not to use eye makeup, towels, washcloths, eye medication of others; reinfection may occur
- That drug container tip should not be touched to eye
- To report itching, increased redness, burning, stinging, swelling; drug should be discontinued
- That drug may cause blurred vision when ointment is applied

bacitracin (topical)

(bass-i-tray'sin)

Baciguent, Bacitin*

Func. class.: Local antiinfective
Chem. class.: Antibacterial

Action: Interferes with bacterial cell wall function by inhibiting protein synthesis

Uses: Topical staphylococci, streptococci

Dosage and routes:

- *Adult and child:* TOP bid-qid or more often if needed

Available forms include: Oint 500 U/g

Side effects/adverse reactions:

INTEG: Rash, urticaria, stinging, burning, contact dermatitis

Contraindications: Hypersensitivity

Precautions: Pregnancy (C), lactation

NURSING CONSIDERATIONS

Administer:

- After C&S is obtained, if lesion is weeping
- Enough medication to completely cover lesions
- After cleansing with soap, water before each application, dry well (as ordered)

Perform/provide:

- Storage at room temperature in dry place

Evaluate:

- Therapeutic response: decrease in size, number of lesions

• Allergic reaction: burning, stinging, swelling, redness
• For systemic effects and superimposed infections

Teach patient/family:

• To use medical asepsis (hand washing) before, after each application to prevent further infection
• To apply with glove to prevent further infection
• To avoid use of OTC creams, ointments, lotions unless directed by physician
• To watch for superimposed infections with long-term use or allergic reaction

---

baclofen

(bak'loe-fen)

Lioresal, Lioresal DS

Func. class.: Skeletal muscle relaxant, central acting
Chem. class.: GABA chlorophenyl derivative

Action: Inhibits synaptic responses in CNS by decreasing GABA, which decreases neurotransmitter function; decreases frequency, severity of muscle spasms

Uses: Spinal cord injury, spasticity in multiple sclerosis

Dosage and routes:

• *Adult:* PO 5 mg tid × 3 days, then 10 mg tid × 3 days, then 15 mg tid × 3 days, then 20 mg tid × 3 days, then titrated to response, not to exceed 80 mg/day

Available forms include: Tabs 10, 20 mg

Side effects/adverse reactions:

CNS: Dizziness, weakness, fatigue, drowsiness, headache, disorientation, insomnia, paresthesias, tremors
EENT: Nasal congestion, blurred vision, mydriasis, tinnitus
CV: Hypotension, chest pain, palpitations, edema
GI: Nausea, constipation, vomiting, increased AST, alk phosphatase, abdominal pain, dry mouth, anorexia
GU: Urinary frequency
INTEG: Rash, pruritus

Contraindications: Hypersensitivity

Precautions: Peptic ulcer disease, renal disease, hepatic disease, stroke, seizure disorder, diabetes mellitus, pregnancy (C), elderly

Pharmacokinetics:

PO: Peak 2-3 hr, duration >8 hr, half-life 2½-4 hr, partially metabolized in liver, excreted in urine (unchanged)

Interactions/incompatibilities:

• Increased CNS depression: alcohol, tricyclic antidepressants, narcotics, barbiturates, sedatives, hypnotics

NURSING CONSIDERATIONS

Assess:

• B/P, weight, blood sugar, and hepatic function periodically
• For increased seizure activity in epilepsy patient; this drug decreases seizure threshold
• I&O ratio; check for urinary retention, frequency, hesitancy
• ECG in epileptic patients; poor seizure control has occurred in patients taking this drug

Administer:

• With meals for GI symptoms
• Gum, frequent sips of water for dry mouth

Perform/provide:

• Storage in tight container at room temperature
• Assistance with ambulation if dizziness or drowsiness occurs

Evaluate:

• Therapeutic response: decreased pain, spasticity

---

* Available in Canada only

• Allergic reactions: rash, fever, respiratory distress
• Severe weakness, numbness in extremities
• Psychologic dependency: increased need for medication, more frequent requests for medication, increased pain
• CNS depression: dizziness, drowsiness, psychiatric symptoms
• Dosage, as individual titration is required

Teach patient/family:
• Not to discontinue medication quickly; hallucinations, spasticity, tachycardia will occur; drug should be tapered off over 1-2 wk
• Not to take with alcohol, other CNS depressants
• To avoid altering activities while taking this drug
• To avoid hazardous activities if drowsiness or dizziness occurs
• To avoid using OTC medication: cough preparations, antihistamines, unless directed by physician
• To increase fluid intake >2L/day

Lab test interferences:
Increase: AST, alk phosphatase, blood glucose

Treatment of overdose: Induce emesis of conscious patient, lavage, dialysis

beclomethasone dipropionate

(be-kloe-meth'a-sone)

Beclovent, Vancenase, Vanceril Beconase

Func. class.: Corticosteroid, synthetic

Chem. class.: Glucocorticoid

Action: Prevents inflammation by depression of migration of polymorphonuclear leukocytes, fibroblasts, reversal of increased capillary permeability and lysosomal stabilization; does not suppress hypothalamus and pituitary function

B

Uses: Chronic asthma, rhinitis

Dosage and routes:
• *Adult:* INH 2-4 puffs tid-qid, not to exceed 20 inhalations/day
• *Child:* 6-12 yr: INH 1-2 puffs tid-qid, not to exceed 10 inhalations/day

Available forms include: Aerosol 42 μg/actuation

Side effects/adverse reactions:
RESP: ***Bronchospasm***
GI: Dry mouth
EENT: Hoarseness, candidal infections of oral cavity, sore throat

Contraindications: Hypersensitivity, status asthmaticus (primary treatment), nonasthmatic bronchial disease, bacterial, fungal, or viral infections of mouth, throat, or lungs, children < 3 yr

Precautions: Nasal disease/surgery, pregnancy (C)

Pharmacokinetics:
INH: Onset 10 min, excreted in feces (metabolites), half-life 3-15 hr, crosses placenta, metabolized in lungs, liver, GI system

NURSING CONSIDERATIONS

Assess:
• Adrenal function periodically for HPA axis suppression

Administer:
• INH with water to decrease possibility of fungal infections
• Titrated dose, use lowest effective dose

Perform/provide:
• Gum, rinsing of mouth for dry mouth

Evaluate:
• Therapeutic response: decreased dyspnea, wheezing, dry rales on auscultation

Teach patient/family:
• That ID as steroid user should be carried

• To notify physician if therapeutic response decreases; dosage adjustment may be needed
• Proper administration technique
• To wash inhaler with warm water and dry after each use
• All aspects of drug usage including cushingoid symptoms
• Symptoms of adrenal insufficiency: nausea, anorexia, fatigue, dizziness, dyspnea, weakness, joint pain, depression
• To keep drug out of children's reach

---

beclomethasone dipropionate (nasal)

(be-kloe-meth'a-sone)

Beconase Nasal Inhaler, Beclovent, Vanceril, Vancenase Nasal Inhaler

Func. class.: Synthetic corticosteroid

Chem. class.: Beclomethasone diester

Action: Antiinflammatory, vasoconstrictive properties in nasal passages

Uses: Seasonal or perennial rhinitis

Dosage and routes:

• *Adult and child >12 yr:* INSTILL 1-2 sprays in each nostril bid-qid

Available forms include: Aero 42 μg/spray

Side effects/adverse reactions:

EENT: Dryness, nasal irritation, burning, sneezing, secretions with blood, nasal ulcerations, ***perforation of nasal septum,*** *Candida* infection, earache, hoarseness

ENDO: ***Adrenal suppression***

INTEG: Rash, urticaria, pruritus

CNS: Headache, paresthesia

RESP: ***Acute status asthmaticus***

Contraindications: Hypersensitivity, systemic corticosteroid therapy

Precautions: Pregnancy (C), lactation, children <12, nasal ulcers, recurrent epistaxis respiration

Pharmacokinetics:

INSTILL: Readily absorbed; peak concentration, other data have not been determined

NURSING CONSIDERATIONS

Assess:

• Adrenal function periodically for HPA axis suppression

Administer:

• After cleaning aerosol top daily with warm water, dry thoroughly

Perform/provide:

• Storage in cool environment, do not puncture or incinerate container

Evaluate:

• Therapeutic response: decrease in runny nose
• Adrenal suppression: 17-KS, plasma cortisol for decreased levels
• Nasal passages during long-term treatment for changes in mucus

Teach patient/family:

• To clear nasal passages if sneezing attack occurs, repeat dose
• To continue using product even if mild nasal bleeding occurs, is usually transient
• Method of installation after providing written instructions from manufacturer
• To clear nasal passages before administration, use decongestant if needed; shake inhaler, invert, tilt head backward, insert nozzle into nostril, away from septum; hold other nostril closed and depress activator, inhale through nose, exhale through mouth

---

belladonna alkaloids

(bell-a-don'a)
Bellafoline

Func. class.: Gastrointestinal anticholinergic
Chem. class.: Belladonna alkaloid

Action: Inhibits muscarinic actions of acetylcholine at postganglionic parasympathetic neuron effector sites

Uses: Treatment of peptic ulcer disease, irritable bowel syndrome in combination with other drugs; for other GI disorders

Dosage and routes:
- *Adult:* PO 0.25-0.5 mg tid; SC 0.125-0.5 mg qd or bid
- *Child >6 yr:* PO 0.125-0.25 mg tid

Available forms include: Tabs 0.25 mg; inj SC 0.5 mg/ml

Side effects/adverse reactions:
CNS: Confusion, stimulation in elderly, headache, insomnia, dizziness, drowsiness, anxiety, weakness, hallucination
GI: Dry mouth, constipation, ***paralytic ileus,*** heartburn, nausea, vomiting, dysphagia, absence of taste
GU: Hesitancy, retention, impotence
CV: Palpitations, tachycardia
EENT: Blurred vision, photophobia, mydriasis, cycloplegia, increased ocular tension
INTEG: Urticaria, rash, pruritus, anhidrosis, fever, allergic reactions, flushing

Contraindications: Hypersensitivity to anticholinergics, narrow-angle glaucoma, GI obstruction, myasthenia gravis, paralytic ileus, GI atony, toxic megacolon

Precautions: Hyperthyroidism, coronary artery disease, dysrhythmias, CHF, ulcerative colitis, hypertension, hiatal hernia, hepatic disease, renal disease, pregnancy (C), urinary obstruction

Pharmacokinetics:
PO: Duration 4-6 hr; metabolized by liver, excreted in urine, half-life 13-38 hr

Interactions/incompatibilities:
- Increased anticholinergic effect: amantadine, tricyclic antidepressants, MAOIs
- Increased effect of: nitrofurantoin
- Decreased effect of: phenothiazines, levodopa

NURSING CONSIDERATIONS

Assess:
- VS, cardiac status: checking for dysrhythmias, increased rate, palpitations, flushing
- I&O ratio; check for urinary retention or hesitancy

Administer:
- ½-1 hr ac for better absorption
- Decreased dose to elderly patients; their metabolism may be slowed
- Gum, hard candy, frequent rinsing of mouth for dryness of oral cavity

Perform/provide:
- Storage in tight container protected from light
- Increased fluids, bulk, exercise to patient's lifestyle to decrease constipation

Evaluate:
- Therapeutic response: absence of epigastric pain, bleeding, nausea, vomiting
- GI complaints: pain, bleeding (frank or occult), nausea, vomiting, anorexia, constipation

Teach patient/family:
- To avoid driving or other hazardous activities until stabilized on medication

• To avoid alcohol or other CNS depressants; will enhance sedating properties of this drug
• To avoid hot environments, stroke may occur, drug suppresses perspiration
• To use sunglasses when outside to prevent photophobia

benazepril

(ben-a-ze'prel)
Lotensin

Func. class.: Antihypertensive
Chem. class.: Angiotensin-converting enzyme (ACE) inhibitor

Action: Selectively suppresses renin-angiotensin-aldosterone system; inhibits ACE, prevents conversion of angiotensin I to angiotensin II; results in dilation of arterial, venous vessels
Uses: Hypertension, alone or in combination with thiazide diuretics
Dosage and routes:
• *Adult:* PO 10 mg qd initially, then 20-40 mg/day divided bid or qd
Renal impairment: 5 mg qd with Ccr <30 ml/min/1.73 m^2, increase as needed to maximum of 40 mg/day
Available forms include: tabs 5, 10, 20, 40 mg
Side effects/adverse reactions:
CV: Hypotension, postural hypotension, syncope, palpitations, angina
GU: Increased BUN, creatinine, decreased libido, impotence, urinary tract infection
HEMA: ***Neutropenia, agranulocytosis***
INTEG: ***Angioedema,*** rash, flushing, sweating
RESP: Cough, asthma, bronchitis, dyspnea, sinusitis
META: Hyperkalemia, hyponatremia
GI: Nausea, constipation, vomiting, gastritis, melena
CNS: Anxiety, hypertonia, insomnia, paresthesia, headache, dizziness, fatigue
MS: Arthralgia, arthritis, myalgia
Contraindications: Hypersensitivity to ACE inhibitors, pregnancy (D), lactation, children
Precautions: Impaired renal, liver function, dialysis patients, hypovolemia, blood dyscrasias, CHF, COPD, asthma, elderly
Pharmacokinetics:
PO: Peak ½-1 hr, serum protein binding 97%, half-life 10-11 hr, metabolized by liver (metabolites), excreted in urine
Interactions/incompatibilities:
• Increased hypotension: diuretics, other antihypertensives, ganglionic blockers, adrenergic blockers
• Increased toxicity: vasodilators, hydralazine, prazosin, potassium-sparing diuretics, sympathomimetics
• Decreased absorption: antacids
• Decreased antihypertensive effect: indomethacin
• Increased serum levels of: digoxin, lithium
• Increased hypersensitivity: allopurinol

NURSING CONSIDERATIONS

Assess:
• Blood studies: neutrophils, decreased platelets
• B/P, orthostatic hypotension, syncope
• Renal studies: protein, BUN, creatinine; watch for increased levels that may indicate nephrotic syndrome
• Baselines in renal, liver function tests before therapy begins

• Potassium levels, although hyperkalemia rarely occurs
• Dipstick of urine for protein qd in first morning specimen; if protein is increased, a 24 hr urinary protein should be collected

Administer:
• IV infusion of 0.9% NaCl (as ordered) to expand fluid volume if severe hypotension occurs

Perform/provide:
• Storage in tight container at 30° C or less
• Supine or Trendelenburg position for severe hypotension

Evaluate:
• Therapeutic response: decrease in B/P
• Edema in feet, legs daily
• Allergic reactions: rash, fever, pruritus, urticaria; drugs should be discontinued if antihistamines fail to help
• Renal symptoms: polyuria, oliguria, frequency, dysuria

Teach patient/family:
• Not to discontinue drug abruptly
• Not to use OTC products (cough, cold, allergy) unless directed by physician; do not use salt substitutes containing potassium without consulting physician
• Importance of complying with dosage schedule, even if feeling better
• To rise slowly to sitting or standing position to minimize orthostatic hypotension
• To notify physician of: mouth sores, sore throat, fever, swelling of hands or feet, irregular heartbeat, chest pain
• To report excessive perspiration, dehydration, vomiting, diarrhea; may lead to fall in B/P
• That drug may cause dizziness, fainting, light-headedness; may occur during 1st few days of therapy
• That drug may cause skin rash or impaired perspiration
• How to take B/P, and normal readings for age group

Lab test interferences:
False positive: Urine acetone

Treatment of overdose: 0.9% NaCl IV INF, hemodialysis

---

benzalkonium chloride

(benz-al-koe'nee-um)

Benasept, Benzachlor-50,* Bena-All, Ionax Scrub,* Sabol Shampoo,* Zalkon, Zalkonium Chloride, Zephiran, Zephiran Chloride,* Mercurochrome II, Benza, Dermo-Sterol

Func. class.: Disinfectant
Chem. class.: Quaternary ammonium cationic surfactant

Action: Inhibits and destroys organisms by enzyme inactivation (bactericidal/bacteriostatic)

Uses: Irrigate eye, vagina, body cavities, disinfection of skin before surgery

Dosage and routes:
• *Adult and child:* TOP 1:750 for minor wounds, disinfection before surgery; 1:3000-20,000 deep infected wounds; 1:2000-5000 vaginal irrigation; 1:5000-10,000 denuded skin, eye, mucous membrane irrigation; 1:5000-20,000 bladder, urethral irrigation

Available forms include: Top sol 0.1%, 0.13%, 17%, 17.5%, 50%; tinct 0.13%

Side effects/adverse reactions:
CNS: Confusion, restlessness
INTEG: Irritation, contact dermatitis, hypersensitivity, rash, burning
GI: Nausea, vomiting
RESP: Dyspnea, ***respiratory paralysis, coma*** (if ingested)

Contraindications: Hypersensitivity, occlusive dressing, casts/traction

Interactions/incompatibilities:

- Decreased action of benzalkonium: soap
- Not to be used with fluorescein, nitrates, lanolin, potassium permanganate, kaolin, zinc sulfate, zinc oxide, caramel, aluminum, iodine, peroxide, yellow oxide of mercury, citrates, sulfonamides

NURSING CONSIDERATIONS

Administer:

- After diluting with sterile water for injection for irrigating wounds
- To ⅓ of body or less to avoid chilling

Perform/provide:

- Rust tablets for cleaning metal objects, or instrument will rust
- Wet dressings using clear solution only; discontinue if necrosis occurs

Evaluate:

- Area of body involved: irritation, rash, breaks, dryness, scales, discharge

Teach patient/family:

- To store at room temperature no longer than 1 wk
- To use applicator, insert high into vagina, notify physician of itching, discharge, burning

Treatment of ingestion: Administer milk, soap solution, gastric lavage, supportive care

benzocaine (oral)

(ben-zoe-kane)

Orabase with Benzocaine, Oracin, Ora-Jel, Spec-T Anesthetic, Trocaine, Tyzomint, Solarcaine, Dermoplast, Chiggerex, Benzocal, Americaine

Func. class.: Topical local anesthetic

Chem. class.: Ester

Action: Inhibits conduction of nerve impulses from sensory nerves

Uses: Oral irritation, sore throat, toothache, cold sore, canker sore, sunburn, minor cuts, insect bites, pain, itching

Dosage and routes:

- *Adult and child >12 yr:* TOP apply to affected area; LOZ suck as needed

Available forms include: Cream 1%, 5%; lotion 0.5%, 8%; oint 2%, 5%, 20%; sol 2.1%, 2.5%, 6.3%, 20%; lozenges 3, 5, 6.25, 10 mg; topical aerosol 20%; gel 6.3%, 7.5%, 10%, 20%

Side effects/adverse reactions:

EENT: Itching, irritation in ear

INTEG: Rash, urticaria

Contraindications: Hypersensitivity

Precautions: Pregnancy (C)

Pharmacokinetics:

TOP: Peak 1 min, duration ½-1 hr

NURSING CONSIDERATIONS

Administer:

- To gums as needed for teething pain
- Lozenges for temporary sore throat pain

Perform/provide:

- Storage in tight, light-resistant container; do not freeze, puncture, or incinerate aerosol container

Evaluate:

- Affected area for redness, swelling, pain

Teach patient/family:

- To avoid contact with eyes
- Not to use for prolonged periods of time, use for <1 wk; if condition remains, physician should be contacted

benzonatate

(ben-zoe'na-tate)

Tessalon

Func. class.: Antitussive, nonnarcotic

Chem. class.: Tetracaine derivative

Action: Inhibits cough reflex by anesthetizing stretch receptors in respiratory system, direct action on cough center in medulla

Uses: Nonproductive cough

Dosage and routes:

• *Adult and child:* PO 100 mg tid, not to exceed 600 mg/day

• *Child <10 yr:* PO 8 mg/kg in 3-6 divided doses

Available forms include: Perles 100 mg

Side effects/adverse reactions:

CNS: Dizziness, drowsiness, headache

GI: Nausea, constipation, upset stomach

EENT: Nasal congestion, burning eyes

CV: Increased B/P, chest tightness, numbness

INTEG: Urticaria, rash, pruritus

Contraindications: Hypersensitivity

Precautions: Pregnancy (C), lactation

Pharmacokinetics:

PO: Onset 15-20 min, duration 3-8 hr, metabolized by liver, excreted in urine

NURSING CONSIDERATIONS

Perform/provide:

• Storage in tight, light-resistant containers

• Increased fluids, bulk, exercise to patient's lifestyle to decrease constipation, liquefy sputum

• Chest percussion to bring up secretion if needed

Evaluate:

• Therapeutic response: absence of cough

• Cough: type, frequency, character including sputum

Teach patient/family:

• Avoid driving, other hazardous activities until patient is stabilized on this medication

• Not to chew or break capsules; will anesthetize mouth

• To avoid smoking, smoke-filled rooms, perfumes, dust, environmental pollutants, cleaners

benzoyl peroxide

(ben'zoe-ill per-ox'ide)

Benoxyl, Benzac, Benzagel, Clearasil, Desquam-X,* Oxy-5, Oxy-10, Persadox, Persa-Gel, Xerac BP, Pan Oxyl, Propa P.H. Acne

Func. class.: Antiacne medication

Action: Antibacterial activity especially against predominant bacteria causing acne

Uses: Mild-moderate acne

Dosage and routes:

• *Adult and child:* TOP apply to affected area qd or bid

Available forms include: Topical cleansers, lotions, creams, sticks, pads, gels, bars

Side effects/adverse reactions:

INTEG: Local skin irritation, stinging, warmth (dryness), scaling, erythema, edema, allergic, contact dermatitis

Contraindications: Hypersensitivity to benzoic acid derivatives

Precautions: Pregnancy (C), lactation, children <12 yr

Pharmacokinetics:

TOP: 50% absorbed through skin, metabolized to benzoic acid, excreted in urine

NURSING CONSIDERATIONS

Administer:

• Then wash hands immediately to avoid irritation

Perform/provide:

• Storage at room temperature

Evaluate:

• Therapeutic response: decreased amount of acne on body

• Area of body involved, including time involved, what helps or aggravates condition

• Allergic reaction: rash, irritation, scaling, dermatitis; discontinue use

Teach patient/family:

• To avoid application on normal skin or getting cream in eyes, nose, or other mucous membranes

• To discontinue use if rash or irritation develops

• That may cause transitory warmth or stinging over area treated

• To expect dryness, peeling of area treated

• To avoid contact with hair or clothing; they may stain

• That cosmetics may be used over drug

• That dryness and peeling can be expected

benzquinamide HCl

(benz-kwin'a-mide)

Emete-Con, Quantril

Func. class.: Antiemetic

Chem. class.: Benzoquinolize amide

Action: Acts centrally by blocking chemoreceptor trigger zone, which in turn acts on vomiting center

Uses: To inhibit nausea, vomiting associated with anesthetic, surgery

Dosage and routes:

• *Adult:* IM 50 mg or 0.5-1 mg/kg, may be repeated in 1 hr, then q3-4 hr prn; IV 25 mg or 0.2-0.4 mg/kg as a one-time dose

Available forms include: Inj 50 mg/vial

Side effects/adverse reactions:

CNS: Drowsiness, fatigue, restlessness, tremor, headache, stimulation, dizziness, insomnia, twitching, excitement, nervousness, extrapyramidal symptoms

GI: Nausea, anorexia

CV: ***Premature atrial*** or ***ventricular contractions, atrial fibrillation,*** hypertension, hypotension

INTEG: Rash, urticaria, fever, chills, flushing, hives, shivering, sweating, temperature

EENT: Dry mouth, blurred vision, hiccups, salivation

Contraindications: Hypersensitivity, hypertension

Precautions: Children, pregnancy (C), lactation, elderly

Pharmacokinetics:

IM/IV: Onset 15 min, duration 3-4 hr, metabolized by liver, excreted in urine, feces, half-life 40 min

NURSING CONSIDERATIONS

Assess:

• Vital signs, B/P; check patients with cardiac disease more often; hypotension, hypertension, dysrhythmias may occur

Administer:

• After reconstituting with 2.2 ml sterile water for injection to a concentration of 25 mg/ml; do not use sodium chloride

• Reduced dosage if patient is receiving pressor drugs

• Direct IV 25 mg over ½-1 min by Y-tube; incompatible with saline solutions

Perform/provide:

• Storage of injection before, after reconstitution in light-resistant container, single dose container

Evaluate:

- Therapeutic response: absence of nausea, vomiting
- Observe for drowsiness; instruct patient not to drive, operate machinery

Treatment of overdose:

- Supportive care; atropine may be helpful

---

benztropine mesylate

(benz'troe-peen)

Apo-Benzotropine, Bensylate, Cogentin

Func. class.: Cholinergic blocker
Chem. class.: Tertiary amine

Action: Blockade of central acetylcholine receptors

Uses: Parkinson symptoms, extrapyramidal symptoms associated with neuroleptic drugs

Dosage and routes:

Drug-induced extrapyramidal symptoms

- *Adult:* IM/IV 1-2 mg 1-2× day; give PO dose as soon as possible; PO 1-2 mg bid/tid, increase by 0.5 mg q5-6 days

Parkinson symptoms

- *Adult:* PO 0.5-1 mg qd, increased 0.5 mg q5-6 days titrated to patient response

Available forms include: Tabs 0.5, 1, 2 mg; inj IM, IV 1 mg/ml

Side effects/adverse reactions:

MS: Muscular weakness, cramping
INTEG: Rash, urticaria, dermatoses
MISC: Increased temperature, flushing, decreased sweating, hyperthermia, heat stroke, numbness of fingers
CNS: Confusion, anxiety, restlessness, irritability, delusions, hallucinations, headache, sedation, depression, incoherence, dizziness, memory loss
EENT: Blurred vision, photophobia, dilated pupils, difficulty swallowing, dry eyes, mydriasis
CV: Palpitations, tachycardia, hypotension, bradycardia
GI: Dryness of mouth, constipation, nausea, vomiting, abdominal distress, ***paralytic ileus,*** epigastric distress
GU: Hesitancy, retention

Contraindications: Hypersensitivity, narrow-angle glaucoma, myasthenia gravis, GI/GU obstruction, child <3 yr, peptic ulcer, megacolon

Precautions: Pregnancy (C), elderly, lactation, tachycardia, prostatic hypertrophy, liver, kidney disease, drug abuse history, dysrhythmias, hypotension, hypertension, psychiatric patients

Pharmacokinetics:

IM/IV: Onset 15 min, duration 6-10 hr
PO: Onset 1 hr, duration 6-10 hr

Interactions/incompatibilities:

- Increased anticholinergic effect: antihistamines, phenothiazines, amantadine
- Decreased effect of: levodopa
- Increased schizophrenic symptoms: haloperidol

NURSING CONSIDERATIONS

Assess:

- I&O ratio; retention commonly causes decreased urinary output

Administer:

- With or after meals to prevent GI upset; may give with fluids other than water
- At hs to avoid daytime drowsiness in patient with parkinsonism
- Parenteral dose slowly; keep in bed for at least 1 hr after dose

Perform/provide:

- Storage at room temperature
- Hard candy, frequent drinks, gum to relieve dry mouth

Evaluate:
- Therapeutic response: absence of involuntary movements
- Parkinsonism, extrapyramidal symptoms: shuffling gait, muscle rigidity, involuntary movements
- Urinary hesitancy, retention; palpate bladder if retention occurs
- Constipation; increase fluids, bulk, exercise if this occurs
- For tolerance over long-term therapy; dose may need to be increased or changed
- Mental status: affect, mood, CNS depression, worsening of mental symptoms during early therapy

Teach patient/family:
- Not to discontinue this drug abruptly; to taper off over 1 wk
- To avoid driving or other hazardous activities, drowsiness may occur
- To avoid OTC medication: cough, cold preparations with alcohol, antihistamines unless directed by physician

---

bepridil HCl

(beh'prih-dill)

Vascor

Func. class.: Calcium channel blocker type 4

Action: Inhibits calcium ion influx across cell membrane during cardiac depolarization; produces relaxation of coronary vascular smooth muscle, dilates coronary arteries, decreases SA/AV node conduction, dilates peripheral arteries

Uses: Stable angina, used alone or in combination with propranolol

Dosage and routes:

Angina

Adult: 200-450 mg qd

Available forms include: Tabs, film-coated, 200, 300, 400 mg

Side effects/adverse reactions:

CV: Dysrhythmia, edema, CHF, bradycardia, hypotension, palpitations, AV block

GI: Nausea, vomiting, diarrhea, gastric upset, constipation, increased liver function studies

GU: Nocturia, polyuria

CNS: Headache, fatigue, drowsiness, dizziness, anxiety, depression, weakness, insomnia, confusion, light-headedness, nervousness

Contraindications: Sick sinus syndrome, 2nd or 3rd degree heart block, Wolff-Parkinson-White syndrome, hypotension less than 90 mm Hg systolic, cardiogenic shock

Precautions: CHF, hypotension, hepatic injury, pregnancy (C), lactation, children, renal disease, concomitant β-blocker therapy

Pharmacokinetics: Peak 2-3 hr, 99% plasma protein bound, half-life 42 hr; completely metabolized in the liver and excreted in urine and feces

Interactions/incompatibilities:
- Increased effects: β-blockers
- Decreased effects of: lithium, rifampin
- Increased levels of: digoxin

NURSING CONSIDERATIONS

Administer:
- Before meals, hs

Evaluate:
- Therapeutic response: decreased anginal pain, decreased B/P
- Cardiac status: B/P, pulse, respiration, ECG intervals (PR, QRS, QT), dysrhythmias

Teach patient/family:
- How to take pulse before taking drug; record or graph should be kept
- To avoid hazardous activities until stabilized on drug, dizziness is no longer a problem

---

• To limit caffeine consumption
• To avoid OTC drugs unless directed by a physician
• Importance of patient compliance to all areas of medical regimen: diet, exercise, stress reduction, drug therapy

Lab test interferences:
Increase: Liver function tests

Treatment of overdose: Defibrillation, atropine for AV block, vasopressor for hypotension

---

beractant

(Bear-ac'-tant)
Survanta

Func. class.: Natural lung surfactant

Action: Replenishes surfactant and restores surface activity to the lungs in premature infants

Uses: Prevention and treatment (rescue) of respiratory distress syndrome in premature infants

Dosage and routes:
Intratracheal instill: Four doses can be administered in the first 48 hrs of life; give doses no more frequently than q6h; each dose is 100 mg of phospholipids/kg birth weight (4 ml/kg)

Available forms include: Susp 25 mg phospholipds/ml in 0.9% NaCl in single-use vials containing 8 ml susp

Side effects/adverse reactions:
RESP: ***Pulmonary air leaks, pulmonary interstitial emphysema, apnea, pulmonary hemorrhage***
SYST: ***Patent ductus arteriosus, intracranial hemorrhage, severe intracranial hemorrhage, necrotizing entercolitis, post-treatment sepsis, post-treatment infection,*** bradycardia, oxygen desaturation

Precautions: Bradycardia, rales, infections

Pharmacokinetics: Becomes lung associated within hours of administration

NURSING CONSIDERATIONS

Assess:
• Respiratory rate, rhythm, character, chest expansion, color, transcutaneous saturation, ABGs
• Endotracheal tube placement before dosing; for apnea after endotracheal administration
• Reflux of drug into the endotracheal tube during administration; stop drug administration if this occurs, and if needed, increase peak inspiratory pressure on the ventilator by 4-5 cm H_2O until tube is cleared

Administer:
• After suctioning before administration
• By endotracheal administration only by persons trained in neonatal intubation and ventilation
• After using a No. 5 Fr end-hole catheter inserted into the endotracheal tube with the tip protruding just beyond the end of the endotracheal tube; shorten the length of the catheter before insertion; do not insert the drug into the mainstem bronchus
• Divide each dose into quarters and administer with infant in different positions
• Determine the dosing by weight of infant; slowly withdraw the contents into the plastic syringe through a 20G needle, do not filter or shake; attach the premeasured No. 5 Fr catheter to syringe; fill with drug and discard excess through the catheter so only dose to be given remains in syringe
• For prevention dosing stabilize, weigh, and intubate the infant; give

drug within 15 min of birth if possible; position infant and inject the first quarter dose through catheter over 2-3 sec, remove catheter and manually ventilate with O_2 to prevent cyanosis (60 bpm) and sufficient positive pressure to promote air exchange and chest wall excursion that is adequate

• For rescue dosing give dosing as soon as infant is placed on ventilator after birth; immediately before administering dose change ventilator settings to 60/min, inspiratory time 0.5 sec, FIO_2 1, position infant and inject first quarter through catheter over 2-3 sec, remove catheter, return to mechanical ventilator

• Ventilate infant for >30 sec or until stable after prevention or rescue strategy, resposition for next dose; provide same procedure for subsequent dosing; do not suction for at least 1 hr after dosing unless airway obstruction is evident, resume ventilator therapy after dosing

Perform/provide:

• Reduction in peak venilator inspiratory pressures immediately if chest expansion improves substantially after dose

• Reduction in FIO_2 in small, repeated steps when infant becomes pink and transcutaneous oxygen saturation is in excess of 95%; oxygen saturation should remain between 90% and 95%

• Suctioning of all infants before administration to prevent mucus plugging; if endotracheal tube obstruction is suspected, remove the obstruction and replace tube immediately

• Storage in refrigeration; protect from light, warm to room temperature for >20 min or warm in hand >8 min before giving; do not use artificial warming methods; enter a vial only once; unopened, unused vials that have been warmed to room temperature may be re-refrigerated within 8 hr of warming; do not warm and return to refrigerator more than once

Evaluate:

• Therapeutic response: significant improvement in respiratory status

• Infant for repeat dosing using radiographic confirmation of RDS; repeat doses should be given as above; ventilator settings for repeat doses FIO_2 were decreased by 0.2 or amount to prevent cyanosis; ventilator rate of 30/min; inspiratory time <1 sec; if infant's pretreatment rate was >30, it was left unchanged during dosing; resume usual ventilator management after dosing

---

betamethasone/betamethasone sodium phosphate/betamethasone disodium phosphate/betamethasone acetate, betamethasone sodium phosphate

(bay-ta-meth'a-sone)

Betnelan, Celestone/Celestone Phosphate*/Betnesol/Celestone Soluspan

Func. class.: Corticosteroid, synthetic

Chem. class.: Glucocorticoid, long-acting

Action: Decreases inflammation by suppression of migration of polymorphonuclear leukocytes, fibroblasts, reversal of increased capillary permeability and lysosomal stabilization

Uses: Immunosupression, severe

---

* Available in Canada only

inflammation, prevention of neonatal respiratory distress syndrome (by administering to mothers)

Dosage and routes:

- *Adult:* PO 0.6-7.2 mg qd; IM/IV 0.6-7.2 mg qd in joint or soft tissue (sodium phosphate)
- *Pregnant adult:* IM 12 mg 36-48 hr, before premature delivery, then same dose in 24 hr (betamethasone acetate)

Available forms include: Tabs 0.6 mg; syr 0.6 mg/5 ml; inj 3, 4 mg/ml

Side effects/adverse reactions:

INTEG: Acne, poor wound healing, ecchymosis, bruising, petechiae

CNS: Depression, flushing, sweating, headache, ecchymosis, bruising, mood changes

*CV: Hypertension, **circulatory collapse, thrombophlebitis, embolism,*** tachycardia, ***necrotizing angiitis, CHF***

HEMA: ***Thrombocytopenia***

MS: Fractures, osteoporosis, weakness

*GI: Diarrhea, nausea, abdominal distention, **GI hemorrhage,** increased appetite, **pancreatitis***

EENT: Fungal infections, increased intraocular pressure, blurred vision

Contraindications: Psychosis, hypersensitivity, idiopathic thrombocytopenia, acute glomerulonephritis, amebiasis, fungal infections, nonasthmatic bronchial disease, child <2 yr, AIDS, TB

Precautions: Pregnancy (C), diabetes mellitus, glaucoma, osteoporosis, seizure disorders, ulcerative colitis, CHF, myasthenia gravis, renal disease, esophagitis, peptic ulcer

Pharmacokinetics:

PO: Onset 1-2 hr, peak 1 hr, duration 3 days

IM/IV: Onset 10 min, peak 4-8 hr, duration 1-1½ days

Metabolized in liver, excreted in urine as steroids, crosses placenta

Interactions/incompatibilities:

- Decreased action of betamethasone: cholestyramine, colestipol, barbiturates, rifampin, ephedrine, phenytoin, theophylline
- Decreased effects of: anticoagulants, anticonvulsants, antidiabetics, ambenonium, neostigmine, isoniazid, toxoids, vaccines, anticholinesterases, salicylates, somatrem
- Increased side effects: alcohol, salicylates, indomethacin, amphotericin B, digitalis, cyclosporine, diuretics
- Increased action of betamethasone: salicylates, estrogens, indomethacin, oral contraceptives, ketoconazole, macrolide antibiotics

NURSING CONSIDERATIONS

Assess:

- Potassium, blood sugar, urine glucose while on long-term therapy; hypokalemia and hyperglycemia
- Weight daily, notify physician of weekly gain >5 lb
- B/P q4h, pulse, notify physician if chest pain occurs
- I&O ratio, be alert for decreasing urinary output and increasing edema
- Plasma cortisol levels during long-term therapy (normal level: 138-635 nmol/L SI units when drawn at 8 AM)

Administer:

- IV, only sodium phosphate product; give > 1 min; may be given by IV INF in compatible sol
- After shaking suspension (parenteral)
- Titrated dose, use lowest effective dose

• IM injection deeply in large mass, rotate sites, avoid deltoid, use 21G needle
• In one dose in AM to prevent adrenal suppression, avoid SC administration, may damage tissue
• With food or milk to decrease GI symptoms

Perform/provide:
• Assistance with ambulation in patient with bone tissue disease to prevent fractures

Evaluate:
• Therapeutic response: ease of respirations, decreased inflammation
• Infection: increased temperature, WBC even after withdrawal of medication; drug masks infection symptoms
• Potassium depletion: paresthesias, fatigue, nausea, vomiting, depression, polyuria, dysrhythmias, weakness
• Edema, hypertension, cardiac symptoms
• Mental status: affect, mood, behavioral changes, aggression

Teach patient/family:
• That ID as steroid user should be carried
• To notify physician if therapeutic response decreases; dosage adjustment may be needed
• Not to discontinue this medication abruptly or adrenal crisis can result
• To avoid OTC products: salicylates, alcohol in cough products, cold preparations unless directed by physician
• All aspects of drug usage including cushingoid symptoms
• Symptoms of adrenal insufficiency: nausea, anorexia, fatigue, dizziness, dyspnea, weakness, joint pain

Lab test interferences:
Increase: Cholesterol, sodium, blood glucose, uric acid, calcium, urine glucose
Decrease: Calcium, potassium, T_4, T_3, thyroid ^{131}I uptake test, urine 17-OHCS, 17-KS, PBI
False negative: Skin allergy tests

---

betamethasone benzoate

(bay-ta-meth'a-sone)

Beben, Benisone, Uticort

Func. class.: Topical corticosteroid
Chem. class.: Synthetic fluorinated agent, group III potency

Action: Possesses antipruritic, antiinflammatory actions

Uses: Psoriasis, eczema, contact dermatitis, pruritus

Dosage and routes:
• *Adult and child:* Apply to affected area qid

Available forms include: Oint 0.025%; cream 0.025%; lotion 0.025%; gel 0.025%

Side effects/adverse reactions:
INTEG: Burning, dryness, itching, irritation, acne, folliculitis, hypertrichosis, perioral dermatitis, hypopigmentation, atrophy, striae, miliaria, allergic contact dermatitis, secondary infection

Contraindications: Hypersensitivity to corticosteroids, fungal infections

Precautions: Pregnancy (C), lactation, viral infections, bacterial infections

NURSING CONSIDERATIONS

Assess:
• Temperature; if fever develops, drug should be discontinued

Administer:
• Only to affected areas; do not get in eyes
• Medication, then cover with occlusive dressing (only if pre-

---

* Available in Canada only

scribed), seal to normal skin, change q12h; systemic absorption may occur
• Only to dermatoses; do not use on weeping, denuded, or infected area

Perform/provide:
• Cleansing before application of drug
• Treatment for a few days after area has cleared
• Storage at room temperature

Evaluate:
• Therapeutic response: absence of severe itching, patches on skin, flaking
• For systemic absorption: increased temperature, inflammation, irritation

Teach patient/family:
• To avoid sunlight on affected area; burns may occur

---

betamethasone valerate

(bay-ta-meth'a-sone)

Beta Cort,* Betaderm,* Beta-Val, Betatrex, Valnac, Valisone

Func. class.: Topical corticosteroid
Chem. class.: Synthetic fluorinated agent

Action: Possesses antipruritic, antiinflammatory actions

Uses: Psoriasis, eczema, contact dermatitis, pruritus

Dosage and routes:
• *Adult and child:* Apply to affected area qid

Available forms include: Oint 0.1%; cream 0.01%, 0.1%; lotion 0.1%

Side effects/adverse reactions:
INTEG: Burning, dryness, itching, irritation, acne, folliculitis, hypertrichosis, perioral dermatitis, hypopigmentation, atrophy, striae, miliaria, allergic contact dermatitis, secondary infection

Contraindications: Hypersensitivity to corticosteroids, fungal infections

Precautions: Pregnancy (C), lactation, viral infections, bacterial infections

NURSING CONSIDERATIONS

Assess:
• Temperature; if fever develops, drug should be discontinued

Administer:
• Only to affected areas; do not get in eyes
• Medication, then cover with occlusive dressing (only if prescribed), seal to normal skin, change q12h; systemic absorption may occur
• Only to dermatoses; do not use on weeping, denuded, or infected area

Perform/provide:
• Cleansing before applying drug
• Treatment for a few days after area has cleared
• Storage at room temperature

Evaluate:
• Therapeutic response: absence of severe itching, patches on skin, flaking
• For systemic absorption: increased temperature, inflammation, irritation

Teach patient/family:
• To avoid sunlight on affected area; burns may occur

---

bethanechol chloride

(be-than'e-kile)

Duvoid, Myotonachol, Urecholine, Urabeth

Func. class.: Cholinergic stimulant
Chem. class.: Synthetic choline ester

Action: Stimulates muscarinic

ACh receptors directly; mimics effects of parasympathetic nervous system stimulation; stimulates gastric motility, stimulates ganglia
Uses: Urinary retention (postoperative, postpartum), neurogenic atony of bladder with retention
Dosage and routes:
• *Adult:* PO 10-50 mg bid-qid; SC 2.5-10 mg tid-qid prn
Test dose
• *Adult:* SC 2.5 mg repeated 15-30 min intervals × 4 doses to determine effective dose
Available forms include: Tabs 5, 10, 25, 50 mg; inj SC 5 mg/ml
Side effects/adverse reactions:
INTEG: Rash, urticaria, flushing, increased sweating, hypothermia
CNS: Dizziness, headache, confusion, weakness, ***convulsions***
GI: Nausea, bloody diarrhea, vomiting, cramps, fecal incontinence
CV: Hypotension, bradycardia, orthostatic hypotension, reflex tachycardia, ***cardiac arrest, circulatory collapse***
GU: Frequency, incontinence
RESP: ***Acute asthma, dyspnea***
EENT: Miosis, increased salivation, lacrimation, blurred vision
Contraindications: Hypersensitivity, severe bradycardia, asthma, severe hypotension, hyperthyroidism, peptic ulcer, parkinsonism, seizure disorders, CAD, coronary occlusion, mechanical obstruction
Precautions: Hypertension, pregnancy (C), lactation, child <8 yr, urinary retention
Pharmacokinetics:
PO: Onset 30-90 min, duration 6 hr
SC: Onset 5-15 min, duration 2 hr, excreted by kidneys
Interactions/incompatibilities:
• Increased action of bethanechol: other cholinergics
• Hypotension: ganglionic blockers
• Decreased action of bethanechol: procainamide, quinidine

NURSING CONSIDERATIONS

Assess:
• B/P, pulse; observe after parenteral dose for 1 hr
• I&O ratio; check for urinary retention or incontinence
Administer:
• Parenteral dose by SC route; use of IM, IV may result in cardiac arrest
• Only with atropine sulfate available for cholinergic crisis
• Only after all other cholinergics have been discontinued
• Increased doses if tolerance occurs
• With food or milk to decrease GI symptoms (bilateral vagotomy); may decrease action of this drug
• On empty stomach for better absorption
Perform/provide:
• Storage at room temperature
• Bedpan/urinal if given for urinary retention
• Use of rectal tube if ordered to increase passage of gas when used for abdominal distention
Evaluate:
• Therapeutic response: absence of urinary retention, abdominal distention
• Bradycardia, hypotension, bronchospasm, headache, dizziness, convulsions, respiratory depression; drug should be discontinued if toxicity occurs
Teach patient/family:
• To take drug exactly as prescribed
• To make position changes slowly, orthostatic hypotension may occur
Treatment of overdose: Administer atropine 0.6-1.2 mg IV or IM (adult)

Lab test interferences:
Increase: AST, lipase/amylase, bilirubin, BSP

biperiden HCl, biperiden lactate

(bye-per'i-den)
Akineton
Func. class.: Cholinergic blocker

Action: Centrally acting competitive anticholinergic
Uses: Parkinson symptoms, extrapyramidal symptoms secondary to neuroleptic drug therapy
Dosage and routes:
Extrapyramidal symptoms
• *Adult:* PO 2-6 mg bid-tid; IM/IV 2 mg q30min, if needed, not to exceed 8 mg/24 hr
Parkinson symptoms
• *Adult:* PO 2 mg tid-qid
Available forms include: Tabs 2 mg; inj IM/IV 5 mg/ml (lactate)
Side effects/adverse reactions:
CNS: Confusion, anxiety, restlessness, irritability, delusions, hallucinations, headache, sedation, depression, incoherence, dizziness, euphoria, tremors, memory loss
EENT: Blurred vision, photophobia, dilated pupils, difficulty swallowing, mydriasis
CV: Palpitations, tachycardia, postural hypotension, bradycardia
GI: Dryness of mouth, constipation, nausea, vomiting, abdominal distress, ***paralytic ileus***
GU: Hesitancy, retention
MS: Weakness, cramping
INTEG: Rash, urticaria, dermatoses
MISC: Increased temperature, flushing, decreased sweating, hyperthermia, heat stroke, numbness of fingers
Contraindications: Hypersensitivity, narrow-angle glaucoma, myasthenia gravis, GI/GU obstruction, megacolon, stenosing peptic ulcers
Precautions: Pregnancy (C), elderly, lactation, tachycardia, prostatic hypertrophy, dysrhythmias, liver, kidney disease, drug abuse, hypotension, hypertension, psychiatric patients, children
Pharmacokinetics:
IM/IV: Onset 15 min, duration 6-10 hr
PO: Onset 1 hr, duration 6-10 hr
Interactions/incompatibilities:
• Increased levels of: digoxin, levodopa
• Increased schizophrenic symptoms: haloperidol
• Increased anticholinergic effect: antihistamines, phenothiazines, amantadine

NURSING CONSIDERATIONS

Assess:
• I&O ratio; retention commonly causes decreased urinary output
Administer:
• Parenteral dose with patient recumbent to prevent postural hypotension
• With or after meals to prevent GI upset; may give with fluids other than water
• At hs to avoid daytime drowsiness in patient with parkinsonism
• Parenteral dose slowly (>1 min); keep in bed for at least 1 hr after dose
Perform/provide:
• Storage at room temperature
• Hard candy, frequent drinks, gum to relieve dry mouth
Evaluate:
• Therapeutic response: absence of involuntary movements
• Parkinsonism, extrapyramidal symptoms: shuffling gait, muscle rigidity, involuntary movements

• Urinary hesitancy, retention; palpate bladder if retention occurs
• Constipation; increase fluids, bulk, exercise if this occurs
• For tolerance over long-term therapy; dose may need to be increased or changed
• Mental status: affect, mood, CNS depression, worsening of mental symptoms during early therapy

Teach patient/family:
• Not to discontinue this drug abruptly, to taper off over 1 wk
• To avoid driving or other hazardous activities, drowsiness may occur
• To avoid OTC medication: cough, cold preparations with alcohol, antihistamines unless directed by physician

bisacodyl

(bis-a-koe'dill)

Apo-Bisacodyl,* Bisco-Lax, Dulcolax, Fleet Bisacodyl, Theralax, Dacodyl, Deficol

Func. class.: Laxative, stimulant
Chem. class.: Diphenylmethane

Action: Acts directly on intestine by increasing motor activity, thought to irritate colonic intramural plexus

Uses: Short-term treatment of constipation, bowel or rectal preparation for surgery, examination

Dosage and routes:
• *Adult:* PO 10-15 mg in PM or AM, may use up to 30 mg for bowel or rectal preparation; REC 10 mg; ENEMA 1.25 oz
• *Child >3 yr:* PO 5-10 mg
• *Child >2 yr:* REC 10 mg
• *Child <2 yr:* REC 5 mg
• *Child <6 yr:* ENEMA one-half contents of micro enema

Available forms include: Enteric coated tabs 5 mg; rec supp 10 mg

Side effects/adverse reactions:
CNS: Muscle weakness
GI: Nausea, vomiting, anorexia, cramps, diarrhea, rectal burning (suppositories)
META: Protein-losing enteropathy, alkalosis, hypokalemia, ***tetany,*** electrolyte, fluid imbalances

Contraindications: Hypersensitivity, rectal fissures, abdominal pain, nausea/vomiting, appendicitis, acute surgical abdomen, ulcerated hemorrhoids, acute hepatitis, fecal impaction, intestinal/biliary tract obstruction

Precautions: Pregnancy (C)

Pharmacokinetics:
PO: Onset 6-10 min, acts within 6-12 hr
REC: Onset 15-16 min
Metabolized by liver, excreted in urine, bile, feces, breast milk

Interactions/incompatibilities:
• Gastric irritation: antacids, milk, H_2 blockers

NURSING CONSIDERATIONS

Assess:
• Blood, urine electrolytes if drug is used often by patient
• I&O ratio: to identify fluid loss

Administer:
• Alone only with water for better absorption; do not take within 1 hr of other drugs or within 1 hr of antacids, milk, or cimetidine
• In morning or evening (oral dose)

Evaluate:
• Therapeutic response: decrease in constipation
• Cause of constipation; identify whether fluids, bulk, or exercise is missing from lifestyle
• Cramping, rectal bleeding, nausea, vomiting; if these symptoms occur, drug should be discontinued

Teach patient/family:
• To swallow tabs whole; do not chew

*Available in Canada only

• Not to use laxatives for long-term therapy; bowel tone will be lost
• That normal bowel movements do not always occur daily
• Not to use in presence of abdominal pain, nausea, vomiting
• To notify physician if constipation is unrelieved or if symptoms of electrolyte imbalance occur: muscle cramps, pain, weakness, dizziness

bismuth subsalicylate

(bis-meth)
Pepto-Bismol
Func. class.: Antidiarrheal
Chem. class.: Salicylate

Action: Inhibits prostaglandin synthesis responsible for GI hypermotility, stimulates absorption of fluid and electrolytes
Uses: Diarrhea (cause undetermined), prevention of diarrhea when traveling
Dosage and routes:
• *Adult:* PO 30 ml or 2 tabs q30-60 min, not to exceed 8 doses for >2 days
• *Child 10-14 yr:* PO 15 ml
• *Child 6-10 yr:* PO 10 ml
• *Child 3-6 yr:* PO 5 ml
Available forms include: Chewable tabs 262 mg; susp 262 mg/15 ml
Side effects/adverse reactions:
HEMA: Increased bleeding time
GI: Increased fecal impaction (high doses), dark stools
CNS: Confusion, twitching
EENT: Hearing loss, tinnitus, metallic taste, blue gums
Contraindications: Child <3 yr
Precautions: Anticoagulant therapy
Pharmacokinetics:
PO: Onset 1 hr, peak 2 hr, duration 4 hr
Interactions/incompatibilities:
• Increased side effects: alcohol, aminosalicyclic acid, carbonic anhydrase inhibitors
• Increased action of bismuth: ammonium chloride
• Decreased action of bismuth: antacids, corticosteroids
• Decreased action of: uricosurics, indomethacin, antidiabetics, tetracyclines

NURSING CONSIDERATIONS

Assess:
• Skin turgor; shift if dehydration is suspected
• Electrolytes (K, Na, Cl) if diarrhea is severe or continues for a long term
Administer:
• But stop use if symptoms do not improve within 2 days or become worse, or if diarrhea is accompanied by high fever
• Increased fluids to rehydrate the patient
Evaluate:
• Therapeutic response: decreased diarrhea or absence of diarrhea when traveling
• Bowel pattern before drug therapy, after treatment
Teach patient/family:
• To chew or dissolve in mouth; do not swallow whole
• To avoid other salicylates unless directed by physician
• That stools may turn gray; tongue may darken
Lab test interferences:
Interfere: Radiographic studies of GI system

bitolterol mesylate

(bye-tole'-ter-ol)

Tornalate

Func. class.: Adrenergic β_2-agonist

Chem. class.: Acid ester of colterol

Action: Causes bronchodilation by action on β_2 receptors with increased synthesis of cAMP, relaxes bronchial smooth muscle, inhibits mast cell degranulation, and stimulates cilia to remove secretions with very little effect on heart rate

Uses: Asthma, bronchospasm

Dosage and routes:

• *Adult and child >12 yr:* INH 2 puffs, wait 1-3 min before 3rd puff if needed, not to exceed 3 INH q6h or 2 INH q4h

Available forms include: Aerosol 0.37 mg/actuation

Side effects/adverse reactions:

CNS: Tremors, anxiety, insomnia, headache, dizziness, stimulation, restlessness, hallucinations

EENT: Dry nose, irritation of nose and throat

CV: Palpitations, tachycardia, hypertension, angina, hypotension

GI: Heartburn, nausea, vomiting, anorexia

MS: Muscle cramps

RESP: ***Bronchospasm***, dyspnea

Contraindications: Hypersensitivity to sympathomimetics

Precautions: Lactation, pregnancy (C), cardiac disorders, hyperthyroidism, diabetes mellitus

Pharmacokinetics:

INH: Onset 3 min, peak ½-1 hr, duration 5-8 hr

Interactions/incompatibilities:

• Increased action of: aerosol bronchodilators

• Increased action of bitolterol: tricyclic antidepressants, MAOIs

• May inhibit action when used with other β-blockers

NURSING CONSIDERATIONS

Assess:

• Respiratory function: vital capacity, forced expiratory volume, ABGs

Administer:

• After shaking, exhale, place mouthpiece in mouth, inhale slowly, hold breath, remove, exhale slowly

• Gum, sips of water for dry mouth

Perform/provide:

• Storage in light-resistant container, do not expose to temperatures over 86° F

Evaluate:

• Therapeutic response: absence of dyspnea, wheezing over 1 hr

Teach patient/family:

• Not to use OTC medications; extra stimulation may occur

• To use inhaler, review package insert with patient

• To avoid getting aerosol in eyes

• To wash inhaler in warm water and dry qd

• On all aspects of drug; avoid smoking, smoke-filled rooms, persons with respiratory infections

Treatment of overdose: Administer a β_2 adrenergic blocker

bleomycin sulfate

(blee-oh-mye'sin)

Blenoxane

Func. class.: Antineoplastic, antibiotic

Chem. class.: Glycopeptide

Action: Inhibits synthesis of DNA, RNA, protein; this drug is derived from *Streptomyces verticillus;* replication is decreased by binding to DNA, which causes strand splitting; drug is phase specific in the

G_2 and M phases; a nonvesicant

Uses: Cancer of head, neck, penis, cervix, vulva of squamous cell origin, Hodgkin's disease, lymphosarcoma, reticulum cell sarcoma, testicular carcinoma

Dosage and routes:

• *Adult:* SC/IV/IM 0.25-0.5 U/kg 1-2×/wk or 10-20 U/m^2, then 1 U/day or 5 U/wk; may also be given intraarterially; do not exceed total dose, 400 μg in lifetime

Available forms include: Inj IV, SC, IM 5 units

Side effects/adverse reactions:

SYST: ***Anaphylaxis***

GI: Nausea, vomiting, anorexia, stomatitis, weight loss

INTEG: Rash, hyperkeratosis, nail changes, alopecia, fever and chills

RESP: ***Fibrosis,*** pneumonitis, wheezing, ***pulmonary toxicity***

CNS: Fever, chills

IDIOSYNCRATIC REACTION: Hypotension, confusion, fever, chills, wheezing

Contraindications: Hypersensitivity

Precautions: Renal, hepatic, respiratory disease, pregnancy (D)

Pharmacokinetics: Half-life 2 hr when CrCl >35 ml/min half-life is increased in lower clearance, metabolized in liver, 50% excreted in urine (unchanged)

Interactions/incompatibilities:

• Increased toxicity: other antineoplastics or radiation therapy

• Decreased serum digoxin levels: digoxin

NURSING CONSIDERATIONS

Assess:

• IM test dose

• Pulmonary function tests: chest x-ray before and during therapy; should be obtained q2 wk during treatment

• Temperature q4h; fever may indicate beginning infection

• Serum creatinine

Administer:

• IM/SC after reconstituting 5 U/1-5 ml sterile H_2O, D_5W, 0.9% NaCl, or bacteriostatic water for inj; do not use products containing benzyl alcohol when giving to neonates

• Direct IV after reconstituting 15 U/5 ml of D_5W or 0.9% NaCl; give over 10-15 min

• IV INF after further diluting with 50-100 ml D_5W or 0.9% NaCl

• Two test doses 2-5U before initial dose; monitor for anaphylaxis

• Antiemetic 30-60 min before giving drug to prevent vomiting, continue antiemetics 6-10 hr after treatment

• Topical or systemic analgesics for pain of stomatitis as ordered; antihistamines and antipyretics for fever and chills

• Intraarterial/IV injections over >10 min

Perform/provide:

• Deep breathing exercises with patient tid-qid; place in semi-Fowler's position

• Liquid diet: carbonated beverage, gelatin may be added if patient is not nauseated or vomiting

• Rinsing of mouth tid-qid with water, club soda; brushing of teeth with baking soda bid-tid with soft brush or cotton-tipped applicators for stomatitis; use unwaxed dental floss

• HOB raised to facilitate breathing

Evaluate:

• Therapeutic response: decrease in size of tumor

• Dyspnea, rales, unproductive cough, chest pain, tachypnea, fatigue, increased pulse, pallor, lethargy

• Food preferences; list likes, dislikes
• Effects of alopecia and skin color on body image; discuss feelings about body changes
• Buccal cavity q8h for dryness, sores, ulceration, white patches, oral pain, bleeding, dysphagia
• Local irritation, pain, burning, discoloration at injection site
• Symptoms indicating severe allergic reaction: rash, pruritus, urticaria, purpuric skin lesions, itching, flushing
• Storage for 2 wk after reconstituting at room temperature; discard unused portions

Teach patient/family:
• To report any complaints, side effects to nurse or physician
• To report any changes in breathing, coughing, fever
• That hair may be lost during treatment and wig or hairpiece may make patient feel better; tell patient that new hair may be different in color, texture
• To avoid foods with citric acid, hot or rough texture
• To report any bleeding, white spots, ulcerations in mouth; to examine mouth qd and report symptoms

---

bretylium tosylate

(bre-til'ee-um)

Bretylate,* Bretylol

Func. class.: Antidysrhythmic (Class III)

Chem. class.: Quaternary ammonium compound

Action: After a transient release of norepinephrine, inhibits further release by postganglionic nerve endings; prolongs action potential duration and effective refractory period

Uses: Serious ventricular tachycardia, cardioversion, ventricular fibrillation; for short-term use only

Dosage and routes:

Severe ventricular fibrillation
• *Adult:* IV BOL 5 mg/kg, increase to 10 mg/kg repeated q15 min, up to 30 mg/kg; IV INF 1-2 mg/min or give 5-10 mg/kg over 10 min q6h (maintenance)

Ventricular dysrhythmias
• *Adult:* IV INF 500 mg diluted in 50 ml D_5W or NS, infuse over 10-30 min, may repeat in 1 hr, maintain with 1-2 mg/min or 5-10 mg/kg over 10-30 min q6h; IM 5-10 mg/kg undiluted; repeat in 1-2 hr if needed; maintain with same dose q6-8h

Available forms include: Inj IV 50 mg/ml; 1, 2, 4 mg/ml prefilled syringes

Side effects/adverse reactions:

CNS: Syncope, dizziness, confusion, psychosis, anxiety

GI: Nausea, vomiting

CV: Hypotension, postural hypotension, bradycardia, angina, PVCs, substernal pressure, transient hypertension, precipitation of angina

RESP: ***Respiratory depression***

Contraindications: Hypersensitivity, digitalis toxicity, aortic stenosis, pulmonary hypertension, children

Precautions: Renal disease, pregnancy (C), lactation

Pharmacokinetics:

IV: Onset 5 min

IM: Onset ½-2 hr, peak 6-9 hr

Half-life 4-17 hr, excreted unchanged by kidneys (70%-80% in 24 hr), not metabolized

Interactions/incompatibilities:
• Increased or decreased effects of

---

*Available in Canada only

bretylium: quinidine, procainamide, propranolol or other antidysrhythmics
• Hypotension: antihypertensives
• Toxicity: digitalis
• Incompatible with all medications in solution or syringe

NURSING CONSIDERATIONS

Assess:
• ECG continuously to determine drug effectiveness, PVCs or other dysrhythmias
• IV inf rate to avoid causing nausea, vomiting
• For dehydration or hypovolemia
• B/P continuously for hypotension, hypertension
• I&O ratio

Administer:
• IV INF by diluting 500 mg of drug/50 ml or more compatible solution, give over 15-30 min
• By continuous infusion using an infusion pump
• IM inj, rotate sites, inject <5 ml in any one site
• Reduced dosage slowly with ECG monitoring

Perform/provide:
• Place patient in supine position unless otherwise ordered
• Have suction equipment available

Evaluate:
• Therapeutic response: absence of ventricular tachycardia, fibrillation
• For rebound hypertension after 1-2 hr
• Cardiac status: rate, rhythm, character, continuously

Lab test interferences:
Decrease: Urinary epinephrine, urinary norepinephrine, urinary VMA epinephrine

Treatment of overdose: O_2, artificial ventilation, ECG, administer dopamine for circulatory depression, administer diazepam or thiopental for convulsions

B

bromocriptine mesylate

(broe-moe-krip'teen)
Parlodel

Func. class.: Dopamine receptor agonist; ovulation stimulant
Chem. class.: Ergot alkaloid derivative

Action: Inhibits prolactin release by activating postsynaptic dopamine receptors; activation of striatal dopamine receptors could be reason for improvement in Parkinson's disease

Uses: Female infertility, Parkinson's disease, prevention of postpartum lactation, amenorrhea caused by hyperprolactinemia, acromegaly

Dosage and routes:

Hyperprolactinemic indications
• *Adult:* PO 1.25-2.5 mg with meals; may increase by 2.5 mg q3-7 days, usual 5-7.5 mg

Acromegaly
• *Adult:* PO 1.25-2.5 mg × 3 days hs, may increase by 1.25-2.5 mg q3-7 days, usual range 20-30 mg/day

Postpartum lactation
• *Adult:* PO 2.5 mg qd-tid with meal × 14 or 21 days

Parkinson's disease
• *Adult:* PO 1.25 mg bid with meals, may increase q2-4 wk by 2.5 mg/day, not to exceed 100 mg qd

Available forms include: Caps 5 mg; tabs 2.5 mg

Side effects/adverse reactions:
EENT: Blurred vision, diplopia, burning eyes, nasal congestion
CNS: Headache, depression, restlessness, anxiety, nervousness,

confusion, ***convulsions,*** hallucinations, dizziness, fatigue, drowsiness, abnormal involuntary movements, psychosis

GU: Frequency, retention, incontinence, diuresis

GI: Nausea, vomiting, anorexia, cramps, constipation, diarrhea, dry mouth, GI hemorrhage

INTEG: Rash on face, arms, alopecia

CV: Orthostatic hypotension, decreased B/P, palpitation, extra systole, ***shock,*** dysrhythmias, bradycardia

Contraindications: Hypersensitivity to ergot, severe ischemic disease, pregnancy (D), severe peripheral vascular disease

Precautions: Lactation, hepatic disease, renal disease, children

Pharmacokinetics:

PO: Peak 1-3 hr, duration 4-8 hr, 90%-96% protein bound, half-life 3 hr, metabolized by liver (inactive metabolites), excreted in urine, feces

Interactions/incompatibilities:

• Decreased action of bromocriptine: phenothiazines, imipramine, haloperidol, droperidol, amitriptyline

• Increased action of: antihypertensives

NURSING CONSIDERATIONS

Assess:

• B/P; establish baseline, compare with other reading; this drug decreases B/P

Administer:

• With meal to prevent GI symptoms

• At hs so dizziness, orthostatic hypotension do not occur

Perform/provide:

• Storage at room temperature in tight container

Evaluate:

• Therapeutic response (Parkinson's disease): decreased dyskinesia, decreased slow movements, decreased drooling

Teach patient/family:

• To change position slowly, to prevent orthostatic hypotension

• To use contraceptives during treatment with this drug; pregnancy may occur; to use methods other than oral contraceptives

• That therapeutic effect may take 2 mo: galactorrhea, amenorrhea

• To avoid hazardous activity if dizziness occurs

Lab test interferences:

Increase: Growth hormone, AST/ALT, CPK, BUN, uric acid, alk phosphatase, GGTP

brompheniramine maleate

(brome-fen-ir'a-meen)

Brombay, Dimetane, Dimetane-Ten, Rolabromophen, Spentane, Veltane, and others

Func. class.: Antihistamine

Chem. class.: Alkylamine, H_1-receptor antagonist

Action: Acts on blood vessels, GI, respiratory system by competing with histamine for H_1-receptor site; decreases allergic response by blocking histamine

Uses: Allergy symptoms, rhinitis

Dosage and routes:

• *Adult:* PO 4-8 mg tid-qid, not to exceed 36 mg/day; TIME REL 8-12 mg bid-tid, not to exceed 36 mg/day; IM/IV/SC 5-20 mg q6-12h, not to exceed 40 mg/day

• *Child >6 yr:* PO 2 mg tid-qid, not to exceed 12 mg/day; IM/IV/SC 0.5 mg/kg/day divided tid or qid

• *Child <6 yr:* Only as directed by physician

Available forms include: Tabs 4 mg; tabs, time rel 8, 12 mg; elix 2 mg/5 ml; inj IM/SC/IV 10, 100 mg/ml

Side effects/adverse reactions:

CNS: Dizziness, drowsiness, poor coordination, fatigue, anxiety, euphoria, confusion, paresthesia, neuritis

CV: Hypotension, palpitations, tachycardia

RESP: Increased thick secretions, wheezing, chest tightness

HEMA: ***Thrombocytopenia, agranulocytosis, hemolytic anemia***

GI: Dry mouth, nausea, vomiting, anorexia, constipation, diarrhea

INTEG: Photosensitivity

GU: Retention, dysuria, frequency, impotence

EENT: Blurred vision, dilated pupils, tinnitus, nasal stuffiness, dry nose, throat, mouth

Contraindications: Hypersensitivity to H_1-receptor antagonists, acute asthma attack, lower respiratory tract disease, child <6 yr

Precautions: Increased intraocular pressure, renal disease, cardiac disease, hypertension, bronchial asthma, seizure disorder, stenosed peptic ulcers, hyperthyroidism, prostatic hypertrophy, bladder neck obstruction, pregnancy (C)

Pharmacokinetics:

PO: Peak 2-5 hr, duration to 48 hr; metabolized in liver, excreted by kidneys, excreted in breast milk, half-life 12-34 hr

Interactions/incompatibilities:

• Increased CNS depression: barbiturates, narcotics, hypnotics, tricyclic antidepressants, alcohol

• Decreased effect of: oral anticoagulants, heparin

• Increased drying effect: MAOIs

NURSING CONSIDERATIONS

Assess:

• I&O ratio; be alert for urinary retention, frequency, dysuria; drug should be discontinued if these occur

• CBC during long-term therapy

Administer:

• Direct IV undiluted or diluted with 10 ml 0.9% NaCl, given over 1 min or more

• IV INF by diluting in D_5W, 0.9% NaCl

• With meals if GI symptoms occur; absorption may slightly decrease

Perform/provide:

• Hard candy, gum, frequent rinsing of mouth for dryness

• Storage in tight container at room temperature

Evaluate:

• Therapeutic response: absence of running or congested nose or rashes

• Blood dyscrasias: thrombocytopenia, agranulocytosis (rare)

• Respiratory status: rate, rhythm, increase in bronchial secretions, wheezing, chest tightness

Teach patient/family:

• Not to crush or chew sustained release forms

• All aspects of drug use; to notify physician if confusion, sedation, hypotension occurs

• To avoid driving or other hazardous activities if drowsiness occurs

• To avoid use of alcohol or other CNS depressants while taking drug

Lab test interferences:

False negative: Skin allergy tests

Treatment of overdose: Administer ipecac syrup or lavage, diazepam, vasopressors, barbiturates (short-acting)

buclizine HCl

(byoo'kli-zeen)

Bucladin-S, Softran, Equivert, Vibazine

Func. class.: Antiemetic, antihistamine, anticholinergic

Chem. class.: H_1-receptor antagonist (piperazine)

Action: Acts centrally by blocking chemoreceptor trigger zone, which in turn acts on vomiting center

Uses: Motion sickness, dizziness, nausea, vomiting

Dosage and routes:

• *Adult:* PO 25-50 mg prn ½ hr before travel; may be repeated q4-6h prn

Available forms include: Tabs 50 mg

Side effects/adverse reactions:

CNS: Drowsiness, dizziness, fatigue, restlessness, headache, insomnia

GI: Nausea, anorexia, bitterness

EENT: Dry mouth, blurred vision

Contraindications: Hypersensitivity to cyclizines, shock

Precautions: Children, narrow-angle glaucoma, lactation, prostatic hypertrophy, elderly, pregnancy (C)

Pharmacokinetics:

PO: Duration 4-6 hr, other pharmacokinetics not known

NURSING CONSIDERATIONS

Assess:

• VS, B/P

Administer:

• Tablets may be swallowed whole, chewed, or allowed to dissolve

Evaluate:

• Therapeutic response: absence of dizziness, nausea, vomiting

• Signs of toxicity of other drugs or masking of symptoms of disease: brain tumor, intestinal obstruction

• Drowsiness, dizziness

Teach patient/family:

• To avoid hazardous activities or activities requiring alertness; dizziness may occur; instruct patient to request assistance with ambulation

• To avoid alcohol, other depressants

bumetanide

(byoo-met'a-nide)

Bumex

Func. class.: Loop diuretic

Chem. class.: Sulfonamide derivative

Action: Acts on ascending loop of Henle by increasing excretion of chloride, sodium

Uses: Edema in CHF, liver disease, renal disease (nephrotic syndrome), pulmonary edema, ascites (nephrotic syndrome), hypertension

Dosage and routes:

• *Adult:* PO 0.5-2.0 mg qd, may give 2nd or 3rd dose at 4-5 hr intervals, not to exceed 20 mg/day, may be given on alternate days or intermittently; IV/IM 0.5-1.0 mg/day, may give 2nd or 3rd dose at 2-3 hr intervals, not to exceed 20 mg/day

Available forms include: Tabs 0.5, 1, 2 mg; inj IV, IM 0.25 mg/ml

Side effects/adverse reactions:

GU: Polyuria, ***renal failure,*** glycosuria

ELECT: Hypokalemia, hypochloremic alkalosis, hypomagnesemia, hyperuricemia, hypocalcemia, hyponatremia

CNS: Headache, fatigue, weakness, vertigo

GI: Nausea, diarrhea, dry mouth,

* Available in Canada only

vomiting, anorexia, cramps, upset stomach, abdominal pain, ***acute pancreatitis, jaundice***
EENT: ***Loss of hearing,*** ear pain, tinnitus, blurred vision
INTEG: *Rash, pruritus,* purpura, ***Stevens-Johnson syndrome,*** sweating, photosensitivity
MS: Cramps, arthritis, stiffness
ENDO: *Hyperglycemia*
HEMA: ***Thrombocytopenia, agranulocytosis, neutropenia***
CV: Chest pain, hypotension, ***circulatory collapse,*** ECG changes
Contraindications: Hypersensitivity to sulfonamides, anuria, hepatic coma, hypovolemia, lactation
Precautions: Dehydration, ascites, severe renal disease, pregnancy (C)
Pharmacokinetics:
PO: Onset ½-1 hr, duration 4 hr
IM: Onset 40 min, duration 4 hr
IV: Onset 5 min, duration 2-3 hr, Excreted by kidneys, crosses placenta, excreted by breast milk
Interactions/incompatibilities:
• Decreased diuretic effect: indomethacin
• Ototoxicity: cisplatin, aminoglycosides, vancomycin
• Increased effect: antihypertensives
• Increased toxicity: lithium, nondepolarizing skeletal muscle relaxants, digitalis
• Decreased effects of: antidiabetics

NURSING CONSIDERATIONS
Assess:
• Hearing with high IV doses
• Weight, I&O daily to determine fluid loss; effect of drug may be decreased if used qd
• Rate, depth, rhythm of respiration, effect of exertion
• B/P lying, standing; postural hypotension may occur
• Electrolytes: potassium, sodium, chloride; include BUN, blood sugar, CBC, serum creatinine, blood pH, ABGs, uric acid, calcium, magnesium
• Glucose in urine if patient is diabetic
Administer:
• Direct IV over at least 1 min
• INT IV after dilution in LR, D_5W, 0.9% NaCl
• In AM to avoid interference with sleep if using drug as a diuretic
• Potassium replacement if potassium is less than 3.0
• With food if nausea occurs; absorption may be decreased slightly
Evaluate:
• Therapeutic response: decreased edema, B/P
• Improvement in edema of feet, legs, sacral area daily if medication is being used in CHF
• Improvement in CVP q8h
• Signs of metabolic alkalosis: drowsiness, restlessness
• Signs of hypokalemia: postural hypotension, malaise, fatigue, tachycardia, leg cramps, weakness
• Rashes, temperature elevation qd
• Confusion, especially in elderly; take safety precautions if needed
Teach patient/family:
• To increase fluid intake 2-3 L/day unless contraindicated; to rise slowly from lying or sitting position
• Adverse reactions: muscle cramps, weakness, nausea, dizziness
• To take with food or milk for GI symptoms
• To take early in day to prevent nocturia
Treatment of overdose: Lavage if taken orally, monitor electrolytes, administer dextrose in saline, monitor hydration, CV, renal status

bupivacaine HCl

(byoop-a-va'caine)
Marcaine, Sensorcaine
Func. class.: Local anesthetic
Chem. class.: Amide

Action: Competes with calcium for sites in nerve membrane that control sodium transport across cell membrane; decreases rise of depolarization phase of action potential
Uses: Epidural anesthesia, peripheral nerve block, caudal anesthesia
Dosage and routes:
Varies depending on route of anesthesia
Available forms include: Inj 0.25%, 0.5%, 0.75%; inj with epinephrine 0.25%, 0.5%, 0.75%
Side effects/adverse reactions:
CNS: Anxiety, restlessness, ***convulsions, loss of consciousness,*** drowsiness, disorientation, tremors, shivering
CV: ***Myocardial depression, cardiac arrest, dysrhythmias,*** bradycardia, hypotension, hypertension, fetal bradycardia
GI: Nausea, vomiting
EENT: Blurred vision, tinnitus, pupil constriction
INTEG: Rash, urticaria, allergic reactions, edema, burning, skin discoloration at injection site, tissue necrosis
RESP: ***Status asthmaticus, respiratory arrest, anaphylaxis***
Contraindications: Hypersensitivity, child <12 yr, elderly, severe liver disease
Precautions: Elderly, severe drug allergies, pregnancy (C)
Pharmacokinetics:
Onset 4-17 min, duration 4-8 hr, excreted in urine (metabolites), metabolized by liver
Interactions/incompatibilities:
• Dysrhythmias: epinephrine, halothane, enflurane
• Hypertension: MAOIs, tricyclic antidepressants, phenothiazines
• Decreased action of bupivacaine: chloroprocaine

NURSING CONSIDERATIONS
Assess:
• B/P, pulse, respiration during treatment
• Fetal heart tones if drug is used during labor
Administer:
• Only with crash cart, resuscitative equipment nearby
• Only drugs without preservatives for epidural or caudal anesthesia
Perform/provide:
• Use of new solution, discard unused portions
Evaluate:
• Therapeutic response: anesthesia necessary for procedure
• Allergic reactions: rash, urticaria, itching
• Cardiac status: ECG for dysrhythmias, pulse, B/P during anesthesia
Treatment of overdose: Airway, O_2, vasopressor, IV fluids, anticonvulsants for seizures

buprenorphine HCl

(byoo-preen'or-feen)
Buprenex
Func. class.: Narcotic analgesics
Chem. class.: Opiate, thebaine derivative

Controlled Substance Schedule V
Action: Depresses pain impulse transmission at the spinal cord level by interacting with opioid receptors
Uses: Moderate to severe pain
Dosage and routes:
• *Adult:* IM/IV 0.3-0.6 mg q6h prn, reduce dosage in elderly

Available forms include: Inj IM, IV 1, 2 mg/ml, 0.3 mg/ml (1 ml vials)

Side effects/adverse reactions:

CNS: Drowsiness, dizziness, confusion, headache, sedation, euphoria

GI: Nausea, vomiting, anorexia, constipation, cramps

GU: Increased urinary output, dysuria

INTEG: Rash, urticaria, bruising, flushing, diaphoresis, pruritus

EENT: Tinnitus, blurred vision, miosis, diplopia

CV: Palpitations, bradycardia, change in B/P

*RESP: **Respiratory depression***

Contraindications: Hypersensitivity, addiction (narcotic)

Precautions: Addictive personality, pregnancy (C), lactation, increased intracranial pressure, MI (acute), severe heart disease, respiratory depression, hepatic disease, renal disease

Pharmacokinetics:

IM: Onset 10-30 min, peak ½ hr, duration 3-4 hr

IV: Onset 1 min, peak 5 min, duration 2-5 hr

REC: Onset slow, duration 4-6 hr; metabolized by liver, excreted by kidneys, crosses placenta, excreted in breast milk, half-life 2½-3½ hr, 96% bound to plasma proteins

Interactions/incompatibilities:

- Effects may be increased with other CNS depressants: alcohol, narcotics, sedative/hypnotics, antipsychotics, skeletal muscle relaxants

NURSING CONSIDERATIONS

Assess:

- I&O ratio; check for decreasing output; may indicate urinary retention

Administer:

- IV slowly over 2-3 min
- With antiemetic if nausea, vomiting occur
- When pain is beginning to return; determine dosage interval by patient response

Perform/provide:

- Assistance with ambulation
- Safety measures: siderails

Evaluate:

- Therapeutic response: decrease in pain, absence of grimacing
- CNS changes, dizziness, drowsiness, hallucinations, euphoria, LOC, pupil reaction
- Allergic reactions: rash, urticaria
- Respiratory dysfunction: respiratory depression, character, rate, rhythm; notify physician if respirations are <12/min
- Need for pain medication, physical dependence

Teach patient/family:

- To report any symptoms of CNS changes, allergic reactions
- That physical dependency may result when used for extended periods of time

Treatment of overdose: Narcan 0.2-0.8 mg IV, O_2, IV fluids, vasopressors

bupropion

(byoo-proe' pee-on)
Wellbutrin

Func. class.: Misc. antidepressant

Action: Inhibits reuptake of dopamine, serotonin, norepinephrine

Uses: Depression

Dosage and routes:

Adult: PO 100 mg bid initially, then increase after 3 day to 100 mg tid if needed; may increase after 1 month to 150 mg tid

Available forms: 75, 100 mg

Side effects/adverse reactions: *CNS: Headache, agitation, confusion,* ***seizures,*** akathisia, delusions, insomnia, sedation, tremors
CV: Dysrhythmias, hypertension, palpitations, tachycardia, hypotension
GI: Nausea, vomiting, dry mouth, increased appetite, constipation
GU: Impotence, frequency, retention
INTEG: Rash, pruritus, sweating
EENT: Blurred vision, auditory disturbance

Contraindications: Hypersensitivity, seizure disorder, eating disorders

Precautions: Renal and hepatic disease, recent MI, cranial trauma, pregnancy (B), lactation, children

Pharmacokinetics: Onset 2-4 wk, half-life 12-14 hr, metabolized by liver

Interactions/incompatibilities:
• Increased adverse reactions: levodopa, MAOIs, phenothiazines, tricyclic antidepressants, benzodiazepines, alcohol

NURSING CONSIDERATIONS

Assess:
• Blood studies: CBC, leukocytes, differential, cardiac enzymes if patient is on long-term therapy
• Liver function tests before, during therapy: bilirubin, AST, ALT, creatinine
• ECG: watch for flattening of T wave, bundle branch block, AV block, dysrhythmias in cardiac patients

Administer:
• Increased fluids, bulk in diet if constipation, urinary retention occur
• With food or milk for GI symptoms
• Gum, hard candy, or frequent sips of water for dry mouth

Perform/provide:
• Assistance with ambulation during beginning therapy, since sedation occurs
• Safety measures, including siderails, primarily in elderly
• Checking to see PO medication is swallowed

Evaluate:
• Therapeutic response: decreased depression, ability to function in daily activities, ability to sleep throughout the night
• Mental status: mood sensorium, affect, suicidal tendencies, increase in psychiatric symptoms
• EPS primarily in elderly: akathisia
• Withdrawal symptoms: headache, nausea, vomiting, muscle pain, weakness occurs if drug is discontinued abruptly
• Alcohol consumption: if alcohol is consumed, hold dose until morning

Teach patient/family:
• Therapeutic effects may take 2-4 wk
• To use caution in driving or other activities requiring alertness; sedation and blurred vision may occur
• To avoid alcohol ingestion, other CNS depressants
• Not to discontinue medication quickly after long-term use, may cause nausea, headache, malaise

Treatment of overdose: ECG monitoring; induce emesis, lavage, activated charcoal; administer anticonvulsant

buspirone HCl

(byoo-spear'own)

BuSpar

Func. class.: Antianxiety agent
Chem. class.: Azaspirodecanedione

Action: Unknown; may act by inhibiting 5-HT, a receptor in brain tissue

Uses: Management and short-term relief of anxiety disorders

Dosage and routes:

• *Adult:* PO 5 mg tid, may increase by 5 mg/day q2-3d, not to exceed 60 mg/day

Available forms include: Tabs 5, 10 mg

Side effects/adverse reactions:

CNS: Dizziness, headache, depression, stimulation, insomnia, nervousness, lightheadedness, numbness, paresthesia, incoordination, tremors, excitement, involuntary movements, confusion, akathisia

GI: Nausea, dry mouth, diarrhea, constipation, flatulence, increased appetite, rectal bleeding

CV: Tachycardia, palpitations, hypotension, hypertension, ***CVA, CHF, MI***

EENT: Sore throat, tinnitus, blurred vision, nasal congestion, red, itching eyes, change in taste, smell

GU: Frequency, hesitancy, menstrual irregularity, change in libido

MS: Pain, weakness, muscle cramps, spasms

RESP: Hyperventilation, chest congestion, shortness of breath

INTEG: Rash, edema, pruritus, alopecia, dry skin

MISC: Sweating, fatigue, weight gain, fever

Contraindications: Hypersensitivity, child <18 yr

Precautions: Pregnancy (B), lactation, elderly, impaired hepatic/renal function

Interactions/incompatibilities:

• Increased B/P: MAOIs; do not use together
• Increased effects: psychotropic drugs, alcohol (avoid use)
• Increased ALT: trazodone

NURSING CONSIDERATIONS

Assess:

• B/P (lying, standing), pulse; if systolic B/P drops 20 mm Hg, hold drug, notify physician
• Blood studies: CBC during long-term therapy; blood dyscrasias have occurred rarely
• Hepatic studies: AST, ALT, bilirubin, creatinine, LDH, alk phosphatase
• I&O; may indicate renal dysfunction
• Mental status: mood, sensorium, affect, sleeping pattern, drowsiness, dizziness

Administer:

• With food or milk for GI symptoms
• Crushed if patient unable to swallow medication whole
• Sugarless gum, hard candy, frequent sips of water for dry mouth

Perform/provide:

• Assistance with ambulation during beginning therapy; drowsiness, dizziness occur
• Safety measures, including siderails if drowsiness occurs
• Check to see PO medication swallowed

Evaluate:

• Therapeutic response: decreased anxiety, restlessness, sleeplessness
• Suicidal tendencies

Teach patient/family:

• That drug may be taken with food
• To avoid OTC preparations unless approved by physician

• To avoid driving, activities requiring alertness, since drowsiness may occur
• To avoid alcohol ingestion or other psychotropic medications, unless prescribed by physician
• Not to discontinue medication abruptly after long-term use
• To rise slowly or fainting may occur, especially elderly
• That drowsiness might worsen at beginning of treatment
• 1-2 wk of therapy may be required before therapeutic effects occur

Treatment of overdose: Gastric lavage, VS, supportive care

---

busulfan

(byoo-sul'fan)

Myleran

Func. class.: Antineoplastic alkylating agent

Chem. class.: Nitrosurea

Action: Changes essential cellular ions to covalent bonding with resultant alkylation; this interferes with normal biologic function of DNA; activity is not phase specific, action is due to myelosuppression

Uses: Chronic myelocytic leukemia

Dosage and routes:

• *Adult:* PO 4-12 mg/day initially until WBC levels fall to 10,000/mm^3, then drug is stopped until WBC levels raise over 50,000/mm^3, then 1-3 mg/day
• *Child:* PO 0.06-0.12 mg/kg or 1.8-4.6 mg/m^2 day; dose is titrated to maintain WBC levels at 20,000/mm^3

Available forms include: Tab 2 mg

Side effects/adverse reactions:

HEMA: ***Thrombocytopenia, leukopenia, pancytopenia, severe bone marrow depression***

GI: Nausea, vomiting, *diarrhea, weight loss*

GU: Impotence, sterility, amenorrhea, gynecomastia, ***renal toxicity,*** hyperuremia

INTEG: Dermatitis, hyperpigmentation

RESP: ***Fibrosis,*** pneumonitis

OTHER: ***Chromosomal aberrations***

Contraindications: Radiation, chemotherapy, lactation, pregnancy (3rd trimester) (D), "blastic" phase of chronic myelocytic leukemia, hypersensitivity

Precautions: Childbearing age men, women, leukopenia, thrombocytopenia, anemia, hepatotoxicity, renal toxicity

Pharmacokinetics:

Well absorbed orally, excreted in urine, crosses placenta, excreted in breast milk

Interactions/incompatibilities:

Increased toxicity: other antineoplastics or radiation

NURSING CONSIDERATIONS

Assess:

• CBC, differential, platelet count weekly; withhold drug if WBC is <4000 or platelet count is <75,000; notify physician of results
• Pulmonary function tests, chest x-ray films before, during therapy; chest film should be obtained q2wk during treatment
• Renal function studies: BUN, serum uric acid, urine CrCl before, during therapy
• I&O ratio; report fall in urine output of 30 ml/hr
• Monitor for cold, fever, sore throat (may indicate beginning infection)
• For decreased hyperuricemia

---

* Available in Canada only

Administer:
• Antacid before oral agent, give drug after evening meal, before bedtime
• Antiemetic 30-60 min before giving drug to prevent vomiting
• Allopurinol or sodium bicarbonate to maintain uric acid levels, alkalinization of urine
• Antibiotics for prophylaxis of infection

Perform/provide:
• Comprehensive oral hygiene
• Strict medical asepsis, protective isolation if WBC levels are low
• Deep breathing exercises with patient tid-qid; place in semi-Fowler's position for pulmonary reactions
• Increase fluid intake to 2-3 L/day to prevent urate deposits, calculi formation
• Diet low in purines: organ meats (kidney, liver), dried beans, peas to maintain alkaline urine
• Storage in tight container

Evaluate:
• Therapeutic response: decreased exacerbations of chronic myelocytic leukemia
• Bleeding: hematuria, guaiac, bruising or petechiae, mucosa or orifices q8h, no rectal temps
• Dyspnea, rales, unproductive cough, chest pain, tachypnea
• Food preferences; list likes, dislikes
• Edema in feet, joint, stomach pain, shaking
• Inflammation of mucosa, breaks in skin, use viscous xylocaine for oral pain

Teach patient/family:
• About protective isolation precautions
• To avoid use of products containing aspirin or ibuprofen, razors, commercial mouthwash
• To report signs of anemia, (fatigue, headache, irritability, faintness, shortness of breath)
• To report symptoms of bleeding (hematuria, tarry stools)
• That impotence or amenorrhea can occur, are reversible after discontinuing treatment
• To report any changes in breathing or coughing even several months after treatment

---

butoconazole nitrate

(byoo'toe-kone-a-zole)
Femstat

Func. class.: Local antiinfective
Chem. class.: Antifungal

Action: Binds sterols in fungal cell membrane, which increases permeability

Uses: Vulvovaginal infections caused by *Candida*

Dosage and routes:
• *Adult:* INTRA VAG 1 applicatorful hs × 3 days (nonpregnant), 6 days (2nd/3rd trimester pregnancy)

Available forms include: Vaginal cream 2%

Side effects/adverse reactions:
GU: Rash, stinging, burning, vulvovaginal itching, soreness, swelling, discharge

Contraindications: Hypersensitivity

Precautions: Pregnancy (C), lactation

NURSING CONSIDERATIONS

Administer:
• 1 applicatorful every night into vagina

Perform/provide:
• Storage at room temperature in dry place

Evaluate:
• Therapeutic response: decrease in itching, or white discharge

• Allergic reaction: burning, stinging, itching, discharge, soreness

Teach patient/family:

• To use medical asepsis (hand washing) before, after each application

• May experience increased dreaming

• To apply with applicator only

• To avoid use of any other vaginal product unless directed by physician, sanitary napkin may prevent soiling of undergarments

• To abstain from sexual intercourse until treatment is completed

• To notify physician if symptoms persist

---

butorphanol tartrate

(byoo-tor'fa-nole)

Stadol

Func. class.: Narcotic analgesics
Chem. class.: Opiate

Action: Depresses pain impulse transmission at the spinal cord level by interacting with opioid receptors

Uses: Moderate to severe pain

Dosage and routes:

• *Adult:* IM 1-4 mg q3-4h prn; IV 0.5-2 mg q3-4h prn

Available forms include: Inj IM, IV 1, 2 mg/ml

Side effects/adverse reactions:

CNS: Drowsiness, dizziness, confusion, headache, sedation, euphoria, weakness

GI: Nausea, vomiting, anorexia, constipation, cramps

GU: Increased urinary output, dysuria, urinary retention

INTEG: Rash, urticaria, bruising, flushing, diaphoresis, pruritus

EENT: Tinnitus, blurred vision, miosis, diplopia

CV: Palpitations, bradycardia, change in B/P

RESP: ***Respiratory depression,*** pulmonary hypertension

Contraindications: Hypersensitivity, addiction (narcotic), CHF, myocardial infarction

Precautions: Addictive personality, pregnancy (B), lactation, increased intracranial pressure, respiratory depression, hepatic disease, renal disease, child <18 yr

Pharmacokinetics:

IM: Onset 10-30 min, peak ½ hr, duration 3-4 hr

IV: Onset 1 min, peak 5 min, duration 2-4 hr

REC: Onset slow, duration 4-6 hr, metabolized by liver, excreted by kidneys, crosses placenta, excreted in breast milk, half-life 2½-3½ hr

Interactions/incompatibilities:

• Effects may be increased with other CNS depressants: alcohol, narcotics, sedative/hypnotics, antipsychotics, skeletal muscle relaxants

NURSING CONSIDERATIONS

Assess:

• I&O ratio; check for decreasing output; may indicate urinary retention

• For withdrawal symptoms in narcotic dependent patients: pulmonary embolus, vascular occlusion, abscesses, ulcerations

Administer:

• IV over 3-5 min

• IM deeply in large muscle mass

• With antiemetic if nausea, vomiting occur

• When pain is beginning to return; determine dosage interval by patient response

Perform/provide:

• Storage in light-resistant area at room temperature

• Assistance with ambulation

• Safety measures: siderails, night

---

light, call bell within easy reach, especially elderly

Evaluate:

- Therapeutic response: decrease in pain
- CNS changes: dizziness, drowsiness, hallucinations, euphoria, LOC, pupil reaction
- Allergic reactions: rash, urticaria
- Respiratory dysfunction: respiratory depression, character, rate, rhythm; notify physician if respirations are <10/min
- Need for pain medication, physical dependence

Teach patient/family:

- To report any symptoms of CNS changes, allergic reactions
- That physical dependency may result when used for extended periods of time
- That withdrawal symptoms may occur: nausea, vomiting, cramps, fever, faintness, anorexia

Lab test interferences:

Increase: Amylase

Treatment of overdose: Narcan 0.2-0.8 mg IV, O_2, IV fluids, vasopressors

caffeine

(kaf-een)

No-Doz, Tirend, Vivarin, Dexitac, Quick Pep

Func. class.: Analeptic
Chem. class.: Xanthine

Action: Increases calcium permeability in sarcoplasmic reticulum, promotes accumulation of cAMP, and competitively blocks adenosine receptors

Uses: Mild CNS stimulation, in combination with analgesics, diuretics for tension and fluid retention associated with menstruation

Dosage and routes:

- *Adult:* PO 100-200 mg q4h prn; IM 500 mg; timed rel 200-250 mg q4-6h

Available forms include: Tabs 65, 150 mg; time rel caps 200, 250 mg; inj 850 mg/ml

Side effects/adverse reactions:

CNS: Hyperactivity, insomnia, restlessness, talkativeness, dizziness, headache, *stimulation,* irritability, aggressiveness, tremors, twitching, mild delirium, tinnitus

GI: Nausea, vomiting, anorexia, gastric irritation, diarrhea

GU: Diuresis

CV: Tachycardia, extrasystole, dysrhythmias, palpitations

INTEG: Hyperesthesia

Contraindications: Hypersensitivity

Precautions: Dysrhythmias, Gilles de la Tourette's disorder, pregnancy (B), lactation, renal, psychological disorders

Pharmacokinetics:

PO: Onset 15 min, peak ½-1 hr, metabolized by liver, excreted by kidneys, crosses placenta, breast milk, half-life 3-4 hr

Interactions/incompatibilities:

- Increased effect of caffeine: oral contraceptives, cimetidine, theophylline

NURSING CONSIDERATIONS

Assess:

- VS, B/P

Evaluate:

- Therapeutic response: increased CNS stimulation, decreased drowsiness
- Mental status: mood, sensorium, affect, stimulation, insomnia, irritability
- Tolerance or dependency: an increased amount may be used to get same effect

• Overdose: pain, fever, dehydration, insomnia, hyperactivity

Teach patient/family:

• To decrease other caffeine consumption (coffee, tea, cola, chocolate), which may increase irritability, stimulation

• To taper off drug over several weeks if used long-term

Lab test interferences:

Increase: Urinary cathecholamines

False positive: Serum urate

Treatment of overdose: Lavage, activated charcoal, monitor electrolytes, VS, administer anticonvulsants if needed

---

calcifediol

(kal-si-fe-dye′ole)

Calderol

Func. class.: Vitamin D analog

Chem. class.: Sterol

Action: Increases intestinal absorption of calcium for bones; increases renal tubular absorption of phosphate, increases mobilization of calcium from bones, bone resorption

Uses: Metabolic bone disease with chronic renal failure, osteopenia, osteomalacia, hypocalcemia

Dosage and routes:

• *Adult:* PO 300-350 μg qwk divided into qd or qod doses; may increase q4wk

Available forms include: Caps 20, 50 μg

Side effects/adverse reactions:

EENT: Tinnitus

CNS: Drowsiness, headache, vertigo, fever, lethargy

GI: Nausea, diarrhea, vomiting, jaundice, anorexia, dry mouth, constipation, cramps, metallic taste

MS: Myalgia, arthralgia, decreased bone development

GU: Polyuria, hypercalciuria, hyperphosphatemia, hematuria

CV: dysrhythmias

Contraindications: Hypersensitivity, hyperphosphatemia, hypercalcemia

Precautions: Pregnancy (C), renal calculi, lactation, CV disease

Pharmacokinetics:

PO: Peak 4 hr, duration 15-20 days; half-life 12-22 days

Interactions/incompatibilities:

• Decreased absorption of calcifediol: cholestyramine, colestipol HCl, mineral oil

• Hypercalcemia: thiazide diuretics

• Cardiac dysrhythmias: cardiac glycosides

• Decreased effect of this drug: corticosteroids

NURSING CONSIDERATIONS

Assess:

• BUN, urinary calcium, AST, ALT, cholesterol, creatinine, uric acid, chloride, magnesium, electrolytes, urine pH, phosphate; may increase, calcium should be kept at 9-10 mg/dl, vitamin D 50-135 IU/dl, phosphate 70 mg/dl

• Alk phosphatase; may be decreased

• For increased blood level since toxic reactions may occur rapidly

Administer:

• PO may be increased q4wk depending on blood level

Perform/provide:

• Storage in tight, light-resistant containers at room temperature

• Restriction of sodium, potassium if required

• Restriction of fluids if required for chronic renal failure

Evaluate:

• Therapeutic response: calcium levels 9-10 mg/dl, decreasing symptoms of bone disease

• For dry mouth, metallic taste,

---

polyuria, bone pain, muscle weakness, headache, fatigue, tinnitus, change in LOC, irregular pulse, dysrhythmias, increased respirations, anorexia, nausea, vomiting, cramps, diarrhea, constipation; may indicate hypercalcemia

• Renal status: decreased urinary output (oliguria, anuria), edema in extremities, weight gain 5 lb, periorbital edema

• Nutritional status, diet for sources of vitamin D (milk, some seafood), calcium (dairy products, dark green vegetables), phosphates (dairy products)

Teach patient/family:

• The symptoms of hypercalcemia

• About foods rich in calcium

Lab test interferences:

False increase: Cholesterol

---

calcitonin (human)

(kal-si-toe'nin)

Cibacalcin

Func. class.: Parathyroid agents (calcium regulator)

Chem. class.: Polypeptide hormone

Action: Decreases bone resorption, blood calcium levels; increases deposits of calcium in bones

Uses: Paget's disease

Dosage and routes:

Paget's disease

• *Adult:* SC 0.5 mg/day initially; may require 0.5 mg bid × 6 mo, then decrease until symptoms reappear

Available forms include: Inj (SC) 0.5 mg/vial

Side effects/adverse reactions:

INTEG: Rash, flushing, pruritus of ear lobes, edema of feet

CNS: Headache, tetany, chills, weakness, dizziness

GU: Diuresis

GI: Nausea, diarrhea, vomiting, anorexia, abdominal pain, salty taste

MS: Swelling, tingling of hands

CV: Chest pressure

RESP: Dyspnea

Contraindications: Hypersensitivity

Precautions: Renal disease, children, lactation, osteogenic sarcoma, pregnancy (C)

Pharmacokinetics:

IM/SC: Onset 15 min, peak 4 hr, duration 8-24 hr; metabolized by kidneys, excreted as inactive metabolites

NURSING CONSIDERATIONS

Assess:

• GI symptoms, polyuria, flushing, head swelling, tingling, headache; may indicate hypercalcemia

• Nutritional status; diet for sources of vitamin D (milk, some seafood), calcium (dairy products, dark green vegetables), phosphates

Administer:

• By SC route only, rotate injection sites; use within 6 hr of reconstitution, give hs to minimize nausea, vomiting

Perform/provide:

• Store at <77° F, protect from light

Evaluate:

• Therapeutic response: calcium levels 9-10 mg/dl, decreasing symptoms of Paget's disease

• BUN, creatinine, uric acid, chloride, electrolytes, urine pH, urinary calcium, magnesium, phosphate, urinalysis, (calcium should be kept at 9-10 mg/dl, vitamin D 50-135 IU/dl), alk phosphatase baseline and q3-6 mo

• Increased drug level since toxic reactions occur rapidly, have calcium chloride on hand if calcium level drops too low; check for tetany

• Urine for sediment

Teach patient/family:

• Method of injection if patient will be responsible for self-medication

---

calcitonin (salmon)

(kal-si-toe'nin)

Calcimar, Miacalcin

Func. class.: Parathyroid agents (calcium regulator)

Chem. class.: Polypeptide hormone

Action: Decreases bone resorption, blood calcium levels; increases deposits of calcium in bones

Uses: Hypercalcemia, postmenopausal osteoporosis, Paget's disease

Dosage and routes:

Osteoporosis/Paget's disease

• *Adult:* SC/IM 100 IU qd, maintenance for Paget's disease 50-100 IU qd or qod

Hypercalcemia

• *Adult:* IM 4-8 IU/kg q6-12h

Available forms include: Inj SC/IM 200 MRC units/ml, 100 IU/ml

Side effects/adverse reactions:

INTEG: Rash, pruritus of ear lobes, edema of feet

CNS: Headache, flushing, ***tetany,*** chills, weakness, dizziness

GU: Diuresis

GI: Nausea, diarrhea, vomiting, anorexia, abdominal pain, salty taste

MS: Swelling, tingling of hands

Contraindications: Hypersensitivity, children, lactation

Precautions: Renal disease, osteoporosis, pernicious anemia, Zollinger-Ellison syndrome, pregnancy (C)

Pharmacokinetics:

IM/SC: Onset 15 min, peak 4 hr, duration 8-24 hr; metabolized by kidneys, excreted as inactive metabolites

NURSING CONSIDERATIONS

Assess:

• BUN, creatinine, uric acid, chloride, electrolytes, urine pH, urinary calcium, magnesium, phosphatase, urinalysis, calcitonin antibody formation (calcium should be kept at 9-10 mg/dl, vitamin D 50-135 IU/dl), alk phosphatase

• Increased level since toxic reactions may occur rapidly

• Urine for sediment and casts

Administer:

• After test dose of 10 IU/ml, give 0.1 ml intradermally, watch 15 min; give only with epinephrine and emergency meds available

• IM injection in deep muscle mass slowly, rotate sites

Perform/provide:

• Storage in light-resistant area, refrigerate

• Restriction of sodium, potassium if required

Evaluate:

• Therapeutic response: calcium 9-10 mg/dl, decreasing symptoms of bone disease

• GI symptoms, polyuria, flushing, head swelling, tingling, headache; may indicate hypercalcemia

• Nutritional status; diet for sources of vitamin D (milk, some seafood), calcium (dairy products, dark green vegetables), phosphates

• Systemic allergic reaction to drug: skin test before 1st dose

Teach patient/family:

• To avoid OTC products

• To administer drug SC if patient will be responsible for self-medication

---

* Available in Canada only

calcitriol (1,25-Dihydroxycholecalciferol)

(kal-si-tyre'ole)
Rocaltrol

Func. class.: Parathyroid agents (calcium regulator)
Chem. class.: Vitamin D hormone

Action: Increases intestinal absorption of calcium, provides calcium for bones, increases renal tubular resorption of phosphate

Uses: Hypocalcemia in chronic renal dialysis, hypoparathyroidism, pseudohypoparathyroidism

Dosage and routes:

Hypocalcemia

• *Adult:* PO 0.25 μg qd, may increase by 0.25 μg/day q4-8wk, maintenance 0.25 μg qod-1 μg qd

Hypoparathyroidism/pseudohypoparathyroidism

• *Adult and child >1 yr:* PO 0.25 μg qd, may be increased q2-4wk; maintenance 0.25-2 μg qd

Available forms include: Caps 0.25, 0.5 μg

Side effects/adverse reactions:

CNS: Drowsiness, headache, vertigo, fever, lethargy

GI: Nausea, diarrhea, vomiting, jaundice, anorexia, dry mouth, constipation, cramps, metallic taste

MS: Myalgia, arthralgia, decreased bone development

GU: Polyuria, hypercalciuria, hyperphosphatemia, hematuria

Contraindications: Hypersensitivity, hyperphosphatemia, hypercalcemia

Precautions: Pregnancy (C), renal calculi, lactation, CV disease

Pharmacokinetics:

PO: Peak 4 hr, duration 15-20 days, half-life 3-6 hr

Interactions/incompatibilities:

• Decreased absorption of calcitriol: cholestyramine, mineral oil
• Hypercalcemia: thiazide diuretics, calcium supplement
• Cardiac dysrhythmias: cardiac glycosides, verapamil
• Decreased effect of calcifediol: barbiturates, phenytoin, corticosteroids

NURSING CONSIDERATIONS

Assess:

• BUN, urinary calcium, AST, ALT, cholesterol, creatinine, uric acid, chloride, magnesium, electrolytes, urine pH, phosphate; may increase calcium, should be kept at 9-10 mg/dl, vitamin D 50-135 IU/dl, phosphate 70 mg/dl
• Alk phosphatase; may be decreased
• For increased drug level since toxic reactions may occur rapidly

Perform/provide:

• Storage protected from light, heat, moisture
• Restriction of sodium, potassium if required
• Restriction of fluids if required for chronic renal failure

Evaluate:

• Therapeutic response: calcium 9-10 mg/dl, decreasing symptoms of hypocalcemia, hypoparathyroidism
• For dry mouth, metallic taste, polyuria, bone pain, muscle weakness, headache, fatigue, change in LOC, dysrhythmias, increased respirations, anorexia, nausea, vomiting, cramps, diarrhea, constipation; may indicate hypercalcemia
• Renal status: decreased urinary output (oliguria, anuria), edema in extremities, weight gain 75 lb, periorbital edema
• Nutritional status, diet for sources of vitamin D (milk, some seafood), calcium (dairy products, dark green vegetables), phosphates (dairy products) must be avoided

Teach patient/family:
- The symptoms of hypercalcemia
- About foods rich in calcium
- To avoid products with sodium: cured meats, dairy products, cold cuts, olives, beets, pickles, soups, meat tenderizers in chronic renal failure
- To avoid products with potassium: oranges, bananas, dried fruit, peas, dark green leafy vegetables, milk, melons, beans in chronic renal failure
- To avoid OTC products containing calcium, potassium, or sodium in chronic renal failure
- To avoid all preparations containing vitamin D

Lab test interferences:
False increase: Cholesterol

calcium carbonate

Alka-2, Amitone, Apo-Cal, Biocal Calcilac, Calglycine, Chooz, Dicarbosil, El-Da-Minte, Equilet, Gustalac, Mallamint, Os-Cal, P.H. Tablets, Titracid, Titralac, Trialea, Tums, Cal-sup, Caltrate

Func. class.: Antacid, calcium supplement
Chem. class.: Calcium product

Action: Neutralizes gastric acidity
Uses: Antacid, calcium supplement
Dosage and routes:
- *Adult:* PO 1 g 4-6 ×/day, chewed with water; SUSP 1 g 1 hr pc, hs

Available forms include: Chewable tabs 350, 420, 500, 750 mg; tabs 650 mg; gum 500 mg; susp 1 g/5 ml
Side effects/adverse reactions:
GI: Constipation, anorexia, ***obstruction,*** nausea, vomiting, flatulence, diarrhea, rebound hyperacidity, eructation
CV: ***Hemorrhage, rebound hypertension***
META: Hypercalcemia, metabolic alkalosis
GU: Renal dysfunction, renal stones, ***renal failure***
Contraindications: Hypersensitivity, hypercalcemia, hyperparathyroidism, bone tumors
Precautions: Elderly, fluid restriction, decreased GI motility, GI obstruction, dehydration, renal disease, pregnancy (C)
Pharmacokinetics:
PO: Onset 3 min, excreted in feces
Interactions/incompatibilities:
- Increased plasma levels of: quinidine, amphetamines
- Decreased levels of: salicylates, calcium channel blockers, ketoconazole, tetracyclines, iron salts
- Hypercalcemia: thiazide diuretics

NURSING CONSIDERATIONS

Assess:
- Ca^+ (serum, urine), Ca^+ should be 8.5-10.5 mg/dl, urine Ca^+ should be 150 mg/day, monitor weekly

Administer:
- As antacid 1 hr pc and hs
- As supplement 1½ hr pc and hs
- Only with regular tablets or capsules, do not give with enteric-coated tablets
- Laxatives, or stool softeners if constipation occurs

Evaluate:
- Therapeutic response: absence of pain, decreased acidity
- Milk-alkali syndrome: nausea, vomiting, disorientation, headache
- Constipation; increase bulk in the diet if needed
- Hypercalcemia: headache, nausea, vomiting, confusion

Teach patient/family:
- To increase fluids to 2000 ml unless contraindicated

* Available in Canada only

• Not to switch antacids unless directed by physician

calcium chloride/calcium gluceptate/calcium gluconate/calcium lactate

Func. class.: Electrolyte replacement—calcium product

Action: Cation needed for maintenance of nervous, muscular, skeletal, enzyme reactions, normal cardiac contractility, coagulation of blood; affects secretory activity of endocrine, exocrine glands

Uses: Prevention and treatment of hypocalcemia, hypermagnesemia, hypoparathyroidism, neonatal tetany, cardiac toxicity caused by hyperkalemia, lead colic

Dosage and routes:

Calcium chloride

• *Adult:* IV 500 mg-1 g q1-3 days as indicated by serum calcium levels, give at <1 ml/min; IAV 200-800 mg injected in ventricle of heart

• *Child:* IV 25 mg/kg over several min

Calcium gluceptate

• *Adult:* IV 5-20 ml; IM 2-5 ml

• *Newborn:* 0.5 ml/100 ml of blood transfused

Calcium gluconate

• *Adult:* PO 0.5-2 g bid-qid; IV 0.5-2 g at 0.5 ml/min (10% solution)

• *Child:* PO/IV 500 mg/kg/day in divided doses

Calcium lactate

• *Adult:* PO 325 mg-1.3 g tid with meals

• *Child:* PO 500 mg/kg/day in divided doses

Available forms include: Many, check product listings

Side effects/adverse reactions:

INTEG: Pain, burning at IV site, severe venous thrombosis, necrosis, extravasation

Hypercalcemia: Drowsiness, lethargy, muscle weakness, headache, constipation, ***coma,*** anorexia, nausea, vomiting, polyuria, thirst

CV: Shortened Q-T, heart block, hypotension, bradycardia, dysrthymias, ***cardiac arrest***

Contraindications: Hypercalcemia, digitalis toxicity, ventricular fibrillation, renal calculi

Precautions: Pregnancy (C), lactation, children, renal disease, respiratory disease, cor pulmonale, digitalized patient, respiratory failure

Interactions/incompatibilities:

• Increased dysrhythmias: digitalis glycosides

• Decreased action: calcium channel blockers

NURSING CONSIDERATIONS

Assess:

• ECG for decreased QT and T wave inversion: hypercalcemia, drug should be reduced or discontinued

• Calcium levels during treatment (8.5-1.5 g/dl is normal level)

Administer:

• Through small-bore needle into large vein, give over several min, if extravasation occurs, necrosis will result (IV); may be given directly or diluted in compatible IV sol; IM injection may cause severe burning, necrosis, and tissue sloughing, warm sol to body temp before administering

• In large vein, avoiding scalp

• PO with or following meals to enhance absorption

Perform/provide:

• Seizure precautions: padded side rails, decreased stimuli, (noise, light); place airway suction equip-

ment, padded mouth gag if Ca levels are low
• Store at room temperature
Evaluate:
• Therapeutic response: decreased twitching, paresthesias, muscle spasms, absence of tremors, convulsions, dysrhythmias, dyspnea, laryngospasm, negative Chvostek's sign, negative Trousseau's sign
• Cardiac status: rate, rhythm, CVP, (PWP, PAWP if being monitored directly)
Teach patient/family:
• To remain recumbent ½ hr after IV dose
• To add food high in vitamin D content
• To add calcium-rich foods to diet: dairy products, shellfish, dark green leafy vegetables; and decrease oxalate-rich and zinc-rich foods: nuts, legumes, chocolate, spinach, soy
• To prevent injuries, avoid immobilization
Lab test interferences:
Increase: 11-OCHS
False decrease: Magnesium
Decrease: 17-OHCS

calcium polycarbophil

(pol-i-kar'boe-fil)
Mitrolan
Func. class.: Laxative
Chem. class.: Bulk-forming

Action: Attracts water, expands in intestine to increase peristalsis; also absorbs excess water in stool; decreases diarrhea
Uses: Constipation, irritable bowel syndrome (diarrhea), acute, nonspecific diarrhea
Dosage and routes:
• *Adult:* PO 1 g qd-qid prn, not to exceed 6 g/24 hr
• *Child 6-12 yr:* PO 500 mg bid prn, not to exceed 3 g/24 hr
• *Child 3-6 yr:* PO 500 mg bid prn, not to exceed 1.5 g/24 hr
Available forms include: Chew tab 500, 625, 1250 mg
Side effects/adverse reactions:
GI: ***Obstruction,*** abdominal distention, laxative dependency, flatus
Contraindications: Hypersensitivity, GI obstruction
Precautions: Pregnancy (C)
Pharmacokinetics:
PO: Onset 12-24 min, peak 1-3 days

NURSING CONSIDERATIONS

Assess:
• Blood, urine electrolytes if drug is used often by patient
• I&O ratio to identify fluid loss
Administer:
• Alone for better absorption; do not take within 1 hr of other drugs
• In morning or evening (oral dose)
Evaluate:
• Therapeutic response: decreased constipation
• Cause of constipation; identify whether fluids, bulk, or exercise is missing from lifestyle
• Cramping, rectal bleeding, nausea, vomiting; if these symptoms occur, drug should be discontinued
Teach patient/family:
• Not to use laxatives for long-term therapy; bowel tone will be lost
• That normal bowel movements do not always occur daily
• Not to use in presence of abdominal pain, nausea, vomiting
• To notify physician if constipation unrelieved or if symptoms of electrolyte imbalance occur: muscle cramps, pain, weakness, dizziness
• To chew thoroughly and follow with water

capreomycin sulfate

(kap-ree-oh-mye'sin)
Capastat Sulfate
Func. class.: Antitubercular
Chem. class.: *S. carpreolus* polypeptide antibiotic

Action: Inhibits RNA synthesis, decreases tubercle bacilli replication
Uses: Pulmonary tuberculosis as adjunct
Dosage and routes:
• *Adult:* IM 1 g qd × 2-4 mo, then 1 g 2-3 × /wk × 18-24 mo, not to exceed 20 mg/kg/day, must be given with another antitubercular medication
Available forms include: Powder for inj 1 g/10 ml vial
Side effects/adverse reactions:
INTEG: Pain, irritation, sterile abscess at injection site, rash, urticaria
CNS: Vertigo, fever
EENT: Tinnitus, ***deafness, ototoxicity***
GU: ***Proteinuria,*** decreased CrCl, increased BUN, serum Cr, ***tubular necrosis,*** hypokalemia, alkalosis, ***hematuria, albuminuria, nephrotoxicity***
HEMA: ***Eosinophilia, leukocytosis, leukopenia***
Contraindications: Hypersensitivity
Precautions: Renal disease, hearing impairment, allergy history, hepatic disease, pregnancy (C)
Pharmacokinetics:
IM: Peak 1-2 hr, half-life 4-6 hr; excreted in urine unchanged
Interactions/incompatibilities:
• Increased renal toxicity: aminoglycosides, polymyxin, colistin, vancomycin
• Increased neuroblocking action: phenothiazine, tubocurarine, neostigmine

NURSING CONSIDERATIONS
Assess:
• Liver studies qwk: ALT, AST, bilirubin; potassium
• Renal status: before; qwk: BUN, creatinine, output, sp gr, urinalysis
• Blood levels of drug
• Audiometric testing before, during, after treatment
Administer:
• After reconstituting with NS or sterile water for injection, wait 2-3 min before giving
• With other antituberculars
• IM in large muscle mass, rotate sites
• Reduced dosage in renal impairment, if BUN >20 mg/dl, drug should be decreased or discontinued
Evaluate:
• Therapeutic response: decreased dyspnea, fatigue
• Ototoxicity: tinnitus, vertigo, change in hearing
• Hepatic status: decreased appetite, jaundice, dark urine, fatigue
Teach patient/family:
• That compliance with dosage schedule, duration is necessary
• Side effects, adverse reactions: hearing loss, change in urine or urinary habits

captopril

(kap'toe-pril)
Capoten
Func. class.: Antihypertensive
Chem. class.: Renin-angiotensin antagonist

Action: Selectively suppresses renin-angiotensin-aldosterone system; inhibits ACE, prevents conversion of angiotensin I to angiotensin II, results in dilation of arterial, venous vessels

Uses: Hypertension, heart failure not responsive to conventional therapy

Dosage and routes:

Malignant hypertension

• *Adult:* PO 25 mg increasing q2h until desired response, not to exceed 450 mg/day

Hypertension

• *Initial dose:* 12.5 mg 2-3 × daily; may increase to 50 mg bid-tid at 1-2 wk intervals; usual range: 25-150 mg bid-tid; max 450 mg

CHF

• *Adult:* PO 12.5 mg 2-3 × daily given with a diuretic, digitalis; may increase to 50 mg bid-tid, after 14 days, may increase to 150 mg tid if needed

Available forms include: Tabs 12.5, 25, 37.5, 50, 100 mg

Side effects/adverse reactions:

CV: Hypotension

GU: Impotence, dysuria, nocturia, proteinuria, ***nephrotic syndrome, acute reversible renal failure,*** polyuria, oliguria, frequency

HEMA: ***Neutropenia***

INT: Rash, *angioedema*

RESP: ***Bronchospasm,*** dyspnea, cough

META: Hyperkalemia

GI: Loss of taste

CNS: Fever, chills

Contraindications: Hypersensitivity, pregnancy (C), lactation, heart block, children, K-sparing diuretics

Precautions: Dialysis patients, hypovolemia, leukemia, scleroderma, lupus erythematosus, blood dyscrasias, CHF, diabetes mellitus, renal disease, thyroid disease, COPD, asthma

Pharmacokinetics:

PO: Peak 1 hr; duration 2-6 hr; half-life 6-7 hr, metabolized by liver (metabolites), excreted in urine, crosses placenta, excreted in breast milk

Interactions/incompatibilities:

• Increased hypotension: diuretics, other antihypertensives, ganglionic blockers, adrenergic blockers

• Do not use with vasodilators, hydralazine, prazosin, potassium-sparing diuretics, sympathomimetics

NURSING CONSIDERATIONS

Assess:

• Blood studies: neutrophils, decreased platelets

• B/P

• Renal studies: protein, BUN, creatinine, watch for increased levels that may indicate nephrotic syndrome

• Baselines in renal, liver function tests before therapy begins

• K levels, although hyperkalemia rarely occurs

• Dipstick of urine for protein qd in first morning specimen, if protein is increased a 24 hr urinary protein should be collected

Administer:

• IV infusion of 0.9% NaCl (as ordered) to expand fluid volume if severe hypotension occurs

Perform/provide:

• Storage in tight container at 30° C or less

• Supine or Trendelenburg position for severe hypotension

Evaluate:

• Therapeutic response: decrease in B/P in hypertension, decreased B/P, edema, moist rales (CHF)

• Edema in feet, legs daily

• Allergic reaction: rash, fever, pruritus, urticaria; drug should be

discontinued if antihistamines fail to help
• Symptoms of CHF: edema, dyspnea, wet rales, B/P
• Renal symptoms: polyuria, oliguria, frequency
Teach patient/family:
• To administer 1 hr before meals
• Not to discontinue drug abruptly
• Not to use OTC (cough, cold, or allergy) products unless directed by physician
• To avoid sunlight or wear sunscreen if in sunlight, photosensitivity may occur
• To comply with dosage schedule, even if feeling better
• To rise slowly to sitting or standing position to minimize orthostatic hypotension
• To notify physician of mouth sores, sore throat, fever, swelling of hands or feet, irregular heartbeat, chest pain, signs of angioedema
• That excessive perspiration, dehydration, vomiting; diarrhea may lead to fall in blood pressure—consult physician if these occur
• That dizziness, fainting, lightheadedness may occur during 1st few days of therapy
• That skin rash or impaired perspiration may occur
• How to take B/P
Lab test interferences:
False positive: Urine acetone
Treatment of overdose: 0.9% Na Ca IV/INF hemodialysis

carbachol

(kar'ba-kole)

Miostat, Carbacel, Isopto Carbachol, Carcholin, Doryl, Lentin, Mistura C, P.V. Carbachol, Murocarb

Func. class.: Miotic, cholinergic

Action: Contracts spinchter muscle of iris, causes spasms of ciliary muscle, deepening of anterior chamber
Uses: Miosis in ocular surgery, glaucoma (open-angle, narrow-angle)
Dosage and routes:
Ocular surgery
• *Adult:* INSTILL 0.5 ml (intraocular) of 0.01% solution in anterior chamber of eye (done by physician) for miosis during surgery
Glaucoma
• *Adult:* INSTILL 1-2 gtt (topical) of 0.75%-3% solution into eye bid-tid
Available forms include: 0.75%, 1.5%, 2.25%, 3.0% sol for topical use; sol, powders for preparing sol for inj
Side effects/adverse reactions:
CV: ***Marked hypotension,*** bradycardia, headache
GI: Nausea, vomiting, abdominal discomfort, diarrhea, salivation
EENT: Blurred vision, varying degrees of myopia, decreased visual acuity in dim light, slight conjunctival hyperemia, altered distance vision, decreased night vision, eye ache
RESP: Asthma attacks
Contraindications: Hypersensitivity, when miosis is undesirable, corneal abrasions
Precautions: Bradycardia, CAD, hyperthyroidism, asthma, pregnancy, obstruction of GI or urinary tract, peptic ulcer, parkinsonism, epilepsy, peritonitis
Pharmacokinetics:
INSTILL/OINT: Miosis onset 10-20 min, duration 4-8 hr; decreased IOP onset 4 hr duration 8 hr

NURSING CONSIDERATIONS

Assess:
• Heart, respiratory rate, B/P

Perform/provide:
• Use of reconstituted solution immediately, discard unused potion

Evaluate:
• Therapeutic response: decreasing intraocular pressure, miosis during ocular surgery

Teach patient/family:
• To report change in vision, blurring or loss of sight, trouble breathing, sweating, flushing
• Method of instillation, including pressure on lacrimal sac for 1 min, and not to touch dropper to eye
• That long-term therapy may be required in glaucoma
• That blurred vision will decrease with repeated use of drug
• Not to drive during first few days of treatment

---

carbamazepine

(kar-ba-maz'e-peen)

Apo-Carbamazepine,* Epitol, Mazepine,* Tegretol

Func. class.: Anticonvulsant
Chem. class.: Iminostilbene derivative

Action: Inhibits nerve impulses by limiting influx of sodium ions across cell membrane in motor cortex

Uses: Tonic-clonic, complex-partial, mixed seizures; trigeminal neuralgia

Dosage and routes:

Seizures
• *Adult and child >12 yr:* PO 200 mg bid, may be increased by 200 mg/day in divided doses q6-8h; adjustment is needed to minimum dose to control seizures
• *Child <12 yr:* PO 10-20 mg/kg/day in 2-3 divided doses

Trigeminal neuralgia
• *Adult:* PO 100 mg bid, may increase 100 mg q12h until pain subsides, not to exceed 1.2 g/day; maintenance is 200-400 mg bid

Available forms include: Tabs, chewable 100 mg; tabs 200 mg

Side effects/adverse reactions:
HEMA: ***Thrombocytopenia, agranulocytosis, leukocytosis, neutropenia, aplastic anemia, eosinophilia,*** increased pro-time
CNS: Drowsiness, dizziness, confusion, fatigue, ***paralysis,*** headache, hallucinations
GI: Nausea, constipation, diarrhea, anorexia, vomiting, abdominal pain, stomatitis, glossitis, increased liver enzymes, ***hepatitis***
INTEG: Rash, ***Stevens-Johnson syndrome,*** urticaria
EENT: Tinnitus, dry mouth, blurred vision, diplopia, nystagmus, conjunctivitis
CV: ***Hypertension, CHF,*** hypotension, aggravation of cardiac artery disease
RESP: Pulmonary hypersensitivity (fever, dyspnea, pneumonitis)
GU: Frequency, retention, albuminuria, glycosuria, impotence

Contraindications: Hypersensitivity to carbamazepine or tricyclic antidepressants, bone marrow depression, concomitant use of MAOIs

Precautions: Glaucoma, hepatic disease, renal disease, cardiac disease, psychosis, pregnancy (C), lactation, child <6 yr

Pharmacokinetics:
PO: Onset slow, peak 4-8 hr, metabolized by liver, excreted in urine, feces, crosses placenta, excreted in breast milk, half-life 14-16 hr

Interactions/incompatibilities:
• Toxicity: troleandomycin, eryth-

---

* Available in Canada only

romycin, cimetidine, isoniazid, propoxyphene, lithium
• Decreased effects of: phenobarbital, phenytoin, primidone
• Increased effects of: vasopressin, lypressin, desmopressin

NURSING CONSIDERATIONS

Assess:
• Renal studies: urinalysis, BUN, urine creatinine q3mo
• Blood studies: RBC, Hct, Hgb, reticulocyte counts qwk for 4 wk then qmo; if myelosupression occurs, drug should be discontinued
• Hepatic studies: ALT, AST, bilirubin, creatinine
• Drug levels during initial treatment; should remain at 3-9 μg/ml; anorexia may indicate increased blood levels
• Description of seizures

Administer:
• With food, milk to decrease GI symptoms
• Chewable tablets; tell patient to chew tablet, not swallow it whole

Perform/provide:
• Storage at room temperature
• Hard candy, frequent rinsing of mouth, gum for dry mouth
• Assistance with ambulation during early part of treatment; dizziness occurs

Evaluate:
• Therapeutic response: decreased seizure activity, document on patient's chart
• Mental status: mood, sensorium, affect, behavioral changes; if mental status changes notify physician
• Eye problems: need for ophthalmic examinations before, during, after treatment (slit lamp, fundoscopy, tonometry)
• Allergic reaction: purpura, red raised rash, if these occur, drug should be discontinued
• Blood dyscrasias: fever, sore throat, bruising, rash, jaundice
• Toxicity: bone marrow depression, nausea, vomiting, ataxia, diplopia, cardiovascular collapse, Stevens-Johnson syndrome

Teach patient/family:
• To carry Medic-Alert ID stating drugs taken, condition, physician's name, phone number
• To avoid driving, other activities that require alertness
• To avoid alcohol ingestion; convulsions may result
• Not to discontinue medication quickly after long-term use
• That urine may turn pink to brown

Lab test interferences:
Decrease: Thyroid function tests

Treatment of overdose: Lavage, VS

---

carbamide peroxide (otic)

(kar'ba-mide per-ox'ide)

Debrox, Murine Ear Drops

Func. class.: Otic

Chem. class.: Urea compound, hydrogen peroxide

Action: Foaming action facilitates removal of impacted cerumen

Uses: Impacted cerumen, prevention of ceruminosis

Dosage and routes:
• *Adult and child:* INSTILL 5-10 gtts bid × 3-4 days

Available forms include: Sol 6.5%

Side effects/adverse reactions:
EENT: Itching, irritation in ear, redness

Contraindications: Hypersensitivity, otic surgery, perforated eardrum

Precautions: Pregnancy (C)

NURSING CONSIDERATIONS
Administer:
• Drug, then irrigate to remove cerumen
• By allowing drops to enter ear canal, do not touch dropper to ear
Evaluate:
• Therapeutic response: loosened cerumen, ability to hear better
Teach patient/family:
• Method of instillation, using aseptic technique

---

carbarsone

(kar-bar'sone)

Func. class.: Amebicide
Chem. class.: Pentavalent organic arsenic

Action: Organism death occurs in intestinal lumen by inhibition of sulfhydryl enzymes
Uses: Intestinal amebiasis
Dosage and routes:
• *Adult:* PO 250 mg bid-tid × 10 days; REC 2 g/200 ml warm 2% $NaHCO_3$ sol, qod × 5 doses
• *Child:* PO 75 mg/kg/day in 3 divided doses × 10 days
Available forms include: Caps 250 mg; powder
Side effects/adverse reactions:
RESP: Congestion
HEMA: ***Agranulocytosis, aplastic anemia***
INTEG: Rash, pruritus, ***exfoliative dermatitis***
CNS: Neuritis, ***convulsion, hemorrhagic encephalitis, coma***
EENT: Blurred vision, sore throat, retinal edema
GI: *Nausea, vomiting,* diarrhea, epigastric distress, anorexia, constipation, abdominal cramps, irritation, hepatomegaly, jaundice, ***hepatitis, gastric necrosis,*** weight decrease
GU: Polyuria, albuminuria, ***nephrotoxicity***
CV: Tachycardia, hypotension, edema
Contraindications: Hypersensitivity to this drug or arsenic, renal disease, hepatic disease, contracted visual or color fields
Precautions: Pregnancy (D), elderly
Pharmacokinetics:
PO: Slowly excreted by kidneys, accumulation may occur

NURSING CONSIDERATIONS
Assess:
• Stools during entire treatment; should be clear at end of therapy; stools must be clear for 1 yr before patient is considered cured
• ECG before, during, after therapy; be aware that T wave inversion occurs
• Vision by ophthalmologic exam during, after therapy; vision problems often occur
• I&O; stools for number, frequency, character
• Blood studies: CBC as dyscrasias occur
Administer:
• Dimercaprol for arsenic toxicity as ordered
• PO after meals to avoid GI symptoms
Perform/provide:
• Storage in tight container
Evaluate:
• Therapeutic response: decreasing diarrhea, absence of amebiasis on culture
• Allergic reaction: fever, rash, itching, chills; drug should be discontinued if these occur
• Nephrotoxicity: polyuria, albuminuria, hematuria
• Arsenic toxicity: sore throat, edema, pruritus, nausea, vomiting, dizziness, anorexia, epigastric

---

* Available in Canada only

pain, weight decrease, gastritis, hepatitis, visual problems, convulsions, polyuria, agranulocytosis
• Superimposed infection: fever, monilial growth, fatigue, malaise
• Tachycardia, decreasing B/P, GI symptoms, weakness, neuromuscular symptoms
• Diarrhea for 2-3 days

Teach patient/family:
• To report any side effects
• Proper hygiene after BM: handwashing technique
• To avoid contact of drug with eyes, mouth, nose, other mucous membranes
• Need for compliance with dosage schedule, duration of treatment

Treatment of overdose: Administer dimercaprol, gastric lavage, O_2, IV fluids

---

carboplatin

(kar-boe'-pla-tin)
Paraplatin

Func. class.: Antineoplastic-alkylating agent
Chem. class.: Platinum coordination compound

Action: Produces interstrand DNA cross-links and, to a lesser extent, DNA-protein cross-links

Uses: Palliative treatment of ovarian carcinoma recurrent after treatment with other antineoplastic agents, including cisplatin

Dosage and routes (single agent):
• *Adult:* IV INF 360 mg/m^2 given over >15 min on day 1 q4wk; do not repeat single intermittent courses until neutrophil count is >2,000/mm^3 and platelet count is >100,000/mm^3

Available forms: Inj 50, 150, 450 mg/vial

Side effects/adverse reactions:
EENT: Tinnitus, hearing loss, ***vestibular toxicity***
HEMA: ***Thrombocytopenia, leukopenia, pancytopenia, neutropenia,*** anemia, bleeding
CV: Cardiac abnormalities
GI: Severe nausea, vomiting, diarrhea, weight loss
GU: ***Renal tubular damage,*** renal insufficiency, impotence, sterility, amenorrhea, gynecomastia
INTEG: Alopecia, dermatitis, rash, erythema, pruritus, urticaria
CNS: ***Convulsions, central neurotoxicity,*** peripheral neuropathy
RESP: Mucositis
META: Hypomagnesemia, hypocalcemia, hypokalemia, hyponatremia, hyperuremia

Contraindications: Hypersensitivity to this drug, platinum products, mannitol; severe bone marrow depression, significant bleeding, pregnancy (D)

Precautions: Radiation therapy with 1 mo, chemotherapy within 1 mo, lactation, liver disease

Pharmacokinetics: Initial half-life 1-2 hr, postdistribution half-life 2½-6 hr, not bound to plasma proteins, excreted by the kidneys

Interactions/incompatibilities:
• Increased nephrotoxicity or ototoxicity: aminoglycosides

NURSING CONSIDERATIONS

Assess:
• CBC, differential, platelet count weekly; withhold drug if WBC count is <4000/mm^3 or platelet count is <100,000/mm^3; notify physician of results
• Renal function studies: BUN, creatinine, serum uric acid, urine CrCl before and during therapy
• I&O ratio; report fall in urine output of <30 ml/hr
• Monitor temperature q4h (may

indicate beginning of infection)
• Liver function tests before and during therapy (bilirubin, AST, ALT, LDH) as needed or monthly

Administer:
• IV after reconstituting to a concentration of 10 mg/ml (INT INF) or 0.5 mg/ml (direct IV)
• IV INF over 5-6 hr; do not use needles or IV administration sets containing aluminum, may cause precipitate
• Antiemetic 30-60 min before giving drug to prevent vomiting, and PRN
• Allopurinol or sodium bicarbonate to maintain uric acid levels, alkalinization of urine
• Antibiotics for prophylaxis of infection
• Diuretic (furosemide 40 mg IV) after infusion

Perform/provide:
• Storage protected from light at room temperature; reconstituted solutions are stable for 8 hr at room temperature
• Deep breathing exercises with patient tid-qid; place in semi-Fowler's position
• Increase fluid intake 2-3 L/day to prevent urate deposits and calculi formation and to speed elimination of drug
• Diet low in purines: organ meats (kidney, liver), dried beans, peas to maintain alkaline urine

Evaluate:
• Therapeutic response: decreasing size of tumor; spread of malignancy
• Bleeding: hematuria, stool guaiac, bruising or petechiae, mucosa or orifices q8h
• Dyspnea, rales, unproductive cough, chest pain, tachypnea
• Food preferences; list likes, dislikes
• Effects of alopecia on body image, discuss feelings about body changes
• Yellowing of skin, sclera, dark urine, clay-colored stools, itchy skin, abdominal pain, fever, diarrhea
• Edema in feet, joint pain, stomach pain, shaking
• Inflammation of mucosa, breaks in skin

Teach patient/family:
• To report any complaints or side effects to nurse or physician
• That impotence or amenorrhea can occur, reversible after treatment is discontinued
• To report any changes in breathing or coughing
• That hair may be lost during treatment; a wig or hairpiece may make patient feel better; new hair may be different in color, texture

carboprost tromethamine

(kar'boe-prost)
Prostin/M15

Func. class.: Oxytocic
Chem. class.: Prostaglandin

Action: Stimulates uterine contractions causing complete abortion in approximately 16 hr

Uses: Abortion between 13-20 wk gestation

Dosage and routes:
• *Adult:* IM 250 μg, then 250 μg q1½-3½ hr, may increase to 500 μg if no response, not to exceed 12 mg total dose

Available forms include: Inj IM 250 μg/ml carboprost, 83 μg/ml tromethamine

Side effects/adverse reactions:
CNS: Fever, chills, headache
GI: Nausea, vomiting, diarrhea

Contraindications: Hypersensitiv-

* Available in Canada only

ity, severe hepatic disease, severe renal disease, PID, respiratory disease, cardiac disease
Precautions: Asthma, anemia, jaundice, diabetes mellitus, convulsive disorders, past uterine surgery
Pharmacokinetics: Onset: 15 min, peak 2 hr; metabolized in lungs, liver, excreted in urine (metabolites)

NURSING CONSIDERATIONS

Assess:
- B/P, pulse; watch for change that may indicate hemorrhage
- Respiratory rate, rhythm, depth; notify physician of abnormalities

Administer:
- IM in deep muscle mass, rotate injection sites if additional doses are given
- After having crash cart available on unit

Perform/provide:
- Emotional support before and after the abortion

Evaluate:
- Therapeutic response: expulsion of fetus
- For length, duration of contraction; notify physician of contractions lasting over 1 min or absence of contractions
- For incomplete abortion, pregnancy must be terminated by another method, drug is teratogenic

Teach patient/family:
- To report increased blood loss, abdominal cramps, increased temperature or foul-smelling lochia
- Methods of comfort control and pain control

carisoprodol

(kar-eye-soe-proe'dole)
Rela, Soma

Func. class.: Skeletal muscle relaxant, central acting
Chem. class.: Meprobamate congener

Action: Depresses CNS by blocking interneuronal activity in descending reticular formation, spinal cord, producing sedation
Uses: Relieving pain, stiffness in musculoskeletal conditions
Dosage and routes:
- *Adult and child >12 yr:* PO 350 mg tid, hs

Available forms include: Tabs 350 mg
Side effects/adverse reactions:
CNS: Dizziness, weakness, drowsiness, headache, tremor, depression, insomnia, ataxia, irritability
EENT: Diplopia, temporary loss of vision
CV: Postural hypotension, tachycardia
GI: Nausea, vomiting, hiccups, epigastric discomfort
INTEG: Rash, pruritus, fever, facial flushing
Contraindications: Hypersensitivity, child <12 yr, intermittent porphyria
Precautions: Renal disease, hepatic disease, addictive personalities, pregnancy (C), elderly
Pharmacokinetics:
PO: Onset ½ hr, duration 4-6 hr, metabolized by liver, excreted in urine, crosses placenta, excreted in breast milk (large amounts), half-life 8 hr
Interactions/incompatibilities:
- Increased CNS depression: alcohol, tricyclic antidepressants, nar-

cotics, barbiturates, sedatives, hypnotics

NURSING CONSIDERATIONS

Assess:

- Blood studies: CBC, WBC, differential; blood dyscrasias may occur
- Liver function studies: AST, ALT, alk phosphatase; hepatitis may occur
- ECG in epileptic patients; poor seizure control has occurred with patients taking this drug
- Idiosyncratic reaction, anaphylaxis within a few min or hr of first to fourth dose

Administer:

- With meals for GI symptoms

Perform/provide:

- Storage in tight container at room temperature
- Assistance with ambulation if dizziness, drowsiness occurs, especially elderly

Evaluate:

- Therapeutic response: decreased pain, spasticity
- Allergic reactions: rash, fever, respiratory distress
- Severe weakness, numbness in extremities
- Psychologic dependency: increased need for medication, more frequent requests for medication, increased pain
- CNS depression: dizziness, drowsiness, psychiatric symptoms

Teach patient/family:

- Not to discontinue the medication quickly; insomnia, nausea, headache, spasticity, tachycardia will occur; drug should be tapered off over 1-2 wk
- Not to take with alcohol, other CNS depressants
- To avoid altering activities while taking this drug
- To avoid hazardous activities if drowsiness, dizziness occurs
- To avoid using OTC medication: cough preparations, antihistamines, unless directed by physician

Treatment of overdose: Induce emesis of conscious patient, lavage, dialysis

---

carmustine (BCNU)

(kar-mus'teen)

BiCNU

Func. class.: Antineoplastic alkylating agent

Chem. class.: Nitrosourea

Action: Alkylates DNA, RNA; is able to inhibit enzymes that allow synthesis of amino acids in proteins

Uses: Brain tumors such as glioblastoma, medulloblastoma, astrocytoma; multiple myeloma, Hodgkin's disease, other lymphomas

Dosage and routes:

- *Adult:* IV 75-100 mg/m^2 over 1-2 hr × 2 days or 200 mg/m^2 × 1 dose q6-8wk; if leukocytes fall below 2000 or platelets below 25,000 only 50% of dose should be given

Available forms include: Inj IV 100 mg; powder

Side effects/adverse reactions:

HEMA: ***Thrombocytopenia, leukopenia, myelosuppression, anemia***

GI: Nausea, vomiting, anorexia, stomatitis, ***hepatotoxicity***

GU: Azotemia, ***renal failure***

INTEG: Burning, hyperpigmentation at injection site

RESP: ***Fibrosis, pulmonary infiltrate***

Contraindications: Hypersensitivity, leukopenia, thrombocytopenia

Precautions: Pregnancy (D)

Pharmacokinetics:

Degraded within 15 min, crosses blood-brain barrier; 70% excreted in urine within 96 hr, 10% excreted as CO_2, fate of 20% is unknown

Interactions/incompatibilities:

- Increased toxicity: other antineoplastics, or radiation
- Enhanced action: Vitamin A or caffeine
- Increased toxicity: cimetidine, other antineoplastics or radiation

NURSING CONSIDERATIONS

Assess:

- CBC, differential, platelet count weekly; withhold drug if WBC is <4000 or platelet count is <75,000; notify physician of results
- Liver function tests: AST, ALT, bilirubin
- Pulmonary function tests, chest x-ray films before, during therapy; chest film should be obtained q2wk during treatment
- Renal function studies: BUN, serum uric acid, urine CrCl before, during therapy
- I&O ratio; report fall in urine output of 30 ml/hr
- Monitor for cold, cough, fever (may indicate beginning infection)

Administer:

- IV after diluting 100 mg drug/3 ml ethyl alcohol (provided); then further dilute 27 ml sterile H_2O for INJ; then dilute with 500 ml 0.9% NaCl or D_5W
- Antiemetic 30-60 min before giving drug to prevent vomiting
- Antibiotics for prophylaxis of infection

Perform/provide:

- Storage in refrigerator
- Strict medical asepsis, protective isolation if WBC levels are low
- Special skin care
- Deep breathing exercises with patient tid-qid; place in semi-Fowler's position
- Increase fluid intake to 2-3 L/day to prevent urate deposits, calculi formation
- Rinsing of mouth tid-qid with water or club soda; brushing of teeth bid-tid with soft brush or cotton-tipped applicators for stomatitis; use unwaxed dental floss, use viscous Xylocaine
- Warm compresses at injection site for inflammation

Evaluate:

- Therapeutic response: decreasing size of tumor, spread of malignancy
- Bleeding: hematuria, guaiac, bruising or petechiae, mucosa or orifices q8h
- Dyspnea, rales, unproductive cough, chest pain, tachypnea
- Food preferences; list likes, dislikes
- Inflammation of mucosa, breaks in skin

Teach patient/family:

- Protective isolation precautions
- To report any changes in breathing or coughing
- To avoid foods with citric acid, hot or rough texture
- To report any bleeding; white spots, or ulceration in mouth to physician; tell patient to examine mouth qd
- To avoid use of aspirin, ibuprofen; razors, commercial mouthwash
- To report signs of anemia (fatigue, irritability, shortness of breath, faintness)
- To report signs of infection (sore throat, fever)

carteolol

(kar-tee'oe-lole)

Cartrol

Func. class.: Antihypertensive

Chem. class.: Nonselective β-blocker

Action: Produces fall in B/P without reflex tachycardia or significant reduction in heart rate through mixture of α-blocking, β-blocking effects; elevated plasma renins are reduced

Uses: Mild to moderate hypertension

Dosage and routes:

• *Adult:* PO 2.5 mg tid initially, may gradually increase to desired response

Available forms include: Tabs 2.5, 5, 10 mg

Side effects/adverse reactions:

CV: Orthostatic hypotension, ***bradycardia, CHF, chest pain, ventricular dysrhythmias, AV block, peripheral vascular insufficiency,*** palpitations

CNS: Dizziness, mental changes, drowsiness, fatigue, headache, catatonia, depression, anxiety, nightmares, paresthesia, lethargy, insominia, decreased concentration

GI: Nausea, vomiting, diarrhea, dry mouth, flatulence, constipation, anorexia

INTEG: Rash, alopecia, urticaria, pruritus, fever

HEMA: ***Agranulocytosis, thrombocytopenic purpura (rare)***

EENT: Tinnitus, visual changes, sore throat, double vision, dry burning eyes

GU: Impotence, dysuria, ejaculatory failure, urinary retention

RESP: ***Bronchospasm,*** dyspnea, wheezing, nasal stuffiness, pharyngitis

MS: Joint pain, arthralgia, muscle cramps, pain

OTHER: Facial swelling, decreased exercise tolerance, weight change, Raynaud's disease

Contraindications: Hypersensitivity to β-blockers, cardiogenic shock, heart block (2nd or 3rd degree), sinus bradycardia, CHF, bronchial asthma

Precautions: Major surgery, pregnancy (C), lactation, diabetes mellitus, renal disease, thyroid disease, COPD, well-compensated heart failure, CAD, nonallergic bronchospasm

Pharmacokinetics:

PO: Onset 1-2 hr, peak 2-4 hr, duration 8-12 hr, half-life 6-8 hr, metabolized by liver (metabolites inactive), excreted in urine, bile, crosses placenta, excreted in breast milk

Interactions/incompatibilities:

• Increased hypotension: diuretics, other antihypertensives, halothane, cimetidine, nitroglycerin, prazosin

• Decreased β-blocker effects: sympathomimetics, nonsteroidal antiinflammatory agents, salicylates

• Increased hypoglycemia effect: insulin

• Increased effects of: lidocaine

• Decreased bronchodilating effects of: theophylline

NURSING CONSIDERATIONS

Assess:

• I&O, weight daily

• B/P, pulse q4h; note rate, rhythm, quality

• Apical/radial pulse before administration; notify physician of any significant changes

• Baselines in renal, liver function tests before therapy begins

Administer:

• PO: ac, hs; tablet may be crushed or swallowed whole

• Reduced dosage in renal dysfunction

Perform/provide:

• Storage in dry area at room temperature, do not freeze

Evaluate:

• Therapeutic response: decreased B/P after 1-2 wk

---

* Available in Canada only

- Edema in feet, legs daily
- Skin turgor, dryness of mucous membranes for hydration status

Teach patient/family:

- Not to discontinue drug abruptly; taper over 2 wk or may precipitate angina
- Not to use OTC products containing α-adrenergic stimulants (nasal decongestants, OTC cold preparations) unless directed by physician
- To report bradycardia, dizziness, confusion, depression, fever
- To take pulse at home, advise when to notify physician
- To avoid alcohol, smoking, sodium intake
- To comply with weight control, dietary adjustments, modified exercise program
- To carry Medic Alert ID to identify drug being taken, allergies
- To avoid hazardous activities if dizziness is present
- To report symptoms of CHF: difficult breathing, especially on exertion or when lying down, night cough, swelling of extremities
- To take medication hs to minimize orthostatic hypotension
- To wear support hose to minimize effects of orthostatic hypotension

Lab test interferences:

False increase: Urinary catecholamines

Interference: Glucose, insulin tolerance tests

Treatment of overdose: Lavage, IV atropine for bradycardia, IV theophylline for bronchospasm, digitalis, O_2, diuretic for cardiac failure; hemodialysis is useful for removal; administer vasopressor (norepinephrine) for hypotension, isoproterenol for heart block

cascara sagrada/cascara sagrada aromatic fluid extract/cascara sagrada fluid extract

(kas-kar'a)

Func. class.: Laxative
Chem. class.: Anthraquinone

Action: Direct chemical irritation in colon; increases propulsion of stool

Uses: Constipation, bowel, or rectal preparation for surgery or examination

Dosage and routes:

- *Adult:* PO 325 mg hs; FLUID 1 ml qd; AROMATIC FLUID 5 ml qd
- *Child 2-12 yr:* PO/FLUID/AROMATIC FLUID ½ adult dose
- *Child <2 yr:* PO/FLUID/AROMATIC FLUID ¼ adult dose

Available forms include: Powder, tabs 325 mg; oral sol

Side effects/adverse reactions:

GI: Nausea, vomiting, anorexia, cramps, diarrhea

META: Hypocalcemia, enteropathy, alkalosis, hypokalemia, ***tetany***

Contraindications: Hypersensitivity, GI bleeding, obstruction, CHF, lactation, abdominal pain, nausea/vomiting, appendicitis, acute surgical abdomen, alcoholics (aromatic form)

Precautions: Pregnancy (C)

Pharmacokinetics:

PO: Peak 6-12 hr; metabolized by liver, excreted by kidneys, in feces

Interactions/incompatibilities:

- Decreased absorption: antibiotics, digitalis, nitrofurantoin, salicylates, tetracyclines, oral anticoagulants

NURSING CONSIDERATIONS

Assess:

- Blood, urine electrolytes if drug is used often by patient

• I&O ratio to identify fluid loss

Administer:

• Alone for better absorption; do not take within 1 hr of other drugs or within 1 hr of antacids, milk

• In morning or evening (oral dose)

Evaluate:

• Therapeutic response: decrease in constipation

• Cause of constipation; identify whether fluids, bulk, or exercise is missing from lifestyle

• Cramping, rectal bleeding, nausea, vomiting; if these symptoms occur, drug should be discontinued

Teach patient/family:

• To swallow tabs whole; do not chew

• Not to use laxatives for long-term therapy; bowel tone will be lost

• That normal bowel movements do not always occur daily

• Not to use in presence of abdominal pain, nausea, vomiting

• To notify physician if constipation unrelieved or if symptoms of electrolyte imbalance occur: muscle cramps, pain, weakness, dizziness

---

castor oil

Alphamul, Emulsoil, Fleet Castor Oil, Kelloff's Castor Oil, Neoloid, Purge

Func. class.: Laxative

Action: Directly acts on intestine by increasing motor activity, thought to irritate colonic intramural plexus

Uses: Bowel, rectal preparation for surgery or examination

Dosage and routes:

• *Adult:* PO LIQ 15-60 ml

• *Child >2 yr:* LIQ 5-15 ml

• *Child <2 yr:* LIQ 1.25-7.5 ml

• *Infants:* LIQ 1-4 ml

Available forms include: Liq 36.4%, 60%, 64%, 95%; caps 0.62 ml/cap

Side effects/adverse reactions:

GI: Nausea, vomiting, anorexia, cramps, diarrhea, rebound constipation, colon irritation, flatus

META: Alkalosis, hypokalemia, electrolytes, fluid imbalance

Contraindications: Hypersensitivity, fecal impaction, GI bleeding, pregnancy (X), lactation, abdominal pain, nausea/vomiting, appendicitis, acute surgical abdomen

Pharmacokinetics:

PO: Peak 2-3 hr; excreted in breast milk

NURSING CONSIDERATIONS

Assess:

• Blood, urine electrolytes if drug is used often by patient

• I&O ratio to identify fluid loss

Administer:

• Alone for better absorption; do not take within 1 hr of other drugs or within 1 hr of antacids, milk

• In morning or evening (oral dose)

Perform/provide:

• Storage in cool environment, do not freeze

Evaluate:

• Therapeutic response: decrease in constipation

• Cause of constipation; identify whether fluids, bulk, or exercise is missing from lifestyle

• Cramping, rectal bleeding, nausea, vomiting; if these symptoms occur, drug should be discontinued

Teach patient/family:

• To swallow tabs whole; do not chew

• Not to use laxatives for long-term therapy; bowel tone will be lost

• That normal bowel movements do not always occur daily

• Not to use in presence of abdominal pain, nausea, vomiting

---

* Available in Canada only

• To notify physician if constipation unrelieved or if symptoms of electrolyte imbalance occur: muscle cramps, pain, weakness, dizziness, severe thirst
• To keep out of children's reach

cefaclor

(sef'a-klor)
Ceclor

Func. class.: Antibiotic
Chem. class.: Cephalosporin (2nd generation)

Action: Inhibits bacterial cell wall synthesis, which renders cell wall osmotically unstable
Uses: Gram-negative bacilli: *H. influenzae, E. coli, P. mirabilis, Klebsiella;* gram-positive organisms: *S. pneumoniae, S. pyogenes, S. aureus;* upper and lower respiratory tract, urinary tract, skin infections, otitis media
Dosage and routes:
• *Adult:* PO 250-500 mg q8h, not to exceed 4 g/day
• *Child >1 mo:* PO 20-40 mg/kg/qd in divided doses q8h, not to exceed 1 g/day
Available forms include: Caps 250, 500 mg; oral susp 125, 250 mg/5 ml
Side effects/adverse reactions:
CNS: Headache, dizziness, weakness, paresthesia, fever, chills
GI: Nausea, vomiting, *diarrhea, anorexia,* pain, glossitis, bleeding, increased AST, ALT, bilirubin, LDH, alk phosphatase, abdominal pain
GU: Proteinuria, vaginitis, pruritus, candidiasis, increased BUN, ***nephrotoxicity, renal failure***
HEMA: ***Leukopenia, thrombocytopenia, agranulocytosis,*** anemia, ***neutropenia, lymphocytosis, eosinophilia, pancytopenia, hemolytic anemia***
INTEG: Rash, urticaria, dermatitis, ***anaphylaxis***
RESP: Dyspnea
Contraindications: Hypersensitivity to cephalosporins, infants <1 mo
Precautions: Hypersensitivity to penicillins, pregnancy (B), lactation, renal disease
Pharmacokinetics:
Peak ½-1 hr, half-life 36-54 min, 25% bound by plasma proteins, 60%-85% eliminated unchanged in urine in 8 hr, crosses placenta, excreted in breast milk
Interactions/incompatibilities:
• Decreased effects: tetracyclines, erythromycins
• Increased toxicity: aminoglycosides, furosemide, probenecid, sulfinpyrazone, colistin, ethacrynic acid, vancomycin

NURSING CONSIDERATIONS

Assess:
• Sensitivity to penicillins and other cephalosporins
Nephrotoxicity: increased BUN, creatinine
• I&O daily
• Blood studies: AST, ALT, CBC, Hct, bilirubin, LDH, alk phosphatase, Coombs' test monthly if patient is on long-term therapy
• Electrolytes: potassium, sodium, chloride monthly if patient is on long-term therapy
• Bowel pattern qd; if severe diarrhea occurs, drug should be discontinued; may indicate pseudomembranous colitis
Administer:
• For 10-14 days to ensure organism death, prevent superimposed infection
• With food if needed for GI symptoms
• After C&S completed

Evaluate:
- Therapeutic response: decreased symptoms of infection
- Urine output; if decreasing, notify physician (may indicate nephrotoxicity)
- Allergic reactions: rash, urticaria, pruritus, chills, fever, joint pain; angioedema may occur a few days after therapy begins
- Bleeding: ecchymosis, bleeding gums, hematuria, stool guaiac daily
- Overgrowth of infection: perineal itching, fever, malaise, redness, pain, swelling, drainage, rash, diarrhea, change in cough, sputum

Teach patient/family:
- If diabetic, to use Clinistix or Ketodiastix, blood glucose level
- Not to drink alcohol or meds with alcohol or reaction may occur
- To use yogurt or buttermilk to maintain intestinal flora, decrease diarrhea
- To take all medication prescribed for length of time ordered
- To report sore throat, bruising, bleeding, joint pain; may indicate blood dyscrasias (rare)

Lab test interferences:
Increase (false): Creatinine (serum urine), urinary 17-KS
False positive: Urinary protein, direct Coombs', urine glucose
Interference: Cross-matching
Treatment of overdose: Epinephrine, antihistamines, resuscitate if needed (anaphylaxis)

---

cefadroxil

(sef-a-drox'ill)
Duricef, Ultracef

Func. class.: Antibiotic
Chem. class.: Cephalosporin (1st generation)

Action: Inhibits bacterial cell wall synthesis, rendering cell wall osmotically unstable
Uses: Gram-negative bacilli: *E. coli, P. mirabilis, Klebsiella (UTI only);* gram-positive organisms: *S. pneumoniae, S. pyogenes, S. aureus;* upper, lower respiratory tract, urinary tract, skin infections, otitis media; tonsillitis; particularly for urinary tract infections
Dosage and routes:
- *Adult:* PO 1-2 g qd or q12h, give a loading dose of 1 g initially; dosage reduction indicated in renal impairment (CrCl < 50 ml/min)
- *Child:* 30 mg/kg/day

Available forms include: Caps 500 mg; tabs 1 g; oral susp 125, 250, 500 mg/5 ml
Side effects/adverse reactions:
CNS: Headache, dizziness, weakness, paresthesia, fever, chills
GI: Nausea, vomiting, *diarrhea, anorexia,* pain, glossitis, bleeding, increased AST, ALT, bilirubin, LDH, alk phosphatase, abdominal pain, ***pseudomembranous colitis***
GU: Proteinuria, vaginitis, pruritus, candidiasis, increased BUN, ***nephrotoxicity, renal failure***
HEMA: ***Leukopenia, thrombocytopenia, agranulocytosis,*** anemia, ***neutropenia, lymphocytosis, eosinophilia, pancytopenia, hemolytic anemia***
INTEG: Rash, urticaria, dermatitis, ***anaphylaxis***
RESP: Dyspnea
Contraindications: Hypersensitivity to cephalosporins, infants <1 mo
Precautions: Hypersensitivity to penicillins, pregnancy (B), lactation, renal disease
Pharmacokinetics:
Peak 1-1½ hr, half-life 1-2 hr, 20% bound by plasma proteins, crosses placenta, excreted in breast milk

---

Interactions/incompatibilities:
• Decreased effects: tetracyclines, erythromycins
• Increased toxicity: aminoglycosides, furosemide, probenecid, sulfinpyrazone, colistin, ethacrynic acid, vancomycin

NURSING CONSIDERATIONS

Assess:
• Sensitivity to penicillin and other cephalosporins
• Nephrotoxicity: increased BUN, creatinine
• I&O daily
• Blood studies: AST, ALT, CBC, Hct, bilirubin, LDH, alk phosphatase, Coombs' test monthly if patient is on long-term therapy
• Electrolytes: potassium, sodium, chloride monthly if patient is on long-term therapy
• Bowel pattern qd; if severe diarrhea occurs drug should be discontinued; may indicate pseudomembranous colitis

Administer:
• For 10-14 days to ensure organism death, prevent superimposed infection
• With food if needed for GI symptoms
• After C&S completed

Evaluate:
• Therapeutic response: decreased symptoms of infection
• Urine output; if decreasing, notify physician; may indicate nephrotoxicity
• Allergic reactions: rash, urticaria, pruritus, chills, fever, joint pain; angioedema; may occur few days after therapy begins
• Bleeding: ecchymosis, bleeding gums, hematuria, stool guaiac daily
• Overgrowth of infection: perineal itching, fever, malaise, redness, pain, swelling, drainage, rash, diarrhea, change in cough, sputum

Teach patient/family:
• If diabetic to use Clinistix or Ketodiastix, blood glucose level
• Not to drink alcohol or use meds with alcohol or reaction may occur
• To use yogurt or buttermilk to maintain intestinal flora, decrease diarrhea
• To take all medication prescribed for length of time ordered
• To report sore throat, bruising, bleeding, joint pain; may indicate blood dyscrasias (rare)

Lab test interferences:
Increase (false): Creatinine (serum urine), urinary 17-KS
False positive: Urinary protein, direct Coombs', urine glucose
Interference: Cross-matching

Treatment of overdose: Epinephrine, antihistamines, resuscitate if needed (anaphylaxis)

---

cefamandole nafate

(sef-a-man'dole)
Mandol

Func. class.: Antibiotic
Chem. class.: Cephalosporin (2nd generation)

Action: Inhibits bacterial cell wall synthesis, rendering cell wall osmotically unstable

Uses: Gram-negative bacilli: *H. influenzae, E. coli, P. mirabilis, Klebsiella;* gram-positive organisms: *S. pneumoniae, S. pyogenes, S. aureus;* upper, lower respiratory tract, urinary tract, skin infections, peritonitis, septicemia, surgical prophylaxis

Dosage and routes:
• *Adult:* IM/IV 500 mg-1 g q4-8h; may give up to 2 g q4h for severe infections
• *Child >1 mo:* IM/IV 50-100 mg/

kg/day in divided doses q4-8h, not to exceed adult dose
• Dosage reduction indicated in renal impairment (CrCl < 5 ml/min)
Available forms include: Inj IM, IV 500 mg, 1, 2, 10 g; IV 1, 2 g
Side effects/adverse reactions:
CNS: Headache, dizziness, weakness, paresthesia, fever, chills
GI: Nausea, vomiting, diarrhea, anorexia, pain, glossitis, bleeding, increased AST, ALT, bilirubin, LDH, alk phosphatase, abdominal pain
GU: Proteinuria, vaginitis, pruritus, candidiasis, increased BUN, ***nephrotoxicity, renal failure***
HEMA: ***Leukopenia, thrombocytopenia, agranulocytosis,*** anemia, ***neutropenia, lymphocytosis, eosinophilia, pancytopenia, hemolytic anemia,*** bleeding, ***hypoprothrombinemia***
INTEG: Rash, urticaria, dermatitis, ***anaphylaxis***
RESP: Dyspnea
Contraindications: Hypersensitivity to cephalosporins, infants <1 mo
Precautions: Hypersensitivity to penicillins, pregnancy, lactation, renal disease
Pharmacokinetics:
Peak 1-1½ hr, half-life ½-1 hr, 60%-75% bound by plasma proteins, crosses placenta, excreted in breast milk
Interactions/incompatibilities:
• Do not mix with tetracyclines, erythromycins, calcium chloride, magnesium salts, aminoglycosides, cimetidine in same parenteral fluid
• Decreased effects: tetracyclines, erythromycins
• Increased toxicity: aminoglycosides, furosemide, probenecid, sulfinpyrazone, colistin, ethacrynic acid, vancomycin
• Disulfiram reaction: disulfiram

NURSING CONSIDERATIONS

Assess:
• Sensitivity to penicillin or other cephalosporins
• Nephrotoxicity: increased BUN, creatinine
• I&O daily
• Blood studies: AST, ALT, CBC, Hct, bilirubin, LDH, alk phosphatase, Coombs' test, pro-time monthly if patient is on long-term therapy
• Electrolytes: potassium, sodium, chloride monthly if patient is on long-term therapy
• Bowel pattern qd, if severe diarrhea occurs drug should be discontinued; may indicate pseudomembranous colitis
• IV site for extravasation or phlebitis, change site q72h
Administer:
• IV, check often for irritation, extravasation, dilute 1 g of drug/10 ml normal saline or sterile H_2O for inj, run over 3-5 min; may be further diluted with 100 ml of compatible sol and run over 15-30 min; may also be diluted in 1000-ml compatible sol
• For 10-14 days to ensure organism death, prevent superimposed infection
• After C&S completed
Evaluate:
• Therapeutic response: decreased symptoms of infection
• Urine output, if decreasing, notify physician; may indicate nephrotoxicity
• Allergic reactions: rash, urticaria, pruritus, chills, fever, joint pain, angioedema; may occur few days after therapy begins
• Bleeding: ecchymosis, bleeding gums, hematuria, stool guaiac daily
• Overgrowth of infection: perineal itching, fever, malaise, redness,

pain, swelling, drainage, rash, diarrhea, change in cough, sputum

Teach patient/family:

- If diabetic, to use Clinistix or Ketodiastix, blood glucose level
- Not to drink alcohol or meds with alcohol or reaction may occur
- To report sore throat, bruising, bleeding, joint pain; may indicate blood dyscrasias (rare)

Lab test interferences:

Increase (false): Urinary 17-KS
False positive: Urinary protein, direct Coombs', urine glucose
Interference: Cross-matching

Treatment of overdose: Epinephrine, antihistamines, resuscitate if needed (anaphylaxis)

---

cefazolin sodium

(sef-a'zoe-lin)

Ancef, Kefzol

Func. class.: Antibiotic
Chem. class.: Cephalosporin (1st generation)

Action: Inhibits bacterial cell wall synthesis rendering cell wall osmotically unstable

Uses: Gram-negative bacilli: *H. influenzae, E. coli, P. mirabilis, Klebsiella;* gram-positive organisms: *S. pneumoniae, S. pyogenes, S. aureus;* upper, lower respiratory tract, urinary tract, skin infections, bone, joint, biliary, genital infections, endocarditis, surgical prophylaxis, septicemia

Dosage and routes:

Life-threatening infections

- *Adult:* IM/IV 1-1.5 g q6h
- *Child >1 mo:* IM/IV 100 mg/kg in 3-4 equal doses

Mild/moderate infections

- *Adult:* IM/IV 250-500 mg q8h
- *Child >1 mo:* IM/IV 25-50 mg/kg in 3-4 equal doses
- Dosage reduction indicated in renal impairment (CrCl < 54 ml/min)

Available forms include: Inj IM, IV, 250, 500 mg, 1, 5, 10 g

Side effects/adverse reactions:

CNS: Headache, dizziness, weakness, paresthesia, fever, chills

GI: Nausea, vomiting, *diarrhea, anorexia,* pain, glossitis, bleeding, increased AST, ALT, bilirubin, LDH, alk phosphatase, abdominal pain, oral candidiasis

GU: Proteinuria, vaginitis, pruritus, candidiasis, increased BUN, ***nephrotoxicity, renal failure***

HEMA: ***Leukopenia, thrombocytopenia, agranulocytosis,*** anemia, ***neutropenia, lymphocytosis, eosinophilia, pancytopenia, hemolytic anemia***

INTEG: Rash, urticaria, dermatitis, ***anaphylaxis***

Contraindications: Hypersensitivity to cephalosporins, infants <1 mo

Precautions: Hypersensitivity to penicillins, pregnancy (B), lactation, renal disease

Pharmacokinetics:

IM: Peak ½-2 hr, half-life 1½-2¼ hr

IV: Peak 10 min, eliminated unchanged in urine 70% to 86% protein bound

Interactions/incompatibilities:

- Do not mix with tetracyclines, erythromycins, calcium salts, magnesium salts, barbiturates, aminoglycosides in same parenteral fluid
- Decreased effects: tetracyclines, erythromycins
- Increased toxicity: aminoglycosides, furosemide, probenecid, sulfinpyrazone, colistin, ethacrynic acid

NURSING CONSIDERATIONS

Assess:

• Sensitivity to penicillin or other cephalosporins
• Nephrotoxicity: increased BUN, creatinine
• I&O daily
• Blood studies: AST, ALT, CBC, Hct, alk phosphatase, bilirubin, LDH, Coombs' test monthly if patient is on long-term therapy
• Electrolytes: potassium, sodium, chloride monthly if patient is on long-term therapy
• Bowel pattern qd; if severe diarrhea occurs drug should be discontinued; may indicate pseudomembranous colitis
• IV site for extravasation or phlebitis, change site q72h

Administer:

• IV, check for irritation, extravasation often, dilute in 10 ml sterile H_2O for inj and run over 3-5 min; may be further diluted with 50-100 ml of compatible sol and run over ½-1 hr
• For 10-14 days to ensure organism death, prevent superimposed infection
• After C&S completed

Evaluate:

• Therapeutic response: decreased fever, malaise, chills
• Urine output, if decreasing, notify physician; may indicate nephrotoxicity
• Allergic reactions: rash, urticaria, pruritus, chills, fever, joint pain, angioedema; may occur few days after therapy begins
• Bleeding: ecchymosis, bleeding gums, hematuria, stool guaiac daily
• Overgrowth of infection: perineal itching, fever, malaise, redness, pain, swelling, drainage, rash, diarrhea, change in cough, sputum

Teach patient/family:

• If diabetic, to use Clinistix or Ketodiastix, blood glucose level
• Not to use alcohol or meds with alcohol or reaction may occur

Lab test interferences:

Increase (false): Urinary 17-KS
False positive: urinary protein, direct Coombs', urine glucose
Interference: Cross-matching

Treatment of overdose: Epinephrine, antihistamines, resuscitate if needed (anaphylaxis)

---

cefixime

(sef-ex'ime)
Suprax

Func. class.: Broad-spectrum antibiotic
Chem. class.: Cephalosporin (3rd generation)

Action: Inhibits bacterial cell wall synthesis, rendering cell wall osmotically unstable

Uses: Uncomplicated UTI *(E. coli, P. mirabilis)*, pharyngitis and tonsillitis *(S. pyogenes)*, otitis media *(H. influenzae)*, *M. catarrhalis*, acute bronchitis, and acute exacerbations of chronic bronchitis *(S. pneumoniae, H. influenzae)*

Dosage and routes:

• *Adult:* PO 400 mg qd as a single dose or 200 mg q12h
• *Child >50 kg or >12 yrs:* PO use adult dosage
• *Child: <50 kg or <12 years:* PO 8 mg/kg/day as a single dose or 4 mg/kg q12h
•*Available forms include:* Tabs 200, 400 g; powder for oral susp 100 mg/5 ml

Side effects/adverse reactions:

CNS: Headache, dizziness, paresthesia, fever, chills, lethargy, fatigue, confusion

---

* Available in Canada only

GI: Nausea, vomiting, diarrhea, anorexia, pain, glossitis, bleeding, increased AST, ALT, bilirubin, LDH, alk phosphatase, heartburn, dysgeusia, flatulence
GU: ***Proteinuria,*** vaginitis, pruritus, increased BUN, ***nephrotoxicity, renal failure,*** pyuria, dysuria
HEMA: ***Leukopenia, thrombocytopenia, agranulocytosis,*** anemia, ***neutropenia, lymphocytosis, eosinophilia, pancytopenia, hemolytic anemia***
INTEG: Rash, urticaria, ***exfoliative dermatitis, anaphylaxis***
RESP: ***Bronchospasm,*** dyspnea, tight chest

Contraindications: Hypersensitivity to cephalosporins, infants <6 mo

Precautions: Hypersensitivity to penicillins, pregnancy (B), lactation, renal disease

Pharmacokinetics:
PO: Peak 1 hr
Half-life 3-4 hr, 65% bound by plasma proteins, 50% eliminated unchanged in urine; crosses placenta, excreted in breast milk

Interactions/incompatibilities:
• Decreased bactericidal effects: tetracyclines, erythromycins, chloramphenicol
• Increased renal toxicity: aminoglycosides, furosemide, colistin, ethacrynic acid, vancomycin

NURSING CONSIDERATIONS

Assess:
• Sensitivity to penicillin or other cephalosporins
• Nephrotoxicity: increased BUN, creatinine
• I&O daily
• Blood studies: AST, ALT, CBC, Hct, bilirubin, LDH, alk phosphatase; Coombs' test monthly if patient is on long-term therapy
• Bowel pattern qd; if severe diarrhea occurs, drug should be discontinued (may indicate pseudomembranous colitis)

Administer:
• For 10-14 days to ensure organism death, prevent superimposed infection
• After C&S completed

Evaluate:
• Therapeutic response: decreased fever, malaise, chills
• Urine output, if decreasing, notify physician (may indicate nephrotoxicity)
• Allergic reactions: rash, urticaria, pruritus, chills, fever, joint pain, angioedema; may occur a few days after therapy begins
• Bleeding: ecchymosis, bleeding, itching, fever, malaise, redness, pain, swelling, drainage, rash, diarrhea, change in cough, sputum

Teach patient/family:
• To report sore throat, bruising, bleeding, joint pain (may indicate blood dyscrasias [rare])
• If diabetic, to use Clinistix or Ketodiastix, blood glucose level
• Not to use alcohol or meds with alcohol or reaction may occur

Lab test interferences:
Increase (false): Urinary 17-KS
False positive: Urinary protein, direct Coombs', urine glucose
Interference: Cross-matching

Treatment of overdose: Epinephrine, antihistamines, resuscitate if needed (anaphylaxis)

---

cefmetazole

(sef-met'a-zole)
Zefazone

Func. class.: Broad-spectrum antibiotic
Chem. class.: Cephalosporin (2nd generation)

Action: Inhibits bacterial cell wall

synthesis, rendering cell wall osmotically unstable

Uses: Gram-negative bacilli: *H. influenzae, E. coli, Proteus, Klebsiella, B. fragilis;* gram-positive organisms: *S. pneumoniae, S. pyogenes, S. aureus;* anaerobes, including *Clostridium;* infections of lower respiratory tract, urinary tract, skin, bone; septicemia; intraabdominal infections

Dosage and routes:

• *Adult:* IV 1-8 g divided q6-12h × 5-14 days

• *Available forms include:* Powder for inj 1, 2 gm/vial

Side effects/adverse reactions:

CNS: Headache, dizziness, paresthesia, fever, chills, lethargy, fatigue, confusion

GI: Nausea, vomiting, diarrhea, anorexia, pain, glossitis, bleeding, increased AST, ALT, bilirubin, LDH, alk phosphatase, heartburn, flatulence

GU: ***Proteinuria,*** vaginitis, pruritus, candidiasis, increased BUN, ***nephrotoxicity, renal failure***

HEMA: ***Leukopenia, thrombocytopenia, agranulocytosis,*** anemia, ***neutropenia, lymphocytosis, eosinophilia, pancytopenia, hemolytic anemia***

INTEG: Rash, urticaria, ***exfoliative dermatitis,*** thrombophlebitis ***angioedema,*** erythema, pruritus

SYST: ***Anaphylaxis***

Contraindications: Hypersensitivity to cephalosporins, infants <1 mo

Precautions: Hypersensitivity to penicillins, pregnancy (B), lactation, renal disease

Pharmacokinetics:

IM: Peak 30-45 min, 68% bound by plasma proteins, excreted by kidneys, half-life 1-3 hr

Interactions/incompatibilities:

• Do not mix with aminoglycosides in same parenteral fluid

• Decreased bactericidal effects: tetracyclines, erythromycins, chloramphenicol

• Increased renal toxicity and ototoxicity: aminoglycosides, furosemide, colistin, ethacrynic acid, vancomycin

• Increased plasma level of cefmetazole

NURSING CONSIDERATIONS

Assess:

• Sensitivity to penicillin and other cephalosporins

• Nephrotoxicity: increased BUN, creatinine

• I&O daily

• Blood studies: AST, ALT, CBC, Hct, bilirubin, LDH, alk phosphatase, Coombs' test monthly if patient is on long-term therapy

• Electrolytes: potassium, sodium, chloride monthly if patient is on long-term therapy

• Bowel pattern qd, if severe diarrhea occurs drug should be discontinued (may indicate pseudomembranous colitis)

• IV site for extravasation or phlebitis, change site q72h

Administer:

• IV after reconstituting with diluent specified on package, give over 3-5 min

• For 10-14 days to ensure organism death, prevent superimposed infection

• After C&S completed

Evaluate:

• Therapeutic response: decreased fever, malaise, chills

• Urine output; if decreasing, notify physician (may indicate nephrotoxicity)

• Allergic reactions: rash, urticaria, pruritis, chills, fever, joint

pain, 7-10 days after therapy begins
• Bleeding: ecchymosis, bleeding gums, hematuria, stool guaiac daily
• Overgrowth of infection: perineal itching, fever, malaise, redness, pain, swelling, drainage, rash, diarrhea, change in cough, sputum

Teach patient/family:
• If diabetic, to use Clinistix or Ketodiastix, blood glucose level
• Not to use alcohol or meds with alcohol or reaction may occur
• To report sore throat, bruising, bleeding, joint pain (may indicate blood dyscrasias [rare])

Lab test interferences:
Increase (false): Creatinine (serum urine), urinary 17-KS
False positive: Urinary protein, direct Coombs', urine glucose
Interference: Cross-matching

Treatment of overdose: Epinephrine, antihistamines, resuscitate if needed (anaphylaxis)

---

cefonicid sodium

(se-fon'i-sid)
Monocid

Func. class.: Antibiotic
Chem. class.: Cephalosporin (2nd generation)

Action: Inhibits bacterial cell wall synthesis rendering cell wall osmotically unstable

Uses: Gram-negative bacilli: *H. influenzae, E. coli, P. mirabilis, Klebsiella;* gram-positive organisms: *S. pneumoniae, S. pyogenes, S. aureus;* lower respiratory tract, urinary tract, skin infections, otitis media, peritonitis, septicemia

Dosage and routes:
Life-threatening infections
• *Adult:* IM/IV BOL or INF 1-2 g/24 hr; divide in two doses if giving 2 g
• Dosage reduction indicated in renal impairment

Available forms include: Inj IM, IV, 500 mg, 1, 10 g

Side effects/adverse reactions:
CNS: Headache, dizziness, weakness, paresthesia, fever, chills
GI: Nausea, vomiting, diarrhea, anorexia, pain, glossitis, bleeding, increased AST, ALT, bilirubin, LDH, alk phosphatase, abdominal pain
GU: Proteinuria, vaginitis, pruritus, candidiasis, increased BUN, ***nephrotoxicity, renal failure***
HEMA: ***Leukopenia, thrombocytopenia, agranulocytosis,*** anemia, ***neutropenia, lymphocytosis, eosinophilia, pancytopenia, hemolytic anemia***
INTEG: Rash, urticaria, dermatitis, ***anaphylaxis***

Contraindications: Hypersensitivity to cephalosporins, infants <1 mo

Precautions: Hypersensitivity to penicillins, pregnancy (B), lactation, renal disease

Pharmacokinetics:
IV: Onset 5 min
IM: Peak 1 hr
Half-life 4½ hr, excreted in breast milk, 98% protein bound

Interactions/incompatibilities:
• Decreased effects: tetracyclines, erythromycins
• Increased toxicity: aminoglycosides, furosemide, probenecid, sulfinpyrazone, colistin, ethacrynic acid, vancomycin, other cephalosporins

NURSING CONSIDERATIONS

Assess:
• Sensitivity to penicillin and other cephalosporins
• Nephrotoxicity: increased BUN, creatinine
• I&O daily

• Blood studies: AST, ALT, CBC, Hct, bilirubin, LDH, alk phosphatase, Coombs' test monthly if patient is on long-term therapy
• Electrolytes: potassium, sodium, chloride monthly if patient is on long-term therapy
• Bowel pattern qd; if severe diarrhea occurs, drug should be discontinued; may indicate pseudomembranous colitis

Administer:
• IV bolus over 3-5 min
• IV diluted in 50-100 ml compatible IV sol, slight yellowing of sol does not affect potency
• IV, check for irritation, extravasation often
• For 10-14 days to ensure organism death, prevent superimposed infection
• After C&S completed

Evaluate:
• Therapeutic response: decreased symptoms of infection
• Urine output; if decreasing, notify physician; may indicate nephrotoxicity
• Allergic reactions: rash, urticaria, pruritus, chills, fever, joint pain, angioedema; may occur few days after therapy begins
• Bleeding: ecchymosis, bleeding gums, hematuria, stool guaiac daily
• Overgrowth of infection: perineal itching, fever, malaise, redness, pain, swelling, drainage, rash, diarrhea, change in cough, sputum

Teach patient/family:
• If diabetic, to use Clinistix or Ketodiastix, blood glucose level
• Not to use alcohol or meds with alcohol or reaction may occur
• To report sore throat, bruising, bleeding, joint pain; may indicate blood dyscrasias (rare)

Lab test interferences:
Increase (false): Urinary 17-KS
False positive: Urinary protein, direct Coombs', urine glucose
Interference: Cross-matching

Treatment of overdose: Epinephrine, antihistamines, resuscitate if needed (anaphylaxis)

---

cefoperazone sodium

(sef-oh-per'a-zone)
Cefobid

Func. class.: Antibiotic, broad-spectrum
Chem. class.: Cephalosporin (3rd generation)

Action: Inhibits bacterial cell wall synthesis rendering cell wall osmotically unstable

Uses: Gram-negative bacilli: *H. influenzae, E. coli, P. mirabilis, Klebsiella, Enterobacter, Serratia, Citrobacter, Providencia, P. aeruginosa;* lower respiratory tract, urinary tract, skin, bone infections, bacterial septicemia, peritonitis, pelvic inflammatory disease (PID)

Dosage and routes:
Mild/moderate infections
• *Adult:* IM/IV 1-2 g q12h
Severe infections
• *Adult:* IM/IV 6-12 g/day divided in 2-4 equal doses

Available forms include: Inj IM, IV, 1, 2 g

Side effects/adverse reactions:
CNS: Headache, dizziness, weakness, paresthesia, fever, chills
GI: Nausea, vomiting, diarrhea, anorexia, pain, glossitis, bleeding, increased AST, ALT, bilirubin, LDH, alk phosphatase, abdominal pain, pseudomembranous colitis
GU: Proteinuria, vaginitis, pruritus, candidiasis, increased BUN, ***nephrotoxicity, renal failure***
HEMA: ***Leukopenia, thrombocytopenia, agranulocytosis,*** anemia,

*Available in Canada only

neutropenia, lymphocytosis, eosinophilia, pancytopenia, hemolytic anemia, bleeding, hypoprothrombinemia
INTEG: Rash, urticaria, dermatitis, ***anaphylaxis***
RESP: Dyspnea
Contraindications: Hypersensitivity to cephalosporins, infants <1 mo
Precautions: Hypersensitivity to penicillins, pregnancy (B), lactation, renal disease
Pharmacokinetics:
IV: Onset 5 min, peak 5-20 min, duration 6-8 hr
IM: Peak 1-2 hr, duration 6-8 hr
Half-life 2 hr, 70%-75% is eliminated unchanged in bile, 20%-30% unchanged in urine, excreted in breast milk (small amounts)
Interactions/incompatibilities:
• Do not mix with aminoglycosides in same parenteral fluid
• Decreased effects: tetracyclines, erythromycins
• Increased toxicity: aminoglycosides, furosemide, probenecid, sulfinpyrazone, colistin, ethacrynic acid, vancomycin
• Disulfiram-like reactions if alcohol ingested within 24-72 hr of cefoperazone administration

NURSING CONSIDERATIONS

Assess:
• Sensitivity to penicillin or other cephalosporins
• Nephrotoxicity: increased BUN, creatinine
• I&O daily
• Blood studies: AST, ALT, CBC, Hct, bilirubin, LDH, alk phosphatase, Coombs' test pro-time monthly if patient is on long-term therapy
• Electrolytes: potassium, sodium, chloride monthly if patient is on long-term therapy
• Bowel pattern qd; if severe diarrhea occurs, drug should be discontinued; may indicate pseudomembranous colitis
• IV site for extravasation or phlebitis, change site q72h
Administer:
• IV after diluting 1 g/2.8 ml sterile H_2O for Inj, or 0.9% NaCl; shake; run over 15-30 min; may be further diluted to a concentration of no greater than 25 mg/ml
• IM for concentration of >250 mg/ml, dilute in sterile water, then lidocaine, inject deeply
• For 10-14 days to ensure organism death, prevent superimposed infection
• After C&S completed
Evaluate:
• Therapeutic response: decreased symptoms of infection
• Urine output, if decreasing, notify physician; may indicate nephrotoxicity
• Allergic reactions: rash, urticaria, pruritus, chills, fever, joint pain, angioedema; may occur few days after therapy begins
• Bleeding: ecchymosis, bleeding gums, hematuria, stool guaiac daily
• Overgrowth of infection: perineal itching, fever, malaise, redness, pain, swelling, drainage, rash, diarrhea, change in cough, sputum
Teach patient/family:
• Not to drink alcohol during or for 3 days after use
• To report sore throat, bruising, bleeding, joint pain; may indicate blood dyscrasias (rare)
Lab test interferences:
Increase (false): Urinary 17-KS
False positive: Urinary protein, direct Coombs', urine glucose
Interference: Cross-matching
Treatment of overdose: Epineph-

rine, antihistamines, resuscitate if needed (anaphylaxis)

ceforanide

(sef-or-aa-nide)
Precef

Func. class.: Antibiotic, broad-spectrum
Chem. class.: Cephalosporin (2nd generation)

Action: Inhibits bacterial cell wall synthesis, rendering cell wall osmotically unstable
Uses: Gram-negative bacilli: *H. influenzae, E. coli, P. mirabilis, Klebsiella;* gram-positive organisms: *S. pneumoniae, S. aureus;* lower respiratory tract, urinary tract, skin, bone infections, septicemia, endocarditis
Dosage and routes:
- *Adult:* IM/IV 0.5-1 g q12h
- *Child:* IM/IV 20-40 mg/kg/day in 2 equal doses q12h
- Dosage reduction indicated in renal impairment (CrCl < 59 ml/min)

Available forms include: Powder for inj IM, IV 500 mg, 1, 10 g
Side effects/adverse reactions:
CNS: Headache, dizziness, weakness, paresthesia, fever, chills
GI: Nausea, vomiting, diarrhea, anorexia, pain, glossitis, bleeding, increased AST, ALT, bilirubin, LDH, alk phosphatase, abdominal pain
GU: Proteinuria, vaginitis, pruritus, increased BUN, ***nephrotoxicity, renal failure***
HEMA: ***Leukopenia, thrombocytopenia, agranulocytosis,*** anemia, ***neutropenia, lymphocytosis, eosinophilia, pancytopenia, hemolytic anemia***
INTEG: Rash, urticaria, dermatitis, ***anaphylaxis***
RESP: Dyspnea
Contraindications: Hypersensitivity to cephalosporins, infants <1 mo
Precautions: Hypersensitivity to penicillins, pregnancy (B), lactation, renal disease
Pharmacokinetics:
IV: Peak 2 hr
IM: Peak 1 hr
Half-life 2½-3 hr, 80% is bound by plasma proteins, 90% is eliminated unchanged in urine; crosses placenta, excreted in breast milk
Interactions/incompatibilities:
- Do not mix with aminoglycosides in same parenteral fluid
- Decreased effects: tetracyclines, erythromycins
- Increased toxicity: aminoglycosides, furosemide, probenecid, sulfinpyrazone, colistin, ethacrynic acid, vancomycin

NURSING CONSIDERATIONS

Assess:
- Sensitivity to penicillin or other cephalosporins
- Nephrotoxicity: increased BUN, creatinine
- I&O daily
- Blood studies: AST, ALT, CBC, Hct, bilirubin, LDH alk phosphatase, Coombs' test monthly if patient is on long-term therapy
- Electrolytes: potassium, sodium, chloride monthly if patient is on long-term therapy
- Bowel pattern qd; if severe diarrhea occurs, drug should be discontinued; may indicate pseudomembranous colitis
- IV site for extravasation or phlebitis; change site q72h

Administer:
- IV INF diluted 1 g of drug/10 ml of diluent, shake, give over 3-5 min

directly or run over 15-30 min as an infusion
• For 10-14 days to ensure organism death, prevent superimposed infection
• After C&S completed

Evaluate:
• Therapeutic response: decreased symptoms of infection
• Urine output, if decreasing, notify physician; may indicate nephrotoxicity
• Allergic reactions: rash, urticaria, pruritus, chills, fever, joint pain, angioedema; may occur few days after therapy begins
• Bleeding: ecchymosis, bleeding gums, hematuria, stool guaiac daily
• Overgrowth of infection: perineal itching, fever, malaise, redness, pain, swelling, drainage, rash, diarrhea, change in cough, sputum

Teach patient/family:
• If diabetic, to use Clinistix, Ketodiastix, blood glucose level
• Not to drink alcohol or meds with alcohol as reaction may occur
• To report sore throat, bruising, bleeding, joint pain; may indicate blood dyscrasias (rare)

Lab test interferences:
Increase (false): Urinary 17-KS
False positive: Urinary protein, direct Coombs', urine glucose
Interference: Cross-matching

Treatment of overdose: Epinephrine, antihistamines, resuscitate if needed (anaphylaxis)

cefotaxime sodium

(sef-oh-taks'eem)
Claforan
Func. class.: Antibiotic, broad-spectrum
Chem. class.: Cephalosporin (3rd generation)

Action: Inhibits bacterial cell wall synthesis, rendering cell wall osmotically unstable

Uses: Gram-negative organisms: *H. influenzae, E. coli, N. gonorrhoeae,*
N. meningitidis, P. mirabilis, Klebsiella, Citrobacter, Serratia, Salmonella, Shigella, gram-positive organisms: *S. pneumoniae, S. pyogenes, S. aureus,* lower serious respiratory tract, urinary tract, skin, bone, gonococcal infections, bacteremia, septicemia, meningitis

Dosage and routes:
• *Adult:* IM/IV 1 g q8-12h

Severe infections
• *Adult:* IM/IV 2 g q4h, not to exceed 12 g/day
• Uncomplicated gonorrhea, 1 g IM
• Dosage reduction indicated for severe renal impairment (CrCl < 10 ml/min)

Available forms include: Powder for inj IM, IV, 1, 2, 10 g, frozen inj/IV 20, 40 mg/ml

Side effects/adverse reactions:
CNS: Headache, dizziness, weakness, paresthesia, fever, chills
GI: Nausea, vomiting, diarrhea, anorexia, pain, glossitis, bleeding, increased AST, ALT, bilirubin, LDH, alk phosphatase, abdominal pain
GU: Proteinuria, vaginitis, pruritus, candidiasis, increased BUN, ***nephrotoxicity, renal failure***
HEMA: ***Leukopenia, thrombocytopenia, agranulocytosis,*** anemia, ***neutropenia, lymphocytosis, eosinophilia, pancytopenia, hemolytic anemia***
INTEG: Rash, urticaria, dermatitis, ***anaphylaxis,*** pain, induration (IM), inflammation (IV)

Contraindications: Hypersensitivity to cephalosporins, infants <1 mo

Precautions: Hypersensitivity to penicillins, pregnancy (B), lactation, renal disease

Pharmacokinetics:

IV: Onset 5 min

IM: Onset 30 min

Half-life 1 hr, 35%-65% is bound by plasma proteins, 40%-65% is eliminated unchanged in urine in 24 hr, 25% metabolized to active metabolites, excreted in breast milk (small amounts)

Interactions/incompatibilities:

• Do not mix with aminoglycosides, aminophylline, HCO_3, erythromycins in same parenteral fluid

• Decreased effects: tetracyclines, erythromycins

• Increased toxicity: aminoglycosides, furosemide, probenecid, sulfinpyrazone, colistin, ethacrynic acid, vancomycin

NURSING CONSIDERATIONS

Assess:

• Sensitivity to penicillin or other cephalosporins

• Nephrotoxicity: increased BUN, creatinine

• I&O daily

• Blood studies: AST, ALT, CBC, Hct, bilirubin, LDH, alk phosphatase, Coombs' test monthly if patient is on long-term therapy

• Electrolytes: potassium, sodium, chloride monthly if the patient is on long-term therapy

• Bowel pattern qd; if severe diarrhea occurs, drug should be discontinued; may indicate pseudomembranous colitis

• IV site for extravasation or phlebitis, change site q72h

Administer:

• IV after diluting 1g/10 ml and give over 3-5 min; may be diluted further with 50-100 ml of normal saline or D_5W; run over ½-1 hr

• For 10-14 days to ensure organism death, prevent superimposed infection

• After C&S completed

Evaluate:

• Therapeutic response: decreased symptoms of infection

• Urine output; if decreasing, notify physician; may indicate nephrotoxicity

• Allergic reactions: rash, urticaria, pruritis, chills, fever, joint pain, angioedema; may occur few days after therapy begins

• Bleeding: ecchymosis, bleeding gums, hematuria, stool guaiac daily

• Overgrowth of infection: perineal itching, fever, malaise, redness, pain, swelling, drainage, rash, diarrhea, change in cough, sputum

Teach patient/family:

• To report sore throat, bruising, bleeding, joint pain; may indicate blood dyscrasias (rare)

• If diabetic, to use Clinistix or Ketodiastix, blood gluose level

• Not to use alcohol or meds with alcohol or reaction may occur

Lab test interferences:

Increase (false): Urinary 17-KS

False positive: Urinary protein, direct Coombs', urine glucose

Interference: Cross-matching

Treatment of overdose: Epinephrine, antihistamines, resuscitate if needed (anaphylaxis)

cefotetan disodium

(sef'oh-tee-tan)

Cefotan

Func. class.: Antibiotic, broad-spectrum

Chem. class.: Cephalosporin (3rd generation)

Action: Inhibits bacterial cell wall

* Available in Canada only

synthesis, which renders cell osmotically unstable

Uses: Gram-negative organisms: *H. influenzae, E. coli, E. aerogenes, P. mirabilis, Klebsiella, Citrobacter, Enterobacter, Salmonella, Shigella, Acinetobacter, B. fragilis, Neisseria, Serratia;* gram-positive organisms: *S. pneumoniae, S. pyogenes, S. aureus;* upper, lower, serious respiratory tract, urinary tract, skin, gonococcal, intraabdominal infections, septicemia, meningitis

Dosages and routes:

• *Adult:* IV/IM 1-2g q12h × 5-10 days

Perioperative prophylaxis

• *Adult:* IV 1-2 g ½-1 hr before surgery

Available forms include: Inj (IV, IM)

Side effects/adverse reactions:

CNS: Headache, dizziness, weakness, paresthesia, fever, chills

GI: Nausea, vomiting, diarrhea, anorexia, pain, glossitis, bleeding, increased AST, ALT, bilirubin, LDH, alk phosphatase, ***pseudomembranous colitis***

GU: Proteinuria, vaginitis, pruritus, candidiasis, increased BUN, ***nephrotoxicity, renal failure***

HEMA: ***Leukopenia, thrombocytopenia, agranulocytosis,*** anemia, ***neutropenia, lymphocytosis, eosinophilia, pancytopenia, hemolytic anemia***

INTEG: Rash, urticaria, dermatitis

RESP: Dyspnea, ***anaphylaxis***

Contraindications: Hypersensitivity to cephalosporins, children

Precautions: Hypersensitivity to penicillins, pregnancy (B), lactation, renal disease

Pharmacokinetics:

IV/IM: Peak 1½-3 hr; half-life 3-5 hr, 70%-90% bound by plasma proteins, 50%-80% eliminated unchanged in urine, crosses placenta, excreted in milk

Interactions/incompatibilities:

• Do not mix with tetracyclines, erythromycins, aminoglycosides in same parenteral fluid

• Increased toxicity: aminoglycosides

NURSING CONSIDERATIONS

Assess:

• Sensitivity to penicillin or other cephalosporins

• Nephrotoxicity: increased BUN, creatinine

• I&O daily

• Blood studies: AST, ALT, CBC, Hct, bilirubin, LDH, alk phosphatase, Coombs' test monthly if patient is on long-term therapy

• Electrolytes: potassium, sodium, chloride monthly if patient is on long-term therapy

• Bowel pattern qd; if severe diarrhea occurs, drug should be discontinued; may indicate pseudomembranous colitis

• IV site for extravasation, phlebitis, change site q72h

Administer:

• IV after diluting 1 g/10 ml and give over 3-5 min; may be diluted further with 50-100 ml of normal saline or D_5W; run over ½-1 hr

• For 5-10 days to ensure organism death, prevent superimposed infection

• After C&S is taken

Evaluate:

• Therapeutic response: decreased symptoms of infection

• Urine output: if decreasing, notify physician, may indicate nephrotoxicity

• Allergic reactions: rash, urticaria, pruritus, chills, fever; may occur a few days after therapy begins

• Bleeding: ecchymosis, bleeding gums, hematuria, stool guaiac daily
• Overgrowth of infection: perineal itching, fever, malaise, redness, swelling, drainage, rash, diarrhea, change in cough, sputum

Teach patient/family:
• To report sore throat, bruising, bleeding, joint pain; may indicate blood dyscrasias
• To report severe diarrhea; may indicate pseudomembranous colitis
• To avoid use of alcohol during and for 3 days after use

Lab test interferences:
Increase (false): Urinary 17-KS
False positive: Urinary protein, direct Coombs' test, urine glucose
Interference: Cross-matching

Treatment of overdose: Epinephrine, antihistamines; resuscitate if needed (anaphylaxis)

cefoxitin sodium

(se-fox'i-tin)
Mefoxin

Func. class.: Antibiotic, broad-spectrum
Chem. class.: Cephamycin (2nd generation)

Action: Inhibits bacterial cell wall synthesis rendering cell wall osmotically unstable

Uses: Gram-negative bacilli: *H. influenzae, E. coli, Proteus, Klebsiella, B. fragilis, N. gonorrhoeae;* gram-positive organisms: *S. pneumoniae, S. pyogenes, S. aureus;* anaerobes including *Clostridium,* lower respiratory tract, urinary tract, skin, bone, gonococcal infections, septicemia, peritonitis

Dosage and routes:
• *Adult:* IM/IV 1-2 g q6-8h
• Dosage reduction indicated in renal impairment (CrCl <50 ml/min)
• Uncomplicated gonorrhea 2 g IM as single dose with 1 g PO probenecid at same time

Severe infections
• *Adult:* IM/IV 2 g q4h

Available forms include: Powder for inj IM, IV 1, 2, 10 g

Side effects/adverse reactions:
CNS: Headache, dizziness, weakness, paresthesia, fever, chills
GI: Nausea, vomiting, diarrhea, anorexia, pain, glossitis, bleeding, increased AST, ALT, bilirubin, LDH, alk phosphatase, abdominal pain
GU: Proteinuria, vaginitis, pruritus, candidiasis, increased BUN, ***nephrotoxicity, renal failure***
HEMA: ***Leukopenia, thrombocytopenia, agranulocytosis,*** anemia, ***neutropenia, lymphocytosis, eosinophilia, pancytopenia, hemolytic anemia***
INTEG: Rash, urticaria, dermatitis, thrombophlebitis
SYST: ***Anaphylaxis***

Contraindications: Hypersensitivity to cephalosporins, infants <1 mo

Precautions: Hypersensitivity to penicillins, pregnancy (B), lactation, renal disease

Pharmacokinetics:
IV: Peak 3 min
IM: Peak 15-60 min
Half-life 1 hr, 55%-75% bound by plasma proteins, 90%-100% eliminated unchanged in urine; crosses placenta, blood-brain barrier, eliminated in milk, not metabolized

Interactions/incompatibilities:
• Do not mix with aminoglycosides in same parenteral fluid
• Decreased effects: tetracyclines, erythromycins
• Increased toxicity: aminoglycosides, furosemide, probenecid,

* Available in Canada only

sulfinpyrazone, colistin, ethacrynic acid, vancomycin

NURSING CONSIDERATIONS

Assess:

- Sensitivity to penicillin or other cephalosporins
- Nephrotoxicity: increased BUN, creatinine
- I&O daily
- Blood studies: AST, ALT, CBC, Hct, bilirubin, LDH, alk phosphatase, Coombs' test monthly if patient is on long-term therapy
- Electrolytes: potassium, sodium, chloride monthly if patient is on long-term therapy
- Bowel pattern qd, if severe diarrhea occurs drug should be discontinued (may indicate pseudomembranous colitis)
- IV site for extravasation or phlebitis, change site q72h

Administer:

- IV after diluting 1 g/10 ml and give over 3-5 min; may be diluted further with 50-100 ml of normal saline or D_5W; run over ½-1 hr
- For 10-14 days to ensure organism death, prevent superimposed infection
- After C&S completed

Evaluate:

- Therapeutic response: decreased symptoms of infection
- Urine output; if decreasing, notify physician; may indicate nephrotoxicity
- Allergic reactions: rash, urticaria, pruritis, chills, fever, joint pain, angioedema; may occur few days after therapy begins
- Bleeding: ecchymosis, bleeding gums, hematuria, stool guaiac daily
- Overgrowth of infection: perineal itching, fever, malaise, redness, pain, swelling, drainage, rash, diarrhea, change in cough, sputum

Teach patient/family:

- If diabetic, to use Clinistix or Ketodiastix, blood glucose level
- Not to use alcohol or meds with alcohol or reaction can occur
- To report severe diarrhea; may indicate pseudomembranous colitis
- To report sore throat, bruising, bleeding, joint pain; may indicate blood dyscrasias (rare)

Lab test interferences:

Increase (false): Creatinine (serum urine), urinary 17-KS

False positive: Urinary protein, direct Coombs', urine glucose

Interference: Cross-matching

Treatment of overdose: Epinephrine, antihistamines, resuscitate if needed (anaphylaxis)

cefprozil monohydrate

(sef-pro'zil)

Cefzil

Func. class.: Antibiotic broad-spectrum

Chem. class.: Cephalosporin

Action: Inhibits bacterial cell wall synthesis, which renders cell wall osmotically unstable

Uses: Pharyngitis/tonsillitis, otitis media, secondary bacterial infection of acute bronchitis, and acute bacterial exacerbation of chronic bronchitis and uncomplicated skin and skin structure infections

Dosage and routes:

Upper respiratory infections

- *Adult:* PO 500 mg qd × 10 days

Otitis media

- *Child:* (6 mo-12 yr) PO 15mg/kg q12h × 10 days

Lower respiratory infections

- *Adult:* PO 500 mg bid × 10 days

Skin/skin structure infections

- *Adult:* PO 250-500 mg q12h × 10 days

Available forms include: Tabs 250, 500 mg; susp. 125, 250 mg/5ml

Side effects/adverse reactions:

CNS: Dizziness, headache, weakness, paresthesia, fever, chills

GU: ***Nephrotoxicity, proteinuria, increased BUN, renal failure, hematuria,*** vaginitis, genitoanal pruritus, candidiasis

GI: Diarrhea, nausea, vomiting, pain, glossitis, anorexia, bleeding, increased AST, ALT, bilirubin, LDH, alk phosphatse, abdominal pain, ***pseudomembranous colitis,*** flatulence

HEMA: ***Leukopenia, thrombocytopenia, agranulocytosis, anemia, neutropenia, lymphocytosis, eosinophilia, pancytopenia, hemolytic anemia***

INTEG: Rash, urticaria, dermatitis

RESP: ***Anaphylaxis,*** dyspnea

Contraindications: Hypersensitivity to cephalosporins

Precautions: Pregnancy (B), lactation, elderly, hypersensitivity to penicillins, renal disease

Pharmacokinetics:

PO: Peak 6-10 hr, plasma protein binding 99%, elimination half-life 25 hr, extensively metabolized to an active metabolite

Interactions/incompatibilities:

- Decreased effects of: tetracyclines, erythromycins, chloramphenicol
- Increased toxicity of: aminoglycosides, probenecid, sulfinpyrazone, colistin

NURSING CONSIDERATIONS

Assess:

- Sensitivity to penicillin or other cephalosporins
- Nephrotoxicity: increased BUN, creatinine
- I&O daily
- Blood studies: AST, ALT, CBC, Hct, bilirubin, LDH, alk phosphatase, Coombs' test monthly, bowel pattern qd; if severe diarrhea occurs, drug should be discontinued; may indicate pseudomembranous colitis

Administer:

- For 10-14 days to ensure organism death, prevent superimposed infection
- After C&S is taken

Evaluate:

- Therapeutic response: negative C&S
- Urine output; if decreasing, notify physician; may indicate nephrotoxicity
- Allergic reactions: rash, urticaria, pruritus, chills, fever, joint pain, angioedema; may occur few days after therapy begins
- Bleeding: ecchymosis, bleeding gums, hematuria, stool guaiac daily
- Overgrowth of infection: perineal itching, fever, malaise, redness, pain, swelling, drainage, rash, diarrhea, change in cough, sputum

Teach patient/family:

- Not to use alcohol or meds with alcohol or reaction may occur
- To report severe diarrhea; may indicate pseudomembranous colitis
- To report sore throat, bruising, bleeding, joint pain; may indicate blood dyscrasias (rare)

Lab test interferences:

Increase (false): Urinary 17-KS

False positive: Urinary protein, direct Coombs', urine glucose

Interference: Cross-matching

Treatment of overdose: Epinephrine, antihistamines, resuscitate if needed (anaphylaxis)

ceftazidime

(sef'tay-zi-deem)

Fortaz, Manacef, Tazicef, Tazidime

Func. class.: Antibiotic, broad-spectrum

Chem. class.: Cephalosporin (3rd generation)

Action: Inhibits bacterial cell wall synthesis, which renders cell osmotically unstable

Uses: Gram-negative organisms: *H. influenzae, E. coli, E. aerogenes, P. mirabilis, Klebsiella, Citrobacter, Enterobacter, Salmonella, Shigella, Acinetobacter, B. fragilis, Neisseria, Serratia;* gram-positive organisms: *S. pneumoniae, S. pyogenes, S. aureus;* upper, lower, serious respiratory tract, urinary tract, skin, gonococcal, intraabdominal infections; septicemia, meningitis

Dosage and routes:

- *Adult:* IV/IM 1 g q8-12h × 5-10 days
- *Children:* IV 30-50 mg/kg/day, not to exceed 6 g/day
- *Neonates:* IV 30 mg/kg q12h

Available forms include: Inj (IV, IM)

Side effects/adverse reactions:

CNS: Headache, dizziness, weakness, paresthesia, fever, chills

GI: Nausea, vomiting, diarrhea, anorexia, pain, glossitis, bleeding, increased AST, ALT, bilirubin, LDH, alk phosphatase

GU: Proteinuria, vaginitis, pruritus, candidiasis, increased BUN, ***nephrotoxicity, renal failure***

HEMA: ***Leukopenia, thrombocytopenia, agranulocytosis,*** anemia, ***neutropenia, lymphocytosis, eosinophilia, pancytopenia, hemolytic anemia***

INTEG: Rash, urticaria, dermatitis, ***anaphylaxis***

RESP: Dyspnea

Contraindications: Hypersensitivity to cephalosporins, children

Precautions: Hypersensitivity to penicillins, pregnancy (B), lactation, renal disease

Pharmacokinetics:

IV/IM: Peak 1 hr, half-life ½-1 hr, 90% bound by plasma proteins, 80% eliminated unchanged in urine, crosses placenta, excreted in breast milk

Interactions/incompatibilities:

- Do not mix with tetracyclines, erythromycins, aminoglycosides in same parenteral fluid
- Increased toxicity: aminoglycosides

NURSING CONSIDERATIONS

Assess:

- Sensitivity to penicillin or other cephalosporins
- Nephrotoxicity: increased BUN, creatinine
- I&O daily
- Blood studies: AST, ALT, CBC, Hct, bilirubin, LDH, alk phosphatase, Coombs' test monthly if patient is on long-term therapy
- Electrolytes: potassium, sodium chloride monthly if patient is on long-term therapy
- Bowel pattern qd; if severe diarrhea occurs, drug should be discontinued; may indicate pseudomembranous colitis
- IV site for extravasation, phlebitis, change site q72h

Administer:

- IV after diluting 1 g/10 ml and give over 3-5 min; may be diluted further with 50-100 ml of normal saline or D_5W; run over ½-1 hr
- For 5-10 days to ensure organism death, prevent superimposed infection
- After C&S is taken

Evaluate:
• Therapeutic response: decreased symptoms of infection
• Urine output: if decreasing, notify physician, may indicate nephrotoxicity
• Allergic reactions: rash, urticaria, pruritus, chills, fever; may occur a few days after therapy begins
• Bleeding: ecchymosis, bleeding gums, hematuria, stool guaiac daily
• Overgrowth of infection: perineal itching, fever, malaise, redness, swelling, drainage, rash, diarrhea, change in cough, sputum

Teach patient/family:
• To report sore throat, bruising, bleeding, joint pain; may indicate blood dyscrasias
• To report severe diarrhea; may indicate pseudomembranous colitis
• If diabetic, to use Clinistix or Ketodiastix, blood glucose level
• Not to use alcohol or meds with alcohol or reaction may occur

Lab test interferences:
Increase (false): Urinary 17-KS
False positive: Urinary protein, direct Coombs' test, urine glucose
Interference: Cross-matching

Treatment of overdose: Epinephrine, antihistamines, resuscitate if needed (anaphylaxis)

ceftizoxime sodium

(sef-ti-zox'eem)

Cefizox

Func. class.: Antibiotic, broad-spectrum

Chem. class.: Cephalosporin (3rd generation)

Action: Inhibits bacterial cell wall synthesis, which renders cell wall osmotically unstable

Uses: Gram-negative organisms: *H. influenzae, E. coli, E. aerogenes, P. mirabilis, Klebsiella, Enterobacter;* gram-positive organisms: *S. pneumoniae, S. pyogenes, S. aureus;* lower serious respiratory tract, urinary tract, skin, intraabdominal infections, septicemia, meningitis, bone, joint infections

Dosage and routes:
• *Adult:* IM/IV 1-2 g q8-12h, may give up to 2g q4h in life-threatening infections.

Available forms include: Inj 1, 2g

Side effects/adverse reactions:
CNS: Headache, dizziness, paresthesia, fever
GI: Nausea, vomiting, diarrhea, anorexia, pain, glossitis, bleeding, increased AST, ALT, bilirubin, LDH, alk phosphatase, abdominal pain, ***pseudomembranous colitis***
GU: Proteinuria, vaginitis, pruritus, candidiasis
HEMA: ***Leukopenia, thrombocytopenia, agranulocytosis,*** anemia, ***neutropenia, eosinophilia, hemolytic anemia***
INTEG: Rash, urticaria, dermatitis
RESP: Dyspnea, ***anaphylaxis***

Contraindications: Hypersensitivity to cephalosporins, infants <1 mo

Precautions: Hypersensitivity to penicillins, pregnancy (B), lactation, renal disease

Pharmacokinetics:
IV: Onset 5 min
IM: Peak 1 hr
Half-life 5-8 hr, 90% bound by plasma proteins, 36%-60% is eliminated unchanged in urine, crosses placenta, excreted in milk

Interactions/incompatibilities:
• Do not mix with tetracyclines, erythromycins, aminoglycosides in same parenteral fluid
• Decreased effects: tetracyclines, erythromycins

• Increased toxicity: aminoglycosides, furosemide, probenecid, sulfinpyrazone, colistin, ethacrynic acid

NURSING CONSIDERATIONS

Assess:

• Sensitivity to penicillin or other cephalosporins
• Nephrotoxicity: increased BUN, creatinine
• I&O daily
• Blood studies: AST, ALT, CBC, Hct, bilirubin, LDH, alk phosphatase, Coombs' test monthly if patient is on long-term therapy
• Electrolytes: potassium, sodium, chloride monthly if patient is on long-term therapy
• Bowel pattern qd; if severe diarrhea occurs, drug should be discontinued; may indicate pseudomembranous colitis
• IV site for extravasation, phlebitis; change site q72h

Administer:

• IV after diluting 1 g/10 ml and give over 3-5 min; may be diluted further with 50-100 ml of normal saline or D_5W; run over ½-1 hr
• For 10-14 days to ensure organism death, prevent superimposed infection
• After C&S

Evaluate:

• Therapeutic response: decreased symptoms of infection
• Allergic reactions: rash, urticaria, pruritus, chills, fever, joint pain, angioedema; may occur few days after therapy begins
• Bleeding: ecchymosis, bleeding gums, hematuria, stool guaiac daily
• Overgrowth of infection: perineal itching, fever, malaise, redness, pain, swelling, drainage, rash, diarrhea, change in cough, sputum

Teach patient/family:

• If diabetic, to use Clinistix or Ketodiastix, blood glucose level
• Not to use alcohol or meds with alcohol or reaction can occur
• To report sore throat, bruising, bleeding, joint pain; may indicate blood dyscrasias (rare)

Lab test interferences:

Increase (false): Urinary 17-KS
False positive: Urinary protein, direct Coombs', urine glucose
Interference: Cross-matching

Treatment of overdose: Epinephrine, antihistamines, resuscitate if needed (anaphylaxis)

---

ceftriaxone sodium

Rocephin

Func. class.: Antibiotic, broad-spectrum
Chem. class.: Cephalosporin (3rd generation)

Action: Inhibits bacterial cell wall synthesis, which renders cell wall osmotically unstable

Uses: Gram-negative organisms: *H. influenzae, E. coli, E. aerogenes, P. mirabilis, Klebsiella, Citrobacter, Enterobacter, Salmonella, Shigella, Acinetobacter, B. fragilis, Neisseria, Serratia;* gram-positive organisms: *S. pneumoniae, S. pyogenes, S. aureus;* lower serious respiratory tract, urinary tract, skin, gonococcal, intraabdominal infections, septicemia, meningitis, bone, joint infections

Dosage and routes:

• *Adult:* IM/IV 1-2 g qd or in two equal doses
• *Child:* IM/IV 50-75 mg/kg/day in equal doses q12h

Uncomplicated gonorrhea

• 250 mg IM as single dose
• Dosage reduction may be indicated in severe renal impairment (CrCl < 10 ml/min)

Meningitis
• *Adult and child:* IM/IV 100 mg/kg/day in equal doses q12h
Surgical prophylaxis
• Adult: IV 1 g ½-2 hr preop
Available forms include: Inj IM, IV 250, 500 mg, 1, 2, 10 g
Side effects/adverse reactions:
CNS: Headache, dizziness, weakness, paresthesia, fever, chills
GI: Nausea, vomiting, diarrhea, anorexia, pain, glossitis, bleeding, increased AST, ALT, bilirubin, LDH, alk phosphatase, abdominal pain, ***pseudomembranous colitis***
GU: Proteinuria, vaginitis, pruritus, candidiasis, increased BUN, ***nephrotoxicity, renal failure***
HEMA: ***Leukopenia, thrombocytopenia, agranulocytosis,*** anemia, ***neutropenia, lymphocytosis, eosinophilia, pancytopenia, hemolytic anemia***
INTEG: Rash, urticaria, dermatitis
RESP: Dyspnea, ***anaphylaxis***
Contraindications: Hypersensitivity to cephalosporins, infants <1 mo
Precautions: Hypersensitivity to penicillins, pregnancy (B), lactation, renal disease
Pharmacokinetics:
IV: Onset 5 min
IM: Peak 1 hr
Half-life 5-8 hr, 90% bound by plasma proteins, 35%-60% is eliminated unchanged in urine, crosses placenta, excreted in milk
Interactions/incompatibilities:
• Do not mix with tetracyclines, erythromycins, aminoglycosides in same parenteral fluid
• Decreased effects: tetracyclines, erythromycins
• Increased toxicity: aminoglycosides, furosemide, probenecid, sulfinpyrazone, colistin, ethacrynic acid

NURSING CONSIDERATIONS
Assess:
• Sensitivity to penicillin or other cephalosporins
• Nephrotoxicity: increased BUN, creatinine
• I&O daily
• Blood studies: AST, ALT, CBC, Hct, bilirubin, LDH, alk phosphatase, Coombs' test monthly if patient is on long-term therapy
• Electrolytes: potassium, sodium, chloride monthly if patient is on long-term therapy
• Bowel pattern qd; if severe diarrhea occurs, drug should be discontinued; may indicate pseudomembranous colitis
• IV site for extravasation, phlebitis; change site q72h
Administer:
• For 10-14 days to ensure organism death, prevent superimposed infection
• IV after diluting 250 mg/2.4 ml of D_5W, H_2O for inj, 0.9% NaCl; may be further diluted with 50-100 ml of compatible sol; run over ½-1 hr
• IV after diluting 1 g/10 ml and give over 3-5 min; may be diluted further with 50-100 ml of normal saline or D_5W; run over ½-1 hr
• After C&S
Evaluate:
• Therapeutic response: decreased symptoms of infection
• Urine output; if decreasing, notify physician; may indicate nephrotoxicity
• Allergic reactions: rash, urticaria, pruritus, chills, fever, joint pain, angioedema; may occur few days after therapy begins
• Bleeding: ecchymosis, bleeding gums, hematuria, stool guaiac daily
• Overgrowth of infection: perineal itching, fever, malaise, redness,

pain, swelling, drainage, rash, diarrhea, change in cough, sputum

Teach patient/family:

- If diabetic, to use Clinistix or Ketodiastix, blood glucose level
- Not to use alcohol or meds with alcohol or reaction may occur
- To report severe diarrhea; may indicate pseudomembranous colitis
- To report sore throat, bruising, bleeding, joint pain; may indicate blood dyscrasias (rare)

Lab test interferences:

Increase (false): Urinary 17-KS
False positive: Urinary protein, direct Coombs', urine glucose
Interference: Cross-matching

Treatment of overdose: Epinephrine, antihistamines, resuscitate if needed (anaphylaxis)

---

cefuroxime axetil

(sef-fyoor-ox'eem)
Ceftin

Func. class.: Antibiotic, broad-spectrum
Chem. class.: Cephalosporin (2nd generation)

Action: Inhibits bacterial cell wall synthesis, rendering cell wall osmotically unstable

Uses: Gram-negative bacilli *(H. influenzae, E. coli, Neisseria, P. mirabilis, Klebsiella);* gram-positive organisms *(S. pneumoniae, S. pyogenes, S. aureus);* serious lower respiratory tract, urinary tract, skin, gonococcal infections; septicemia; meningitis

Dosage and routes:

- *Adult and child:* PO 250 mg q12h, may increase to 500 mg q12h in serious infections

Urinary tract infections

- *Adult:* PO 125 mg q12h, may increase to 250 q12h if needed

Otitis media

- Child <2 yr: PO 125 mg bid
- Child >2 yr: PO 250 mg bid

Available forms include: Tabs 125, 250, 500 mg

Side effects/adverse reactions:

CNS: Headache, dizziness, weakness, paresthesia, fever, chills
GI: Nausea, vomiting, diarrhea, anorexia, pain, glossitis, bleeding, increased AST, ALT, bilirubin, LDH, alk phosphatase, abdominal pain, ***pseudomembranous colitis***
GU: Proteinuria, vaginitis, pruritus, candidiasis, increased BUN, ***nephrotoxicity, renal failure***
HEMA: ***Leukopenia, thrombocytopenia, agranulocytosis,*** anemia, ***neutropenia, lymphocytosis, eosinophilia, pancytopenia, hemolytic anemia***
INTEG: Rash, urticaria, dermatitis
RESP: ***Anaphylaxis***

Contraindications: Hypersensitivity to cephalosporins, infants <1 mo

Precautions: Hypersensitivity to penicillins, pregnancy (B), lactation, renal disease

Pharmacokinetics:
65% excreted unchanged in urine, half-life 1-2 hr in normal renal function

Interactions/incompatibilities:

- Decreased effects: tetracyclines, erythromycins
- Increased side effects: aminoglycosides, furosemide, probenecid, sulfinpyrazone, colistin, ethacrynic acid

NURSING CONSIDERATIONS

Assess:

- Sensitivity to penicillin or other cephalosporins
- Nephrotoxicity: increased BUN, creatinine
- I&O daily
- Blood studies: AST, ALT, CBC,

Hct, bilirubin, LDH, alk phosphatase, Coombs' test monthly if patient is on long-term therapy
• Electrolytes: potassium, sodium, chloride monthly if patient is on long-term therapy
• Bowel pattern qd; if severe diarrhea occurs, drug should be discontinued; may indicate pseudomembranous colitis
• IV site for extravasation, phlebitis; change site q72h

Administer:
• For 10-14 days to ensure organism death, prevent superimposed infection
• With food if needed for GI symptoms
• After C&S

Evaluate:
• Therapeutic response: decreased symptoms of infection
• Urine output: if decreasing, notify physician; may indicate nephrotoxicity
• Allergic reactions: rash, urticaria, pruritus, chills, fever, joint pain, angioedema; may occur a few days after therapy begins
• Bleeding: ecchymosis, bleeding gums, hematuria, stool guaiac daily
• Overgrowth of infection: perineal itching, fever, malaise, redness, pain, swelling, drainage, rash, diarrhea, change in cough, sputum

Teach patient/family:
• To use yogurt or buttermilk to maintain intestinal flora, decrease diarrhea
• To take all medication prescribed for length of time ordered
• To report sore throat, bruising, bleeding, joint pain; may indicate blood dyscrasias (rare)
• If diabetic, to use Clinistix or Ketodiastix, blood glucose level
• Not to use alcohol or meds with alcohol or reaction may occur

Lab test interferences:
Increase (false): Creatinine (serum urine), urinary 17-KS
False positive: Urinary protein, direct Coombs', urine glucose
Interferences: Cross-matching

Treatment of overdose: Epinephrine, antihistamine, resuscitate if needed (anaphylaxis)

cefuroxime sodium

(se-fyoor-ox'eem)
Zinacef, Kefurox
Func. class.: Antibiotic, broad-spectrum
Chem. class.: Cephalosporin (2nd generation)

Action: Inhibits bacterial cell wall synthesis, rendering cell wall osmotically unstable

Uses: Gram-negative organisms: *H. influenzae, E. coli, Neisseria, P. mirabilis, Klebsiella;* gram-positive organisms: *S. pneumoniae, S. pyogenes, S. aureus;* serious lower respiratory tract, urinary tract, skin, gonococcal infections, septicemia, meningitis

Dosage and routes:
• *Adult:* IM/IV 750 mg-1.5 g q8h for 5-10 days

Surgical prophylaxis
• *Adult:* IV 1.5 g ½-1 hr preop

Severe infections
• *Adult:* IM/IV 1.5 g q6h; may give up to 3 g q8h for bacterial meningitis
• *Child >3 mo:* IM/IV 50-100 mg/kg/day; may give up to 200-240 mg/kg/day IV in divided doses for bacterial meningitis
• Dosage reduction indicated in severe renal impairment (CrCl < 20 ml/min)
• ***Uncomplicated gonorrhea:*** 1.5 g

IM as single dose with oral probenecid
Available forms include: Inj IM, IV 750 mg, 1.5 g, powder
Side effects/adverse reactions:
CNS: Headache, dizziness, weakness, paresthesia, fever, chills
GI: Nausea, vomiting, diarrhea, anorexia, pain, glossitis, bleeding, increased AST, ALT, bilirubin, LDH, alk phosphatase, abdominal pain, ***pseudomembranous colitis***
GU: Proteinuria, vaginitis, pruritus, candidiasis, increased BUN, ***nephrotoxicity, renal failure***
HEMA: ***Leukopenia, thrombocytopenia, agranulocytosis,*** anemia, ***neutropenia, lymphocytosis, eosinophilia, pancytopenia, hemolytic anemia***
INTEG: Rash, urticaria, dermatitis
RESP: Dyspnea, ***anaphylaxis***
Contraindications: Hypersensitivity to cephalosporins, infants <1 mo
Precautions: Hypersensitivity to penicillins, pregnancy (B), lactation, renal disease
Pharmacokinetics:
IV: Peak 3 min
IM: Peak 15-60 min
Half-life 1-2 hr, 33%-50% bound by plasma proteins, 70%-100% eliminated unchanged in urine, crosses placenta, blood-brain barrier, excreted in breast milk, not metabolized
Interactions/incompatibilities:
- Do not mix with aminoglycosides in the same parenteral fluid
- Decreased effects: tetracyclines, erythromycins
- Increased toxicity: aminoglycosides, furosemide, probenecid, sulfinpyrazone, colistin, ethacrynic acid, vancomycin

NURSING CONSIDERATIONS

Assess:
- Sensitivity to penicillin or other cephalosporins
- Nephrotoxicity: increased BUN, creatinine
- I&O daily
- Blood studies: AST, ALT, CBC, Hct, bilirubin, LDH, alk phosphatase, Coombs' test monthly if patient is on long-term therapy
- Electrolytes: potassium, sodium, chloride monthly if patient is on long-term therapy
- Bowel pattern qd; if severe diarrhea occurs, drug should be discontinued; may indicate pseudomembranous colitis
- IV site for extravasation, phlebitis; change site q72h

Administer:
- IV after diluting 8 ml/750 mg of sterile H_2O for Inj and give over 3-5 min; may be further diluted with 100 ml of compatible sol; run over ½ hr; may also be given by continuous infusion
- For 10-14 days to ensure organism death, prevent superimposed infection
- After C&S

Evaluate:
- Therapeutic response: decreased symptoms of infection
- Urine output: if decreasing, notify physician; may indicate nephrotoxicity
- Allergic reactions: rash, urticaria, pruritus, chills, fever, joint pain, angioedema; may occur few days after therapy begins
- Bleeding: ecchymosis, bleeding gums, hematuria, stool guaiac daily
- Overgrowth of infection: perineal itching, fever, malaise, redness, pain, swelling, drainage, rash, diarrhea, change in cough, sputum

Teach patient/family:
- To report severe diarrhea; may indicate pseudomembranous colitis
- If diabetic, to use Clinistix or Ketodiastix, blood glucose level
- Not to use alcohol or meds with alcohol or reaction can occur
- To report sore throat, bruising, bleeding, joint pain; may indicate blood dyscrasias (rare)

Lab test interferences:
Increase (false): Urinary 17-KS
False positive: Urinary protein, direct Coombs', urine glucose
Interference: Cross-matching
Treatment of overdose: Epinephrine, antihistamines, resuscitate if needed (anaphylaxis)

cellulose sodium phosphate

Calcibind, Calcisorb*

Func. class.: Antihypercalcemia
Chem. class.: Phosphorylated cellulose

Action: Decreases hypercalcium by binding with calcium in bowel, facilitates excretion
Uses: Calcium oxalate or phosphate renal stones associated with absorptive hypercalciuria type I
Dosage and routes:
- *Adult:* PO 15 g/day divided between each meal, then 10 g/day when urine Ca <150 mg/day

Available forms include: Powder 2.5 g packets
Side effects/adverse reactions:
GU: Hypomagnesuria, hyperoxaluria
GI: Nausea, anorexia, diarrhea, dyspepsia
Contraindications: Hypersensitivity, hyperparathyroidism, hypomagnesium, enteric hyperoxaluria, bone disease, hypocalcemia
Precautions: CHF, ascites, liver disease, pregnancy (C), children, elderly
Pharmacokinetics:
Not known
Interactions/incompatibilities:
- Decreased action of cellulose: magnesium preparations

NURSING CONSIDERATIONS

Assess:
- Calcium levels (serum, urinary) throughout treatment (therapeutic values: 2.3-2.8 mmol/L, serum; <3.75 mmol/24 hr, urine)

Administer:
- Powder with water, juice; take within 30 min of meals
- Increase fluids to 3 L/day; urinary output should be >2 L/day

Evaluate:
- Therapeutic response: absence of renal stone formation

Teach patient/family:
- To decrease calcium in diet: dairy products; decrease sodium, citrus fruits in diet; increased excretion of drug will occur; decrease oxalate (chocolate, tea, spinach)
- To increase fluid intake to 3-4 L/day

cephalexin

(sef-a-lex'in)

Ceporex,* Keftab, Keflex, Keflet, Novolexin*

Func. class.: Antibiotic
Chem. class.: Cephalosporin (1st generation)

Action: Inhibits bacterial cell wall synthesis, rendering cell wall osmotically unstable
Uses: Gram-negative bacilli: *H. influenzae, E. coli, P. mirabilis, Klebsiella;* gram-positive organisms: *S. pneumoniae, S. pyogenes, S. aureus;* upper, lower respiratory

* Available in Canada only

tract, urinary tract, skin, bone infections, otitis media

Dosage and routes:

- *Adult:* PO 250-500 mg q6h
- *Child:* PO 25-50 mg/kg/day in 4 equal doses

Moderate skin infections

500 mg q12h

Severe infections

- *Adult:* PO 500 mg-1 g q6h
- *Child:* PO 50-100 mg/kg/day in 4 equal doses
- Dosage reduction indicated in renal impairment (CrCl < 50 ml/min)

Available forms include: Caps 250, 500 mg; tabs 250, 500, 1000 mg; pulvules 250 mg; oral susp 125, 250 mg/5 ml; pediatric susp 100 mg/5 ml

Side effects/adverse reactions:

CNS: Headache, dizziness, weakness, paresthesia, fever, chills

GI: Nausea, vomiting, diarrhea, anorexia, pain, glossitis, bleeding, increased AST, ALT, bilirubin, LDH, alk phosphatase, abdominal pain, ***pseudomembranous colitis***

GU: Proteinuria, vaginitis, pruritus, candidiasis, increased BUN, ***nephrotoxicity, renal failure***

HEMA: ***Leukopenia, thrombocytopenia, agranulocytosis,*** anemia, ***neutropenia, lymphocytosis, eosinophilia, pancytopenia, hemolytic anemia***

INTEG: Rash, urticaria, dermatitis

RESP: Dyspnea, ***anaphylaxis***

Contraindications: Hypersensitivity to cephalosporins, infants <1 mo.

Precautions: Hypersensitivity to penicillins, pregnancy (B), lactation, renal disease

Pharmacokinetics:

PO: Peak 1 hr, duration 6-8 hr, half-life 30-72 min, 5%-15% bound by plasma proteins, 90%-100% eliminated unchanged in urine, crosses placenta, excreted in breast milk

Interactions/incompatibilities:

- Decreased effects: tetracyclines, erythromycins
- Increased toxicity: aminoglycosides, furosemide, probenecid, sulfinpyrazone, colistin, ethacrynic acid, vancomycin

NURSING CONSIDERATIONS

Assess:

- Sensitivity to penicillin or other cephalosporins
- Nephrotoxicity: increased BUN, creatinine
- I&O daily
- Blood studies: AST, ALT, CBC, Hct, bilirubin, LDH, alk phosphatase, Coombs' test monthly if patient is on long-term therapy
- Electrolytes: potassium, sodium, chloride monthly if patient is on long-term therapy
- Bowel pattern qd; if severe diarrhea occurs, drug should be discontinued; may indicate pseudomembranous colitis

Administer:

- For 10-14 days to ensure organism death, prevent superimposed infection
- With food if needed for GI symptoms
- After C&S

Evaluate:

- Therapeutic response: decreased symptoms of infection
- Urine output: if decreasing, notify physician; may indicate nephrotoxicity
- Allergic reactions: rash, urticaria, pruritus, chills, fever, joint pain, angioedema; may occur few days after therapy begins
- Bleeding: ecchymosis, bleeding gums, hematuria, stool guaiac daily
- Overgrowth of infection: perineal itching, fever, malaise, redness,

pain, swelling, drainage, rash, diarrhea, change in cough, sputum

Teach patient/family:

- If diabetic, to use Clinistix or Ketodiastix, blood glucose level
- Not to use alcohol or meds with alcohol or reaction may occur
- To use yogurt or buttermilk to maintain intestinal flora, decrease diarrhea
- To take all medication prescribed for length of time ordered
- To report sore throat, bruising, bleeding, joint pain; may indicate blood dyscrasias (rare)
- To report severe diarrhea; may indicate pseudomembranous colitis

Lab test interferences:
Increase (false): Creatinine (serum urine), urinary 17-KS
False positive: Urinary protein, direct Coombs', urine glucose
Interference: Cross-matching

Treatment of overdose: Epinephrine, antihistamines, resuscitate if needed (anaphylaxis)

---

cephalothin sodium

(sef-a'loe-thin)

Ceporacin,* Keflin, Seffin

Func. class.: Antibiotic, broad-spectrum
Chem. class.: Cephalosporin (1st generation)

Action: Inhibits bacterial cell wall synthesis, rendering cell wall osmotically unstable

Uses: Gram-negative bacilli: *H. influenzae, E. coli, P. mirabilis, Klebsiella, Salmonella, Shigella;* gram-positive organisms: *S. pneumoniae, S. pyogenes, S. aureus;* lower respiratory tract, urinary tract, skin, bone infections, septicemia, endocarditis, bacterial peritonitis

Dosage and routes:

- *Adult:* IM/IV 500 mg-1 g q4-6h
- *Child:* IM/IV 14-27 mg/kg q4h or 20-40 mg/kg, q6h
- Dosage reduction indicated in renal impairment (CrCl < 50 ml/min)
- Uncomplicated gonorrhea 2 g IM as single dose

Severe infections

- *Adult:* IM/IV 1-2 g q4h

Available forms include: Powder for inj IM, IV 1, 2, 4, 10, 20 g; frozen IV 20, 30, 40 mg/ml

Side effects/adverse reactions:
CNS: Headache, dizziness, weakness, paresthesia, fever, chills
GI: Nausea, vomiting, diarrhea, anorexia, pain, glossitis, bleeding, increased AST, ALT, bilirubin, LDH, alk phosphatase, abdominal pain, ***pseudomembranous colitis***
GU: Proteinuria, vaginitis, pruritus, candidiasis, increased BUN, ***nephrotoxicity, renal failure***
HEMA: ***Leukopenia, thrombocytopenia, agranulocytosis,*** anemia, ***neutropenia, lymphocytosis, eosinophilia, pancytopenia, hemolytic anemia***
INTEG: Rash, urticaria, dermatitis
RESP: Dyspnea, ***anaphylaxis***

Contraindications: Hypersensitivity to cephalosporins

Precautions: Hypersensitivity to penicillins, pregnancy (B), lactation, renal disease

Pharmacokinetics:
IV: Peak 15 min
IM: Peak 30 min
Half-life ½-1 hr, 65%-80% bound by plasma proteins, 50%-75% eliminated unchanged in urine in 8 hr, crosses placenta, excreted in breast milk, deacetylated in kidneys, liver

Interactions/incompatibilities:

- Do not mix with tetracyclines,

---

* Available in Canada only

erythromycins, calcium chloride, magnesium salts, aminoglycosides, barbiturates, aminophylline in same parenteral fluid
• Decreased effects: tetracyclines, erythromycins
• Increased toxicity: aminoglycosides, furosemide, probenecid, sulfinpyrazone, colistin, ethacrynic acid, vancomycin

NURSING CONSIDERATIONS

Assess:
• Nephrotoxicity: increased BUN, creatinine
• Sensitivity to penicillin or other cephalosporins
• I&O daily
• Blood studies: AST, ALT, CBC, Hct, bilirubin, LDH, alk phosphatase, Coombs' test monthly if patient is on long-term therapy
• Electrolytes: potassium, sodium, chloride monthly if patient is on long-term therapy
• Bowel pattern qd; if severe diarrhea occurs, drug should be discontinued; may indicate pseudomembranous colitis
• IV site for extravasation, phlebitis; change site q72h

Administer:
• IV after diluting 1 g/10 ml of D_5W normal saline, sterile H_2O for inj; give over 3-5 min; may be further diluted with 50 ml of compatible sol, run over 15-30 min; may also be given by continuous infusion
• For 10-14 days to ensure organism death, prevent superimposed infection
• After C&S

Evaluate:
• Therapeutic response: decreased symptoms of infection
• Urine output: if decreasing, notify physician; may indicate nephrotoxicity
• Allergic reactions: rash, urticaria, pruritus, chills, fever, joint pain, angioedema; may occur few days after therapy begins
• Bleeding: ecchymosis, bleeding gums, hematuria, stool guaiac daily
• Overgrowth of infection: perineal itching, fever, malaise, redness, pain, swelling, drainage, rash, diarrhea, change in cough, sputum

Teach patient/family:
• If diabetic, to use Clinistix or Ketodiastix, blood glucose level
• Not to use alcohol or meds with alcohol or reaction can occur
• To report sore throat, bruising, bleeding, joint pain; may indicate blood dyscrasias (rare)
• To report severe diarrhea; may indicate pseudomembranous colitis

Lab test interferences:
Increase (false): Creatinine (serum urine), urinary 17-KS
False positive: Urinary protein, direct Coombs', urine glucose
Interference: Cross-matching

Treatment of overdose: Epinephrine, antihistamines, resuscitate if needed (anaphylaxis)

cephapirin sodium

(sef-a-pye'rin)
Cefadyl

Func. class.: Antibiotic, broad-spectrum
Chem. class.: Cephalosporin (1st generation)

Action: Inhibits bacterial cell wall synthesis, rendering cell wall osmotically unstable
Uses: Gram-negative bacilli: *H. influenzae, E. coli, P. mirabilis, Klebsiella;* gram-positive organisms: *S. pneumoniae, S. viridans, S. aureus;* lower respiratory tract, urinary tract, skin infections, sep-

ticemia, endocarditis, bacterial peritonitis

Dosage and routes:

- *Adult:* IM/IV 500 mg-1 g q4-6h
- *Child:* IM/IV 20-30 mg/kg, q6h
- Dosage reduction indicated in renal impairment (CrCl < 50 ml/min)

Available forms include: Powder for inj IM, IV 500 mg, 1, 2, 20 g; IV only 1, 2, 4 g

Side effects/adverse reactions:

CNS: Headache, dizziness, weakness, paresthesia, fever, chills

GI: Nausea, vomiting, diarrhea, anorexia, pain, glossitis, bleeding, increased AST, ALT, bilirubin, LDH, alk phosphatase, abdominal pain, ***pseudomembranous colitis***

GU: Proteinuria, vaginitis, pruritus, candidiasis, increased BUN, ***nephrotoxicity, renal failure***

HEMA: ***Leukopenia, thrombocytopenia, agranulocytosis,*** anemia, ***neutropenia, lymphocytosis, eosinophilia, pancytopenia, hemolytic anemia***

INTEG: Rash, urticaria, dermatitis

RESP: Dyspnea, **anaphylaxis**

Contraindications: Hypersensitivity to cephalosporins, infants <1 mo

Precautions: Hypersensitivity to penicillins, pregnancy (B), lactation, renal disease

Pharmacokinetics:

IV: Peak 5 min

IM: Peak 30 min

Half-life 21-47 min, 44%-50% bound by plasma proteins, 40%-70% eliminated unchanged in urine, crosses placenta, excreted in breast milk, metabolized in liver

Interactions/incompatibilities:

- Do not mix with tetracyclines, aminoglycosides in same parenteral fluid
- Decreased effects: tetracyclines, erythromycins
- Increased toxicity: aminoglycosides, furosemide, probenecid, sulfinpyrazone, colistin, ethacrynic acid

NURSING CONSIDERATIONS

Assess:

- Sensitivity to penicillin or other cephalosporins
- Nephrotoxicity: increased BUN, creatinine
- I&O daily
- Blood studies: AST, ALT, CBC, Hct, bilirubin, LDH, alk phosphatase, Coombs' test monthly if patient is on long-term therapy
- Electrolytes: potassium, sodium, chloride monthly if patient is on long-term therapy
- Bowel pattern qd; if severe diarrhea occurs drug should be discontinued; may indicate pseudomembranous colitis
- IV site for extravasation, phlebitis; change site q72h

Administer:

- IV after diluting 1 g/10 ml or more normal saline, D_5W or bacteriostatic H_20 for inj; may be further diluted in 50-100 ml of compatible sol; run over 15 min; may also be given by continuous infusion
- For 10-14 days to ensure organism death, prevent superimposed infection
- After C&S

Evaluate:

- Therapeutic response: decreased symptoms of infection
- Urine output: if decreasing, notify physician; may indicate nephrotoxicity
- Allergic reactions: rash, urticaria, pruritus, chills, fever, joint pain, angioedema; may occur few days after therapy begins

- Bleeding: ecchymosis, bleeding gums, hematuria, stool guaiac daily
- Overgrowth of infection: perineal itching, fever, malaise, redness, pain, swelling, drainage, rash, diarrhea, change in cough, sputum

Teach patient/family:

- If diabetic, to use Clinistix or Ketodiastix, blood glucose level
- Not to use alcohol or meds with alcohol or reaction may occur
- To report severe diarrhea; may indicate pseudomembranous colitis
- To report sore throat, bruising, bleeding, joint pain; may indicate blood dyscrasias (rare)

Lab test interferences:
Increase (false:) Creatinine (serum urine), urinary 17-KS
False positive: Urinary protein, direct Coombs', urine glucose
Interference: Cross-matching

Treatment of overdose: Epinephrine, antihistamines, resuscitate if needed (anaphylaxis)

---

cephradine

(sef'ra-deen)
Anspor, Velosef

Func. class.: Antibiotic
Chem. class.: Cephalosporin (1st generation)

Action: Inhibits bacterial cell wall synthesis, rendering cell wall osmotically unstable

Uses: Gram-negative bacilli: *H. influenzae, E. coli, P. mirabilis, Klebsiella;* gram-positive organisms: *S. pneumoniae, S. pyogenes, S. aureus;* serious respiratory tract, urinary tract, skin infections, otitis media

Dosage and routes:

- *Adult:* IM/IV 500 mg-1 g q4-6h not to exceed 8 g/day; PO 250 mg-1 g q6-12h
- *Child >1 yr.:* IM/IV 12-25 mg/kg q6h; PO 6-12 mg/kg q6h

Available forms include: Powder for inj IM, IV 250, 500 mg, 1 g; caps 250, 500 mg; oral susp 125, 250 mg/5 ml

C

Side effects/adverse reactions:
CNS: Headache, dizziness, weakness, paresthesia, fever, chills
GI: Nausea, vomiting, diarrhea, anorexia, pain, glossitis, bleeding, increased AST, ALT, bilirubin, LDH, alk phosphatase, abdominal pain, ***pseudomembranous colitis***
GU: Proteinuria, vaginitis, pruritus, candidiasis, increased BUN, ***nephrotoxicity, renal failure***
HEMA: ***Leukopenia, thrombocytopenia, agranulocytosis,*** anemia, ***neutropenia, lymphocytosis, eosinophilia, pancytopenia, hemolytic anemia***
INTEG: Rash, urticaria, dermatitis
RESP: Dyspnea, ***anaphylaxis***

Contraindications: Hypersensitivity to cephalosporins, infants <1 mo

Precautions: Hypersensitivity to penicillins, pregnancy (B), lactation, renal disease

Pharmacokinetics:
PO: Peak 1 hr
IV: Peak 5 min
IM: Peak 1 hr
Half-life 0.75-1.5 h, 20% bound by plasma proteins, 80%-90% eliminated unchanged in urine, crosses placenta, excreted in breast milk

Interactions/incompatibilities:

- Do not mix with tetracyclines, erythromycins, calcium chloride, magnesium salts, aminoglycosides in same parenteral fluid
- Decreased effects: tetracyclines, erythromycins
- Increased toxicity: aminoglycosides, furosemide, probenecid,

sulfinpyrazone, colistin, ethacrynic acid, vancomycin

NURSING CONSIDERATIONS

Assess:

• Sensitivity to penicillin or other cephalosporins

• Nephrotoxicity: increased BUN, creatinine

• I&O daily

• Blood studies: AST, ALT, CBC, Hct, bilirubin, LDH, alk phosphatase, Coombs' test monthly if patient is on long-term therapy

• Electrolytes: potassium, sodium, chloride monthly if patient is on long-term therapy

• Bowel pattern qd; if severe diarrhea occurs, drug should be discontinued; may indicate pseudomembranous colitis

• IV site for extravasation, phlebitis; change site q72h

Administer:

• IV after diluting 1 g/10 ml of D_5W or normal saline; give over 3-5 min; may be further diluted 1 g/10 ml of compatible sol, run over ½-1 hr

• For 10-14 days to ensure organism death, prevent superimposed infection

• With food if needed for GI symptoms

• After C&S

Evaluate:

• Therapeutic response: decreased symptoms of infection

• Urine output: if decreasing, notify physician; may indicate nephrotoxicity

• Allergic reactions: rash, urticaria, pruritus, chills, fever, joint pain, angioedema; may occur few days after therapy begins

• Bleeding: ecchymosis, bleeding gums, hematuria, stool guaiac daily

• Overgrowth of infection: perineal itching, fever, malaise, redness, pain, swelling, drainage, rash, diarrhea, change in cough, sputum

Teach patient/family:

• If diabetic, to use Clinistix or Ketodiastix, blood glucose level

• Not to use alcohol or meds with alcohol or reaction can occur

• To use yogurt or buttermilk to maintain intestinal flora, decrease diarrhea

• To take all medication prescribed for length of time ordered

• To report sore throat, bruising, bleeding, joint pain; may indicate blood dyscrasias (rare)

Lab test interferences:

Increase (false): Creatinine (serum urine), urinary 17-KS

False positive: Urinary protein, direct Coombs', urine glucose

Interference: Cross-matching

Treatment of overdose: Epinephrine, antihistamines, resuscitate if needed (anaphylaxis)

---

chenodiol

(kee-noe-dye'ole)

Chenix

Func. class.: Antilithic

Chem. class.: Chenodeoxycholic acid

Action: Suppresses synthesis of cholesterol, cholic acid, replacing cholic acid with drug metabolite, which leads to the degradation of gallstones

Uses: Dissolving gallstones instead of surgery

Dosage and routes:

• *Adult:* PO 250 mg bid × 2 wk, then increased by 250 mg/day, not to exceed 16 mg/kg/day × 24 mo

Available forms include: Tabs 250 mg

Side effects/adverse reactions:

HEMA: ***Leukopenia***

GI: Diarrhea, fecal urgency, heartburn, nausea, cramps, increased ALT, AST, LDH, vomiting, dysphagia, absence of taste, ***hepatotoxicity,*** flatulence, dyspepsia
Contraindications: Hypersensitivity, hepatic disease, bile duct obstruction, biliary GI fistula, pregnancy (X)
Precautions: Lactation, children, atherosclerosis, elderly
Pharmacokinetics:
Metabolized by liver, excreted in feces (metabolite/unchanged drug), crosses placenta
Interactions/incompatibilities:
• Decreased action of chenodiol: cholestyramine, colestipol, aluminum antacids, estrogens, clofibrate

NURSING CONSIDERATIONS
Assess:
• Vital signs, cardiac status: checking for dysrhythmias increased rate, palpitations
• I&O ratio; check for urinary retention or hesitancy, especially elderly
• Oral cholecystogram or ultrasonogram q6-9 mo
Administer:
• With meals for better absorption
• Antidiarrheals if diarrhea occurs
Perform/provide:
• Storage at room temperature
• Increased fluids, bulk, exercise to patient's lifestyle to decrease constipation
Evaluate:
• Therapeutic response: absence of pain (epigastric), gallstones on diagnostic testing
• GI complaints: nausea, vomiting, anorexia, diarrhea; if diarrhea is severe dosage may need to be decreased
Teach patient/family:
• That stone dissolution may take 6-24 mo, therapy is discontinued in 18 mo if gallstones are still intact
• To notify physician if pregnancy is suspected, birth defects may occur

C

chloral hydrate

(klor-al hye'drate)
Aquachloral Supprettes, Cohidrate, Noctec, Novochlorhydrate*
Func. class.: Sedative-hypnotic
Chem. class.: Chloral derivative

Controlled Substance Schedule IV (USA), Schedule F (Canada)
Action: Reduction product trichloroethanol produces mild cerebral depression, which causes sleep
Uses: Sedation, insomnia
Dosage and routes:
Sedation
• *Adult:* PO/REC 250 mg tid pc
• *Child:* PO 8 mg/kg tid, not to exceed 500 mg tid
Insomnia
• *Adult:* PO/REC 500 mg-1g ½ hr before hs
• *Child:* PO/REC 50 mg/kg in one dose, up to 1
Available forms include: Caps 250, 500 mg; syr 250, 500 mg/5 ml; supp 325, 500, 650 mg
Side effects/adverse reactions:
HEMA: ***Eosinophilia, leukopenia***
CNS: Drowsiness, dizziness, stimulation, nightmares, ataxia, hangover (rare), light-headedness, headache, paranoia
GI: Nausea, vomiting, flatulence, diarrhea, unpleasant taste, ***gastric necrosis***
INTEG: Rash, urticaria, angioedema, fever, purpura, eczema
CV: Hypotension, dysrhythmias
RESP: ***Depression***
Contraindications: Hypersensitivity to this drug or triclofos, severe renal disease, severe hepatic dis-

ease, GI disorders (oral forms), gastritis

Precautions: Severe cardiac disease, depression, suicidal individuals, asthma, intermittent porphyria, pregnancy (C), lactation, elderly

Pharmacokinetics:

PO: Onset 30 min-1 hr, duration 4-8 hr

REC: Onset slow, duration 4-6 hr; metabolized by liver, excreted by kidneys (inactive metabolite) and feces, crosses placenta, excreted in breast milk; metabolite is highly protein bound

Interactions/incompatibilities:

- Increased action of: oral anticoagulants, furosemide
- Increased action of both drugs: alcohol, CNS depressants

NURSING CONSIDERATIONS

Assess:

- Blood studies: Hct, Hgb, RBCs serum folate (if on long-term therapy), pro-time in patients receiving anticoagulants

Administer:

- After removal of cigarettes, to prevent fires
- After trying conservative measures for insomnia
- ½-1 hr before hs for sleeplessness
- On empty stomach with full glass of water or juice for best absorption and decrease corrosion (do not chew); after meals to decrease GI symptoms if using for sedation

Perform/provide:

- Assistance with ambulation after receiving dose, especially elderly
- Safety measure: siderails, nightlight, callbell within easy reach
- Checking to see PO medication swallowed
- Storage in dark container, suppositories in refrigerator

Evaluate:

- Therapeutic response: ability to sleep at night, decreased amount of early morning awakening if taking drug for insomnia
- Mental status: mood, sensorium, affect, memory (long, short)
- Physical dependency: more frequent requests for medication, shakes, anxiety
- Respiratory dysfunction: respiratory depression, character, rate, rhythm; hold drug if respirations are <10/min or if pupils are dilated (rare)
- Blood dyscrasias: fever, sore throat, bruising, rash, jaundice, epistaxis (rare)
- Previous history of substance abuse, cardiac disease, or gastritis

Teach patient/family:

- To avoid driving or other activities requiring alertness
- To avoid alcohol ingestion or CNS depressants; serious CNS depression may result
- Not to discontinue medication quickly after long-term use; drug should be tapered over 1-2 wk
- That effects may take 2 nights for benefits to be noticed
- Alternate measures to improve sleep (reading, exercise several hours before hs, warm bath, warm milk, TV, self-hypnosis, deep breathing)

Lab test interferences:

Interferences: Urine catecholamines, urinary 17-OHCS

False Positive: Urine glucose (copper sulfate test)

Treatment of overdose: Lavage, activated charcoal, monitor electrolytes, vital signs

* Available in Canada only

chlorambucil

(klor-am'byoo-sil)
Leukeran
Func. class.: Antineoplastic alkylating agent
Chem. class.: Nitrogen mustard

Action: Alkylates DNA, RNA; inhibits enzymes that allow synthesis of amino acids in proteins
Uses: Chronic lymphocytic leukemia, Hodgkin's disease, other lymphomas, macroglobulinemia, nephrotic syndrome, breast carcinoma, choreocarcinoma, ovarian carcinoma
Dosage and routes:
• *Adult:* PO 0.1-0.2 mg/kg/day for 3-6 wk initially, then 2-6 mg/day; maintenance 0.2 mg/kg for 2-4 wk, course may be repeated at 2-4 wk intervals
• *Child:* PO 0.1-0.2 mg/kg/day in divided doses or 4.5 mg/m^2/day as 1 dose or in divided doses
Available forms include: Tabs 2 mg
Side effects/adverse reactions:
CNS: ***Convulsions in children***
HEMA: ***Thrombocytopenia, leukopenia, pancytopenia*** (prolonged use), ***permanent bone marrow depression***
GI: Nausea, vomiting, diarrhea, weight loss
GU: Hyperuremia
INTEG: Alopecia (rare), dermatitis, rash
RESP: ***Fibrosis, pneumonitis***
Contraindications: Radiation therapy within 1 mo, chemotherapy within 1 mo, thrombocytopenia, smallpox vaccination, pregnancy (1st trimester) (D)
Precautions: Pneumococcus vaccination
Pharmacokinetics:
Well absorbed orally, metabolized in liver, excreted in urine; half-life 2 hr
Interactions/incompatibilities:
• Increased toxicity: other antineoplastics, or radiation

NURSING CONSIDERATIONS

Assess:
• CBC, differential, platelet count weekly; withhold drug if WBC is <4000 or platelet count is <75,000; notify physician of results
• Pulmonary functions test, chest x-ray films before, during therapy; chest film should be obtained q2wk during treatment
• Renal function studies: BUN, serum uric acid, urine CrCl before, during therapy
• I&O ratio; report fall in urine output of 30 ml/hr
• Monitor temperature q4h (may indicate beginning infection)
• Liver function tests before, during therapy (bilirubin, AST, ALT, LDH) as needed or monthly
Administer:
• Antacid before oral agent, give drug after evening meal, before bedtime
• Antiemetic 30-60 min before giving drug to prevent vomiting
• Allopurinol or sodium bicarbonate to maintain uric acid levels, alkalinization of urine
• Antibiotics for prophylaxis of infection
Perform/provide:
• Storage in tight container
• Strict medical asepsis, protective isolation if WBC levels are low
• Increase fluid intake to 2-3 L/day to prevent urate deposits, calculi formation
• Diet low in purines: organ meats (kidney, liver), dried beans, peas to maintain alkaline urine

Evaluate:

- Therapeutic response: decreased size of tumor, spread of malignancy
- Bleeding: hematuria, guaiac, bruising or petechiae, mucosa or orifices q8h
- Food preferences; list likes, dislikes
- Yellowing of skin, sclera, dark urine, clay-colored stools, itchy skin, abdominal pain, fever, diarrhea
- Dyspnea, rales, unproductive cough, chest pain, tachypnea
- Effects of alopecia on body image; discuss feelings about body changes (rare)

Teach patient/family:

- To report signs of infection: increased temperature, sore throat, flu symptoms
- To report signs of anemia: fatigue, headache, faintness, shortness of breath, irritability
- To report bleeding; avoid use of razors or commercial mouthwash
- To avoid use of aspirin products or ibuprofen
- About protective isolation precautions
- To report any changes in breathing or coughing
- That hair may be lost during treatment; a wig or hairpiece may make patient feel better; new hair may be different in color, texture (rare)

---

chloramphenicol/chloramphenicol palmitate/chloramphenicol sodium succinate

Chloromycetin, Mychel, Novochlorocap*

Func. class.: Antibacterial/antirickettsial

Chem. class.: Dichloroacetic acid derivative

Action: Binds to 50S ribosomal subunit, which interferes with or inhibits protein synthesis

Uses: Infections caused by *H. influenzae, S. typhi, Rickettsia, Neisseria,* mycoplasma

Dosage and routes:

- *Adult and child:* PO/IV 50-100 mg/kg/day in divided doses q6h, not to exceed 100 mg/kg/day
- *Premature infants and neonates:* IV/PO 25 mg/kg/day in divided doses q6h

Available forms include: Inj (IV) 1 g; caps 250, 500 mg; oral susp 150 mg/5 ml

Side effects/adverse reactions:

HEMA: ***Anemia, bone marrow depression, thrombocytopenia, aplastic anemia, granulocytopenia, leukopenia*** (rare)

EENT: Optic neuritis, blindness

GI: Nausea, vomiting, diarrhea, abdominal pain, xerostomia, glossitis, colitis, pruritus ani

INTEG: Itching, urticaria, contact dermatitis, rash

CV: ***Gray syndrome in newborns: failure to feed, pallid, cyanosis, abdominal distention, irregular respiration, vasomotor collapse***

CNS: Headache, ***depression,*** confusion

Contraindications: Hypersensitivity, severe renal disease, severe hepatic disease, minor infections

Precautions: Hepatic disease, renal disease, infants, children, bone marrow depression (drug-induced), pregnancy (C), lactation

Pharmacokinetics:

PO/IV: Peak 1-2 hr, duration 8 hr, half-life 1½-4 hr, conjugated in liver, excreted in urine (up to 15% as free drug), breast milk, feces, crosses placenta

Interactions/incompatibilities:

- Increased action of: dicumarol,

---

* Available in Canada only

phenytoin, tolbutamide, chlorpropamide, phenobarbital
• Increased prothrombin time: anticoagulants
• Decreased action of: iron, vitamin B_{12}, folic acid, penicillins
• Do not mix with any drug before consulting package inserts; incompatible with many drugs
• Avoid use with myelosuppressive drugs

NURSING CONSIDERATIONS

Assess:
• Signs of infections, anemia
• Any patient with compromised renal system; drug is excreted slowly in poor renal system function; toxicity may occur rapidly
• Liver studies: AST, ALT
• Blood studies: WBC, RBC, Hct, Hgb, platelets, serum iron, reticulocytes; drug should be discontinued if bone marrow depression occurs
• Renal studies: urinalysis, protein, blood, BUN, creatinine
• C&S before drug therapy; may be taken as soon as culture is taken
• Drug level in impaired hepatic, renal systems

Administer:
• IV after diluting 1 g/10 ml of sterile H_2O for inj or D_5W, give over >1 min; may be further diluted in 50-100 ml of compatible sol; run over ½-1 hr
• Oral form on empty stomach with full glass of water

Perform/provide:
• Storage of capsules in tight container at room temperature, reconstituted solution at room temperature for up to 30 days
• Adrenalin, suction, tracheostomy set, endotracheal intubation equipment on unit
• Adequate intake of fluids (2000 ml) during diarrhea episodes

Evaluate:
• Therapeutic response: decreased symptoms of infection
• Bowel pattern before, during treatment
• Skin eruptions, itching, dermatitis after administration
• Respiratory status: rate, character, wheezing, tightness in chest
• Allergies before treatment, reaction of each medication; place allergies on chart, Kardex in bright red letters; notify all people giving drugs
• Neonates for beginning gray syndrome: cyanosis, abdominal distention, irregular respiration, failure to feed; drug should be discontinued immediately

Teach patient/family:
• Aspects of drug therapy: need to complete entire course of medication to ensure organism death (10-14 days); culture may be taken after complete course of medication
• To report sore throat, fever, fatigue, unusual bleeding, bruising; could indicate bone marrow depression (may occur weeks or months after termination of drug)
• That drug must be taken in equal intervals around clock to maintain blood levels

Treatment of overdose: Withdraw drug, maintain airway, administer epinephrine, aminophylline, O_2, IV corticosteroids

chloramphenicol (ophthalmic)

(klor-am-fen'i-kole)

Antibiopto, Chloromycetin Ophthalmic, Chloroptic, Chloroptic SOP, Econochlor Ophthalmic, Fenicol,* Isopto Fenical,* Ophthoclor Ophthalmic, Pentamycin*

Func. class.: Antiinfective

Action: Inhibits bacterial protein synthesis

Uses: Infection of eye

Dosage and routes:

• *Adult and child:* INSTILL 2 gtts in eye qd-qid until desired response; TOP apply oint to conjunctival sac q3-6h as needed or hs if using gtts also

Available forms include: Oint 1%; sol 0.25, 0.5%, 25 mg

Side effects/adverse reactions:

EENT: Poor corneal wound healing, temporary visual haze, overgrowth of nonsusceptible organisms

Contraindications: Hypersensitivity

Precautions: Antibiotic hypersensitivity, pregnancy (C)

NURSING CONSIDERATIONS

Administer:

• After washing hands, cleanse crusts or discharge from eye before application

• Apply pressure to lacrimal sac for 1 min to prevent systemic absorption

Perform/provide:

• Storage at room temperature, protect from light

Evaluate:

• Therapeutic response: absence of redness, inflammation, tearing

• Allergy: itching, lacrimation, redness, swelling

Teach patient/family:

• To use drug exactly as prescribed

• Not to use eye makeup, towels, washcloths, eye medication of others; reinfection may occur

• That drug container tip should not touch eye

• To report itching, increased redness, burning, stinging, swelling; drug should be discontinued

• That drug may cause blurred vision when ointment is applied

• That prolonged or frequent use may lead to serious reactions: hypersensitivity, bone marrow depression

chloramphenicol (otic)

(klor-am-fen'i-kole)

Chloromycetin Otic, Sopamycetin*

Func. class.: Otic, broad-spectrum antibiotic

Chem. class: Antibacterial

Action: Inhibits protein synthesis in susceptible gram-positive, gram-negative microorganisms

Uses: Ear infection (external)

Dosage and routes:

• *Adult and child:* INSTILL 2-3 gtts tid

Available forms include: Sol 0.5%

Side effects/adverse reactions:

EENT: Itching, irritation in ear

INTEG: Rash, urticaria, contact dermatitis, burning, ***angioedema***

HEMA: ***Bone marrow hypoplasia, aplastic anemia***

Contraindications: Hypersensitivity, perforated eardrum

NURSING CONSIDERATIONS

Administer:

• After removing impacted cerumen by irrigation

• After cleaning stopper with alcohol

*Available in Canada only

• After restraining child if necessary
• Warming solution to body temperature; do not warm above body temperature; loss of potency will occur

Perform/provide:
• Storage at room temperature, protection from light

Evaluate:
• Therapeutic response: decreased ear pain
• For redness, swelling, pain in ear, which indicates superimposed infection

Teach patient/family:
• Method of instillation, using aseptic technique, including not touching dropper to ear
• That dizziness may occur after instillation

chloramphenicol (topical)

(klor-am-fen'i-kole)
Chloromycetin
Func. class.: Local antiinfective
Chem. class.: Antibacterial

Action: Interferes with bacterial protein synthesis
Uses: Skin infections (bacterial)
Dosage and routes:
• *Adult and child:* TOP apply to affected area bid-qid
Available forms include: Cream 1%
Side effects/adverse reactions:
HEMA: ***Blood dyscrasias***
INTEG: Rash, urticaria, stinging, burning, vesicular, maculopapular dermatitis, ***angioedema***
Contraindications: Hypersensitivity
Precautions: Pregnancy (C), lactation

NURSING CONSIDERATIONS

Administer:
• Enough medication to completely cover lesions
• After cleansing with soap, water before each application, dry well

Perform/provide:
• Storage at room temperature in dry place, protect from light

Evaluate:
• Therapeutic response: decrease in size, number of lesions
• Allergic reaction: burning, stinging, swelling, redness
• Signs and symptoms of blood dyscrasias

Teach patient/family:
• To use medical asepsis (hand washing) before, after each application to prevent further infection
• To apply with glove to prevent further infection
• To avoid use of OTC creams, ointments, lotions unless directed by physician
• To notify physician if conditions worsen or if rash or irritation develops
• To watch for superimposed infections with diarrhea

chlordiazepoxide HCl

(klor-dye-az-e-pox'ide)
A-poxide, Libritabs, Librium, Medilium,* Novopoxide,* Relaxil, Solium,* Lipoxide, SK-Lygen
Func. class.: Antianxiety
Chem. class.: Benzodiazepine

Controlled Substance Schedule IV
Action: Depresses subcortical levels of CNS, including limbic system, reticular formation
Uses: Short-term management of anxiety, acute alcohol withdrawal, preoperatively for relaxation

Dosage and routes:
Mild anxiety
• *Adult:* PO 5-10 mg tid-qid
• *Child >6 yr:* 5 mg bid-qid, not to exceed 10 mg bid-tid
Severe anxiety
• *Adult:* PO 20-25 mg tid-qid
Preoperatively
• *Adult:* PO 5-10 mg tid-qid on day before surgery; IM 50-100 mg 1 hr before surgery
Alcohol withdrawal
• *Adult:* PO/IM/IV 50-100 mg, not to exceed 300 mg/day
Available forms include: Caps 5, 10, 25 mg; tabs 5, 10, 25 mg; powder for IM inj 100 mg
Side effects/adverse reactions:
CNS: Dizziness, drowsiness, confusion, headache, anxiety, tremors, stimulation, fatigue, depression, insomnia, hallucinations
GI: Constipation, dry mouth, nausea, vomiting, anorexia, diarrhea
INTEG: Rash, dermatitis, itching
CV: Orthostatic hypotension, ***ECG changes, tachycardia,*** hypotension
EENT: Blurred vision, tinnitus, mydriasis
Contraindications: Hypersensitivity to benzodiazepines, narrow-angle glaucoma, psychosis, pregnancy (D), child <18 yr
Precautions: Elderly, debilitated, hepatic disease, renal disease
Pharmacokinetics:
PO: Onset 30 min, peak ½ hr, duration 4-6 hr, metabolized by liver, excreted by kidneys, crosses placenta, breast milk, half-life 5-30 hr
Interactions/incompatibilities:
• Decreased effects of chlordiazepoxide: oral contraceptives, rifampin, valproic acid
• Increased effects of chlordiazepoxide: CNS depressants, alcohol, cimetidine, disulfiram, oral contraceptives

NURSING CONSIDERATIONS
Assess:
• B/P (lying, standing), pulse; if systolic B/P drops 20 mm Hg, hold drug, notify physician
• Blood studies: CBC during long-term therapy, blood dyscrasias have occurred rarely
• Hepatic studies: AST, ALT, bilirubin, creatinine, LDH, alk phosphatase
• I&O; may indicate renal dysfunction
• For ataxia, oversedation in elderly, debilitated patients
Administer:
• By IV 5 ml saline 100 mg/powder, agitate ampule gently; do not use IM diluent for IV use
• With food or milk for GI symptoms
• Crushed if patient is unable to swallow medication whole
• Sugarless gum, hard candy, frequent sips of water for dry mouth
Perform/provide:
• Assistance with ambulation during beginning therapy, since drowsiness/dizziness occurs
• Safety measure, including siderails
• Check to see PO medication has been swallowed
Evaluate:
• Therapeutic response: decreased anxiety, restlessness, sleeplessness
• Mental status: mood, sensorium, affect, sleeping pattern, drowsiness, dizziness
• Physical dependency, withdrawal symptoms: headache, nausea, vomiting, muscle pain, weakness after long-term use
• Suicidal tendencies, paradoxical reactions such as excitement, stimulation, and acute rage
Teach patient/family:
• That drug may be taken with food

* Available in Canada only

- Not to be used for everyday stress or used longer than 4 mo, unless directed by physician
- Not to take more than prescribed amount, may be habit-forming
- To avoid OTC preparations unless approved by physician
- To avoid driving, activities that require alertness; drowsiness may occur
- To avoid alcohol ingestion or other psychotropic medications, unless prescribed by physician
- Not to discontinue medication abruptly after long-term use, may precipitate convulsions
- To rise slowly or fainting may occur, especially elderly
- That drowsiness might worsen at beginning of treatment

Lab test interferences:
Increase: AST/ALT, serum bilirubin
False increase: 17-OHCS
Decrease: RAIU
Treatment of overdose: Lavage, VS, supportive care

---

chloroprocaine HCl

(klor'-oh-pro-kane)
Nesacaine, Nesacaine-CE
Func. class.: Local anesthetic
Chem. class.: Ester

Action: Competes with calcium for sites in nerve membrane that control sodium transport across cell membrane; decreases rise of depolarization phase of action potential
Uses: Epidural anesthesia, peripheral nerve block, caudal anesthesia, infiltration block
Dosage and routes:
Varies depending on route of anesthesia
Available forms include: Inj 1%, 2%, 3%

Side effects/adverse reactions:
CNS: Anxiety, restlessness, ***convulsions, loss of consciousness,*** drowsiness, disorientation, tremors, shivering
CV: ***Myocardial depression, cardiac arrest, dysrhythmias,*** bradycardia, hypotension, hypertension, fetal bradycardia
GI: Nausea, vomiting
EENT: Blurred vision, tinnitus, pupil constriction
INTEG: Rash, urticaria, allergic reactions, edema, burning, skin discoloration at injection site, tissue necrosis
RESP: ***Status asthmaticus, respiratory arrest, anaphylaxis***
Contraindications: Hypersensitivity, child <12 yr, elderly, severe liver disease
Precautions: Elderly, severe drug allergies, pregnancy (C)
Pharmacokinetics:
Duration ½-1 hr, metabolized by liver, excreted in urine (metabolites)
Interactions/incompatibilities:
- Dysrhythmias: epinephrine, halothane, enflurane
- Hypertension: MAOIs, tricyclic antidepressants, phenothiazines

NURSING CONSIDERATIONS

Assess:
- B/P, pulse, respiration during treatment
- Fetal heart tones if drug is used during labor

Administer:
- Only with crash cart, resuscitative equipment nearby
- Only drugs without preservatives for epidural or caudal anesthesia

Perform/provide:
- Use of new solution, discard unused portions

Evaluate:
- Therapeutic response: anesthesia necessary for procedure

• Allergic reactions: rash, urticaria, itching
• Cardiac status: ECG for dysrhythmias, pulse, B/P during anesthesia

Treatment of overdose: Airway, O_2, vasopressor, IV fluids, anticonvulsants for seizures

---

chloroquine HCl/ chloroquine phosphate

(klor'oh-kwin)

Aralen HCl, Aralen Phosphate, Chlorocon, Novochloroquine*

Func. class.: Antimalarial
Chem. class.: Synthetic 4-aminoquinoline derivative

Action: Inhibits parasite replications, transcription of DNA to RNA by forming complexes with DNA of parasite

Uses: Malaria caused by *Plasmodium vivax, P. malariae, P. ovale, P. falciparum* (some strains), rheumatoid arthritis, amebiasis

Dosage and routes:

Malaria suppression

• *Adult and child:* PO 5 mg/kg/wk on same day of week, not to exceed 500 mg; treatment should begin 2 wk before exposure and for 8 wk after; if treatment begins after exposure, 600 mg for adult and 10 mg/kg for children in 2 divided doses 6 hr apart

Extraintestinal amebiasis

• *Adult:* IM 160-200 mg qd (HCl) up to 12 days, then 1 g (phosphate) qd × 2 days, then 500 mg qd × 2-3 wk; PO 600 mg qd × 2 days, then 300 mg qd × 2-3 wk
• *Child:* IM/PO 10 mg/kg qd (HCl) × 2-3 wk, not to exceed 300 mg/day

Rheumatoid arthritis

• *Adult:* PO 250 mg (phosphate) qd with evening meal

Available forms include: Tabs 250, 500 mg; inj IM 40 mg/ml

Side effects/adverse reactions:

CV: Hypotension, heart block, asystole with syncope, ECG changes

INTEG: Pruritus, pigmentary changes, skin eruptions, lichen planuslike eruptions, eczema, ***exfoliative dermatitis,*** alopecia

CNS: Headache, stimulation, fatigue, irritability, ***convulsion,*** bad dreams, dizziness, confusion, psychosis, decreased reflexes

EENT: Blurred vision, corneal changes, retinal changes, difficulty focusing, tinnitus, vertigo, deafness, photophobia, corneal edema

GI: Nausea, vomiting, anorexia, diarrhea, cramps, weight loss, stomatitis

HEMA: ***Thrombocytopenia, agranulocytosis, hemolytic anemia, leukopenia***

Contraindications: Hypersensitivity, retinal field changes, porphyria, children (long-term)

Precautions: Pregnancy (C), children, blood dyscrasias, severe GI disease, neurologic disease, alcoholism, hepatic disease, G-6-PD deficiency, psoriasis, eczema

Pharmacokinetics:

PO: Peak 1-2 hr, half-life 3-5 days, metabolized in the liver, excreted in urine, feces, breast milk, crosses placenta

Interactions/incompatibilities:

• Decreased action of chloroquine: magnesium aluminum compounds, kaolin

NURSING CONSIDERATIONS

Assess:

• Ophthalmic test if long-term treatment or drug dosage >150 mg/day

---

* Available in Canada only

• Liver studies qwk: AST, ALT, bilirubin
• Blood studies: CBC, since blood dyscrasias occur
• For decreased reflexes: knee, ankle
• ECG during therapy
• Watch for depression of T waves, widening of QRS complex

Administer:
• Before or after meals at same time each day to maintain drug level
• IM after aspirating to avoid injection into blood system, which may cause hypotension, asystole, heart block; rotate injection sites

Perform/provide:
• Storage in tight, light-resistant containers at room temperature; injection should be kept in cool environment

Evaluate:
• Therapeutic response: decreased symptoms of infection
• Allergic reactions: pruritus, rash, urticaria
• Blood dyscrasias: malaise, fever, bruising, bleeding (rare)
• For ototoxicity (tinnitus, vertigo, change in hearing); audiometric testing should be done before, after treatment
• For toxicity: blurring vision, difficulty focusing, headache, dizziness, knee, ankle reflexes; drug should be discontinued immediately

Teach patient/family:
• To use sunglasses in bright sunlight to decrease photophobia
• That urine may turn rust or brown color
• To report hearing, visual problems, fever, fatigue, bruising, bleeding, which may indicate blood dyscrasias

Treatment of overdose: Induce vomiting, gastric lavage, administer barbiturate (ultrashort-acting), vasopressin; tracheostomy may be necessary

chlorothiazide

(klor-oh-thye'a-zide)

Diachlor, Diurigen, Diuril, Ro-Chlorozide, SK-Chlorothiazide

Func. class.: Diuretic
Chem. class.: Thiazide; sulfonamide derivative

Action: Acts on distal tubule by increasing excretion of water, sodium, chloride, potassium

Uses: Edema, hypertension, diuresis

Dosage and routes:

Edema, hypertension
• *Adult:* PO/IV 500 mg-2 g qd in 2 divided doses

Diuresis
• *Child >6 mo:* PO 20 mg/kg/day in divided doses
• *Child <6 mo:* PO up to 30 mg/kg/day in 2 divided doses

Available forms include: Tabs 250, 500 mg; oral susp 250 mg/5 ml; inj 500 mg

Side effects/adverse reactions:

GU: Frequency, polyuria, ***uremia,*** glucosuria

CNS: Drowsiness, paresthesia, anxiety, depression, headache, *dizziness, fatigue, weakness*

GI: Nausea, vomiting, anorexia, constipation, diarrhea, cramps, pancreatitis, GI irritation, ***hepatitis***

EENT: Blurred vision

INTEG: Rash, urticaria, purpura, photosensitivity, fever

META: Hyperglycemia, hyperuricemia, hypomagnesemia, increased creatinine, BUN

HEMA: ***Aplastic anemia, hemolytic anemia, leukopenia, agranulocy-***

tosis, thrombocytopenia, neutropenia

CV: Irregular pulse, orthostatic hypotension, palpitations, volume depletion

ELECT: Hypokalemia, hypercalcemia, hyponatremia, hypochloremia

Contraindications: Hypersensitivity to thiazides or sulfonamides, anuria, renal decompensation, pregnancy (D)

Precautions: Hypokalemia, renal disease, hepatic disease, gout, COPD, lupus erythematosus, diabetes mellitus, elderly

Pharmacokinetics:

PO: Onset 2 hr, peak 4 hr, duration 6-12 hr; crosses placenta, excreted in breast milk

Interactions/incompatibilities:

- Increased toxicity: lithium, nondepolarizing skeletal muscle relaxants, digitalis
- Decreased effects of: antidiabetics, sulfonylureas
- Decreased absorption of thiazides: cholestyramine, colestipol
- Decreased hypotensive response: indomethacin
- Hyperglycemia, hyperuricemia, hypotension: diazoxide

NURSING CONSIDERATIONS

Assess:

- Weight, I&O daily to determine fluid loss; effect of drug may be decreased if used qd
- Rate, depth, rhythm of respiration, effect of exertion
- B/P lying, standing; postural hypotension may occur, especially elderly
- Electrolytes: potassium, sodium, chloride; include BUN, blood sugar, CBC, serum creatinine, blood pH, ABGs, uric acid, calcium, magnesium
- Glucose in urine if patient is diabetic

Administer:

- IV after diluting 0.5 g/18 ml of sterile water for inj or more; may be diluted further with compatible IV sol; give over 5 min
- In AM to avoid interference with sleep if using drug as a diuretic
- Potassium replacement if potassium is less than 3.0
- With food if nausea occurs; absorption may be decreased slightly

Evaluate:

- Therapeutic response: improvement in edema of feet, legs, sacral area daily if medication is being used in CHF
- Improvement in CVP q8h
- Signs of metabolic alkalosis: drowsiness, restlessness
- Signs of hypokalemia: postural hypotension, malaise, fatigue, tachycardia, leg cramps, weakness
- Rashes, temperature elevation qd
- Confusion, especially in elderly; take safety precautions if needed

Teach patient/family:

- To increase fluid intake 2-3 L/day unless contraindicated, to rise slowly from lying or sitting position
- To notify physician of muscle weakness, cramps, nausea, dizziness
- That drug may be taken with food or milk
- That blood sugar may be increased in diabetics
- To take early in day to avoid nocturia

Lab test interferences:

Increase: BSP retention, calcium, amylase, parathyroid test

Decrease: PBI, PSP

Treatment of overdose: Lavage if taken orally, monitor electrolytes, administer dextrose in saline, monitor hydration, CV, renal status

chlorotrianisene

(klor-oh-trye-an'i-seen)
TACE

Func. class.: Estrogen
Chem. class.: Nonsteroidal synthetic estrogen

Action: Needed for adequate functioning of female reproductive system, it affects release of pituitary gonadotropins, inhibits ovulation, adequate calcium use in bone structures

Uses: Prostatic cancer, menopause, female hypogonadism, atrophic vaginitis, kraurosis vulvae

Dosage and routes:

Prostatic cancer

- *Adult:* PO 12-25 mg qd

Menopause

- *Adult:* PO 12-25 mg qd × 30 days or 3 wk on 1 wk off

Female hypogonadism

- *Adult:* PO 12-25 mg × 21 days, then progesterone 100 mg IM or 5 days of progesterone PO given with last 5 days of medroxyprogesterone 5-10 mg

Vaginitis

- *Adult:* PO 12-25 mg qd × 30-60 days

Available forms include: Caps 12, 25, 72 mg

Side effects/adverse reactions:

CNS: Dizziness, headache, migraines, depression

CV: Hypotension, ***thrombophlebitis***, edema, ***thromboembolism, stroke, pulmonary embolism, myocardial infarction***

GI: Nausea, vomiting, diarrhea, anorexia, pancreatitis, cramps, constipation, increased appetite, increased weight, ***cholestatic jaundice***

EENT: Contact lens intolerance, increased myopia, astigmatism

GU: Amenorrhea, cervical erosion, breakthrough bleeding, dysmenorrhea, vaginal candidiasis, breast changes, *gynecomastia, testicular atrophy, impotence*

INTEG: Rash, urticaria, acne, hirsutism, alopecia, oily skin, seborrhea, purpura, melasma

META: Folic acid deficiency, hypercalcemia, hyperglycemia

Contraindications: Breast cancer, thromboembolic disorders, reproductive cancer, genital bleeding (abnormal, undiagnosed), pregnancy (X)

Precautions: Hypertension, asthma, blood dyscrasias, gallbladder disease, CHF, diabetes mellitus, bone disease, depression, migraine headache, convulsive disorders, hepatic disease, renal disease, family history of cancer of the breast or reproductive tract

Pharmacokinetics:

PO: Degraded in liver, excreted in urine, crosses placenta, excreted in breast milk

Interactions/incompatibilities:

- Decreased action of: anticoagulants, oral hypoglycemics
- Toxicity: tricyclic antidepressants
- Decreased action of chlorotrianisene: anticonvulsants, barbiturates, phenylbutazone, rifampin
- Increased action of: corticosteroids

NURSING CONSIDERATIONS

Assess:

- Urine glucose in patient with diabetes, increased urine glucose may occur
- Weight daily, notify physician if weekly weight gain is >5 lb, if increase, diuretic may be ordered
- B/P q4h, watch for increase caused by water and sodium retention
- I&O ratio; be alert for decreasing

urinary output and increasing edema
• Liver function studies, including AST, ALT, bilirubin, alk phosphatase
Administer:
• Titrated dose, use lowest effective dose
• In one dose in AM, for prostatic cancer, vaginitis, hypogonadism
• With food or milk to decrease GI symptoms
Evaluate:
• Therapeutic response: reversal of menopause or decrease in tumor size in prostatic cancer
• Edema, hypertension, cardiac symptoms, jaundice
• Mental status: affect, mood, behavioral changes, aggression
• Hypercalcemia
Teach patient/family:
• To weigh weekly, report gain >5 lb
• To report breast lumps, vaginal bleeding, edema, jaundice, dark urine, clay colored stools, dyspnea, headache, blurred vision, abdominal pain, numbness, stiffness, or pain in legs, chest pain; male to report impotence or gynecomastia
• To check with physician before using OTC drugs
Lab test interferences:
Increase: BSP retention test, PBI, T_4, serum sodium, platelet aggressability, thyroxine-binding globulin (TBG), prothrombin, factors VII, VIII, IX, X, triglycerides
Decrease: Serum folate, serum triglyceride, T_3 resin uptake test, glucose tolerance test, antithrombin III, pregnanediol, metyrapone test
False positive: LE prep, antinuclear antibodies

chlorphenesin carbamate

(klor-fen'e-sin)
Maolate, Mycil*
Func. class.: Skeletal muscle relaxant, central acting
Chem. class.: Carbamate

Action: Unknown; may be related to sedative properties; does not directly relax muscle or depress nerve conduction
Uses: Adjunct for relieving pain in acute, painful musculoskeletal conditions
Dosage and routes:
• *Adult:* PO 800 mg tid, maintenance 400 mg qid, not to exceed 8 wk
Available forms include: Tabs 400 mg
Side effects/adverse reactions:
CNS: Dizziness, weakness, drowsiness, headache, tremor, depression, insomnia, confusion
EENT: Diplopia, temporary loss of vision
HEMA: ***Blood dyscrasias***
CV: Postural hypotension, tachycardia
GI: Nausea, vomiting, hiccups
INTEG: Rash, pruritus, fever, facial flushing
SYST: Anaphylaxis
Contraindications: Hypersensitivity, child <12 yr, intermittent porphyria
Precautions: Renal disease, hepatic disease, addictive personalities, pregnancy (C), elderly
Pharmacokinetics:
PO: Onset ½ hr, peak 1-2 hr, duration 4-6 hr, metabolized by liver, excreted in urine, crosses placenta, excreted in breast milk (large amounts), half-life 4 hr

* Available in Canada only

Interactions/incompatibilities:
• Increased CNS depression: alcohol, tricyclic antidepressants, narcotics, barbiturates, sedatives, hypnotics

NURSING CONSIDERATIONS

Assess:
• Blood studies: CBC, WBC, differential; blood dyscrasias may occur
• Liver function studies: AST, ALT, alk phosphatase; hepatitis may occur
• Kidney function studies
• ECG in epileptic patients; poor seizure control has occurred with patients taking this drug
• B/P lying and standing, postural hypotension may occur

Administer:
• With meals for GI symptoms

Perform/provide:
• Storage in tight container at room temperature
• Assistance with ambulation if dizziness, drowsiness occurs, especially elderly

Evaluate:
• Therapeutic response: decreased pain, spasticity
• Allergic reactions: rash, fever, respiratory distress
• Severe weakness, numbness in extremities
• Psychologic dependency: increased need for medication, more frequent requests for medication, increased pain
• CNS depression: dizziness, drowsiness, psychiatric symptoms

Teach patient/family:
• Not to discontinue medication quickly, insomnia, nausea, headache, spasticity, tachycardia will occur; drug should be tapered off over 1-2 wk
• Not to take with alcohol, other CNS depressants
• To avoid altering activities while taking this drug
• To avoid hazardous activities if drowsiness, dizziness occurs
• To avoid using OTC medication: cough preparations, antihistamines, unless directed by physician

Treatment of overdose: Give physostigmine IV; monitor cardiac function

---

chlorpheniramine maleate

(klor-fen-eer'a-meen)

Alleroid-OD, AL-R, Chlormene, Chlortab, Chlor-Trimeton, Chlor-Tripolon, Novopheniram, Teldrin

Func. class.: Antihistamine
Chem. class.: Alkylamine, H_1-receptor antagonist

Action: Acts on blood vessels, GI system, respiratory system, by competing with histamine for H_1-receptor site; decreases allergic response by blocking histamine

Uses: Allergy symptoms, rhinitis

Dosage and routes:
• *Adult:* PO 2-4 mg tid-qid, not to exceed 36 mg/day; TIME-REL 8-12 mg bid-tid, not to exceed 36 mg/day; IM/IV/SC 5-40 mg/day
• *Child 6-12 yr:* PO 2 mg q4-6h, not to exceed 12 mg/day; SUS REL 8 mg hs or qd, SUS REL not recommended for child <6 yr
• *Child 2-5 yr:* PO 1 mg q4-6h, not to exceed 4 mg/day

Available forms include: Tabs, chewable 2 mg; tabs 4 mg; tabs, time-rel 8, 12 mg, caps, time-rel 8, 12 mg; syr 2 mg/5 ml; inj IM, SC, IV 10, 100 mg/ml

Side effects/adverse reactions:
CNS: Dizziness, drowsiness, poor

coordination, fatigue, anxiety, euphoria, confusion, paresthesia, neuritis
RESP: Increased thick secretions, wheezing, chest tightness
HEMA: ***Thrombocytopenia, agranulocytosis, hemolytic anemia***
GI: Dry mouth, nausea, anorexia, diarrhea
INTEG: Photosensitivity
GU: Retention, dysuria, frequency
EENT: Blurred vision, dilated pupils, tinnitus, nasal stuffiness, dry nose, throat, mouth
Contraindications: Hypersensitivity to H_1-receptor antagonists, acute asthma attack, lower respiratory tract disease
Precautions: Increased intraocular pressure, renal disease, cardiac disease, hypertension, bronchial asthma, seizure disorder, stenosed peptic ulcers, hyperthyroidism, prostatic hypertrophy, bladder neck obstruction, pregnancy (B), elderly
Pharmacokinetics:
PO: Onset 20-60 min, duration 8-12 hr; detoxified in liver, excreted by kidneys, (metabolites/free drug), half-life 20-24 hr
Interactions/incompatibilities:
• Increased CNS depression: barbiturates, narcotics, hypnotics, tricyclic antidepressants, alcohol
• Decreased effect of: oral anticoagulants, heparin
• Increased effect of chlorpheniramine: MAOIs

NURSING CONSIDERATIONS
Assess:
• I&O ratio; be alert for urinary retention, frequency, dysuria; drug should be discontinued if these occur
• CBC during long-term therapy
Administer:
• IV undiluted at a rate of 10 mg/1 min or longer
• With meals if GI symptoms occur; absorption may slightly decrease
Perform/provide:
• Hard candy, gum, frequent rinsing of mouth for dryness
• Storage in tight container at room temperature
Evaluate:
• Therapeutic response: absence of running or congested nose or rashes
• Blood dyscrasias: thrombocytopenia, agranulocytosis (rare)
• Respiratory status: rate, rhythm, increase in bronchial secretions, wheezing, chest tightness
Teach patient/family:
• Not to chew or crush sustained release forms
• All aspects of drug use; to notify physician if confusion, sedation, hypotension occurs
• To avoid driving or other hazardous activity if drowsiness occurs, especially elderly
• To avoid concurrent use of alcohol or other CNS depressants
Lab test interferences:
False negative: Skin allergy tests
Treatment of overdose: Administer ipecac syrup or lavage, diazepam, vasopressors, barbiturates (short-acting)

chlorpromazine HCl

(klor-proe'ma-zeen)
Chlor-Promanyl, Chlorpromanyl,* Largactil, Promaz, Thorazine
Func. class.: Antipsychotic/neuroleptic
Chem. class.: Phenothiazine-aliphatic

Action: Depresses cerebral cortex, hypothalamus, limbic system, which control activity aggression; blocks neurotransmission produced

*Available in Canada only

by dopamine at synapse; exhibits a strong α-adrenergic, anticholinergic blocking action; mechanism for antipsychotic effects is unclear

Uses: Psychotic disorders, mania, schizophrenia, anxiety, intractable hiccups, nausea, vomiting, preoperatively for relaxation, and acute intermittent porphyria, behavioral problems in children

Dosage and routes:

Psychiatry

- *Adult:* PO 10-50 mg q1-4h initially, then increase up to 2000 mg/day if necessary
- *Adult:* IM 10-50 mg q1-4h
- *Child:* PO 0.25 mg/lb q4-6h or 0.5 mg/kg
- *Child:* IM 0.25 mg/lb q6-8h or 0.5 mg/kg
- *Child:* REC 0.5 mg/lb q6-8h or 1 mg/kg

Nausea and vomiting

- *Adult:* PO 10-25 mg q4-6h prn; IM 25-50 mg q3h prn; REC 50-100 mg q6-8h prn, not to exceed 400 mg/day
- *Child:* PO 0.25 mg/lb q4-6h prn, IM 0.25 mg/lb q6-8h prn not to exceed 40 mg/day (<5 yr) or 75 mg/day (5-12 yr); REC 0.5 mg/lb q6-8h prn
- *Adult:* IV 25-50 mg qd-qid
- *Child:* IV 0.55 mg/kg q6-8h

Intractable hiccups

- *Adult:* PO 25-50 mg tid-qid; IM 25-50 mg (used only if PO dose does not work); IV 25-50 mg in 500-1000 ml saline (only for severe hiccups)

Available forms include: Tabs 10, 25, 50, 100, 200 mg; time-release caps 30, 75, 150, 200, 300 mg; syr 10 mg/5ml; conc 30, 100 mg/ml; supp 25, 100 mg; inj IM, IV 25 mg/ml

Side effects/adverse reactions:

RESP: ***Laryngospasm,*** dyspnea, ***respiratory depression***

CNS: Extrapyramidal symptoms: pseudoparkinsonism, akathisia, dystonia, tardive dyskinesia, seizures, *headache*

HEMA: Anemia, ***leukopenia, leukocytosis, agranulocytosis***

INTEG: Rash, photosensitivity, dermatitis

EENT: Blurred vision, glaucoma, dry eyes

GI: Dry mouth, nausea, vomiting, anorexia, constipation, diarrhea, jaundice, weight gain

GU: Urinary retention, urinary frequency, enuresis, impotence, amenorrhea, gynecomastia, breast engorgement

CV: Orthostatic hypotension, hypertension, ***cardiac arrest,*** ECG changes, ***tachycardia***

Contraindications: Hypersensitivity, circulatory collapse, liver damage, cerebral arteriosclerosis, coronary disease, severe hypertension/hypotension, blood dyscrasias, coma, child <2 years, brain damage, bone marrow depression, alcohol and barbiturate withdrawal states

Precautions: Pregnancy (C), lactation, seizure disorders, hypertension, hepatic disease, cardiac disease, elderly

Pharmacokinetics:

PO: Onset erratic, peak 2-4 hr, duration may be detected for up to 6 mo after last dose

IM: Onset 15-30 min, peak 15-20 min, duration may be detected for up to 6 mo after last dose

IV: Onset 5 min, peak 10 min, duration may be detected for up to 6 mo after last dose

REC: Onset erratic, peak 3 hr; metabolized by liver, excreted in urine (metabolites), crosses placenta, enters breast milk; 95% bound to plasma proteins; elimination half-life 10-30 hr

Interactions/incompatibilities:

- Oversedation: other CNS depressants, alcohol, barbiturate anesthetics
- Toxicity: epinephrine
- Decreased absorption: aluminum hydroxide or magnesium hydroxide antacids
- Decreased effects of: levodopa, phenobarbital
- Decreased serum chlorpromazine: lithium
- Increased effects of both drugs: β-adrenergic blockers, alcohol
- Increased anticholinergic effects: anticholinergics

NURSING CONSIDERATIONS

Assess:

- Mental status before initial administration
- Swallowing of PO medication; check for hoarding or giving of medication to other patients
- I&O ratio; palpate bladder if low urinary output occurs, especially elderly
- Bilirubin, CBC, liver function studies monthly
- Urinalysis is recommended before, during prolonged therapy

Administer:

- IV after diluting 1 mg/1 ml with normal saline, give 1 mg/2 min; may be further diluted in 500-1000 ml of compatible sol
- Antiparkinsonian agent, to be used if extrapyramidal symptoms occur
- Drug in liquid form mixed in glass of juice or cola, if hoarding is suspected
- Decreased dose in elderly

Perform/provide:

- Decreased stimuli by dimming lights, avoiding loud noises
- Supervised ambulation until stabilized on medication; do not involve in strenuous exercise program because fainting is possible; patient should not stand still for long periods of time
- Increased fluids to prevent constipation
- Sips of water, candy, gum for dry mouth
- Storage in tight, light-resistant container, oral solutions in amber bottles

Evaluate:

- Therapeutic response: decrease in emotional excitement, hallucinations, delusions, paranoia, reorganization of patterns of thought, speech
- Affect, orientation, LOC, reflexes, gait, coordination, sleep pattern disturbances
- B/P standing and lying; take pulse and respirations q4h during initial treatment; establish baseline before starting treatment; report drops of 30 mm Hg
- Dizziness, faintness, palpitations, tachycardia on rising
- For neuroleptic malignant syndrome: hyperpyrexia, muscle rigidity, increased CPK, altered mental status
- Extrapyramidal symptoms including akathisia (inability to sit still, no pattern to movements), tardive dyskinesia (bizarre movements of the jaw, mouth, tongue, extremities), pseudoparkinsonism (rigidity, tremors, pill rolling, shuffling gait)
- Skin turgor daily
- Constipation, urinary retention daily; if these occur, increase bulk, water in diet

Teach patient/family:

- That orthostatic hypotension occurs often, and to rise from sitting or lying position gradually

* Available in Canada only

• To remain lying down after IM injection for at least 30 min
• To avoid hot tubs, hot showers, or tub baths since hypotension may occur
• To avoid abrupt withdrawal of this drug or extrapyramidal symptoms may result; drug should be withdrawn slowly
• To avoid OTC preparations (cough, hayfever, cold) unless approved by physician since serious drug interactions may occur; avoid use with alcohol or CNS depressants; increased drowsiness may occur
• To use a sunscreen and sunglasses during sun exposure to prevent burns
• Regarding compliance with drug regimen
• About extrapyramidal symptoms and necessity for meticulous oral hygiene since oral candidiasis may occur
• To report sore throat, malaise, fever, bleeding, mouth sores; if these occur, CBC should be drawn and drug discontinued
• That in hot weather, heat stroke may occur; take extra precautions to stay cool

Lab test interferences:
Increase: Liver function tests, cardiac enzymes, cholesterol, blood glucose, prolactin, bilirubin, PBI, cholinesterase, ^{131}I
Decrease: Hormones (blood and urine)
False positive: Pregnancy tests, PKU
False negative: Urinary steroids, 17-OHCS

Treatment of overdose: Lavage, if orally ingested, provide an airway; *do not induce vomiting or use epinephrine*

chlorpropamide

(klor-proe'pa-mide)
Chloronase,* Diabinese, Novopropamide*

Func. class.: Antidiabetic
Chem. class.: Sulfonylurea (1st generation)

Action: Causes functioning β-cells in pancreas to release insulin, leading to drop in blood glucose levels; may improve insulin binding to insulin receptors or increase the number of insulin receptors; not effective if patient lacks functioning β-cells

Uses: Stable adult-onset diabetes mellitus (type II) NIDDM

Dosage and routes:
• *Adult:* PO 100-250 mg qd, initially, then 100-500 mg maintenance according to response; not to exceed 750 mg/day

Available forms include: Tabs 100, 250 mg

Side effects/adverse reactions:
CNS: Headache, weakness, dizziness, drowsiness, tinnitus, fatigue, vertigo
GI: ***Hepatotoxicity, cholestatic jaundice,*** nausea, vomiting, diarrhea, heartburn
HEMA: ***Leukopenia, thrombocytopenia, agranulocytosis, aplastic anemia, pancytopenia, hemolytic anemia***
INTEG: Rash, allergic reactions, pruritus, urticaria, eczema, photosensitivity, erythema
ENDO: ***Hypoglycemia***

Contraindications: Hypersensitivity to sulfonylureas, juvenile or brittle diabetes, pregnancy (D)

Precautions: Elderly, cardiac disease, thyroid disease, renal disease, hepatic disease, severe hypoglycemic reactions

Pharmacokinetics:
PO: Completely absorbed by GI route, onset 1 hr, peak 3-6 hr, duration 60 hr, half-life 36 hr, metabolized in liver, excreted in urine (metabolites and unchanged drug), breast milk, 90%-95% is plasma protein bound

Interactions/incompatibilities:
- Increased hypoglycemic effects: oral anticoagulants, salicylates, sulfonamides, nonsteroidal antiinflammatories, chloramphenicol, cimetidine, MAOIs, insulin, guanethidine, methyldopa, probenecid, ranitidine
- Increased effects of chlorpropamide: insulin, MAOIs
- Decreased digoxin levels: digoxin
- Decreased effect of both drugs; diazoxide
- Dilsulfirm-like reaction: alcohol
- Decreased action of chlorpropamide: calcium channel blockers, corticosteroids, oral contraceptives, thiazide diuretics, thyroid preparations, estrogens, phenobarbital, phenytoin, rifampin, sympathomimetics

NURSING CONSIDERATIONS

Administer:
- Drug 30 min before meals

Perform/provide:
- Storage in tight container in cool environment

Evaluate:
- Therapeutic response: decrease in polyuria, polydipsia, polyphagia, clear sensorium, absence of dizziness, stable gait
- Hypoglycemic/hyperglycemic reaction that can occur soon after meals

Teach patient/family:
- To check for symptoms of cholestatic jaundice: dark urine, pruritus, yellow sclera; if these occur, physician should be notified
- To use capillary blood glucose test or Chemstrip 3 × /day
- Symptoms of hypo/hyperglycemia, what to do about each
- That this drug must be continued on daily basis; explain consequence of discontinuing drug abruptly
- To take drug in morning to prevent hypoglycemic reactions at night
- To avoid OTC medications unless prescribed by physician
- That diabetes is life-long illness, drug will not cure disease
- That all food included in diet plan must be eaten to prevent hypoglycemia
- To carry Medic-Alert ID for emergency purposes
- Not to drink alcohol

Treatment of overdose: 10%-50% glucose solution IV

---

chlortetracycline HCl (topical)

(klor-te-tra-sye'kleen)
Aureomycin

Func. class.: Local antiinfective
Chem. class.: Antibacterial

Action: Interferes with bacterial protein cell synthesis

Uses: Pyogenic skin infections

Dosage and routes:
- *Adult and child:* TOP rub into affected area bid-qid

Available forms include: Oint 3%

Side effects/adverse reactions:
INTEG: Rash, urticaria, stinging, burning, dry skin, photosensitivity, tooth discoloration

Contraindications: Hypersensitivity to this drug or wool

Precautions: Pregnancy (D), lactation

* Available in Canada only

NURSING CONSIDERATIONS

Administer:
- Enough medication to completely cover lesions
- After cleansing with soap, water before each application, dry well

Perform/provide:
- Storage at room temperature in dry place, in light-resistant container

Evaluate:
- Allergic reaction: burning, stinging, swelling, redness
- Therapeutic response: decrease in size, number of lesions

Teach patient/family:
- To watch for superimposed infections
- To use medical asepsis (hand washing) before, after each application
- To apply with glove to prevent further infection
- To avoid use of OTC creams, ointments, lotions unless directed by physician
- To avoid squeezing or poking lesions or spreading may occur
- To notify physician if condition worsens, or rash, irritation, or swelling occurs
- To avoid sunlight or ultraviolet light
- That skin may be stained
- That long-term use may cause tooth discoloration

chlorthalidone

(klor-thal'i-done)

Hygroton, Hylidone, Novothalidone,* Thalitone

Func. class.: Diuretic

Chem. class.: Thiazide-like; phthalimidine derivative

Action: Acts on distal tubule by increasing excretion of water, sodium, chloride, potassium

Uses: Edema, hypertension, diuresis, CHF

Dosage and routes:
- *Adult:* PO 25-100 mg/day or 100 mg every other day
- *Child:* PO 2 mg/kg 3 ×/wk

Available forms include: Tabs 25, 50, 100 mg

Side effects/adverse reactions:

GU: Frequency, polyuria, ***uremia,*** glucosuria

CNS: Drowsiness, paresthesia, anxiety, depression, headache, *dizziness, fatigue, weakness*

GI: Nausea, vomiting, anorexia, constipation, diarrhea, cramps, pancreatitis, GI irritation, ***hepatitis***

EENT: Blurred vision

INTEG: Rash, urticaria, purpura, photosensitivity, fever

META: Hyperglycemia, hyperuremia, increased creatinine, BUN

HEMA: ***Aplastic anemia, hemolytic anemia, leukopenia, agranulocytosis, thrombocytopenia, neutropenia***

CV: Irregular pulse, orthostatic hypotension, palpitations, volume depletion

ELECT: Hypokalemia, hypomagnesemia, hypercalcemia, hyponatremia, hypochloremia

Contraindications: Hypersensitivity to thiazides or sulfonamides, anuria, renal decompensation

Precautions: Hypokalemia, renal disease, pregnancy (C), hepatic disease, gout, diabetes mellitus, elderly

Pharmacokinetics:

PO: Onset 2 hr, peak 6 hr, duration 24-72 hr; excreted unchanged by kidneys, crosses placenta, enters breast milk, half-life 40 hr

Interactions/incompatibilities:
- Increased toxicity: lithium, non-

depolarizing skeletal muscle relaxants
• Decreased effects of: antidiabetics
• Decreased absorption of thiazides: cholestyramine, colestipol
• Decreased hypotensive response: indomethacin
• Hyperglycemia, hyperuricemia, hypotension: diazoxide

NURSING CONSIDERATIONS

Assess:
• Weight, I&O daily to determine fluid loss; effect of drug may be decreased if used qd
• Rate, depth, rhythm of respiration, effect of exertion
• B/P lying, standing; postural hypotension may occur
• Electrolytes: potassium, magnesium, sodium chloride; include BUN, blood sugar, CBC, serum creatinine, blood pH, ABGs, uric acid, calcium
• Glucose in urine if patient is diabetic

Administer:
• In AM to avoid interference with sleep if using drug as a diuretic
• Potassium replacement if potassium is less than 3.0
• With food if nausea occurs; absorption may be decreased slightly

Evaluate:
• Therapeutic response: improvement in edema of feet, legs, sacral area daily if medication is being used in CHF
• Improvement in CVP q8h
• Signs of metabolic alkalosis: drowsiness, restlessness
• Signs of hypokalemia: postural hypotension, malaise, fatigue, tachycardia, leg cramps, weakness
• Rashes, temperature elevation qd
• Confusion, especially in elderly; take safety precautions if needed

Teach patient/family:
• To increase fluid intake 2-3 L/day unless contraindicated, to rise slowly from lying or sitting position
• To notify physician of muscle weakness, cramps, nausea, dizziness
• That drug may be taken with food or milk
• That blood sugar may be increased in diabetics
• To take early in day to avoid nocturia

Lab test interferences:
Increase: BSP retention, calcium, cholesterol, triglycerides, amylase
Decrease: PBI, PSP, parathyroid test

Treatment of overdose: Lavage if taken orally, monitor electrolytes, administer dextrose in saline, monitor hydration, CV, renal status

---

chlorzoxazone

(klor-zox'a-zone)
Paraflex, Oxyren

Func. class.: Skeletal muscle relaxant
Chem. class.: Benzoxazole derivative

Action: Inhibits multisynaptic reflex arcs
Uses: Relieving pain, spasm in musculoskeletal conditions
Dosage and routes:
• *Adult:* PO 250-750 mg tid-qid
• *Child:* PO 20 mg/kg/day in divided doses bid-tid
Available forms include: Tabs 250 mg
Side effects/adverse reactions:
GU: Urine discoloration
HEMA: ***Granulocytopenia, anemia***
CNS: Dizziness, drowsiness, headache, insomnia, stimulation, malaise

---

* Available in Canada only

GI: Nausea, vomiting, anorexia, diarrhea, constipation, ***hepatotoxicity, jaundice***
INTEG: Rash, pruritus, petechiae, ecchymoses, ***angioedema***
SYST: ***Anaphylaxis***
Contraindications: Hypersensitivity, impaired hepatic function
Precautions: Pregnancy (C), lactation, hepatic disease, elderly
Pharmacokinetics:
PO: Onset 1 hr, peak 3-4 hr, duration 6 hr, half-life 1 hr, metabolized in liver, excreted in urine (metabolites)
Interactions/incompatibilities:
• Increased CNS depression: alcohol, tricyclic antidepressants, narcotics, barbiturates, sedatives, hypnotics

NURSING CONSIDERATIONS

Assess:
• Blood studies: CBC, WBC, differential; blood dyscrasias may occur
• Liver function studies: AST, ALT, alk phosphatase; hepatitis may occur; hold dose and notify physician if signs of hepatotoxicity occur
• EEG in epileptic patients; poor seizure control has occurred with patients taking this drug
Administer:
• With meals for GI symptoms
Perform/provide:
• Storage in tight container at room temperature
• Assistance with ambulation if dizziness or drowsiness occurs, especially elderly
Evaluate:
• Therapeutic response: decreased pain, spasticity
• Allergic reactions: rash, fever, respiratory distress
• Severe weakness, numbness in extremities
• Psychologic dependency: increased need for medication, more frequent requests for medication, increased pain
• CNS depression: dizziness, drowsiness, psychiatric symptoms
Teach patient/family:
• Not to discontinue the medication quickly; insomnia, nausea, headache, spasticity, tachycardia will occur; drug should be tapered off over 1-2 wk
• Not to take with alcohol, other CNS depressants
• To avoid altering activities while taking this drug
• To avoid hazardous activities if drowsiness, dizziness occurs
• To avoid using OTC medication: cough preparations, antihistamines, unless directed by physician
• That urine may be orange or purple
Treatment of overdose: Gastric lavage or induce emesis, then administer activated charcoal; use other supportive treatment as necessary; monitor cardiac function

---

cholestyramine

(koe-less-tir'a-meen)
Questran
Func. class.: Antilipemic
Chem. class.: Bile acid sequestrant

Action: Absorbs, combines with bile acids to form insoluble complex that is excreted through feces; loss of bile acids lowers cholesterol levels
Uses: Primary hypercholesterolemia, pruritus associated with biliary obstruction, diarrhea caused by excess bile acid, digitalis toxicity xanthomas
Dosage and routes:
• *Adult:* PO 4 g ac, and hs, not to exceed 32 g/day

• *Child:* PO 240 mg/kg/day in 3 divided doses; administer with food or drink

Available forms include: Powd 9 g/4 g cholestyramine

Side effects/adverse reactions:

CNS: Headache, dizziness, drowsiness, vertigo, tinnitus

MS: Muscle, joint pain

GI: Constipation, abdominal pain, nausea, fecal impaction, hemorrhoids, flatulence, vomiting, steatorrhea, peptic ulcer

INTEG: Rash, irritation of perianal area, tongue, skin

HEMA: Decreased vitamin A, D, K, red cell folate content, ***hyperchloremic acidosis, bleeding,*** decreased pro-time

Contraindications: Hypersensitivity, biliary obstruction

Precautions: Pregnancy (C), lactation, children

Pharmacokinetics:

PO: Excreted in feces, maximum effect in 2 wk

Interactions/incompatibilities:

• Decreased absorption of: phenylbutazone, warfarin, thiazides, digitalis, penicillin G, tetracyclines, cephalexin, phenobarbital, folic acid, corticosteroids, iron, thyroid, clindamycin, trimethoprim, chenodiol, fat-soluble vitamins

NURSING CONSIDERATIONS

Assess:

• Cardiac glycoside level, if both drugs are being administered

• For signs of vitamin A, D, K deficiency

• Serum cholesterol, triglyceride levels, electrolytes if on extended therapy

Administer:

• Drug ac, hs; give all other medications 1 hr before cholestyramine or 4 hr after cholestyramine to avoid poor absorption

• Drug mixed/applesauce or stirred into beverage (2-6 oz), do not take dry, let stand for 2 min

• Supplemental doses of vitamins A, D, K, if levels are low

Evaluate:

• Therapeutic response: decreased cholesterol level (hyperlipidemia); diarrhea, pruritus (excess bile area)

• Bowel pattern daily; increase bulk, water in diet if constipation develops

Teach patient/family:

• Symptoms of hypothrombinemia: bleeding mucous membranes, dark tarry stools, hematuria, petechiae; report immediately

• Importance of compliance since toxicity may result if doses are missed

• That risk factors should be decreased: high fat diet, smoking, alcohol consumption, absence of exercise

Lab test interferences:

Increase: Liver function studies, chloride, PO_4

---

choline salicylate

(koe'leen)

Arthropan, Teejel*

Func. class.: Nonnarcotic analgesic

Chem. class.: Salicylate

Action: Blocks pain impulses in CNS that occur in response to inhibition of prostaglandin synthesis; antipyretic action results from inhibition of hypothalamic heat-regulating center to produce vasodilation to allow heat dissipation

Uses: Mild to moderate pain or fever including arthritis, juvenile rheumatoid arthritis

*Available in Canada only

Dosage and routes:
Arthritis
• *Adult:* PO 870-1740 mg qid
Pain/fever
• *Adult:* PO 870 mg q3-4h prn
• *Child 3-6 yr:* PO 105-210 mg q4h prn
Available forms include: Liq 870 mg/5 ml
Side effects/adverse reactions:
HEMA: ***Thrombocytopenia, agranulocytosis, leukopenia, neutropenia, hemolytic anemia,*** increased pro-time
CNS: Stimulation, drowsiness, dizziness, confusion, ***convulsion,*** headache, flushing, hallucinations, ***coma***
GI: Nausea, vomiting, GI bleeding, diarrhea, heartburn, anorexia, ***hepatitis***
INTEG: Rash, urticaria, bruising
EENT: Tinnitus, hearing loss
CV: Rapid pulse, pulmonary edema
RESP: Wheezing, hyperpnea
ENDO: Hypoglycemia, hyponatremia, hypokalemia
Contraindications: Hypersensitivity to salicylates, GI bleeding, bleeding disorders, children < 3 yr, vitamin K deficiency, children with flulike symptoms
Precautions: Anemia, hepatic disease, renal disease, Hodgkin's disease, pregnancy (C), lactation
Pharmacokinetics:
PO: Onset 15-30 min, metabolized by liver, excreted by kidneys, crosses placenta, excreted in breast milk
Interactions/incompatibilities:
• Decreased effects of choline: antacids, steroids, urinary alkalizers
• Increased blood loss: alcohol, heparin
• Increased effects of: anticoagulants, insulin, methotrexate
• Decreased effects of: probenecid, spironolactone, sulfinpyrazone, sulfonylamides
• Toxic effects: PABA, furosemide, carbonic anhydrase inhibitors
• Decreased blood sugar levels: salicylates
• GI bleeding: steroids, antiinflammatories

NURSING CONSIDERATIONS

Assess:
• Liver function studies: AST, ALT, bilirubin, creatinine if patient is on long-term therapy
• Renal function studies: BUN, urine creatinine if patient is on long-term therapy
• Blood studies: CBC, Hct, Hgb, pro-time if patient is on long-term therapy
• I&O ratio; decreasing output may indicate renal failure (long-term therapy)
Administer:
• Mixed with fruit juice, carbonated beverage, water
Evaluate:
• Therapeutic response: decreased pain, fever, stiffness of joints
• Hepatotoxicity: dark urine, clay-colored stools, yellowing of skin, sclera, itching, abdominal pain, fever, diarrhea if patient is on long-term therapy
• Allergic reactions: rash, urticaria; if these occur, drug may need to be discontinued
• Renal dysfunction: decreased urine output
• Ototoxicity: tinnitus, ringing, roaring in ears; audiometric testing needed before, after long-term therapy
• Visual changes: blurring, halos, corneal, retinal damage
• Edema in feet, ankles, legs
• Prior drug history; there are many drug interactions

Teach patient/family:
- To report any symptoms of hepatotoxicity, renal toxicity, visual changes, ototoxicity, allergic reactions, bleeding (long-term therapy)
- Not to exceed recommended dosage; acute poisoning may result
- To read label on other OTC drugs; many contain aspirin
- That therapeutic response takes 2 wk (arthritis)
- To avoid alcohol ingestion; GI bleeding may occur
- That if anticoagulants are given with this drug, this drug should be decreased 2 wk before surgery

Lab test interferences:
Increase: Coagulation studies, liver function studies, serum uric acid, amylase, CO_2, urinary protein
Decrease: Serum potassium, PBI, cholesterol
Interfere: Urine catecholamines, pregnancy test
Treatment of overdose: Lavage, activated charcoal, monitor electrolytes, VS

chorionic gonadotropin, human

(go-nad'oh-troe-pin)
Android HCG, APL, Chorex, Follutein, Glukor, Gonic, Libigen, Pregnyl, Profasi HP, Stemutrolin
Func. class.: Human chorionic gonadotropin
Chem. class.: Polypeptide hormone

Action: Stimulates production of gonadal steroids, androgens; stimulates corpus luteum to produce progesterone
Uses: Infertility, anovulation, hypogonadism, nonobstructive cryptorchidism

Dosage and routes:
Infertility/anovulation
- *Adult:* IM 10,000 U 1 day after last dose of menotropins

Hypogonadism
- *Adult:* IM 500-1000 U 3 × wk × 3 wk, then 2 × wk × 3 wk, or 4000 U 3 × wk × 6-9 mo, then 2000 U 3 × wk × 3 mo

Cryptorchidism
- *Child (boy 4-9 yr):* IM 5000 U qod × 4 doses

Available forms include: Powder for inj 200, 1000, 2000 U/ml
Side effects/adverse reactions:
CNS: Headache, depression, fatigue, anxiety, irritability
GU: Gynecomastia, early puberty, edema, ***ectopic pregnancy***
INTEG: Pain at injection site
Contraindications: Hypersensitivity, pituitary hypertrophy/tumor, early puberty, prostatic CA
Precautions: Asthma, migraine headache, convulsive disorders, cardiac disease, renal disease
Pharmacokinetics:
IM: Peak 6 hr, half-life 11-24 hr, excreted by kidneys

NURSING CONSIDERATIONS

Assess:
- Weight weekly; notify physician if weekly weight gain is >5 lb
- B/P before, during treatment
- Be alert for decreasing urinary output, increasing edema

Administer:
- Only after clomiphene citrate has been tried on anovulatory client
- After reconstitution with diluent enclosed in package

Perform/provide:
- Refrigeration for up to 2 mo

Evaluate:
- Therapeutic response: ovulation, fertility
- Edema, hypertension

* Available in Canada only

Teach patient/family:
• To report facial, axillary, pubic hair, change in voice, penile enlargement, acne in male, abdominal pain, distention, vaginal bleeding in women
• To report symptoms of ectopic pregnancy: dizziness, pain on one side, shoulder, pallor, weak thready pulse, hemorrhage; shock may proceed rapidly

---

chymopapain

(kye'moe-pa-pane)
Chymodiactin, Discase
Func. class.: Enzyme
Chem. class.: Proteolytic

Action: Hydrolyzes noncollagenous polypeptides that maintain structure of chondromucoprotein; this activity decreases pressure on disk
Uses: Herniated lumbar intervertebral disk
Dosage and routes:
• *Adult:* Inj 2000-4000 U/disk injected intradiskally, not to exceed 10,000 U in a multiple herniation
Available forms include: Powder for inj 4000, 10,000 U/vial
Side effects/adverse reactions:
CNS: ***Paraplegia, cerebral hemorrhage,*** headache, dizziness, paresthesia, numbness of extremities
INTEG: Rash, urticaria, itching
GI: Nausea, paralytic ileus
MS: Back pain, stiffness, spasm, acute transverse myelitis, weakness, leg pain
SYSTEM: ***Anaphylaxis***
GU: Urinary retention
Contraindications: Hypersensitivity to this drug, papaya, meat tenderizer; severe spondylolisthesis; severe progressing paralysis; spinal cord tumor; cauda equina lesion, previous use
Precautions: Pregnancy, (C) children
Pharmacokinetics:
Onset 30 min, duration 24 hr
Interactions/incompatibilities:
• Dysrhythmias: halothane anesthetics plus epinephrine

NURSING CONSIDERATIONS
Assess:
• RBCs, ESR before treatment
• Respiratory rate, rhythm, depth; notify physician of abnormalities
• Anaphylaxis for several days after injection
• Neuro status after surgery; elimination status, since paralytic ileus can occur
Administer:
• Only with epinephrine available for anaphylaxis
• Only in lumbar spine by physician
• After diluting with sterile water for injection, use within 60 min
• After completing allergy test (ChymoFAST)
Evaluate:
• Therapeutic response: absence of back pain, increased mobility
• For allergies: iodine, papaya, meat tenderizer; if allergies are identified, drug should not be used
Teach patient/family
• To report allergic reactions that have occurred up to 2 wk after injection
• To be aware of possible infection; redness, swelling, pain

---

ciclopirox olamine (topical)

(sye-kloe-peer'ox)
Loprox
Func. class.: Local antiinfective
Chem. class.: Antifungal

Action: Interferes with fungal cell

membrane, which increases permeability, leaking of cell nutrients
Uses: Tinea cruris, tinea corporis, tinea pedis, tinea versicolor, cutaneous candidiasis
Dosage and routes:
• *Adult and child >10 yr:* TOP rub into affected area bid
Available forms include: Cream 1%
Side effects/adverse reactions:
INTEG: Rash, urticaria, stinging, burning, pruritus, pain
Contraindications: Hypersensitivity
Precautions: Pregnancy (B), lactation, child <10 yr
NURSING CONSIDERATIONS
Administer:
• Enough medication to completely cover lesions
• After cleansing with soap, water before each application, dry well
Perform/provide:
• Storage at room temperature in dry place
Evaluate:
• Therapeutic response: decrease in size, number of lesions
• Allergic reaction: burning, stinging, swelling, redness
Teach patient/family:
• To apply with glove to prevent further infection
• To avoid use of OTC creams, ointments, lotions unless directed by physician
• To continue even though condition improves
• To use medical asepsis (hand washing) before, after each application
• Not to cover with occlusive dressing
• To change shoes and socks once a day during treatment of tinea pedis
• To report blisters, burning, oozing, swelling

cimetidine

(sye-met'i-deen)
Tagamet
Func. class.: H_2 Histamine receptor antagonist
Chem. class.: Imidazole derivative

Action: Inhibits histamine at H_2 receptor site in parietal cells, which inhibits gastric acid secretion
Uses: Short-term treatment of duodenal and gastric ulcers and maintenance
Dosage and routes:
• *Adult and child: PO* 300 mg qid with meals, hs × 8 wk or 400 mg bid, 800 mg hs; after 8 wk give hs dose only; IV BOL 300 mg/20 ml 0.9% NaCl over 1-2 min q6h; IV INF 300 mg/50 ml D_5W over 15-20 min; IM 300 mg q6h, not to exceed 2400 mg
Prophylaxis of duodenal ulcer
• *Adult and child >16 yr:* 400 mg hs
Available forms include: Tabs 200, 300, 400, 800 mg; liq 300 mg/5 ml; inj IV 300 mg/2 ml, 300 mg/50 ml 0.9% NaCl
Side effects/adverse reactions:
CNS: Confusion, headache, depression, dizziness, anxiety, weakness, psychosis, tremors, ***convulsions***
GI: Diarrhea, abdominal cramps, ***paralytic ileus, jaundice***
GU: Gynecomastia, galactorrhea, impotence, increase in BUN, creatinine
CV: Bradycardia, tachycardia
HEMA: ***Agranulocytosis, thrombocytopenia, neutropenia, aplastic anemia, increase in pro-time***
INTEG: Urticaria, rash, alopecia,

* Available in Canada only

sweating, flushing, ***exfoliative dermatitis***

Contraindications: Hypersensitivity

Precautions: Pregnancy (B), lactation, child <16 yr, organic brain syndrome, hepatic disease, renal disease

Pharmacokinetics:

PO: Peak 1-1½ hr, half-life 1½ hr; metabolized by liver, excreted in urine (unchanged), crosses placenta, enters breast milk

Interactions/incompatibilities:

- Increased toxicity: anticoagulants, benzodiazepines, metoprolol, propranolol, phenytoins, quinidine, theophyllines, tricyclic antidepressants, lidocaine, procainamide
- Decreased absorption of cimetidine: antacids
- Decreased absorption: ketoconazole

NURSING CONSIDERATIONS

Assess:

- Gastric pH (>5 should be maintained)
- I&O ratio, BUN, creatinine

Administer:

- IV after diluting 300 mg/20 ml of normal saline for inj; give over 2 min; may be diluted; 300 mg/50 ml of compatible sol run over 15-20 min
- With meals for prolonged drug effect
- Antacids 1 hr before or 1 hr after cimetidine
- IV slowly, bradycardia may occur, give over 30 min

Perform/provide:

- Storage of diluted solution at room temperature for up to 48 hr

Evaluate:

- Therapeutic response: decreased pain in abdomen

Teach patient/family:

- That gynecomastia, impotence may occur, but is reversible
- To avoid driving or other hazardous activities until patient is stabilized on this medication
- To avoid black pepper, caffeine, alcohol, harsh spices, extremes in temperature of food
- To avoid OTC preparations: aspirin, cough, cold preparations
- That drug must be continued for prescribed time to be effective
- To report bruising, fatigue, malaise; blood dyscrasias may occur

Lab test interferences:

Increase: Alk phosphatase, AST, creatinine

False positive: Gastric bleeding test

cinoxacin

(sin-ox'a-sin)

Cinobac

Func. class.: Urinary tract antibacterial

Action: Interferes with conversion of intermediate DNA fragments into high-molecular-weight DNA in bacteria

Uses: Urinary tract infections caused by *E. coli, Klebsiella, Enterobacter, P. mirabilis, P. vulgaris, P. morgani, Serratia, Citrobacter*

Dosage and routes:

- *Adult and child >12 yr:* PO 1 g/day in 2-4 divided doses × 1-2 wk

Available forms include: Caps 250, 500 mg

Side effects/adverse reactions:

INTEG: Pruritus, rash, urticaria, photosensitivity, edema

CNS: Dizziness, headache, agitation, insomnia, confusion

GI: Nausea, vomiting, anorexia, abdominal cramps, diarrhea

EENT: Sensitivity to light, visual disturbances, blurred vision, tinnitus

Contraindications: Hypersensitivity to this drug, anuria, CNS damage

Precautions: Renal disease, hepatic disease, pregnancy (B), nursing mothers

Pharmacokinetics:

PO: Duration 6-8 hr, half-life 1½ hr, excreted in urine (unchanged/inactive metabolites)

Interactions/incompatibilities:

• Increased levels of cinoxacin: probenecid

NURSING CONSIDERATIONS

Assess:

• Kidney, liver function studies: BUN, creatinine, AST, ALT

• I&O ratio, urine pH; <5.5 is ideal

Administer:

• After clean-catch urine is obtained for C&S

• Two daily doses if urine output is high or if patient has diabetes

Perform/provide:

• Limited intake of alkaline foods, drugs: milk, dairy products, peanuts, vegetables, alkaline antacids, sodium bicarbonate

Evaluate:

• Therapeutic response: decreased pain, frequency, urgency, C&S absence of infection

• CNS symptoms: insomnia, vertigo, headache, agitation, confusion

• Allergic reactions: fever, flushing, rash, urticaria, pruritus

Teach patient/family:

• That photophobic reactions occur; that patient should avoid sunlight or use sunglasses, sunscreen

• That fluids must be increased to 3 L/day to avoid crystallization in kidneys

• That if dizziness occurs, ambulate/activities with assistance

• Complete full course of drug therapy

• To contact physician if adverse reactions occur

• To take with food/milk to decrease GI irritation

Lab test interferences:

Increase: AST/ALT, BUN, creatinine, alk phosphatase

ciprofloxacin

(sip-ro-floks'a-sin)

Cipro

Func. class.: Urinary antiinfectives

Chem. class.: Fluoroquinolone antibacterial

Action: Interferes with conversion of intermediate DNA fragments into high-molecular-weight DNA in bacteria; DNAgyrase inhibitor

Uses: Adult urinary tract infections (including complicated) caused by *E. coli, E. cloacae, P. mirabilis, K. pneumoniae, P. vulgans, C. freusdil,* group D strep

Dosage and routes:

Uncomplicated urinary tract infections

• *Adult:* PO 250 mg q12h; IV 200 mg q12h

Complicated/severe urinary tract infections

• *Adult:* PO 500 mg q12h; IV 400 mg q12h

Respiratory, bone, skin, joint infections

• *Adult:* PO 500 mg q12h

Available forms include: Tabs 250, 500, 750 mg; IV 200 mg/100 ml D_5, 400 mg/200 ml D_5; 200, 400 mg vial

Side effects/adverse reactions:

CNS: Headache, dizziness, fatigue, insomnia, depression, restlessness

* Available in Canada only

GI: Nausea, constipation, increased ALT, AST, flatulence, insomnia, heartburn, vomiting, diarrhea, oral candidiasis, dysphagia
INTEG: Rash, pruritus, urticaria, photosensitivity, flushing, fever, chills
MS: Blurred vision, tinnitus
Contraindications: Hypersensitivity to quinolones
Precautions: Pregnancy (C), lactation, children, renal disease
Pharmacokinetics:
PO: Peak 1 hr, half-life 3-4 hr; steady state 2 days; excreted in urine as active drug, metabolites
Interactions/incompatibilities:
- Decreased absorption: magnesium antacids, aluminum hydroxide
- Increased serum levels of ciprofloxacin: probenecid
- Increased theophylline levels when used with ciprofloxacin

NURSING CONSIDERATIONS

Assess:
- CNS symptoms: headache, dizziness, fatigue, insomnia, depression
- Kidney, liver function studies: BUN, creatinine, AST, ALT
- I&O ratio, urine pH <5.5 is ideal

Administer:
- After clean-catch urine is obtained for C&S
- Two daily doses if urine output is high or if patient has diabetes

Perform/provide:
- Limited intake of alkaline foods, drugs: milk, dairy products, peanuts, vegetables, alkaline antacids, sodium bicarbonate

Evaluate:
- Therapeutic response: decreased pain, frequency, urgency, C&S—absence of infection
- Allergic reactions: fever, flushing, rash, urticaria, pruritus

Teach patient/family:
- Not to take antacids containing magnesium or aluminum with this drug or within 2 hr of drug
- That photosensitivity occurs; patient should avoid sunlight or use sunscreen to prevent burns
- That fluids must be increased to 3 L/day to avoid crystallization in kidneys
- If dizziness occurs, to ambulate, perform activities with assistance
- To complete full course of drug therapy
- To contact physician if adverse reaction occurs
- To take with food, milk to decrease GI irritation

Lab test interferences:
Increase: AST, ALT, BUN, creatinine, alk phosphatase

---

cisplatin

(sis'pla-tin)
Platinol
Func. class.: Antineoplastic alkylating agent
Chem. class.: Inorganic heavy metal

Action: Alkylates DNA, RNA; inhibits enzymes that allow synthesis of amino acids in proteins
Uses: Advanced bladder cancer, adjunctive in metastatic testicular cancer, adjunctive in metastatic ovarian cancer, head, neck cancer, esophagus, prostate, lung and cervical cancer, lymphoma
Dosage and routes:
Testicular cancer
- *Adult:* IV 20 mg/m^2 qd $\times$ 5 days, repeat q3wk for 3 cycles or more, depending on response

Bladder cancer
- *Adult:* IV 50-70 mg/m^2 q3-4wk

Ovarian cancer

• *Adult:* IV 100 mg/m^2 q4wk or 50 mg/m^2 q3wk with doxorubicin therapy; mix with 2 L of NaCl and 37.5 g mannitol over 6 hr

Available forms include: Inj IV 10, 50 mg

Side effects/adverse reactions:

EENT: Tinnitus, hearing loss, vestibular toxicity

HEMA: ***Thrombocytopenia, leukopenia, pancytopenia***

CV: Cardiac abnormalities

GI: Severe nausea, vomiting, diarrhea, weight loss

GU: ***Renal tubular damage,*** renal insufficiency, impotence, sterility, amenorrhea, gynecomastia, hyperuremia

INTEG: Alopecia, dermatitis

CNS: ***Convulsions,*** peripheral neuropathy

RESP: ***Fibrosis***

META: Hypomagnesemia, hypocalcemia, hypokalemia, hypophosphatemia

SYST: ***Hypersensitivity reaction***

Contraindications: Radiation therapy within 1 mo, chemotherapy within 1 mo, thrombocytopenia, smallpox vaccination

Precautions: Pneumococcus vaccination, pregnancy (D)

Pharmacokinetics:

Well absorbed orally, metabolized in liver, excreted in urine; half-life 2 hr

Interactions/incompatibilities:

• Increased toxicity: aminoglycosides

• Decreased effects of: phenytoin

NURSING CONSIDERATIONS

Assess:

• CBC, differential, platelet count weekly; withhold drug if WBC is <4000 or platelet count is <75,000; notify physician of results

• Renal function studies: BUN, creatinine, serum uric acid, urine CrCl before, electrolytes during therapy

• I&O ratio; report fall in urine output of 30 ml/hr

• Monitor temperature q4h (may indicate beginning infection)

• Liver function tests before, during therapy (bilirubin, AST, ALT, LDH) as needed or monthly

Administer:

• IV after diluting 10 mg/10 ml sterile H_2O for inj; IV INF is given over 3-4 hr; check site for irritation; phlebitis; do not use equipment containing aluminum

• Hydrate patient with 1-2 L of fluids over 8-12 hr before treatment

• Epinephrine for hypersensitivity reaction

• Antiemetic 30-60 min before giving drug to prevent vomiting, and PRN

• Allopurinol or sodium bicarbonate to maintain uric acid levels, alkalinization of urine

• Antibiotics for prophylaxis of infection

• Diuretic (furosemide 40 mg IV) or mannitol after infusion

Perform/provide:

• Strict medical asepsis, protective isolation if WBC levels are low

• Comprehensive oral hygiene

• Storage protected from light in refrigerator (dry powder)

• Deep breathing exercises with patient tid-qid; place in semi-Fowler's position

• Increase fluid intake to 2-3 L/day to prevent urate deposits, calculi formation, elimination of drug

• Diet low in purines: organ meats (kidney, liver), dried beans, peas to maintain alkaline urine

Evaluate:

• Therapeutic response: decreased tumor size, spread of malignancy

• Bleeding: hematuria, guaiac, bruising or petechiae, mucosa or orifices q8h, obtain prescription for viscous Xylocaine
• Dyspnea, rales, unproductive cough, chest pain, tachypnea
• Food preferences; list likes, dislikes
• Effects of alopecia on body image, discuss feelings about body changes
• Yellowing of skin, sclera, dark urine, clay-colored stools, itchy skin, abdominal pain, fever, diarrhea
• Edema in feet, joint pain, stomach pain, shaking
• Inflammation of mucosa, breaks in skin

Teach patient/family:
• To report signs of infection: increased temperature, sore throat, flu symptoms
• To report signs of anemia: fatigue, headache, faintness, shortness of breath, irritability
• To report bleeding: avoid use of razors or commercial mouthwash
• To avoid use of aspirin or ibuprofen
• About protective isolation precautions
• To report any complaints or side effects to nurse or physician
• That impotence or amenorrhea can occur, reversible after discontinuing treatment
• To report any changes in breathing or coughing
• That hair may be lost during treatment; a wig or hairpiece may make patient feel better; new hair may be different in color, texture

clarithromycin

(clare-i-thro-mye'sin)
Biaxin

Func. class.: Antibacterial
Chem. class.: Macrolide antibiotic

Action: Binds to 50S ribosomal subunits of susceptible bacteria and suppresses protein synthesis
Uses: Mild to moderate infections of the upper respiratory tract, lower respiratory tract, uncomplicated skin and skin structure infections caused by *S. pneumoniae, M. pneumoniae, C. diphtheriae, B. pertussis, L. monocytogenes, H. influenzae, S. pyogenes, S. aureus*
Dosage and routes:
• *Adult:* PO 250-500 mg bid for 7-14 days
Available forms include: Tabs 250, 500 mg
Side effects/adverse reactions:
INTEG: Rash, urticaria, pruritus
GI: Nausea, vomiting, diarrhea, ***hepatotoxicity,*** abdominal pain, stomatitis, heartburn, anorexia, abnormal taste
GU: Vaginitis, moniliasis
MISC: Headache
Contraindications: Hypersensitivity
Precautions: pregnancy (C), lactation, hepatic, renal disease
Pharmacokinetics: Peak 2 hr, duration 12 hr, half-life 4-6 hr, metabolized by the liver, excreted in bile, feces
Interactions/incompatibilities:
• Increased effects of: oral anticoagulants, digoxin, theophylline, methylprednisolone, cyclosporine, bromocriptine, disopyramide
• Decreased action of: clindamycin
• Toxicity: carbamazepine
• Increased or decreased action of: penicillins

NURSING CONSIDERATIONS

Assess:

• I&O ratio; report hematuria, oliguria in renal disease
• Liver studies: AST, ALT
• Renal studies: urinalysis, protein, blood
• C&S before drug therapy; drug may be taken as soon as culture is taken; C&S may be repeated after treatment

Administer:

• Adequate intake of fluids (2000 ml) during diarrhea episodes

Perform/provide:

• Storage at room temperature

Evaluate:

• Therapeutic response: C&S negative for infection
• Bowel pattern before, during treatment
• Skin eruptions, itching
• Respiratory status: rate, character, wheezing, tightness in chest; discontinue drug if these occur
• Allergies before treatment, reaction of each medication; place allergies on chart, notify all people giving drugs

Teach patient/family:

• To take with a full glass of water; may give with food if GI symptoms occur
• Do not take with fruit juices
• To report sore throat, fever, fatigue; could indicate superimposed infection
• To notify nurse of diarrhea stools, dark urine, pale stools, yellow discoloration of eyes or skin, severe abdominal pain
• To take at evenly spaced intervals; complete dosage regimen

Lab test interferences:

False increase: 17-OHCS/17-KS, AST, ALT
Decrease: Folate assay

Treatment of overdose: Withdraw drug, maintain airway, administer epinephrine, aminophylline, O_2, IV corticosteroids

---

clemastine fumarate

(klem'as-teen)

Tavist, Tavist-1

Func. class.: Antihistamine
Chem. class.: Ethanolamine derivative, H_1-receptor antagonist

---

Action: Acts on blood vessels, GI, respiratory system by competing with histamine for H_1-receptor site; decreases allergic response by blocking histamine

Uses: Allergy symptoms, rhinitis, angioedema, urticaria

Dosage and routes:

• *Adult and child >12 yr:* PO 1.34-2.68 mg bid-tid, not to exceed 8.04 mg/day

Available forms include: Tabs 1.34, 2.68 mg; syr 0.67 mg/ml

Side effects/adverse reactions:

CNS: Dizziness, drowsiness, poor coordination, fatigue, anxiety, euphoria, confusion, paresthesia, neuritis

CV: Hypotension, palpitations, tachycardia

RESP: Increased thick secretions, wheezing, chest tightness

HEMA: ***Thrombocytopenia, agranulocytosis, hemolytic anemia***

GI: Constipation, dry mouth, nausea, vomiting, anorexia, diarrhea

INTEG: Rash, urticaria, photosensitivity

GU: Retention, dysuria, frequency

EENT: Blurred vision, dilated pupils, tinnitus, nasal stuffiness, dry nose, throat, mouth

Contraindications: Hypersensitivity to H_1-receptor antagonists, acute asthma attack, lower respiratory tract disease

---

* Available in Canada only

Precautions: Increased intraocular pressure, renal disease, cardiac disease, hypertension, bronchial asthma, seizure disorder, stenosed peptic ulcers, hyperthyroidism, prostatic hypertrophy, bladder neck obstruction, pregnancy (B), elderly

Pharmacokinetics:

PO: Peak 5-7 hr, duration 10-12 hr or more; metabolized in liver, excreted by kidneys

Interactions/incompatibilities:

- Increased CNS depression: barbiturates, narcotics, hypnotics, tricyclic antidepressants, alcohol
- Decreased effect of: oral anticoagulants, heparin
- Increased effect of clemastine: MAOIs

NURSING CONSIDERATIONS

Assess:

- I&O ratio; be alert for urinary retention, frequency, dysuria; drug should be discontinued if these occur
- CBC during long-term therapy

Administer:

- With meals if GI symptoms occur; absorption may slightly decrease

Perform/provide:

- Hard candy, gum, frequent rinsing of mouth for dryness
- Storage in tight container at room temperature

Evaluate:

- Therapeutic response: absence of running or congested nose or rashes
- Blood dyscrasias: thrombocytopenia, agranulocytosis (rare)
- Respiratory status: rate, rhythm, increase in bronchial secretions, wheezing, chest tightness
- Cardiac status: palpitations, increased pulse, hypotension

Teach patient/family:

- All aspects of drug use; to notify physician if confusion, sedation, hypotension occurs
- To avoid driving or other hazardous activity if drowsiness occurs
- To avoid concurrent use of alcohol or other CNS depressants
- To change position slowly, as drug may cause dizziness, hypotension (elderly)

Lab test interferences:

False negative: Skin allergy tests

Treatment of overdose: Administer ipecac syrup or lavage, diazepam, vasopressors, barbiturates (short-acting)

clidinium bromide

(kli'di-nee-um)

Quarzan

Func. class.: GI anticholinergic

Chem. class.: Synthetic quaternary ammonium antimuscarinic

Action: Inhibits muscarinic actions of acetylcholine at postganglionic parasympathetic neuroeffector sites

Uses: Treatment of peptic ulcer disease in combination with other drugs

Dosage and routes:

- *Adult:* PO 2.5-5 mg tid-qid ac, hs
- *Elderly:* PO 2.5 mg tid ac

Available forms include: Caps 2.5, 5 mg

Side effects/adverse reactions:

CNS: Confusion, stimulation in elderly, headache, insomnia, dizziness, drowsiness, anxiety, weakness, hallucination

GI: Dry mouth, constipation, ***paralytic ileus,*** heartburn, nausea, vomiting, dysphagia, absence of taste

GU: Hesitancy, retention, impotence

CV: Palpitations, tachycardia

EENT: Blurred vision, photopho-

bia, mydriasis, cycloplegia, increased ocular tension
INTEG: Urticaria, rash, pruritus, anhidrosis, fever, allergic reactions
Contraindications: Hypersensitivity to anticholinergics, narrow-angle glaucoma, GI obstruction, myasthenia gravis, paralytic ileus, GI atony, toxic megacolon
Precautions: Hyperthyroidism, coronary artery disease, dysrhythmias, CHF, ulcerative colitis, hypertension, hiatal hernia, hepatic disease, renal disease, pregnancy (C), urinary retention, prostatic hypertrophy, elderly
Pharmacokinetics:
PO: Onset 1 hr, duration 3 hr; ionized, excreted in urine
Interactions/incompatibilities:
- Increased anticholinergic effect: amantadine, tricyclic antidepressants, MAOIs
- Decreased effect of: phenothiazines, levodopa, ketoconazole

NURSING CONSIDERATIONS

Assess:
- VS, cardiac status: checking for dysrhythmias, increased rate, palpitations
- I&O ratio; check for urinary retention or hesitancy, especially elderly

Administer:
- ½-1 hr ac for better absorption
- Decreased dose to elderly patients since their metabolism may be slowed
- Gum, hard candy, frequent rinsing of mouth for dryness of oral cavity

Perform/provide:
- Storage in tight container protected from light
- Increased fluids, bulk, exercise to patient's lifestyle to decrease constipation

Evaluate:
- Therapeutic response: absence of epigastric pain, bleeding, nausea, vomiting
- GI complaints: pain, bleeding (frank or occult), nausea, vomiting, anorexia

Teach patient/family:
- To avoid driving or other hazardous activities until stabilized on medication
- To avoid alcohol or other CNS depressants; will enhance sedating properties of this drug
- To avoid hot environments; stroke may occur, drug suppresses perspiration
- To use sunglasses when outside to prevent photophobia, may cause blurred vision
- To drink plenty of fluids
- To report dysphagia

---

clindamycin HCl/clindamycin palmitate HCl/clindamycin phosphate

(klin-da-mye'sin)
Cleocin, Dalacin C*
Func. class.: Antibacterial macrolide
Chem. class.: Lincomycin derivative

Action: Binds to 50S subunit of bacterial ribosomes, suppresses protein synthesis
Uses: Infections caused by staphylococci, streptococci, pneumococci, *Rickettsia, Fusobacterium, Actinomyces, Peptococcus, Clostridium*
Dosage and routes:
- *Adults:* PO 150-450 mg q6h; IM/IV 300 mg q6-12h, not to exceed 4800 mg/day
- *Child >1 mo:* PO 8-25 mg/kg/

* Available in Canada only

day in divided doses q6-8h; IM/IV 15-40 mg/kg/day in divided doses q6-8h 3-4 equal doses
• *PID:* Adult IV 600 mg qid plus gentamicin

Available forms include: Inj 150-300 mg/ml; caps 75, 150-300 mg; oral sol 75 mg/ml

Side effects/adverse reactions:
HEMA: ***Leukopenia, eosinophilia, agranulocytosis, thrombocytopenia***
GI: Nausea, vomiting, abdominal pain, diarrhea, ***pseudomembranous colitis,*** anorexia, weight loss
GU: Increased AST, ALT, bilirubin, alk phosphatase, jaundice, *vaginitis,* urinary frequency
EENT: Rash, urticaria, pruritus, erythema, pain, abscess at injection site

Contraindications: Hypersensitivity to this drug or lincomycin, ulcerative colitis/enteritis, infants <1 mo

Precautions: Renal disease, liver disease, GI disease, elderly, pregnancy (B), lactation, tartrazine sensitivity

Pharmacokinetics:
PO: Peak 45 min, duration 6 hr
IM: Peak 3 hr, duration 8-12 hr
Half-life 2½ hr, metabolized in liver, excreted in urine, bile, feces as active/inactive metabolites, crosses placenta, excreted in breast milk

Interactions/incompatibilities:
• Increased neuromuscular blockage: nondepolarizing muscle relaxants
• Decreased action of: chloramphenicol, erythromycin

NURSING CONSIDERATIONS

Assess:
• Any patient with compromised renal system; drug is excreted slowly in poor renal system function; toxicity may occur rapidly
• Liver studies: AST, ALT
• Blood studies: WBC, RBC, Hct, Hgb, platelets, serum iron, reticulocytes; drug should be discontinued if bone marrow depression occurs
• Renal studies: urinalysis, protein, blood, BUN, creatinine
• C&S before drug therapy; drug may be taken as soon as culture is taken
• Drug level in impaired hepatic, renal systems
• B/P, pulse in patient receiving drug parenterally

Administer:
• IV by infusion only; do not administer bolus dose, dilute 300 mg/50 ml of compatible sol; run over >10 min; no more than 1200 mg in a single 1-hr inf
• IM deep injection; rotate sites
• Orally with at least 8 oz water

Perform/provide:
• Storage at room temperature (capsules) and up to 2 wk (reconstituted solution)
• Adrenalin, suction, tracheostomy set, endotracheal intubation equipment on unit
• Adequate intake of fluids (2000 ml) during diarrhea episodes

Evaluate:
• Therapeutic response: decreased temperature, negative C&S
• Bowel pattern before, during treatment
• Skin eruptions, itching, dermatitis after administration
• Respiratory status: rate, character, wheezing, tightness in chest
• Allergies before treatment, reaction of each medication; place allergies on chart, Kardex in bright red letters; notify all people giving drugs

Teach patient/family:
- To take oral drug with full glass of water; may give with food if GI symptoms occur
- Aspects of drug therapy: need to complete entire course of medication to ensure organism death (10-14 days); culture may be taken after completed medication course
- To report sore throat, fever, fatigue; could indicate superimposed infection
- That drug must be taken in equal intervals around clock to maintain blood levels
- To notify nurse of diarrhea

Lab test interferences:
Increase: Alk phosphatase, bilirubin, CPK, AST, ALT
Treatment of hypersensitivity: Withdraw drug, maintain airway, administer epinephrine, aminophylline, O_2, IV corticosteroids

clioquinol (iodochlorhydroxyquin)

(klee-oh-kwee'nole)

Quin III, Torofor, Vioform

Func. class.: Local antiinfective
Chem. class.: Halogenated hydroxyquinoline

Action: Increases cell membrane permeability is susceptible organisms by binding sterols; decreases potassium, sodium, and nutrients in cell
Uses: Cutaneous infections: athlete's foot, eczema, and other fungal infections
Dosage and routes:
TOP: apply to affected area bid or tid ×7 days only
Available forms include: cream, oint 3%
Side effects/adverse reactions:
INTEG: Rash, urticaria, stinging, burning, dry skin, pruritus, contact dermatitis, erythema, redness, staining of hair and skin
Contraindications: Hypersensitivity to iodine, chloroxine
Precautions: Pregnancy (C), varicella, viral skin conditions, deep or puncture wounds, serious burns
Pharmacokinetics:
Some absorbed through the skin, excreted in urine (conjugated form), the rest excreted slowly

NURSING CONSIDERATIONS

Administer:
- Enough medication to completely cover lesions
- After cleansing with soap and water before each application, dry well

Perform/provide:
- Storage at room temperature in dry place

Evaluate:
- Therapeutic response: decrease in size, number of lesions
- Allergic reaction: burning, stinging, swelling, redness

Teach patient/family:
- To avoid use of OTC creams, ointments, lotions unless directed by physician
- To use medical asepsis (hand washing) before, after each application to prevent further infection
- Not to cover with occlusive dressing
- To continue even if condition improves
- That drug may stain clothing, skin, hair

Lab test interference:
Interference: Thyroid function tests

* Available in Canada only

clobetasol propionate

(klo-bet'-a-sol)

Temovate

Func. class.: Topical corticosteroid
Chem. class.: Synthetic fluorinated agent, group I potency

Action: Possesses antipruritic, antiinflammatory actions

Uses: Psoriasis, eczema, contact dermatitis, pruritus; usually reserved for severe dermatoses that have not responded to less potent formulation

Dosage and routes:

• *Adult and child:* Apply to affected area bid

Available forms include: Oint 0.05%; cream 0.05%

Side effects/adverse reactions:

INTEG: Burning, dryness, itching, irritation, acne, folliculitis, hypertrichosis, perioral dermatitis, hypopigmentation, atrophy, striae, miliaria, allergic contact dermatitis, secondary infection

Contraindications: Hypersensitivity to corticosteroids, fungal infections

Precautions: Pregnancy (C), lactation, viral infections, bacterial infections

NURSING CONSIDERATIONS

Assess:

• Temperature; if fever develops, drug should be discontinued

Administer:

• Only to affected areas; do not get in eyes

• Leaving uncovered or lightly covered; occlusive dressing is not recommended, systemic absorption may occur

• Only to dermatoses; do not use on weeping, denuded, or infected area

Perform/provide:

• Cleansing before application of drug

• Treatment for a few days after area has cleared

• Storage at room temperature

Evaluate:

• Therapeutic response: absence of severe itching, patches on skin, flaking

• For systemic absorption: increased temperature, inflammation, irritation

Teach patient/family:

• To avoid sunlight on affected area; burns may occur

• To limit treatment to 14 days using <50 g/wk

clocortolone pivalate

(klo-kort'-oo-lone)

Cloderm

Func. class.: Topical corticosteroid
Chem. class.: Synthetic fluorinated agent, group IV potency

Action: Possesses antipruritic, antiinflammatory actions

Uses: Psoriasis, eczema, contact dermatitis, pruritus

Dosage and routes:

• *Adult and child:* Apply to affected area tid or qid

Available forms include: Cream 0.1%

Side effects/adverse reactions:

INTEG: Burning, dryness, itching, irritation, acne, folliculitis, hypertrichosis, perioral dermatitis, hypopigmentation, atrophy, striae, miliaria, allergic contact dermatitis, secondary infection

Contraindications: Hypersensitivity to corticosteroids, fungal infections

Precautions: Pregnancy (C), lactation, viral infections, bacterial infections

C

NURSING CONSIDERATIONS
Assess:
• Temperature; if fever develops, drug should be discontinued
Administer:
• Only to affected areas; do not get in eyes
• Medication, then cover with occlusive dressing (only if prescribed), seal to normal skin, change q12h; systemic absorption may occur
• Only to dermatoses; do not use on weeping, denuded, or infected area
Perform/provide:
• Cleansing before application of drug
• Treatment for a few days after area has cleared
• Storage at room temperature
Evaluate:
• Therapeutic response: absence of severe itching, patches on skin, flaking
• For systemic absorption: increased temperature, inflammation, irritation
Teach patient/family:
• To avoid sunlight on affected area; burns may occur

---

clofazimine

(kloe-faaz'-ii-meen)
Lamprene
Func. class.: Leprostatic

Action: Inhibits mycobacterial growth, binds to mycobacterial DNA; exerts antiinflammatory properties in controlling leprosy reactions
Uses: Lepromatous leprosy, dapsone-resistant leprosy, lepromatous leprosy complicated by erythema nodosum leprosum
Dosage and routes:
Erythema nodosum leprosum
• *Adult:* PO: 100-200 mg qd × 3 mo, then taper dosage to 100 mg when disease is controlled, do not exceed 200 mg/day
Dapsone-resistant leprosy
• *Adult:* PO: 100 mg/day in combination with at least one other antileprosy drug × 3 yr, then 100 mg qd clofazimine (only)
Available forms include: Caps 50, 100 mg
Side effects/adverse reactions:
GI: Diarrhea, nausea, vomiting, abdominal pain, intolerance, ***GI bleeding, obstruction,*** anorexia, constipation, ***hepatitis,*** jaundice
EENT: Pigmentation of cornea, conjunctive, drying, burning, itching, irritation
INTEG: Pink or brown discoloration, dryness, pruritus, rash, photosensitivity, acne, monilial cheilosis
CNS: Dizziness, headache, fatigue, drowsiness
MISC: Discolored urine, feces, sputum, sweat
Precautions: Pregnancy (C), lactation, children, abdominal pain, diarrhea, depression
Pharmacokinetics:
Deposited in fatty tissue, reticuloendothelial system; half-life 70 days, small amount excreted in feces, sputum, sweat
NURSING CONSIDERATIONS
Assess:
• Liver studies qwk: ALT, AST, bilirubin
• Renal studies: BUN, creatinine, I&O, sp gr, urinalysis before; qmo
• Blood level of drug
Administer:
• With meals to decrease GI symptoms
• Antiemetic if vomiting occurs
• After C&S is completed; qmo to detect resistance

---

* Available in Canada only

Perform/provide:
• Infants to be kept with mother infected with leprosy; breastfeeding during drug therapy is encouraged
Evaluate:
• Therapeutic response: decreased symptoms of infection
• Mental status often: affect, mood, behavioral changes; psychosis may occur
• Hepatic status: decreased appetite, jaundice, dark urine, fatigue
Teach patient/family:
• That therapeutic effects may occur after 3-6 mo of drug therapy
• That compliance with dosage schedule, length is necessary
• That scheduled appointments must be kept or relapse may occur
• That drug must be taken with meals
• Skin, sweat, sputum, urine, feces discoloration, although reversible, may take several months or years to disappear
Lab test interferences:
Increase: Albumin, bilirubin, AST, eosinophilia, hypokalemia

clofibrate

(kloe-fye'brate)
Atromide-S, Claripen,* Claripex*
Func. class.: Antilipemic
Chem. class.: Aryloxisobutyric acid derivative

Action: Inhibits biosynthesis of VLDL, LDL, which are responsible for triglyceride development, mobilizes triglycerides from tissue, increases excretion of neutral sterols
Uses: Hyperlipidemia; xanthoma tuberosum; types III, IV, V hyperlipidemia
Dosage and routes:
• *Adult:* PO 2 g/day in 4 divided doses
Available forms include: Caps 500 mg
Side effects/adverse reactions:
GI: Nausea, vomiting, dyspepsia, increased liver enzymes, stomatitis, flatulence, hepatomegaly, gastritis, increased cholelithiasis, weight gain
INTEG: Rash, urticaria, pruritus, dry hair and skin, alopecia
HEMA: ***Leukopenia,*** anemia, ***eosinophilia,*** bleeding
CNS: Fatigue, weakness, drowsiness, dizziness
GU: Decreased libido, impotence, dysuria, proteinuria, oliguria, ***hematuria***
MS: Myalgias, arthralgias
CV: Angina, dysrhythmias, thrombophlebitis, ***pulmonary emboli***
MISC: Polyphagia, weight gain
Contraindications: Severe hepatic disease, severe renal disease, primary biliary cirrhosis
Precautions: Peptic ulcer, pregnancy (C), lactation
Pharmacokinetics:
PO: Peak 2-6 hr, plasma protein binding >90%; half-life 6-25 hr, excreted in urine, metabolized in liver
Interactions/incompatibilities:
• Increased effects of: sulfonylureas, insulin
• Increased toxicity of clofibrate: probenecid
• Increased anticoagulant effects of: oral anticoagulants
• Decreased effects of clofibrate: rifampin

NURSING CONSIDERATIONS

Assess:
• Renal and hepatic levels if patient is on long-term therapy
Administer:
• Drug with meals if GI symptoms occur

Evaluate:
• Therapeutic response: decreased triglycerides, diarrhea, pruritus (excess bile area)
• Bowel pattern daily; increase bulk, water in diet if constipation develops

Teach patient/family:
• That patient compliance is needed since toxicity may result if doses are missed
• That risk factors should be decreased: high-fat diet, smoking, alcohol consumption, absence of exercise
• That birth control should be practiced while on this drug
• To report GU symptoms: decreased libido, impotence, dysuria, proteinuria, oliguria, hematuria

Lab test interferences:
Increase: Liver function studies, CPK, BSP, thymol turbidity

---

clomiphene citrate

(kloe'mi-feen)
Clomid, Serophene
Func. class.: Ovulation stimulant
Chem. class.: Nonsteroidal antiestrogenic

Action: Increases LH, FSH release from the pituitary, which increase maturation of ovarian follicle, ovulation, development of corpus luteum

Uses: Female infertility

Dosage and routes:
• *Adult:* PO 50-100 mg qd × 5 days or 50-100 mg qd beginning on day 5 of cycle; may be repeated until conception occurs or 3 cycles of therapy have been completed

Available forms include: Tabs 50 mg

Side effects/adverse reactions:
CV: Vasomotor flushing, phlebitis, deep vein thrombosis
EENT: Blurred vision, diplopia, photophobia
CNS: Headache, depression, restlessness, anxiety, nervousness, fatigue, insomnia, dizziness, flushing
GI: Nausea, vomiting, constipation, abdominal pain, bloating
INTEG: Rash, dermatitis, urticaria, alopecia
GU: Polyuria, frequency, birth defects, spontaneous abortions, multiple ovulation, breast pain, oliguria, abnormal uterine bleeding

Contraindications: Hypersensitivity, pregnancy (X), hepatic disease, undiagnosed vaginal bleeding

Precautions: Hypertension, depression, convulsions, diabetes mellitus

Pharmacokinetics: Metabolized in liver, excreted in feces

NURSING CONSIDERATIONS

Administer:
• After discontinuing estrogen therapy
• At same time qd to maintain drug level

Evaluate:
• Therapeutic response: fertility

Teach patient/family:
• That multiple births are common after drug is taken
• To notify physician if low abdominal pain occurs; may indicate ovarian cyst, cyst rupture
• If dose is missed, double at next time; if more than one dose is missed call physician
• That response usually occurs 4-10 days after last day of treatment
• Method for taking, recording basal body temperature to determine whether ovulation has occurred
• If ovulation can be determined (there is a slight decrease in temperature then a sharp increase for ovulation), to attempt coitus 3 days

before and qod until after ovulation
• If pregnancy is suspected, to notify physician immediately
Lab test interferences:
Increase: FSH/LH, BSP, thyroxine, TBG

clomipramine
(klom-ip′ra-meen)
Anafranil
Func. class.: Tricyclic antidepressant
Chem. class.: Tertiary amine

Action: Not known. Potent inhibitor of serotonin uptake, also increases dopamine metabolism
Uses: Depression, dysphoria, phobias, anxiety, agoraphobia, obsessive-compulsive disorder
Dosage and routes:
Obsessive-compulsive disorder
• *Adult:* PO 25 mg hs and increase gradually over 4 wk to a dose of 75-300 mg/day in divided doses
• *Child (10-18 yr):* PO 50 mg/day gradually increased; not to exceed 200 mg/day
Depression
• *Adult:* PO 50-150 mg/day in a single or divided dose
Anxiety/agoraphobia
• *Adult:* PO 25-75 mg/day
Available forms include: Caps 25, 50, 75 mg
Side effects/adverse reactions:
HEMA: ***Agranulocytosis, neutropenia, pancytopenia***
CV: Hypotension, tachycardia, ***cardiac arrest***
CNS: Dizziness, tremors, mania, ***seizures,*** aggressiveness
ENDO: Galactorrhea, hyperprolactinemia
META: Hyponatremia
GI: Constipation, dry mouth
GU: Delayed ejaculation, anorgasmy, retention
INTEG: Diaphoresis
Contraindications: Pregnancy, hypersensitivity
Precautions: Seizures, suicidal patients, elderly
Pharmacokinetics: Extensively bound to tissue and plasma proteins, demethylated in liver (active metabolites), excreted in urine (metabolites); half-life: 21 hr parent compound, 36 hr metabolite
Interactions/incompatibilities:
• Hypotensive antagonism: bethanidine
• Toxicity: phenothiazines, cimetidine
• Ethanol reaction: disulfiram, guanadrel increased or decreased effects
• Increased or decreased effects of clomipramine: estrogens
• Delirium: ethchlorvynol
• Hypertensive crisis, convulsions, hypertensive episode: MAOIs
• Decreased seizure threshold: phenytoin, phenobarbital

NURSING CONSIDERATIONS
Assess:
• B/P (lying, standing), pulse q4h; if systolic B/P drops 20 mm Hg withhold drug, notify physician; take vital signs q4h in patients with cardiovascular disease
• Blood studies: CBC, leukocytes, differential, cardiac enzymes if patient is receiving long-term therapy
• Hepatic studies: AST, ALT, bilirubin, creatinine
Administer:
• Increased fluids, bulk in diet if constipation, urinary retention occur, especially elderly
• With food or milk for GI symptoms
• Gum, hard candy, or frequent sips of water for dry mouth

Perform/provide:
• Storage in tight container at room temperature, do not freeze
• Assistance with ambulation during beginning therapy since drowsiness/dizziness occurs
• Safety measures, including siderails, primarily in elderly
• Checking to see PO medication swallowed
Evaluate:
• Therapeutic response: decreased anxiety, depression
• Mental status: mood, sensorium, affect, suicidal tendencies; increase in psychiatric symptoms: depression, panic
• Urinary retention, constipation; constipation is more likely to occur in children
• Withdrawal symptoms: headache, nausea, vomiting, muscle pain, weakness; do not usually occur unless drug is discontinued abruptly
• Alcohol consumption; if alcohol is consumed, withhold dose until morning
Teach patient/family:
• That the effects may take 2-3 wk
• To use caution in driving or other activities requiring alertness because of drowsiness, dizziness, blurred vision
• To avoid alcohol ingestion, other CNS depressants
• Not to discontinue medication quickly after long-term use, may cause nausea, headache, malaise
Lab test interferences:
Increase: Prolactin, TBG
Decrease: Serum thryoid hormone
Treatment of overdose: ECG monitoring, induce emesis, lavage, activated charcoal, administer anticonvulsant

clonazepam

(kloe-na'zi-pam)
Klonopin, Rivotril
Func. class.: Anticonvulsant
Chem. class.: Benzodiazapine derivative

Controlled Substance Schedule IV
Action: Inhibits spike, wave formation in absence seizures (petit mal), decreases amplitude, frequency, duration, spread of discharge in minor motor seizures
Uses: Absence, atypical absence, akinetic, myoclonic seizures
Dosage and routes:
• *Adult:* PO Not to exceed 1.5 mg/day in 3 divided doses; may be increased 0.5-1 mg q3 days until desired response, not to exceed 20 mg/day
• *Child <10 yr or 30 kg:* PO 0.01-0.03 mg/kg/day in divided doses q8h, not to exceed 0.05 mg/kg/day; may be increased 0.25-0.5 mg q3 days until desired response, not to exceed 0.1-0.2 mg/kg/day
Available forms include: Tabs 0.5, 1, 2 mg
Side effects/adverse reactions:
HEMA: ***Thrombocytopenia, leukocytosis, eosinophilia***
CNS: Drowsiness, dizziness, confusion, behavioral changes, tremors, insomnia, headache, suicidal tendencies, slurred speech
GI: Nausea, constipation, polyphagia, anorexia, xerostomia, diarrhea, gastritis, sore gums
INTEG: Rash, alopecia, hirsutism
EENT: Increased salivation, nystagmus, diplopia, abnormal eye movements
RESP: ***Respiratory depression,*** dyspnea, congestion

* Available in Canada only

CV: Palpitations, bradycardia
GU: Dysuria, enuresis, nocturia, retention
Contraindications: Hypersensitivity to benzodiazepines, acute narrow-angle glaucoma
Precautions: Open-angle glaucoma, chronic respiratory disease, pregnancy (C), renal, hepatic disease, elderly
Pharmacokinetics:
PO: Peak 1-2 hr, metabolized by liver, excreted in urine, half-life 18-50 hr
Interactions/incompatibilities:
• Increased CNS depression: alcohol, barbiturates, narcotics, antidepressants, other anticonvulsants
• Decreased effect of: carbamazepine
• Seizures: valproic acid

NURSING CONSIDERATIONS

Assess:
• Renal studies: urinalysis, BUN, urine creatinine
• Blood studies: RBC, Hct, Hgb, reticulocyte counts qwk for 4 wk then qmo
• Hepatic studies: ALT, AST, bilirubin, creatinine
• Drug levels during initial treatment
Administer:
• With food, milk to decrease GI symptoms
Perform/provide:
• Storage at room temperature
• Hard candy, frequent rinsing of mouth, gum for dry mouth
• Assistance with ambulation during early part of treatment; dizziness occurs, especially elderly
Evaluate:
• Therapeutic response: decreased seizure activity, document on patient's chart
• Mental status: mood, sensorium, affect, oversedation, behavioral changes; if mental status changes, notify physician
• Eye problems: need for ophthalmic examinations before, during, after treatment (slit lamp, fundoscopy, tonometry)
• Allergic reaction: red raised rash; if this occurs, drug should be discontinued
• Blood dyscrasias: fever, sore throat, bruising, rash, jaundice
• Toxicity: bone marrow depression, nausea, vomiting, ataxia, diplopia, cardiovascular collapse
Teach patient/family:
• To carry ID card to Medic-Alert bracelet stating drugs taken, condition, physician's name, phone number
• To avoid driving, other activities that require alertness
• To avoid alcohol ingestion or CNS depressants, increased sedation may occur
• Not to discontinue medication quickly after long-term use; taper off over several weeks
Lab test interferences:
Increase: AST, alk phosphatase
Treatment of overdose: Lavage, activated charcoal, monitor electrolytes, VS, administer vasopressors

---

clonidine HCl

(kloe'ni-deen)
Catapres, Dixarit*
Func. class.: Antihypertensive
Chem. class.: Central α-adrenergic agonist

Action: Inhibits sympathetic vasomotor center in CNS, which reduces impulses in sympathetic nervous system; blood pressure decreases, pulse rate, cardiac output decreases
Uses: Hypertension

Dosage and routes:
Hypertension
• *Adult:* PO/TRANS 0.1 mg bid, then increase by 0.1 mg/day or 0.2 mg/day until desired response; range 0.2-0.8 mg/day in divided doses
Available forms include: Tabs 0.1, 0.2, 0.3 mg; trans sys 2.5, 5, 7.5 mg delivering 0.1, 0.2, 0.3 mg/24 hr respectively
Side effects/adverse reactions:
CV: Orthostatic hypotension, palpitations, ***CHF,*** ECG abnormalities
CNS: Drowsiness, sedation, headache, fatigue, nightmares, insomnia, mental changes, anxiety, depression, hallucinations, delirium
GI: Nausea, vomiting, malaise, constipation, dry mouth
INTEG: Rash, alopecia, facial pallor, pruritus, hives, edema, burning papules, excoriation (transdermal patches)
EENT: Taste change, parotid pain
ENDO: Hyperglycemia
MS: Muscle/joint pain, leg cramps
GU: Impotence, dysuria, *nocturia,* gynecomastia
Contraindications: Hypersensitivity
Precautions: MI (recent), diabetes mellitus, chronic renal failure, Raynaud's disease, thyroid disease, depression, COPD, child <12 (patches), asthma, pregnancy (C), lactation, elderly
Pharmacokinetics:
PO: Peak 3-5 hr; half-life 12-16 hr, metabolized by liver (metabolites), excreted in urine (unchanged, inactive metabolites, feces), crosses blood-brain barrier, excreted in breast milk
Interactions/incompatibilities:
• Increased CNS depression: narcotics, sedatives, alcohol, anesthetics
• Decreased hypotensive effects: tricyclic antidepressants, MAOIs, appetite suppressants, other antihypertensives
• Increased hypotensive effects: diuretics
• Increased bradycardia: β-blockers, cardiac glycosides

NURSING CONSIDERATIONS

Assess:
• Blood studies: neutrophils, decreased platelets
• Renal studies: protein, BUN, creatinine; watch for increased levels that may indicate nephrotic syndrome
• Baselines in renal, liver function tests before therapy begins
• K levels, although hyperkalemia rarely occurs
• Dipstick of urine for protein qd in first morning specimen, if protein is increased, a 24 hr urinary protein should be collected
Administer:
• IV infusion of 0.9% NaCl (as ordered) to expand fluid volume if severe hypotension occurs
• SL if patient is unable to swallow
Perform/provide:
• Storage of patches in cool environment, tablets in tight containers
Evaluate:
• Therapeutic response: decrease in B/P in hypertension
• Edema in feet, legs daily
• Allergic reaction: rash, fever, pruritus, urticaria; drug should be discontinued if antihistamines fail to help
• Allergic reaction from patches: rash, urticaria, angioedema; should not continue to use
• Symptoms of CHF: edema, dyspnea, wet rales, B/P

• Renal symptoms: polyuria, oliguria, frequency
• For retinal degeneration: periodic eye exam

Teach patient/family:
• To avoid hazardous activities, may cause drowsiness
• To administer 1 hr before meals
• Not to discontinue drug abruptly or withdrawal symptoms may occur: anxiety, increased B/P, headache, insomnia, increased pulse, tremors, nausea, sweating
• Not to use OTC (cough, cold, or allergy) products unless directed by physician
• To avoid sunlight or wear sunscreen if in sunlight, photosensitivity may occur
• To comply with dosage schedule even if feeling better
• To rise slowly to sitting or standing position to minimize orthostatic hypotension, especially elderly
• To notify physician of mouth sores, sore throat, fever, swelling of hands or feet, irregular heartbeat, chest pain, signs of angioedema
• About excessive perspiration, dehydration, vomiting; diarrhea may lead to fall in blood pressure—consult physician if these occur
• That drug may cause dizziness, fainting; light-headedness may occur during 1st few days of therapy
• That drug may cause dry mouth; use hard candy, saliva product
• That compliance is necessary, not to skip or stop drug unless directed by physician
• That drug may cause skin rash or impaired perspiration
• That response may take 2-3 days to occur if drug is given transdermally

Lab test interferences:
Increase: Blood glucose
Decrease: VMA, catecholamines, aldosterone

Treatment of overdose: Supportive treatment, administer tolazdine, atropine, dopamine prn

C

---

clorazepate dipotassium

(klor-az'e-pate)
Tranxene
Func. class.: Antianxiety
Chem. class.: Benzodiazepine

Controlled Substance Schedule IV

Action: Depresses subcortical levels of CNS, including limbic system, reticular formation

Uses: Anxiety, acute alcohol withdrawal, adjunct in seizure disorders

Dosage and routes:

Anxiety
• *Adult:* PO 15-60 mg/day

Alcohol withdrawal
• *Adult:* PO 30 mg then 30-60 mg in divided doses; day 2, 45-90 mg in divided doses; day 3, 22.5-45 mg in divided doses; day 4, 15-30 mg in divided doses; then reduce daily dose to 7.5-15 mg

Seizure disorders
• *Adult and child >12 yr:* PO 7.5 mg tid, may increase by 7.5 mg/wk or less, not to exceed 90 mg/day
• *Child 9-12 yr:* PO 7.5 mg bid, may increase by 7.5 mg/wk or less, not to exceed 60 mg/day

Available forms include: Caps 3.75, 7.5, 15 mg; tabs 3.75, 7.5, 15 mg, single dose tab 11.25, 22.5 mg

Side effects/adverse reactions:
CNS: Dizziness, drowsiness, confusion, headache, anxiety, tremors, stimulation, fatigue, depression, insomnia, hallucinations
GI: Constipation, dry mouth, nausea, vomiting, anorexia, diarrhea

INTEG: Rash, dermatitis, itching
CV: Orthostatic hypotension, ***ECG changes, tachycardia,*** hypotension
EENT: Blurred vision, tinnitus, mydriasis

Contraindications: Hypersensitivity to benzodiazepines, narrow-angle glaucoma, psychosis, pregnancy (D), child <18 yr

Precautions: Elderly, debilitated, hepatic disease, renal disease

Pharmacokinetics:

PO: Onset 15 min, peak 1-2 hr, duration 4-6 hr, metabolized by liver, excreted by kidneys, crosses placenta, breast milk, half-life 30-100 hr

Interactions/incompatibilities:

- Decreased effects of clorazepate: valproic acid
- Increased effects of clorazepate: CNS depressants, alcohol, disulfiram, oral contraceptives, antidepressants, MAOIs

NURSING CONSIDERATIONS

Assess:

- B/P (lying, standing), pulse; if systolic B/P drops 20 mm Hg, hold drug, notify physician
- Blood studies: CBC during long-term therapy, blood dyscrasias have occurred rarely
- Hepatic studies: AST, ALT, bilirubin, creatinine, LDH, alk phosphatase
- I&O; may indicate renal dysfunction

Administer:

- With food or milk for GI symptoms
- Crushed if patient is unable to swallow medication whole
- Sugarless gum, hard candy, frequent sips of water for dry mouth

Perform/provide:

- Assistance with ambulation during beginning therapy, since drowsiness/dizziness occurs, especially elderly
- Safety measures, including siderails
- Check to see PO medication has been swallowed

Evaluate:

- Therapeutic response: decreased anxiety, restlessness, insomnia
- Mental status: mood, sensorium, affect, sleeping pattern, drowsiness, dizziness
- Physical dependency, withdrawal symptoms: headache, nausea, vomiting, muscle pain, weakness after long-term use
- Suicidal tendencies

Teach patient/family:

- That drug may be taken with food
- Not to be used for everyday stress or used longer than 4 mo, unless directed by physician; not to take more than prescribed amount, may be habit forming
- To avoid OTC preparations unless approved by physician
- To avoid driving, activities that require alertness; drowsiness may occur, especially elderly
- To avoid alcohol ingestion or other psychotropic medications, unless prescribed by physician
- Not to discontinue medication abruptly after long-term use
- To rise slowly or fainting may occur
- That drowsiness might worsen at beginning of treatment

Lab test interferences:

Increase: AST/ALT, serum bilirubin

Decrease: RAIU

False increase: 17-OHCS

Treatment of overdose: Lavage, VS, supportive care

---

clotrimazole

(kloe-trim'a-zole)

Canesten,* Gyne-Lotrimin, Mycelex, Mycelex-G

Func. class.: Local antiinfective
Chem. class.: Imidazole derivative

Action: Interferes with fungal DNA replication; binds sterols in fungal cell membrane, which increases permeability, leaking of cell nutrients; fungicidal

Uses: Tinea pedis, tinea cruris, tinea corporis, tinea versicolor, *Candida albicans* infection of the vagina, vulva, throat, mouth

Dosage and routes:

- *Adult and child:* TOP rub into affected area bid × 1-8 wk; LOZ dissolve in mouth 5×/day × 2 wk; INTRA VAG 1 applicator/1 tab × 1-2 wk hs, oral troches 10 mg 5×/day × 14 days

Available forms include: Cream, sol, lotion 1%; vag tabs 100, 500 mg; vag cream 1%, troches 10 mg

Side effects/adverse reactions:

INTEG: Rash, urticaria, stinging, burning, peeling, blistering

OTHER: Abdominal cramps, bloating, urinary frequency, dyspareunia

Contraindications: Hypersensitivity

Precautions: Pregnancy (B), lactation

NURSING CONSIDERATIONS

Administer:

- 1 applicator or 1 tablet intravaginally each night
- Enough medication to completely cover lesions
- After cleansing with soap, water before each application, dry well

Perform/provide:

- Storage at room temperature in dry place

Evaluate:

- Therapeutic response: decrease in size, number of lesions, decrease in itching or white patches around vulva
- Allergic reaction: burning, stinging, swelling, redness

Teach patient/family:

- To apply with glove to prevent further infection
- To avoid use of OTC creams, ointments, lotions unless directed by physician
- To use medical asepsis (hand washing) before, after each application
- To abstain from sexual intercourse during vaginal/vulvular treatment
- To use continuously even during menstrual period
- To report to physician if infection persists

cloxacillin sodium

(klox-a-sill'in)

Apo Cloxi,* Bactopen,* Cloxapen, Novocloxin,* Orbenin,* Tegopen

Func. class.: Broad-spectrum antibiotic
Chem. class.: Penicillinase-resistant penicillin

Action: Interferes with cell wall replication of susceptible organisms; the cell wall, rendered osmotically unstable, swells, bursts from osmotic pressure

Uses: Effective for gram-positive cocci *(S. aureus, S. pyogenes, E. pyogenes, S. pneumoniae)*

Dosage and routes:

- *Adult:* PO 1-4 g/day in divided doses q6h
- *Child:* PO 50-100 mg/kg in divided doses q6h

Available forms include: Caps 250,

500 mg; powder for oral susp 125 mg/5 ml

Side effects/adverse reactions:
HEMA: Anemia, increased bleeding time, ***bone marrow depression, granulocytopenia***
GI: Nausea, vomiting, diarrhea, increased AST, ALT, abdominal pain, glossitis, colitis
GU: Oliguria, proteinuria, hematuria, *vaginitis, moniliasis,* ***glomerulonephritis***
CNS: Lethargy, hallucinations, anxiety, depression, twitching, ***coma, convulsions***

Contraindications: Hypersensitivity to penicillins; neonates

Precautions: Pregnancy (B), hypersensitivity to cephalosporins

Pharmacokinetics:
PO: Peak 1 hr, duration 6 hr; half-life 30-60 min, metabolized in liver, excreted in urine, bile, breast milk, crosses placenta

Interactions/incompatibilities:
- Decreased antimicrobial effectiveness of cloxacillin: tetracyclines, erythromycins
- Increased cloxacillin concentrations: aspirin, probenecid

NURSING CONSIDERATIONS

Assess:
- I&O ratio; report hematuria, oliguria since penicillin in high doses is nephrotoxic
- Any patient with compromised renal system, since drug is excreted slowly in poor renal system function; toxicity may occur rapidly
- Liver studies: AST, ALT
- Blood studies: WBC, RBC, H&H, bleeding time
- Renal studies: urinalysis, protein, blood
- Culture, sensitivity before drug therapy; drug may be taken as soon as culture is taken

Administer:
- After C&S completed

Perform/provide:
- Adrenaline, suction, tracheostomy set, endotracheal intubation equipment on unit
- Adequate intake of fluids (2000 ml) during diarrhea episodes
- Scratch test to assess allergy after securing order from physician; usually done when penicillin is only drug of choice
- Storage in tight container; after reconstituting, store in refrigerator for 2 wk, room temperature 1 wk

Evaluate:
- Therapeutic response: absence of temperature, draining wounds
- Bowel pattern before, during treatment
- Skin eruptions after administration of penicillin to 1 wk after discontinuing drug
- Respiratory status: rate, character, wheezing, tightness in chest
- Allergies before initiation of treatment; reaction of each medication; place allergies on chart, Kardex in bright red

Teach patient/family:
- Aspects of drug therapy including need to complete entire course of medication to ensure organism death (10-14 days); culture may be taken after completed course of medication
- To report sore throat, fever, fatigue (could indicate superimposed infection)
- To wear or carry a Medic Alert ID if allergic to penicillins
- To notify nurse of diarrhea
- To take on an empty stomach with a full glass of water

Lab test interferences:
False positive: Urine glucose, urine protein
Decreased: Uric acid

* Available in Canada only

Treatment of overdose: Withdraw drug, maintain airway, administer epinephrine, aminophylline, O_2, IV corticosteroids for anaphylaxis

clozapine

(kloz-a′pin)

Clozaril

Func. class.: Antipsychotic

Chem. class.: Tricyclic dibenzodiazepine derivative

Action: Interferes with binding of dopamine at D_1 and D_2 receptors with lack of extrapyramidal symptoms, also acts as an adrenergic, cholinergic, histaminergic, serotonergic antagonist

Uses: Management of psychotic symptoms in schizophrenic patients for whom other antipsychotics have failed

Dosage and routes:

• *Adult:* PO 25 mg qd or bid, may increase by 25-50 mg/day, normal range 300-450 mg/day after 2 wk, do not increase dose more than 2 ×/wk, do not exceed 900 mg/day, use lowest dose to control symptoms

Available forms include: Tabs 25, 100 mg

Side effects/adverse reactions:

CNS: Sedation, salivation, dizziness, headache, tremors, sleep problems, akinesia, fever, ***seizures,*** *sweating, akathisia, confusion, fatigue, insomnia,* depression, slurred speech, anxiety

GI: Dry mouth, constipation, nausea, abdominal discomfort, vomiting, diarrhea, anorexia

MS: Weakness; pain in back, neck, legs; spasm

CV: Tachycardia, hypotension, hypertension, chest pain, ECG changes

GU: Urinary abnormalities, incontinence, ejaculation dysfunction, frequency, urgency, retention

RESP: Dyspnea, nasal congestion, throat discomfort

HEMA: ***Leukopenia, neutropenia, agranulocytosis, eosinophilia***

Contraindications: Hypersensitivity, myeloproliferative disorders, severe granulocytopenia, CNS depression, coma, narrow-angle glaucoma

Precautions: Pregnancy (B), lactation, children <16, hepatic, renal, cardiac disease, seizures, prostatic enlargement, elderly

Pharmacokinetics:

Steady state 2.5 hr, 95% protein bound, completely metabolized by the liver, excreted in urine and feces (metabolites), half-life 8-12 hr

Interactions/incompatibilities:

• Increased anticholinergic effects: anticholinergics

• Increased hypotension: antihypertensives

• Increased CNS depression: CNS drugs

• Increased bone marrow suppression: antineoplastics, other drugs suppressing bone marrow

• Increased plasma concentrations: warfarin, digoxin, other highly protein bound drugs

NURSING CONSIDERATIONS

Assess:

• Swallowing of PO medication; check for hoarding or giving of medication to other patients

• I&O ratio; obtain baseline before treatment begins; palpate bladder if low urinary output occurs

• Bilirubin, CBC, liver function studies monthly

• Urinalysis is recommended before, during prolonged therapy

Adminster:

• Antiparkinsonian agent, to be

used if extrapyramidal symptoms occur

Perform/provide:

• Decreased noise input by dimming lights, avoiding loud noises

• Supervised ambulation until stabilized on medication; do not involve in strenuous exercise program because fainting is possible; patient should not stand still for long periods of time

• Increased fluids to prevent constipation

• Sips of water, candy, gum for dry mouth

• Storage in tight, light-resistant container

Evaluate:

• Therapeutic response: decrease in emotional excitement, hallucinations, delusions, paranoia, reorganization of patterns of thought, speech

• Affect, orientation, LOC, reflexes, gait, coordination, sleep pattern disturbances

• B/P standing and lying; take pulse and respirations q4h during initial treatment; establish baseline before starting treatment; report drops of 30 mm Hg

• Dizziness, faintness, palpitations, tachycardia on rising

• EPS including akathisia (inability to sit still, no pattern to movements), tardive dyskinesia (bizarre movements of the jaw, mouth, tongue, extremities), pseudoparkinsonism (rigidity, tremors, pill rolling, shuffling gait)

• Skin turgor daily

• Constipation, urinary retention daily, if these occur, increase bulk, water in diet, especially elderly

Teach patient/family:

• That orthostatic hypotension occurs often, and to rise from sitting or lying position gradually

• To avoid hot tubs, hot showers, or tub baths since hypotension may occur

• To avoid abrupt withdrawal of this drug or EPS may result; drug should be withdrawn slowly

• To avoid OTC preparations (cough, hayfever, cold) unless approved by physician since serious drug interactions may occur; avoid use with alcohol or CNS depressants; increased drowsiness may occur

• Regarding compliance with drug regimen

• About EPS and necessity for meticulous oral hygiene since oral candidiasis may occur

• To report sore throat, malaise, fever, bleeding, mouth sores, if these occur, CBC should be drawn and drug discontinued

• In hot weather, heat stroke may occur; take extra precautions to stay cool

• To avoid driving or other hazardous activities; seizures may occur

• To notify physician if pregnant or if pregnancy is intended

Lab test interferences:

Increase: Liver function tests, cardiac enzymes, cholesterol, blood glucose, bilirubin, PBI, cholinesterase, ^{131}I

False positive: Pregnancy tests, PKU

False negative: Urinary steroids, 17-OHCS

Treatment of overdose: Lavage, activated charcoal, provide an airway; do not induce vomiting

---

* Available in Canada only

codeine sulfate/codeine phosphate

(koe'deen)

Func. class.: Narcotic analgesics
Chem. class.: Opiate, phenathrene derivative

Controlled Substance Schedule II
Action: Depresses pain impulse transmission at the spinal cord level by interacting with opioid receptors
Uses: Moderate to severe pain, nonproductive cough
Dosage and routes:
Pain
• *Adult:* PO 15-60 mg q4h prn; IM/SC 15-60 mg q4h prn
• *Child:* PO 3 mg/kg/day in divided doses q4h prn
Cough
• *Adult:* PO 10-20 mg q4-6h, not to exceed 120 mg/day
• *Child:* PO 1-1.5 mg/kg/day in 4 divided doses, not to exceed 60 mg/day
Available forms include: Inj IM, SC 15, 30, 60 mg/ml; tabs 15, 30, 60 mg
Side effects/adverse reactions:
CNS: Drowsiness, sedation, dizziness, agitation, dependency, lethargy, restlessness
GI: Nausea, vomiting, anorexia, constipation
RESP: ***Respiratory depression, respiratory paralysis***
CV: Bradycardia, palpitations, orthostatic hypotension, tachycardia
GU: Urinary retention
INTEG: Flushing, rash, urticaria
Contraindications: Hypersensitivity to opiates, respiratory depression, increased intracranial pressure, seizure disorders, severe respiratory disorders
Precautions: Elderly, cardiac dysrhythmias, pregnancy (C)
Pharmacokinetics: Onset 15-30 min, peak 1-2 hr, duration 4-6 hr; metabolized by liver, excreted by kidneys, crosses placenta, excreted in breast milk, half-life 2½-4 hr
Interactions/incompatibilities:
• Effects may be increased with other CNS depressants: alcohol, narcotics, sedative/hypnotics, antipsychotics, skeletal muscle relaxants

NURSING CONSIDERATIONS

Assess:
• I&O ratio; check for decreasing output; may indicate urinary retention, especially elderly
Administer:
• With antiemetic if nausea, vomiting occur
• With milk or food for GI symptoms
• When pain is beginning to return; determine dosage interval by patient response
Perform/provide:
• Storage in light-resistant container at room temperature
• Assistance with ambulation
• Safety measures: siderails, night light, call bell
Evaluate:
• Therapeutic response: decrease in pain, absence of grimacing or decreased cough
• Cough: type, duration, ability to raise secretion
• CNS changes, dizziness, drowsiness, hallucinations, euphoria, LOC, pupil reaction
• Allergic reactions: rash, urticaria
• Respiratory dysfunction: respiratory depression, character, rate rhythm; notify physician if respirations are <10/min
• Need for pain medication, physical dependence
Teach patient/family:
• To report any symptoms of CNS changes, allergic reactions

• That physical dependency may result when used for extended periods of time
• To change position slowly, orthostatic hypotension may occur
• To avoid hazardous activities if drowsiness or dizziness occurs
• To avoid alcohol unless directed by physician

colchicine

(kol'chi-seen)
Colsalide, Novocolchine
Func. class.: Antigout agent
Chem. class.: Colchicum autumnale alkaloid

Action: Inhibits microtubule formation of lactic acid in leukocytes, which decreases phagocytosis and inflammation in joints
Uses: Gout, gouty arthritis (prevention, treatment) to arrest progression of neurologic disability in multiple sclerosis
Dosage and routes:
Prevention
• *Adult:* PO 0.5-1.8 mg qd depending on severity; IV 0.5-1 mg 1-2 × day
Treatment
• *Adult:* PO 0.5-1.2 mg, then 0.5-1.2 mg q1h, until pain decreases or side effects occur; IV 2 mg, 0.5 mg q6h, not to exceed 4 mg/24 hr
Available forms include: Tabs 0.5, 0.6 mg; inj IV 1 mg/2 ml
Side effects/adverse reactions:
MISC: Myopathy, alopecia, reversible azoospermia, peripheral neuritis
GU: Hematuria, oliguria, renal damage
HEMA: ***Agranulocytosis, thrombocytopenia, aplastic anemia, pancytopenia***
GI: Nausea, vomiting, anorexia, malaise, metallic taste, cramps, peptic ulcer, diarrhea
INTEG: Chills, dermatitis, pruritus, purpura, erythema
Contraindications: Hypersensitivity, serious GI, renal, hepatic, cardiac disorders; blood dyscrasias
Precautions: Severe renal disease, blood dyscrasias, pregnancy (C), hepatic disease, elderly, lactation, children
Pharmacokinetics:
PO: Peak ½-2 hr, half-life 20 min, deacetylates in liver, excreted in feces (metabolites/active drug)
Interactions/incompatibilities:
• Decreased action of colchicine: acidifying agents
• Decreased action of: vitamin B_{12}
• Increased action of: CNS depressants, sympathomimetics
• Increased action of colchicine: alkalinizers

NURSING CONSIDERATIONS

Assess:
• I&O ratio; observe for decrease in urinary output
• CBC, platelets, reticulocytes before, during therapy (q3mo)
• Coombs' test to determine Coombs' negative hemolytic anemia
Administer:
• IV undiluted or diluted 1 mg/10-20 ml normal saline or sterile H_2O for inj; give over 2-5 min
• On empty stomach only, to facilitate absorption
Evaluate:
• Therapeutic response: decreased stone formation on x-ray, decreased pain in kidney region, absence of hematuria, decreased pain in joints
Teach patient/family:
• To increase fluids to 3-4 L/day
• To avoid alcohol, OTC preparations that contain alcohol; skin rashes have occurred

• To report any pain, redness, or hard area usually in legs
• Importance of complying with medical regimen; bone marrow depression may occur

Lab test interferences:
Increase: Alk phosphatase, AST/ ALT
False positive: RBC, Hgb

colestipol HCl

(koe-les'ti-pole)
Colestid
Func. class.: Antilipemic
Chem. class.: Bile sequestrant, resin exchange agent

Action: Absorbs, combines with bile acids to form insoluble complex that is excreted through feces; loss of bile acids lowers cholesterol levels

Uses: Primary hypercholesterolemia, xanthomas, digitalis toxicity, pruritus due to biliary obstruction, diarrhea due to bile acids

Dosage and routes:
• *Adult:* PO 15-30 g/day in 2-4 divided doses

Available forms include: Granules

Side effects/adverse reactions:
GI: Constipation, abdominal pain, nausea, fecal impaction, hemorrhoids, flatulence, vomiting, steatorrhea, peptic ulcer
INTEG: *Rash,* irritation of perianal area, tongue, skin
HEMA: *Decreased vitamins A, D, K,* red folate content ***hyperchloremic acidosis,*** bleeding, decreased pro-time

Contraindications: Hypersensitivity, biliary obstruction

Precautions: Pregnancy (B), lactation, children, bleeding disorders

Pharmacokinetics:
PO: Excreted in feces

Interactions/incompatibilities:
• May reduce action of: thiazide, digitalis, warfarin, penicillin G, folic acid, phenylbutazone, tetracycline, corticosteroids, iron, thyroid agents, clindamycin, trimethoprim, chenodiol, fat-soluble vitamins, cephalexin, phenobarbital

NURSING CONSIDERATIONS

Assess:
• Cardiac glycoside levels, if both drugs are being administered
• For signs of vitamins A, D, K deficiency
• Serum cholesterol, triglyceride levels, electrolytes if on extended therapy

Administer:
• Drug ac, hs; give all other medications 1 hr before colestipol or 4 hr after colestipol to avoid poor absorption
• Drug mixed in applesauce or stirred into beverage (2-6 oz), do not take dry; let stand for 2 min
• Supplemental doses of vitamins A, D, K if levels are low

Evaluate:
• Therapeutic response: decreased triglycerides, diarrhea, pruritus (excess bile area)
• Bowel pattern daily; increase bulk, water in diet if constipation develops

Teach patient/family:
• Symptoms of hypothrombinemia: bleeding mucous membranes, dark tarry stools, hematuria, petechiae; report immediately
• That patient compliance is needed since toxicity may result if doses are missed
• That risk factors should be decreased: high fat diet, smoking, alcohol consumption, absence of exercise

Lab test interferences:
Increase: Liver function studies, chloride, PO_4

colfosceril palmitate

(kohl-foss'sir-ill)

Exosurf Neonatal

Func. class.: Synthetic lung surfactant

Chem. class.: dipalmitoylphosphatidylcholine (DPPC)

Action: Surfactant maintains lung inflation and prevents collapse by lowering surface tension

Uses: Treatment of respiratory distress syndrome (RDS) in premature infants

Dosage and routes:

Prophylactic treatment

Endotracheally: 5 ml/kg as soon as possible after birth and repeat doses 12 and 24 hr later to infants remaining on mechanical ventilation

Rescue treatment

Endotracheally: administer in two 5 ml/kg doses; give initial dose after treatment of RDS, then second dose in 12 hr

Available forms include: 10 ml/vial with sterile H_2O for inj and 5 endotracheal tube adapters

Side effects/adverse reactions:

RESP: ***Apnea, pulmonary hemorrhage, pulmonary air leak, congenital pneumonia***

SYST: ***Nonpulmonary fatal infections***

Precautions: Congenital anomalies, prophylactic treatment

Pharmacokinetics: Distributed to all lobes, alveolar spaces, distal airways; alveolar half-life 12 hr; 90% of alveolar phospholipids are recycled

NURSING CONSIDERATIONS

Assess:

- Respiratory rate, rhythm, character, chest expansion, color, transcutaneous saturation, ABGs
- Endotracheal tube placement before dosing
- For apnea after endotracheal administration
- Reflux of drug into the endotracheal tube during administration; stop drug administration if this occurs, and, if needed, increase peak inspiratory pressure on the ventilator by 4-5 cm H_2O until tube is cleared

Administer:

- Infants should be suctioned before administration
- After selecting an adapter size that corresponds to the diameter of the endotracheal tube, insert the adapter into the tube by twisting, connect the breathing circuit to the adapter, remove the cap from the adapter sideport, and attach the syringe to the sideport; after dose is completed, remove the syringe and recap the sideport
- After reconstituting each vial with 8 ml preservative-free sterile water for injection, fill a 10-12 ml syringe with 8 ml preservative-free sterile water for injection, using an 18-19 gauge needle; allow the vacuum in the vial to draw the liquid into the vial; aspirate the 8 ml out of the vial into the syringe while maintaining the vacuum and then release the syringe plunger; repeat the aspiration and release until adequately mixed; draw the dose required into the syringe from below the froth in the vial; do not use if large particles are present
- By endotracheal administration only by persons trained in neonatal intubation and ventilation

Perform/provide:

- Reduction in peak ventilator inspiratory pressures immediately if chest expansion improves substantially after dose

* Available in Canada only

• Reduction in FiO_2 in small, repeated steps when infant becomes pink and transcutaneous oxygen saturation is in excess of 95%; oxygen saturation should remain between 90% and 95%
• Suctioning of all infants before administration to prevent mucus plugging; if endotracheal tube obstruction is suspected, remove the obstruction and replace tube immediately
• Storage at room temperature in dry place

Evaluate:
• Therapeutic response: decreased respiratory distress

---

corticotropin (ACTH)

(kor-ti-koe-troe'pin)

ACTHAR, Cortigel-40, Cortigel-80, Cortrophin Gel, Cotropic-Gel-40, Cotropic-Gel-80, Cortrophin Zinc, Duracton,* H.P. Acthar Gel

Func. class.: Pituitary hormone
Chem. class.: Adrenocorticotropic hormone

Action: Stimulates adrenal cortex to produce, secrete corticosterone, cortisol

Uses: Testing adrenocortical function, treatment of adrenal insufficiency caused by administration of corticosteroids (long term), multiple sclerosis

Dosage and routes:

Testing of adrenocortical function
• *Adult:* IM/SC up to 80 units in divided doses; IV 10-25 units in 500 ml D_5W given over 8 hr

Inflammation
• *Adult:* SC/IM 40 units in 4 divided doses (aqueous) or 40 units q12-24h (gel/repository form)

Available forms include: Inj IM, IV, SC 25, 40 U/vial, repository inj IM, SC 40, 80/ml

Side effects/adverse reactions:

INTEG: Impaired wound healing, rash, urticaria, hirsutism, petechiae, ecchymoses, sweating, acne, hyperpigmentation

CNS: ***Convulsions,*** dizziness, euphoria, insomnia, headache, mood swings, behavioral changes, depression, psychosis

GI: Nausea, vomiting, ***peptic ulcer perforation,*** pancreatitis, distention, ulcerative esophagitis

GU: Water, sodium retention, hypokalemia

EENT: Cataracts, glaucoma

MS: Weakness, osteoporosis, compression fractures, muscle atrophy, steroid myopathy, myalgia, arthralgia

ENDO: Cushingoid symptoms, diabetes mellitus, antibody formation, growth retardation in children, menstrual irregularities

Contraindications: Hypersensitivity, scleroderma, osteoporosis, CHF, peptic ulcer disease, hypertension, systemic fungal infections, smallpox vaccination, recent surgery, ocular herpes simplex, primary adrenocortical insufficiency/hyperfunction

Precautions: Pregnancy (C), lactation, latent TB, hepatic disease, hypothyroiditis, child bearing-age women, psychiatric diagnosis, myasthenia gravis, acute gouty arthritis

Pharmacokinetics:

IV/IM/SC: Onset $<$6 hr, duration 2-4 hr, repository duration up to 3 days, half-life $<$20 min, excreted in urine

Interactions/incompatibilities:
• Possible ulceration: salicylates, alcohol, corticosteroids

• Hypokalemia: diuretics (K-depleting), amphotericin B
• Hyperglycemia: insulin, or oral hypoglycemic agents

NURSING CONSIDERATIONS

Assess:
• Baseline ECG, B/P, chest x-ray, GTT
• Pulse, B/P
• I&O ratio; weight qwk, report gain over 5 lb/wk
• 2 hr postprandial, chest x-ray, serum potassium, 17 KS, 17-OHCS, cortisol, during long-term treatment

Administer:
• Test for hypersensitivity for individuals allergic to pork products
• Decreased sodium, increase potassium for dependent edema
• Increase protein diet for nitrogen loss
• Gel at room temperature, give deep IM using 21G needle
• May be used to treat edema
• IV; give over 2 min; dilute 25 U/1 ml sterile H_2O or normal saline or 40 U/2 ml; may dilute 10-25 U/500 ml compatible sol; give over 8 hr

Perform/provide:
• Storage in refrigerator of unused portion; use within 24 hr

Evaluate:
• Therapeutic response: absence of inflammation, pain, increased muscle strength in myasthenia gravis
• Dependent edema, moon face, pulmonary edema, cerebral edema
• Infection; drug may mask infections
• Increased stress in patient's life that may require increased corticosteroids
• Mental status: affect, mood, increased aggressiveness, irritability; a change in mental status may require decreased steroids
• Growth rate of child
• Hypoadrenalism in neonates if drug was given during pregnancy
• Allergic reaction: rash, urticaria, fever, nausea, vomiting, dyspnea; drug should be discontinued immediately, administer epinephrine 1:1000

Teach patient/family:
• To avoid vaccinations during drug treatment
• To maintain adequate hydration up to 2000 ml/day unless contraindicated
• To avoid OTC products: salicylates, products with alcohol
• Not to discontinue medication abruptly, thyroid crisis may occur; drug should be tapered off over several wk
• To wear Medic Alert ID specifying steroid therapy
• That drug does not cure condition, only decreases symptoms
• To notify physician of infection: increased temperature, sore throat, muscular pain
• To tell patient to notify anyone involved in medical or dental care that this drug is being taken

---

cortisone acetate

(kor′-ti-sone)

Cortone

Func. class.: Corticosteroid, synthetic

Chem. class.: Glucocorticoid, short-acting

Action: Decreases inflammation by suppression of migration of polymorphonuclear leukocytes, fibroblasts, reversal of increased capillary permeability and lysosomal stabilization

Uses: Inflammation, severe allergy, adrenal insufficiency, collagen dis-

* Available in Canada only

orders, respiratory, dermatologic disorders

Dosage and routes:

• *Adult:* PO 25-300 mg qd or q2 days, titrated to patient response

Available forms include: Tabs 5, 10, 25 mg

Side effects/adverse reactions:

INTEG: Acne, poor wound healing, ecchymosis, bruising, petechiae

CNS: Depression, flushing, sweating, headache, mood changes

CV: Hypertension, ***circulatory collapse, thrombophlebitis, embolism,*** tachycardia, ***necrotizing angiitis, CHF,*** edema

HEMA: ***Thrombocytopenia***

MS: Fractures, osteoporosis, weakness

GI: Diarrhea, nausea, abdominal distention, ***GI hemorrhage,*** increased appetite, ***pancreatitis***

EENT: Fungal infections, increased intraocular pressure, blurred vision

Contraindications: Psychosis, hypersensitivity, idiopathic thrombocytopenia, acute glomerulonephritis, amebiasis, fungal infections, nonasthmatic bronchial disease, child <2 yr, AIDS, TB

Precautions: Pregnancy (C), diabetes mellitus, glaucoma, osteoporosis, seizure disorders, ulcerative colitis, CHF, myasthenia gravis, renal disease, esophagitis, peptic ulcer

Pharmacokinetics:

PO: Peak 2 hr, duration 1½ days

IM: Peak 20-48 hr, duration 1½ days

Interactions/incompatibilities:

• Decreased action of cortisone: cholestyramine, colestipol, barbiturates, rifampin, ephedrine, phenytoin, theophylline

• Decreased effects of: anticoagulants, anticonvulsants, antidiabetics, ambenonium, neostigmine, isoniazid, toxoids, vaccines, anticholinesterases, salicylates, somatrem

• Increased side effects: alcohol, salicylates, indomethacin, amphotericin B, digitalis, cyclosporine, diuretics

• Increased action of cortisone: salicylates, estrogens, indomethacin, oral contraceptives, ketoconazole, macrolide antibiotics

NURSING CONSIDERATIONS

Assess:

• Potassium, blood sugar, urine glucose while on long-term therapy; hypokalemia and hyperglycemia

• Weight daily, notify physician of weekly gain >5 lb

• B/P q4h, pulse, notify physician if chest pain occurs

• I&O ratio; be alert for decreasing urinary output and increasing edema

• Plasma cortisol levels during long-term therapy (normal level: 138-635 nmol/L SI units if drawn at 8 AM)

Administer:

• After shaking suspension (parenteral)

• Titrated dose, use lowest effective dose

• IM inj deeply in large mass, rotate sites, avoid deltoid, use a 21G needle

• In one dose in AM to prevent adrenal suppression, avoid SC administration, damage may be done to tissue

• With food or milk to decrease GI symptoms

Perform/provide:

• Assistance with ambulation in patient with bone tissue disease to prevent fractures

Evaluate:

• Therapeutic response: ease of res-

pirations, decreased inflammation
• Infection: increased temperature, WBC even after withdrawal of medication; drug masks symptoms of infection
• Potassium depletion: paresthesias, fatigue, nausea, vomiting, depression, polyuria, dysrhythmias, weakness
• Edema, hypertension, cardiac symptoms
• Mental status: affect, mood, behavioral changes, aggression

Teach patient/family:
• That ID as steroid user should be carried at all times
• To notify physician if therapeutic response decreases; dosage adjustment may be needed
• Not to discontinue this medication abruptly or adrenal crisis can result
• To avoid OTC products: salicylates, alcohol in cough products, cold preparations unless directed by physician
• All aspects of drug usage, including cushingoid symptoms
• Symptoms of adrenal insufficiency: nausea, anorexia, fatigue, dizziness, dyspnea, weakness, joint pain

Lab test interferences:
Increase: Cholesterol, sodium, blood glucose, uric acid, calcium, urine glucose
Decrease: Calcium, potassium, T_4, T_3, thyroid ^{131}I uptake test, urine 17-OHCS, 17-KS, PBI
False negative: Skin allergy tests

---

cosyntropin

(koe-sin-troe'pin)
Cortrosyn, Synacthen Depot*
Func. class.: Pituitary hormone
Chem. class.: Synthetic polypeptide

Action: Stimulates adrenal cortex to produce, secrete corticosterone, cortisol
Uses: Testing adrenocortical function
Dosage and routes:
• *Adult and child >2 yr:* IM/IV 0.25-1 mg between blood sampling
• *Child <2 yr:* IM/IV 0.125 mg
Available forms include: Inj IM, IV 0.25 mg/vial
Side effects/adverse reactions:
INTEG: Rash urticaria, pruritus, flushing
Contraindications: Hypersensitivity
Precautions: Pregnancy (C)
Pharmacokinetics:
IV/IM: Onset 5 min, peak 1 hr, duration 2-4 hr

NURSING CONSIDERATIONS

Assess:
• Plasma cortisol levels at ½-1 hr after drug administered (>5 μg/dl is normal), at end of 1 hr, levels should have doubled

Administer:
• After reconstitution with 1 ml 0.9% NaCl/0.25 mg; may be further diluted in D_5 or normal saline; run 40 mg/hr over 6 hr

Perform/provide:
• Storage at room temperature for 24 hr or refrigerated for 3 wk

---

co-trimoxazole (sulfamethoxazole and trimethoprim)

(koe-trye-mox'a-zole)
Apo-Sulfatrim,* Bactrim, Cotrim, Comoxol, Septra, Sulfatrim, Bethaprim
Func. class.: Antibiotic
Chem. class.: Miscellaneous sulfonamide

Action: Sulfamethoxazole inter-

* Available in Canada only

feres with bacterial biosynthesis of proteins by competitive antagonism of PABA when adequate levels are maintained; trimethoprim blocks synthesis of tetrahydrofolic acid; this combination blocks 2 consecutive steps in bacterial synthesis of essential nucleic acids, protein

Uses: Urinary tract infections, otitis media, acute and chronic prostatitis, shigellosis, *Pneumocystis carinii* pneumonitis, chronic bronchitis, chancroid

Dosage and routes:

Urinary tract infections

- *Adult:* PO 160 mg TMP/800 mg SMZ q12h × 10-14 days
- *Child:* PO 8 mg/kg TMP/40 mg/kg SMZ qd in 2 divided doses q12h

Otitis media

- *Child:* PO 8 mg/kg TMP/40 mg/kg SMZ qd in 2 divided doses q12h × 10 days

Chronic bronchitis

- *Adult:* PO 160 mg TMP/800 mg SMZ q12h × 14 days

Pneumocystis carinii pneumonitis

- *Adult and child:* PO 20 mg/kg TMP/100 mg/kg SMZ qd in 4 divided doses q6h × 14 days; IV 15-20 mg/kg/day (based on TMP) in 3-4 divided doses for up to 14 days
- Dosage reduction necessary in moderate to severe renal impairment (CrCL < 30 ml/min)

Available forms include: Tabs 80 mg trimethoprim (TMP)/400 mg sulfamethoxazole (SMZ), 160 mg trimethoprim/800 mg sulfamethoxazole; susp 40 mg/200 mg/5 ml; IV inj 16 mg/80 mg/ml

Side effects/adverse reactions:

SYST: ***Anaphylaxis, SLE***

RESP: Cough, shortness of breath

GI: Nausea, vomiting, abdominal pain, stomatitis, ***hepatitis,*** glossitis, pancreatitis, diarrhea, ***enterocolitis***, anorexia

CNS: Headache, insomnia, hallucinations, depression, vertigo, fatigue, anxiety, convulsions, drug fever, chills, aseptic meningitis

HEMA: ***Leukopenia, neutropenia, thrombocytopenia, agranulocytosis, hemolytic anemia, hypoprothrombinemia, Henoch-Schönlein purpura, methemoglobinemia, eosinophilia***

INTEG: Rash, dermatitis, urticaria, ***Stevens-Johnson syndrome,*** erythema, photosensitivity, pain, inflammation at injection site

GU: ***Renal failure, toxic nephrosis,*** increased BUN, creatinine, crystalluria

CV: ***Allergic myocarditis***

Contraindications: Hypersensitivity to trimethoprim or sulfonamides, pregnancy at term, megaloblastic anemia, infants <2 mo, CrCl <15 ml/min, lactation

Precautions: Pregnancy (C), renal disease, elderly, G-6-PD deficiency, impaired hepatic function, possible folate deficiency, severe allergy, bronchial asthma

Pharmacokinetics:

PO: Rapidly absorbed, peak 1-4 hr; half-life 8-13 hr, excreted in urine (metabolites and unchanged), breast milk, crosses placenta, highly bound to plasma proteins; TMP achieves high levels in prostatic tissue and fluid

Interactions/incompatibilities:

- Increased hypoglycemic response: sulfonylurea agents
- Increased anticoagulant effects: oral anticoagulants
- Decreased hepatic clearance of: phenytoin
- Increased nephrotoxicity: cyclosporine
- Increased bone marrow depressant effects: methotrexate

NURSING CONSIDERATIONS

Assess:

• I&O ratio; note color, character, pH of urine if drug administered for urinary tract infections; output should be 800 ml less than intake; if urine is highly acidic, alkalization may be needed

• Kidney function studies: BUN, creatinine, urinalysis if on long-term therapy

Administer:

• With full glass of water to maintain adequate hydration; increase fluids to 2000 ml/day to decrease crystallization in kidneys

• Medication after C&S; repeat C&S after full course of medication completed

• After diluting 5 ml of drug/125 ml D_5W, run over 1-1½ hr

• With resuscitative equipment available; severe allergic reactions may occur

Perform/provide:

• Storage in tight, light-resistant containers at room temperature

Evaluate:

• Therapeutic response: absence of pain, fever, C&S negative

• Blood dyscrasias: skin rash, fever, sore throat, bruising, bleeding, fatigue, joint pain

• Allergic reaction: rash, dermatitis, urticaria, pruritus, dyspnea, bronchospasm

Teach patient/family:

• To take each oral dose with full glass of water to prevent crystalluria

• To complete full course of treatment to prevent superimposed infection

• To avoid sunlight or use sunscreen to prevent burns

• To avoid OTC medications (aspirin, vitamin C) unless directed by physician

• To use alternative contraceptive measures; decreased effectiveness of oral contraceptives may result

• To notify physician if skin rash, sore throat, fever, mouth sores, unusual bruising, bleeding occur

Lab test interferences:

Increase: Alk phosphatase, creatinine, bilirubin

False positive: Urinary glucose test

---

cromolyn sodium

(kroe'moe-lin)

Opticrom 4%

Func. class.: Ophthalmic

Chem. class.: Mast cell stabilizer

Action: Inhibits degranulation of mast cells after contact with antigens, which decreases release of histamine and SRS-A from mast cell

Uses: Vernal keratoconjunctivitis, conjunctivitis, vernal keratitis, allergic keratoconjunctivitis

Dosage and routes:

• *Adult:* INSTILL 1-2 gtts in both eyes q4-6h

Available forms include: Sol 40 mg/ml

Side effects/adverse reactions:

EENT: Stinging, burning, itching, lacrimation, puffiness

Contraindications: Hypersensitivity

Precautions: Pregnancy (B), lactation, children <4 yrs

NURSING CONSIDERATIONS

Perform/provide:

• Refrigeration; keep out of direct sunlight; discard unused portions after 4 wk

Evaluate:

• Therapeutic response: signs and symptoms will disappear in days but treatment may be required for 6 wk

---

Teach patient/family:
• To report stinging, burning, itching, lacrimation, puffiness
• Method of instillation, including pressure on lacrimal sac for 1 min, and not to touch dropper to eye
• Not to wear soft contact lens, use may be reinstituted 4-6 hr after therapy is discontinued

cromolyn sodium (disodium cromoglycate)

(kroe'moe-lin)

Intal, Intal p,* Nasalcrom, Rynacrom,* Gastrocrom

Func. class.: Antiasthmatic
Chem. class.: Mast cell stabilizer

Action: Stabilizes the membrane of the sensitized mast cell preventing release of chemical mediators after an antigen-IgE interaction

Uses: Allergic rhinitis, severe perennial bronchial asthma, exercise-induced bronchospasm (prevention), prevention of acute bronchospasm induced by environmental pollutants, mastocytosis

Dosage and routes:

Allergic rhinitis
• *Adult and child >6 yr:* nasal sol 1 spray in each nostril tid-qid, not to exceed 6 doses/day

Bronchospasm
• *Adult and child >5 yr:* INH 20 mg <1 hr before exercise

Bronchial asthma
• *Adult and child >5 yr:* INH 20 mg qid; NEB 20 mg qid by nebulization

Available forms include: Sol 40 mg/ml; inh, caps for inh, 20 mg; oral caps 100 mg, neb sol 20 mg, aerosol 800 μg/actuation

Side effects/adverse reactions:
EENT: Throat irritation, cough, nasal congestion, burning eyes
CNS: *Headache, dizziness,* neuritis
GU: Frequency, dysuria
GI: Nausea, vomiting, anorexia, dry mouth, bitter taste
INTEG: Rash, urticaria, angioedema
MS: Joint pain/swelling

Contraindications: Hypersensitivity to this drug or lactose, status asthmaticus

Precautions: Pregnancy (B), lactation, renal disease, hepatic disease, child <5 yr

Pharmacokinetics:
INH: Peak 15 min, duration 4-6 hr, excreted unchanged in feces, half-life 80 min

NURSING CONSIDERATIONS

Assess:
• Eosinophil count during treatment

Administer:
• By inhalation/nebulizer only
• Gargle, sip of water to decrease irritation in throat

Evaluate:
• Therapeutic response: decrease in asthmatic symptoms, congested, runny nose
• Respiratory status: respiratory rate, rhythm, characteristics, cough, wheezing, dyspnea

Teach patient/family:
• To clear mucus before using
• Proper inhalation technique: exhale, using inhaler, inhale deeply with head tipped back to open airway, remove, hold breath, exhale, repeat until all of drug is inhaled
• That therapeutic effect may take up to 4 wk
• Not to swallow capsule
• That drug is preventative only, not restorative

crotamiton

(kroe-tam'i-tonn)
Eurax
Func. class.: Scabicide
Chem. class.: Synthetic chloroformate salt

Action: Unknown, toxic to *Sarcoptes scabiei*
Uses: Scabies, pruritus
Dosage and routes:
Scabies
• *Adult and child:* CREAM wash area with soap, water; remove visible crusts, apply cream, apply another coat in 24 hr, remove with soap, water in 48 hr; for pruritus, massage into affected area, repeat as necessary
Available forms include: Cream 10%; lotion 10%
Side effects/adverse reactions:
INTEG: Itching, rash, irritation, contact dermatitis
Contraindications: Hypersensitivity, inflammation of skin, abrasions, or breaks in skin, mucous membranes
Precautions: Children, pregnancy (C)

NURSING CONSIDERATIONS
Administer:
• After patient bathes with soap, water; remove all crusts
• From chin down, do not apply to face, lips, mouth, eyes, any mucous membrane, anus, or meatus
• Topical corticosteroids as ordered to decrease contact dermatitis
• Lotions of menthol or phenol to control itching
• Topical antibiotics for infection
Perform/provide:
• Storage in tight, light-resistant container
• Isolation until areas on skin, scalp have cleared; treatment is completed
Evaluate:
• Therapeutic response: decreased itching after several wk, decreased redness
• Area of body involved, including crusts, brownish trails on skin, itching papules in skin folds
Teach patient/family:
• To change clothing and bed linen the morning after treatment
• To shake well before using
• To wash all inhabitants' clothing, using hot water, dried in hot dryers for >20 min; preventive treatment may be required of all persons living in same house to decrease spread of infection
• That itching may continue for 4-6 wk
• That drug must be reapplied if accidentally washed off or treatment will be ineffective
• To avoid contact with eyes, face, meatus or mucous membranes or irritation may occur
• To discontinue use and notify physician if irritation or sensitization occurs

cyanocobalamin (vitamin B_{12})/hydroxocobalamin (vitamin $B_{12}a$)

(sye-an-oh-koe-bal'a-min)
Anacobin,* Bedoce, Bedoz,* Berubigen, Betalin-12, Crystimin, Cyanabin,* Kaybovit, Pernavite, Poyamin, Rubesol, Rubion,* Rubramin, Sigamine/Alpha Rediso, Alpha-Ruvite, Codroxomin, Droxomin, Neo-Betalin 12, Rubesol-LA, Vibedoz
Func. class.: Vitamin B_{12}, water-soluble vitamin

Action: Needed for adequate nerve

* Available in Canada only

functioning, protein and carbohydrate metabolism, normal growth, RBC development and cell reproduction

Uses: Vitamin B_{12} deficiency, pernicious anemia, vitamin B_{12} malabsorption syndrome, Schilling test, increased requirements with pregnancy thyrotoxicosis, hemolytic anemia, hemorrhage, renal and hepatic disease

Dosage and routes:

• *Adult:* PO 25 μg qd × 5-10 days, maintenance 100-200 mg IM q mo; IM/SC 30-100 μg qd × 5-10 days, maintenance 100-200 μg IM qmo

• *Child:* PO 1 μg qd × 5-10 days, maintenance 60 μg IM qmo or more; IM/SC 1-30 μg qd × 5-10 days, maintenance 60 μg IM qmo or more

Pernicious anemia/malabsorption syndrome

• *Adult:* IM 100-1000 μg qd × 2 wk, then 100-1000 μg IM qmo

• *Child:* IM 100-500 μg over 2 wk or more given in 100-500 μg doses, then 60 μg IM/SC monthly

Schilling test

• *Adult and child:* IM 1000 μg in one dose

Available forms include: Tabs 25, 50, 100, 250, 500, 1000 μg; inj IM 100, 120, 1000 μg/ml

Side effects/adverse reactions:

CNS: Flushing, optic nerve atrophy

GI: Diarrhea

CV: ***CHF,*** peripheral vascular thrombosis, ***pulmonary edema***

INTEG: Itching, rash, pain at site

META: Hypokalemia

Contraindications: Hypersensitivity, optic nerve atrophy

Precautions: Pregnancy (A), lactation, children

Pharmacokinetics: Stored in liver, kidneys, stomach; 50%-90% excreted in urine; crosses placenta, breast milk

Interactions/incompatibilities:

• Decreased absorption: aminoglycosides, anticonvulsants, colchicine, chloramphenicol, aminosalicylic acid, potassium preparation, cimetidine

• Increased absorption: prednisone

NURSING CONSIDERATIONS

Assess:

• GI function: diarrhea, constipation

• Potassium levels during beginning treatment

• CBC for increase in reticulocyte count during 1st week of therapy, then increase in RBC and hemoglobin

Administer:

• With fruit juice to disguise taste

• With meals if possible for better absorption

• By IM injection for pernicious anemia for life unless contraindicated

Perform/provide:

• Protection from light and heat

Evaluate:

• Therapeutic response: decreased anorexia, dyspnea on exertion, palpitations, paresthesias, psychosis, visual disturbances

• Nutritional status: egg yolks, fish, organ meats, dairy products, clams, oysters, which are good sources for vitamin B_{12}

• For pulmonary edema, or worsening of CHF in cardiac patients

Teach patient/family

• That treatment must continue for life if diagnosed as having pernicious anemia

• To eat well-balanced diet

• To avoid contact with persons with infection since infections are more common

Lab test interferences:
False positive: Intrinsic factor
Treatment of overdose: Discontinue drug

cyclandelate

(sye-klan'da-late)
Cyclospasmol, Cyclan
Func. class.: Peripheral vasodilator
Chem. class.: Nonnitrate

Action: Relaxes vascular smooth muscle, dilates peripheral vascular smooth muscle by direct action
Uses: Intermittent claudication, thrombophlebitis, Raynaud's phenomenon, ischemic cerebrovascular disease, arteriosclerosis obliterans, nocturnal leg cramps
Dosage and routes:
- *Adult:* PO 200 mg qid, not to exceed 400 mg qid; maintenance dose is 400-800 mg/day in 2-4 divided doses

Available forms include: Tabs 200, 400 mg; caps 200, 400 mg
Side effects/adverse reactions:
HEMA: Increased bleeding time (rare)
CV: ***Tachycardia***
CNS: Headache, paresthesias, dizziness, weakness
GI: Heartburn, eructation, nausea, pyrosis
INTEG: Sweating, flushing
Contraindications: Hypersensitivity
Precautions: Glaucoma, pregnancy (C), lactation, recent MI, hypertension, severe obliterative coronary artery or cerebrovascular disease
Pharmacokinetics:
PO: Onset 15 min, peak 1½ hr, duration 4 hr

NURSING CONSIDERATIONS

Assess:
- Bleeding time in individuals with bleeding disorders

Administer:
- With meals to reduce GI symptoms

Perform/provide:
- Storage in tight container at room temperature

Evaluate:
- Therapeutic response: ability to walk without pain, increased temperature in extremities, increased pulse volume
- Cardiac status: B/P, pulse, rate, rhythm, character; watch for increasing pulse

Teach patient/family:
- That medication is not cure, may need to be taken continuously
- That it is necessary to quit smoking to prevent excessive vasoconstriction
- That improvement may be sudden, but usually occurs gradually over several weeks
- To report headache, weakness, increased pulse, as drug may need to be decreased or discontinued
- To avoid hazardous activities until stabilized on medication; dizziness may occur

cyclizine HCl/ cyclizine lactate

(sye'kli-zeen)
Marezine, Marzine
Func. class.: Antiemetic, antihistamine, anticholinergic
Chem. class.: H_2-receptor antagonist, piperazine derivative

Action: Acts centrally by blocking chemoreceptor trigger zone, which in turn acts on vomiting center

Uses: Motion sickness, prevention of postoperative vomiting
Dosage and routes:
Vomiting
• *Adult:* IM 50 mg ½ hr before termination of surgery, then q4-6h prn (lactate)
• *Child:* IM 3 mg/kg divided in 3 equal doses
Motion sickness
• *Adult:* PO 50 mg then q4-6h prn, not to exceed 200 mg/day (HCl)
• *Child:* PO 25 mg q4-6h prn
Available forms include: Tabs 50 mg; inj 50 mg/ml
Side effects/adverse reactions:
CNS: Drowsiness, dizziness, vertigo, fatigue, restlessness, headache, insomnia, hallucinations (auditory/visual), hallucinations and ***convulsions*** in children
GI: Nausea, anorexia
EENT: Dry mouth, blurred vision, tinnitus
Contraindications: Hypersensitivity to cyclizines, shock
Precautions: Children, narrow-angle glaucoma, urinary retention, lactation, prostatic hypertrophy, elderly, pregnancy (B), lactation
Pharmacokinetics:
PO: Duration 4-6 hr, other pharmacokinetics not known
Interactions/incompatibilities:
• May increase effect of: alcohol, tranquilizers, narcotics

NURSING CONSIDERATIONS
Assess:
• VS, B/P
Administer:
• IM injection in large muscle mass, aspirate to avoid IV administration
• Tablets may be swallowed whole, chewed, or allowed to dissolve
Evaluate:
• Therapeutic response: absence of motion sickness, vomiting
• Signs of toxicity of other drugs or masking of symptoms of disease: brain tumor, intestinal obstruction
• Observe for drowsiness, dizziness
Teach patient/family:
• That a false-negative result may occur with skin testing; skin testing procedures should not be scheduled for 4 days after discontinuing use
• To avoid hazardous activities or activities requiring alertness; dizziness may occur; instruct patient to request assistance with ambulation
• To avoid alcohol, other depressants
Lab test interferences:
False negative: Allergy skin testing

---

cyclobenzaprine
(sye-kloe-ben'za-preen)
Flexeril

Func. class.: Skeletal muscle relaxant, central acting
Chem. class.: Tricyclic amine salt

Action: Unknown; may be related to antidepressant effects
Uses: Adjunct for relief of muscle spasm and pain in musculoskeletal conditions
Dosage and routes:
• *Adult:* PO 10 mg tid × 1 wk, not to exceed 60 mg/day × 3 wk
Side effects/adverse reactions:
CNS: Dizziness, weakness, drowsiness, headache, tremor, depression, insomnia, confusion, paresthesia
EENT: Diplopia, temporary loss of vision
CV: Postural hypotension, tachycardia, dysrhythmias
GI: Nausea, vomiting, hiccups, dry mouth

INTEG: Rash, pruritus, fever, facial flushing, sweating
GU: Urinary retention, frequency, change in libido

Contraindications: Acute recovery phase of myocardial infarction, dysrhythmias, heart block, CHF, hypersensitivity, child <12 yr, intermittent porphyria, thyroid disease

Precautions: Renal disease, hepatic disease, addictive personalities, pregnancy (B), elderly

Pharmacokinetics:
PO: Onset 1 hr, peak 3-8 hr, duration 12-24 hr, half-life 1-3 days, metabolized by liver, excreted in urine, crosses placenta, excreted in breast milk

Interactions/incompatibilities:
- Decreased effects of: guanethidine
- Increased CNS depression: alcohol, tricyclic antidepressants, narcotics, barbiturates, sedatives, hypnotics
- Do not use within 14 days of MAOI

NURSING CONSIDERATIONS

Assess:
- Blood studies: CBC, WBC, differential; blood dyscrasias may occur
- Liver function studies: AST, ALT, alk phosphatase; hepatitis may occur
- ECG in epileptic patients; poor seizure control has occurred with patients taking this drug

Administer:
- With meals for GI symptoms

Perform/provide:
- Storage in tight container at room temperature
- Assistance with ambulation if dizziness, drowsiness occur, especially elderly

Evaluate:
- Therapeutic response: decreased pain, spasticity; muscle spasms of acute, painful musculoskeletal conditions are generally short term; long-term therapy is seldom warranted
- Allergic reactions: rash, fever, respiratory distress
- Severe weakness, numbness in extremities
- Psychologic dependency: increased need for medication, more frequent requests for medication, increased pain
- CNS depression: dizziness, drowsiness, psychiatric symptoms

Teach patient/family:
- Not to discontinue medication quickly; insomnia, nausea, headache, spasticity, tachycardia will occur; drug should be tapered off over 1-2 wk
- Not to take with alcohol, other CNS depressants
- To avoid altering activities while taking this drug
- To avoid hazardous activities if drowsiness, dizziness occurs
- To avoid using OTC medication: cough preparations, antihistamines, unless directed by physician
- To use gum, frequent sips of water for dry mouth

Treatment of overdose: Empty stomach with emesis, gastric lavage, then administer activated charcoal; use anticonvulsants if indicated; monitor cardiac function

cyclopentolate HCl (optic)

(sye-kloe-pen'toe-late)
AK-Pentolate, Cyclogyl
Func. class.: Mydriatic, cycloplegic, anticholinergic

Action: Blocks response of iris

sphincter muscle, muscle of accommodation of ciliary body to cholinergic stimulation, resulting in dilation, paralysis of accommodation

Uses: Cycloplegic refraction, mydriasis

Dosage and routes:
- *Adult:* INSTILL SOL 1 gtt of a 1% sol, then 1 gtt in 5 min
- *Child >6 yr:* INSTILL SOL 1 gtt of a 0.5%-2% sol, then 1 gtt in 5 min of a 0.5%-1% sol

Available forms include: Sol 0.5%, 1%, 2%

Side effects/adverse reactions:

SYST: Tachycardia, confusion, fever, flushing, dry skin, dry mouth, abdominal discomfort (infants: bladder distention, irregular pulse, ***respiratory depression***)

EENT: Blurred vision, temporary burning sensation on instillation, eye dryness, photophobia, conjunctivitis, increased intraocular pressure

CNS: Psychotic reaction, behavior disturbances, ataxia, restlessness, hallucinations, somnolence, disorientation, failure to recognize people, ***grand mal seizures***

GI: Abdominal distention, vomiting

Contraindications: Hypersensitivity, infants <3 mo, local or systemic glaucoma, conjunctivitis

Precautions: Pregnancy (C)

Pharmacokinetics:

INSTILL: Peak 30-60 min (mydriasis), 25-74 min (cycloplegia), duration ¼-1 day

NURSING CONSIDERATIONS

Administer:
- After shaking vial to mix drug to clear solution, push stopper to mix sterile water with powder
- After cleaning stopper with alcohol (rubbing)
- Immediately after reconstituting, discard unused portion

Evaluate:
- Therapeutic response: mydriasis

Teach patient/family:
- To report change in vision, blurring, or loss of sight, trouble breathing, sweating, flushing
- Method of instillation: pressure on lacrimal sac for 1 min, do not touch dropper to eye
- That blurred vision will decrease with repeated use of drug
- That drug will burn when instilled
- To wear dark sunglasses for photophobia
- Not to do hazardous duties until able to see

---

cyclophosphamide

(sye-kloe-foss'fa-mide)

Cytoxan, Neosar, Procytox*

Func. class.: Antineoplastic alkylating agent

Chem. class.: Nitrogen mustard

Action: Alkylates DNA, RNA; inhibits enzymes that allow synthesis of amino acids in proteins; is also responsible for cross-linking DNA strands, breast neuroblastoma

Uses: Hodgkin's disease; lymphomas; leukemia; cancer of female reproductive tract, lung, prostate; multiple myeloma; neuroblastoma; retinoblastoma; Ewing's sarcoma

Dosage and routes:
- *Adult:* PO initially 1-5 mg/kg over 2-5 days, maintenance is 1-5 mg/kg; IV initially 40-50 mg/kg in divided doses over 2-5 days, maintenance 10-15 mg/kg q7-10d, or 3-5 mg/kg q3d
- *Child:* PO/IV 2-8 mg/kg or 60-250 mg/m^2 in divided doses for 6 or more days; maintenance 10-15

mg/kg q7-10d or 30 mg/kg q3-4wk; dose should be reduced by half when bone marrow depression occurs

Available forms include: Powder for inj IV 100, 200, 500 mg, 1, 2 g; tabs 25, 50 mg

Side effects/adverse reactions:

CV: ***Cardiotoxicity*** (high doses)

HEMA: ***Thrombocytopenia, leukopenia, pancytopenia; myelosuppression***

GI: Nausea, vomiting, diarrhea, weight loss, colitis, ***hepatotoxicity***

GU: ***Hemorrhagic cystitis,*** *hematuria, neoplasms, amenorrhea, azoospermia, sterility, ovarian fibrosis*

INTEG: Alopecia, dermatitis

RESP: ***Fibrosis***

ENDO: Syndrome of inappropriate antidiuretic hormone (SIADH)

CNS: Headache, dizziness

Contraindications: Lactation, pregnancy (D)

Precautions: Radiation therapy

Pharmacokinetics:

Metabolized by liver, excreted in urine; half-life 4-6½ hr; 50% bound to plasma proteins

Interactions/incompatibilities:

- Increased toxicity: aminoglycosides
- Increased metabolism of cyclophosphamide: phenobarbital
- Potentiation of cyclophosphamide: succinylcholine
- Increased bone marrow depression: allopurinol, thiazides
- Decreased digoxin levels: digoxin

NURSING CONSIDERATIONS

Assess:

- CBC, differential, platelet count weekly; withhold drug if WBC is <4000 or platelet count is <75,000; notify physician of results
- Pulmonary function tests, chest x-ray films before, during therapy; chest film should be obtained q2wk during treatment
- Renal function studies: BUN, serum uric acid, urine CrCl before, during therapy
- I&O ratio; report fall in urine output of 30 ml/hr
- Monitor temperature q4h (may indicate beginning infection)
- Liver function tests before, during therapy (bilirubin, AST, ALT, LDH) as needed or monthly

Administer:

- Fluids IV or PO before chemotherapy to hydrate patient
- Antacid before oral agent, give drug after evening meal, before bedtime
- Antiemetic 30-60 min before giving drug to prevent vomiting, and prn
- Allopurinol or sodium bicarbonate to maintain uric acid levels, alkalinization of urine
- Prevent hyperuricemia
- Antibiotics for prophylaxis of infection
- IV after diluting 100 mg/5 ml of sterile H_2O or bacteriostatic H_2O; shake; may be further diluted in up to 250-ml compatible sol
- Slow (over 3 min) IV infusion using 21-, 23-, 25-gauge needle, check site for irritation, phlebitis
- Topical or systemic analgesics for pain
- Local or systemic drugs for infection
- In AM so drug can be eliminated before hs

Perform/provide:

- Storage in tight container at room temperature
- Strict medical asepsis, protective isolation if WBC levels are low
- Special skin care

* Available in Canada only

• Deep breathing exercises with patient tid-qid; place in semi-Fowler's position
• Increase fluid intake to 2-3 L/day to prevent urate deposits, calculi formation, reduce incidence of hemorrhagic cystitis
• Diet low in purines: organ meats (kidney, liver), dried beans, peas to maintain alkaline urine
• Rinsing of mouth tid-qid with water, club soda; brushing of teeth bid-tid with soft brush or cotton-tipped applicators for stomatitis; use unwaxed dental floss
• Warm compresses at injection site for inflammation

Evaluate:
• Therapeutic response: decreased tumor size, spread of malignancy
• Bleeding: hematuria, guaiac, bruising or petechiae, mucosa or orifices q8h
• Dyspnea, rales, unproductive cough, chest pain, tachypnea
• Food preferences; list likes, dislikes
• Effects of alopecia on body image, discuss feelings about body changes
• Yellowing of skin, sclera, dark urine, clay-colored stools, itchy skin, abdominal pain, fever, diarrhea
• Edema in feet, joint pain, stomach pain, shaking
• Inflammation of mucosa, breaks in skin
• Buccal cavity q8h for dryness, sores or ulceration, white patches, oral pain, bleeding, dysphagia, obtain prescription for viscous Xylocaine
• Symptoms indicating severe allergic reaction: rash, pruritus, urticaria, purpuric skin lesions, itching, flushing
• Tachypnea, ECG changes, dyspnea, edema, fatigue

Teach patient/family:
• Of protective isolation precautions
• That amenorrhea can occur, reversible after discontinuing treatment
• To report any changes in breathing or coughing
• That hair may be lost during treatment; a wig or hairpiece may make patient feel better; new hair may be different in color, texture
• To avoid foods with citric acid, hot or rough texture
• To report any bleeding, white spots, ulcerations in mouth to physician; tell patient to examine mouth qd
• To report signs of infection: increased temperature, sore throat, flu symptoms
• To report signs of anemia: fatigue, headache, faintness, shortness of breath, irritability
• To report bleeding: avoid use of razors, or commercial mouthwash
• To avoid use of aspirin products or ibuprofen

Lab test interferences:
Increase: Uric acid
False positive: Pap test
False negative: PPD, mumps trichophytin, *Candida*
Decrease: Pseudocholinesterase

cycloserine

(sye-kloe-ser'een)
Seromycin Pulvules

Func. class.: Antitubercular
Chem. class.: *S. oichidaceus*, antibiotic

Action: Inhibits cell wall synthesis, analog of D-alanine

Uses: Pulmonary tuberculosis, extrapulmonary as adjunctive
Dosage and routes:
• *Adult:* PO 250 mg q12h × 14 days, then 250 mg q8h × 2 wk if there are no signs of toxicity, then 250 mg q6h if there are no signs of toxicity, not to exceed 1 g/day
• *Child:* PO 10-20 mg/kg/day (max 0.75-1 g) individual doses
Available forms include: Caps 250 mg
Side effects/adverse reactions:
INTEG: Dermatitis, photosensitivity
CV: ***CHF***
CNS: Headache, anxiety, drowsiness, tremors, ***convulsions,*** lethargy, depression, confusion, psychosis, aggression
HEMA: ***Megaloblastic anemia,*** vitamin B_{12}, folic acid deficiency, leukocytosis
Contraindications: Hypersensitivity, seizure disorders, renal disease, alcoholism (chronic), depression, severe anxiety, lactation, anemia
Precautions: Pregnancy (C), children
Pharmacokinetics:
PO: Peak 3-8 hr; excreted unchanged in urine, crosses placenta, excreted in breast milk
Interactions/incompatibilities:
• Seizures: alcohol
• May increase CNS toxicity: isoniazid

NURSING CONSIDERATIONS

Assess:
• Liver studies qwk: ALT, AST, bilirubin
• Blood levels of drug; keep at <30 μg/ml or toxicity may occur
Administer:
• Using pipette provided; use glass container to prevent adherence to sides
• After C&S is completed, qmo to detect resistance
• Pyridoxine (200-300 mg/day) if ordered to prevent neurotoxicity
Perform/provide:
• Storage in tight container at room temperature
Evaluate:
• Therapeutic response: decreased symptoms of TB
• Mental status often: affect, mood, behavioral changes, psychosis may occur
Teach patient/family:
• To avoid alcohol while taking drug
• That compliance with dosage schedule, length is necessary
• To report neurotoxicity: confusion, headache, drowsiness, tremors, paresthesias, mental changes
• To avoid hazardous activities if drowsiness or dizziness occurs
Lab test interferences:
Increase: AST/ALT
Treatment of overdose: Administer vitamin B_6, anticonvulsants, lavage, O_2, assisted respiration

---

cyclosporine

(sye'kloe-spor-een)
Sandimmune
Func. class.: Immunosuppressant
Chem. class.: Fungus-derived peptide

Action: Produces immunosuppression by inhibiting lymphocytes (T)
Uses: Organ transplants to prevent rejection
Dosage and routes:
• *Adult and child:* PO 15 mg/kg several hours before surgery, daily for 2 wk, reduce dosage by 2.5 mg/kg/wk to 5-10 mg/kg/day; IV 5-6 mg/kg several hours before surgery, daily, switch to PO form as soon as possible

*Available in Canada only

Available forms include: Oral sol 100 mg/ml; inj IV 50 mg/ml
Side effects/adverse reactions:
GI: Nausea, vomiting, diarrhea, *oral Candida, gum hyperplasia,* ***hepatotoxicity,*** pancreatitis
INTEG: Rash, acne, *hirsutism*
CNS: Tremors, headache
GU: ***Albuminuria, hematuria, proteinuria, renal failure***
Contraindications: Hypersensitivity
Precautions: Severe renal disease, severe hepatic disease, pregnancy (C)
Pharmacokinetics: Peak 4 hr, highly protein bound, half-life (biphasic) 1.2 hr, 25 hr; metabolized in liver, excreted in feces, crosses placenta, excreted in breast milk
Interactions/incompatibilities:
- Increased action of cyclosporine: amphotericin B, cimetidine, ketoconazole
- Decreased action of cyclosporine: phenytoin, rifampin

NURSING CONSIDERATIONS
Assess:
- Renal studies: BUN, creatinine at least monthly during treatment, 3 mo after treatment
- Liver function studies: alk phosphatase, AST, ALT, bilirubin
- Drug blood levels during treatment

Administer:
- IV after diluting each 50 mg/20-100 ml of normal saline or D_5W; run over 2-6 hr; use an infusion pump
- For several days before transplant surgery
- With corticosteroids
- With meals for GI upset or drug placed in chocolate milk
- With oral antifungal for *Candida* infections

Evaluate:
- Therapeutic response: absence of rejection
- Hepatotoxicity: dark urine, jaundice, itching, light-colored stools; drug should be discontinued

Teach patient/family:
- To report fever, chills, sore throat, fatigue since serious infections may occur
- To use contraceptive measures during treatment, for 12 wk after ending therapy

---

cyproheptadine HCl
(si-proe-hep′-ta-deen)
Periactin, Vimicon*
Func. class.: Antihistamine, H_1 receptor antagonist
Chem. class.: Piperidine

Action: Acts on blood vessels, GI, respiratory system by competing with histamine for H_1-receptor site; decreases allergic response by blocking histamine
Uses: Allergy symptoms, rhinitis, pruritus, cold urticaria
Dosage and routes:
- *Adult:* PO 4 mg tid-qid, not to exceed 0.5 mg/kg/day
- *Child 7-14 yr:* PO 4 mg bid-tid, not to exceed 16 mg/day
- *Child 2-6 yr:* PO 2 mg bid-tid, not to exceed 12 mg/day

Available forms include: Tabs 4 mg; syr 2 mg/5 ml
Side effects/adverse reactions:
CNS: Dizziness, drowsiness, poor coordination, fatigue, anxiety, euphoria, confusion, paresthesia, neuritis
CV: Hypotension, palpitations, tachycardia
RESP: Increased thick secretions, wheezing, chest tightness
GI: Constipation, dry mouth, nau-

sea, vomiting, anorexia, diarrhea, weight gain
INTEG: Rash, urticaria, photosensitivity
GU: Retention, dysuria, frequency, increased appetite
EENT: Blurred vision, dilated pupils; tinnitus; nasal stuffiness; dry nose, throat, mouth
Contraindications: Hypersensitivity to H_1-receptor antagonist, acute asthma attack, lower respiratory tract disease
Precautions: Increased intraocular pressure, renal disease, cardiac disease, hypertension, bronchial asthma, seizure disorder, stenosed peptic ulcers, hyperthyroidism, prostatic hypertrophy, bladder neck obstruction, pregnancy (B), elderly
Pharmacokinetics:
PO: Duration 4-6 hr, metabolized in liver, excreted by kidneys, excreted in breast milk
Interactions/incompatibilities:
- Increased CNS depression: barbiturates, narcotics, hypnotics, tricyclic antidepressants, alcohol
- Decreased effect of: oral anticoagulants, heparin
- Increased effect of cyproheptadine: MAOIs

NURSING CONSIDERATIONS
Assess:
- I&O ratio; be alert for urinary retention, frequency, dysuria; drug should be discontinued if these occur
- CBC during long-term therapy

Administer:
- With meals if GI symptoms occur; absorption may slightly decrease

Perform/provide:
- Hard candy, gum, frequent rinsing of mouth for dryness
- Storage in tight container at room temperature

Evaluate:
- Therapeutic response: absence of running or congested nose or rashes
- Respiratory status: rate, rhythm, increase in bronchial secretions, wheezing, chest tightness
- Cardiac status: palpitations, increased pulse, hypotension

Teach patient/family:
- All aspects of drug use; to notify physician if confusion, sedation, hypotension occurs
- To avoid driving or other hazardous activity if drowsiness occurs, especially elderly
- To avoid concurrent use of alcohol or other CNS depressants

Lab test interferences:
False negative: Skin allergy tests
Treatment of overdose: Administer ipecac syrup or lavage, diazepam, vasopressors, barbiturates (short-acting)

cytarabine (ARA-C, cytosine arabinoside)

(sye-tare'a-been)
Cytosar-U
Func. class.: Antineoplastic, antimetabolite
Chem. class.: Pyrimidine nucleoside

Action: Competes with physiologic substrate that inhibits DNA synthesis; interferes with cell replication at S phase, directly before mitosis
Uses: Acute myelocytic leukemia, acute lymphocytic leukemia, chronic myelocytic leukemia, and in combination for non-Hodgkin's lymphomas in children
Dosage and routes:
Acute myelocytic leukemia
- *Adult:* IV INF 200 mg/m^2/day × 5 days; INTRATHECAL 5-

50 mg/m^2/day × 3 days/wk or 30 mg/m^2/day q4d

In combination

• *Child:* IV INF 100 mg/m^2/day × 5-10 days

Available forms include: Inj IV, intrathecal 100, 500 mg, 1, 2 g

Side effects/adverse reactions:

HEMA: Thrombophlebitis, bleeding, ***thrombocytopenia, leukopenia, myelosuppression, anemia***

GI: Nausea, vomiting, anorexia, diarrhea, stomatitis, ***hepatotoxicity,*** abdominal pain, hematemesis, ***GI hemorrhage***

EENT: Sore throat, conjunctivitis

GU: Urinary retention, ***renal failure, hyperuricemia***

INTEG: Rash, fever, freckling, cellulitis

RESP: ***Pneumonia,*** dyspnea

CV: Chest pain, ***cardiopathy***

CNS: Neuritis, dizziness, headache, personality changes, ataxia, mechanical dysphasia, ***coma***

CYTARABINE SYNDROME: Fever, myalgia, bone pain, chest pain, rash, conjunctivitis, malaise (6-12 hr after administration)

Contraindications: Hypersensitivity, infants, pregnancy (1st trimester)

Precautions: Renal disease, hepatic disease, pregnancy (C)

Pharmacokinetics:

INTRATHECAL: Half-life 2 hr, metabolized in liver, excreted in urine (primarily inactive metabolite), crosses blood-brain barrier, placenta

IV: Distribution half-life 10 min, elimination half-life 1-3 hr

Interactions/incompatibilities:

• Increased toxicity: radiation or other antineoplastics

• Decreased effects of: oral digoxin

NURSING CONSIDERATIONS

Assess:

• CBC (RBC, Hct, Hgb), differential, platelet count weekly; withhold drug if WBC is <4000/mm,^{3} platelet count is <75,000/mm,^{3} or RBC, Hct, Hgb are low; notify physician of these results

• Renal function studies: BUN, serum uric acid, urine creatinine clearance, electrolytes before and during therapy

• I&O ratio; report fall in urine output to <30 ml/hr

• Monitor temperature q4h; fever may indicate beginning infection; no rectal temperatures

• Liver function tests before and during therapy: bilirubin, ALT, AST, alk phosphatase, as needed or monthly

• Blood uric acid levels during therapy

Administer:

• Antiemetic 30-60 min before giving drug to prevent vomiting, and prn

• Allopurinol or sodium bicarbonate to maintain uric acid levels and alkalinization of the urine

• Prevent hyperuricemia

• Antibiotics for prophylaxis of infection

• IV after diluting 100 mg/5 ml of sterile H_2O for inj; may be further diluted in 50-100 ml normal saline or D_5W

• Slow IV infusion using 21-, 23-, 25-gauge needle

• Topical or systemic analgesics for pain

• Transfusion for anemia

• Antispasmodic for GI symptoms

Perform/provide:

• Strict medical asepsis and protective isolation if WBC levels are low

• Increase fluid intake to 2-3 L/day to prevent urate deposits and calculi formation, unless contraindicated

• Diet low in purines: absence of organ meats (kidney, liver), dried

beans, peas to prevent increased urate deposits
• Rinsing of mouth tid-qid with water, club soda; brushing of teeth bid-tid with soft brush or cotton-tipped applicators for stomatitis; use unwaxed dental floss
• HOB increased to facilitate breathing if dyspnea or pneumonia occurs

Evaluate:
• Therapeutic response: decreased tumor size, spread of malignancy
• Cytarabine syndrome: fever, myalgia, bone pain, chest pain, rash, conjunctivitis, malaise; corticosteroids may be ordered
• Bleeding: hematuria, guaiac, bruising or petechiae, mucosa or orifices q8h
• Dyspnea, rales, unproductive cough, chest pain, tachypnea, fatigue, increased pulse, pallor, lethargy, personality changes, with high doses
• Food preferences; list likes, dislikes
• Edema in feet, joint pain, stomach pain, shaking
• Inflammation of mucosa, breaks in skin
• Yellowing of skin, sclera, dark urine, clay-colored stools, itchy skin, abdominal pain, fever, diarrhea
• Buccal cavity q8h for dryness, sores or ulceration, white patches, oral pain, bleeding, dysphagia
• Local irritation, pain, burning, discoloration at injection site
• GI symptoms: frequency of stools, cramping
• Acidosis, signs of dehydration: rapid respirations, poor skin turgor, decreased urine output, dry skin, restlessness, weakness

Teach patient/family:
• Why protective isolation precautions are necessary
• To report any coughing, chest pain, or changes in breathing, which may indicate beginning pneumonia
• To avoid foods with citric acid, hot or rough texture if stomatitis is present
• To report stomatitis: any bleeding, white spots, ulcerations in mouth; tell patient to examine mouth qd, report any symptoms
• To report signs of infection: increased temperature, sore throat, flu symptoms
• To report signs of anemia: fatigue, headache, faintness, shortness of breath, irritability
• To report bleeding; avoid use of razors or commercial mouthwash
• To avoid use of aspirin products or ibuprofen

dacarbazine (DTIC)

(da-kar'ba-zeen)

DTIC-Dome

Func. class.: Antineoplastic alkylating agent
Chem. class.: Cytotoxic triazine

Action: Alkylates DNA, RNA; inhibits enzymes that allow synthesis of amino acids in proteins; also responsible for cross-linking DNA strands

Uses: Hodgkin's disease, sarcomas, neuroblastoma, malignant melanoma

Dosage and routes:
• *Adult:* IV 2-4.5 mg/kg or 70-160 mg/m^2 qd × 10 days, repeat q4wk depending on response or 250 mg/m^2 qd × 5 days, repeat q3wk

Available forms include: Inj IV 100, 200 mg

Side effects/adverse reactions:
HEMA: ***Thrombocytopenia, leukopenia,*** anemia

GI: Nausea, anorexia, vomiting, ***hepatotoxicity***
CNS: Facial paresthesia, flushing, fever, malaise
INTEG: Alopecia, dermatitis, pain at injection site
Contraindications: Lactation
Precautions: Radiation therapy, pregnancy (1st trimester) (C)
Pharmacokinetics:
Metabolized by liver, excreted in urine; half-life 35 min, terminal 5 hr, 5% protein bound
Interactions/incompatibilities:
Decreased effectiveness of dacarbazine: phenytoin, phenobarbital

NURSING CONSIDERATIONS

Assess:
- CBC, differential, platelet count weekly; withhold drug if WBC is <4000 or platelet count is <75,000; notify physician of results
- Monitor temperature q4h (may indicate beginning infection)
- Liver function tests before, during therapy (bilirubin, AST, ALT, LDH) as needed or monthly

Administer:
- Antiemetic 30-60 min before giving drug to prevent vomiting
- Antibiotics for prophylaxis of infection
- After diluting 100 mg/9.9 ml of sterile H_2O for inj; may be further diluted in 50-250 ml of D_5W or normal saline for inj
- Slow IV infusion using 21-, 23-, 25-gauge needle, watch for extravasation

Perform/provide:
- Storage in light-resistant container, dry area
- Strict medical asepsis, protective isolation if WBC levels are low
- Increase fluid intake to 2-3 L/day to prevent urate deposits, calculi formation
- Warm compresses at injection site for inflammation

Evaluate:
- Therapeutic response: decreased tumor size, spread of malignancy
- Bleeding: hematuria, guaiac, bruising or petechiae, mucosa or orifices q8h
- Food preferences; list likes, dislikes
- Effects of alopecia on body image, discuss feelings about body changes
- Yellowing of skin, sclera, dark urine, clay-colored stools, itchy skin, abdominal pain, fever, diarrhea
- Inflammation of mucosa, breaks in skin

Teach patient/family:
- Of protective isolation precautions
- That hair may be lost during treatment; a wig or hairpiece may make the patient feel better; new hair may be different in color, texture
- To report signs of infection: increased temperature, sore throat, flu symptoms
- To report signs of anemia: fatigue, headache, faintness, shortness of breath, irritability
- To report bleeding; avoid use of razors or commercial mouthwash
- To avoid use of aspirin products or ibuprofen

---

dactinomycin (actinomycin D)

(dak-ti-noe-mye'sin)
Cosmegen
Func. class.: Antineoplastic, antibiotic

Action: Inhibits DNA, RNA, protein synthesis; derived from *Streptomyces parrullus;* replication is decreased by binding to DNA, which causes strand splitting; cell cycle nonspecific; a vesicant

Uses: Sarcomas, melanomas, trophoblastic tumors in women, testicular cancer, Wilms' tumor, rhabdomyosarcoma

Dosage and routes:

• *Adult:* IV 500 μg/m²/day × 5 days; stop drug for 2-4 wk; then repeat cycle

• *Child:* IV 15 μg/kg/day × 5 days, not to exceed 500 μg/day; stop drug until bone marrow recovery, then repeat cycle

Available forms include: Inj IV 500 μg

Side effects/adverse reactions:

HEMA: ***Thrombocytopenia, leukopenia, aplastic anemia***

GI: Nausea, vomiting, anorexia, stomatitis, ***hepatotoxicity,*** abdominal pain, diarrhea

INTEG: Rash, alopecia, pain at injection site, folliculitis, acne, desquamation, ***extravasation***

EENT: Chelitis, dysphagia, esophagitis

CNS: Malaise, fatigue, lethargy, fever

MS: Myalgia

Contraindications: Hypersensitivity, herpes infections, child <6 months

Precautions: Renal disease, hepatic disease, pregnancy (C), lactation, bone marrow depression

Pharmacokinetics: Half-life 36 hr; IV: onset 2-5 min, concentrates in kidneys, liver, spleen; does not cross blood-brain barrier, excreted in feces and urine

Interactions/incompatibilities:

• Increased toxicity: other antineoplastics or radiation

NURSING CONSIDERATIONS

Assess:

• CBC, differential, platelet count weekly; withhold drug if WBC is <4000/mm³ or platelet count is <75,000/mm³; notify physician of these results

• Renal function studies: BUN, serum uric acid, urine CrCl, electrolytes before, during therapy

• I&O ratio; report fall in urine output to <30 ml/hr

• Monitor temperature q4h; fever may indicate beginning infection

• Liver function tests before, during therapy: bilirubin, AST, ALT, alk phosphatase, as needed or monthly

Administer:

• Antiemetic 30-60 min before giving drug to prevent vomiting

• Antibiotics as ordered for prophylaxis of infection

• After diluting 0.5 mg/1.1 ml of sterile H_2O for inj without preservative, may be further diluted in 50 ml D_5W or normal saline for infusion; run over 10-15 min

• Slow IV infusion using 21-, 23-, 25-gauge needle, check for extravasation

• Topical or systemic analgesics for pain

• Local or systemic drugs for infection

• Hydrocortisone, sodium thiosulfate to infiltration area, and ice compress after stopping infusion

• Antispasmodic for GI symptoms

Perform/provide:

• Strict handwashing technique, gloves and protective covering

• Liquid diet: carbonated beverages, gelatin may be added if patient is not nauseated or vomiting

• Rinsing of mouth tid-qid with water, club soda; brushing of teeth bid-qid with soft brush or cotton-tipped applicators for stomatitis; use unwaxed dental floss

---

• Storage in darkness in cool environment

Evaluate:

• Therapeutic response: decreased tumor size, spread of malignancy

• Bleeding: hematuria, guaiac stools, bruising, petechiae, mucosa or orifices q8h

• Food preferences; list likes, dislikes

• Effects of alopecia on body image; discuss feelings about body changes

• Inflammation of mucosa, breaks in skin

• Yellowing of skin, sclera, dark urine, clay-colored stools, itchy skin, abdominal pain, fever, diarrhea

• Buccal cavity q8h for dryness, sores, ulceration, white patches, oral pain, bleeding, dysphagia

• Local irritation, pain, burning at injection site

• Symptoms indicating severe allergic reaction: rash, pruritus, urticaria, purpuric skin lesions, itching, flushing

• GI symptoms: frequency of stools, cramping

• Acidosis, signs of dehydration: rapid respirations, poor skin turgor, decreased urine output, dry skin, restlessness, weakness

Teach patient/family:

• To report any complaints, side effects to nurse or physician

• That hair may be lost during treatment and wig or hairpiece may make patient feel better; tell patient that new hair may be different in color, texture

• To avoid foods with citric acid, hot or rough texture

• To report any bleeding, white spots, ulcerations in mouth to physician; tell patient to examine mouth qd

• To avoid crowds and sources of infection when granulocyte count is low

Lab test interferences:

Increase: Uric acid

---

danazol

(da'na-zole)

Cyclomen,* Danocrine

Func. class.: Androgen

Chem. class.: α-Ethinyl testosterone derivative

Action: Atrophy of endometrial tissue, decreases FSH, LH, which are controlled by pituitary; this leads to amenorrhea/anovulation

Uses: Endometriosis, prevention of hereditary angioedema, fibrocystic breast disease

Dosage and routes:

Endometriosis

• *Adult:* PO initial dose 500 mg bid then decreased to 400 mg bid × 3-9 mo

Fibrocystic breast disease

• *Adult:* PO 100-400 mg qd in 2 divided doses × 2-6 mo

Hereditary angioedema

• *Adult:* PO 200 mg bid-tid until desired response, then decrease dose to 100 mg at 1-3 mo intervals

Available forms include: Caps 50, 100, 200 mg

Side effects/adverse reactions:

INTEG: Rash, acneiform lesions, oily hair, skin, flushing, sweating, acne vulgaris, alopecia, hirsutism

CNS: Dizziness, headache, fatigue, tremors, paresthesias, flushing, sweating, anxiety, lability, insomnia

MS: Cramps, spasms

CV: Increased B/P

GU: Hematuria, amenorrhea, atrophic vaginitis, decreased libido, de-

creased breast size, clitoral hypertrophy, testicular atrophy
GI: Nausea, vomiting, constipation, weight gain, ***cholestatic jaundice***
EENT: Carpal tunnel syndrome, conjunctional edema, nasal congestion
ENDO: Abnormal GTT
Contraindications: Severe renal disease, severe cardiac disease, severe hepatic disease, hypersensitivity, genital bleeding (abnormal)
Precautions: Migraine headaches, seizure disorders, pregnancy (C)
Interactions/incompatibilities:
• Increased effects of: oral antidiabetics, oxyphenbutazone
• Increased prothrombin time: anticoagulants
• Edema: ACTH, adrenal steroids
• Decreased effects of: insulin

NURSING CONSIDERATIONS

Assess:
• Potassium, blood sugar, urine glucose while on long-term therapy
• Weight daily; notify physician if weekly weight gain is >5 lb
• I&O ratio; be alert for decreasing urinary output, increasing edema
Administer:
• With food or milk to decrease GI symptoms
Perform/provide:
• Storage in tight container at room temperature
• ROM exercise for patients who are immobile
Evaluate:
• Therapeutic response: decreased pain in endometriosis, decreased size, pain in fibrocystic breast disease
• Edema, hypertension, cardiac symptoms, jaundice
• Mental status: affect, mood, behavioral changes, aggression, sleep disorders, depression
• Signs of virilization: deepening of voice, decreased libido, facial hair (may not be reversible)
• Hypercalcemia: GI symptoms, polydipsia, polyuria, increased calcium levels, decrease in muscle tone
Teach patient/family:
• To notify physician if therapeutic response decreases
• Not to discontinue medication abruptly but to taper over several weeks
• To report menstrual irregularities; that amenorrhea usually occurs but menstruation resumes 2-3 mo after termination of therapy
• About routine breast self-exam, report any increase in nodule size
• That drug should induce anovulation; reversible within 60-90 days after drug is discontinued
• That endometriosis tends to recur after drug is discontinued
Lab test interferences:
Increase: Cholesterol
Decrease: Cholesterol, T_4, T_3, thyroid ^{131}I uptake test, 17-KS, PBI
Interferes: GTT

dantrolene sodium

(dan'troe-leen)
Dantrium, Dantrium IV
Func. class.: Skeletal muscle relaxant, direct acting
Chem. class.: Hydantoin

Action: Interferes with intracellular release of calcium necessary to initiate contraction
Uses: Spasticity in multiple sclerosis, stroke, spinal cord injury, cerebral palsy, malignant hyperthermia
Dosage and routes:
Spasticity
• *Adult:* PO 25 mg/day; may in-

* Available in Canada only

crease by 25-100 mg bid-qid, not to exceed 400 mg/day × 1 wk
• *Child:* PO 1 mg/kg/day given in divided doses bid-tid; may increase gradually, not to exceed 100 mg qid
Malignant hyperthermia
• *Adult and child:* IV 1 mg/kg, may repeat to total dose of 10 mg/kg; PO 4-8 mg/kg/day in 4 divided doses × 3 days to prevent further hyperthermia
Available forms include: Caps 25, 50, 100 mg; powder for inj IV 20 mg/vial
Side effects/adverse reactions:
CNS: Dizziness, weakness, fatigue, drowsiness, headache, disorientation, insomnia, paresthesias, tremors
EENT: Nasal congestion, blurred vision, mydriasis
HEMA: ***Eosinophilia***
CV: Hypotension, chest pain, palpitations
GI: Nausea, constipation, vomiting, increased AST, alk phosphatase, abdominal pain, dry mouth, anorexia, hepatitis
GU: Urinary frequency, nocturia, impotence, crystalluria
INTEG: Rash, pruritus, photosensitivity
Contraindications: Hypersensitivity, compromised pulmonary function, active hepatic disease, impaired myocardial function
Precautions: Peptic ulcer disease, renal disease, hepatic disease, stroke, seizure disorder, diabetes mellitus, pregnancy (C) elderly
Pharmacokinetics:
PO: Peak 5 hr, highly protein bound, half-life 8 hr, metabolized in liver, excreted in urine (metabolites)
Interactions/incompatibilities:
• Increased CNS depression: alcohol, tricyclic antidepressants, narcotics, barbiturates, sedatives, hypnotics

NURSING CONSIDERATIONS

Assess:
• For increased seizure activity in epilepsy patient
• I&O ratio; check for urinary retention, frequency, hesitancy, especially elderly
• ECG in epileptic patients; poor seizure control has occurred with patients taking this drug
• Hepatic function by frequent determination of AST, ALT, renal function studies, CBC
Administer:
• With meals for GI symptoms
• Gum, frequent sips of water for dry mouth
• IV after diluting 20 mg/60 ml sterile H_2O for inj without bacteriostatic agent; shake; give by rapid IV push through Y-tube or 3-way stopcock
Perform/provide:
• Storage in tight container at room temperature
• Assistance with ambulation if dizziness, drowsiness occurs
Evaluate:
• Therapeutic response: decreased pain, spasticity
• Allergic reactions: rash, fever, respiratory distress
• Severe weakness, numbness in extremities
• Psychologic dependency: increased need for medication, more frequent requests for medication, increased pain
• CNS depression: dizziness, drowsiness, psychiatric symptoms
• Signs of hepatitis: jaundice, yellow sclera, pain in abdomen, nausea, fever
Teach patient/family:
• Not to discontinue medication quickly; hallucinations, spasticity,

tachycardia will occur; drug should be tapered off over 1-2 wk, notify physician of abdominal pain, jaundiced sclera, clay-colored stools, change in color of urine
• Not to take with alcohol, other CNS depressants
• That if improvement does not occur within 6 wk physician may discontinue
• To avoid altering activities while taking this drug
• To avoid hazardous activities if drowsiness, dizziness occurs
• To avoid using OTC medication: cough preparations, antihistamines, unless directed by physician

Treatment of overdose: Induce emesis of conscious patient, lavage, dialysis

---

dapiprazole HCl

Rev-Eyes

Func. class.: Ophthalmic alpha-adrenergic blocking agents

Action: Blocks alpha-adrenergic receptors in smooth muscle in the eye; miosis occurs through effect on the iris dilator muscle

Uses: Iatrogenically induces mydriasis produced by adrenergic or parasympatholytic agents

Dosage and routes:
• *Adult:* Instill 2 gtts, then 2 gtts 5 min later applied to the conjunctiva; do not use more than once a week

Available forms include: Pwd for lyophilized 25 mg (0.5% sol reconstituted)

Side effects/adverse reactions:
EENT: Burning, ptosis, lid erythema, lid edema, itching, keratitis, corneal edema; browache, photophobia, headaches, eye dryness, tearing, blurring vision

Contraindications: Hypersensitivity, acute iritis

Precautions: Pregnancy (B), lactation, children, severe cardiovascular disease

NURSING CONSIDERATIONS

Assess:
• Cardiac status; watch for bradycardia, palpitations, especially in cardiac disease (including hypertension)

Administer:
• By instillation after tearing off aluminum seals; remove and discard rubber plugs from drugs and diluent; remove dropper and attach to vial; shake

Perform/provide:
• Storage at room temperature after reconstituting × 21 days

Teach patient/family:
• That drug may cause burning, itching, blurring dryness of eye

---

dapsone (DDS)

(dap'sone)

Avlosulfon*

Func. class.: Leprostatic
Chem. class.: Sulfone

Action: Bactericidal and bacteriostatic against *M. leprae*

Uses: Hansen's disease

Dosage and routes:
• *Adult:* PO 100 mg qd with rifampin 600 mg qd × 6 mo

Available forms include: Tabs 25, 100 mg

Side effects/adverse reactions:
INTEG: ***Exfoliative dermatitis,*** photosensitivity
CNS: Peripheral neuropathy, headache, anxiety, drowsiness, tremors, ***convulsions,*** lethargy, depression, confusion, psychosis, aggression
GI: Nausea, vomiting, abdominal pain, anorexia

---

* Available in Canada only

GU: Proteinuria, nephrotic syndrome, renal papillary necrosis
EENT: Blurred vision, optic neuritis, photophobia
HEMA: ***Megaloblastic anemia***
Contraindications: Hypersensitivity to sulfones, severe anemia
Precautions: Renal disease, hepatic disease, G-6-PD deficiency, pregnancy (A), lactation
Pharmacokinetics:
Rapid complete absorption; half-life 25-31 hr; highly bound to plasma protein, metabolized in liver, excreted in urine
Interactions/incompatibilities:
- Increased side effects: hemolytic agents
- Increased action of dapsone: probenecid, folic acid antagonists
- Decreased blood levels of dapsone: rifampin
- Decreased bactericidal action: PABA
- Decreased GI absorption of dapsone: activated charcoal

NURSING CONSIDERATIONS

Assess:
- Temperature, if $<101°$ F, drug should be reduced
- Liver studies qwk: ALT, AST, bilirubin
- Renal status: BUN, creatinine, output, sp gr, urinalysis before; qmo
- Blood levels of drug
- For anemia: Hct, Hgb, fatigue; for peripheral neuritis; or exfoliative dermatitis

Administer:
- With meals to decrease GI symptoms
- Antiemetic if vomiting occurs
- After C&S is completed; qmo to detect resistance

Perform/provide:
- Infants to be kept with mothers infected with leprosy, breastfeeding during drug therapy is encouraged

Evaluate:
- Therapeutic response: decreased symptoms of Hansen's disease
- Mental status often: affect, mood, behavioral changes; psychosis may occur
- Hepatic status: decreased appetite, jaundice, dark urine, fatigue

Teach patient/family:
- That therapeutic effects may occur after 3-6 mo of drug therapy
- That compliance with dosage schedule, duration is necessary
- To avoid hazardous machinery if drowsiness occurs

---

daunorubicin HCl

(daw-noe-roo'bi-sin)
Cerubidine
Func. class.: Antineoplastic, antibiotic
Chem. class.: Anthracycline glycoside

Action: Inhibits DNA synthesis, primarily; derived from *S. verticillus;* replication is decreased by binding to DNA, which causes strand splitting; cell cycle specific (S phase); a vesicant
Uses: Myelogenous, monocytic leukemia, acute nonlymphocytic leukemia, Ewing's sarcoma, Wilms' tumor, neuroblastoma, rhabdomyosarcoma
Dosage and routes:
Single agent
- *Adult:* IV 60 mg/m^2/day × 3-5 day q4wk

In combination
- *Adult:* IV 45 mg/m^2/day × 3 days, then 2 days of subsequent courses with cytosine arabinoside

Available forms include: Inj IV 20 mg

D

Side effects/adverse reactions:
HEMA: ***Thrombocytopenia, leukopenia, anemia***
GI: Nausea, vomiting, anorexia, mucositis, ***hepatotoxicity***
GU: Impotence, sterility, amenorrhea, gynecomastia, hyperuricemia
INTEG: Rash, ***extravasation,*** dermatitis, reversible alopecia, cellulitis, thrombophlebitis at injection site
CV: ***Dysrhythmias, CHF, pericarditis, myocarditis,*** peripheral edema
CNS: Fever, chills

Contraindications: Hypersensitivity, pregnancy (1st trimester) (D), lactation, systemic infections, cardiac disease

Precautions: Renal, hepatic, gout, bone marrow depression

Pharmacokinetics: Half-life 18½ hr, metabolized by liver, crosses placenta, appears in breast milk, excreted in urine, bile

Interactions/incompatibilities:
- Increased toxicity: other antineoplastics or radiation
- Do not mix with other drugs in solution or syringe

NURSING CONSIDERATIONS

Assess:
- CBC, differential, platelet count weekly; withhold drug if WBC is <4000/mm^3 or platelet count is <75,000/mm^3; notify physician of these results
- Blood, urine uric acid levels
- Renal function studies: BUN, serum uric acid, urine CrCl, electrolytes before, during therapy
- I&O ratio; report fall in urine output to <30 ml/hr
- Monitor temperature q4h; fever may indicate beginning infection
- Liver function tests before, during therapy: bilirubin, AST, ALT, alk phosphatase as needed or monthly
- ECG; watch for ST-T wave changes, low QRS and T, possible dysrhythmias (sinus tachycardia, heart block, PVCs)

Administer:
- Antiemetic 30-60 min before giving drug and 6-10 hr after treatment to prevent vomiting
- Antibiotics for prophylaxis of infection
- Allopurinol or sodium bicarbonate to reduce uric acid levels, alkalinization of urine
- IV after diluting 20 mg/4 ml sterile H_2O for inj; further dilute in 10-15 ml normal saline; give over 3-5 min; may be further diluted in 50 ml of compatible sol and run over 10-15 min
- Transfusion for anemia
- Antispasmodic for GI symptoms
- Hydrocortisone for extravasation, apply ice compress after stopping infusion

Perform/provide:
- Strict handwashing technique, gloves, protective clothing
- Liquid diet: carbonated beverages, gelatin may be added if patient is not nauseated or vomiting
- Increased fluid intake to 2-3 L/day to prevent urate and calculi formation
- Diet low in purines: absence of organ meats (kidney, liver), dried beans, peas to reduce uric acid level
- Rinsing of mouth tid-qid with water, club soda; brushing of teeth bid-qid with soft brush or cotton-tipped applicators for stomatitis; use unwaxed dental floss
- Storage at room temperature for 24 hr after reconstituting or 48 hr refrigerated

Evaluate:
- Therapeutic response: decreased

* Available in Canada only

tumor size, spread of malignancy
• Bleeding: hematuria, guaiac stools, bruising or petechiae, mucosa or orifices q8h
• Food preferences; list likes, dislikes
• Effects of alopecia on body image; discuss feelings about body changes
• Inflammation of mucosa, breaks in skin
• Yellowing of skin, sclera, dark urine, clay-colored stools, itchy skin, abdominal pain, fever, diarrhea
• Buccal cavity q8h for dryness, sores or ulceration, white patches, oral pain, bleeding, dysphagia
• Local irritation, pain, burning at injection site
• GI symptoms: frequency of stools, cramping
• Acidosis, signs of dehydration: rapid respirations, poor skin turgor, decreased urine output, dry skin, restlessness, weakness
• Cardiac status: B/P, pulse, character, rhythm, rate

Teach patient/family:
• To report any complaints, side effects to nurse or physician
• That hair may be lost during treatment and wig or hairpiece may make patient feel better; tell patient that new hair may be different in color, texture
• To avoid foods with citric acid, hot or rough texture
• To report any bleeding, white spots, ulcerations in mouth; tell patient to examine mouth qd
• That urine and other body fluids may be red-orange for 48 hr

Lab test interferences:
Increase: Uric acid

deferoxamine mesylate

(de-fer-ox'a-meen)
Desferal
Func. class.: Heavy metal antagonist
Chem. class.: Chelating agent

D

Action: Binds iron ions (ferric ions) to form water-soluble complex that is removed by kidneys
Uses: Acute, chronic iron intoxication, hemochromatosis, hemosiderosis
Dosage and routes:
Acute
• *Adult and child:* IM/IV 1 g, then 500 mg q4h × 2 doses, then 500 mg q4-12h × 2 doses, not to exceed 15 mg/kg/hr or 6 g/24 hr
Chronic
• *Adult and child:* IM 500 mg-1 g/day plus IV INF 2 g given by separate line with each blood transfusion, not to exceed 15 mg/kg/hr or 6 g/24 hr; SC 1-2 g over 8-24 hr by SC infusion pump
Available forms include: Powder for inj IV, IM, SC 500 mg/vial
Side effects/adverse reactions:
INTEG: Urticaria, erythema, pruritus, pain at injection site, fever
CV: Hypotension, tachycardia
GI: Diarrhea, abdominal cramps
EENT: Blurred vision, cataracts, decreased healing, ***ototoxicity***
MS: Leg cramps
GU: Dysuria, pyelonephritis
SYST: ***Anaphylaxis***
Contraindications: Hypersensitivity, anuria, severe renal disease, child <3 yr
Precautions: Pregnancy (C), lactation
Pharmacokinetics:
Metabolized by plasma enzymes, excreted by kidneys as complex, unchanged drug

NURSING CONSIDERATIONS

Assess:

- Inj site for redness, inflammation, pain
- For blood in stools
- Vision and hearing periodically
- VS
- I&O, kidney function studies: BUN, creatinine, CrCl, serum iron levels

Administer:

- IV (used for shock) after diluting in 500 mg/2 ml H_2O for inj; may be further diluted with D_5W or LR or NS; run at <15 mg/kg/hr; to be used only for short time; IM is preferred route
- IM after diluting with 2 ml sterile water for injection per 500 mg of drug; rotate injection sites
- Only when epinephrine 1 : 1000 is on unit for anaphylaxis

Evaluate:

- Therapeutic response: decreased symptoms of heavy metal intoxication
- Allergic reactions: rash, urticaria; if these occur, drug should be discontinued

Teach patient/family:

- That urine may turn red

---

demeclocycline HCl

(dem-e-kloe-sye'kleen)

Declomycin, DMCT, Ledermycin

Func. class.: Broad-spectrum antibiotic/antiinfective

Chem. class.: Tetracycline

Action: Inhibits protein synthesis, phosphorylation in microorganisms by binding to 30S ribosomal subunits, reversibly binding to 50S ribosomal subunits; bacteriostatic

Uses: Uncommon gram-positive/gram-negative bacteria, protozoa, *Rickettsia, Mycoplasma*

Dosage and routes:

- *Adult:* PO 150 mg q6h or 300 mg q12h
- *Child >8 yr:* PO 6-12 mg/kg/day in divided doses q6-12h

Gonorrhea

- *Adult:* PO 600 mg, then 300 mg q12h × 4 days, total 3 g

Inappropriate ADH syndrome

- *Adult:* PO 600-1200 mg/day in divided doses

Available forms include: Tabs 150, 300 mg; caps 150 mg

Side effects/adverse reactions:

CNS: Fever, headache, paresthesia

HEMA: ***Eosinophilia, neutropenia, thrombocytopenia, leukocytosis, hemolytic anemia***

EENT: Dysphagia, glossitis, decreased calcification of deciduous teeth, abdominal pain, oral candidiasis

GI: Nausea, vomiting, diarrhea, anorexia, enterocolitis, ***hepatotoxicity,*** flatulence, abdominal cramps, epigastric burning, stomatitis, ***psuedomembranous colitis***

CV: Pericarditis

GU: Increased BUN, polyuria, polydipsia, ***renal failure, nephrotoxicity***

INTEG: Rash, urticaria, photosenitivity, increased pigmentation, ***exfoliative dermatitis,*** pruritus, angioedema

Contraindications: Hypersensitivity to tetracyclines, children <8 yr, pregnancy (D)

Precautions: Renal disease, hepatic disease, lactation, nephrogenic diabetes insipidus

Pharmacokinetics:

PO: Peak 3-6 hr, duration 48-72 hr, half-life 10-17 hr, excreted in urine, crosses placenta, excreted in breast milk, 36%-91% bound to serum protein

---

* Available in Canada only

Interactions/incompatibilities:

• Decreased effect of demeclocycline: antacids, $NaHCO_3$, dairy, alkali products, iron, kaolin, pectin, cimetidine

• Increased effect: anticoagulants

• Decreased effect: penicillins, oral contraceptives

• Nephrotoxicity: methoxyflurane

NURSING CONSIDERATIONS

Assess:

• I&O ratio

• Blood studies: PT, CBC, AST, ALT, BUN, creatinine

• Urine sp gr, sodium

• Signs of infection

Administer:

• On empty stomach 1 hr ac or 2 hr pc with 8 oz of water

• After C&S obtained

• 2 hr before or after laxative or ferrous products; 3 hr after antacid or kaolin-pectin products

Perform/provide:

• Storage in tight, light-resistant container at room temperature

Evaluate:

• Therapeutic response: decreased temperature, absence of lesions, negative C&S

• Allergic reactions: rash, itching, pruritus, angioedema

• Nausea, vomiting, diarrhea; administer antiemetic, antacids as ordered

• Overgrowth of infection: increased temperature, malaise, redness, pain, swelling, drainage, perineal itching, diarrhea, changes in cough, sputum

Teach patient/family:

• To avoid sun exposure since burns may occur; sunscreen does not seem to decrease photosensitivity

• If diabetic, to avoid use of Clinistix, Diastix, or Tes-Tape for urine glucose testing

• That all prescribed medication must be taken to prevent superimposed infection

• To avoid milk products, take with full glass of water

Lab test interferences:

False negative: Urine glucose with Clinistix or Tes-Tape

False increase: Urinary catecholamines, AST, ALT, BUN

---

desipramine HCl

(dess-ip'ra-meen)

Norpramin, Pertofrane

Func. class.: Antidepressant, tricyclic

Chem. class.: Dibenzazepine, secondary amine

Action: Blocks reuptake of norepinephrine, serotonin into nerve endings, increasing action of norepinephrine, serotonin in nerve cells

Uses: Depression

Dosage and routes:

• *Adult:* PO 75-150 mg/day in divided doses, may increase to 300 mg/day or may give daily dose hs

• *Adolescent/geriatric:* PO 25-50 mg/day, may increase to 100 mg/day

Available forms include: Tabs 10, 25, 50, 75, 100, 150 mg; caps 25, 50 mg

Side effects/adverse reactions:

HEMA: ***Agranulocytosis, thrombocytopenia, eosinophilia, leukopenia***

CNS: Dizziness, drowsiness, confusion, headache, anxiety, tremors, stimulation, weakness, insomnia, nightmares, EPS (elderly), increased psychiatric symptoms, paresthesia

GI: Diarrhea, dry mouth, nausea, vomiting, ***paralytic ileus,*** in-

creased appetite, cramps, epigastric distress, jaundice, ***hepatitis,*** stomatitis
GU: Retention, ***acute renal failure***
INTEG: Rash, urticaria, sweating, pruritus, photosensitivity
CV: Orthostatic hypotension, ECG changes, tachycardia, ***hypertension,*** palpitations
EENT: Blurred vision, tinnitus, mydriasis, ophthalmoplegia
Contraindications: Hypersensitivity to tricyclic antidepressants, recovery phase of myocardial infarction, narrow-angle glaucoma, convulsive disorders, prostatic hypertrophy, child <12 yr
Precautions: Suicidal patients, severe depression, increased intraocular pressure, narrow-angle glaucoma, elderly, pregnancy (C)
Pharmacokinetics:
PO: Steady state 2-11 days; metabolized by liver, excreted by kidneys, crosses placenta, half-life 14-62 hr
Interactions/incompatibilities:
- Decreased effects of: guanethidine, clonidine, indirect acting sympathomimetics (ephedrine)
- Increased effects of: direct acting sympathomimetics (epinephrine) alcohol, barbiturates, benzodiazepines, CNS depressants
- Hyperpyretic crisis, convulsions, hypertensive episode: MAOI (pargyline [Eutonyl])

NURSING CONSIDERATIONS

Assess:
- B/P (lying, standing), pulse q4h; if systolic B/P drops 20 mm Hg hold drug, notify physician; take vital signs q4h in patients with cardiovascular disease
- Blood studies: CBC, leukocytes, differential, cardiac enzymes if patient is receiving long-term therapy
- Hepatic studies: AST, ALT, bilirubin, creatinine
- Weight qwk, appetite may increase with drug
- ECG for flattening of T wave, bundle branch block, AV block, dysrhythmias in cardiac patients

Administer:
- Increased fluids, bulk in diet if constipation, urinary retention occur, especially in elderly
- With food or milk for GI symptoms
- Crushed if patient is unable to swallow medication whole
- Dosage hs if oversedation occurs during day; may take entire dose hs; elderly may not tolerate once/day dosing
- Gum, hard candy, or frequent sips of water for dry mouth

Perform/provide:
- Storage at room temperature
- Assistance with ambulation during beginning therapy since drowsiness/dizziness occurs
- Safety measures including siderails primarily in elderly
- Checking to see PO medication swallowed

Evaluate:
- Therapeutic response: decreased depression
- EPS primarily in elderly: rigidity, dystonia, akathisia
- Mental status: mood, sensorium, affect, suicidal tendencies, an increase in psychiatric symptoms: depression, panic
- Urinary retention, constipation; constipation is more likely to occur in children
- Withdrawal symptoms: headache, nausea, vomiting, muscle pain, weakness; do not usually occur unless drug was discontinued abruptly
- Alcohol consumption; if alco-

* Available in Canada only

hol is consumed, hold dose until morning

Teach patient/family:

- That therapeutic effects may take 2-3 wk
- To use caution in driving or other activities requiring alertness because of drowsiness, dizziness, blurred vision
- To avoid alcohol ingestion, other CNS depressants
- Not to discontinue medication quickly after long-term use; may cause nausea, headache, malaise
- To wear sunscreen or large hat since photosensitivity occurs

Lab test interferences:

Increase: Serum bilirubin, blood glucose, alk phosphatase

False increase: Urinary catecholamines

Decrease: VMA, 5-HIAA

Treatment of overdose: ECG monitoring, induce emesis, lavage, activated charcoal, administer anticonvulsant

desmopressin acetate

(des-moe-press'in)

DDAVP, Stimate

Func. class.: Pituitary hormone

Chem. class.: Synthetic antidiuretic hormone

Action: Promotes reabsorption of water by action on renal tubular epithelium; causes smooth muscle constriction, resulting in vasopressor effect

Uses: Hemophilia A, von Willebrand's disease Type 1, nonnephrogenic diabetes insipidus, symptoms of polyuria/polydipsia caused by pituitary dysfunction

Dosage and routes:

Diabetes insipidus

- *Adult:* INTRANASAL 0.1-0.4 ml qd in divided doses: IV/SC 0.5-1 ml qd in divided doses
- *Child 3 mo to 12 yr:* INTRANASAL 0.05-0.3 ml qd in divided doses

Hemophilia/von Willebrand's disease

- *Adult and child:* IV 0.3 μg/kg in NaCl over 15-30 min; may repeat if needed

Available forms include: INTRANASAL 0.1 mg/ml; inj IV, SC 4 μg/ml

Side effects/adverse reactions:

EENT: Nasal irritation, congestion, rhinitis

CNS: Drowsiness, headache, lethargy, flushing

GU: Vulval pain

GI: Nausea, heartburn, cramps

CV: Increased B/P

Contraindications: Hypersensitivity, nephrogenic diabetes insipidus

Precautions: Pregnancy (B), CAD, lactation, hypertension, coronary artery disease

Pharmacokinetics:

NASAL: Onset 1 hr, peak 1-2 hr, duration 8-20 hr, half-life 8 min, 76 min (terminal)

Interactions/incompatibilities:

- Increased response: carbamazepine, chlorpropamide, clofibrate

NURSING CONSIDERATIONS

Assess:

- Pulse, B/P when giving drug IV or SC
- I&O ratio, weight daily; check for edema in extremities; if water retention is severe, diuretic may be prescribed

Perform/provide:

- Storage in refrigerator or cool environment

Evaluate:

- Therapeutic response: absence of severe thirst, decreased urine output, osmolality

• Water intoxication: lethargy, behavioral changes, disorientation, neuromuscular excitability
• Intranasal use: nausea, congestion, cramps, headache, usually decreased with decreased dose

Teach patient/family:
• Technique for nasal instillation: to insert tube into nasal cavity to instill drug
• To avoid OTC products: cough, hayfever products since these preparations may contain epinephrine, decrease drug response; do not use with alcohol
• To wear Medic Alert ID specifying therapy

---

desonide

(dess'oh-nide)
DesOwen, Tridesilon

Func. class.: Topical corticosteroid
Chem. class.: Synthetic nonfluorinated agent, group IV potency

Action: Possesses antipruritic, antiinflammatory actions
Uses: Psoriasis, eczema, contact dermatitis, pruritus
Dosage and routes:
• *Adult and child:* Apply to affected area bid-tid
Available forms include: Cream 0.05%; oint 0.05%
Side effects/adverse reactions:
INTEG: Burning, dryness, itching, irritation, acne, folliculitis, hypertrichosis, perioral dermatitis, hypopigmentation, atrophy, striae, miliaria, allergic contact dermatitis, secondary infection
Contraindications: Hypersensitivity to corticosteroids, fungal infections
Precautions: Pregnancy (C), lactation, viral infections, bacterial infections

NURSING CONSIDERATIONS

Assess:
• Temperature; if fever develops, drug should be discontinued

Administer:
• Only to affected areas; do not get in eyes
• Medication, then cover with occlusive dressing (only if prescribed), seal to normal skin, change q12h; systemic absorption may occur
• Only to dermatoses; do not use on weeping, denuded, or infected area

Perform/provide:
• Cleansing before application of drug
• Treatment for a few days after area has cleared
• Storage at room temperature

Evaluate:
• Therapeutic response: absence of severe itching, patches on skin, flaking
• For systemic absorption: increased temperature, inflammation, irritation

Teach patient/family:
• To avoid sunlight on affected area; burns may occur

---

desoximetasone

(des-ox-i-met'a-sone)
Topicort, Topicort LP

Func. class.: Topical corticosteroid
Chem. class.: Synthetic fluorinated agent, group II potency (0.25%), group III potency (0.05%)

Action: Possesses antipruritic, antiinflammatory actions
Uses: Psoriasis, eczema, contact dermatitis, pruritus
Dosage and routes:
• *Adult and child:* TOP apply to affected area bid-tid

Available forms include: Cream 0.05% (LP), 0.25%; oint 0.25%; gel 0.05%
Side effects/adverse reactions: *INTEG:* Burning, dryness, itching, irritation, acne, folliculitis, hypertrichosis, perioral dermatitis, hypopigmentation, atrophy, striae, miliaria, allergic contact dermatitis, secondary infection
Contraindications: Hypersensitivity to corticosteroids, fungal infections
Precautions: Pregnancy (C), lactation, viral infections, bacterial infections

NURSING CONSIDERATIONS

Assess:
- Temperature; if fever develops, drug should be discontinued

Administer:
- Only to affected areas; do not get in eyes
- Medication, then cover with occlusive dressing (only if prescribed), seal to normal skin, change q12h; use occlusive dressing with extreme caution (group II potency), systemic absorption may occur
- Only to dermatoses; do not use on weeping, denuded, or infected area

Perform/provide:
- Cleansing before application of drug
- Treatment for a few days after area has cleared
- Storage at room temperature

Evaluate:
- Therapeutic response: absence of severe itching, patches on skin, flaking
- For systemic absorption: increased temperature, inflammation, irritation

Teach patient/family:
- To avoid sunlight on affected area; burns may occur

dexamethasone

(dex-a-meth'a-sone)
Aeroseb-Dex, Decaderm, Decaspray
Func. class.: Topical corticosteroid
Chem. class.: Synthetic fluorinated agent

Action: Possesses antipruritic, antiinflammatory actions
Uses: Corticosteroid-responsive dermatoses
Dosage and routes:
- *Adult and child:* TOP apply to affected area bid-qid

Available forms include: Gel 0.1%; aerosol 0.01%, 0.04%
Side effects/adverse reactions: *INTEG:* Burning, dryness, itching, irritation, acne, folliculitis, hypertrichosis, perioral dermatitis, hypopigmentation, atrophy, striae, miliaria, allergic contact dermatitis, secondary infection
Contraindications: Hypersensitivity to corticosteroids, fungal infections, viral infections
Precautions: Pregnancy (C), lactation, viral infections, bacterial infections

NURSING CONSIDERATIONS

Assess:
- Temperature, if fever develops drug should be discontinued

Administer:
- Only to affected areas, do not get in eyes
- Then cover with occlusive dressing if ordered, seal to normal skin, change q12h, systemic absorption may occur
- Only to dermatoses, do not use on weeping, denuded or infected area

Perform/provide:
- Cleansing before application of drug

• Treatment for a few days after area has cleared
• Storage at room temperature

Evaluate:
• Therapeutic response: absence of severe itching, patches on skin, flaking
• Systemic absorption: fever, infection, irritation

Teach patient/family:
• To avoid sunlight on affected area; burns may occur

---

dexamethasone/dexamethasone acetate/dexamethasone sodium phosphate

(dex-a-meth'a-sone)

Decadron, Dexamethasone Intensol, Dexasone,* Dexone, Hexadrol/Dalalone-LA, Decadron-LA, Decaject-LA, Decameth-LA, Dexcen-LA, Dexasone-LA, Dexone-LA/Decadron Phosphate, Decaject, Decameth, Dexacen-4, Dexasone, Dexone, Hexadrol Phosphate

Func. class.: Corticosteroid
Chem. class.: Glucocorticoid, long-acting

Action: Decreases inflammation by suppression of migration of polymorphonuclear leukocytes, fibroblasts, reversal of increased capillary permeability and lysosomal stabilization

Uses: Inflammation, allergies, neoplasms, cerebral edema, shock, collagen disorders

Dosage and routes:

Inflammation
• *Adult:* PO 0.25-4 mg bid-qid
IM 4-16 mg q1-3 wk (acetate)

Shock
• *Adult:* IV 1-6 mg/kg or 40 mg q2-6h (phosphate)

Cerebral edema
• *Adult:* IV 10 mg, then 4-6 mg IM q6h × 2-4 days, then taper over 1 wk
• *Child:* PO 0.2 mg/kg/day in divided doses

Available forms include: Tabs 0.25, 0.5, 0.75, 1, 1.5, 3, 4, 6 mg; inj IM acetate 8, 16 mg/ml; inj IV phosphate 4, 10 mg/ml; elix 0.5 mg/5 ml; oral sol 0.5 mg/5 ml, 0.5 mg/1 ml

Side effects/adverse reactions:
INTEG: Acne, poor wound healing, ecchymosis, petechiae
CNS: Depression, flushing, sweating, headache, mood changes
CV: Hypertension, ***circulatory collapse, thrombophlebitis, embolism,*** tachycardia, edema
HEMA: ***Thrombocytopenia***
MS: Fractures, osteoporosis, weakness
GI: Diarrhea, nausea, abdominal distention, ***GI hemorrhage,*** *increased appetite,* ***pancreatitis***
EENT: Fungal infections, increased intraocular pressure, blurred vision

Contraindications: Psychosis, hypersensitivity, idiopathic thrombocytopenia, acute glomerulonephritis, amebiasis, fungal infections, nonasthmatic bronchial disease, child <2 yr, AIDS, TB

Precautions: Pregnancy (C), diabetes mellitus, glaucoma, osteoporosis, seizure disorders, ulcerative colitis, CHF, myasthenia gravis, renal disease, peptic ulcer, esophagitis

Pharmacokinetics:
PO: Peak 1-2 h, duration 2⅓ days
IM: Peak 8 h, duration 6 days
Half-life 3-4½ hr

Interactions/incompatibilities:
• Decreased action of dexamethasone: cholestyramine, colestipol, barbiturates, rifampin, ephedrine,

---

* Available in Canada only

phenytoin, theophylline, antacids
• Decreased effects of: anticoagulants, anticonvulsants, antidiabetics, ambenonium, neostigmine, isoniazid, toxoids, vaccines, anticholinesterases, salicylates, somatrem
• Increased side effects: alcohol, salicylates, indomethacin, amphotericin B, digitalis, cyclosporine, diuretics
• Increased action of dexamethasone: salicylates, estrogens, indomethacin, oral contraceptives, ketoconazole, macrolide antibiotics

NURSING CONSIDERATIONS

Assess:
• Potassium, blood sugar, urine glucose while on long-term therapy; hypokalemia and hyperglycemia
• Weight daily, notify physician of weekly gain >5 lb
• B/P q4h, pulse; notify physician if chest pain occurs
• I&O ratio; be alert for decreasing urinary output and increasing edema
• Plasma cortisol levels during long-term therapy (normal level: 138-635 nmol/L SI units when drawn at 8 AM)

Administer:
• IV after diluting or undiluted; give over 1 min; may be further diluted with normal saline or D_5W
• After shaking suspension (parenteral); do not give suspension IV
• Titrated dose, use lowest effective dose
• IM inj deeply in large mass, rotate sites, avoid deltoid, use 21G needle
• In one dose in AM to prevent adrenal suppression; avoid SC administration, damage may be done to tissue
• With food or milk to decrease GI symptoms

Perform/provide:
• Assistance with ambulation in patient with bone tissue disease to prevent fractures

Evaluate:
• Therapeutic response: ease of respirations, decreased inflammation
• Infection: increased temperature, WBC even after withdrawal of medication; drug masks symptoms of infection
• Potassium depletion: paresthesias, fatigue, nausea, vomiting, depression, polyuria, dysrhythmias, weakness
• Edema, hypertension, cardiac symptoms
• Mental status: affect, mood, behavioral changes, aggression

Teach patient/family:
• That ID as steroid user should be carried
• To notify physician if therapeutic response decreases; dosage adjustment may be needed
• Not to discontinue this medication abruptly or adrenal crisis can result
• To avoid OTC products: salicylates, alcohol in cough products, cold preparations unless directed by physician
• To teach patient all aspects of drug usage, including cushingoid symptoms
• Symptoms of adrenal insufficiency: nausea, anorexia, fatigue, dizziness, dyspnea, weakness, joint pain

Lab test interferences:
Increase: Cholesterol, sodium, blood glucose, uric acid, calcium, urine glucose
Decrease: Calcium, potassium, T_4, T_3, thyroid ^{131}I uptake test, urine 17-OHCS, 17-KS, PBI

D

False negative: Skin allergy tests

dexamethasone/dexamethasone sodium phosphate

(dex-a-meth'a-sone)

Ophthalmic Suspension/Decadron Phosphate Ophthalmics, Maxidex Ophthalmic

Func. class.: Ophthalmic antiinflammatory

Action: Results in decreased inflammation, resulting in decreased pain, photophobia, hyperemia, cellular infiltration

Uses: Inflammation of eye, lids, conjunctiva, cornea, uveitis, iridocyclitis, allergic condition, burns, foreign bodies

Dosage and routes:

• *Adult and child:* Instill 1-2 gtts into conjunctival sac q1-4h depending on condition

Available forms include: Oint 0.05%; ophthalmic sol 0.1%

Side effects/adverse reactions:

EENT: ***Increased intraocular pressure,*** poor corneal wound healing, increased possibility of corneal infection, glaucoma exacerbation, ***optic nerve damage,*** decreased acuity, visual field, cataracts

Contraindications: Hypersensitivity, acute superficial herpes simplex, fungal/viral diseases of the eye or conjunctiva, active diabetes mellitus, ocular TB, infections of the eye

Precautions: Corneal abrasions, glaucoma, pregnancy (C)

NURSING CONSIDERATIONS

Perform/provide:

• Storage in light-resistant container

Evaluate:

• Therapeutic response: absence of swelling, redness, exudate

Teach patient/family:

• Instillation method: pressure on lacrimal duct for 1 min

• Not to share eye medications with others

• Not to use if purulent drainage is present

• To shake before using

• Not to discontinue abruptly, taper over 1-2 wk

dexamethasone sodium phosphate

(dex-a-meth'a-sone)

Decadron Phosphate

Func. class.: Topical corticosteroid
Chem. class.: Synthetic fluorinated agent, group VI potency

Action: Possesses antipruritic, antiinflammatory actions

Uses: Psoriasis, eczema, contact dermatitis, pruritus

Dosage and routes:

• *Adult and child:* Apply to affected area tid-qid

Available forms include: Cream 0.1%

Side effects/adverse reactions:

INTEG: Burning, dryness, itching, irritation, acne, folliculitis, hypertrichosis, perioral dermatitis, hypopigmentation, atrophy, striae, miliaria, allergic contact dermatitis, secondary infection

Contraindications: Hypersensitivity to corticosteroids, fungal infections

Precautions: Pregnancy (C), lactation, viral infections, bacterial infections

NURSING CONSIDERATIONS

Assess:

• Temperature; if fever develops, drug should be discontinued

Administer:

• Only to affected areas; do not get in eyes

• Medication, then cover with occlusive dressing (only if prescribed), seal to normal skin, change q12h, systemic absorption may occur
• Only to dermatoses; do not use on weeping, denuded, or infected area

Perform/provide:
• Cleansing before application of drug
• Treatment for a few days after area has cleared
• Storage at room temperature

Evaluate:
• Therapeutic response: absence of severe itching, patches on skin, flaking
• For systemic absorption: increased temperature, inflammation, irritation

Teach patient/family:
• To avoid sunlight on affected area; burns may occur

---

dexamethasone sodium phosphate (nasal)

(dex-a-meth'a-sone)

Decadron Phosphate Turbinaire

Func. class.: Steroid, intranasal
Chem. class.: Glucocorticoid

Action: Long-acting synthetic adrenocorticoid with antiinflammatory activity, minimal mineralocorticoid properties

Uses: Inflammation (not within sinuses), nasal polyps, allergic conditions of nose

Dosage and routes:
• *Adult:* SPRAY 1-2 sprays bid-tid, not to exceed 12/day
• *Child 6-12 yr:* SPRAY 1-2 sprays bid, not to exceed 8/day

Available forms include: 84 μg/metered spray

Side effects/adverse reactions:
EENT: Nasal irritation, dryness, rebound congestion, epistaxis, sneezing, ***infarction of nasal mucosa***
INTEG: Urticaria
CNS: Headache, dizziness
SYSTEMIC: ***CHF, convulsions,*** increased sodium, hypertension

Contraindications: Hypersensitivity, child <12 yr, localized infection of nose, acute status asthmaticus

Precautions: Lactation, nasal trauma, pregnancy (C)

NURSING CONSIDERATIONS

Administer:
• After cleaning spray container daily with warm water, dry thoroughly

Perform/provide:
• Storage in cool environment, do not puncture or incinerate container

Evaluate:
• Therapeutic response: decreased inflammation, redness
• Adrenal suppression: 17-KS, plasma cortisol for decreased levels
• Nasal passages during long-term treatment for changes in mucus
• For edema, increased B/P, increase in K^+ during treatment, which indicates systemic absorption

Teach patient/family:
• To clear nasal passages if sneezing attack occurs, repeat dose
• To continue using product even if mild nasal bleeding occurs, is usually transient
• Method of instillation after providing written instructions from manufacturer
• To clear nasal passages before administration, use decongestant if needed, shake inhaler, invert, tilt head backward, insert nozzle into nostril, away from septum, hold other nostril closed, depress acti-

vator, inhale through nose, exhale through mouth

- To decrease gradually if drug has been used consistently
- That only 1 person should use a single-container drug
- If irritation, dryness, epistaxis occur, that drug may need to be discontinued
- That benefit requires regular use, will not occur after several days

dexchlorpheniramine maleate

(dex-klor-fen-eer'a-meen)

Polaramine

Func. class.: Antihistamine
Chem. class.: Alkylamine derivative, H_1-receptor antagonist

Action: Acts on blood vessels, GI, respiratory system by competing with histamine for H_1-receptor site; decreases allergic response by blocking histamine

Uses: Allergy symptoms, rhinitis, pruritus, contact dermatitis

Dosage and routes:

- *Adult:* PO 1-2 mg tid-qid; REPEAT ACTION 4-6 mg bid-tid
- *Child 6-11 yr:* PO 1 mg q4-6h, or TIME REL 4 mg hs
- *Child 2-5 yr:* PO 0.5 mg q4-6h; do not use repeat action form

Available forms include: Tabs 2 mg; repeat-action tab 4, 6 mg; syr 2 mg/5 ml

Side effects/adverse reactions:

CNS: Dizziness, drowsiness, poor coordination, fatigue, anxiety, euphoria, confusion, paresthesia, neuritis

CV: Hypotension, palpitations, tachycardia

RESP: Increased thick secretions, wheezing, chest tightness

GI: Constipation, dry mouth, nausea, vomiting, anorexia, diarrhea

INTEG: Rash, urticaria, photosensitivity

GU: Retention, dysuria, frequency

EENT: Blurred vision, dilated pupils, tinnitus, nasal stuffiness, dry nose, throat, mouth

Contraindications: Hypersensitivity to H_1-receptor antagonist; acute asthma attack, lower respiratory tract disease

Precautions: Increased intraocular pressure, renal disease, cardiac disease, hypertension, bronchial asthma, seizure disorder, stenosed peptic ulcers, hyperthyroidism, prostatic hypertrophy, bladder neck obstruction, pregnancy (B), elderly

Pharmacokinetics:

PO: Onset 15 min, peak 3 hr, duration 3-6 hr, metabolized in liver, excreted by kidneys (inactive metabolites), excreted in breast milk (small amounts)

Interactions/incompatibilities:

- Increased CNS depression: barbiturates, narcotics, hypnotics, tricyclic antidepressants, alcohol
- Decreased effect of: oral anticoagulants, heparin
- Increased effect of dexchlorpheniramine: MAOIs

NURSING CONSIDERATIONS

Assess:

- I&O ratio; be alert for urinary retention, frequency, dysuria; drug should be discontinued if these occur
- CBC during long-term therapy

Administer:

- With meals if GI symptoms occur, absorption may slightly decrease

Perform/provide:

- Hard candy, gum, frequent rinsing of mouth for dryness
- Storage in tight container at room temperature

* Available in Canada only

Evaluate:
• Therapeutic response: absence of running or congested nose or rashes
• Respiratory status: rate, rhythm, increase in bronchial secretions, wheezing, chest tightness
• Cardiac status: palpitations, increased pulse, hypotension

Teach patient/family:
• All aspects of drug use; to notify physician if confusion, sedation, hypotension occurs
• To avoid driving or other hazardous activity if drowsiness occurs, especially elderly
• To avoid concurrent use of alcohol or other CNS depressants

Lab test interferences:
False negative: Skin allergy tests

Treatment of overdose: Administer ipecac syrup or lavage, diazepam, vasopressors, barbiturates (short-acting)

dextran 40

Gentran 40, LMD, Rheomacrodex

Func. class.: Plasma volume expander

Chem. class.: Low molecular weight polysaccharide

Action: Similar to human albumin, which expands plasma volume by drawing fluid from interstitial space to intravascular space

Uses: Expand plasma volume, prophylaxis of embolism, thrombosis

Dosage and routes:

Shock
• *Adult:* IV INF 500 ml over 15-30 min, total dose in 24 hr not to exceed 20 ml/kg then subsequent doses given slowly, if given >24 hr, not to exceed 10 ml/kg/day, not to exceed therapy >5 days

Thrombosis/embolism
• *Adult:* IV INF 500-1000 ml, then 500 ml/day × 3 days, then 500 ml q2-3 days × 2 wk if needed

Available forms include: 10% dextran 40/5% dextrose, 10% dextran 40/0.9% sodium chloride

Side effects/adverse reactions:
HEMA: Decreased hematocrit, platelet function, increased bleeding/coagulation times
INTEG: Rash, urticaria, pruritus, angioedema, chills, fever, flushing
RESP: Wheezing, dyspnea, ***bronchospasm, pulmonary edema***
CV: Hypotension, ***cardiac arrest***
GU: ***Osmotic nephrosis, renal failure, stasis,*** hyponatremia
GI: Nausea, vomiting, increased AST, ALT
SYST: ***Anaphylaxis***

Contraindications: Hypersensitivity, renal failure, CHF (severe), extreme dehydration

Precautions: Active hemorrhage, pregnancy (C)

Pharmacokinetics:
IV: Expands blood volume 1-2 × amount infused, excreted in urine and feces

NURSING CONSIDERATIONS

Assess:
• VS q5min × 30 min
• CVP during infusion (5-10 cm H_2O—normal range)
• Urine output q1h; watch for increase in urinary output, which is common; if output does not increase, infusion should be decreased or discontinued
• I&O ratio and specific gravity, urine osmolarity; if specific gravity is very low, renal clearance is low, drug should be discontinued

Administer:
• After crossmatch is drawn, if blood is to be given also
• Dextran 1 (Promit) to prevent anaphylaxis if ordered

Perform/provide:

- Storage at constant temperature 15° C (59° F) to 30° C (86° F); discard unused portions, protect from freezing

Evaluate:

- Therapeutic response: increased plasma volume
- Allergy: rash, urticaria, pruritus, wheezing, dyspnea, bronchospasm, drug should be discontinued immediately
- Circulatory overload: increased pulse, respirations, SOB, wheezing, chest tightness, chest pain
- Dehydration after infusion: decreased output, decreased sp. gravity of urine, increased temperature, poor skin turgor, increased specific gravity, dry skin

Lab test interferences:

False increase: Blood glucose, urinary protein, bilirubin, total protein

Interference: Rh test, blood typing/crossmatching

---

dextran 70/75

Gentran 75, Macrodex

Func. class.: Plasma volume expander

Chem. class.: High molecular weight polysaccharide

Action: Similar to human albumin, which expands plasma volume by drawing fluid from interstitial spaces to intravascular space

Uses: Expand plasma volume in hypovolemic shock or impending shock

Dosage and routes:

- *Adult:* IV INF 500-1000 ml not to exceed 20-40 ml/min, not to exceed 10 ml/kg/24 hr if therapy >24 hr

Available forms include: 70/75 dextran in 0.9% NaCl, D_5%

Side effects/adverse reactions:

HEMA: Decreased hematocrit, platelet function, increased bleeding/coagulation times

INTEG: Rash, urticaria, pruritus, angioedema, chills, fever, flushing

RESP: Wheezing, dyspnea, ***bronchospasm, pulmonary edema***

CV: Hypotension, ***cardiac arrest***

GU: ***Osmotic nephrosis, renal failure, stasis,*** hypernatremia

GI: Nausea, vomiting, increase AST, ALT

SYST: ***Anaphylaxis***

Contraindications: Hypersensitivity, renal failure, CHF (severe), extreme dehydration

Precautions: Active hemorrhage, pregnancy (C)

Pharmacokinetics:

IV: Expands blood volume 1-2 × amount infused, excreted in urine and feces

NURSING CONSIDERATIONS

Assess:

- VS q5min × 30 min
- CVP during infusion (5-10 cm H_2O—normal range)
- Urine output q1h, watch for increase in urinary output, which is common; if output does not increase, infusion should be decreased or discontinued
- I&O ratio and specific gravity, urine osmolarity; if specific gravity is very low, renal clearance is low, drug should be discontinued

Administer:

- After crossmatch is drawn, if blood is to be given also
- Dextran 1 (Promit) to prevent anaphylaxis

Perform/provide:

- Storage at constant temperature <25° C (77° F); discard unused portions, do not use unless clear

Evaluate:

- Therapeutic response: increased plasma volume

---

* Available in Canada only

• Allergy: rash, urticaria, pruritus, wheezing, dyspnea, bronchospasm, drug should be discontinued immediately
• Circulatory overload: increased pulse, respirations, SOB, wheezing, chest tightness, chest pain
• Dehydration after infusion: decreased output, increased temperature, poor skin turgor, increased specific gravity, dry skin

Lab test interferences:
False increase: Blood glucose, urinary protein, bilirubin, total protein
Interferes: Rh test, blood typing/crossmatching

---

dextroamphetamine sulfate

(dex-troe-am-fet'a-meen)

Dexedrine, Ferndex, Oxydess II, Spancap #1

Func. class.: Cerebral stimulant
Chem. class.: Amphetamine

Controlled Substance Schedule II

Action: Increases release of norepinephrine, dopamine in cerebral cortex to reticular activating system

Uses: Narcolepsy, exogenous obesity, attention deficit disorder with hyperactivity

Dosage and routes:

Narcolepsy
• *Adult:* PO 5-60 mg qd in divided doses
• *Child >12 yr:* PO 10 mg qd increasing by 10 mg/day at weekly intervals
• *Child 6-12 yr:* PO 5 mg qd increasing by 5 mg/wk (max 60 mg/day)

Attention deficit disorder
• *Child >6 yr:* PO 5 mg qd-bid increasing by 5 mg/day at weekly intervals
• *Child 3-6 yr:* PO 2.5 mg qd increasing by 2.5 mg/day at weekly intervals

Obesity
• *Adult:* PO 10-30 mg/day (sus rel) or 5-10 mg qd 30-60 min before meals

Available forms include: Tabs 5, 10 mg; caps sus rel 5, 10, 15 mg; elix 5 mg/5 ml

Side effects/adverse reactions:
CNS: Hyperactivity, insomnia, restlessness, talkativeness, dizziness, headache, chills, stimulation, dysphoria, irritability, aggressiveness, tremor
GI: Anorexia, dry mouth, diarrhea, constipation, weight loss, metallic taste
GU: Impotence, change in libido
CV: Palpitations, tachycardia, hypertension, decrease in heart rate, dysrhythmias
INTEG: Urticaria

Contraindications: Hypersensitivity to sympathomimetic amines, hyperthyroidism, hypertension, glaucoma hypertrophy, severe arteriosclerosis, drug abuse, cardiovascular disease, anxiety

Precautions: Gilles de la Tourette's disorder, pregnancy (C), lactation, child <3 yr

Pharmacokinetics:
PO: Onset 30 min, peak 1-3 hr, duration 4-20 hr, metabolized by liver, urine excretion pH dependent, crosses placenta, breast milk, half-life 10-30 hr

Interactions/incompatibilities:
• Hypertensive crisis: MAOIs or within 14 days of MAOIs
• Increased effect of dextroamphetamine: acetazolamide, antacids, sodium bicarbonate, phenothiazines, haloperidol
• Decreased effect of dextroamphetamine: barbiturates, ascorbic acid, ammonium chloride
• Decreased effect of: guanethidine

NURSING CONSIDERATIONS

Assess:

• VS, B/P since this drug may reverse antihypertensives check patients with cardiac disease more often

• CBC, urinalysis; in diabetes: blood sugar, urine sugar; insulin changes may need to be made since eating will decrease

• Height, growth rate in children; growth rate may be decreased

Administer:

• At least 6 hr before hs to avoid sleeplessness

• For obesity only if the patient is on a weight reduction program including dietary changes and exercise; patient will develop tolerance and weight loss won't occur without additional methods, give 30-60 min before meals

• Gum, hard candy, frequent sips of water for dry mouth

Evaluate:

• Therapeutic response: increased CNS stimulation, decreased drowsiness

• Mental status: mood, sensorium, affect, stimulation, insomnia, irritability

• Tolerance or dependency: an increased amount may be used to get same effect; will develop after long-term use

• Overdose: pain, fever, dehydration, insomnia, hyperactivity

Teach patient/family:

• Not to crush or chew sus rel forms

• To decrease caffeine consumption (coffee, tea, cola, chocolate), which may increase irritability, stimulation

• To avoid OTC preparations unless approved by the physician

• To taper off drug over several weeks or depression, increased sleeping, lethargy

• To avoid alcohol ingestion

• To avoid hazardous activities until patient is stabilized on medication

• To get needed rest, patients will feel more tired at end of day

Treatment of overdose: Administer fluids, hemodialysis or peritoneal dialysis; antihypertensive for increased B/P, ammonium Cl for increased excretion

---

dextromethorphan hydrobromide

(dex-troe-meth-or'fan)

Creamcoat, Pertussin 8-hour, Mediquell, Robitussin DM, Sucrets, Hold

Func. class.: Antitussive, nonnarcotic

Chem. class.: Levorphanol derivative

Action: Depresses cough center in medulla

Uses: Nonproductive cough

Dosage and routes:

• *Adult:* PO 10-20 mg q4h, or 30 mg q6-8h, not to exceed 120 mg/day; CON-REL LIQ 60 mg bid, not to exceed 120 mg/day

• *Child 6-12 yr:* PO 5-10 mg q4h; CON-REL LIQ 30 mg bid, not to exceed 60 mg/day

• *Child 2-6 yr:* PO 2.5-5 mg q4h, or 7.5 mg q6-8h, not to exceed 30 mg/day

Available forms include: Loz 5 mg; sol 5, 7.5, 10, 15 mg/5 ml

Side effects/adverse reactions:

CNS: Dizziness

GI: Nausea

Contraindications: Hypersensitivity, asthma/emphysema, productive cough

Precautions: Nausea/vomiting,

*Available in Canada only

increased temperature, persistent headache, pregnancy (C)

Pharmacokinetics:

PO: Onset 15-30 min, duration 3-6 hr

Interactions/incompatibilities:

• Do not give with MAOIs, penicillins, salicylates, tetracyclines, phenobarbital, iodines (high doses)

NURSING CONSIDERATIONS

Administer:

• Decreased dose to elderly patients; their metabolism may be slowed

Perform/provide:

• Increased fluids to liquefy secretions

• Humidification of patient's room

Evaluate:

• Therapeutic response: absence of cough

• Cough: type, frequency, character including sputum

Teach patient/family:

• To avoid driving or other hazardous activities until patient is stabilized on this medication

• To avoid smoking, smoke-filled rooms, perfumes, dust, environmental pollutants, cleaners that increase cough

---

dextrose (*D*-glucose)

Func. class.: Caloric

Action: Needed for adequate utilization of amino acids, decreases protein, nitrogen loss, prevents ketosis

Uses: Increases intake of calories, increases fluids in patients unable to take adequate fluids, calories orally

Dosage and routes:

• *Adult and child:* IV depends on individual requirements

Available forms include: Inj IV 2.5%, 5%, 10%, 20%, 40%, 50%

Side effects/adverse reactions:

CNS: Confusion, ***loss of consciousness,*** dizziness

CV: Hypertension, ***CHF, pulmonary edema***

GU: ***Glycosuria, osmotic diuresis***

ENDO: Hyperglycemia, rebound hypoglycemia, hyperosmolar syndrome, hyperglycemic nonketotic syndrome

INTEG: Chills, flushing, warm feeling, rash, urticaria, extravasation necrosis

Contraindications: Hyperglycemia, delirium tremens, hemorrhage (cranial/spinal), CHF

Precautions: Renal, liver, cardiac disease, diabetes mellitus

NURSING CONSIDERATIONS

Assess:

• Electrolytes (K, Na, Ca, Cl, Mg), blood glucose, ammonia, phosphate

• Renal, liver function studies: BUN, creatinine, ALT, AST, bilirubin

• Injection site for extravasation: redness along vein, edema at site, necrosis, pain, hard tender area; site should be changed immediately

• Monitor respiratory function q4h: auscultate lung fields bilaterally for crackles, respirations, quality, rate, rhythm

• Monitor temperature q4h for increased fever, indicating infection; if infection suspected, infusion is discontinued, tubing, bottle, catheter tip cultured

• Urine glucose q6h using Chemstrips, which are not affected by infusion substances

Administer:

• After changing IV catheter, dressing q24h with aseptic technique

Evaluate:
- Therapeutic response: increased weight
- Nutritional status: calorie count by dietitian

Teach patient/family
- Reason for dextrose infusion

---

dextrothyroxine sodium

(dex-troe-thye-rox'een)

Choloxin

Func. class.: Antilipemic
Chem. class.: Hormone isomer

Action: Stimulates hepatic catabolism, excretion of cholesterol; increases bile products into feces

Uses: Hyperlipidemia in euthyroid patients with no evidence of organic heart disease

Dosage and routes:
- *Adult:* PO 1-2 mg/day, may increase 1-2 mg/day qmo, not to exceed 8 mg/day
- *Child:* PO 0.05 mg/kg/day, may increase 0.05 mg/kg/day qmo, not to exceed 4 mg/day

Available forms include: Tabs 1, 2, 4, 6 mg

Side effects/adverse reactions:

GI: Nausea, vomiting, diarrhea, constipation, anorexia, weight loss, jaundice, gallstones

INTEG: Flushing, alopecia, sweating, hyperthermia

CV: Palpitations, dysrhythmias, ***myocardial infarction, ischemic myocardial changes,*** angina

EENT: Visual disturbances, ptosis, retinopathy, lid lag

GU: Menstrual irregularities, change in libido

CNS: Insomnia, tremors, headache, dizziness, paresthesia, decreased sensorium

Contraindications: Severe hepatic disease, severe renal disease, organic heart disease, Hx of myocardial infarction, cardiac dysrhythmias, rheumatic heart disease, CHF, hypertension, iodism, angina, obesity

Precautions: Hepatic disease, renal disease, pregnancy (C), lactation, surgery

Interactions/incompatibilities:
- Decreased effects of dextrothyroxine: cholestyramine, colestipol
- Increased effects of: digitalis, oral anticoagulants, sympathomimetics
- Increased CNS stimulation: tricyclic antidepressants
- Increased blood sugar levels in patients with diabetes
- Decreased effects of: beta blockers

NURSING CONSIDERATIONS

Assess:
- Renal and hepatic function tests, if patient is on long-term therapy
- CV status: rate, rhythm, character, chest pain

Evaluate:
- Therapeutic response: decreased cholesterol levels, (hyperlipidemia); diarrhea, pruritus (excess bile area)
- Bowel pattern daily; increase bulk, water in diet if constipation develops

Teach patient/family:
- That compliance is needed since toxicity may result if doses are missed
- That risk factors should be decreased: high fat diet, smoking, alcohol consumption, absence of exercise
- That birth control should be practiced while on this drug
- That if anticoagulants are given with this drug, this drug should be discontinued 2 wks before surgery

---

dezocine

Dalgan

Func. class.: Narcotic agonist-antagonist analgesic

Chem. class.: Opioid, synthetic

Action: Depresses pain impulse transmission at the spinal cord level by interacting with opioid receptors

Uses: Severe pain

Dosage and routes:

Adult: IM 5-20 mg q3-6h, not to exceed 120 mg/day; IV 2.5-10 mg q2-4h

Available forms include: IM, IV inj 5, 10, 15 mg single-dose vials, multiple dose 10 mg/ml

Side effects/adverse reactions:

CV: Hypotension, pulse irregularity, hypertension, chest pain, pallor, edema, thrombophlebitis

CNS: Drowsiness, dizziness, confusion, sedation, anxiety, headache, depression, delirium, sleep disturbances

GI: Nausea, vomiting, anorexia, constipation, cramps, abdominal pain, dry mouth, diarrhea

INTEG: Injection site reactions, pruritus, rash, sweating, chills

RESP: ***Respiratory depression,*** hiccups

GU: Urinary frequency, hesitancy, retention

Contraindications: Hypersensitivity

Precautions: Addictive personality, pregnancy (C), lactation, increased intracranial pressure, respiratory depression, hepatic disease, renal disease, child <18 yr, elderly, biliary surgery, COPD, sulfite sensitivity

Pharmacokinetics: IM: Onset 30 min, peak 50-90 min, duration 2-4 hr; IV: Onset 10 min, peak 30 min, duration 2-4 hr; metabolized by liver, excreted by kidneys, may cross placenta

Interactions/incompatibilities:

- Increased CNS depression: alcohol, narcotics, sedative/hypnotics, antipsychotics, skeletal muscle relaxants, general anesthetics, tranquilizers

NURSING CONSIDERATIONS

Assess:

- I&O ratio; check for decreasing output; may indicate urinary retention

Administer:

- With antiemetic if nausea, vomiting occur
- When pain is beginning to return; determine dosage interval by patient response

Perform/provide:

- Storage in light-resistant area at room temperature
- Assistance with ambulation
- Safety measures: siderails, night light, call bell within easy reach

Evaluate:

- Therapeutic response: decrease in pain
- CNS changes: dizziness, drowsiness, hallucinations, euphoria, LOC, pupil reaction
- Allergic reactions: rash, urticaria
- Respiratory dysfunction: respiratory depression, character, rate, rhythm of respirations; notify physician if respirations are <10/min
- Need for pain medication, physical dependence

Teach patient/family:

- To report any symptoms of CNS changes, allergic reactions
- That physical dependency may result when used for extended periods of time
- That withdrawal symptoms may occur: nausea, vomiting, cramps, fever, faintness, anorexia

Treatment of overdose: Naloxone

0.2-0.8 IV, O_2, IV fluids, vasopressors

diazepam

(dye-az'-e-pam)

D-Tran,* E-Pam,* Meval,* Novodipam,* Stress-Pam,* Valium, Valrelease, Vivol*

Func. class.: Antianxiety
Chem. class.: Benzodiazepine

Controlled Substance Schedule IV

Action: Depresses subcortical levels of CNS, including limbic system, reticular formation

Uses: Anxiety, acute alcohol withdrawal, adjunct in seizure disorders, preoperatively

Dosage and routes:

Anxiety/convulsive disorders

• *Adult:* PO 2-10 mg tid-qid; EXT REL 15-30 mg qd

• *Child >6 mo:* PO 1-2.5 mg tid-qid

Tetanic muscle spasms

• *Child >5 yr:* IM/IV 5-10 mg q3-4 hr prn

• *Infants >30 days:* IM/IV 1-2 mg q 3-4 hr prn

Status epilepticus

• *Adult:* IV BOLUS 5-20 mg, 2 mg/min, may repeat q5-10 min, not to exceed 60 mg, may repeat in 30 min if seizures reappear

• *Child:* IV BOLUS 0.1-0.3 mg/kg (1 mg/min over 3 min), may repeat q15 min × 2 doses

Available forms include: Tabs 2, 5, 10 mg; caps ext rel 15 mg, IM/IV inj

Side effects/adverse reactions:

CNS: Dizziness, drowsiness, confusion, headache, anxiety, tremors, stimulation, fatigue, depression, insomnia, hallucinations

GI: Constipation, dry mouth, nausea, vomiting, anorexia, diarrhea

INTEG: Rash, dermatitis, itching

CV: Orthostatic hypotension, ***ECG changes, tachycardia,*** hypotension

EENT: Blurred vision, tinnitus, mydriasis

Contraindications: Hypersensitivity to benzodiazepines, narrow-angle glaucoma, psychosis, pregnancy (D), child <18 yr

Precautions: Elderly, debilitated, hepatic disease, renal disease

Pharmacokinetics:

PO: Onset ½, duration 2-3 hr

IM: Onset 15-30 min, duration 1-1½ hr

IV: Onset 1-5 min, duration 15 min; metabolized by liver, excreted by kidneys, crosses placenta, breast milk, half-life 20-50 hr, more effective by mouth

Interactions/incompatibilities:

• Decreased effects of diazepam: oral contraceptives, rifampin, valproic acid

• Increased effects of diazepam: CNS depressants, alcohol, cimetidine, disulfiram, oral contraceptives

• Incompatible with all drugs in solution or syringe

NURSING CONSIDERATIONS

Assess:

• B/P (lying, standing), pulse; if systolic B/P drops 20 mm Hg, hold drug, notify physician; respirations q5-15 min if given IV

• Blood studies: CBC during long-term therapy, blood dyscrasias have occurred rarely

• Hepatic studies: AST, ALT, bilirubin, creatinine, LDH, alk phosphatase

Administer:

• IV into large vein; do not dilute or mix with any other drug; give IV 5 mg or less/1 min

* Available in Canada only

• With food or milk for GI symptoms
• Crushed if patient is unable to swallow medication whole
• Sugarless gum, hard candy, frequent sips of water for dry mouth
• Reduced narcotic dose by ⅓ if given concomitantly with diazepam

Perform/provide:
• Assistance with ambulation during beginning therapy, since drowsiness/dizziness occurs
• Safety measures, including siderails
• Check to see PO medication has been swallowed

Evaluate:
• Therapeutic response: decreased anxiety, restlessness, insomnia
• Mental status: mood, sensorium, affect, sleeping pattern, drowsiness, dizziness
• Physical dependency, withdrawal symptoms: headache, nausea, vomiting, muscle pain, weakness after long-term use
• Suicidal tendencies

Teach patient/family:
• That drug may be taken with food
• Not to be used for everyday stress or used longer than 4 mo, unless directed by physician; not to take more than prescribed amount, may be habit forming
• To avoid OTC preparations unless approved by physician
• To avoid driving, activities that require alertness; drowsiness may occur
• To avoid alcohol ingestion or other psychotropic medications, unless prescribed by physician
• Not to discontinue medication abruptly after long-term use
• To rise slowly or fainting may occur, especially in elderly
• That drowsiness might worsen at beginning of treatment

Lab test interferences:
Increase: AST/ALT, serum bilirubin
False increase: 17-OHCS
Decrease: RAIU

Treatment of overdose: Lavage, VS, supportive care

diazoxide

(dye-az-ox'ide)
Hyperstat
Func. class.: Antihypertensive
Chem. class.: Vasodilator

Action: Vasodilates arteriolar smooth muscle by direct relaxation; a reduction in blood pressure with concomitant increases in heart rate, cardiac output

Uses: Hypertensive crisis when urgent decrease of diastolic pressure required, increase blood glucose levels in hyperinsulinism

Dosage and routes:
• *Adult:* IV BOL 1-3 mg/kg rapidly up to a max of 150 mg in a single injection, dose may be repeated at 5-15 min intervals until desired response is achieved; give IV in 30 sec or less
• *Child:* IV BOL 1-2 mg/kg rapidly; administration same as adult, not to exceed 150 mg

Available forms include: Inj IV 15 mg/ml

Side effects/adverse reactions:
CV: ***Hypotension,*** T-wave changes, angina pectoris, palpitations, ***supraventricular tachycardia, edema,*** rebound hypertension
CNS: *Headache,* sleepiness, euphoria, anxiety, extrapyramidal symptoms, confusion, tinnitus, blurred vision, dizziness, weakness
GI: Nausea, vomiting, dry mouth
INTEG: Rash

HEMA: Decreased hemoglobin, hematocrit, ***thrombocytopenia***
GU: Breast tenderness, increased BUN, fluid, electrolyte imbalances, sodium, water retention
ENDO: Hyperglycemia in diabetics, transient hyperglycemia in nondiabetics
Contraindications: Hypersensitivity to thiazides, sulfonamides, hypertension associated with aortic coarctation or AV shunt, pheochromocytoma, dissecting aortic aneurysm
Precautions: Tachycardia, fluid, electrolyte imbalances, pregnancy (B), lactation, impaired cerebral or cardiac circulation, children
Pharmacokinetics:
IV: Onset 1-2 min, peak 5 min, duration 3-12 hr
Half-life 20-36 hr, excreted slowly in urine, crosses blood-brain barrier, placenta
Interactions/incompatibilities:
• Increased effects: thiazide diuretics, antihypertensives, coumadin, guanethidine, sympathomimetics
• Do not mix with any drug in syringe or solution
• Increased effects of: warfarin, other coumarins
• Hyperglycemia/hyperuricemia: thiazides, diuretics
• Decreased pharmacologic effects of both: sulfonylureas
NURSING CONSIDERATIONS
Assess:
• B/P q5min × 2 hr, then q1h × 2 hr, then q4h
• Pulse, jugular venous distention q4h
• Electrolytes, blood studies: potassium, sodium, chloride, CO_2, CBC, serum glucose
• Weight daily, I&O
Administer:
• Undiluted; give over ½ min or less
• To patient in recumbent position, keep in that position for 1 hr after administration
Perform/provide:
• Protection from light
Evaluate:
• Therapeutic response: decreased B/P, primarily diastolic pressure
• Edema in feet, legs daily
• Skin turgor, dryness of mucous membranes for hydration status
• Rales, dyspnea, orthopnea
• IV site for extravasation, rate
• Signs of CHF: dyspnea, edema, wet rales
• Postural hypotension, take B/P sitting, standing
Teach patient/family:
• That hirsutism is reversible after drug is discontinued
Treatment of overdose: Administer levarterenol, dopamine, or norepinephrine for hypotension, dialysis

diazoxide (oral)

(dye-az-ox'ide)
Proglycem
Func. class.: Hyperglycemic
Chem. class.: Benzothiadiazine

Action: Decreases release of insulin from β-cells in pancreas, resulting in an increase in blood glucose
Uses: Hypoglycemia caused by hyperinsulinism
Dosage and routes:
• *Adult and child:* PO 3-8 mg/kg/day in 3 divided doses q8-12h
• *Infants and neonates:* PO 8-15 mg/kg/day in 2-3 divided doses q8-12h
Available forms include: Caps 50 mg; oral susp 50 mg/ml
Side effects/adverse reactions:
CNS: Headache, weakness, mal-

aise, anxiety, dizziness, insomnia, paresthesia
EENT: Diplopia, cataracts, ring scotoma
HEMA: ***Thrombocytopenia, leukopenia,*** eosinophilia, decreased hemoglobulin, hematocrit
INTEG: Increased hair growth
GI: Nausea, vomiting, anorexia
CV: Dysrhythmias, tachycardia, palpitations, hypotension
META: Hyperuricemia, sodium/fluid retention, ketoacidosis, hyperglycemia
Contraindications: Hypersensitivity to this drug or thiazides, functional hypoglycemia
Precautions: Pregnancy (C), lactation, renal disease, diabetes mellitus, CV disease, gout
Pharmacokinetics:
PO: Onset 1 hr, duration 8 hr, half-life 20-36 min, excreted unchanged by kidneys, crosses blood-brain barrier, placenta
Interactions/incompatibilities:
- Increased effects of diazoxide: phenothiazines
- Decreased effects of: phenytoin
- Increased effects of: antihypertensives, oral anticoagulants
- Decreased effects of diazoxide: α-adrenergic blockers, sulfonylureas

NURSING CONSIDERATIONS
Assess:
- I&O ratio, weight weekly
- Electrolytes (K, Na, Cl), glucose, Hct, Hgb, platelets, differential
- Urine for glucose, ketones qd

Administer:
- Shake before using

Perform/provide:
- Sus storage: protect from light

Evaluate:
- Therapeutic response: adequate blood, urine glucose, absence of ketones in urine

Teach patient/family:
- That if drug is not effective within 2-3 wk, drug may be discontinued
- That if hirsutism occurs, it is reversible after discontinuing treatment

Lab test interferences:
Increase: Bilirubin, uric acid, blood glucose
Decrease: Creatinine, Hgb, Hct, plasma-free fatty acids

---

dibucaine HCl (topical)

(dye'byoo-kane)
D-Caine, Nupercainal
Func. class.: Topical anesthetic
Chem. class.: Amide

Action: Inhibits nerve impulses from sensory nerves, which produces anesthesia
Uses: Pruritus, sunburn, toothache, sore throat, cold sores, oral pain, rectal pain and irritation
Dosage and routes:
- *Adult and child:* TOP apply qid as needed; REC insert tid and after each BM

Available forms include: Cream 0.5%; rec or top oint 1%
Side effects/adverse reactions:
INTEG: Rash, irritation, sensitization
Contraindications: Hypersensitivity, infants <1 yr, application to large areas
Precautions: Child <6 yr, sepsis, pregnancy (C), denuded skin

NURSING CONSIDERATIONS
Administer:
- After cleansing and drying of affected area

Evaluate:
- Therapeutic response: absence of pain, itching of affected area

• Allergy: rash, irritation, reddening, swelling
• Infection: if affected area is infected, do not apply

Teach patient/family:
• To report rash, irritation, redness, swelling
• How to apply cream, ointment

---

diclofenac

(dye-kloe'-fen-ac)
Voltaren

Func. class.: Nonsteroidal antiinflammatory
Chem. class.: Phenylacetic acid

Action: Inhibits prostaglandin synthesis by decreasing enzyme needed for biosynthesis; possesses analgesic, antiinflammatory, antipyretic properties

Uses: Acute, chronic rheumatoid arthritis, osteoarthritis, ankylosing spondylitis

Dosage and routes:

Osteoarthritis
• *Adult:* PO 100-150 mg/day in divided doses

Rheumatoid arthritis
• *Adult:* PO 150-200 mg/day in divided doses

Ankylosing spondylitis
• *Adult:* PO 100-125 mg/day; give 25 mg qid and 25 mg hs if needed

Available forms include: Tabs enteric coated 25, 50, 75 mg

Side effects/adverse reactions:

GI: Nausea, anorexia, vomiting, diarrhea, ***jaundice, cholestatic hepatitis,*** constipation, flatulence, cramps, dry mouth, peptic ulcer, GI bleeding

CNS: Dizziness, drowsiness, fatigue, tremors, confusion, insomnia, anxiety, depression, nervousness, paresthesia, muscle weakness

CV: ***CHF,*** tachycardia, peripheral edema, palpitations, ***dysrhythmias,*** hypotension, hypertension, fluid retention

INTEG: Purpura, rash, pruritus, sweating, erythema, petechiae, photosensitivity, alopecia

GU: ***Nephrotoxicity: dysuria, hematuria, oliguria, azotemia, cystitis, UTI***

HEMA: ***Blood dyscrasias,*** epistaxis, bruising

EENT: Tinnitus, hearing loss, blurred vision

RESP: Dyspnea, hemoptysis, pharyngitis, ***bronchospasm, laryngeal edema,*** rhinitis, shortness of breath

Contraindications: Hypersensitivity to aspirin, iodides, other nonsteroidal antiinflammatory agents, asthma

Precautions: Pregnancy (B) 1st, 2nd trimester, lactation, children, bleeding disorders, GI disorders, cardiac disorders, hypersensitivity to other antiinflammatory agents

Pharmacokinetics:

PO: Peak 2-3 hr, elimination half-life 1-2 hr, 90% bound to plasma proteins, metabolized in liver to metabolite, excreted in urine

Interactions/incompatibilities:
• Decreased antihypertensive effect: β-blockers, diuretics
• Increased anticoagulant effect: coumarin
• Increased toxicity: phenytoin, sulfonamides, sulfonylurea
• Increased plasma levels of diclofenac: probenecid, potassium-sparing diuretics

NURSING CONSIDERATIONS

Assess:
• Blood counts during therapy, watch for decreasing platelets, if low, therapy may need to be discontinued, restarted after hematologic recovery

---

* Available in Canada only

Evaluate:
- Therapeutic response: decreased inflammation in joints
- Blood dyscrasias (thrombocytopenia): bruising, fatigue, bleeding, poor healing

Teach patient/family:
- That drug must be continued for prescribed time to be effective
- To report bleeding, bruising, fatigue, malaise since blood dyscrasias do occur
- To avoid aspirin, alcoholic beverages
- To take with food, milk, or antacids to avoid GI upset, to swallow whole
- To use caution when driving; drowsiness, dizziness may occur
- To take with a full glass of water to enhance absorption

---

dicloxacillin sodium

(dye-klox-a-sill'-in)

Dycill, Dynapen, Pathocil

Func. class.: Broad-spectrum antibiotic

Chem. class.: Penicillinase-resistant penicillin

Action: Interferes with cell wall replication of susceptible organisms; osmotically unstable cell wall swells, bursts from osmotic pressure

Uses: Effective for gram-positive cocci *(S. aureus, S. pyogenes, S. viridans, S. faecalis, S. bovis, S. pneumoniae)*, infections caused by penicillinase-producing *Staphylococcus*

Dosage and routes:
- *Adult:* PO 0.5-4 g/day in divided doses q6h
- *Child:* PO 12.5-25 mg/kg in divided doses q6h

Available forms include: Caps 125, 250, 500 mg; powder for oral susp 62.5 mg/5 ml

Side effects/adverse reactions:

HEMA: Anemia, increased bleeding time, ***bone marrow depression, granulocytopenia***

GI: Nausea, vomiting, diarrhea, increased AST, ALT, abdominal pain, glossitis, colitis

GU: ***Oliguria, proteinuria, hematuria,*** *vaginitis, moniliasis,* ***glomerulonephritis***

CNS: Lethargy, hallucinations, anxiety, depression, twitching, ***coma, convulsions***

Contraindications: Hypersensitivity to penicillins; neonates

Precautions: Hypersensitivity to cephalosporins, pregnancy (B)

Pharmacokinetics:

PO: Peak 1 hr, duration 4-6 hr, half-life 30-60 min, metabolized in liver, excreted in urine, bile, breast milk, crosses placenta

Interactions/incompatibilities:
- Decreased antimicrobial effectiveness of dicloxacillin: tetracyclines, erythromycins
- Increased dicloxacillin concentrations: aspirin, probenecid

NURSING CONSIDERATIONS

Assess:
- I&O ratio; report hematuria, oliguria since penicillin in high doses is nephrotoxic
- Any patient with compromised renal system since drug is excreted slowly in poor renal system function; toxicity may occur rapidly
- Liver studies: AST, ALT
- Blood studies: WBC, RBC, H&H, bleeding time
- Renal studies: urinalysis, protein, blood
- C&S before drug therapy; drug may be taken as soon as culture is taken

Administer:
- Drug after C&S has been completed
- On an empty stomach with a full glass of water

Perform/provide:
- Adrenalin, suction, tracheostomy set, endotracheal intubation equipment
- Adequate fluid intake (2000 ml) during diarrhea episodes
- Scratch test to assess allergy, after securing order from physician; usually done when penicillin is only drug of choice
- Storage in tight container; after reconstituting, store in refrigerator up to 2 wk

Evaluate:
- Therapeutic response: absence of fever, draining wounds
- Bowel pattern before, during treatment
- Skin eruptions after administration of penicillin to 1 wk after discontinuing drug
- Respiratory status: rate, character, wheezing, tightness in chest
- Allergies before initiation of treatment, reaction of each medication; highlight allergies on chart, Kardex

Teach patient/family:
- Aspects of drug therapy, including need to complete course of medication to ensure organism death (10-14 days); culture may be taken after completed course
- To report sore throat, fever, fatigue (could indicate superimposed infection)
- To wear or carry Medic Alert ID if allergic to penicillins
- To notify nurse of diarrhea

Lab test interferences:
False positive: Urine glucose, urine protein

Treatment of overdose: Withdraw drug, maintain airway, administer epinephrine, aminophylline, O_2, IV corticosteroids for anaphylaxis

---

dicyclomine HCl

(dye-sye'kloe-meen)

Antispas, Bentyl, Bentylol,* Dibent, Formulex,* Neoquess, Viserol*

Func. class.: Gastrointestinal anticholinergic

Chem. class.: Synthetic tertiary amine

Action: Inhibits muscarinic actions of acetylcholine at postganglionic parasympathetic neuroeffector sites

Uses: Treatment of peptic ulcer disease in combination with other drugs; infant colic

Dosage and routes:
- *Adult:* PO 10-20 mg tid-qid; IM 20 mg q4-6h
- *Child >2 yr:* PO 10 mg tid-qid
- *Child 6 mo-2 yr:* PO 5 mg tid-qid

Available forms include: Caps 10, 20 mg; tabs 20 mg; syr 10 mg/5 ml; inj IM 10 mg/ml

Side effects/adverse reactions:
CNS: Confusion, stimulation in elderly, headache, insomnia, dizziness, drowsiness, anxiety, weakness, hallucination; ***seizures, coma*** (child <3 mo)
GI: Dry mouth, constipation, ***paralytic ileus,*** heartburn, nausea, vomiting, dysphagia, absence of taste
GU: Hesitancy, rentention, impotence
CV: Palpitations, tachycardia
EENT: Blurred vision, photophobia, mydriasis, cycloplegia, increased ocular tension
INTEG: Urticaria, rash, pruritus, anhidrosis, fever, allergic reactions

Contraindications: Hypersensitiv-

---

* Available in Canada only

ity to anticholinergics, narrow-angle glaucoma, GI obstruction, myasthenia gravis, paralytic ileus, GI atony, toxic megacolon
Precautions: Hyperthyroidism, coronary artery disease, dysrhythmias, CHF, ulcerative colitis, hypertension, hiatal hernia, hepatic disease, renal disease, pregnancy (B), urinary retention, prostatic hypertrophy
Pharmacokinetics:
PO: Onset 1-2 hr, duration 3-4 hr; metabolized by liver, excreted in urine
Interactions/incompatibilities:
• Increased anticholinergic effect: amantadine, tricylic antidepressants, MAOIs, H_1 antihistamines
• Decreased effect of: phenothiazines, levodopa, ketoconazole

NURSING CONSIDERATIONS

Assess:
• VS, cardiac status: checking for dysrhythmias, increased rate, palpitations
• I&O ratio; check for urinary retention or hesitancy
Administer:
• ½-1 hr ac for better absorption
• Decreased dose to elderly patients; their metabolism may be slowed
• Gum, hard candy, frequent rinsing of mouth for dryness of oral cavity
Perform/provide:
• Storage in tight container protected from light
• Increased fluids, bulk, exercise to patient's lifestyle to decrease constipation
Evaluate:
• Therapeutic response: absence of epigastric pain, bleeding, nausea, vomiting
• GI complaints: pain, bleeding (frank or occult), nausea, vomiting, anorexia
Teach patient/family:
• To avoid driving or other hazardous activities until stabilized on medication, may cause blurred vision
• To avoid alcohol or other CNS depressants; will enhance sedating properties of this drug
• To avoid hot environments, stroke may occur, drug suppresses perspiration
• To use sunglasses when outside to prevent photophobia
• To drink plenty of fluids
• To report dysphagia

didanosine

(dye-dan'-o-seen)
Videx, ddI, Dideoxyinosine
Func. class.: Antiviral
Chem. class.: Synthetic purine nucleoside of deoxyadenosine

Action: Inhibits HIV by the conversion of this drug by cellular enzymes to activate antiviral metabolite
Uses: Advanced HIV infections in adults and children who have been unable to use zidovudine or who have not responded to treatment
Dosage and routes:
• *Adult:* PO >75 kg, 300 mg bid tabs, or 375 mg bid buffered powder
50-74 kg, 200 mg bid tabs, or 250 mg bid buffered powder
35-49 kg, 125 mg bid tabs, or 167 mg bid buffered powder
• *Child:* PO 1.1-1.4 m^2, 100 mg bid tabs, or 125 mg bid pedi powder
0.8-1 m^2, 75 mg bid tabs, or 94 mg bid pedi powder
0.5-0.7 m^2, 50 mg bid tabs, or 62 mg bid pedi powder

< 0.4 m^2, 25 mg bid tabs, or 31 mg bid pedi powder
Available forms include: Tabs, buffered, chewable/dispersible 25, 50, 100, 150 mg; powder for oral sol, buffered 100, 167, 250, 375 mg; powder for oral sol, pedi 2, 4 g
Side effects/adverse reactions:
GI: ***Pancreatitis,*** diarrhea, nausea, vomiting, abdominal pain, constipation, stomatitis, dyspepsia, liver abnormalities, flatulence, taste perversion, dry mouth, oral thrush, melena, increased ALT, AST, Alk phosphatase, amylase
GU: Increased bilirubin, uric acid
CNS: ***Peripheral neuropathy, seizures,*** confusion, anxiety, hypertonia, abnormal thinking, asthenia, insomnia, ***CNS depression,*** pain, dizziness, chills, fever
RESP: Cough, pneumonia, dyspnea, asthma, epistaxis, hypoventilation, sinusitis
INTEG: Rash, pruritus, alopecia, ecchymosis, hemorrhage, petechiae, sweating
MS: Myalgia, arthritis, myopathy, muscular atrophy
CV: Hypertension, vasodilation, dysrhythmia, syncope, CHF, palpitation
EENT: Ear pain, otitis, photophobia, visual impairment
HEMA: ***Leukopenia, granulocytopenia, thrombocytopenia, anemia***
Contraindications: Hypersensitivity
Precautions: Renal, hepatic disease, pregnancy (B), lactation, children, sodium-restricted diets
Pharmacokinetics:
PO: Elimination half-life 1.62 hr, extensive metabolism is thought to occur; administration within 5 min of food will decrease absorption
Interactions/incompatibilities:
• Decreased absorption: ketoconazole, dapsone, food
• Do not administer with tetracyclines
• Decreased concentrations of: fluoroquinolone antibiotics

NURSING CONSIDERATIONS

Assess:
• Neuropathy: tingling or pain in hands and feet, distal numbness
• Pancreatitis: Abdominal pain, nausea, vomiting, elevated liver enzymes; drug should be discontinued since condition can be fatal
• Children by dilated retinal examination q6mo to rule out retinal depigmentation
• CBC, differential, platelet count weekly, withhold drug if WBC is <4000 or platelet count is <75,000; notify physician of results
• Renal function studies: BUN, serum uric acid, urine CrCl before, during therapy
• Temperature q4h, may indicate beginning infection
• Liver function tests before, during therapy (bilirubin, AST, ALT) as needed or monthly
Administer:
• Antibiotics for prophylaxis of infection
Perform/provide:
• Strict medical asepsis, protective isolation if WBC levels are low
• Clean-up of powdered products; use wet mop or damp sponge
Evaluate:
• Therapeutic response: Absence of infection; symptoms of HIV
Teach patient/family:
• To report signs of infection: increased temperature, sore throat, flu symptoms
• To report signs of anemia: fatigue, headache, faintness, shortness of breath, irritability
• To report bleeding; avoid use of razors or commercial mouthwash

• That hair may be lost during therapy; a wig or hairpiece may make patient feel better

dienestrol

(dye-en-ess'trole)

DV, Estraguard, Ortho Dienestrol

Func. class.: Estrogen

Chem. class.: Nonsteroidal synthetic estrogen

Action: Needed for adequate functioning of female reproductive system, it affects release of pituitary gonadotropins, inhibits ovulation, adequate calcium use in bone structures

Uses: Atrophic vaginitis, kraurosis vulvae

Dosage and routes:

• *Adult:* VAG CREAM 1-2 applications qd × 2 wk, then ½ dose × 2 wk, then 1 application

Available forms include: Vag cream 0.01%

Side effects/adverse reactions:

CNS: Dizziness, headache, migraines, depression

CV: Hypotension, thrombophlebitis, edema, ***thromboembolism, stroke, pulmonary embolism, myocardial infarction***

GI: Nausea, vomiting, diarrhea, anorexia, pancreatitis, cramps, constipation, increased appetite, increased weight, ***cholestatic jaundice***

EENT: Contact lens intolerance, increased myopia, astigmatism

GU: Amenorrhea, cervical erosion, breakthrough bleeding, dysmenorrhea, vaginal candidiasis, breast changes, gynecomastia, testicular atrophy, impotence

INTEG: Rash, urticaria, acne, hirsutism, alopecia, oily skin, seborrhea, purpura, melasma

META: Folic acid deficiency, hypercalcemia, hyperglycemia

Contraindications: Breast cancer, thromboembolic disorders, reproductive cancer, genital bleeding (abnormal, undiagnosed), pregnancy (X)

Precautions: Hypertension, asthma, blood dyscrasias, gallbladder disease, CHF, diabetes mellitus, bone disease, depression, migraine headache, convulsive disorders, hepatic disease, renal disease, family history of cancer of the breast or reproductive tract

Pharmacokinetics:

TOP: Degraded in liver, excreted in urine, crosses placenta, excreted in breast milk

Interactions/incompatibilities:

• Decreased action of: anticoagulants, oral hypoglycemics

• Toxicity: tricyclic antidepressants

• Decreased action of dienestrol: anticonvulsants, barbiturates, phenylbutazone, rifampin

• Increased action of: corticosteroids

NURSING CONSIDERATIONS

Assess:

• Weight daily; notify physician of weekly weight gain >5 lb

• B/P q4h

• I&O ratio; be alert for decreasing urinary output and increasing edema

• Liver function studies including ALT, AST, bilirubin

Administer:

• At hs for better absorption

• Titrated dose, use lowest effective dose, to prevent adverse reactions

• Dosage reduction should continue at 3-6 month intervals

Perform/provide:

• Storage in tight, light-resistant container in refrigerator

Evaluate:
• Therapeutic response: decreased symptoms of vaginitis, kraurosis
• Edema, hypertension, cardiac symptoms, jaundice
• Mental status: affect, mood, behavioral changes, aggression
• Hypercalcemia

Teach patient/family:
• How to fill applicator and insert cream
• To check with physician before using any OTC drugs
• To report breast lumps, vaginal bleeding, edema, jaundice, dark urine, clay-colored stools, dyspnea, headache, blurred vision, abdominal pain, numbness or stiffness in legs, chest pain

---

diethylpropion HCl

Dospan, Nobesine, Nu-Dispoz, Regibon, Ro-Diet, Tenuate, Tepanil, Ten-Tab, Tepanic

Func. class.: Anorexant
Chem. class.: Amphetamine-like analog

Controlled Substance Schedule IV

Action: Direct stimulation of partial adrenergic pathways to suppress appetite

Uses: Exogenous obesity

Dosage and routes:
• *Adult:* PO 25 mg/hr ac, or 75 mg controlled release qd midmorning

Available forms include: Tabs 25 mg, tabs susp rel 75 mg

Side effects/adverse reactions:
HEMA: ***Bone marrow depression,*** leukopenia, agranulocytosis
CNS: Hyperactivity, restlessness, anxiety, insomnia, dizziness, dysphonia, depression, tremors, headache, blurred vision, incoordination, fatigue, malaise, euphoria, depression, tremor, confusion
GI: Nausea, vomiting, anorexia, dry mouth, diarrhea, constipation
GU: Impotence, change in libido, menstrual irregularities, dysuria, polyuria
CV: Palpitations, tachycardia, hypertension, dysrhythmias, pulmonary hypertension, BCG changes
INTEG: Urticaria

Contraindications: Hypersensitivity, hyperthyroidism, hypertension, glaucoma, angina pectoris, drug abuse, cardiovascular disease, children <12 yr, severe arteriosclerosis, agitated states

Precautions: Convulsive disorders, pregnancy (B), lactation

Pharmacokinetics:
PO: Duration 4 hr
CONT REL: Duration 10-14 hr; metabolized by liver, excreted by kidneys, crosses placenta, breast milk, half-life 1-3½ hr

Interactions/incompatibilities:
• Hypertensive crisis: MAOIs or within 14 days of MAOIs
• Increased effect of diethylpropion: acetazolamide, antacids, sodium bicarbonate, ascorbic acid, ammonium chloride
• Decreased effects of diethylpropion: barbiturates, tricyclics, ascorbic acid, ammonium chloride
• Decreased effects of: guanethidine, other antihypertensives

NURSING CONSIDERATIONS

Assess:
• VS, B/P since this drug may reverse antihypertensives; check patients with cardiac disease more often
• CBC, urinalysis, in diabetes: blood sugar, urine sugar; insulin changes may need to be made since eating will decrease

---

* Available in Canada only

• Height, growth rate in children; growth rate may be decreased

Administer:

• At least 6 hr before hs to avoid sleeplessness

• For obesity only if patient is on weight reduction program, including dietary changes, exercise; patient will develop tolerance, and weight loss won't occur without additional methods; give 1 hour before meals

• Gum, hard candy, frequent sips of water for dry mouth

Evaluate:

• Therapeutic response: decreased weight

• Mental status: mood, sensorium, affect, stimulation, insomnia, aggressiveness

• Physical dependency: should not be used for extended time; dose should be discontinued gradually, drug tolerance occurs after long-term use

• Withdrawal symptoms: headache, nausea, vomiting, muscle pain, weakness

Teach patient/family:

• To not crush or chew sus rel preps; not to take more frequently than prescribed

• To decrease caffeine consumption (coffee, tea, cola, chocolate); may increase irritability, stimulation

• To avoid OTC preparations unless approved by physician

• To taper off drug over several weeks, or depression, increased sleeping, lethargy will occur

• To avoid alcohol ingestion

• To avoid hazardous activities until patient is stabilized on medication

• To get needed rest, patients will feel more tired at end of day

Treatment of overdose: Administer fluids, hemodialysis for peritoneal dialysis; antihypertensive for increased B/P; ammonium Cl for increased excretion

---

diethylstilbestrol/diethylstilbestrol diphosphate

(dye-eth-il-stil-bess'trole)

DES, Stilboestrol*/Honvol,* Stilphostrol

Func. class.: Estrogen

Chem. class.: Nonsteroidal synthetic estrogen

Action: Needed for adequate functioning of female reproductive system, it affects release of pituitary gonadotropins, inhibits ovulation, adequate calcium use in bone structures

Uses: Atrophic vaginitis, kraurosis vulvae, menopause, postcoital contraception, hypogonadism, castration, primary ovarian failure, breast engorgement, breast cancer, prostatic cancer

Dosage and routes:

Atrophic vaginitis/kraurosis vulvae

• *Adult:* VAG SUPP 0.1-1 mg qd × 10-14 days with oral therapy or up to 5 mg qwk

Menopause

• *Adult:* PO 0.1-2 mg qd3wk on, 1 wk off

Contraception

• *Adult:* PO 25 mg bid × 5 days, within 72 hr of intercourse

Hypogonadism/castration/ovarian failure

• *Adult:* PO 0.2-0.5 mg qd

Breast engorgement

• *Adult:* PO 5 mg qd-tid, not to exceed 30 mg

Prostatic cancer

• *Adult:* PO 1-3 mg qd, then 1 mg qd; PO 50-200 mg tid (diphosphate); IM 5 mg 2×/wk, then 4 mg 2×/wk; IV 0.25-1 g qd × 5 days, then 1-2×/wk

Breast cancer

• *Adult:* PO 15 mg qd

Available forms include: Tabs 1, 5 mg; tabs enteric coated 0.1, 0.25, 0.5, 1, 5 mg; vag supp 0.1, 0.5 mg

Side effects/adverse reactions:

CNS: Dizziness, headache, migraines, depression

CV: Hypotension, thrombophlebitis, edema, ***thromboembolism, stroke, pulmonary embolism, myocardial infarction***

GI: Nausea, vomiting, diarrhea, anorexia, pancreatitis, cramps, constipation, increased appetite, increased weight, ***cholestatic jaundice***

EENT: Contact lens intolerance, increased myopia, astigmatism

GU: Amenorrhea, cervical erosion, breakthrough bleeding, dysmenorrhea, vaginal candidiasis, breast changes, *gynecomastia, testicular atrophy, impotence*

INTEG: Rash, urticaria, acne, hirsutism, alopecia, oily skin, seborrhea, purpura, melasma

META: Folic acid deficiency, hypercalcemia, hyperglycemia

Contraindications: Breast cancer, thromboembolic disorders, reproductive cancer, genital bleeding (abnormal, undiagnosed), pregnancy (X)

Precautions: Hypertension, asthma, blood dyscrasias, gallbladder disease, CHF, diabetes mellitus, bone disease blocking agents

Interactions/incompatibilities:

• Decreased action of: anticoagulants, oral hypoglycemics

• Toxicity: tricyclic antidepressants

• Decreased action of diethylstilbestrol: anticonvulsants, barbiturates, phenylbutazone, rifampin

• Increased action of: corticosteroids

NURSING CONSIDERATIONS

Assess:

• Urine glucose in patient with diabetes; increased urine glucose may occur

• Weight daily, notify physician of weekly weight gain >5 lb; if increase, diuretic may be ordered

• B/P q4h, watch for increase caused by water and sodium retention

• I&O ratio; be alert for decreasing urinary output and increasing edema

• Liver function studies, including AST, ALT, bilirubin, alk phosphatase

Administer:

• IV after diluting in 300 ml of dextrose or saline sol; give at a rate of 20 g hs/min × 15 min; may increase rate to complete infusion 1 hr after starting

• Titrated dose, use lowest effective dose

• IM injection deeply in large muscular mass

• In one dose in AM for prostatic cancer, vaginitis, hypogonadism

• With food or milk to decrease GI symptoms

Evaluate:

• Therapeutic response: absence of breast engorgement, reversal of menopause or decrease in tumor size in prostatic cancer

• Edema, hypertension, cardiac symptoms, jaundice

• Mental status: affect, mood, behavioral changes, aggression

• Hypercalcemia

Teach patient/family:

• To weigh weekly, report gain >5 lb

• To report breast lumps, vaginal

* Available in Canada only

bleeding, edema, jaundice, dark urine, clay-colored stools, dyspnea, headache, blurred vision, abdominal pain, numbness or stiffness in legs, chest pain; male to report impotence or gynecomastia
• To check with physician before taking any OTC drugs

Lab test interferences:
Increase: BSP retention test, PBI, T_4, serum sodium, platelet aggressability, thyroxine-binding globulin (TBG), prothrombin, factors VII, VIII, IX, X, triglycerides
Decrease: Serum folate, serum triglyceride, T_3 resin uptake test, glucose tolerance test, antithrombin III, pregnanediol, metyraponetest
False positive: LE prep, antinuclear antibodies

difenoxin HCl with atropine sulfate

(dye-fen-ox' -in)
Motofen

Func. class.: Antidiarrheal
Chem. class.: Phenylpiperidine derivative, opiate agonist

Controlled Substance Schedule IV

Action: Inhibits gastric motility by acting on mucosal receptors responsible for peristalsis
Uses: Acute nonspecific and acute exacerbations of chronic functional diarrhea
Dosage and routes:
• *Adult:* PO 2 mg, then 1 mg after each loose stool or 1 mg q3-4h as needed, not to exceed 8 mg/24 hr
Available forms include: Tab 1 mg difenoxin HCl, 0.025 mg atropine sulfate
Side effects/adverse reactions:
CNS: Dizziness, drowsiness, headache, fatigue, nervousness, insomnia, confusion
GI: Nausea, vomiting, dry mouth, epigastric distress, constipation
EENT: Burning eyes, blurred vision
Contraindications: Hypersensitivity, pseudomembranous enterocolitis, jaundice, glaucoma, child <2 yr, severe electrolyte imbalances, diarrhea associated with organisms that penetrate intestinal mucosa
Precautions: Hepatic disease, renal disease, ulcerative colitis, pregnancy (C), lactation, severe liver disease
Pharmacokinetics:
PO: Peak 40-60 min, duration 3-4 hr, terminal half-life 12-14 hr; metabolized in liver to inactive metabolite; excreted in urine, feces
Interactions/incompatibilities:
• Do not use with MAOIs; hypertensive crisis may occur
• Increased action of: alcohol, narcotics, barbituates, other CNS depressants, anticholinergics

NURSING CONSIDERATIONS

Assess:
• Electrolytes (K, Na, Cl) if on long-term therapy
Administer:
• For 48 hr only
Evaluate:
• Therapeutic response: decreased diarrhea
• Bowel pattern before; for rebound constipation after termination of medication
• Response after 48 hr; if no response, drug should be discontinued
• Abdominal distention, toxic megacolon, which may occur in ulcerative colitis
Teach patient/family:
• To avoid OTC products unless directed by physician; may contain alcohol

• Not to exceed recommended dose
• That drug may be habit forming

diflorasone diacetate

(die-floor'-a-sone)

Florone, Futone, Maxiflor, Psorcon

Func. class.: Topical corticosteroid
Chem. class.: Synthetic fluorinated agent, group II potency

Action: Possesses antipruritic, antiinflammatory actions
Uses: Psoriasis, eczema, contact dermatitis, pruritus
Dosage and routes:
• *Adult and child:* Apply to affected area qd-tid
Available forms include: Cream 0.05%; oint 0.05%
Side effects/adverse reactions:
INTEG: Burning, dryness, itching, irritation, acne, folliculitis, hypertrichosis, perioral dermatitis, hypopigmentation, atrophy, striae, miliaria, allergic contact dermatitis, secondary infection
Contraindications: Hypersensitivity to corticosteroids, fungal infections
Precautions: Pregnancy (C), lactation, viral infections, bacterial infections

NURSING CONSIDERATIONS
Assess:
• Temperature; if fever develops, drug should be discontinued
Administer:
• Only to affected areas; do not get in eyes
• Medication, then cover with occlusive dressing (only if prescribed), seal to normal skin, change q12h; use occlusive dressing with extreme caution, systemic absorption may occur
• Only to dermatoses; do not use on weeping, denuded, or infected area
Perform/provide:
• Cleansing before application of drug
• Treatment for a few days after area has cleared
• Storage at room temperature
Evaluate:
• Therapeutic response: absence of severe itching, patches on skin, flaking
• For systemic absorption: increased temperature, inflammation, irritation
Teach patient/family:
• To avoid sunlight on affected area; burns may occur

diflunisal

(dye-floo'ni-sal)

Dolobid

Func. class.: Nonsteroidal antiinflammatory
Chem. class.: Salicylate derivative

Action: May block pain impulses in CNS that occur in response to inhibition of prostaglandin synthesis; antipyretic action results from inhibition of hypothalamic heat-regulating center to produce vasodilation to allow heat dissipation
Uses: Mild to moderate pain or fever including arthritis, juvenile rheumatoid arthritis, 3-4 times more potent than aspirin
Dosage and routes:
Pain/fever
• *Adult:* PO loading dose 1 g then 500-1000 mg/day in 2 divided doses, q12h, not to exceed 1500 mg/day
Available forms include: Tabs 250, 500 mg
Side effects/adverse reactions:
HEMA: ***Thrombocytopenia, agran-***

* Available in Canada only

ulocytosis, leukopenia, neutropenia, hemolytic anemia, increased pro-time
CNS: Stimulation, drowsiness, dizziness, confusion, ***convulsion,*** headache, flushing, hallucinations, coma
GI: Nausea, vomiting, GI bleeding, diarrhea, heartburn, anorexia, ***hepatitis***
INTEG: Rash, urticaria, bruising
EENT: Blurred vision, decreased acuity, corneal deposits
CV: Rapid pulse, ***pulmonary edema***
RESP: Wheezing, hyperpnea
ENDO: Hypoglycemia, hyponatremia, hypokalemia

Contraindications: Hypersensitivity to salicylates, GI bleeding, bleeding disorders, children <3 yr, vitamin K deficiency

Precautions: Anemia, hepatic disease, renal disease, Hodgkin's disease, pregnancy (C), lactation

Pharmacokinetics:
PO: Onset 15-30 min, peak 2-3 hr, half-life 10-12 hr, metabolized by liver, excreted by kidneys, crosses placenta, 99% protein bound, excreted in breast milk

Interactions/incompatibilities:
• Decreased effects of diflunisal: antacids, steroids, urinary alkalizers
• Increased blood loss: alcohol, heparin
• Increased effects of: anticoagulants, insulin, methotrexate, hydrochlorothiazide, acetaminophen
• Decreased effects of: probenecid, spironolactone, sulfinpyrazone, sulfonylmides
• Toxic effects: PABA
• Decreased blood sugar levels: salicylates

NURSING CONSIDERATIONS

Assess:
• Liver function studies: AST, ALT, bilirubin, creatinine if patient is on long-term therapy
• Renal function studies: BUN, urine creatinine if patient is on long-term therapy
• Blood studies: CBC, Hct, Hgb, pro-time if patient is on long-term therapy
• I&O ratio; decreasing output may indicate renal failure (long-term therapy)

Administer:
• To patient whole
• With food or milk to decrease gastric symptoms

Evaluate:
• Therapeutic response: decreased pain, stiffness of joints
• Hepatotoxicity: dark urine, clay-colored stools, yellowing of skin, sclera, itching, abdominal pain, fever, diarrhea if patient is on long-term therapy
• Allergic reactions: rash, urticaria; if these occur, drug may need to be discontinued
• Renal dysfunction: decreased urine output
• Ototoxicity: tinnitus, ringing, roaring in ears; audiometric testing is needed before, after long-term therapy
• Visual changes: blurring, halos, corneal, retinal damage
• Edema in feet, ankles, legs
• Prior drug history; there are many drug interactions

Teach patient/family:
• To report any symptoms of hepatotoxicity, renal toxicity, visual changes, ototoxicity, allergic reactions (long-term therapy)
• Not to exceed recommended dosage; acute poisoning may result
• To read label on other OTC drugs; many contain aspirin
• That therapeutic response takes 2 wk (arthritis)

• To avoid alcohol ingestion; GI bleeding may occur

Lab test interferences:
Increase: Coagulation studies, liver function studies, serum uric acid, amylase, CO_2, urinary protein
Decrease: Serum potassium, PBI, cholesterol
Interfere: Urine catecholamines, pregnancy test

Treatment of overdose: Lavage, activated charcoal, monitor electrolytes, VS

---

digitoxin

(di-ji-tox'in)

Crystodigin, Digitaline,* Purodigin*

Func. class.: Antidysrhythmic, cardiac glycoside cardiotonic
Chem. class.: Digitalis preparation

Action: Acts by increased influx of calcium ions from extracellular to intracellular cytoplasm, increasing force of contraction and cardiac output; decreases conduction velocity through AV node; prolongs effective refractory period

Uses: Congestive heart failure, atrial fibrillation, atrial flutter, atrial tachycardia, rapid digitalization in these disorders

Dosage and routes:
• *Adult and child >12 yr:* 1.2-1.6 initially; give in divided doses over 24 hr; 150 μg qd
• *Neonates:* 22 μg/kg; 2 wk-1 yr: 45 μg/kg; 1-2 yr: 40 μg/kg; 2-12 yr: 30 μg/kg
Maintenance dose: 10% initial dose

Available forms include: Powder, tabs 50, 100, 150, 200 μg

Side effects/adverse reactions:
CNS: Headache, drowsiness, apathy, confusion, disorientation, fatigue, depression, hallucinations
*CV: **Dysrhythmias,** hypotension,* bradycardia, AV block
GI: Nausea, vomiting, anorexia, abdominal pain, diarrhea
EENT: Blurred vision, yellow-green halos, photophobia, diplopia
MS: Muscular weakness

Contraindications: Hypersensitivity to digitalis, ventricular fibrillation, ventricular tachycardia, carotid sinus syndrome, 2nd or 3rd degree heart block

Precautions: Hepatic disease, acute MI, AV block, hypokalemia, hypomagnesemia, sinus node disease, lactation, severe respiratory disease, hypothyroidism, elderly, pregnancy (C)

Pharmacokinetics:
PO: Onset ½-2 hr, peak 4-12 hr; duration 2-3 wk, half-life 4-20 days; metabolized in liver; excreted in urine

Interactions/incompatibilities:
• Hypokalemia: diuretics
• Increased blood levels: spironolactone
• Decreased effects: hydantoins, aminoglutethimide, rifampin, phenylbutazone, barbiturates, cholestyramine, colestipol
• Toxicity: adrenergics, diuretics, succinylcholine, quinidine, thioamines
• Decreased level of digitoxin: thyroid agents

NURSING CONSIDERATIONS

Assess:
• Apical pulse for 1 min before giving drug; if pulse <60, take again in 1 hr; if <60, call physician
• Electrolytes: potassium, sodium, chloride, calcium; renal function studies: BUN, creatinine; blood studies: ALT, AST, bilirubin
• Monitor drug levels (therapeutic level 25-35 ng/ml)

---

* Available in Canada only

Administer:
- Potassium supplements if ordered for potassium levels <3.0

Evaluate:
- Therapeutic response: decreased weight, edema, pulse, respiration and increased urine output
- Cardiac status: apical pulse, character, rate, rhythm

Teach patient/family:
- Not to stop drug abruptly; teach all aspects of drug
- To avoid OTC medications, since many adverse drug interactions may occur

Lab test interferences:
Increase: CPK

Treatment of overdose: Discontinue drug, administer potassium, digoxin immune FAB, monitor EKG

digoxin

(di-jox'in)

Lanoxicaps, Lanoxin

Func. class.: Antidysrhythmic, cardiac glycoside

Chem. class.: Digitalis preparation

Action: Acts by inhibiting the sodium-potassium ATPase, which makes more calcium available for contractile proteins, resulting in increased cardiac contractility and cardiac output

Uses: CHF, atrial fibrillation, atrial flutter, atrial tachycardia, rapid digitalization in these disorders

Dosage and routes:
- *Adult:* IV 0.5 mg given over >5 min then PO 0.125-0.5 mg qd in divided doses q4-6h as needed
- *Elderly:* PO 0.125 qd maintenance
- *Child >2 yr:* PO 0.02-0.04 mg/kg divided q8h over 24 hr, maintenance 0.006-0.012 mg/kg qd in divided doses q12hr; IV loading dose 0.015-0.035 mg/kg over >5 min
- *Child 1 mo-2 yr:* IV 0.03-0.05 mg/kg in divided doses over >5 min q4-8h; change to PO as soon as possible; PO 0.035-0.060 mg/kg divided in 3 doses over 24 hr; maintenance 0.01-0.02 mg/kg in divided doses q12h
- *Neonates:* IV loading dose 0.02-0.03 mg/kg over >5 min in divided doses q4-8h; change to PO as soon as possible; PO loading dose 0.035 mg/kg divided q8h, over 24h, maintenance 0.01 mg/kg in divided doses q12h
- *Premature infants:* IV 0.015-0.025 mg/kg divided in 3 doses over 24 hr, given over >5 min maintenance 0.003-0.009 mg/kg in divided doses q12h

Available forms include: Caps 50, 100, 200 μg; elix 50 μg/ml; tabs 125, 250, 500 μg; inj 100, 250 μg/ml

Side effects/adverse reactions:
CNS: Headache, drowsiness, apathy, confusion, disorientation, fatigue, depression, hallucinations
CV: ***Dysrhythmias,*** *hypotension,* bradycardia, ***AV block***
GI: Nausea, vomiting, anorexia, abdominal pain, diarrhea
EENT: Blurred vision, yellow-green halos, photophobia, diplopia
MS: Muscular weakness

Contraindications: Hypersensitivity to digitalis, ventricular fibrillation, ventricular tachycardia, carotid sinus syndrome, 2nd or 3rd degree heart block

Precautions: Renal disease, acute MI, AV block, severe respiratory disease, hypothyroidism, elderly, pregnancy (C), sinus nodal disease, lactation, hypokalemia

Pharmacokinetics:
IV: Onset 5-30 min, peak 1-5 hr, duration variable, half-life 1.5 days excreted in urine

Interactions/incompatibilities:
• Hypokalemia: diuretics, amphotericin B, carbenicillin, ticarcillin, corticosteroids
• Decreased digoxin level: thyroid agents
• Increased blood levels: propantheline bromide, spironolactone quinidine, verapamil, aminoglycosides PO, amiodarone, anticholinergics, quinine
• Toxicity: adrenergics, amphotericin, corticosteroids, diuretics, glucose, insulin, reserpine, succinylcholine, quinidine, thioamines
• Incompatible with all medications in syringe or solution

NURSING CONSIDERATIONS

Assess:
• Apical pulse for 1 min before giving drug; if pulse <60, take again in 1 hr; if <60, call physician
• Electrolytes: potassium, sodium chloride, magnesium, calcium; renal function studies: BUN, creatinine; blood studies: ALT, AST, bilirubin
• I&O ratio, daily weights
• Monitor drug levels (therapeutic level 0.5-2 ng/ml)

Administer:
• Potassium supplements if ordered for potassium levels <3.0
• IV undiluted or 1 ml of drug/4 ml sterile H_2O, D_5, or normal saline; give over >5 min through Y-tube or 3-way stopcock

Evaluate:
• Therapeutic response: decreased weight, edema, pulse, respiration and increased urine output
• Cardiac status: apical pulse, character, rate, rhythm

Teach patient/family:
• Not to stop drug abruptly; teach all aspects of drug
• To avoid OTC medications, since many adverse drug interactions may occur; do not take antacid at same time
• To notify physician if loss of appetite, lower stomach pain, diarrhea, weakness, drowsiness, headache, blurred or yellow vision, rash, depression; toxicity is occurring

Lab test interferences:
Increase: CPK

Treatment of overdose: Discontinue drug, administer potassium, monitor EKG, administer an adrenergic blocking agent, digoxin immune FAB

---

digoxin immune FAB (ovine)

Digibind

Func. class.: Antidote—digoxin specific

Action: Fragments bind to free digoxin to reverse digoxin toxicity by not allowing digoxin to bind to sites of action

Uses: Life-threatening digoxin or digitoxin toxicity

Dosage and routes:

Digoxin
• *Adult:* IV dose (mg) =
Dose ingested (mg) × 0.8 × 66.7; if ingested amount is unknown, give 800 mg IV
If digoxin liquid caps or digitoxin used, do not multiply ingested dose by 0.8

Available forms include: Inj 40 mg/vial (binds 0.6 mg digoxin or digitoxin)

Side effects/adverse reactions:
CV: ***CHF,*** ventricular rate increase,

atrial fibrillation, low cardiac output

RESP: ***Impaired respiratory function, rapid respiratory rate***

META: Hypokalemia

INTEG: Hypersensitivity, allergic reactions

Contraindications: Mild digoxin toxicity

Precautions: Children, lactation, cardiac disease, renal disease, pregnancy (C)

Pharmacokinetics:

IV: Peaks after completion of infusion, onset 30 min (variable); not known if crosses placenta, breast milk; half-life biphasic—14-20 hr; prolonged in renal disease; excreted by kidneys

NURSING CONSIDERATIONS

Assess:

• Potassium levels, may decrease rapidly

Administer:

• After diluting 40 mg/4 ml of sterile H_2O for inj; mix; may be further diluted with normal saline

• By bolus if cardiac arrest is eminent, or IV over 30 min using a 0.22 μm filter

Perform/provide:

• Storage of reconstituted solution for up to 4 hr, in refrigerator

Evaluate:

• Therapeutic response: correction of digoxin toxicity, check digoxin levels

Lab test interferences:

Interfere: Immunoassay digoxin

dihydroergotamine mesylate

(dye-hye-droe-er-got'a-meen)

D.H.E. 45

Func. class.: α-Adrenergic blocker

Chem. class.: Ergot alkaloid (dihydrogenated)

Action: Constricts smooth muscle in periphery, cranial blood vessels; inhibits norepinephrine uptake

Uses: Vascular headache (migraine or histamine)

Dosage and routes:

• *Adult:* IM/IV 1 mg, may repeat q1-2h if needed, not to exceed 3 mg/day or 6 mg/wk

Available forms include: Inj 1 mg/ml

Side effects/adverse reactions:

CNS: Numbness in fingers, toes, weakness

CV: Transient tachycardia, chest pain, bradycardia, increase or decrease in B/P, *gangrene*

GI: Nausea, vomiting

MS: Muscle pain

Contraindications: Hypersensitivity to ergot preparations, occlusion (peripheral, vascular), CAD, hepatic disease, pregnancy (X), renal disease, peptic ulcer, hypertension, lactation, children, uremia

Pharmacokinetics:

IM: Onset 15-30 min, peak 2 hr, duration 3-4 hr

IV: Onset 5 min, peak 45 min, duration 3-4 hr

Half-life 1.3-4 hr

Interactions/incompatibilities:

• Increased effects: troleandomycin

• Increased vasoconstriction: β-blockers

NURSING CONSIDERATIONS

Assess:

• Weight daily, check for peripheral edema in feet, legs

Administer:

• IV undiluted; give 1 mg or less/min

• IM dose, which takes 20 min for effect, or use IV for immediate effect

• At beginning of headache, dose must be titrated to patient response

• Only to women who are not pregnant; harm to fetus may occur

Perform/provide:

• Storage in dark area, do not use discolored solutions

• Quiet, calm environment with decreased stimulation for noise, or bright light or excessive talking

Evaluate:

• Therapeutic response: decrease in frequency, severity of headache

• For stress level, activity, recreation, coping mechanisms of patient

• Neurologic status: LOC, blurring vision, nausea, vomiting, tingling in extremities that occur preceding the headache

• Ingestion of tyramine foods (pickled products, beer, wine, aged cheese), food additives, preservatives, colorings, artificial sweeteners, chocolate, caffeine, which may precipitate these types of headaches

Teach patient/family:

• Not to use OTC medications; serious drug interactions may occur

• To report side effects: increased vasoconstriction starting with cold extremities, then paresthesia, weakness

• That an increase in headaches may occur when this drug is discontinued after long-term use

• To keep drug out of reach of children; death may occur

---

dihydrotachysterol

(dye-hye-droe-tak-iss'ter-ole)

DHT Intensol, DHT Oral Solution, Hytakerol

Func. class.: Parathyroid agent (calcium regulator)

Chem. class.: Vitamin D analog

Action: Increases intestinal absorption of calcium for bones, increases renal tubular absorption of phosphate

Uses: Renal osteodystrophy, hypoparathyroidism, pseudohypoparathyroidism, familial hypophosphatemia, postoperative tetany

Dosage and routes:

Hypophosphatemia

• *Adult and child:* PO 0.5-2 mg qd, maintenance 0.3-1.5 mg qd

Hypoparathyroidism/pseudohypoparathyroidism

• *Adult:* PO 0.8-2.4 mg qd × 1 wk, maintenance 0.2-2 mg qd regulated by serum Ca levels

• *Child:* PO 1-5 mg qd × 1 wk, maintenance 0.2-1 mg qd regulated by serum Ca levels

Renal osteodystrophy

• *Adult:* PO 0.1-0.6 mg qd

Available forms include: Tabs 0.125, 0.2, 0.4 mg; caps 0.125 mg; oral sol 0.2, 0.25 mg/5 ml

Side effects/adverse reactions:

EENT: Tinnitus

CNS: Drowsiness, headache, vertigo, fever, lethargy

GI: Nausea, diarrhea, vomiting, jaundice, anorexia, dry mouth, constipation, cramps, metallic taste

MS: Myalgia, arthralgia, decreased bone development

GU: ***Polyuria,*** hypercalciuria, hyperphosphatemia, ***hematuria***

Contraindications: Hypersensitivity, renal disease, hyperphosphatemia, hypercalcemia

Precautions: Pregnancy (C), renal calculi, lactation, CV disease

Pharmacokinetics:

PO: Onset 2 wk; metabolized by liver, excreted in feces (active/inactive)

Interactions/incompatibilities:

• Decreased absorption of dihydrotachysterol: cholestyramine, colestipol, HCl, mineral oil

---

• Hypercalcemia: thiazide diuretics, calcium supplements
• Cardiac dysrhythmias: cardiac glycosides, verapamil
• Decreased effect of dihydrotachysterol: corticosteroids, phenytoin, barbiturates

NURSING CONSIDERATIONS

Assess:
• BUN, urinary calcium, AST, ALT, cholesterol, creatinine, uric acid, chloride, magnesium, electrolytes, urine pH, phosphate; may increase calcium, should be kept at 9-10 mg/dl, vitamin D 50-135 IU/dl, phosphate 70 mg/dl
• Alk phosphatase; may be decreased
• For increased blood level since toxic reactions may occur rapidly

Administer:
• PO, may be increased q4wk depending on blood level

Perform/provide:
• Storage in tight, light-resistant containers at room temperature
• Restriction of sodium, potassium if required
• Restriction of fluids if required for chronic renal failure

Evaluate:
• Therapeutic response: prevention of bone deficiencies
• For dry mouth, metallic taste, polyuria, bone pain, muscle weakness, headache, fatigue, tinnitus, change in LOC, irregular pulse, dysrhythmias, increased respirations, anorexia, nausea, vomiting, cramps, diarrhea, constipation; may indicate hypercalcemia
• Renal status: decreased urinary output (oliguria, anuria), edema in extremities, weight gain 5 lb, periorbital edema
• Nutritional status, diet for sources of vitamin D (milk, some seafood), calcium (dairy products, dark green vegetables), phosphates (dairy products) must be avoided

Teach patient/family:
• Symptoms of hypercalcemia
• About foods rich in calcium

Lab test interferences:
False increase: Cholesterol

D

dihydroxyaluminum sodium carbonate

(dye-hye-drox′-ee-a-loom-aa-nim)

Rolaids

Func. class.: Antacid
Chem. class.: Aluminum product

Action: Neutralizes gastric acidity, reduces pepsin

Uses: Antacid

Dosage and routes:
• *Adult:* PO 1-2 as needed; may give up to 2-4 tabs

Available forms include: Chewable tab 334 mg

Side effects/adverse reactions:
GI: Constipation, ***obstruction***

Contraindications: Hypersensitivity to aluminum products

Precautions: Elderly, sodium/fluid restriction, decreased GI motility, GI obstruction, dehydration, severe renal disease, CHF, pregnancy (C)

Pharmacokinetics:
PO: Onset 20-40 min, excreted in feces

Interactions/incompatibilities:
• Decreased effectiveness of: tetracyclines, ketoconazole, isoniazid, phenothiazines, iron salts, digitalis

NURSING CONSIDERATIONS

Administer:
• Laxatives or stool softeners if constipation occurs

Evaluate:
• Therapeutic response: absence of pain, decreased acidity

• Constipation; increase bulk in the diet if needed

Teach patient/family:

• To increase fluids to 2000 ml/day unless contraindicated

• To avoid long-term use

---

diltiazem HCl

(dil-tye'a-zem)

Cardizem, Cardizem SR

Func. class.: Calcium channel blocker

Chem. class.: Benzothiazepine

Action: Inhibits calcium ion influx across cell membrane during cardiac depolarization; produces relaxation of coronary vascular smooth muscle, dilates coronary arteries, slows SA/AV node conduction times, dilates peripheral arteries

Uses: Chronic stable angina pectoris, vasospastic angina, coronary artery spasm, hypertension

Dosage and routes:

• *Adult:* PO 30 mg qid, increasing dose gradually to 180-360 mg/day in divided doses or 60-120 mg bid; may increase to 240-360 mg/day

Available forms include: Tabs 30, 60, 90, 120 mg, sus rel 60, 90, 120, 150 mg

Side effects/adverse reactions:

CV: Dysrhythmia, edema, ***CHF,*** bradycardia, hypotension, palpitations, heart block, peripheral edema, angina

GI: Nausea, vomiting, diarrhea, gastric upset, constipation, increased liver function studies

GU: Nocturia, polyuria, ***acute renal failure***

INTEG: Rash, pruritus, flushing, photosensitivity

CNS: Headache, fatigue, drowsiness, dizziness, depression, weakness, insomnia, tremor, paresthesia

Contraindications: Sick sinus syndrome, 2nd or 3rd degree heart block, hypotension less than 90 mm Hg systolic, acute MI, pulmonary congestion

Precautions: CHF, hypotension, hepatic injury, pregnancy (C), lactation, children, renal disease

Pharmacokinetics: Onset 30-60 min, peak 2-3 hr, immediate rel, 6-11 sus rel, half-life 3½-9 hr; metabolized by liver, excreted in urine (96% as metabolites)

Interactions/incompatibilities:

• Increased effects of: β-blockers, digitalis, lithium, carbamazepine, cyclosporine

• Increased effects of diltiazem: cimetidine

NURSING CONSIDERATIONS

Assess:

• Blood levels (therapeutic levels: 0.025-0.1 μg/ml)

Administer:

• Before meals, hs

Perform/provide:

• Storage in tight container at room temperature

Evaluate:

• Therapeutic response: decreased anginal pain, decreased B/P

• Cardiac status: B/P, pulse, respiration, ECG and intervals PR, QRS, QT

Teach patient/family:

• To carry nitrites at all times

• How to take pulse before taking drug; record or graph should be kept

• To avoid hazardous activities until stabilized on drug; dizziness is no longer a problem

• To limit caffeine consumption

• To avoid OTC drugs unless directed by a physician

• Importance of complying with all areas of medical regimen: diet, ex-

---

ercise, stress reduction, drug therapy

Treatment of overdose: Defibrillation, atropine for AV block, vasopressor for hypotension

---

dimenhydrinate

(dye-men-hye'dri-nate)

Calm-X, Dimen, Dimentabs, Dipendrate, Dramamine, Dramamine Junior, Dymenate, Gravol,* Hydrate, Nauseal,* Nauseatol,* Novodimenate,* Marmine, Reidamine, Travamine,* Vertiban

Func. class.: Antiemetic, antihistamine, anticholinergic

Chem. class.: H_1-receptor antagonist, ethanolamine derivative

---

Action: Acts centrally by blocking chemoreceptor trigger zone, which in turn acts on vomiting center

Uses: Motion sickness, nausea, vomiting

Dosage and routes:

- *Adult:* PO 50-100 mg q4h; REC 100 mg qd or bid; IM/IV 50 mg as needed
- *Child:* IM/PO 5 mg/kg divided in 4 equal doses

Available forms include: Tabs 50 mg; inj 500 mg/ml; liq 12.5/4 ml; supp 50, 100 mg

Side effects/adverse reactions:

CNS: Drowsiness, restlessness, headache, dizziness, insomnia, confusion, nervousness, tingling, vertigo, hallucinations and ***convulsions*** in young children

GI: Nausea, anorexia, diarrhea, vomiting, constipation

CV: Hypertension, hypotension, palpitation

INTEG: Rash, urticaria, fever, chills, flushing

EENT: Dry mouth, blurred vision, diplopia, nasal congestion, photosensitivity

Contraindications: Hypersensitivity to narcotics, shock

Precautions: Children, cardiac dysrhythmias, elderly, asthma, pregnancy (B), prostatic hypertrophy, bladder-neck obstruction, narrow-angle glaucoma, stenosing peptic ulcer, pyloroduodenal obstruction

Pharmacokinetics:

IM/PO: Duration 4-6 hr

Interactions/incompatibilities:

- Increased effect: alcohol, other CNS depressants
- May mask ototoxic symptoms associated with aminoglycosides

NURSING CONSIDERATIONS

Assess:

- VS, B/P; check patients with cardiac disease more often

Administer:

- IV after diluting 50 mg/10 ml of NaCl inj; give 50 mg or less over 2 min
- IM injection in large muscle mass; aspirate to avoid IV administration
- Tablets may be swallowed whole, chewed, or allowed to dissolve

Evaluate:

- Therapeutic response: absence of nausea, vomiting
- Signs of toxicity of other drugs or masking of symptoms of disease: brain tumor, intestinal obstruction
- Observe for drowsiness, dizziness

Teach patient/family:

- That a false-negative result may occur with skin testing; these procedures should not be scheduled for 4 days after discontinuing use
- To avoid hazardous activities, activities requiring alertness; dizziness may occur; instruct patient to request assistance with ambulation

D

• To avoid alcohol, other depressants

Lab test interferences:
False negative: Allergy skin testing

dimercaprol

(dye-mer-kap'role)
BAL in Oil, British Anti-Lewisite*
Func. class.: Heavy metal antagonist
Chem. class.: Chelating agent (dithiol compound)

Action: Binds ions from arsenic, gold, mercury, lead, copper to form water-soluble complex removed by kidneys

Uses: Arsenic, gold, mercury, lead poisoning

Dosage and routes:

Severe gold/arsenic poisoning
• *Adult:* IM 3 mg/kg q4h × 2 days, then qid × 1 day, then bid ×10 days

Mild gold/arsenic poisoning
• *Adult:* IM 2.5 mg/kg qid × 2 days, then bid × 1 day, then qd × 10 days

Acute lead poisoning
• *Adult:* IM 4 mg/kg, then q4h with edetate calcium disodium 12.5 mg/kg IM, not to exceed 5 mg/kg/dose

Mercury poisoning
• *Adult:* IM 5 mg/kg, then 2.5 mg/kg/day or bid × 10 days

Available forms include: Inj IM 100 mg/ml

Side effects/adverse reactions:
CNS: Headache, paresthesia, anxiety, tremors, ***convulsions, shock***
INTEG: Urticaria, erythema, pruritus, pain at injection site, fever
CV: Hypertension, tachycardia
GI: Nausea, vomiting, salivation
EENT: Rhinorrhea, throat pain or constriction, lacrimation
GU: Burning sensation in penis, ***nephrotoxicity***
SYST: ***Anaphylaxis,*** metabolic acidosis

Contraindications: Hypersensitivity, anuria, hepatic insufficiency, poisoning of other metals, severe renal disease, child <3 yr

Precautions: Hypertension, pregnancy (D), lactation

Pharmacokinetics:
Metabolized by plasma enzymes, excreted by kidneys as complex, unchanged drug

Interactions/incompatibilities:
• Increased toxicity: iron, selenium, uranium, cadmium

NURSING CONSIDERATIONS

Assess:
• B/P, increasing B/P or tachycardia, respirations, pulse
• Monitor I&O, kidney function studies: BUN, creatinine, CrCl; report decreases in output
• Urine: pH, albumin, casts, blood
• Metal levels daily, temperature

Administer:
• IM in deep muscle mass; rotate injection sites if giving EDTA also, give in separate site; observe for sterile abscesses
• Only when epinephrine 1 : 1000 is on unit for anaphylaxis
• Being careful not to allow drug to touch skin; contact dermatitis can occur
• Acetazolamide or sodium citrate to decrease pH of urine, which decreases renal damage

Evaluate:
• Therapeutic response: decreasing level of metal exposed to in the blood
• Allergic reactions (rash, urticaria); if these occur, drug should be discontinued

Teach patient/family:
• That breath may be odorous

*Available in Canada only

Lab test interferences:
Decrease: RAIU test

dinoprostone

(dye-noe-prost'one)
PGE_2, Prepidil Gel*, Prostin E_2
Func. class.: Oxytocic
Chem. class.: Prostaglandin E_2

Action: Stimulates uterine contractions causing abortion; acts within 30 hr for complete abortion
Uses: Abortion during 2nd trimester, benign hydatidiform mole, expulsion of uterine contents in fetal deaths to 28 wk, missed abortion
Dosage and routes:
- *Adult:* VAG SUPP 20 mg, repeat q3-5h until abortion occurs

Available forms include: Vag supp 20 mg
Side effects/adverse reactions:
CNS: Headache, dizziness, chills, fever
CV: Hypotension
GI: Nausea, vomiting, diarrhea
GU: Vaginitis, vaginal pain, vulvitis, vaginismus
INTEG: Rash, skin color changes
MS: Leg cramps, joint swelling, weakness
EENT: Blurred vision
Contraindications: Hypersensitivity, uterine fibrosis, cervical stenosis, pelvic surgery, pelvic inflammatory disease (PID), respiratory disease
Precautions: Hepatic disease, renal disease, cardiac disease, asthma, anemia, jaundice, diabetes mellitus, convulsive disorders, hypertension, hypotension
Pharmacokinetics:
SUPP: Onset 10 min, duration 2-3 hr; metabolized in spleen, kidney, lungs, excreted in urine

NURSING CONSIDERATIONS
Assess:
- Respiratory rate, rhythm, depth; notify physician of abnormalities, pulse, B/P, temperature
- Vaginal discharge: check for itching, irritation; indicates vaginal infection

Administer:
- Antiemetic/antidiarrheal before administration of this drug
- High in vagina
- After warming suppository by running warm water over package

Evaluate:
- Therapeutic response: expulsion of fetus
- For length, duration of contraction; notify physician of contractions lasting over 1 min or absence of contractions
- For fever, chills: increase fluids, or give tepid sponge bath or blanket

Teach patient/family:
- To remain supine for 10-15 min after insertion
- To report excessive cramping, bleeding, chills, fever
- Methods of pain, comfort control

diphenhydramine HCl

(dye-fen-hye'dra-meen)
Allerdryl, Baramine, Bax, Benachlor, Benadryl, Benahist, Bendylate, Benylin, Bentract, Compoz, Diphenacen, Fenylhist, Nordryl, Rohydra, Span-Lanin, Valdrene, Wehdryl
Func. class.: Antihistamine
Chem. class.: Ethanolamine derivative, H_1-receptor antagonist

Action: Acts on blood vessels, GI, respiratory system by competing with histamine for H_1-receptor site; decreases allergic response by blocking histamine

Uses: Allergy symptoms, rhinitis, motion sickness, antiparkinsonism, nighttime sedation, infant colic, nonproductive cough

Dosage and routes:

• *Adult:* PO 25-50 mg q4-6h, not to exceed 400 mg/day; IM/IV 10-50 mg, not to exceed 400 mg/day

• *Child >12 kg:* PO/IM/IV 5 mg/kg/day in 4 divided doses, not to exceed 300 mg/day

Available forms include: Caps 25, 50 mg; tabs 50 mg; elix 12.5 mg/5 ml; syr 12.5 mg/5ml; inj IM, IV 10, 50 mg/ml

Side effects/adverse reactions:

CNS: Dizziness, drowsiness, poor coordination, fatigue, anxiety, euphoria, confusion, paresthesia, neuritis

RESP: Increased thick secretions, wheezing, chest tightness

HEMA: ***Thrombocytopenia, agranulocytosis, hemolytic anemia***

GI: Dry mouth, nausea, anorexia, diarrhea

INTEG: Photosensitivity

GU: Retention, dysuria, frequency

EENT: Blurred vision, dilated pupils, tinnitus, nasal stuffiness, dry nose, throat, mouth

Contraindications: Hypersensitivity to H_1-receptor antagonist, acute asthma attack, lower respiratory tract disease

Precautions: Increased intraocular pressure, renal disease, cardiac disease, hypertension, bronchial asthma, seizure disorder, stenosed peptic ulcers, hyperthyroidism, prostatic hypertrophy, bladder neck obstruction, pregnancy (C)

Pharmacokinetics:

PO: Peak 1-3 hr, duration 4-7 hr; *IM:* Onset ½ hr, peak 1-4 hr, duration 4-7 hr; *IV:* Onset immediate, duration 4-7 hr; metabolized in liver, excreted by kidneys; crosses placenta, excreted in breast milk; half-life 2-7 hr

Interactions/incompatibilities:

• Increased CNS depression: barbiturates, narcotics, hypnotics, tricyclic antidepressants, alcohol

• Decreased effect of: oral anticoagulants, heparin

• Increased effect of: diphenhydramine: MAOIs

NURSING CONSIDERATIONS

Assess:

• I&O ratio; be alert for urinary retention, frequency, dysuria; drug should be discontinued if these occur

• CBC during long-term therapy

Administer:

• With meals if GI symptoms occur, absorption may slightly decrease

• IV undiluted; give 25 mg/1 min

• Deep IM in large muscle; rotate site

• hs only if using for sleep aid

Perform/provide:

• Hard candy, gum, frequent rinsing of mouth for dryness

• Storage in tight container at room temperature

Evaluate:

• Therapeutic response: absence of running or congested nose or rashes, improved sleep

• Respiratory status: rate, rhythm, increase in bronchial secretions, wheezing, chest tightness

Teach patient/family:

• All aspects of drug use; to notify physician if confusion, sedation, hypotension occurs

• To avoid driving or other hazardous activity if drowsiness occurs

• To avoid concurrent use of alcohol or other CNS depressants

Lab test interferences:

False negative: Skin allergy tests

Treatment of overdose: Administer ipecac syrup or lavage, diazepam, vasopressors, barbiturates (short-acting)

diphenidol

(dye-fen'-i-dole)

Vontrol

Func. class.: Antiemetic
Chem. class.: Trihexyphenidyl derivative

Action: May act as dopamine antagonist at chemoreceptor trigger zone to inhibit vomiting
Uses: Nausea, vomiting, peripheral dizziness
Dosage and routes:
• *Adult:* PO 25-50 mg q4h
• *Children >23 kg:* PO 25 mg q4h prn; do not exceed 5.5 mg/kg/24 hr
Available forms include: Tabs 25 mg
Side effects/adverse reactions:
CNS: Drowsiness, fatigue, restlessness, tremor, headache, stimulation, dizziness, insomnia, twitching, disorientation, confusion, sleep disturbance, auditory, visual hallucination, depression
GI: Nausea, indigestion
CV: Hypotension
INTEG: Rash
EENT: Dry mouth, blurred vision
Contraindications: Hypersensitivity, psychosis, anuria
Precautions: Children, prostatic hypertrophy, glaucoma, pyloric and duodenal stenosis, elderly, pregnancy (C), lactation
Pharmacokinetics:
PO: Onset 30-45 min, duration 3-6 hr, metabolized by liver, excreted by kidneys

NURSING CONSIDERATIONS

Assess:
• VS, B/P; check patients with cardiac disease more often
• Observe for CNS adverse effects: confusion, hallucination
• Monitor I&O (90% excreted in urine)
Administer:
• Tabs may be swallowed whole, chewed, or allowed to dissolve
Evaluate:
• Therapeutic response: absence of nausea, vomiting
• Signs of toxicity of other drugs or masking of symptoms of disease: brain tumor, intestinal obstruction
• Drowsiness, dizziness
Teach patient/family:
• To avoid alcohol, other depressants
• That drug should be used only under close supervision

diphenoxylate HCl with atropine sulfate

(dye-fen-ox'i-late)

Diphenatol, Lofene, Lomotil, Lo-Trol

Func. class.: Antidiarrheal
Chem. class.: Phenylipeperidine derivative, opiate agonist

Controlled Substance Schedule V
Action: Inhibits gastric motility by acting on mucosal receptors responsible for peristalsis
Uses: Diarrhea (cause undetermined)
Dosage and routes:
• *Adult:* PO 2.5-5 mg qid, titrated to patient response
• *Child 2-12 yr:* PO 0.3-0.4 mg/kg/day in divided doses
Available forms include: Tabs 2.5 mg
Side effects/adverse reactions:
CNS: Drowsiness, headache, sedation, depression, weakness, lethargy, flushing, hyperthermia
GI: Nausea, vomiting, abdominal

pain, glossitis, colitis, ***paralytic ileus, toxic megacolon,*** dry mucous membranes
EENT: Blurred vision, nystagmus, mydriasis
INTEG: Rash, urticaria, pruritus, ***angioneurotic edema***
CV: Tachycardia
GU: Urine retention
Contraindications: Hypersensitivity, severe liver disease, pseudomembranous enterocolitis, glaucoma, child <2 yr, electrolyte imbalances
Precautions: Hepatic disease, renal disease, ulcerative colitis, pregnancy (C), lactation, elderly
Pharmacokinetics:
PO: Onset 45-60 min, peak 2 hr, duration 3-4 hr, half-life 2½ hr; metabolized in liver to active, terminal half-life 12-14 hr, excreted in urine, feces, breast milk
Interactions/incompatibilities:
- Do not use with MAOIs; hypertensive crisis may occur
- Increased action of: alcohol, narcotics, barbiturates, other CNS depressants, anticholinergics

NURSING CONSIDERATIONS

Assess:
- Electrolytes (K, Na, Cl) if on long-term therapy

Administer:
- For 48 hr only

Evaluate:
- Therapeutic response: decreased diarrhea
- Bowel pattern before; for rebound constipation after termination of medication
- Response after 48 hr; if no response, drug should be discontinued
- Dehydration in children
- Abdominal distention, toxic megacolon, which may occur in ulcerative colitis

Teach patient/family:
- To avoid OTC products unless directed by physician; may contain alcohol
- Not to exceed recommended dose
- That drug may be habit forming

---

diphtheria and tetanus toxoids and pertussis vaccine (DPT)

Tri-Immunol

Func. class.: Vaccine/toxoid

Action: Provide immunity to diphtheria, tetanus, pertussis by stimulating antibody/antitoxin production
Uses: Prevention of diphtheria, tetanus, pertussis
Dosage and routes:
- *Child >6 wk-6 yr:* IM 0.5 ml at 2, 4, 6 mos, 1½ yr; booster needed 0.5 ml at age 6

Available forms include: Inj IM diphtheria 12.5 LfU, tetanus 5 LfU, pertussis 4 U/0.5 ml
Side effects/adverse reactions:
GI: Nausea, vomiting, anorexia
INTEG: Skin abscess, urticaria, itching, swelling, erythema, edema at site
CV: Tachycardia, hypotension
SYST: Lymphadenitis, ***anaphylaxis,*** fever, chills, malaise
CNS: Crying, fretfulness, fever, drowsiness, ***seizures***
MS: Osteomyelitis
Contraindications: Hypersensitivity, active infection, poliomyelitis outbreak, immunosuppression, febrile illness
Precautions: Pregnancy
Interactions/incompatibilities:
- Decreased response to toxoid: immunosuppressive agents: antineoplastics, corticosteroids, radiation therapy; alkylating agents

---

* Available in Canada only

NURSING CONSIDERATIONS

Assess:

- For skin reactions: swelling, rash, urticaria

Administer:

- At least 4 wk apart × 3 doses
- Only with epinephrine 1:1000 on unit to treat laryngospasm
- IM only; not to be given SC (vastus lateralis in infants)

Perform/provide:

- Storage in refrigerator, do not freeze
- Written record of immunization

Evaluate:

- For history of allergies, skin conditions (eczema, psoriasis, dermatitis), reactions to vaccinations
- For anaphylaxis: inability to breathe, bronchospasm

Teach patient/family:

- That doses are given at least 4 wk apart × 3 doses, booster needed at 10 yr intervals, diphtheria/tetanus

---

dipivefrin HCl

(dye-pi've-frin)

Propine

Func. class.: Adrenergic agonist
Chem. class.: Diesterified epinephrine

Action: Converted to epinephrine, which decreases aqueous production and increases outflow

Uses: Open-angle glaucoma

Dosage and routes:

- *Adult:* INSTILL 1 gtt q12h

Available forms include: Sol 0.1%

Side effects/adverse reactions:

CV: Hypertension, tachycardia, dysrhythmias

EENT: Burning, stinging, mydriasis, photophobia

Contraindications: Hypersensitivity, narrow-angle glaucoma

Precautions: Pregnancy (B), lactation, children, aphakia

Pharmacokinetics:

INSTILL: Onset 30 min, peak 1 hr, duration 12 hr

NURSING CONSIDERATIONS

Perform/provide:

- Storage at room temperature

Evaluate:

- Therapeutic response: decrease in aqueous humor of eye

Teach patient/family:

- To report stinging, burning, itching, lacrimation, puffiness
- Method of instillation, including pressure on lacrimal sac for 1 min and not to touch dropper to eye

---

dipyridamole

(dye-peer-id'a-mole)

Persantine, Pyridamole

Func. class.: Coronary vasodilator, antiplatelet
Chem. class.: Nonnitrate

Action: Increases oxygen saturation in coronary tissues, coronary blood flow; acts on small resistance vessels with little effect on vascular resistance; may increase development of collateral circulation

Uses: Prevention of transient ischemic attacks, inhibition of platelet adhesion to prevent myocardial reinfarction, thromboembolism, with warfarin in prosthetic heart valves, prevention of coronary bypass graft occlusion with aspirin; possibly effective for long-term therapy of chronic angina pectoris

Dosage and routes:

TIA

- *Adult:* PO 50 mg tid, 1 hr ac, not to exceed 400 mg qd

Inhibition of platelet adhesion

- *Adult:* PO 50-75 mg qid in combination with aspirin or warfarin

Available forms include: Tabs 25, 50, 75 mg
Side effects/adverse reactions:
CV: Postural hypotension
CNS: Headache, dizziness, weakness, fainting, syncope
GI: Nausea, vomiting, anorexia, diarrhea
INTEG: Rash, flushing
Contraindications: Hypersensitivity, hypotension
Precautions: Pregnancy (C)
Pharmacokinetics:
PO: Peak 2-2½ hr, duration 6 hr; therapeutic response may take several months, metabolized in liver, excreted in bile, undergoes enterohepatic recirculation
Interactions/incompatibilities:
• Additive antiplatelet effects: ASA, NSAID
• Increased bleeding: Coumadin
NURSING CONSIDERATIONS
Assess:
• B/P, pulse during treatment until stable; take B/P lying, standing; orthostatic hypotension is common
Administer:
• On an empty stomach: 1 hr before meals or 2 hr after
Perform/provide:
• Storage at room temperature
Evaluate:
• Therapeutic response: decreased chest pain (angina), decreased platelet adhesion
• Cardiac status: chest pain, what aggravates or ameliorates condition
Teach patient/family:
• That medication is not cure, may need to be taken continuously
• That it is necessary to quit smoking to prevent excessive vasoconstriction
• To avoid hazardous activities until stabilized on medication; dizziness may occur
Treatment of overdose: Administer IV phenylephrine

disopyramide

(dye-soe-peer'a-mide)
Rythmodan, Norpace, DSP, Napamide, Norpace CR, Norpaceor
Func. class.: Antidysrhythmic (Class IA)
Chem. class.: Nonnitrate

Action: Prolongs action potential duration and effective refractory period; reduces disparity in refractory between normal and infarcted myocardium
Uses: PVCs, ventricular tachycardia, atrial flutter, fibrillation
Dosage and routes:
• *Adult:* PO 100-200 mg q6h, in renal dysfunction 100 mg q6h; SUS REL CAPS 200 mg q12h
• *Child 12-18 yr:* PO 6-15 mg/kg/day, in divided doses q6h
• *Child 4-12 yr:* PO 10-15 mg/kg/day, in divided doses q6h
• *Child 1-4 yr:* PO 10-20 mg/kg/day, in divided doses q6h
• *Child <1 yr:* PO 10-30 mg/kg/day, in divided doses q6h
Available forms include: Caps 100, 150 mg (as phosphate), caps, sus rel 100, 150 mg
Side effects/adverse reactions:
GU: Retention, hesitancy, impotence, urinary frequency, urgency
CNS: Headache, dizziness, psychosis, fatigue, depression, paresthesias, anxiety, insomnia
GI: Dry mouth, constipation, nausea, anorexia, flatulence, diarrhea, vomiting
CV: Hypotension, bradycardia, angina, PVCs, tachycardia, increases QRS, QT segments, ***cardiac arrest,*** edema, weight gain, AV block, ***CHF***, syncope, chest pain

* Available in Canada only

META: Hypoglycemia
INTEG: Rash, pruritus, urticaria
MS: Weakness, pain in extremities
EENT: *Blurred vision, dry nose, throat, eyes,* narrow-angle glaucoma
HEMA: ***Thrombocytopenia, agranulocytosis,*** anemia (rare), decreased hemoglobin, hematocrit

Contraindications: Hypersensitivity, 2nd or 3rd degree block, cardiogenic shock, CHF (uncompensated), sick sinus syndrome, QT prolongation

Precautions: Pregnancy (C), lactation, diabetes mellitus, renal disease, children, hepatic disease, myasthenia gravis, narrow-angle glaucoma, cardiomyopathy, conduction abnormalities

Pharmacokinetics:
PO: Peak 30 min-3 hr, duration 6-12 hr
Half-life 4-10 hr, metabolized in liver, excreted in feces, urine, breast milk, crosses placenta

Interactions/incompatibilities:
- Increased effects of disopyramide: quinidine, procainamide, propranolol, lidocaine, atenolol, other antidysrhythmics
- Do not administer within 48 hr of verapamil
- Increased side effects of disopyramide: anticholinergics
- Decreased effects of disopyramide: phenytoin, rifampin

NURSING CONSIDERATIONS

Assess:
- Apical pulse for 1 min, if less than 60 check again in 1 hr; if still less than 60, notify physician
- ECG, check for increased QT, widening QRS; drug should be discontinued
- Blood level during treatment (therapeutic level 2-8 μg/ml)
- Weight daily, a rapid weight gain should be reported
- For dehydration or hypovolemia, I&O ratio, electrolytes (Na, K, Cl)
- Liver, kidney function studies (AST, ALT, bilirubin, BUN, creatinine) during treatment
- Diabetics for signs of hypoglycemia
- B/P continuously for hypotension, hypertension

Administer:
- Sugar-free gum, frequent sips of water for dry mouth
- Reduced dosage slowly with ECG monitoring

Evaluate:
- Therapeutic response: decreased dysrhythmias
- Increase in QRS, QT; drug should be discontinued
- For rebound hypertension after 1-2 hr
- Constipation, increase bulk in diet, water, stool softeners or laxatives needed
- Cardiac rate, respiration: rate, rhythm, character
- Urinary hesitancy, frequency or a change in I&O ratio; check for edema daily; check for toxicity

Teach patient/family:
- To take drug exactly as prescribed
- To avoid alcohol or severe hypotension may occur; to avoid OTC drugs or serious drug interactions may occur
- To make position change slowly during early therapy to prevent fainting
- To avoid hazardous activities if dizziness or blurred vision occurs
- Importance of complying with drug regimen; tell patient that this drug does not cure condition

Treatment of overdose: O_2, artificial ventilation, ECG, administer dopamine for circulatory depression, administer diazepam or thiopental for convulsions, gastric lavage

Lab test interferences:

Increase: Liver enzymes, lipids, BUN, creatinine

Decrease: Hgb/Hct, blood glucose

---

disulfiram

(dye-sul'fi-ram)

Antabuse, Cronetal, Ro-Sulfiram

Func. class.: Alcohol deterrent

Chem. class.: Aldehyde dehydrogenase inhibitor

Action: Blocks oxidation of alcohol at acetaldehyde stage; accumulation of acetaldehyde produces the disulfiram-alcohol reaction

Uses: Chronic alcoholism (as adjunct)

Dosage and routes:

• *Adult:* PO 250-500 mg qd × 1-2 wk, then 125-500 mg qd until fully socially recovered

Available forms include: Tabs 250, 500 mg

Side effects/adverse reactions:

CNS: Headache, drowsiness, restlessness, dizziness, fatigue, tremors, psychosis, neuritis, sweating, ***convulsions, death,*** peripheral neuropathy

GI: Nausea, vomiting, anorexia, severe thirst, ***hepatotoxicity,*** metallic, garliclike aftertaste

INTEG: Rash, dermatitis, urticaria

RESP: ***Respiratory depression,*** hyperventilation, dyspnea

CV: Tachycardia, chest pain, hypotension, ***dysrhythmias***

Disulfiram: Alcohol reaction: flushing, throbbing, headache, respiratory difficulty, nausea, vomiting, sweating, thirst, chest pain, palpitations, dyspnea, hyperventilation, tachycardia, confusion, CV collapse, MI, CHF, convulsions, death

Contraindications: Hypersensitivity, alcohol intoxication, psychoses, CV disease, pregnancy (X)

Precautions: Hypothyroidism, hepatic disease, diabetes mellitus, seizure disorders, nephritis, cerebral damage

Pharmacokinetics:

PO: Onset 12 hr, oxidized by liver, excreted unchanged in feces

Interactions/incompatibilities:

• Increased effects of: tricyclic antidepressants, diazepam, oral anticoagulants, paraldehyde, phenytoin, chlordiazepoxide, isoniazid, caffeine

• Disulfiram reaction: alcohol

• Psychosis: metronidazole

NURSING CONSIDERATIONS

Assess:

• Liver function studies q2wk during therapy: AST, ALT

• CBC, SMA q3-6 mo to detect any abnormality including increased cholesterol

Administer:

• Only with patient's knowledge; do not give to intoxicated individuals

• Once per day in the AM or hs if drowsiness occurs

• Only after patient has not been drinking for >12 hr

Evaluate:

• Therapeutic response: prevention of alcohol intake

• Mental status: affect, mood, drug history, ability to follow treatment, abstain from alcohol

• For signs of hepatotoxicity: jaundice, dark urine, clay-colored stools, abdominal pain

Teach patient/family:

• Effect of this drug if alcohol is taken; written consent for disulfi-

---

ram therapy should be obtained
- That shaving lotions, creams, lotin, cough preparations, skin products must be checked for alcohol content; even in small amount, alcohol can produce a reaction
- That tolerance will not develop if treatment is prolonged
- That reaction may occur for 2 wk after last dose
- That tablets can be crushed, mixed with beverage
- To carry ID listing disulfiram therapy
- To avoid driving or hazardous tasks if drowsiness occurs
- That disulfiram reaction can be fatal, occurs 15 min after drinking

Lab test interferences:
Increase: Cholesterol
Decrease: ^{131}I uptake, PBI, VMA
Treatment of overdose: IV vitamin C, ephedrine sulfate, antihistamines, O_2

---

dobutamine HCl

(doe-byoo'ta-meen)
Dubutrex

Func. class.: Adrenergic direct-acting β_1-agonist
Chem. class.: Catecholamine

Action: Causes increased contractility, increased coronary blood flow and heart rate by acting on β-1 receptors in heart
Uses: Cardiac surgery, refractory heart failure
Dosage and routes:
- *Adult:* IV INF 2.5-10 μg/kg/min, may increase to 40 μg/kg/min if needed

Available forms include: Inj 250 mg vial IV
Side effects/adverse reactions:
CNS: *Anxiety,* headache, dizziness
CV: Palpitations, tachycardia, hypertension, PVCs, angina
GI: Heartburn, nausea, vomiting
MS: Muscle cramps (leg)
Contraindications: Hypersensitivity, idiopathic hypertropic subaortic stenosis
Precautions: Pregnancy (C), lactation, children, hypertension
Pharmacokinetics:
IV: Onset 1-5 min, peak 10 min, half-life 2 min, metabolized in liver (inactive metabolites), excreted in urine
Interactions/incompatibilities:
- Dysrhythmias: general anesthetics
- Decreased action of dobutamine: other β-blockers
- Increased B/P: oxytocics
- Increased pressor effect and dysrhythmias: tricyclic antidepressant, MAOIs
- Incompatible with alkaline solutions: Na HCO_3

NURSING CONSIDERATIONS

Assess:
- I&O ratio
- ECG during administration continuously; if B/P increases, drug is decreased
- B/P and pulse q5min after parenteral route
- CVP or PWP during infusion if possible

Administer:
- IV diluting each 250 mg/10 ml of sterile H_2O or D_5 for inj; may be further diluted to 50 ml or more
- Plasma expanders for hypovolemia
- Parenteral (IV) dose slowly, after reconstituting, then diluting with at least 50 ml of D_5W, 0.9% NS, or Na lactate

Perform/provide:
- Storage of reconstituted solution

if refrigerated for no longer than 24 hr

Evaluate:

• Therapeutic response: increased B/P with stabilization

Teach patient/family:

• Reason for drug administration

Treatment of overdose: Administer a β-1 adrenergic blocker

docusate calcium/docusate potassium/docusate sodium

(dok'yoo-sate)

Surfak/Kasof/Bu-lax, Colace, Dialose, Diocto, DioSul, Doxinate, D.S.S., Laxinate, Regulex*, Regutol, Roctate, Sulfolax

Func. class.: Laxative, emollient
Chem. class.: Anionic surface

Action: Increases water, fat penetration in intestine; allows for easier passage of stool

Uses: To soften stools

Dosage and routes:

• *Adult:* PO 50-300 mg qd (sodium) or 240 mg (calcium or potassium) prn; ENEMA 5 ml (sodium)

• *Child >12 yr:* ENEMA 2 ml (sodium)

• *Child 6-12 yr:* PO 40-120 mg qd (sodium)

• *Child 3-6 yr:* PO 20-60 mg qd (sodium)

• *Child <3 yr:* PO 10-40 mg qd (sodium)

Available forms include: Caps 50, 100, 240, 250, 300 mg; tabs 50, 100 mg; oral sol 10, 50 mg/ml, 16.7, 20 mg/5 ml, enema conc 18 g/100 ml

Side effects/adverse reactions:

GI: Nausea, anorexia, cramps, diarrhea

INTEG: Rash

EENT: Bitter taste, throat irritation

Contraindications: Hypersensitivity, obstruction, fecal impaction, nausea/vomiting

Precautions: Pregnancy (C)

NURSING CONSIDERATIONS

Assess:

• Blood, urine electrolytes if drug is used often by patient

• I&O ratio to identify fluid loss

Administer:

• Alone with 8 oz H_2O only for better absorption; do not take within 1 hr of other drugs or within 1 hr of antacids, milk, or H_2 blockers

• In morning or evening (oral dose)

Perform/provide:

• Storage in cool environment; do not freeze

Evaluate:

• Therapeutic response: decrease in constipation

• Cause of constipation; identify whether fluids, bulk, or exercise is missing from lifestyle

• Cramping, rectal bleeding, nausea, vomiting; if these symptoms occur, drug should be discontinued

Teach patient/family:

• To swallow tabs whole; do not chew

• That normal bowel movements do not always occur daily

• Do not use in presence of abdominal pain, nausea, vomiting

• To notify physician if constipation unrelieved or if symptoms of electrolyte imbalance occur: muscle cramps, pain, weakness, dizziness, excessive thirst

• To keep out of children's reach

dopamine HCl

(doe'pa-meen)

Dopastat, Intropin, Revimine*

Func. class.: Agonist
Chem. class.: Catecholamine

Action: Causes increased cardiac

* Available in Canada only

output; acts on α-receptors, causing vasoconstriction in blood vessels; when low doses are administered, causes renal and mesenteric vasodilation

Uses: Shock, increase perfusion, hypotension

Dosage and routes:

• *Adult:* IV INF 2-5 μg/kg/min, not to exceed 50 μg/kg/min, titrate to patient's response

Available forms include: Inj 0.8, 1.6, 40, 80, 160 mg/ml

Side effects/adverse reactions:

CNS: Headache

CV: Palpitations, tachycardia, hypertension, ectopic beats, angina, wide QRS complex, peripheral vasoconstriction

GI: Nausea, vomiting, diarrhea

INTEG: Necrosis, tissue sloughing with extravasation, ***gangrene***

RESP: Dyspnea

Contraindications: Hypersensitivity, ventricular fibrillation, tachydysrhythmias, pheochromocytoma

Precautions: Pregnancy (C), lactation, arterial embolism, peripheral vascular disease

Pharmacokinetics:

IV: Onset 5 min, duration <10 min, metabolized in liver, excreted in urine (metabolites)

Interactions/incompatibilities:

• Do not use within 2 wk of MAOIs, phenytoin, barbiturates, or hypertensive crisis may result

• Dysrhythmias: general anesthetics

• Decreased action of dopamine: other β-blockers

• Increased B/P: oxytocics

• Increased pressor effect: tricyclic antidepressant, MAOIs

• Incompatible with alkaline solutions: Na HCO_3

• Additive effect: diuretics

NURSING CONSIDERATIONS

Assess:

• I&O ratio

• ECG during administration continuously; if B/P increases, drug is decreased

• B/P and pulse q5min after parenteral route

• CVP or PWP during infusion if possible

Administer:

• Plasma expanders for hypovolemia

• IV after diluting 200 mg/250-500 ml of compatible sol

• Parenteral IV dose slowly, after reconstituting, use infusion pump, flush line before infusing, infuse as secondary IV line

Perform/provide:

• Storage of reconstituted solution if refrigerated for no longer than 24 hr

• Do not use discolored solutions

Evaluate:

• Therapeutic response: increased B/P with stabilization

• Paresthesias and coldness of extremities, peripheral blood flow may decrease

• Injection site: tissue sloughing; if this occurs, administer phentolamine mixed with NS

Teach patient/family:

• Reason for drug administration

Treatment of overdose: Administer a β-1 adrenergic blocker

---

doxacurium chloride

(dox'a-cure-ee-um)

Nuromax

Func. class.: Neuromuscular blocker (nondepolarizing)

Action: Inhibits transmission of nerve impulses by binding with cholinergic receptor sites, antagonizing action of acetylcholine

Uses: Facilitation of endotracheal intubation, skeletal muscle relaxation during mechanical ventilation, surgery or general anesthesia

Dosage and routes:

• *Adult:* IV 0.05 mg/kg; 0.08 mg/kg is used for prolonged neuromuscular blockade, maintenance 0.025 mg/kg

Available forms include: Inj 1 mg/ml

Side effects/adverse reactions:

CV: ***Decreased B/P, ventricular fibrillation, myocardial infarction, cardiovascular accident***

RESP: ***Prolonged apnea, bronchospasm, wheezing, respiratory depression***

EENT: Diplopia

MS: Weakness, prolonged skeletal muscle relaxation, ***paralysis***

INTEG: Rash, urticaria

Contraindications: Hypersensitivity

Precautions: Pregnancy (C), renal, hepatic disease, lactation, children <3 mo, fluid and electrolyte imbalances, neuromuscular disease, respiratory disease, obesity, elderly

Pharmacokinetics: Not metabolized, excretion of unchanged drug in urine and bile

Interactions/incompatibilities:

• Increased neuromuscular blockade: Aminoglycosides, quinidine, local anesthetics, polymyxin antibiotics, enflurane, isoflurane, tetracyclines, halothane, magnesium, colistin, procainamide, bacitracin, lincomycin, clindamycin, lithium

• Longer onset and shorter duration of doxacurium: phenytoin, carbamazepine

NURSING CONSIDERATIONS

Assess:

• For electrolyte imblances (K, Mg); may lead to increased action of this drug

• Vital signs (B/P, pulse, respirations, airway) until fully recovered; rate, depth, pattern of respirations, strength of hand grip

• I&O ratio; check for urinary retention, frequency, hesitancy

Administer:

• Using nerve stimulator by anesthesiologist to determine neuromuscular blockade

• After succinylcholine effects subside

• Anticholinesterase to reverse neuromuscular blockade

• By slow IV over 1-2 min (only by qualified persons, usually an anesthesiologist)

• Only fresh solution

Perform/provide:

• Storage at room temperature; do not freeze

• Reassurance if communication is difficult during recovery from neuromuscular blockade

• Use reconstituted solution within 24 hr

• Frequent (q2h) instillation of artificial tears and covering eyes to prevent drying of cornea

Evaluate:

• Therapeutic response: paralysis of jaw, eyelid, head, neck, rest of body

• Recovery: decreased paralysis of face, diaphragm, leg, arm, rest of body

• Allergic reactions: if rash, fever, respiratory distress, pruritus, drug should be discontinued

Treatment of overdose: Neostigmine, monitor VS; may require mechanical ventilation

doxapram HCl

(dox'a-pram)

Dopram

Func. class.: Analeptic

Action: Respiratory stimulation through activation of peripheral carotid chemoreceptor; with higher doses medullary respiratory centers are stimulated

Uses: Chronic obstructive pulmonary disease (COPD), postanesthesia respiratory stimulation, acute hypercapnia, drug-induced CNS depression

Dosage and routes:

Postanesthesia

• *Adult:* IV inj 0.5-1 mg/kg, not to exceed 1.5 mg/kg total as a single injection; IV inf 250 mg in 250 ml sol, not to exceed 4 mg/kg, run at 1-3 mg/min

Drug-induced CNS depression

Priming IV dose of 2mg/kg, repeated in 5 min. Repeat q1-2 h till pt awakes; IV inf priming dose 2mg/kg at 1-3 mg/min, not to exceed 3 g/day

COPD

• *Adult:* IV inf 1-2 mg/min, not to exceed 3 mg/min for no longer than 2 hr

Available forms include: Inj IV 20 mg/ml

Side effects/adverse reactions:

CNS: ***Convulsions,*** (clonus/generalized), *headache,* restlessness, dizziness, confusion, paresthesias, flushing, sweating, bilateral Babinski's sign, rigidity, depression

GI: Nausea, vomiting, diarrhea, hiccups

GU: Retention, incontinence

CV: Chest pain, hypertension, change in heart rate, lowered T waves, tachycardia

INTEG: Pruritus, irritation at injection site

EENT: Pupil dilation, sneezing

RESP: ***Laryngospasm, bronchospasm,*** rebound hypoventilation, dyspnea, cough, tachypnea

Contraindications: Hypersensitivity, seizure disorders, severe hypertension, severe bronchial asthma, severe dyspnea, severe cardiac disorders, pneumothorax, pulmonary embolism, severe respiratory disease, newborns

Precautions: Bronchial asthma, pheochromocytoma, severe tachycardia, dysrhythmias, pregnancy (C), hypertension, lactation, children

Pharmacokinetics:

IV: Onset 20-40 sec, peak 1-2 min, duration 5-10 min; metabolized by liver, excreted by kidneys (metabolites), half-life 2.5-4 hr

Interactions/incompatibilities:

• Synergistic pressor effect: MAOIs, sympathomimetics

• Cardiac dysrhythmias: halothane, cyclopropane, enflurane

• Do not mix in alkaline solution including thiopental sodium, bicarbonate, aminophylline

NURSING CONSIDERATIONS

Assess:

• BP, HR, deep tendon reflexes, ABGs before administration, q30min

• PO_2, PCO_2, O_2 saturation during treatment

Administer:

• IV undiluted or diluted with equal parts of sterile H_2O for inj; may be diluted 250 mg/250 ml of D_5W, $D_{10}W$ and run as infusion

• IV at 1-3 mg/min, adjust for desired respiratory response, using infusion pump IV

• Only after adequate airway is established

• After O_2, IV barbiturates, resuscitative equipment is available

Perform/provide:

• Placing patient in Sims' position to prevent aspiration of vomitus

• Discontinue infusion if side effects occur; narrow margin of safety

Evaluate:

• Therapeutic response: increased breathing capacity

• Hypertension, dysrhythmias, tachycardia, dyspnea, skeletal muscle hyperactivity; may indicate overdosage; discontinue if these occur

• Respiratory stimulation: increased respiratory rate, abnormal rhythm

• Extravasation, change IV site q48h

Treatment of overdose: Lavage, activated charcoal, monitor electrolytes, vital signs

---

doxazosin mesylate

Cardura

Func. class.: Peripheral α-adrenergic blocker

Chem. class.: Quinozoline

Action: Peripheral blood vessels are dilated, peripheral resistance lowered; reduction in blood pressure results from α-adrenergic receptors being blocked

Uses: Hypertension

Dosage and routes:

**Adult:* PO 1 mg qd, increasing up to 16 mg qd if required; usual range 4-16 mg/day

Available forms include: Tabs 1, 2, 4, 8 mg

Side effects/adverse reactions:

CV: Palpitations, orthostatic hypotension, tachycardia, edema, dysrhythmias, chest pain

CNS: Dizziness, headache, drowsiness, anxiety, depression, vertigo, weakness, fatigue, asthenia

GI: Nausea, vomiting, diarrhea, constipation, abdominal pain

GU: Incontinence, polyuria

EENT: Epistaxis, tinnitus, dry mouth, red sclera, pharyngitis, rhinitis

Contraindications: Hypersensitivity to quinazolines

Precautions: Pregnancy (C), children, lactation, hepatic disease

Pharmacokinetics:

PO: Onset 2 hr, peak 2-6 hr, duration 6-12 hr; half-life 22 hr, metabolized in liver, excreted via bile/feces (<63%) and in urine (9%); extensively protein bound (98%)

Interaction/incompatibilities:

• Increased hypotensive effects: Beta blockers, indomethacin, verapamil

NURSING CONSIDERATIONS

Assess:

• B/P 2-6 hr after each dose and with each increase; postural effects may occur

• Pulse, jugular venous distention q4h

• BUN, uric acid if on long-term therapy

• I&O, weight daily

Administer:

• Whole; do not chew or crush tablets

Perform/provide:

• Storage in tight containers in cool environment

Evaluate:

• Therapeutic response: decreased B/P

• Edema in feet, legs daily

• Skin turgor, dryness of mucous membranes for hydration status

• Rales, dyspnea, orthopnea q30min

---

* Available in Canada only

Teach patient/family:
• That fainting occasionally occurs after 1st dose; do not drive or operate machinery for 4 hr after 1st dose or take 1st dose hs
Treatment of overdose: Administer volume expanders or vasopressors; discontinue drug; place in supine position

doxepin HCl

(dox'e-pin)
Adapin, Sinequan, Triadapin*
Func. class.: Antidepressant, tricyclic
Chem. class.: Dibenzoxepin, tertiary amine

Action: Blocks reuptake of norepinephrine, serotonin into nerve endings, increasing action of norepinephrine, serotonin in nerve cells
Uses: Major depression, anxiety
Dosage and routes:
• *Adult:* PO 50-75 mg/day in divided doses, may increase to 300 mg/day or may give daily dose hs
Available forms include: Caps 10, 25, 50, 75, 100, 150 mg; oral conc 10 mg/ml
Side effects/adverse reactions:
HEMA: ***Agranulocytosis, thrombocytopenia, eosinophilia, leukopenia***
CNS: Dizziness, drowsiness, confusion, headache, anxiety, tremors, stimulation, weakness, insomnia, nightmares, EPS (elderly), increased psychiatric symptoms, paresthesia
GI: Diarrhea, dry mouth, nausea, vomiting, ***paralytic ileus,*** increased appetite, cramps, epigastric distress, jaundice, ***hepatitis,*** stomatitis
GU: Retention, ***acute renal failure***
INTEG: Rash, urticaria, sweating, pruritus, photosensitivity
CV: Orthostatic hypotension, ECG changes, tachycardia, ***hypertension,*** palpitations
EENT: Blurred vision, tinnitus, mydriasis, ophthalmoplegia, glossitis
Contraindications: Hypersensitivity to tricyclic antidepressants, urinary retention, narrow-angle glaucoma, prostatic hypertrophy
Precautions: Suicidal patients, elderly, pregnancy (C)
Pharmacokinetics:
PO: Steady state 2-8 days; metabolized by liver, excreted by kidneys, crosses placenta, excreted in breast milk, half-life 8-24 hr
Interactions/incompatibilities:
• Decreased effects of: guanethidine, clonidine, indirect acting sympathomimetics (ephedrine)
• Increased effects of: direct acting sympathomimetics (epinephrine), alcohol, barbiturates, benzodiazepines, CNS depressants
• Hyperpyretic crisis, convulsions, hypertensive episode: MAOI (pargyline [Eutonyl])

NURSING CONSIDERATIONS

Assess:
• B/P (lying, standing), pulse q4h; if systolic B/P drops 20 mm Hg hold drug, notify physician; take vital signs q4h in patients with cardiovascular disease
• Blood studies: CBC, leukocytes, differential, cardiac enzymes if patient is receiving long-term therapy
• Hepatic studies: AST, ALT, bilirubin, creatinine
• Weight qwk, appetite may increase with drug
• ECG for flattening of T wave, bundle branch block, AV block, dysrhythmias in cardiac patients
Administer:
• Increased fluids, bulk in diet

if constipation, urinary retention occur
• With food or milk for GI symptoms
• Dosage hs if oversedation occurs during day; may take entire dose hs; elderly may not tolerate once/day dosing
• Gum, hard candy, or frequent sips of water for dry mouth
• Concentrate with fruit juice, water, or milk to disguise taste

Perform/provide:
• Storage protected from direct sunlight, in tight container
• Assistance with ambulation during beginning therapy since drowsiness/dizziness occurs
• Safety measures including siderails primarily in elderly
• Checking to see PO medication swallowed

Evaluate:
• Therapeutic response: decreased anxiety, depression
• EPS primarily in elderly: rigidity, dystonia, akathisia
• Mental status: mood, sensorium, affect, suicidal tendencies, an increase in psychiatric symptoms: depression, panic
• Urinary retention, constipation; constipation is more likely to occur in children
• Withdrawal symptoms: headache, nausea, vomiting, muscle pain, weakness; do not usually occur unless drug is discontinued abruptly
• Alcohol consumption; if alcohol is consumed, hold dose until morning

Teach patient/family:
• That therapeutic effects may take 2-3 wk
• To use caution in driving or other activities requiring alertness because of drowsiness, dizziness, blurred vision
• To avoid alcohol ingestion, other CNS depressants
• Not to discontinue medication quickly after long-term use; may cause nausea, headache, malaise
• To wear sunscreen or large hat since photosensitivity occurs

Lab test interferences:
Increase: Serum bilirubin, blood glucose, alk phosphatase
False increase: Urinary catecholamines
Decrease: VMA, 5-HIAA

Treatment of overdose: ECG monitoring, induce emesis, lavage, activated charcoal, administer anticonvulsant

doxorubicin HCl

(dox-oh-roo'bi-sin)
Adriamycin

Func. class.: Antineoplastic, antibiotic
Chem. class.: Anthracycline glycoside

Action: Inhibits DNA synthesis, primarily; derived from *Streptomyces peucetius;* replication is decreased by binding to DNA, which causes strand splitting; active throughout entire cell cycle, a vesicant

Uses: Wilms' tumor, bladder, breast, cervical, head, neck, liver, lung, ovarian, prostatic, stomach, testicular, thyroid cancer, Hodgkin's disease, acute lymphoblastic leukemia, myeloblastic leukemia, neuroblastomas, lymphomas, sarcomas

Dosage and routes:
• *Adult:* 60-75 mg/m^2 q3 wk, or 30 mg/m^2 on days 1-3 of 4-wk cycle,

* Available in Canada only

not to exceed 550 mg/m² cumulative dose

Available forms include: Inj IV 10, 20, 50 mg

Side effects/adverse reactions:
HEMA: ***Thrombocytopenia, leukopenia, anemia***
GI: Nausea, vomiting, anorexia, mucositis, ***hepatotoxicity***
GU: Impotence, sterility, amenorrhea, gynecomastia, hyperuricemia
INTEG: Rash, necrosis at injection site, dermatitis, reversible alopecia, cellulitis, thrombophlebitis at injection site
CV: Increased B/P, ***sinus tachycardia, PVCs,*** chest pain, ***bradycardia, extra systoles***

Contraindications: Hypersensitivity, pregnancy (1st trimester) (D), lactation, systemic infections

Precautions: Renal, hepatic, cardiac disease, gout, bone marrow depression (severe)

Pharmacokinetics: Triphasic pattern of elimination; half-life 12 min, 3⅓ hr, 29⅔ hr, metabolized by liver, crosses placenta, appears in breast milk, excreted in urine, bile

Interactions/incompatibilities:
- Increased toxicity: other antineoplastics or radiation
- Do not mix with other drugs in solution or syringe or use same IV tubing
- Decreased serum digoxin levels: digoxin

NURSING CONSIDERATIONS

Assess:
- CBC, differential, platelet count weekly; withhold drug if WBC is <4000/mm³ or platelet count is <75,000/mm³; notify physician of these results
- Blood, urine uric acid levels
- Renal function studies: BUN, serum uric acid, urine CrCl, electrolytes before, during therapy
- I&O ratio; report fall in urine output to <30 ml/hr
- Monitor temperature q4h; fever may indicate beginning infection
- Liver function tests before, during therapy: bilirubin, AST, ALT, alk phosphatase as needed or monthly
- ECG; watch for ST-T wave changes, low QRS and T, possible dysrhythmias (sinus tachycardia, heart block, PVCs)

Administer:
- Hydrocortisone, dexamethasone or sodium bicarbonate (1 mEq/1 ml) for extravasation, apply ice compresses
- Antiemetic 30-60 min before giving drug to prevent vomiting
- Allopurinol or sodium bicarbonate to maintain uric acid levels, alkalinization of urine
- IV after diluting 10 mg/5 ml of NaCl for inj; shake; give over 3-5 min; give through Y-tube or 3-way stopcock
- Slow IV infusion using 20-, 21-gauge needle
- Topical or systemic analgesics for pain
- Transfusion for anemia
- Antispasmodic for GI symptoms

Perform/provide:
- Strict handwashing technique, gloves, protective clothing
- Liquid diet: carbonated beverages, Jello may be added if patient is not nauseated or vomiting
- Increased fluid intake to 2-3 L/day to prevent urate, calculi formation
- Diet low in purines: absence of organ meats (kidney, liver), dried beans, peas to maintain alkaline urine
- Rinsing of mouth tid-qid with

water, club soda; brushing of teeth bid-tid with soft brush or cotton-tipped applicators for stomatitis; use unwaxed dental floss
• Storage at room temperature for 24 hr after reconstituting or 48 hr refrigerated

Evaluate:
• Therapeutic response: decreased tumor size, spread of malignancy
• Bleeding: hematuria, guaiac, bruising or petechiae, mucosa or orifices q8h
• Food preferences; list likes, dislikes
• Effects of alopecia on body image; discuss feelings about body changes
• Inflammation of mucosa, breaks in skin
• Yellowing of skin, sclera, dark urine, clay-colored stools, itchy skin, abdominal pain, fever, diarrhea
• Buccal cavity q8h for dryness, sores, ulceration, white patches, oral pain, bleeding, dysphagia
• Alkalosis if severe vomiting is present
• Local irritation, pain, burning at injection site
• GI symptoms: frequency of stools, cramping
• Acidosis, signs of dehydration: rapid respirations, poor skin turgor, decreased urine output, dry skin, restlessness, weakness
• Cardiac status: B/P, pulse, character, rhythm, rate, ABGs, ECG

Teach patient/family:
• To report any complaints, side effects to nurse or physician
• That hair may be lost during treatment and wig or hairpiece may make the patient feel better; tell patient that new hair may be different in color, texture
• To avoid foods with citric acid, hot or rough texture
• To report any bleeding, white spots, ulcerations in mouth to physician; tell patient to examine mouth qd
• That urine and other body fluids may be red-orange for 48 hr
• To avoid crowds and persons with infections when granulocyte count is low

Lab test interferences:
Increase: Uric acid

doxycycline hyclate

(dox-i-sye'kleen)

Doryx, Doxy-Caps, Doxychel, Doxycin,* Doxy-Tabs, Vibramycin, Vibra-Tabs, Vivox

Func. class.: Broad-spectrum antibiotic/antiinfective
Chem. class.: Tetracycline

Action: Inhibits protein synthesis, prosphorylation in microorganisms by binding to 30S ribosomal subunits, reversibly binding to 50S ribosomal subunits, bacteriostatic

Uses: Syphilis, *Chlamydia trachomatis*, gonorrhea, lymphogranuloma venereum, uncommon gram-negative/positive organisms

Dosage and routes:
• *Adult:* PO 100 mg q12h on day 1, then 100 mg/day; IV 200 mg in 1-2 inf on day 1, then 100-200 mg/day
• *Child >8 yr:* PO/IV 4.4 mg/kg/day in divided doses q12h on day 1, then 2.2-4.4 mg/kg/day

Gonorrhea (uncomplicated)
• *Adult:* PO 200 mg, then 100 mg hs and 100 mg bid × 3 days or 300 mg, then 300 mg in 1 hr
• Disseminated; 100 mg PO bid × at least 7 days

Chlamydia trachomatis

* Available in Canada only

• *Adult:* PO 100 mg bid × 7 days
Syphilis
• *Adult:* PO 300 mg/day in divided doses × 10 days
Available forms include: Tabs 50, 100 mg; caps 50, 100 mg; syr 50 mg/ml; powder for inj IV 100, 200 mg, powder for oral susp 25 mg/5 ml
Side effects/adverse reactions:
CNS: Fever
HEMA: ***Eosinophilia, neutropenia, thrombocytopenia, hemolytic anemia***
EENT: Dysphagia, glossitis, decreased calcification of deciduous teeth, oral candidiasis
GI: Nausea, abdominal pain, vomiting, diarrhea, anorexia, enterocolitis, ***hepatotoxicity,*** flatulence, abdominal cramps, gastric burning, stomatitis
CV: Pericarditis
GU: Increased BUN
INTEG: Rash, urticaria, photosensitivity, increased pigmentation, ***exfoliative dermatitis,*** pruritus, ***angioedema***
Contraindications: Hypersensitivity to tetracyclines, children <8 yr, pregnancy (D)
Precautions: Hepatic disease, lactation
Pharmacokinetics:
PO: Peak 1½-4 hr, half-life 15-22 hr; excreted in bile, 25%-93% protein bound
Interactions/incompatibilities:
• Do not mix with other drugs
• Decreased effects of doxycycline: antacids, $NaHCO_3$, dairy products, alkali products, iron, kaolin/pectin, barbiturates, carbemazine, phenytoin, cimetidine
• Increased effect: anticoagulants
• Decreased effects: penicillins, oral contraceptives

NURSING CONSIDERATIONS
Assess:
• I&O ratio
• Blood studies: PT, CBC, AST, ALT, BUN, creatinine
• Signs of infection
Administer:
• IV after diluting 100 mg or less/10 ml of sterile H_2O or normal saline for inj; further dilute with 100-1000 ml of compatible sol; run 100 mg or less over 1-4 hr; do not give IM/SC
• After C&S obtained
• 2 hr before or after laxative or ferrous products; 3 hr after antacid or kaolin-pectin products
Perform/provide:
• Storage in tight, light-resistant container at room temperature
Evaluate:
• Therapeutic response: decreased temperature, absence of lesions, negative C&S
• Allergic reactions: rash, itching, pruritus, angioedema
• Nausea, vomiting, diarrhea; administer antiemetic, antacids as ordered
• Overgrowth of infection: increased temperature, malaise, redness, pain, swelling, drainage, perineal itching, diarrhea, changes in cough or sputum
• IV site for phlebitis/thrombosis; drug is highly irritating
Teach patient/family:
• To avoid sun exposure since burns may occur; sunscreen does not seem to decrease photosensitivity
• If diabetic to avoid use of Clinistix, Diastix, or Tes-Tape for urine glucose testing
• That all prescribed medication must be taken to prevent superimposed infection

• To take with a full glass of water; may take with food or milk

Lab test interferences:

False negative: Urine glucose with Clinistix or Tes-Tape

False increase: Urinary catecholamines; ALT, AST

D-penicillamine

(pen-i-sill'a-meen)

Cuprimine, Depen

Func. class.: Heavy metal antagonist

Chem. class.: Chelating agent (thiol compound)

Action: Binds with ions of lead, mercury, copper, iron, zinc to form a water-soluble complex excreted by kidneys

Uses: Wilson's disease, rheumatoid arthritis, cystinuria, lead poisoning

Dosage and routes:

Cystinuria

• *Adult:* PO 250 mg qid ac, not to exceed 5 g/day

• *Child:* PO 30 mg/kg/day in divided doses qid ac

Wilson's disease

• *Adult:* PO 250 mg qid ac

• *Child:* PO 20 mg/kg/day in divided doses ac

Rheumatoid arthritis

• *Adult:* PO 125-250 mg/day, then increased 250 mg q2-3 mo if needed, not to exceed 1 g/day

Available forms include: Caps 125, 250 mg; tabs 250 mg

Side effects/adverse reactions:

HEMA: ***Thrombocytopenia, granulocytopenia, leukopenia, eosinophilia,*** Lupus syndrome, increased sedimentation rate

INTEG: Urticaria, erythema, pruritus, fever, ecchymosis

CV: Hypotension, tachycardia

GI: Diarrhea, abdominal cramping, nausea, vomiting, ***hepatotoxicity***

EENT: Tinnitus, optic neuritis

MS: Arthralgia

GU: ***Proteinuria, nephrotic syndrome, glomerulonephritis***

SYST: ***Anaphylaxis***

RESP: Pneumonitis

Contraindications: Hypersensitivity to penicillins, anuria, agranulocytosis, severe renal disease, pregnancy (D)

Pharmacokinetics:

PO: Peak 1 hr, metabolized in liver, excreted in urine

Interactions/incompatibilities:

• Increased side effects: oxyphenbutazone, phenylbutazone, gold salts, antimalarials, cytotoxics

• Decreased absorption of D-penicillamine: oral iron

NURSING CONSIDERATIONS

Assess:

• Monitor hepatic, renal studies: AST/ALT, alk phosphatase, BUN, creatinine

• Monitor I&O, temperature

• Monitor platelet, neutropenia, WBC, H&H; if WBC $<3500/mm^3$ or if platelets $<100,000/mm^3$, drug should be discontinued

Administer:

• On an empty stomach, ½-1 hr before meals or at least 2 hr after meals

• Vitamin B_6 daily, depleted when this drug is used

• Only when epinephrine 1:1000 is on unit for anaphylaxis

• Fluids to 3 L/day to prevent renal failure

Evaluate:

• Therapeutic response: absence of pain, rigidity in joints (rheumatoid arthritis)

• Allergic reactions (rash, urticaria); if these occur, drug should be discontinued

Teach patient/family:

- That urine may be red in color
- That therapeutic effect may take 1-3 mo
- To report sore throat, easy bruising, bleeding from mucous membranes; may indicate bone marrow depression

---

droperidol

(droe-per'i-dole)

Inapsine

Func. class.: Neuroleptic
Chem. class.: Butyrophenone derivative

Action: Acts on CNS at subcortical levels, produces tranquilization, sleep, antiemetic

Uses: Premedication for surgery, induction, maintenance in general anesthesia

Dosage and routes:

Induction

- *Adult:* IV 2.5 mg/20-25 lb given with analgesic or general anesthetic
- *Child 2-12 yr:* IV 1-1.5 mg/20-25 lb, titrated to response needed

Premedication

- *Adult:* IM 2.5-10 mg ½-1 hr before surgery
- *Child 2-12 yr:* IM 1-1.5 mg/20-25 lb

Maintaining general anesthesia

- *Adult:* IV 1.25-2.5 mg

Available forms include: Inj IM, IV 2.5 mg/ml

Side effects/adverse reactions:

RESP: ***Laryngospasm, bronchospasm***

CNS: Dystonia, akathisia, flexion of arms, fine tremors, dizziness, anxiety, drowsiness, restlessness, hallucination, depression

CV: Tachycardia, hypotension

EENT: Upward rotation of eyes, oculogyric crisis

INTEG: Chills, facial sweating, shivering

Contraindications: Hypersensitivity, child <2 yr, pregnancy (C)

Precautions: Elderly, cardiovascular disease (hypotension, bradydysrhythmias), renal disease, liver disease, Parkinson's disease

Pharmacokinetics:

IM/IV: Onset 3-10 min, peak ½ hr, duration 3-6 hr; metabolized in liver, excreted in urine as metabolites, crosses placenta

Interactions/incompatibilities:

- Increased CNS depression: alcohol, narcotics, barbiturates, antipsychotics or other CNS depressants
- Decreased effects of: amphetamines, anticonvulsants, anticoagulants, when given with this drug
- Increased intraocular pressure: anticholinergics, antiparkinson drugs
- Increased side effects of: lithium
- Do not mix with barbiturates in solution

NURSING CONSIDERATIONS

Assess:

- VS q10 min during IV administration, q30 min after IM dose

Administer:

- IV undiluted; give through Y-tube or 3-way stopcock; may be given as an infusion by adding dose to 250 ml LR, D_5W, 0.9% NaCl
- Anticholinergics (benztropine, diphenhydramine) for extrapyramidal reaction
- Only with crash cart, resuscitative equipment nearby
- IV slowly only

Perform/provide:

- Slow movement of patient to avoid orthostatic hypotension

D

Evaluate:

• Therapeutic response: decreased anxiety, absence of vomiting during and after surgery

• Extrapyramidal reactions: dystonia, akathisia

• For increasing heart rate or decreasing B/P, notify physician at once; do not place patient in Trendelenburg position or sympathetic blockade may occur causing respiratory arrest

---

dyphylline

(dye'fi-lin)

Asminyl, Dilin, Dilor, Dyflex, Dylline, Lufyllin, Neothylline, Oxystat, Protophylline*

Func. class.: Spasmolytic

Chem. class.: Xanthine, ethylenediamide

Action: Relaxes smooth muscle of respiratory system by blocking phosphodiesterase, which increases cyclic AMP

Uses: Bronchial asthma, bronchospasm in chronic bronchitis, COPD

Dosage and routes:

• *Adult:* PO 200-800 mg q6h; IM 250-500 mg q6h injected slowly

• *Child >6 yr:* PO 4-7 mg/kg/day in 4 divided doses

Available forms include: Tabs 200, 400 mg; elix 100, 160 mg/15 ml; inj IM 250 mg/ml

Side effects/adverse reactions:

CNS: Anxiety, restlessness, insomnia, dizziness, ***convulsions,*** headache, light-headedness, muscle twitching

CV: Palpitations, sinus tachycardia, hypotension, flushing, dysrhythmias

GI: Nausea, vomiting, anorexia, dyspepsia, epigastric pain

INTEG: Flushing, urticaria

RESP: Tachypnea

Other: Fever, dehydration, ***albuminuria,*** hyperglycemia

Contraindications: Hypersensitivity to xanthines, tachydysrhythmias

Precautions: Elderly, CHF, cor pulmonale, hepatic disease, active peptic ulcer disease, diabetes mellitus, hyperthyroidism, hypertension, children, renal disease, pregnancy (C), glaucoma

Pharmacokinetics: Peak 1 hr, half-life 2 hr, excreted in urine unchanged

Interactions/incompatibilities:

• Do not mix in syringe with other drugs

• Increased action of dyphylline: cimetidine, propranolol, erythromycin, troleandomycin

• May increase effects of: anticoagulants

• Cardiotoxicity: β-blockers

• Increased metabolism: barbiturates, phenytoin

• Decreased elimination of dyphylline: uricosurics

NURSING CONSIDERATIONS

Assess:

• Dyphylline blood levels; toxicity may occur with small increase above 20 μg/ml

• Monitor I&O; diuresis occurs, dehydration may result in elderly or children

• Whether theophylline was given recently

Administer:

• PO after meals to decrease GI symptoms; absorption may be affected

• Avoid IM injection; pain occurs

Perform/provide

• Storage protected from light, at room temperature

Evaluate:

• Therapeutic response: decreased dyspnea, respiratory rate, rhythm

---

* Available in Canada only

• Auscultate lung fields bilaterally; notify physician of abnormalities
• Allergic reactions: rash, urticaria; if these occur, drug should be discontinued

Teach patient/family
• To check OTC medications, current prescription medications for ephedrine; will increase stimulation; not to drink alcohol or caffeine
• To avoid hazardous activities; dizziness, drowsiness, blurred vision may occur
• If GI upset occurs, to take drug with 8 oz of water; avoid food, since absorption may be decreased

echothiophate iodide

(ek-oh-thye'oh-fate)

Phospholine Iodide, Echodide

Func. class.: Miotic

Chem. class.: Cholinesterase inhibitor, irreversible

Action: Prevents breakdown of neurotransmitter acetylcholine, which then accumulates, causing enhancement, prolongation of its physiologic effects

Uses: Glaucoma (open-angle), accommodative esotropia, treatment of obstructed aqueous outflow; extremely effective in control of chronic wide-angle glaucoma, aphakic glaucoma, congenital glaucoma

Dosage and routes:
• *Adult and child:* INSTILL 1 gtt of 0.03%, or 0.125% sol qd in conjunctival sac, not to exceed 1 gtt bid

Available forms include: Powder for reconstitution, 1.5 mg (0.03%), 3 mg (0.06%), 6.25 mg (0.125%), 12.5 mg (0.25%) with 5 ml diluent

Side effects/adverse reactions:
GU: Frequency
CV: Hypotension, bradycardia, ***cardiac arrest***
INTEG: Sweating, pallor, cyanosis
RESP: ***Bronchospasm***
GI: Nausea, vomiting, abdominal cramps, diarrhea
EENT: *Blurred vision, stinging, burning, lacrimination,* lid muscle twitching, conjunctival, ciliary redness, browache, headache, induced myopia, iris cysts, hyperemia, hyphema

Contraindications: Hypersensitivity, ureitis

Precautions: Asthma, bradycardia, parkinsonism, peptic ulcer, pregnancy (C)

Interactions/incompatibilities:
• Decreased effect of echothiophate: pilocarpine
• Increased effect of both drugs: ambenonium, edrophonium, neostigmine, physostigmine, pyridostigmine
• Increased effects of: general anesthetics

NURSING CONSIDERATIONS

Administer:
• After checking vial for concentration
• Immediately after reconstituting; discard unused portion
• After reconstituting powder with diluent provided

Evaluate:
• Therapeutic response: decreased aqueous humor in eye
• Specific condition being treated
• History of patient's previous/current conditions (e.g., asthma, cardiac), possible sensitivity, contraindications, drug interactions

Teach patient/family:
• Why patient is receiving medication; patient, family should have a clear regimen as well as name of medication
• To report change in vision, blur-

ring or loss of sight, trouble breathing, sweating, flushing
• Method of instillation, including pressure on lacrimal sac for 1 min, not to touch dropper to eye
• That long-term therapy may be required
• That blurred vision will decrease with repeated use of drug
• That patient may experience stinging sensation, dull ache or tearing, which should subside in a few minutes; if it persists, contact physician
• That patient may experience decreased visual ability at night; instruct not to drive
• To use drops at night to eliminate hazardous, transient blurring

---

econazole nitrate (topical)

(e-kone'a-zole)

Ecostatin, Spectazole

Func. class.: Local antiinfective
Chem. class.: Imidazole derivative, antifungal

Action: Interferes with fungal cell membrane, which increases permeability, leaking of cell nutrients
Uses: Tinea pedis, tinea cruris, tinea corporis, tinea versicolor, cutaneous candidiasis
Dosage and routes:
• *Adult and child:* TOP apply to affected area bid-qid depending on condition
Available forms include: Cream 1%
Side effects/adverse reactions:
INTEG: Rash, urticaria, stinging, burning, pruritus
Contraindications: Hypersensitivity
Precautions: Pregnancy (C), lactation

NURSING CONSIDERATIONS
Administer:
• Enough medication to completely cover lesions
• After cleansing with soap, water before each application, dry well
• For 2 wk in tinea cruris, tinea corporis, *Candida* infections; 1 month tinea pedis
Perform/provide:
• Storage at room temperature in dry place
Evaluate:
• Therapeutic response: decrease in size, number of lesions
• Allergic reaction: burning, stinging, swelling, redness
Teach patient/family:
• To use medical asepsis (hand washing) before, after each application
• To apply with glove to prevent further infection
• To avoid use of OTC creams, ointments, lotions unless directed by physician
• Not to cover with occlusive dressing
• To continue even though condition improves
• To notify physician if condition worsens

---

edetate calcium disodium

(ed'e-tate)

Calcium Disodium Versenate, Calcium EDTA

Func. class.: Heavy metal antagonist
Chem. class.: Chelating agent

Action: Binds ions of lead to form a water-soluble complex that is removed by kidneys
Uses: Lead poisoning, acute lead encephalopathy

Dosage and routes:
Acute lead encephalopathy
• *Adult and child:* 1.5 g/m²/day × 3-5 days, with dimercaprol, may be given again after 4 days off drug
Lead poisoning
• *Adult:* IV 1 g/250-500 ml D_5W or 0.9% NaCl over 1-2 hr or q12h × 3-5 days, may repeat after 2 days, not to exceed 50 mg/kg/day, may be given as a continuous infusion over 8-24 hr
• *Child:* IM 35 mg/kg/day in divided doses q8-12h, not to exceed 50 mg/kg/day
Available forms include: Inj IM, IV 200 mg/ml
Side effects/adverse reactions:
CNS: Headache, paresthesia, numbness
INTEG: Urticaria, erythema, pruritus, pain at injection site, fever, cheilosis
CV: Hypotension, dysrhythmias, thrombophlebitis
GI: Vomiting, *diarrhea, abdominal cramps, anorexia,* cheilosis, histamine-like reaction with GI distress
EENT: Nasal congestion, sneezing
MS: Leg cramps, myalgia, arthralgia, weakness
GU: ***Hematuria, renal tubular necrosis, proteinuria***
Contraindications: Hypersensitivity, anuria, hepatic insufficiency, poisoning of other metals, severe renal disease, child <3 yr
Precautions: Hypertension, pregnancy (C), lactation, gout, active TB
Pharmacokinetics:
Not metabolized, excreted in urine, half-life: 20-60 min (IV), 90 min (IM)

NURSING CONSIDERATIONS
Assess:
• VS, B/P, pulse, respirations, weigh daily
• Monitor I&O, kidney function studies: BUN, creatinine, CrCl; watch for decreasing urine output
• Neuro status: Watch for paresthesias, beginning convulsions
• Urine: pH, albumin, casts, blood, coproporphyrins, calcium
• For febrile reactions that may occur 4-8 hr following drug therapy
Administer:
• EDTA, BAL separately
• IV slowly, IM is preferred route
• IM in large muscle mass; rotate injection sites, procaine HCl should be added to IM injection (1 ml of procaine 1% to each ml of concentrated drug) to minimize pain at injection site
• Only when epinephrine 1:1000 is on unit for anaphylaxis
• IV fluids to ensure adequate hydration before administration of drug
Evaluate:
• Therapeutic response: decreased symptoms of lead poisoning
• Cardiac abnormalities: dysrhythmias, hypotension, tachycardia
• Allergic reactions (rash, urticaria); if these occur drug should be discontinued
Teach patient/family:
• That compliance to dosage schedule must be followed
Lab test interferences:
Decrease: Cholesterol/triglycerides, potassium

edetate disodium
(ed'e-tate)
Disodium EDTA, Disotate, Endrate
Func. class.: Metal antagonist
Chem. class.: Chelating agent

Action: Binds with ions of cal-

cium, zinc, magnesium to form a water-soluble complex excreted from kidneys
Uses: Hypercalcemic crisis
Dosage and routes:
• *Adult and child:* IV INF 15-50 mg/kg/500 ml of D_5W or 0.9% NaCl, given over 3-4 hr, not to exceed 3 g/day (adult) or 70 mg/kg/day (child)
Available forms include: Inj conc 150 mg/ml
Side effects/adverse reactions:
CNS: Headache, paresthesia, ***convulsions***
INTEG: Urticaria, erythema, pain at injection site, hypertension
CV: Hypotension, ***exfoliative dermatitis,*** thrombophlebitis
GI: Nausea, vomiting, anorexia, diarrhea, abdominal cramps
GU: Dysuria, pyelonephritis, ***nephrotoxicity,*** hyperuricemia, hypomagnesemia, polyuria, ***proteinuria, renal tubular necrosis, hypocalcemia***
Contraindications: Hypersensitivity, anuria, hepatic insufficiency, poisoning of other metals, severe renal disease, child <3 yr, seizure disorders, active/inactive TB
Precautions: Hypertension, pregnancy (C), lactation
Pharmacokinetics:
Excreted in urine as calcium chelate

NURSING CONSIDERATIONS
Assess:
• VS, B/P, pulse; if hypotension occurs, drug should be discontinued
• Monitor I&O, kidney function studies: BUN, creatinine, CrCl, calcium (must be done following each administration)
Administer:
• Only when IV calcium preparation is on unit for emergency use
• EDTA, BAL separately
• IV slowly, use infusion pump, rotate infusion sites, observe site for redness, inflammation
• IV fluids to ensure adequate hydration before administration of drug
Perform/provide:
• Assistance with ambulation
Evaluate:
• Therapeutic response: calcium levels between 9-10 mg/dl; absence of hypercalcemic symptoms
• Hypocalcemia: numbness of feet, hands, tongue, lips; positive Chvostek's, Trousseau's signs; convulsions; stupor
• Cardiac abnormalities: dysrhythmias, hypotension, tachycardia
• Allergic reactions (rash, urticaria); if these occur, drug should be discontinued
Teach patient/family:
• To remain recumbent for ½ hr to prevent postural hypotension
• To make position changes slowly to prevent fainting
• That compliance to dosage schedule must be followed
• That breath may be odorous
Lab test interferences:
False decrease: Calcium
Decrease: Magnesium, alk phosphatase

edrophonium chloride

(ed-roe-foe'nee-um)
Enlon, Tensilon
Func. class.: Cholinergics, anticholinesterase
Chem. class.: Quaternary ammonium compound

Action: Inhibits destruction of acetylcholine, which increases concentration at sites where acetylcholine is released; this facilitates transmission of impulses across myoneural junction

Uses: To diagnose myasthenia gravis, curare antagonist, differentiation of myasthenic crisis from cholinergic crisis

Dosage and routes:

Tensilon test

• *Adult:* IV 1-2 mg over 15-30 sec, then 8 mg if no response, IM: 10 mg; if cholinergic reaction occurs, retest after ½ hr with 2 mg IM

• *Child >34 kg:* IV 2 mg, if no response in 45 sec then 1 mg q45 sec, not to exceed 10 mg

• *Child <34 kg:* IV 1 mg, if no response in 45 sec, then 1 mg q45 sec, not to exceed 5 mg

• *Infant:* IV 0.5 mg

Curare antagonist

• *Adult:* IV 10 mg over 30-45 sec, may repeat, not to exceed 40 mg

Differentiation of myasthenic crisis from cholinergic crisis

• *Adult:* IV 1 mg, if no response in 1 min, may repeat

Available forms include: Inj IV 10 mg/ml

Side effects/adverse reactions:

INTEG: Rash, urticaria

CNS: Dizziness, headache, sweating, confusion, weakness, ***convulsions,*** incoordination, ***paralysis***

GI: Nausea, diarrhea, vomiting, cramps

CV: Tachycardia, dysrhythmias, bradycardia, hypotension AV block, ECG changes, ***cardiac arrest***

GU: Frequency, incontinence

RESP: ***Respiratory depression, bronchospasm, constriction, laryngospasm, respiratory arrest***

EENT: Miosis, blurred vision, lacrimation

Contraindications: Obstruction of intestine, renal system, hypersensitivity

Precautions: Seizure disorders, bronchial asthma, coronary occlusion, hyperthyroidism, dysrhythmias, peptic ulcer, megacolon, poor GI motility, pregnancy (C), bradycardia, hypotension

Pharmacokinetics:

IV: Onset 30-60 sec, duration 6-24 min

IM: Onset 2-10 min, duration 12-45 min

Interactions/incompatibilities:

• Decreased action of edrophonium: procainamide, quinidine, aminoglycosides, anesthetics, mecamylamine, polymyxin, magnesium, corticosteroids, antidysrythmics

• Bradycardia: digitalis

NURSING CONSIDERATIONS

Assess:

• VS, respiration during test

• Diabetic patient carefully since this drug lowers blood glucose

Administer:

• IV undiluted or given as continuous infusion

• Only with atropine sulfate available for cholinergic crisis

• Only after all other cholinergics have been discontinued

Perform/provide:

• Storage at room temperature

Evaluate:

• Therapeutic response: increased muscle strength, hand grasp, improved gait, absence of labored breathing (if severe)

Teach patient/family:

• To wear Medic Alert ID specifying myasthenia gravis, drugs taken

Treatment of overdose:

Respiratory support, atropine 1-4 mg (IV)

emetine HCl

(em′e-teen)

Func. class.: Amebicide
Chem. class.: Ipecac alkaloid

Action: Inhibits protein synthesis in developing trophozoites

Uses: Amebic dysentery (acute fulminating), amebic hepatitis, amebic abscess

Dosage and routes:

Amebic dysentery

• *Adult:* SC/IM 1 mg/kg/day, not to exceed 60 mg/day × 3-5 days simultaneously with another amebicide

• *Child:* IM 1 mg/kg/day in 2 divided doses × 5 days, not to exceed 20 mg/day >8 yr, 10 mg/day <8 yr

Amebic hepatitis/abscess

• *Adult:* SC/IM 60 mg/day × 10 days

• *Child:* IM 1 mg/kg in 2 doses × 5 days, not to exceed 20 mg/day >8 yr, 10 mg/day <8 yr (use only if other amebicides have failed)

Available forms include: Inj SC/IM 65 mg/ml

Side effects/adverse reactions:

CV: Hypotension, tachycardia, dysrhythmia, pericarditis, ECG abnormalities, ***CHF,*** chest pain, gallop rhythm, palpitations, hypotension, myocarditis, ***cardiac arrest,*** T-wave inversion, increased QT, widening QRS

HEMA: ***Thrombocytopenia***

INTEG: Rash, pruritus, necrosis, abscess

GI: Nausea, vomiting, diarrhea, epigastric distress, anorexia

CNS: Weakness, tremors, aching, fatigue, depression, paresthesia, ***paralysis,*** encephalitis

Contraindications: Hypersensitivity, renal disease, hepatic disease, pregnancy (X)

Precautions: Elderly, lactation, surgery patients, hypotension, children

Pharmacokinetics:

SC/IM: Metabolized in liver, excreted in urine slowly over 40-60 days

NURSING CONSIDERATIONS

Assess:

• Stools during entire treatment; should be clear at end of therapy; stools must be clear for 1 yr before patient is considered cured

• ECG q2-3d before, after 5th dose, after last therapy dose, 1 wk after; be aware that inversion of T waves occurs

• Vision by ophthalmologic exam during, after therapy; vision problems occur often

• Injection site for irritation, absence of necrosis q8h

• I&O, stools for number, frequency, character

• B/P, pulse q4h; watch for decrease in B/P; discontinue

Administer:

• Being careful not to get drug in eyes; causes mucous membrane irritation

• Cleansing enema if ordered before beginning treatment

• SC or IM, never IV; rotate injection sites

• PO after meals to avoid GI symptoms

Perform/provide:

• Storage in tight, light-resistant container

Evaluate:

• Therapeutic response: decreased diarrhea, symptoms of amebiasis

• Allergic reaction: fever, rash, itching, chills; drug should be discontinued if these occur

• Superimposed infection, fever,

monilial growth, fatigue, malaise
• Tachycardia, decreasing B/P, GI symptoms, weakness, neuromuscular symptoms
• Diarrhea for 2-3 days

Teach patient/family:
• Proper hygiene after BM: hand-washing technique
• To avoid contact of drug with eyes, mouth, nose, other mucous membranes
• Need for compliance with dosage schedule, duration of treatment

---

enalapril maleate

(en-al-a'prel)
Vasotec, Vasotec IV

Func. class.: Antihypertensive
Chem. class.: Renin-angiotensin antagonist

Action: Selectively suppresses renin-angiotensin-aldosterone system; inhibits ACE, prevents conversion of angiotensin I to angiotensin II, dilation of arterial, venous vessels

Uses: Hypertension

Dosage and routes:
• *Adult:* PO 5 mg/day, may increase or decrease to desired response range 10-40 mg/day

Hypertension
• *Adult:* IV 1.25 mg q6h over 5 min

Patients on diuretics
• *Adult:* IV 0.625 over 5 min, may give additional doses of 1.25 mg q6h

Renal impairment
• *Adult:* 1.25 mg q6h with CrCl <3 mg/dl or 0.625 mg if CrCl >3 mg/dl

Available forms include: Tabs 5, 10, 20 mg, inj 1.25 mg/ml

Side effects/adverse reactions:
CV: Hypotension, chest pain, tachycardia, dysrhythmias
CNS: Insomnia, dizziness, paresthesias, headache, fatigue, anxiety
GI: Nausea, vomiting, colitis, cramps, diarrhea, constipation flatulence, dry mouth, loss of taste
INTEG: Rash, purpura, alopecia, hyperhidrosis
HEMA: ***Agranulocytosis, neutropenia***
EENT: Tinnitus, visual changes, sore throat, double vision, dry burning eyes
GU: ***Proteinuria, renal failure,*** increased frequency of polyurea or oliguria
RESP: Dyspnea, cough, rales, angioedema
META: Hyperkalemia

Contraindications: Pregnancy (C), lactation

Precautions: Renal disease, hyperkalemia

Pharmacokinetics:
PO: Peak 4-6 hr; half-life 1½ hr; metabolized by liver to active metabolite, excreted in urine
IV: Onset 5-15 min, peak up to 4 hr

Interactions/incompatibilities:
• Hypersensitivity: allopurinol
• Severe hypotension: diuretics, other antihypertensives
• Decreased effects of enalapril: aspirin, antacids
• Increased potassium levels: salt substitutes, potassium-sparing diuretics, potassium supplements
• May increase effects of: ergots, neuromuscular blocking agents, antihypertensives, hypoglycemics, barbiturates, reserpine, levodopa
• Effects may be increased by phenothiazines, diuretics, phenytoin, quinidine, nifedipine

NURSING CONSIDERATIONS

Assess:
• B/P, pulse q4h; note rate, rhythm, quality

• Electrolytes: K, Na, Cl
• Baselines in renal, liver function tests before therapy begins

Administer:
• By slow IV, over 5 min, use diluent provided or 50 ml of D_5W, 0.9% NaCl, 0.9% NaCl in D_5W or LR, Isolyte E

Evaluate:
• Therapeutic response: decreased B/P
• Edema in feet, legs daily
• Skin turgor, dryness of mucous membranes for hydration status
• Symptoms of CHF: edema, dyspnea, wet rales

Teach patient/family:
• To administer 1 hr before meals
• Not to use OTC (cough, cold, or allergy) products unless directed by physician
• To avoid sunlight or wear sunscreen if in sunlight, photosensitivity may occur
• To comply with dosage schedule, even if feeling better
• To notify physician of: mouth sores, sore throat, fever, swelling of hands or feet, irregular heartbeat, chest pain, signs of angioedema
• Excessive perspiration, dehydration, vomiting, diarrhea may lead to fall in blood pressure—consult physician if these occur
• That drug may cause dizziness, fainting; light-headedness may occur during 1st few days of therapy
• That drug may cause skin rash or impaired perspiration
• Not to discontinue drug abruptly
• Not to use OTC products unless directed by physician
• To rise slowly to sitting or standing position to minimize orthostatic hypotension

Lab test interferences:
Interference: Glucose/insulin tolerance tests

Treatment of overdose: Lavage, IV atropine for bradycardia, IV theophylline for bronchospasm, digitalis, O_2, diuretic for cardiac failure, hemodialysis

enoxacin

(en-ox'aa-sin)
Penetrex

Func. class.: Antiinfective
Chem. class.: Fluoroquinolone

Action: Inhibits the enzyme that repairs bacterial DNA, thereby preventing bacterial replication

Uses: Uncomplicated urethral or cervical gonorrhea, uncomplicated and complicated urinary tract infections (UTI)

Dosage and routes:
Gonorrhea
• *Adult:* PO 400 mg as a single dose
Uncomplicated UTI
• *Adult:* PO 200 mg bid × 7 days
Complicated UTI
• *Adult:* PO 400 mg bid × 14 days

Available forms include: Tabs 200, 400 mg

Side effects/adverse reactions:
CNS: Dizziness, headache, fatigue, somnolence, depression, insomnia
GI: Diarrhea, nausea, vomiting, anorexia, flatulence, heartburn, dry mouth, increased AST, ALT
INTEG: Rash
EENT: Visual disturbances

Contraindications: Hypersensitivity to quinolones

Precautions: Pregnancy (C), lactation, children, elderly, renal disease, seizure disorders

Pharmacokinetics:
PO: Peak 1 hr, half-life 3-6 hr, steady state 2 days; excreted in urine as unchanged drug, metabolites

Interactions/incompatibilities:
• Decreased effects of enoxacin: antacids, nitrofurantoin
• Increased enoxacin levels: probenecid
• Increased toxicity: theophylline

NURSING CONSIDERATIONS

Assess:
• Kidney, liver function studies: BUN, creatinine, AST, ALT
• I&O ratio, urine pH; <5.5 is ideal

Administer:
• After clean-catch urine is obtained for C&S

Perform/provide:
• Limited intake of alkaline foods, drugs; milk, dairy products, peanuts, vegetables, alkaline actacids, sodium bicarbonate

Evaluate:
• Therapeutic response: negative C&S
• CNS symptoms: insomnia, vertigo, headache, agitation, confusion
• Allergic reactions: rash, flushing, urticaria, pruritus

Teach patient/family:
• Fluids must be increased to 3L/day to avoid crystallization in kidneys
• If dizziness occurs, to ambulate, perform activities with assistance
• To complete full course of drug therapy
• To contact physician if adverse reactions occur

ephedrine sulfate (nasal)

(e-fed'rin)

Vatronol Nose Drops, Efedron Nasal

Func. class.: Nasal decongestant
Chem. class.: Indirect/direct sympathomimetic amine

Action: Relaxes bronchial smooth muscle, increases diameter of nasal passage by action on β_2-adrenergic receptors

Uses: Nasal congestion associated with colds, hayfever, sinusitis, other allergic conditions, adjunct in middle ear infections

Dosage and routes:
• *Adult and child:* Instill 3-4 gtts, q4h or small amount of gel in each nostril q4h

Available forms include: Sol 0.5% sulfate, gel 0.6% HCl

Side effects/adverse reactions:
GI: Nausea, vomiting, anorexia
EENT: Irritation, burning, sneezing, stinging, dryness, rebound congestion
INTEG: Contact dermatitis
CNS: Anxiety, restlessness, tremors, weakness, insomnia, dizziness, fever, headache

Contraindications: Hypersensitivity to sympathomimetic amines

Precautions: Child <6 yr, elderly, diabetes, cardiovascular disease, hypertension, hyperthyroidism, increase ICP, prostatic hypertrophy, pregnancy (C)

Interactions/incompatibilities:
• Hypertension: MAOIs, β-adrenergic blockers
• Hypotension: methyldopa, mecamylamine, reserpine

NURSING CONSIDERATIONS

Administer:
• No more than q4h
• For <4 consecutive days

Perform/provide:
• Environmental humidification to decrease nasal congestion, dryness
• Storage in light-resistant containers; do not expose to high temperatures

Evaluate:
• Therapeutic response: decreased congestion, runny nose

• Redness, swelling, pain in nasal passages

Teach patient/family:

• That stinging may occur for a few applications; drying of mucosa may be decreased by environmental humidification

• To notify physician if irregular pulse, insomnia, dizziness, or tremors occur

• Proper administration to avoid systemic absorption

ephedrine sulfate

(e-fed'rin)

Efedrin, Vatronol

Func. class.: Adrenergic, mixed direct and indirect effects

Chem. class.: Phenylisopropylamine

Action: Causes increased contractility and heart rate by acting on β-receptors in the heart; also, acts on α-receptors, causing vasoconstriction in blood vessels

Uses: Shock, increase perfusion, hypotension, bronchodilation

Dosage and routes:

• *Adult:* IM/SC 25-50 mg, not to exceed 150 mg/24 hr

IV 10-25 mg, not to exceed 150 mg/24 hr

• *Child:* SC/IV 3 mg/kg/day in divided doses q4-6h

Bronchodilator

• *Adult:* PO 12.5-50 mg bid-qid, not to exceed 400 mg/day

• *Child:* PO 2-3 mg/kg/day in 4-6 divided doses

Available forms include: Inj 25, 50 mg/ml, IM, SC, IV; caps 25, 50 mg; syr 11, 20 mg/5 ml

Side effects/adverse reactions:

CNS: Tremors, anxiety, insomnia, headache, dizziness, confusion, hallucinations, ***convulsions, CNS depression***

GU: Dysuria, urinary retention

CV: Palpitations, tachycardia, hypertension, chest pain, ***dysrhythmias***

GI: Anorexia, nausea, vomiting

RESP: ***Dyspnea***

Contraindications: Hypersensitivity to sympathomimetics, narrow-angle glaucoma

Precautions: Pregnancy (C), cardiac disorders, hyperthyroidism, diabetes mellitus, prostatic hypertrophy

Pharmacokinetics:

PO: Onset 15-60 min, duration 2-4 hr

IV: Onset 5 min, duration 2 hr

Metabolized in liver, excreted in urine (unchanged), crosses blood-brain barrier, placenta, breast milk

Interactions/incompatibilities:

• Do not use with MAOIs or tricyclic antidepressants; hypertensive crisis may occur

• Decreased effect of ephedrine: methyldopa, urinary acidifiers, rauwolfia alkaloids

• Increased effect of this drug: urinary alkalizers

• Dysrhythmia: halothane, anesthetics, digitalis

• Decreased effect of: guanethidine

NURSING CONSIDERATIONS

Assess:

• I&O ratio

• ECG during administration continuously, if B/P increases, drug is decreased

• B/P and pulse q5min after parenteral route

• CVP or PWP during infusion if possible

Administer:

• IV undiluted given through Y-

tube or 3-way stopcock; give 10 mg or less over 1 min
• Plasma expanders for hypovolemia

Perform/provide:
• Storage of reconstituted solution if refrigerated for no longer than 24 hr
• Do not use discolored solutions

Evaluate:
• Therapeutic response: increased B/P with stabilization
• For paresthesias and coldness of extremities, peripheral blood flow may decrease
• Injection site: tissue sloughing; if this occurs administer phentolamine mixed with NS

Teach patient/family:
• Reason for drug administration

Treatment of overdose: Administer phentolamine for hypertension, diazepam for convulsions

---

epinephrine/ epinephrine bitartrate/ epinephrine HCl

(ep-i-nef'rin)

Bronkaid Mist, Epi Pen, Epi Pen Jr Sus-Phrine (parenteral) Primatene Mist AsthmaHaler, Medihaler-Epi Adrenalin, Sus-Phrine, Vaponefrin*

Func. class.: Adrenergic
Chem. class.: Catecholamine

Action: β_1- and β_2-agonist causing increased levels of cyclic AMP producing bronchodilation, cardiac, and CNS stimulation; large doses cause vasoconstriction; small doses can cause vasodilation via β_2-vascular receptors

Uses: Acute asthmatic attacks, hemostasis, bronchospasm, anaphylaxis, allergic reactions, cardiac arrest

Dosage and routes:
• *Adult:* IM/SC 0.1-0.5 ml of 1:1000 sol, may repeat q10-15 min IV 0.1-0.25 ml of 1:1000 sol
• *Child:* SC 0.01 ml of 1:1000/kg, may repeat q20min to 4 hr; INH 0.005 ml/kg of 1:200 solution, may repeat q8-12h

Asthma
• *Adult and child:* INH 1-2 puffs of 1:100 or 2.25% racemic q1-5min

Hemostasis
• *Adult:* TOP 1:50,000-1:1000 applied as needed to stop bleeding

Cardiac arrest
• *Adult:* IC, IV, endotracheal 0.1-1 mg repeat q5min PRN
• *Child:* IC, IV, endotracheal 5-10 μg q5min, may use 0.1 μ/kg/min IV inf after inital dose

Available forms include: Aerosol 0.16 mg/spray, 0.2 mg/spray, 0.25 mg/spray, inj 1:1000 (1 mg/ml), 1:200 (5 mg/ml), 0.01 mg/ml (1:100,000), 0.1 mg/ml (1:10,000), 0.5 mg/ml (1:2,000); IM, IV, SC; sol for nebulization 1:100, 1.25% 2.25% (base)

Side effects/adverse reactions:
GU: Urinary retention
CNS: Tremors, anxiety, insomnia, headache, dizziness, confusion, hallucinations, ***cerebral hemorrhage***
CV: Palpitations, tachycardia, hypertension, *dysrhythmias,* increase T wave
GI: Anorexia, nausea, vomiting
RESP: Dyspnea

Contraindications: Hypersensitivity to sympathomimetics, narrow-angle glaucoma

Precautions: Pregnancy (C), cardiac disorders, hyperthyroidism, diabetes mellitus, prostatic hypertrophy

Pharmacokinetics:
SC: Onset 3-5 min, duration 20 min
PO, INH: Onset 1 min

Interactions/incompatibilities:
• Do not use with MAOIs or tricyclic antidepressants; hypertensive crisis may occur
• Decreased effect of epinephrine: methyldopa, urinary acidifiers, rauwolfia alkaloids
• Increased effect of epinephrine: urinary alkalizers

NURSING CONSIDERATIONS

Assess:
• ECG during administration continuously; if B/P increases, drug is decreased
• B/P and pulse q5min after parenteral route
• CVP or PCWP during infusion if possible

Administer:
• Parenteral IV dose slowly, after reconstituting 1 mg (1:1000 sol)/ 10 ml or more normal saline; to prepare a 1:10,000 sol for maintenance may be further diluted in 500 ml D_5W; give 1 mg or less over 1 min or more through Y-tube or 3-way stopcock; 1 mg = 1 ml of 1:1,000 or 10 ml of 1:10,000

Perform/provide:
• Storage of reconstituted sol if refrigerated for no longer than 24 hr
• Do not use discolored solutions

Evaluate:
• Therapeutic response: increased B/P with stabilization or ease of breathing
• Injection site: tissue sloughing; if this occurs administer phentolamine mixed with NS

Teach patient/family:
• Reason for drug administration
• To rinse mouth after use to prevent dryness
• Not to take OTC preparations

Treatment of overdose: Administer an α-blocker, and a β-blocker

epinephrine bitartrate/ epinephrine HCl/ epinephryl borate (optic)

(ep-i-nef'rin)

Epitrate, Mytrate/Epifrin, Glaucon/Epinal, Eppy*

Func. class.: Mydriatic
Chem. class.: Sympathomimetic amine

Action: Blocks response of iris sphincter muscle, muscle of accommodation of ciliary body to cholinergic stimulation, resulting in dilation, paralysis of accommodation

Uses: During ocular surgery, open-angle glaucoma

Dosage and routes:
• *Adult and child:* INTRAOCULAR INJ 0.1-0.2 ml of a 0.01 or 0.1% sol (HCl); INSTILL SOL 1-2 gtts of a 1%-2% sol, determined by tonometric reading (Bitartrate); 1 gtt of a 0.5%-2% sol (HCl) or 0.5%-1% (Borate)

During surgery
• *Adult and child:* INSTILL SOL 1 or more gtts of a 0.1% sol (HCl) up to 3 ×/day

Available forms include: Sol 0.1% (HCl)

Side effects/adverse reactions:
CV: Palpitations, tachycardia
EENT: Blurred vision, eye pain, ocular irritation, and tearing

Contraindications: Hypersensitivity to sympathomimetic amines, narrow-angle glaucoma, dysrhythmias, cardiogenic shock, cerebral arteriosclerosis

Precautions: Elderly, prostatic hy-

* Available in Canada only

pertrophy, diabetes mellitus, hyperthymus, TB, Parkinson's disease, pregnancy (C)
Pharmacokinetics:
INSTILL: Onset 1 hr, peak 4-8 hr, duration 12-24 hr
Interactions/incompatibilities:
- Dysrhythmias: cyclopropane, halogenated hydrocarbons
- Increased pressor effects: tricyclic antidepressants, antihistamines, beta blockers, MAOIs

NURSING CONSIDERATIONS
Assess:
- Tonometer readings during long-term treatment
- B/P, pulse, respirations

Evaluate:
- Therapeutic response: mydriasis
- Allergic reaction: itching, edema of eyelids, eye discharge; drug should be discontinued

Teach patient/family:
- To report change in vision, blurring or loss of sight, trouble breathing, sweating, pallor
- Method of instillation: pressure on lacrimal sac for 1 min, do not touch dropper to eye
- That long-term therapy may be required if using for glaucoma
- To check OTC drugs for other sympathetic nervous system stimulants (e.g., phenylephrine)

---

epinephrine HCl (nasal)
(ep-i-nef'rin)
Adrenalin Chloride
Func. class.: Nasal decongestant
Chem. class.: Sympathomimetic amine

Action: Relaxes bronchial smooth muscle, increases diameter of nasal passage by action on β-adrenergics
Uses: Nasal congestion, superficial bleeding
Dosage and routes:
- *Adult and child >6 yr old:* TOP apply to affected area with sterile swab

Available forms include: Sol 0.1%
Side effects/adverse reactions:
GI: Nausea, vomiting, anorexia
EENT: Irritation, burning, sneezing, stinging, dryness, rebound congestion
INTEG: Contact dermatitis
CNS: Anxiety, restlessness, tremors, weakness, insomnia, dizziness, fever, headache
Contraindications: Hypersensitivity to sympathomimetic amines
Precautions: Child <6 yr, elderly, diabetes, cardiovascular disease, hypertension, hyperthyroidism, increased ICP, prostatic hypertrophy, pregnancy (C)
Interactions/incompatibilities:
- Hypertension: MAOIs, β-adrenergic blockers
- Hypotension: methyldopa, mecamylamine, reserpine

NURSING CONSIDERATIONS
Administer:
- No more than q4h
- For <4 consecutive days

Perform/provide:
- Environmental humidification to decrease nasal congestion, dryness
- Storage in light-resistant containers; do not expose to high temperatures

Evaluate:
- Therapeutic response: decreased congestion, bleeding
- For redness, swelling, pain in nasal passages

Teach patient/family:
- That stinging may occur for a few applications; drying of mucosa may be decreased by environmental humidification
- To notify physician if irregular

pulse, insomnia, dizziness, or tremors occur
• Proper administration to avoid systemic absorption

ergoloid mesylate

(er'goe-loid mess'i-late)
Deapril-ST, Gerimal, Hydergine, Hydroloid-G, Niloric
Func. class.: Migraine agent
Chem. class.: Ergot alkaloid–amino acid

Action: May increase cerebral metabolism and blood flow
Uses: Senile dementia, Alzheimer's dementia, multiinfarct dementia, primary progressive dementia
Dosage and routes:
• *Adult:* PO/SL 1 mg tid, may increase to 4.5-12 mg/day
Available forms include: Tabs SL 0.5, 1 mg, tabs 1 mg, cap 1 mg, liquid 1 mg/ml
Side effects/adverse reactions:
GI: Nausea, vomiting, sublingual irritation
Contraindications: Hypersensitivity to ergot preparations; psychosis
Precautions: Acute intermittent porphyria, pregnancy (C)
Pharmacokinetics:
PO: Peak 1 hr; metabolized in liver, excreted as metabolites in feces, crosses blood-brain barrier; half-life 3½ hr

NURSING CONSIDERATIONS
Assess:
• Weigh daily, check for peripheral edema in feet, legs
• B/P and pulse, check regularly
Administer:
• With meals or after meals to avoid GI symptoms; do not crush or chew SL tab
Perform/provide:
• Storage in well-closed container at room temperature
Evaluate:
• Therapeutic response: decreased forgetfulness, increased mental alertness and ability for self-care
• Neurologic status: LOC, blurring vision, nausea, vomiting, tingling in extremities that occur preceding the headache
• Toxicity: dyspnea; hypotension or hypertension; rapid, weak pulse; delirium; nausea; vomiting; bradycardia
Teach family/patient:
• To change positions slowly, and to move extremities before walking
• To maintain dosage at approved level, not to increase drug
• To report side effects, including increased vasoconstriction starting with cold extremities, then paresthesia, weakness
• That 6 months of treatment may be required, some improvement occurs in 1 month
• To keep drug out of reach of children, death may occur
Treatment of overdose: Induce emesis if orally ingested, or gastric lavage; administer saline cathartic, keep warm

ergonovine maleate

(er-goe-noe'veen)
Ergotrate Maleate
Func. class.: Oxytocic
Chem. class.: Ergot alkaloid

Action: Stimulates uterine contractions, decreases bleeding
Uses: Treatment of hemorrhage associated with postpartum or postabortion
Dosage and routes:
• *Adult:* IM 0.2 mg q2-4h, not to

exceed 5 doses; IV 0.2 mg given over 1 min; PO 0.2-0.4 mg q6-12h × 2-7 days after initial IM or IV dose

Available forms include: Inj IM, IV 0.2 mg/ml; tabs 0.2 mg

Side effects/adverse reactions:

CNS: Headache, dizziness, fainting

CV: Hypertension, chest pain

GI: Nausea, vomiting

INTEG: Sweating

RESP: Dyspnea

EENT: Tinnitus

GU: Cramping

Contraindications: Hypersensitivity to ergot medication, augmentation of labor, before delivery of placenta, spontaneous abortion (threatened), pelvic inflammatory disease (PID)

Precautions: Hepatic disease, renal disease, cardiac disease, asthma, anemia, convulsive disorders, hypertension, glaucoma, obliterative vascular disease

Pharmacokinetics:

PO: Onset 5-25 min, duration 3 hr

IM: Onset 2-5 min, duration 3 hr

IV: Onset immediate, duration 45 min

Metabolized in liver, excreted in urine

Interactions/incompatibilities:

• Hypertension: sympathomimetics, ergots

NURSING CONSIDERATIONS

Assess:

• B/P, pulse; watch for change that may indicate hemorrhage

• Respiratory rate, rhythm, depth; notify physician of abnormalities

• Fundal tone, nonphasic contractions, check for relaxation

Administer:

• IV undiluted through Y-tube or 3-way stopcock

• IM in deep muscle mass, rotate injection sites if additional doses are given

• After having crash cart available on unit

Evaluate:

• Therapeutic response: decreased blood loss, severe cramping

Teach patient/family:

• To report increased blood loss, increased temperature or foul-smelling lochia, that cramping is normal

---

ergotamine tartrate

(er-got'a-meen)

Ergomar, Ergostat, Gynergen, Medihaler-Ergotamine, Wigraine

Func. class.: α-Adrenergic blocker

Chem. class.: Ergot alkaloid-amino acid

Action: Constricts smooth muscle in peripheral, cranial blood vessels, relaxes uterine muscle

Uses: Vascular headache (migraine or histamine)

Dosage and routes:

• *Adult:* 2 mg, then 1-2 mg qh or q½ hr for SL, not to exceed 6 mg/day or 10 mg/wk; INH 1 puff, may repeat in 5 min, not to exceed 6/24 hr

Available forms include: SL tabs 2 mg; tabs 1 mg; oral inh 360 μg/dose

Side effects/adverse reactions:

CNS: Numbness in fingers, toes, headache, weakness

CV: Transient tachycardia, chest pain, bradycardia, edema, claudication, increase or decrease in B/P

GI: Nausea, vomiting

MS: Muscle pain

Contraindications: Hypersensitivity to ergot preparations, occlusion (peripheral, vascular), CAD, hepatic disease, renal disease, peptic

ulcer, hypertension, pregnancy (X)
Precautions: Lactation, children, anemia
Pharmacokinetics:
PO: Peak 30 min-3 hr; metabolized in liver, excreted as metabolites in feces, crosses blood-brain barrier, excreted in breast milk
Interactions/incompatibilities:
• Increased effects: troleandomycin
• Increased vasoconstriction: β-blockers

NURSING CONSIDERATIONS

Assess:
• Weight daily, check for peripheral edema in feet, legs
• Check for coldness of extremities and tingling of fingers, drug should be discontinued
Administer:
• At beginning of headache, dose must be titrated to patient response
• By SL route if possible for better, faster absorption
• With meals or after meals to avoid GI symptoms
• Only to women who are not pregnant, harm to fetus may occur
Perform/provide:
• Quiet, calm environment with decreased stimulation for noise, or bright light or excessive talking
Evaluate:
• Therapeutic response: decrease in frequency, severity of headache
• For stress level, activity, recreation, coping mechanisms of patient
• Neurologic status: LOC, blurring vision, nausea, vomiting, tingling in extremities that occur preceding the headache
• Ingestion of tyramine foods (pickled products, beer, wine, aged cheese), food additives, preservatives, colorings, artificial sweeteners, chocolate, caffeine, which may precipitate these types of headaches
• Toxicity: dyspnea, hypotension or hypertension, rapid, weak pulse, delirium, nausea, vomiting
Teach patient/family:
• Not to use OTC medications, serious drug interactions may occur
• To maintain dose at approved level, not to increase even if drug does not relieve headache
• To report side effects including increased vasoconstriction starting with cold extremities, then paresthesia, weakness
• That an increase in headaches may occur when this drug is discontinued after long-term use
• To keep drug out of reach of children, death may occur
Treatment of overdose: Induce emesis if orally ingested, orgastric lavage, administer saline cathartic, keep warm

---

erythrityl tetranitrate

(e-ri'thri-till)
Cardilate
Func. class.: Vasodilator, coronary
Chem. class.: Nitrate

Action: Decreases preload, afterload, which is responsible for decreasing left ventricular end diastolic pressure, systemic vascular resistance, improve exercise tolerance
Uses: Chronic stable angina pectoris, prophylaxis of angina pain
Dosage and routes:
• *Adult:* PO 10-30 mg tid; SL 5-15 mg before stressful activity
Available forms include: Chew tabs 10 mg; tabs PO, SL 5, 10 mg
Side effects/adverse reactions:
CV: Postural hypotension, tachycardia, ***collapse,*** syncope

* Available in Canada only

GI: Nausea, vomiting
INTEG: Pallor, sweating, rash
CNS: Headache, flushing, dizziness ***weakness, fainting***
MISC: Twitching, hemolytic anemia, ***methemoglobinemia***
Contraindications: Hypersensitivity to this drug or nitrites, severe anemia, increased intracranial pressure, cerebral hemorrhage, acute MI
Precautions: Postural hypotension, pregnancy (C), lactation, children
Pharmacokinetics:
PO: Onset 30 min, peak 1-1½ hr, duration 6 hr
SL: Onset 5-10 min, peak 30-45 min, duration 3 hr; metabolized by liver, excreted in urine
Interactions/incompatibilities:
• Increased effects: β-blockers, diuretics, antihypertensives, alcohol

NURSING CONSIDERATIONS
Assess:
• For orthostatic B/P, pulse during beginning therapy
Administer:
• With 8 oz of water on empty stomach (oral tablet)
• After checking expiration date
Evaluate:
• Therapeutic response: decrease or prevention of anginal pain
• Pain: duration, time started, activity being performed, character
• Tolerance if taken over long period of time
• Headache, light-headedness, decreased B/P; may indicate a need for decreased dosage
Teach patient/family:
• To keep tabs in original container
• If 3 SL tabs do not relieve pain, activate EMS
• To avoid alcohol
• That drug may cause headache; tolerance occurs over time
• That drug may be taken before stressful activity: exercise, sexual activity
• That SL may sting when drug comes in contact with mucous membranes
• To avoid hazardous activities if dizziness occurs
• Importance of complying with complete medical regimen
• To make position changes slowly to prevent fainting

---

erythromycin (ophthalmic)

(er-ith-roe-mye'sin)
Ilotycin Ophthalmic
Func. class.: Antiinfective

Action: Inhibits bacterial protein synthesis
Uses: Infection of external eye
Dosage and routes:
• *Adult and child:* Apply oint qd-qid as needed
Ophthalmia neonatorum
• *Neonates:* Apply oint to conjunctival sacs immediately after delivery
Available forms include: Oint 0.5%
Side effects/adverse reactions:
EENT: Poor corneal wound healing, temporary visual haze, overgrowth of nonsusceptible organisms
Contraindications: Hypersensitivity
Precautions: Antibiotic hypersensitivity

NURSING CONSIDERATIONS
Administer:
• After washing hands, cleanse crusts or discharge from eye before application
Perform/provide:
• Storage at room temperature, in tight container

Evaluate:
- Therapeutic response: absence of redness, inflammation, tearing
- Allergy: itching, lacrimation, redness, swelling

Teach patient/family:
- To use drug exactly as prescribed
- Not to use eye makeup, towels, washcloths, eye medication of others; reinfection may occur
- That drug container tip should not be touched to eye
- To report itching, increased redness, burning, stinging, swelling; drug should be discontinued
- That drug may cause blurred vision when ointment is applied

erythromycin (topical)

(er-ith-roe-mye'sin)

Akne-mycin, A/T/S, Eryderm, Staticin

Func. class.: Local antiinfective
Chem. class.: Macrolide antibacterial

Action: Interferes with bacterial protein synthesis
Uses: Pyoderma, acne vulgaris
Dosage and routes:
- Adult and child: TOP apply to affected area tid-qid

Available forms include: Top sol, ointment 1.5%, 2%
Side effects/adverse reactions:
INTEG: Rash, urticaria, stinging, burning, pruritus, dry, scaly, oily skin
EENT: Eye irritation, tenderness
Contraindications: Hypersensitivity
Precautions: Pregnancy (C), lactation
Interactions/incompatibilities: Avoid use with clindamycin, abrasive agents, acids, alkaline media

NURSING CONSIDERATIONS

Administer:
- Enough medication to completely cover lesions
- After cleansing with soap, water before each application, dry well

Perform/provide:
- Storage at room temperature in dry place

Evaluate:
- Therapeutic response: decrease in size, number of lesions
- Allergic reaction: burning, stinging, swelling, redness

Teach patient/family:
- To use medical asepsis (hand washing) before, after each application
- To apply with glove to prevent further infection
- To avoid use of OTC creams, ointments, lotions unless directed by physician
- To avoid use near eyes, nose, mouth
- To monitor for superimposed infection
- To report skin irritation to physician

erythromycin base, erythromycin estolate, erythromycin ethylsuccinate, erythromycin gluceptate, erythromycin lactobionate, erythromycin stearate

(er-ith-roe-mye'sin)

E-Mycin, ERYC, Ery-Tab, Erythromid,* Ethril, Ilotycin, Novorythro,* Robimycin, Staticin, Ilosone, E.E.S., Erythrocin, Pediamycin, Wyamycin Liquid, E-Biotic, Erypar, PCE Dispersatabs, Wintrocin, Wyamycin

Func. class.: Antibacterial
Chem. class.: Macrolide antibiotic

Action: Binds to 50S ribosomal

* Available in Canada only

subunits of susceptible bacteria and suppresses protein synthesis

Uses: Infections caused by *N. gonorrhoeae,* mild to moderate respiratory tract, skin, soft tissue infections caused by *D. pneumoniae, M. pneumoniae, C. diphtheriae, B. pertussis, B. burgdorferi, L. monocytogenes,* syphilis, Legionnaire's disease, *C. trachomatis, H. influenzae*

Dosage and routes:

Soft tissue infections

• *Adult:* PO 250-500 mg q6h (base, estolate, stearate); PO 400-800 mg q6h (ethylsuccinate); IV INF 15-20 mg/kg/day (lactobionate)

• *Child:* PO 30-50 mg/kg/day in divided doses q6h (salts); IV 15-20 mg/kg/day in divided doses q4-6h (lactobionate)

N. gonorrhoeae/PID

• *Adult:* IV 500 mg q6h × 3 days (gluceptate, lactobionate), then PO 250 mg (base, estolate, stearate) or 400 mg (ethylsuccinate) q6h × 1 wk

Syphilis

Adult: PO 20 g in divided doses over 15 days (base, estolate, stearate)

Chlamydia

• *Adult:* PO 500 mg q6h × 1 wk or 250 mg qid × 2 wk

• *Infant:* PO 50 mg/kg/day in 4 divided doses × 3 wk or more

• *Newborn:* PO 50 mg/kg/day in 4 divided doses × 2 wk or more

Intestinal amebiasis

• *Adult:* PO 250 mg q6h × 10-14 days (base, estolate, stearate)

• *Child:* PO 30-50 mg/kg/day in divided doses q6h × 10-14 days (base, estolate, stearate)

Available forms include: Base: tabs, enteric-coated 250, 333, 500 mg; tabs film-coated 250, 500 mg; caps, enteric-coated 125, 250 mg; estolate: tabs chewable 125, 250 mg; tabs 500 mg; caps 125, 250 mg; drops 100 mg/ml; susp 125, 250 mg/5ml; stearate: tabs, film-coated 250, 500 mg; ethylsuccinate: tabs, chewable 200 mg; 100 mg/2.5 ml, 200, 400 mg/5 ml; susp 200, 400 mg powder for suspension 100 mg/2.5 ml, 200 and 400 mg/5 ml powder for inj; 500 mg and 1 g (lactobionate), 250 mg, 500 mg, 1 g (as gluceptate)

Side effects/adverse reactions:

INTEG: Rash, urticaria, pruritus, thrombophlebitis (IV site)

GI: Nausea, vomiting, diarrhea, ***hepatotoxicity,*** abdominal pain, stomatitis, heartburn, anorexia, pruritus ani

GU: Vaginitis, moniliasis

EENT: Hearing loss, tinnitus

Contraindications: Hypersensitivity

Precautions: Pregnancy (C), hepatic disease, lactation

Pharmacokinetics: Peak 4 hr, duration 6 hr, half-life 1-3 hr, metabolized in liver, excreted in bile, feces

Interactions/incompatabilities:

• Increased action of: oral anticoagulants, digitalis, theophylline, methylprednisolone, cyclosporine

• Decreased action of: clindamycin, penicillins

• Toxicity: carbamazepine

NURSING CONSIDERATIONS

Assess:

• I&O ratio; report hematuria, oliguria in renal disease

• Liver studies: AST, ALT

• Renal studies: urinalysis, protein, blood

• C&S before drug therapy; drug may be taken as soon as culture is taken; C&S may be repeated after treatment

Administer:
• IV after diluting 500 mg or less/10 ml sterile H_2O without preservatives; dilute further in 80-250 ml of compatible sol; may be further diluted to 1 mg/ml and given as continuous infusion; run 1 g or less/100 ml over ½-1 hr; continuous infusion over 6 hr, may require buffers to neutralize pH
• Enteric-coated tablets may be given with food

Perform/provide:
• Storage at room temperature
• Adequate intake of fluids (2000 ml) during diarrhea episodes

Evaluate:
• Therapeutic response: decreased symptoms of infection
• Bowel pattern before, during treatment
• Skin eruptions, itching
• Respiratory status: rate, character, wheezing, tightness in chest; discontinue drug if these occur
• Allergies before treatment, reaction of each medication; place allergies on chart, Kardex in bright red letters; notify all people giving drugs

Teach patient/family:
• To take oral drug with full glass of water; may give with food if GI symptoms occur
• Do not take with fruit juice
• To report sore throat, fever, fatigue; could indicate superimposed infection
• To notify nurse of diarrhea stools, dark urine, pale stools, yellow discoloration of eyes or skin, and severe abdominal pain
• To take at evenly spaced intervals; complete dosage regimen

Lab test interferences:
False increase: 17-OHCS/17-KS, AST/ALT
Decrease: Folate assay

Treatment of overdose: Withdraw drug, maintain airway, administer epinephrine, aminophylline, O_2, IV corticosteroids

---

erythropoietin recombinant

(er-ith-row-poe′-ee-tin)
rHU-EPO, eprex*

Func. class.: Hormone
Chem. class.: Amino acid polypeptide

Action: Erythropoietin is one factor controlling rate of red cell production; drug is developed by recombinant DNA technology

Uses: Anemia caused by reduced endogenous erythropoietin production, primarily end-stage renal disease; to correct hemostatic defect in uremia

Dosage and routes:
• *Adult:* IV 5-500 U/kg 3 ×/wk

Side effects/adverse reactions:
CV: Hypertension, ***hypertension encephalopathy***
CNS: ***Seizures,*** coldness, sweating
MS: Bone pain

Contraindications: Hypersensitivity

Pharmacokinetics:
IV: Metabolized in body, extent of metabolism unknown, onset of increased reticulocyte count 1-2 wk

NURSING CONSIDERATIONS

Assess:
• Renal studies: urinalysis, protein, blood, BUN, creatinine
• Blood studies: reticulocyte count weekly
• I&O; report drop in output to <50 ml/hr
• CNS symptoms: coldness, sweating
• CV status: B/P; hypertension

---

* Available in Canada only

may occur rapidly leading to hypertension encephalopathy

Evaluate:

• Therapeutic response: increase in reticulocyte count in 1-2 wk, increased appetite, enhanced sense of well-being

esmolol HCl

(ess'moe-lol)

Brevibloc

Func. class.: β-Adrenergic blocker

Action: Competitively blocks stimulation of β_1-adrenergic receptors in the myocardium; produces negative chronotropic, inotropic activity (decreases rate of SA node discharge, increases recovery time), slows conduction of AV node, decreases heart rate, decreases O_2 consumption in myocardium; also, decreases renin-aldosterone-angiotensin system at high doses, inhibits β_2-receptors in bronchial system slightly

Uses: Supraventricular tachycardia, noncompensatory tachycardia

Dosage and routes:

• *Adult:* IV loading dose—500 μg/kg/min for 1 min; maintenance—50 μg/kg/min for 4 min; may repeat q5min, increasing maintenance inf by 50 μg/kg/min (max of 200 μg/kg/min

Available forms include: Inj IV 10 mg, conc 250 mg/ml

Side effects/adverse reactions:

INTEG: Induration, inflammation at site, discoloration, edema, erythema, burning pallor, flushing, rash, pruritus, dry skin, alopecia

CNS: Confusion, lightheadedness, paresthesia, somnolence, fever, dizziness, fatigue, headache, depression, anxiety

GI: Nausea, vomiting, anorexia, gastric pain, flatulence, constipation, heartburn, bloating

CV: Hypotension, bradycardia, chest pain, peripheral ischemia, shortness of breath, CHF, conduction disturbances

GU: Urinary retention, impotence, dysuria

RESP: ***Bronchospasm,*** dyspnea, cough, wheeziness, nasal stuffiness

Contraindications: 2nd or 3rd degree heart block, cardiogenic shock, CHF, cardiac failure, hypersensitivity

Precautions: Hypotension, pregnancy (C), peripheral vascular disease, diabetes, hypoglycemia, thyrotoxicosis, renal disease, lactation

Pharmacokinetics: Onset very rapid, duration short, half-life 9 min; metabolized by hydrolysis of the ester linkage; excreted via kidneys

Interactions/incompatibilities:

• Increased digoxin levels: digoxin

• Increased esmolol levels: morphine

• Do not mix with other drugs in syringe or solution

• Reversal of esmolol effects: isoproterenol, norepinephrine, dopamine, dobutamine

• Increased effects of both drugs: disopyramide

• Increased effects of lidocaine

NURSING CONSIDERATIONS

Assess:

• I&O ratio, weight daily

• B/P, pulse q4h; note rate, rhythm, quality; rapid changes can cause shock; if systolic <100 or diastolic <60, notify physician before giving drug

• Apical/radial pulse before administration; notify physician if less than 60 bpm

• Baselines in renal, liver function tests before therapy begins

• Breath sounds and respiratory pattern

Administer:

• Reduced dosage in cool environment

• IV diluted 5 g/20 ml of compatible sol; further dilute in the remaining 480 ml (10 mg/ml) and give as infusion

Perform/provide:

• Storage protected from light, moisture; place in cool environment

Evaluate:

• Therapeutic response: decreased B/P immediately

• Respiratory pattern: wheezing from bronchospasm

• Edema in feet, legs daily

• Skin turgor, dryness of mucous membranes for hydration status

Lab test interferences:

Interference: Glucose/insulin tolerance test

Treatment of overdose: Discontinue drug

essential crystalline amino acid solution

Aminosyn-RF, Nephramine, Ren-Amine 6.5

Func. class.: Nitrogen product

Action: Needed for anabolism to maintain structure, decrease catabolism, promote healing

Uses: Renal decompensation

Dosage and routes:

• *Adult:* CENT IV 0.3-0.5 g/kg, 250 ml of amino acid/500 ml D70, given at rate of 20-30 ml/hr, increased by 10 ml/hr q24h, not to exceed 100 ml/hr

• *Child:* CENT IV 1 g/kg/day or less, depending on patient's needs

Available forms include: Inj central line only, many types

Side effects/adverse reactions:

CNS: Dizziness, headache, confusion, ***loss of consciousness***

CV: Hypertension, ***CHF, pulmonary edema***

GI: Nausea, vomiting, liver fat deposits, abdominal pain

GU: ***Glycosuria, osmotic diuresis***

ENDO: Hyperglycemia, rebound hypoglycemia, electrolyte imbalances, hyperosmolar syndrome, hyperosmolar hyperglycemic nonketotic syndrome, alkalosis, acidosis, hypophosphatemia, hyperammonemia, dehydration, hypocalcemia

INTEG: Chills, flushing, warm feeling, rash, urticaria, extravasation necrosis, phlebitis at injection site

Contraindications: Hypersensitivity, severe electrolyte imbalances, anuria, severe liver damage, maple syrup urine disease, PKU

Precautions: Renal disease, pregnancy (C), children, diabetes mellitus, CHF

NURSING CONSIDERATIONS

Assess:

• Electrolytes (K, Na, Ca, Cl, Mg), blood glucose, ammonia, phosphate

• Renal, liver function studies: BUN, creatinine, ALT, AST, bilirubin

• Injection site for extravasation: redness along vein, edema at site, necrosis, pain, hard tender area, site should be changed immediately

• Monitor respiratory function q4h: auscultate lung fields bilaterally for crackles, respirations, quality, rate, rhythm

• Monitor temperature q4h for increased fever, indicating infection; if infection suspected, infusion is discontinued, tubing, bottle, catheter tip cultured

• Urine glucose q6h using Tes-

Tape, Clinistix, Keto-Diastix, which are not affected by infusion substances

Administer:

• TPN must be used only mixed with dextrose to promote protein synthesis

• Immediately after mixing in pharmacy under strict aseptic technique using laminar flowhood; use infusion pump, in-line filter

• Using careful monitoring technique; do not speed up infusion; pulmonary edema, glucose overload will result

Perform/provide:

• Storage depends on type of solution, consult manufacturer

• Changing dressing, IV tubing to prevent infection q24-48h

Evaluate:

• Therapeutic response: weight gain, decreased jaundice in liver disorders, increased serum albumin

• Hyperammonemia: nausea, vomiting, malaise, tremors, anorexia, convulsions

Teach patient/family:

• Reason for use of TPN

• To report chills, sweating at once

estazolam

ProSom

Func. class.: Sedative-hypnotic
Chem. class.: Benzodiazepine derivative

Controlled Substance Schedule IV (US)

Action: Produces CNS depression at the limbic, thalamic, hypothalamic levels of the CNS; may be mediated by neurotransmitter γ-aminobutyric acid (GABA); results are sedation, hypnosis, skeletal muscle relaxation, anticonvulsant activity, anxiolytic action

Uses: Insomnia

Dosage and routes:
Adult: PO 1-2 mg hs

Available forms include: Tabs 1 mg

Side effects/adverse reactions:

INTEG: Dermatitis, allergy, sweating, flushing, pruritus

HEMA: ***Leukopenia, granulocytopenia (rare)***

CNS: Lethargy, drowsiness, daytime sedation, dizziness, confusion, light-headedness, headache, anxiety, irritability, weakness, tremors, depression, lack of coordination

GI: Nausea, vomiting, diarrhea, heartburn, abdominal pain, constipation, anorexia, taste alteration

CV: Chest pain, pulse changes, palpitations, tachycardia

MISC: Joint pain, congestion

Contraindications: Hypersensitivity to benzodiazepines, pregnancy (X), sleep apnea

Precautions: Hepatic disease, renal disease, suicidal individuals, drug abuse, elderly, psychosis, child <18, lactation, depression, pulmonary insufficiency

Pharmacokinetics: Onset 15-45 min, peaks 1½-2 hr, duration 7-8 hr; metabolized by liver, excreted by kidneys (inactive/active metabolites), crosses placenta, excreted in breast milk

Interactions/incompatibilities:

• Increased effects of estazolam: cimetidine, disulfiram, isoniazid, probenecid

• Increased CNS depression: alcohol, CNS depressants

• Decreased effect of estazolam: theophylline, rifampin

NURSING CONSIDERATIONS

Assess:

• Blood studies: Hct, Hgb, RBCs (if on long-term therapy)

- Hepatic studies: AST, ALT, bilirubin

Administer:

- After removal of cigarettes, to prevent fire
- After trying conservative measures for insomnia
- ½-1 hr before hs for sleeplessness
- On empty stomach for fast onset, but may be taken with food if GI symptoms occur

Perform/provide:

- Assistance with ambulation after receiving dose
- Safety measures: siderails, night light, call bell within easy reach
- Checking to see PO medication has been swallowed
- Storage in tight container in cool environment

Evaluate:

- Therapeutic response: ability to sleep at night, decreased amount of early morning awakenings
- Mental status: mood, sensorium, affect, memory (long, short)
- Blood dyscrasias: fever, sore throat, bruising, rash, jaundice, epistaxis (rare)
- Type of sleep problem: falling asleep, staying asleep

Teach patient/family:

- To avoid driving or other activities requiring alertness until drug is stabilized

esterified estrogens

Climestrone,* Estabs, Estratab, Menest, Ms-Med, Neo-Estrone*

Func. class.: Estrogen
Chem. class.: Nonsteroidal synthetic estrogen

Action: Needed for adequate functioning of female reproductive system; affects release of pituitary gonadotropins, inhibits ovulation, adequate calcium use in bone structures

Uses: Menopause, breast cancer, prostatic cancer hypogonadism, castration, primary ovarian failure

Dosage and routes:

Menopause

- *Adult:* PO 0.3-3.75 mg qd3wk on, 1 wk off

Hypogonadism/castration/ovarian failure

- *Adult:* PO 2.5 mg qd-tid3wk on, 1 wk off

Prostatic cancer

- *Adult:* PO 1.25-2.5 mg tid

Breast cancer

- *Adult:* PO 10 mg tid × 3 months or longer

Available forms include: Tabs 0.3, 0.625, 1.25, 2.5 mg

Side effects/adverse reactions:

CNS: Dizziness, headache, migraines, depression

CV: Hypotension, thrombophlebitis, edema, ***thromboembolism, stroke, pulmonary embolism, myocardial infarction***

GI: *Nausea,* vomiting, diarrhea, anorexia, pancreatitis, cramps, constipation, increased appetite, increased weight, ***cholestatic jaundice***

EENT: Contact lens intolerance, increased myopia, astigmatism

GU: Amenorrhea, cervical erosion, breakthrough bleeding, dysmenorrhea, vaginal candidiasis, breast changes, *gynecomastia, testicular atrophy, impotence*

INTEG: Rash, urticaria, acne, hirsutism, alopecia, oily skin, seborrhea, purpura, melasma

META: Folic acid deficiency, hypercalcemia, hyperglycemia

Contraindications: Breast cancer, thromboembolic disorders, reproductive cancer, genital bleeding

* Available in Canada only

(abnormal, undiagnosed), pregnancy (X)

Precautions: Hypertension, asthma, blood dyscrasias, gallbladder disease, CHF, diabetes mellitus, bone disease, depression, migraine headache, convulsive disorders, hepatic disease, renal disease, family history of cancer of breast or reproductive tract

Pharmacokinetics:

PO: Degraded in liver, excreted in urine, crosses placenta, excreted in breast milk

Interactions/incompatibilities:

- Decreased action of: anticoagulants, oral hypoglycemics
- Toxicity: tricyclic antidepressants
- Decreased action of estrogens: anticonvulsants barbiturates, phenylbutazone, rifampin
- Increased action of: corticosteroids

NURSING CONSIDERATIONS

Assess:

- Urine glucose in patient with diabetes, increased urine glucose may occur
- Weight daily, notify physician of weekly weight gain >5 lb; if increase, diuretic may be ordered
- B/P q4h, watch for increase caused by water and sodium retention
- I&O ratio; be alert for decreasing urinary output and increasing edema
- Liver function studies, including AST, ALT, bilirubin, alk phosphatase

Administer:

- Titrated dose, use lowest effective dose
- With food or milk to decrease GI symptoms

Evaluate:

- Therapeutic response: reversal of menopause or decrease in tumor size in prostatic cancer
- Edema, hypertension, cardiac symptoms, jaundice
- Mental status: affect, mood, behavioral changes, aggression
- Hypercalcemia

Teach patient/family:

- To weigh weekly, report gain >5 lb
- To check with physician before using OTC drugs
- To report breast lumps, vaginal bleeding, edema, jaundice, dark urine, clay-colored stools, dyspnea, headache, blurred vision, abdominal pain, numbness or stiffness in legs, chest pain, male to report impotence or gynecomastia

---

estradiol/estradiol cypionate/estradiol valerate

(ess-tra-dye'ole)

Estrace/Depo-Estradiol Cypionate, Depogen, Dura Estrin, E-Ionate PA, Estro-Cyp, Estroject-LA/ Delestrogen,* Dioval Duragen, Estradiol LA, Estraval, Retestrin, Valergen, Hormogen Depot, Deladiol

Func. class.: Estrogen

Chem. class.: Nonsteroidal synthetic estrogen

Action: Needed for adequate functioning of female reproductive system; affects release of pituitary gonadotropins, inhibits ovulation, adequate calcium use in bone structures

Uses: Menopause, breast cancer, prostatic cancer, atrophic vaginitis, kraurosis vulvae, hypogonadism, castration, primary ovarian failure

Dosage and routes:
Menopause/hypogonadism/castration/ovarian failure
• *Adult:* PO 1-2 mg qd3wk on, 1 wk off or 5 days on, 2 days off; IM 0.2-1 mg qwk
Prostatic cancer
• *Adult:* IM 30 mg q1-2wk (valerate); PO 1-2 mg tid (oral estradiol)
Breast cancer
• *Adult:* PO 10 mg tid × 3 mo or longer
Atropic vaginitis
• *Adult:* VAG CREAM 2-4 g qd × 1-2 wk, then 1 g 1-3 ×/wk
Kraurosis valvae
• *Adult:* IM 1-1.5 mg 1-2 ×/wk
Available forms include: Estradiol-tabs 1, 2 mg; cypionate-injection IM 1, 5 mg/ml; valerate-injection IM 10, 20, 40 mg/ml
Side effects/adverse reactions:
CNS: Dizziness, headache, migraines, depression
CV: Hypotension, thrombophlebitis, edema, ***thromboembolism, stroke, pulmonary embolism, myocardial infarction***
GI: Nausea, vomiting, diarrhea, anorexia, pancreatitis, cramps, constipation, increased appetite, increased weight, ***cholestatic jaundice***
EENT: Contact lens intolerance, increased myopia, astigmatism
GU: Amenorrhea, cervical erosion, breakthrough bleeding, dysmenorrhea, vaginal candidiasis, breast changes, *gynecomastia, testicular atrophy, impotence*
INTEG: Rash, urticaria, acne, hirsutism, alopecia, oily skin, seborrhea, purpura, melasma
META: Folic acid deficiency, hypercalcemia, hyperglycemia
Contraindications: Breast cancer, thromboembolic disorders, reproductive cancer, genital bleeding (abnormal, undiagnosed), pregnancy (X)
Precautions: Hypertension, asthma, blood dyscrasias, gallbladder disease, CHF, diabetes mellitus, bone disease, depression, migraine headache, convulsive disorders, hepatic disease, renal disease, family history of cancer of breast or reproductive tract
Pharmacokinetics:
PO/IH/TOP: Degraded in liver, excreted in urine, crosses placenta, excreted in breast milk
Interactions/incompatibilities:
• Decreased action of: anticoagulants, oral hypoglycemics
• Toxicity: tricyclic antidepressants
• Decreased action of estramustine: anticonvulsants, barbiturates, phenylbutazone, rifampin, milk products, calcium
• Increased action of: corticosteroids

NURSING CONSIDERATIONS

Assess:
• Urine glucose in patient with diabetes, increased urine glucose may occur
• Weight daily, notify physician of weekly weight gain >5 lb; if increase, diuretic may be ordered
• B/P q4h, watch for increase caused by water and sodium retention
• I&O ratio; be alert for decreasing urinary output and increasing edema
• Liver function studies, including AST, ALT, bilirubin, alk phosphatase
Administer:
• Titrated dose, use lowest effective dose

* Available in Canada only

• IM injection deeply in large muscle mass
• With food or milk to decrease GI symptoms (oral)

Evaluate:
• Therapeutic response: reversal of menopause or decrease in tumor size in prostatic cancer
• Edema, hypertension, cardiac symptoms, jaundice, hypercalcemia
• Mental status: affect, mood, behavioral changes, aggression

Teach patient/family:
• To weigh weekly, report gain >5 lb
• To report breast lumps, vaginal bleeding, edema, jaundice, dark urine, clay-colored stools, dyspnea, headache, blurred vision, abdominal pain, numbness or stiffness in legs, chest pain; male to report impotence or gynecomastia

Lab test interferences:
Increase: BSP retention test, PBI, T_4, serum sodium, platelet aggregation, thyroxine-binding globulin (TBG), prothrombin, factors VII, VIII, IX, X, triglycerides
Decrease: Serum folate, serum triglyceride, T_3 resin uptake test, glucose tolerance test, antithrombin III, pregnanediol, metyrapone test
False positive: LE prep, antinuclear antibodies

estramustine phosphate sodium

(ess-tra-muss'teen)
Emcyt
Func. class.: Antineoplastic
Chem. class.: Hormone: estrogen

Action: Precise actions unknown
Uses: Metastatic prostate cancer

Dosage and routes:
• *Adult:* PO 10-16 mg/kg in 3-4 divided doses; treatment may continue for 3 mo or more

Available forms include: Caps 140 mg (12.5 mg sodium/cap)

Side effects/adverse reactions:
GI: Nausea, vomiting, anorexia, ***hepatotoxicity***
GU: ***Renal failure,*** impotence, gynecomastia
INTEG: Rash, urticaria, pruritus, flushing, alopecia
RESP: Dyspnea, ***emboli,*** hoarseness
CV: ***Myocardial infarction,*** hypertension, ***CHF, CVA***
CNS: Headache, anxiety, seizures, insomnia, mood swings

Contraindications: Hypersensitivity to estradiol, thromboembolic disorders, pregnancy (D)

Precautions: Edema, hepatic disease, CVA, MI, seizures, hypertension, diabetes mellitus

Pharmacokinetics:
PO: Peak 1-2 hr, metabolized in liver, excreted in bile, half-life 20 hr (terminal)

NURSING CONSIDERATIONS

Assess:
• Renal function studies: BUN, serum uric acid, urine CrCl, electrolytes before, during therapy
• I&O ratio; report fall in urine output of 30 ml/hr
• Liver function tests before, during therapy (bilirubin, AST, ALT, LDH) as needed or monthly

Administer:
• Antacid before oral agent; give drug after evening meal before bedtime

Evaluate:
• Therapeutic response: decreased tumor size, spread of malignancy
• Dyspnea, chest pain, tachypnea, fatigue, increased pulse, pallor, lethargy

• Food preferences; list likes, dislikes
• Edema in feet, joint, stomach pain, shaking
• Inflammation of mucosa, breaks in skin
• Yellowing of skin and sclera, dark urine, clay-colored stools, itchy skin, abdominal pain, fever, diarrhea
• Symptoms indicating severe allergic reaction: rash, pruritus, urticaria, purpuric skin lesions, itching, flushing
• Tachycardia, ECG changes, dyspnea, edema, fatigue, leg cramps; may indicate cardiac toxicity

Teach patient/family:
• To report any complaints, side effects to nurse or physician
• That gynecomastia, impotence can occur and are reversible after discontinuing treatment
• To report any changes in breathing, coughing
• Importance of immediately reporting GI bleeding
• To use contraception during use, positive mutagenic effects

estrogenic substances, conjugated

C.E.S.,* Estrocon, Premarin, Progens

Func. class.: Estrogen
Chem. class.: Nonsteroidal synthetic estrogen

Action: Needed for adequate functioning of female reproductive system; it affects release of pituitary gonadotropins, inhibits ovulation, adequate calcium use in bone structures

Uses: Menopause, breast cancer, prostatic cancer, abnormal uterine bleeding, hypogonadism, castration, primary ovarian failure, osteoporosis

Dosage and routes:

Menopause
• *Adult:* PO 0.3-1.25 mg qd3wk on, 1 wk off

Prostatic cancer
• *Adult:* PO 1.25-2.5 mg tid

Breast cancer
• *Adult:* PO 10 mg tid × 3 mo or longer

Abnormal uterine bleeding
• *Adult:* IV/IM 25 mg, repeat in 6-12 hr

Castration/primary ovarian failure/osteoporosis
• *Adult:* PO 1.25 mg qd3wk on, 1 wk off

Hypogonadism
• *Adult:* PO 2.5 mg bid-tid × 20 days/mo

Available forms include: Tabs 0.3, 0.625, 0.9, 1.25, 2.5 mg

Side effects/adverse reactions:
CNS: Dizziness, headache, migraine, depression
CV: Hypotension, thrombophlebitis, edema, ***thromboembolism, stroke, pulmonary embolism, myocardial infarction***
GI: Nausea, vomiting, diarrhea, anorexia, pancreatitis, cramps, constipation, increased appetite, increased weight, ***cholestatic jaundice***
EENT: Contact lens intolerance, increased myopia, astigmatism
GU: Amenorrhea, cervical erosion, breakthrough bleeding, dysmenorrhea, vaginal candidiasis, breast changes, *gynecomastia, testicular atrophy, impotence*
INTEG: Rash, urticaria, acne, hirsutism, alopecia, oily skin, seborrhea, purpura, melasma
META: Folic acid deficiency, hypercalcemia, hyperglycemia

Contraindications: Breast cancer,

*Available in Canada only

thromboembolic disorders, reproductive cancer, genital bleeding (abnormal, undiagnosed), pregnancy (X), lactation

Precautions: Hypertension, asthma, blood dyscrasias, gallbladder disease, CHF, diabetes mellitus, bone disease, depression, migraine headache, convulsive disorders, hepatic disease, renal disease, family history of cancer of breast or reproductive tract

Pharmacokinetics:

PO/IV/IM: Degraded in liver, excreted in urine, crosses placenta, excreted in breast milk

Interactions/incompatibilities:

- Decreased action of: anticoagulants, oral hypoglycemics
- Toxicity: tricyclic antidepressants
- Decreased action of estrogens: anticonvulsants, barbiturates, phenylbutazone, rifampin
- Increased action of: corticosteroids

NURSING CONSIDERATIONS

Assess:

- Urine glucose in patient with diabetes; increased urine glucose may occur
- Weight daily, notify physician of weekly weight gain >5 lb; if increase, diuretic may be ordered
- B/P q4h; watch for increase caused by water and sodium retention
- I&O ratio; be alert for decreasing urinary output and increasing edema
- Liver function studies, including AST, ALT, bilirubin, alk phosphatase

Administer:

- Titrated dose, use lowest effective dose
- IM injection deeply in large muscle mass
- With food or milk to decrease GI symptoms PO

Evaluate:

- Therapeutic response: absence of breast engorgement, reversal of menopause, or decrease in tumor size in prostatic cancer
- Edema, hypertension, cardiac symptoms, jaundice, hypercalcemia
- Mental status: affect, mood, behavioral changes, aggression

Teach patient/family:

- To avoid breastfeeding, since drug is secreted in breast milk
- To weigh weekly, report gain >5 lb
- To report breast lumps, vaginal bleeding, edema, jaundice, dark urine, clay-colored stools, dyspnea, headache, blurred vision, abdominal pain, numbness or stiffness in legs, chest pain; male to report impotence or gynecomastia
- To avoid sunlight or wear sunscreen; burns may occur

estrone

(ess'trone)

Bestrone, Femogen Forte,* Kestrone-5, Theelin Aqeous, Esmone A

Func. class.: Estrogen
Chem. class.: Nonsteroidal synthetic estrogen

Action: Needed for adequate functioning of female reproductive system; affects release of pituitary gonadotropins, inhibits ovulation, promotes adequate calcium use in bone structures

Uses: Menopause, prostatic cancer, atrophic vaginitis, hypogonadism, primary ovarian failure

Dosage and routes:

Menopause/atrophic vaginitis

• *Adult:* IM 0.1-0.5 mg 2-3 × /wk
Prostatic cancer
• *Adult:* IM 2-4 mg 2-3 × /wk
Female hypogonadism/primary ovarian failure
• *Adult:* IM 0.1-1 mg qwk in one dose or divided doses
Available forms include: Inj IM 2, 5 mg/ml
Side effects/adverse reactions:
CNS: Dizziness, headache, migraine, depression
CV: Hypotension, thrombophlebitis, edema, ***thromboembolism, stroke, pulmonary embolism, myocardial infarction***
GI: Nausea, vomiting, diarrhea, anorexia, pancreatitis, cramps, constipation, increased appetite, increased weight, ***cholestatic jaundice***
EENT: Contact lens intolerance, increased myopia, astigmatism
GU: Amenorrhea, cervical erosion, breakthrough bleeding, dysmenorrhea, vaginal candidiasis, breast changes, *gynecomastia, testicular atrophy, impotence*
INTEG: Rash, urticaria, acne, hirsutism, alopecia, oily skin, seborrhea, purpura, melasma
META: Folic acid deficiency, hypercalcemia, hyperglycemia
Contraindications: Breast cancer, thromboembolic disorders, reproductive cancer, genital bleeding (abnormal, undiagnosed), pregnancy (X)
Precautions: Hypertension, asthma, blood dyscrasias, gallbladder disease, CHF, diabetes mellitus, bone disease, depression, migraine headache, convulsive disorders, hepatic disease, renal disease, family history of cancer of the breast or reproductive tract
Pharmacokinetics:
IM: Degraded in liver, excreted in urine, crosses placenta, excreted in breast milk
Interactions/incompatibilities:
• Decreased action of: anticoagulants, oral hypoglycemics
• Toxicity: tricyclic antidepressants
• Decreased action of estrone: anticonvulsants, barbiturates, phenylbutazone, rifampin
• Increased action of: corticosteroids

NURSING CONSIDERATIONS

Assess:
• Urine glucose in patient with diabetes; increased urine glucose may occur
• Weight daily, notify physician of weekly weight gain >5 lb; if increase, diuretic may be ordered
• B/P q4h, watch for increase caused by water and sodium retention
• I&O ratio; be alert for decreasing urinary output and increasing edema
• Liver function studies, including AST, ALT, bilirubin, alk phosphatase
Administer:
• Titrated dose, use lowest effective dose
• IM injection deeply in large muscle mass
Evaluate:
• Therapeutic response: absence of breast engorgement, reversal of menopause, or decrease in tumor size in prostatic cancer
• Edema, hypertension, cardiac symptoms, jaundice, hypercalcemia
• Mental status: affect, mood, behavioral changes, aggression
Teach patient/family:
• To weigh weekly, report gain >5 lb
• To report breast lumps, vaginal

bleeding, edema, jaundice, dark urine, clay-colored stools, dyspnea, headache, blurred vision, abdominal pain, numbness or stiffness in legs, chest pain; male to report impotence or gynecomastia
• To avoid sunlight or wear sunscreen, burns may occur

ethacrynate sodium/ ethacrynic acid

(eth-a-kri'nate)

Edecrin Sodium

Func. class.: Loop diuretic
Chem. class.: Ketone derivative

Action: Acts on loop of Henle by increasing excretion of chloride, sodium

Uses: Pulmonary edema, edema in CHF, liver disease, nephrotic syndrome, ascites

Dosage and routes:

• *Adult:* PO 50-200 mg/day may give up to 200 mg bid
• *Child:* PO 25 mg, increased by 25 mg/day until desired effect occurs

Pulmonary edema

• *Adult:* IV 50 mg given over several minutes or 0.5-1 mg/kg

Available forms include: Tabs 25, 50 mg; powder for inj 50 mg

Side effects/adverse reactions:

GU: Polyuria, ***renal failure,*** glycosuria

ELECT: Hypokalemia, hypochloremic alkalosis, hypomagnesemia, hyperuricemia, hypocalcemia, hyponatremia

CNS: Headache, fatigue, weakness, vertigo

GI: Nausea, ***severe diarrhea,*** dry mouth, vomiting, anorexia, cramps, upset stomach, abdominal pain, ***acute pancreatitis,*** jaundice, ***GI bleeding***

EENT: ***Loss of hearing,*** ear pain, tinnitus, blurred vision

INTEG: Rash, pruritus, purpura, ***Stevens-Johnson syndrome,*** sweating, photosensitivity

MS: Cramps, arthritis, stiffness

ENDO: Hyperglycemia

HEMA: ***Thrombocytopenia, agranulocytosis, leukopenia, neutropenia***

CV: Chest pain, hypotension, ***circulatory collapse,*** ECG changes

Contraindications: Hypersensitivity to sulfonamides, anuria, hypovolemia, lactation, electrolyte depletion, infants

Precautions: Dehydration, ascites, severe renal disease, pregnancy (D), hypoproteinemia

Pharmacokinetics:

PO: Onset ½ hr, peak 2 hr, duration 6-8 hr

IV: Onset 5 min, peak 15-30 min, duration 2 hr

Excreted by kidneys, crosses placenta, half-life 30-70 min

Interactions/incompatibilities:

• Increased hypotension: antihypertensives
• Decreased diuretic effect: indomethacin
• Increased ototoxicity: cisplatin, aminoglycosides, rancomycin
• Increased toxicity: lithium, nondepolarizing skeletal muscle relaxants, digitalis
• Increased anticoagulant activity: warfarin

NURSING CONSIDERATIONS

Assess:

• Weight, I&O daily to determine fluid loss; effect of drug may be decreased if used qd
• Rate, depth, rhythm of respiration, effect of exertion
• B/P lying, standing; postural hypotension may occur
• Electrolytes: potassium, sodium,

chloride; include BUN, blood sugar, CBC, serum creatinine, blood pH, ABGs, uric acid, calcium, magnesium
• Glucose in urine if patient is diabetic
• Hearing when giving high IV doses

Administer:
• IV after diluting with 50 ml NaCl inj; give through Y-tube or 3-way stopcock, give 10 mg or less over 1 min or run infusion over ½ hr
• In AM to avoid interference with sleep if using drug as a diuretic
• Potassium replacement if potassium is less than 3.0
• With food, if nausea occurs, absorption may be decreased slightly
• PO, IV only, do not give IM/SC

Evaluate:
• Therapeutic response: improvement in edema of feet, legs, sacral area daily if medication is being used in CHF
• Improvement in CVP q8h
• Signs of metabolic alkalosis: drowsiness, restlessness
• Signs of hypokalemia: postural hypotension, malaise, fatigue, tachycardia, leg cramps, weakness
• Rashes, temperature elevation qd
• Confusion, especially in elderly, take safety precautions if needed

Teach patient/family:
• To increase fluid intake 2-3 L/day unless contraindicated; to rise slowly from lying or sitting position
• About adverse reactions: muscle cramps, weakness, nausea, dizziness
• To take with food or milk for GI symptoms
• To take early in day to prevent nocturia

Treatment of overdose: Lavage if taken orally, monitor electrolytes, administer dextrose in saline, monitor hydration, CV, renal status

---

ethambutol HCl

(e-tham'byoo-tole)
Etibi,* Myambutol
Func. class.: Antitubercular
Chem. class.: Diisopropylethylene diamide derivative

Action: Inhibits RNA synthesis, decreases tubercle bacilli replication

Uses: Pulmonary tuberculosis, as an adjunct

Dosage and routes:
• *Adult and child >13 yr:* PO 15 mg/kg/day as a single dose

Retreatment
• *Adult and child >13 yr:* PO 25 mg/kg/day as single dose × 2 mo with at least 1 other drug, then decrease to 15 mg/kg/day as single dose

Available forms include: Tabs 100, 400 mg

Side effects/adverse reactions:
GI: Abdominal distress, anorexia, nausea, vomiting
INTEG: Dermatitis, pruritis
CNS: Headache, confusion, fever, malaise, dizziness, disorientation, hallucinations
EENT: Blurred vision, optic neuritis, photophobia, decreased visual acuity
META: Elevated uric acid, acute gout, liver function impairment
MISC: *Thrombocytopenia,* joint pain

Contraindications: Hypersensitivity, optic neuritis, child <13 yr

Precautions: Pregnancy (D), renal disease, diabetic retinopathy, cataracts, ocular defects, hepatic, hematopoietic disorders

---

*Available in Canada only

Pharmacokinetics:
PO: Peak 2-4 hr, half-life 3 hr; metabolized in liver, excreted in urine (unchanged drug/inactive metabolites, unchanged drug in feces)
Interactions/incompatibilities:
• Increased renal toxicity: aminoglycosides, cisplatin
• Delayed absorption of ethambutol: aluminum salts

NURSING CONSIDERATIONS
Assess:
• Liver studies qwk: ALT, AST, bilirubin
• Signs of anemia: Hct, Hgb, fatigue
Administer:
• With meals to decrease GI symptoms
• Antiemetic if vomiting occurs
• After C&S is completed; qmo to detect resistance
Evaluate:
• Therapeutic response: decreased symptoms of TB
• Mental status often: affect, mood, behavioral changes; psychosis may occur
• Hepatic status: decreased appetite, jaundice, dark urine, fatigue
Teach patient/family:
• That compliance with dosage schedule, duration is necessary
• That scheduled appointments must be kept or relapse may occur

---

ethchlorvynol
(eth-klor-vi'nole)
Placidyl
Func. class.: Sedative-hypnotic
Chem. class.: Tertiary acetylenic alcohol

Controlled Substance Schedule IV (USA), Schedule F (Canada)
Action: Produces cerebral depression, exact action is unknown
Uses: Sedation, insomnia
Dosage and routes:
Sedation
• *Adult:* PO 100-200 mg bid or tid
Insomnia
• *Adult:* PO 500 mg-1g ½ hr before hs, may repeat 100-200 mg if needed
Medication for EEG
• *Child:* PO 25 mg/kg in one dose not to exceed 1 g
Available forms include: Caps 100, 200, 500, 750 mg
Side effects/adverse reactions:
HEMA: ***Thrombocytopenia***
CNS: Fatigue, drowsiness, dizziness, sedation, ataxia, nightmares, hangover, giddiness, weakness, hysteria
GI: Nausea, vomiting
INTEG: *Rash,* urticaria
EENT: Blurred vision, bitter aftertaste
CV: Hypotension
Contraindications: Hypersensitivity to this drug, severe pain, porphyria, pregnancy (C)
Precautions: Depression, hepatic disease, renal disease, suicidal individual, pregnancy (3rd trimester) (C), elderly
Pharmacokinetics:
PO: Onset 15-30 min, peak 1-1½ hr, duration 5 hr; metabolized by liver, excreted by kidneys; half-life 10-20 hr, 21-100 hr terminal
Interactions/incompatibilities:
• Decreased hypoprothrombinemic effect: dicumarol, warfarin
• Increased CNS effects of ETOH, barbiturates, other CNS depressants, MAOIs

NURSING CONSIDERATIONS
Assess:
• Blood studies: Hct, Hgb, RBCs before and after treatment if blood dyscrasias are suspected
• Hepatic studies: AST, ALT, bilirubin if hepatic disease is present

Administer:
• After removal of cigarettes, to prevent fires
• After trying conservative measures for insomnia
• ½-1 hr before hs for sleeplessness
• With food or meals to decrease dizziness, giddiness
• For only 1 wk, not intended for long-term treatment

Perform/provide:
• Assistance with ambulation after receiving dose, especially elderly
• Safety measures: siderails, nightlight, call bell within easy reach
• Checking to see PO medication swallowed
• Storage in tight, light-resistant container in cool environment

Evaluate:
• Therapeutic response: ability to sleep at night, decreased amount of early morning awakenings if taking drug for insomnia
• Mental status: mood, sensorium, affect, memory (long, short)
• Physical dependency: more frequent requests for medication, shakes, anxiety
• Toxicity: hypotension, hypothermia, weakness, poor muscle coordination, visual problems; drug should be discontinued
• Respiratory dysfunction: respiratory depression, character, rate, rhythm; hold drug if respirations are <10/min or if pupils are dilated (rare)
• Blood dyscrasias: fever, sore throat, bruising, rash, jaundice, epistaxis (rare)
• Allergy to tartrazine: this drug contains tartrazine and should not be used in patients allergic to this dye

Teach patient/family:
• To avoid driving or other activities requiring alertness
• To avoid alcohol ingestion or CNS depressants; serious CNS depression may result
• That effects may take 2 nights for benefits to be noticed
• Alternate measures to improve sleep: reading, exercise several hours before hs, warm bath, warm milk, TV, self-hypnosis, deep breathing

Treatment of overdose: Lavage, activated charcoal, monitor electrolytes, vital signs

Lab test interferences:
Interferes: Clinitest

---

ethinyl estradiol

(eth'in-il ess-tra-dye'ole)
Estinyl, Feminone
Func. class.: Estrogen
Chem. class.: Nonsteroidal synthetic estrogen

Action: Needed for adequate functioning of female reproductive system; affects release of pituitary gonadotropins, inhibits ovulation, promotes adequate calcium use in bone structures

Uses: Menopause, prostatic cancer, breast cancer, breast engorgement, hypogonadism

Dosage and routes:

Menopause
• *Adult:* PO 0.02-0.5 mg qd3wk on, 1 wk off

Prostatic cancer
• *Adult:* PO 0.15-2 mg qd

Hypogonadism
• *Adult:* PO 0.05 mg qd-tid × 2 wk/mo, then 2 wk progesterone, then 3-6 mo cycles, then 2 mo off

Breast cancer
• *Adult:* PO 1 mg tid

Breast engorgement
• *Adult:* PO 0.5-1 mg qd × 3 days, then tapered off over 7 days

Available forms include: Tabs 0.02, 0.05, 0.5 mg

Side effects/adverse reactions:

CNS: Dizziness, headache, migraine, depression

CV: Hypotension, thrombophlebitis, edema, ***thromboembolism, stroke, pulmonary embolism, myocardial infarction***

GI: Nausea, vomiting, diarrhea, anorexia, pancreatitis, cramps, constipation, increased appetite, increased weight, ***cholestatic jaundice***

EENT: Contact lens intolerance, increased myopia, astigmatism

GU: Amenorrhea, cervical erosion, breakthrough bleeding, dysmenorrhea, vaginal candidiasis, breast changes, *gynecomastia, testicular atrophy, impotence*

INTEG: Rash, urticaria, acne, hirsutism, alopecia, oily skin, seborrhea, purpura, melasma

META: Folic acid deficiency, hypercalcemia, hyperglycemia

Contraindications: Breast cancer, thromboembolic disorders, reproductive cancer, genital bleeding (abnormal, undiagnosed), pregnancy (X)

Precautions: Hypertension, asthma, blood dyscrasias, gallbladder disease, CHF, diabetes mellitus, bone disease, depression, migraine headache, convulsive disorders, hepatic disease, renal disease, family history of cancer of breast or reproductive tract

Pharmacokinetics:

PO: Degraded in liver, excreted in urine, crosses placenta, excreted in breast milk

Interactions/incompatibilities:

- Decreased action of: anticoagulants, oral hypoglycemics
- Toxicity: tricyclic antidepressants
- Decreased action of estradiol: anticonvulsants, barbiturates, phenylbutazone, rifampin
- Increased action of: corticosteroids

NURSING CONSIDERATIONS

Assess:

- Urine glucose in patient with diabetes; increased urine glucose may occur
- Weight daily, notify physician of weekly weight gain >5 lb; if increase, diuretic may be ordered
- B/P q4h; watch for increase caused by water and sodium retention
- I&O ratio; be alert for decreasing urinary output and increasing edema
- Liver function studies: AST, ALT, bilirubin, alk phosphatase

Administer:

- Titrated dose, use lowest effective dose
- IM injection deeply in large muscle mass
- With food or milk to decrease GI symptoms

Evaluate:

- Therapeutic response: absence of breast engorgement, reversal of menopause, or decrease in tumor size in prostatic cancer
- Edema, hypertension, cardiac symptoms, jaundice, hypercalcemia
- Mental status: affect, mood, behavioral changes, aggression

Teach patient/family:

- To weigh weekly, report gain >5 lb
- To report breast lumps, vaginal bleeding, edema, jaundice, dark urine, clay-colored stools, dyspnea, headache, blurred vision, abdominal pain, numbness or stiffness in legs, chest pain; male to report impotence or gynecomastia

ethionamide

(e-thye-on-am-ide)
Trecator-SC

Func. class.: Antitubercular
Chem. class.: Thiomine derivative

Action: Bacteriostatic against *M. tuberculosis*
Uses: Pulmonary, extrapulmonary tuberculosis when other antitubercular drugs have failed
Dosage and routes:
• *Adult:* PO 500 mg-1 g qd in divided doses, with another antitubercular drug and pyridoxine
• *Child:* PO 15-20 mg/kg/day in 3-4 doses, not to exceed 1g
Available forms include: Tabs 250 mg
Side effects/adverse reactions:
INTEG: Dermatitis, alopecia, acne
CV: Severe postural hypotension
CNS: Headache, drowsiness, tremors, ***convulsions,*** depression, psychosis, dizziness, peripheral neuritis
GI: ***Anorexia, nausea, vomiting, diarrhea,*** metallic taste
EENT: Blurred vision, optic neuritis
HEMA: ***Thrombocytopenia,*** purpura
MISC: Gynecomastia, impotence, menorrhagia, difficulty managing diabetes mellitus
Contraindications: Hypersensitivity, severe hepatic disease
Precautions: Pregnancy (D), renal disease, diabetic retinopathy, cataracts, ocular defects, child <13 yr
Pharmacokinetics:
PO: Peak 3 hr, duration 9 hr, half-life 3 hr; metabolized in liver, excreted in urine (unchanged drug/inactive), crosses placenta
Interactions/incompatibilities:
• Increased neurotoxicity: cycloserine, ethyl alcohol
• Increased adverse reactions: TB test agents, anti-TB drugs

NURSING CONSIDERATIONS

Assess:
• Signs of anemia: Hgb, Hct, fatigue
• Liver studies qwk: ALT, AST, bilirubin
Administer:
• With meals to decrease GI symptoms
• Antiemetic if vomiting occurs
• After C&S is completed, qmo to detect resistance
• Pyridoxine to prevent neuritis
Evaluate:
• Therapeutic response: decreased symptoms of TB
• Mental status often: affect, mood, behavioral changes; psychosis may occur
• Hepatic status: decreased appetite, jaundice, dark urine, fatigue
Teach patient/family:
• That compliance with dosage schedule, duration are necessary
• To avoid alcohol while taking this drug
• To notify physician of depression, mood changes, which are symptoms of toxicity

ethosuximide

(eth-oh-sux'i-mide)
Zarontin

Func. class.: Anticonvulsant
Chem. class.: Succinimide

Action: Inhibits spike, wave formation in absence seizures (petit mal), decreases amplitude, frequency, duration, spread of discharge in minor motor seizures
Uses: Absence seizures, partial seizures, tonic-clonic seizures
Dosage and routes:
• *Adult and child >6 yr:* PO 250

mg bid initially; may increase by 250 mg q4-7d, not to exceed 1.5 g/day
• *Child 3-6 yr:* PO 250 mg/day or 125 mg bid; may increase by 250 mg q4-7d, not to exceed 1.5 g/day
Available forms include: Caps 250 mg, syr 250 mg/5 ml
Side effects/adverse reactions:
HEMA: ***Agranulocytosis, aplastic anemia, thrombocytopenia, leukocytosis, eosinophilia, pancytopenia***
CNS: Drowsiness, dizziness, fatigue, euphoria, lethargy, anxiety, aggressiveness, irritability, depression, insomnia, headache
GI: Nausea, vomiting, heartburn, anorexia, diarrhea, abdominal pain, cramps, constipation, hiccups, weight loss, gum hypertrophy, tongue swelling
GU: Vaginal bleeding, ***hematuria, renal damage***
INTEG: Urticaria, pruritic erythema, hirsutism, ***Stevens-Johnson syndrome***
EENT: Myopia, blurred vision
Contraindications: Hypersensitivity to succinimide derivatives
Precautions: Lactation, pregnancy (C), hepatic disease, renal disease
Pharmacokinetics:
PO: Peak 1-7 hr, steady state 4-7 days, metabolized by liver, excreted in urine, bile, feces, half-life 24-60 hr
Interactions/incompatibilities:
• Antagonist effect: tricyclic antidepressants (imipramine, doxepin)
• Decreased effects of: estrogens, oral contraceptives

NURSING CONSIDERATIONS

Assess:
• Renal studies: urinalysis, BUN, urine creatinine
• Blood studies: CBC, Hct, Hgb, reticulocyte counts qwk for 4 wk, then qmo
• Hepatic studies: AST, ALT, bilirubin, creatinine
• Drug levels during initial treatment, therapeutic range (40-80 μg/ml
Administer:
• With food, milk to decrease GI symptoms
Perform/provide:
• Hard candy, frequent rinsing of mouth, gum for dry mouth
• Assistance with ambulation during early part of treatment; dizziness occurs
Evaluate:
• Therapeutic response: decreased seizure activity, document on patient's chart
• Mental status: mood, sensorium, affect, behavioral changes; if mental status changes, notify physician
• Eye problems: need for ophthalmic examinations before, during, after treatment (slit lamp, fundoscopy, tonometry)
• Allergic reaction: red raised rash, exfoliative dermatitis; if these occur, drug should be discontinued
• Blood dyscrasias: fever, sore throat, bruising, rash, jaundice
• Toxicity: bone marrow depression, nausea, vomiting, ataxia, diplopia, cardiovascular collapse, Stevens-Johnson syndrome
Teach patient/family:
• To carry ID card or Medic-Alert bracelet stating drugs taken, condition, physician's name, phone number
• To avoid driving, other activities that require alertness
• To avoid alcohol ingestion, CNS depressants; increased sedation may occur
• Not to discontinue medication quickly after long-term use

Lab test interferences:
False positive: Direct Coombs' test
Treatment of overdose: Lavage, activated charcoal, monitor electrolytes, VS

ethotoin

(eth'oh-toyin)
Peganone
Func. class.: Anticonvulsant
Chem. class.: Hydantoin derivative

Action: Inhibits nerve in impulses in the motor cortex by decreasing sodium ion influx, limiting tetanic stimulation
Uses: Generalized tonic-clonic or complex-partial seizures
Dosage and routes:
• *Adult:* PO 250 mg qid initially; may increase over several days to 3 g/day in divided doses
• *Child:* PO 250 mg bid; may increase by 250 mg qid
Available forms include: Tabs 250, 500 mg
Side effects/adverse reactions:
HEMA: ***Agranulocytosis, thrombocytopenia, leukopenia, pancytopenia, megaloblastic anemia,*** lymphadenopathy
CNS: Fatigue, insomnia, numbness, fever, headache, dizziness
GI: Nausea, vomiting, diarrhea, gingival hypertrophy
INTEG: Rash
EENT: Nystagmus, diplopia
CV: Chest pain
Contraindications: Hypersensitivity to hydantoins, blood dyscrasias, hematologic disease, hepatic disease, pregnancy (D)
Pharmacokinetics: Metabolized by liver, excreted in urine, half-life 3-9 hr
Interactions/incompatibilities:
• Decreased effects of: rifampin, chronic alcohol, barbiturates, antihistamines, antacids, other anticonvulsants antineoplastics, calcium products, folic acid, oxacillin
• Increased effects of: benzodiazepines, cimetidine, salicylates, sulfonamide, pyrazolones, phenothiazines, estrogens, disulfiram, chloramphenicol, anticoagulants
• Seizures: valproic acid
• Myocardial depressions: lidocaine, propranolol, sympathomimetics

NURSING CONSIDERATIONS

Assess:
• Renal studies: urinalysis, BUN, urine creatinine
• Blood studies: RBC, Hct, Hgb, reticulocyte counts qwk for 4 wk then qmo
• Hepatic studies: AST, ALT, bilirubin, creatinine periodically
• Drug levels during initial treatment, therapeutic level (15-50 μg/ml)
Administer:
• With food, milk to decrease GI symptoms
• After meals
Perform/provide:
• Hard candy, frequent rinsing of mouth, gum for dry mouth
• Assistance with ambulation during early part of treatment; dizziness occurs
Evaluate:
• Therapeutic response: decreased seizure activity, document on patient's chart
• Mental status: mood, sensorium, affect, behavioral changes; if mental status changes, notify physician
• Eye problems: need for ophthalmic examinations before, during, after treatment (slit lamp, fundoscopy, tonometry)
• Allergic reaction: red raised rash;

if this occurs, drug should be discontinued
• Blood dyscrasias: fever, sore throat, bruising, rash, jaundice
• Toxicity: bone marrow depression, nausea, vomiting, ataxia, diplopia, cardiovascular collapse, Stevens-Johnson syndrome, lupuslike syndrome

Teach patient/family:
• To carry ID card or Medic-Alert bracelet stating drugs taken, condition, physician's name, phone number
• To avoid driving, other activities that require alertness
• To avoid alcohol ingestion, CNS depressants; increased sedation may occur
• Not to discontinue medication quickly after long-term use, taper off over several weeks

Lab test interferences:
Increase: Serum glucose, BSP, alk phosphatase
Decrease: Urinary steroids, PBI, dexamethasone/metyrapone tests

Treatment of overdose: Lavage, activated charcoal, monitor electrolytes, VS

---

ethylestrenol

(eth-il-ess'tre-nole)
Maxibolin

Func. class.: Androgenic anabolic steroid
Chem. class.: Hydantoin derivative

Action: Increases weight by building body tissue, increases potassium, phosphorus, chloride, and nitrogen levels, increases bone development

Uses: To increase weight, combat tissue depletion, osteoporosis, immobility, refractory anemias, catabolic effects of corticosteroid therapy

Dosage and routes:
• *Adult:* PO 4-8 mg qd, decreased at beginning clinical response
• *Child:* PO 1-3 mg qd, not to exceed treatment of 6 wk, lupuslike syndrome

Available forms include: Tabs 2 mg; elix 2 mg/5 ml

Side effects/adverse reactions:
INTEG: Rash, acneiform lesions, oily hair, skin, flushing, sweating, acne vulgaris, alopecia, hirsutism
CNS: Dizziness, headache, fatigue, tremors, paresthesias, flushing, sweating, anxiety, lability, insomnia
MS: Cramps, spasms
CV: Increased B/P
GU: ***Hematuria,*** amenorrhea, vaginitis, decreased libido, decreased breast size, clitoral hypertrophy, testicular atrophy
GI: Nausea, vomiting, constipation, weight gain, ***cholestatic jaundice***
EENT: Carpal tunnel syndrome, conjunctional edema, nasal congestion
ENDO: Abnormal GTT

Contraindications: Severe renal disease, severe cardiac disease, severe hepatic disease, hypersensitivity, pregnancy (C), lactation, genital bleeding (abnormal)

Precautions: Migraine headaches, seizure disorders

Pharmacokinetics:
PO: Metabolized in liver, excreted in urine, crosses placenta, excreted in breast milk

Interactions/incompatibilities:
• May increase effects of: oral anticoagulants, antidiabetics, oxyphenbutazone, phenylbutazone
• May decrease effect of ethylestrenol: barbiturates

NURSING CONSIDERATIONS

Assess:

- Weight daily, notify physician if weekly weight gain is >5 lb
- B/P q4h
- I&O ratio; be alert for decreasing urinary output, increasing edema
- Growth rate in children since growth rate may be uneven (linear/bone growth) used for extended periods of time; periodic x-rays are done to assure changes in bone growth
- Electrolytes: K, Na, Cl; cholesterol
- Liver function studies; ALT, AST, bilirubin
- Blood sugar in diabetes (may become hypoglycemic)

Administer:

- Increased calcium, Vitamin D in diet for osteoporosis, decrease in high phosphorus foods (bread, soft drinks, phosphate-based preservatives)
- Titrated dose, use lowest effective dose
- With food or milk to decrease GI symptoms

Perform/provide:

- Diet with increased calories, protein; decrease sodium if edema occurs

Evaluate:

- Therapeutic response: increased appetite, increased stamina
- Edema, hypertension, cardiac symptoms, jaundice
- Mental status: affect, mood, behavioral changes, aggression
- Signs of masculinization in female: increased libido, deepening of voice, breast tissue, enlarged clitoris, menstrual irregularities; male: gynecomastia, impotence, testicular atrophy
- Hypercalcemia: lethargy, polyuria, polydipsia, nausea, vomiting, constipation, drug may need to be decreased
- Hypoglycemia in diabetics, since oral anticoagulant action is decreased

Teach patient/family:

- Drug needs to be combined with complete health plan: diet, rest, exercise
- To notify physician if therapeutic response decreases
- Not to discontinue medication abruptly
- About change in sex characteristics

Lab test interferences:

Increase: Cholesterol

Decrease: Cholesterol, T_4, T_3, thyroid ^{131}I uptake test, 17-KS, PBI

Interferes: GTT

---

ethylnorepinephrine HCl

(eth-il-nor-ep-i-nef'rin)

Bronkephrine

Func. class.: Adrenergic

Chem. class.: Catecholamine

Action: α-Stimulation with vasoconstriction, pressor response, nasal decongestion and β_2-stimulation with vasodilation and bronchial dilation

Uses: Bronchospasm

Dosage and routes:

- *Adult:* IM/SC 0.5-1 ml
- *Child:* IM/SC 0.1-0.5 ml

Available forms include: Inj 2 mg/ml IM, SC

Side effects/adverse reactions:

CNS: Tremors, anxiety, insomnia, headache, dizziness, confusion,

CV: Palpitations, tachycardia, hypertension, chest pain, ***dysrhythmias***

GI: Anorexia, nausea, vomiting

Contraindications: Hypersensitiv-

*Available in Canada only

ity to sympathomimetics, narrow-angle glaucoma
Precautions: Pregnancy (C), cardiac disorders, hyperthyroidism, diabetes mellitus, prostatic hypertrophy
Pharmacokinetics:
IM/SC: Onset 6-12 min, duration 1-2 hr
Interactions/incompatibilities:
• Do not use with MAOIs or tricyclic antidepressants; hypertensive crisis may occur
• Decreased effect of ethylnorepinephrine when used with methyldopa, urinary acidifiers, rauwolfia alkaloids
• Increased effect of ethylnorepinephrine when used with urinary alkalizers

NURSING CONSIDERATIONS
Assess:
• B/P and pulse q5min after parenteral route
Perform/provide:
• Storage of reconstituted solution if refrigerated for no longer than 24 hr
• Do not use discolored solutions
Evaluate:
• Therapeutic response: ease of breathing after several min
Teach patient/family:
• The reason for drug administration

---

etidocaine HCl

(et-ee′-doe-kane)
Duranest
Func. class.: Local anesthetic
Chem. class.: Amide

Action: Competes with calcium for sites in nerve membrane that control sodium transport across cell membrane; decreases rise of depolarization phase of action potential
Uses: Peripheral nerve block, caudal anesthesia, central neural block, vaginal block
Dosage and routes:
Varies depending on route of anesthesia
Available forms include: Inj 1%, 1.5%
Side effects/adverse reactions:
CNS: Anxiety, restlessness, ***convulsions, loss of consciousness,*** drowsiness, disorientation, tremors, shivering
CV: ***Myocardial depression, cardiac arrest, dysrhythmias,*** bradycardia, hypotension, hypertension, fetal bradycardia
GI: Nausea, vomiting
EENT: Blurred vision, tinnitus, pupil constriction
INTEG: Rash, urticaria, allergic reactions, edema, burning, skin discoloration at injection site, tissue necrosis
RESP: ***Status asthmaticus, respiratory arrest, anaphylaxis***
Contraindications: Hypersensitivity, child <12 yr, elderly, severe liver disease
Precautions: Elderly, severe drug allergies, pregnancy (B)
Pharmacokinetics: Onset 2-8 min, duration 3-6 hr; metabolized by liver, excreted in urine (metabolites)
Interactions/incompatibilities:
• Dysrhythmias: epinephrine, halothane, enflurane
• Hypertension: MAOIs, tricyclic antidepressants, phenothiazines
• Decreased action of etidocaine: chloroprocaine

NURSING CONSIDERATIONS
Assess:
• B/P, pulse, respiration during treatment

• Fetal heart tones if drug is used during labor

Administer:

• Only with crash cart, resuscitative equipment nearby

• Only drugs without preservatives for epidural or caudal anesthesia

Perform/provide:

• Use of new solution, discard unused portions

Evaluate:

• Therapeutic response: anesthesia necessary for procedure

• Allergic reactions: rash, urticaria, itching

• Cardiac status: ECG for dysrhythmias, pulse, B/P during anesthesia

Treatment of overdose: Airway, O_2, vasopressor, IV fluids, anticonvulsants for seizures

etidronate disodium

(e-ti-droe'nate)

Didronel, Didronel IV

Func. class.: Parathyroid agents (calcium regulator)

Chem. class.: Diphosphate

Action: Decreases bone resorption and new bone development (accretion)

Uses: Paget's disease, heterotopic ossification, hypercalcemia of malignancy

Dosage and routes:

Paget's disease

• *Adult:* PO 5-10 mg/kg/day 2 hr ac with water, not to exceed 20 mg/kg/day, max 6 mo

Heterotropic ossification

• *Adult:* PO 20 mg/kg qd × 2 wk, then 10 mg/kg/day for 10 wk, total 12 wk

Available forms include: Tabs 200, 400 mg

Side effects/adverse reactions:

GI: Nausea, diarrhea

MS: Bone pain, hypocalcemia, decreased mineralization of nonaffected bones

Contraindications: Pathologic fractures, children, colitis, severe renal disease with creatinine >5 mg/dl

Precautions: Pregnancy (B), renal disease, lactation, restricted vitamin D/calcium

Pharmacokinetics: Not metabolized, excreted in urine/feces, therapeutic response: 1-3 mo

NURSING CONSIDERATIONS

Assess:

• I&O ratio; check for decreased output in renal patients

• BUN, creatinine, uric acid, phosphate chloride, electrolytes, pH, urine calcium, magnesium, alk phosphatase, urinalysis, calcium should be kept at 9-10 mg/dl, vitamin D 50-135 IU/dl

Administer:

• On empty stomach with water 2 hr ac

• Drug therapy should not last longer than 6 mo

• IV after diluting in 250 ml or more of normal saline; give over 2 hr or longer

• Food, especially high in calcium and vitamins with mineral supplements or antacids high in metals should not be given within 2 hr of dose

Evaluate:

• Therapeutic response: prevention of bone deficiencies

• Muscle spasm, laryngospasm, paresthesias, facial twitching, colic; may indicate hypocalcemia

• Nutritional status, diet for sources of vitamin D (milk, some seafood), calcium (dairy products,

dark green vegetables), phosphates—adequate intake is necessary
• Persistent nausea or diarrhea

Teach patient/family:
• To avoid OTC products
• That therapeutic response may take 1-3 mo, effects persist for months after drug is discontinued
• That adequate intake of Ca^+, vitamin D is necessary

---

etodolac

(e-toe-doe'lack)
Lodine

Func. class.: Nonsteroidal antiinflammatory

Action: Inhibits prostaglandin synthesis by decreasing an enzyme needed for biosynthesis; possesses analgesic, antiinflammatory, antipyretic properties

Uses: Mild to moderate pain, osteoarthritis

Dosage and routes:

Osteoarthritis
• *Adult:* PO 800-1200 mg/day in divided doses, initially, then adjust dose to 600-1200 mg/day in divided doses; do not exceed 1200 mg/day; patients <60 kg, not to exceed 20 mg/kg

Analgesia
• *Adult:* PO 200-400 mg q6-8h prn for acute pain; do not exceed 1200 mg/day; patients 60 kg, not to exceed 20 mg/kg
• ***Available forms include:*** Caps 200, 300 mg

Side effects/adverse reactions:
CV: Tachycardia, peripheral edema, fluid retention, palpitations, dysrhythmias, CHF
GU: ***Nephrotoxicity: dysuria, hematuria, oliguria, azotemia,*** cystitis, urinary tract infection
HEMA: ***Blood dyscrasias***
INTEG: Erythema, urticaria, purpura, rash, pruritus, sweating
GI: Nausea, anorexia, vomiting, diarrhea, jaundice, ***cholestatic hepatitis,*** constipation, flatulence, cramps, dry mouth, peptic ulcer, dyspepsia, ***GI bleeding***
CNS: Dizziness, headache, drowsiness, fatigue, tremors, confusion, insomnia, anxiety, depression, light-headedness, vertigo
EENT: Tinnitus, hearing loss, blurred vision

Contraindications: Hypersensitivity; patients in whom aspirin, iodides, or other nonsteroidal antiinflammatories have produced asthma, rhinitis, urticaria, nasal polyps, angioedema, bronchospasm

Precautions: Pregnancy (C), lactation, children, bleeding disorders, GI disorders, cardiac disorders, elderly, renal, hepatic disorders

Pharmacokinetics:
PO: Peak 1-2 hr, serum protein binding >90%, half-life 7 hr; metabolized by liver (metabolites excreted in urine)

Interactions/incompatibilities:
• Increased action of: coumarin, phenytoin, cyclosporin, lithium
• Decreased antihypertensive effects: β-blockers
• Decreased plasma concentration of etodolac: salicylates
• Increased concentration and toxicity of etodolac: probenecid

NURSING CONSIDERATIONS

Assess:
• Blood, renal, liver studies: BUN, creatinine, AST, ALT, Hgb, before treatment, periodically thereafter
• Audiometric, ophthalmic examination before, during, after treatment

Administer:
• With food to decrease Gi symptoms since extent of absorption is not affected by food
Perform/provide:
• Storage at room temperature
Evaluate:
• Therapeutic response: decreased pain, stiffness, swelling in joints, ability to move more easily
• For eye, ear problems: blurred vision, tinnitus; may indicate toxicity
Teach patient/family:
• To report blurred vision or ringing, roaring in ears; may indicate toxicity
• To avoid driving or other hazardous activities if dizziness or drowsiness occurs
• To report change in urine pattern, weight increase, edema, pain increase in joints, fever, blood in urine; indicates nephrotoxicity
• That therapeutic effects may take up to 1 mo
• To avoid aspirin, alcoholic beverages while taking this medication

etomidate

(e-tom'i-date)
Amidate, Hypnomidate
Func. class.: General anesthetic
Chem. class.: Nonbarbiturate hypnotic

Action: Acts at level of reticular-activating system to produce anesthesia
Uses: Induction of general anesthesia
Dosage and routes:
• *Adult and child >10 yr:* IV 0.2-0.6 mg/kg over ½-1 min
Available forms include: Inj IV 2 mg/ml
Side effects/adverse reactions:
GI: Nausea, vomiting (postoperatively)
CNS: Tonic movements, myoclonic movements, averting movements
CV: Tachycardia, hypotension, hypertension, bradycardia
ENDO: Decreases steroid production
RESP: ***Laryngospasm***
INTEG: Pain on administration
Contraindications: Hypersensitivity, labor/delivery
Precautions: Pregnancy (C), child <10 yr, lactation
Pharmacokinetics:
IV: Onset 20 sec, peak 1 min, duration 3-5 min; half-life 75 min, metabolized in liver, excreted in urine

NURSING CONSIDERATIONS

Assess:
• I&O ratio for increasing urine output
• VS q10min during IV administration, q30min after IM dose
• Plasma cortisol levels if administered over several hours (5-20 μg/100 ml normal level of cortisol)
Administer:
• Corticosteroids for severe hypotension
• Only with crash cart, resuscitative equipment nearby
• IV slowly only, muscular twitching is reduced with fentanyl before anesthesia induction
Evaluate:
• Therapeutic response: induction of anesthesia
• Increasing or decreasing heart rate or dysrhythmias shown on ECG

etoposide (VP-16)

(e-toe-poe'side)
VePesid
Func. class.: Antineoplastic
Chem. class.: Semisynthetic podophyllotoxin

Action: Inhibits mitotic activity

through metaphase to mitosis; also inhibits cells from entering mitosis, depresses DNA, RNA synthesis

Uses: Leukemias, lung, testicular cancer, lymphomas, neuroblastoma, melanoma, ovarian cancer

Dosage and routes:

• *Adult:* IV 45-75 mg/m²/day × 3-5 days given q3-5wk or 200-250 mg/m²/wk, or 125-140 mg/m²/day 3 × wk, q5wk

Available forms include: Inj IV 20 mg/ml, caps 50 mg

Side effects/adverse reactions:

HEMA: ***Thrombocytopenia, leukopenia, myelosuppression, anemia***

GI: Nausea, vomiting, anorexia, ***hepatotoxicity***

INTEG: Rash, alopecia, phlebitis

RESP: ***Bronchospasm***

CV: Hypotension

CNS: Headache, *fever*

GU: ***Nephrotoxicity***

Contraindications: Hypersensitivity, bone marrow depression, severe hepatic disease, severe renal disease, bacterial infection, pregnancy (D)

Precautions: Renal disease, hepatic disease, lactation, children, gout

Pharmacokinetics: Half-life 3 hr, terminal 15 hr, metabolized in liver, excreted in urine, crosses placental barrier

Interactions/incompatibilities:

• Do not use with radiation
• Do not use with dextrose solution
• Increased pro-time: warfarin

NURSING CONSIDERATIONS

Assess:

• CBC, differential, platelet count weekly; withhold drug if WBC is <4000 or platelet count is <75,000; notify physician of results
• Renal function studies: BUN, serum uric acid, urine CrCl, electrolytes before, during therapy
• I&O ratio; report fall in urine output of 30 ml/hr
• Monitor temperature q4h; may indicate beginning infection
• Liver function tests before, during therapy (bilirubin, AST, ALT, LDH) as needed or monthly
• RBC, Hct, Hgb since these may be decreased

Administer:

• After diluting 100 mg/250 ml or more D_5W or NaCl to a concentration of 0.2-0.4 mg/ml, infuse over 30-60 min
• Antiemetic 30-60 min before giving drug and prn to prevent vomiting
• Allopurinol or sodium bicarbonate to maintain uric acid levels, alkalinization of urine
• Hyaluronidase 150 U/ml to 1 ml NaCl to infiltration area, ice compress
• Transfusion for anemia
• Antispasmodic

Perform/provide:

• Liquid diet: cola, Jell-O; dry toast or crackers may be added if patient is not nauseated or vomiting
• Increase fluid intake to 2-3 L/day to prevent urate deposits, calculi formation
• Diet low in purines: organ meats (kidney, liver), dried beans, peas to maintain alkaline urine
• Nutritious diet with iron, vitamin supplements
• HOB raised to facilitate breathing

Evaluate:

• Therapeutic response: decreased tumor size, spread of malignancy
• Bleeding: hematuria, guaiac stools, bruising or petechiae, mucosa or orifices q8h
• Food preferences; list likes, dislikes

• Effects of alopecia on body image; discuss feelings about body changes
• Yellowing of skin and sclera, dark urine, clay-colored stools, itchy skin, abdominal pain, fever, diarrhea
• Buccal cavity q8h for dryness, sores or ulceration, white patches, oral pain, bleeding, dysphagia
• Local irritation, pain, burning, discoloration at injection site
• Symptoms indicating severe allergic reaction: rash, pruritus, urticaria, purpuric skin lesions, itching, flushing
• Symptoms of anaphylaxis: flushing, restlessness, coughing, difficulty breathing
• Frequency of stools, characteristics: cramping, acidosis; signs of dehydration: rapid respirations, poor skin turgor, decreased urine output, dry skin, restlessness, weakness

Teach patient/family:
• To report any complaints or side effects to nurse or physician
• To report any changes in breathing or coughing
• That hair may be lost during treatment, a wig or hairpiece may make patient feel better; tell patient that new hair may be different in color, texture
• To make position changes slowly to prevent fainting

etretinate

(e-tret'-in-ate)
Tegison
Func. class.: Systemic antipsoriatic
Chem. class.: Retinol derivative

Action: Unknown; drug is related to retinol

Uses: Severe recalcitrant psoriasis, including erythrodermic and generalized pustular types

Dosage and routes:
• *Adult:* PO 0.75-1 mg/kg/day in divided doses, not to exceed 1.5 mg/kg/day; maintenance dose 0.5-0.75 mg/kg/day

Available forms include: Caps 10, 25 mg

Side effects/adverse reactions:
INTEG: Alopecia; peeling of palms, soles, fingertips; itching; rash; dryness; red scaling face; bruising; sunburn; pyogenic granuloma; paronychia; onycholysis; perspiration change, nail changes
CNS: Fatigue, headache, dizziness, fever, pain, anxiety, amnesia, depression
EENT: Eye irritation, pain, double vision, change in lacrimation, earache, otitis externa, dry nose, eyes, mouth, nosebleed, cheilitis, sore tongue
GI: Anorexia, abdominal pain, nausea, ***hepatitis,*** constipation, diarrhea, flatulence, weight loss
CV: Edema, ***CV obstruction, atrial fibrillation,*** chest pain, coagulation disorders
RESP: Dyspnea, cough
GU: WBC in urine, ***proteinuria,*** glycosuria, *increased BUN, creatinine,* ***hematuria,*** *casts,* ***acetonuria, hemoglobinuria***
MET: Increase or decrease potassium, calcium, phosphate, sodium, chloride
MS: Hyperostosis, bone pain, cramps, myalgia, gout, hypertonia

Contraindications: Pregnancy (X)

Precautions: Lactation, children, hepatic disease

Pharmacokinetics: 99% plasma protein binding; excreted in bile, urine; terminal half-life 120 days; stored in fatty tissue

Interactions/incompatibilities:

- Increased absorption of etretinate: milk

NURSING CONSIDERATIONS

Assess:

- For pseudotumor cerebri: headache, nausea, vomiting, visual problems, papilledema
- Hepatic studies: AST, ALT, LDH, since hepatotoxicity may occur
- Visual problems: blurring, decreased night vision, poor visual acuity; drug should be discontinued and ophthalmologist consulted
- Lipids before, q1-2wk during treatment; after discontinuing treatment, lipids will return to normal

Evaluate:

- Therapeutic response: decrease in scaling, itching, amount of psoriasis

Teach patient/family:

- To take with food
- Not to use during pregnancy; contraception must be used for 1 mo before or after therapy
- Not to take vitamin A supplements
- That contact lens intolerance is common

factor IX complex (human)

Konyne HT, Profilnine Heat-Treated, Proplex T, Proplex SX-T

Func. class.: Hemostatic

Chem. class.: Factors II, VII, IX, X

Action: Causes an increase in blood levels of clotting factors II, VII, IX, X

Uses: Hemophilia B (Christmas disease), factor IX deficiency, anticoagulant reversal, control bleeding in factor VIII inhibitors

Dosage and routes:

- *Adult and child:* IV 1 U/kg × desired % increase

Available forms include: Inj IV (number of units noted on label)

Side effects/adverse reactions:

GI: Nausea, vomiting, abdominal cramps, jaundice, ***viral hepatitis***

INTEG: Rash, flushing, *urticaria*

CNS: Headache, dizziness, malaise, paresthesia, *lethargy, chills, fever, flushing*

HEMA: ***Thrombosis, hemolysis, AIDS, DIC***

CV: Hypotension, tachycardia, *MI,* ***venous thrombosis, pulmonary embolism***

RESP: ***Bronchospasm***

Contraindications: Hypersensitivity, hepatic disease, DIC, elective surgery, mild factor IX deficiency

Precautions: Neonates/infants, pregnancy (C)

Pharmacokinetics:

IV: Half-life factor VII—3-6 hr, factor IX—24-36 hr, rapidly cleared from plasma

NURSING CONSIDERATIONS

Assess:

- Blood studies (coagulation factors assays by % normal: 5% prevents spontaneous hemorrhage, 30%-50% for surgery, 80%-100% for severe hemorrhage)
- Increased B/P, pulse
- For bleeding q15-30min, immobilize and apply ice to affected joints
- I&O; if urine becomes orange or red notify physician

Administer:

- IV 3 ml/min or less, with plastic syringe only
- After dilution with provided diluent, 50 U/ml or 25 U/ml; give not to exceed 10 ml/min

• After crossmatch is completed if patient has blood type A, B, AB, to determine incompatibility with factor

Perform/provide:

• Storage of reconstituted solution for 3 hr at room temp or up to 2 yr refrigeration (powder); check expiration date

Evaluate:

• Therapeutic response: prevention of hemorrhage

• Allergic or pyrogenic reaction: fever, chills, rash, itching, slow infusion rate if not severe

• DIC: bleeding, ecchymosis, hypersensitivity, changes in coagulation tests

Teach patient/family:

• To report any signs of bleeding: gums, under skin, urine, stools, emesis

• Risk of viral hepatitis, AIDS

• That immunization for hepatitis B may be given first

• To be tested q2-3mo for HIV

• To carry ID identifying disease; avoid salicylates, to inform other health professional about condition

famotidine

(fam-oo'-te-dine)

Pepcid, Pepcid IV

Func. class.: H_2 histamine receptor antagonist

Action: Competitively inhibits histamine at histamine H_2 receptor site, decreasing gastric secretion while pepsin remains at stable level

Uses: Short-term treatment of active duodenal ulcer, maintenance therapy for duodenal ulcer, Zollinger-Ellison syndrome, multiple endocrine adenomas, gastric ulcers

Dosage and routes:

Duodenal ulcer

• *Adult:* PO 40 mg qd hs × 4-8 wk, then 20 mg qd hs if needed (maintenance); IV 20 mg q12h if unable to take PO

Hypersecretory conditions

• *Adult:* PO 20 mg q6h, may give 160 mg q6h if needed; IV 20 mg q12h if unable to take PO

Available forms include: Tabs 20, 40 mg; powder for oral susp 40 mg/5 ml; inj IV 10 mg/ml

Side effects/adverse reactions:

HEMA: ***Thrombocytopenia***

CNS: Headache, dizziness, paresthesia, seizure, depression, anxiety, somnolence, insomnia, fever

GI: Constipation, nausea, vomiting, anorexia, cramps, abnormal liver enzymes

RESP: ***Bronchospasm***

EENT: Taste change, tinnitus, orbital edema

INTEG: Rash

MS: Myalgia, arthralgia

Contraindications: Hypersensitivity

Precautions: Pregnancy (B), lactation, children, severe renal disease, severe hepatic function, elderly

Pharmacokinetics:

PO: Peak 1-3 hr, plasma protein-binding 15%-20%; metabolized in liver (active metabolites), excreted by kidneys, half-life 2.5-3.5 hr

Interactions/incompatibilities:

• Decreased absorption: ketoconazole

• Decreased absorption of famotidine: antacids

NURSING CONSIDERATIONS

Assess:

• Blood counts during therapy, watch for decreasing platelets, if low, therapy may need to be discontinued and restarted after hematologic recovery

Administer:
• Antacids 1 hr before or 2 hr after famotidine
• IV after diluting with water for injection
• IV after diluting 2 ml of drug in IV solution to total volume of 5-10 ml, inject over >2 min
• IV infusion after diluting 2 ml of drug in 100 ml of IV solution and run over 15-30 min
Perform/provide:
• Storage in cool environment (oral), IV solution is stable for 48 hr at room temperature
Evaluate:
• Therapeutic response: decreased abdominal pain
• Blood dyscrasias (thrombocytopenia): bruising, fatigue, bleeding, poor healing
Teach patient/family:
• That drug must be continued for prescribed time to be effective
• To report bleeding, bruising, fatigue, malaise since blood dyscrasias do occur
• About possibility of decreased libido, reversible after discontinuing therapy
• To avoid irritating foods and extreme temperatures of foods

fat emulsions

Intralipid 10%, 20%; Liposyn 10%, 20%; Soyacal 10%, 20%; Travamulsion 10%, 20%

Func. class.: Caloric
Chem. class.: Fatty acid, long chain

Action: Needed for energy, heat production; consist of neutral triglycerides, primarily unsaturated fatty acids
Uses: Increase calorie intake, fatty acid deficiency, prevention
Dosage and routes:
Deficiency
• *Adult and child:* IV 8%-10% of required calorie intake (intralipid)
Adjunct to TPN
• *Adult:* IV 1 ml/min over 15-30 min (10%) or 0.5 ml/min over 15-30 min (20%); may increase to 500 ml over 4-8 hr if no adverse reactions occur, not to exceed 2.5 g/kg
• *Child:* IV 0.1 ml/min over 10-15 min (10%) or 0.05 ml/min over 10-15 min (20%); may increase to 1 g/kg over 4 hr if no adverse reactions occur, not to exceed 4 g/kg
Prevention of deficiency
• *Adult:* IV 500 ml twice a wk (10%), given 1 ml/min for 30 min, not to exceed 500 ml over 6 hr
• *Child:* IV 5-10 ml/kg/day (10%), given 0.1 ml/min for 30 min, not to exceed 100 ml/hr
Available forms include: Inj IV many types
Side effects/adverse reactions:
CNS: Dizziness, headache, drowsiness, focal seizures
CV: ***Shock***
GI: Nausea, vomiting, ***hepatomegaly***
RESP: Dyspnea, ***fat in lung tissue***
HEMA: ***Hyperlipemia, hypercoagulation, thrombocytopenia, leukopenia, leukocytosis***
Contraindications: Hypersensitivity, hyperlipemia, lipid necrosis, acute pancreatitis accompanied by hyperlipemia, hyperbilirubinemia of the newborn
Precautions: Severe liver disease, diabetes mellitus, thrombocytopenia, gastric ulcers, premature, term newborns, pregnancy (C), sepsis
Interactions/incompatibilities:
• Do not mix with any drug, elec-

trolytes, solutions, vitamin, unless added to TPN

NURSING CONSIDERATIONS

Assess:

• Triglycerides, free fatty acid levels, platelet counts daily to prevent fat overload, thrombocytopenia

• Liver function studies: AST, ALT

Administer:

• After changing IV tubing at each infusion: infection may occur with old tubing

• With infusion pump at prescribed rate; do not use in-line filter; clogging will occur

Perform/provide:

• Use of mixed solutions that are not separated or oily looking

Evaluate:

• Therapeutic response: increased weight

• Nutritional status: calorie count by dietician

Teach patient/family

• Reason for use of lipids

felodipine

(fell-od'a-pine)

Plendil

Func. class.: Calcium-channel blocker

Chem. class.: Dihydropyridine

Action: Inhibits calcium ion influx across cell membrane, resulting in dilation of peripheral arteries

Uses: Essential hypertension, alone or with other antihypertensives

Dosage and routes:

• *Adult:* PO 5 mg qd initially, usual range 5-10 mg qd; do not exceed 20 mg qd; do not adjust dosage at intervals of <2 wk

Available forms include: Ext rel tabs 5, 10 mg

Side effects/adverse reactions:

CV: Dysrhythmia, edema, CHF, hypotension, palpitations, ***MI, pulmonary edema,*** tachycardia, syncope, AV block, angina

GI: Nausea, vomiting, diarrhea, gastric upset, constipation, increased liver function studies, dry mouth

GU: Nocturia, polyuria

INTEG: Rash, pruritus

MISC: Flushing, sexual difficulties, cough, nasal congestion, shortness of breath, wheezing, epistaxis, respiratory infection, chest pain

CNS: Headache, fatigue, drowsiness, dizziness, anxiety, depression, nervousness, insomnia, lightheadedness, paresthesia, tinnitus, psychosis, somnolence

HEMA: Anemia

Contraindications: Hypersensitivity, sick sinus syndrome, 2nd or 3rd degree heart block

Precautions: CHF, hypotension <90 mm Hg systolic, hepatic injury, pregnancy (C), lacatation, children, renal disease, elderly

Pharmacokinetics: Peak plasma levels 2.5-5 hr; highly protein bound, >99% metabolized in liver, 0.5% excreted unchanged in urine; elimination half-life 11-16 hr

Interactions/incompatibilities:

• Increased effects of: β-blockers, antihypertensives, digitalis

• Increased felodipine level: cimetidine, ranitidine

NURSING CONSIDERATIONS

Administer:

• Once daily as whole tablet

Evaluate:

• Therapeutic response: decreased B/P

• Cardiac status: B/P, pulse, respiration, ECG

Teach patient/family:

• To swallow whole; do not crush or chew

* Available in Canada only

• To avoid hazardous activities until stabilized on drug, dizziness is no longer a problem
• To limit caffeine consumption
• To avoid OTC drugs unless directed by a physician
• Importance of complying with all areas of medical regimen: diet, exercise, stress reduction, drug therapy

Treatment of overdose: Defibrillation, atropine for AV block, vasopressor for hypotension

---

fenfluramine HCl

(fen-fluer'a-meen)

Pondimin

Func. class.: Anorexant
Chem. class.: Amphetamine derivative

Controlled Substance Schedule IV

Action: Influences serotonin pathways in CNS

Uses: Exogenous obesity

Dosage and routes:
• *Adult:* PO 20 mg ac, not to exceed 40 mg tid

Available forms include: Tabs 20 mg

Side effects/adverse reactions:
HEMA: Bone marrow depression, leukopenia, agranulocytosis
MISC: Hair loss, flushing, fever
EENT: Mydriasis, blurred vision
CNS: Insomnia, talkativeness, dizziness, drowsiness, headache, irritability, confusion, mood changes, anxiety, weakness, vivid dreams, uncoordination, depression, fatigue, malaise, euphoria, tremor, confusion
GI: Nausea, vomiting, anorexia, *dry mouth, diarrhea,* constipation, abdominal pain
GU: Impotence, change in libido, dysuria, urinary frequency
CV: Palpitations, tachycardia, hypertension, hypotension, dysrythmias, pulmonary hypertension
INTEG: Urticaria, rash, burning, sweating, chills, fever, erythma

Contraindications: Hypersensitivity to sympathomimetic amine, glaucoma, drug abuse, cardiovascular disease, alcoholism, children <12 yr, hypertension, hyperthyroidism, severe arteriosclerosis

Precautions: Diabetes mellitus, hypertension, depression, pregnancy (C), lactation

Pharmacokinetics:
PO: Onset 1-2 min, duration 4-6 hr, metabolized by liver, excreted by kidneys, half-life 20 hr

Interactions/incompatibilities:
• Hypertensive crisis: MAOIs or within 14 days of MAOIs
• Increased effect of fenfluramine: acetazolamide, antacids, sodium bicarbonate
• Decreased effects of fenfluramine: tricyclics, ascorbic acid, ammonium chloride
• Decrease effects of: guanethidine, other antihypertensives

NURSING CONSIDERATIONS

Assess:
• VS, B/P since this drug may reverse antihypertensives; check patients with cardiac disease more often
• CBC, urinalysis, in diabetes: blood sugar, urine sugar; insulin changes may need to be made since eating will decrease
• Height, growth rate in children; growth rate may be decreased

Administer:
• At least 6 hr before hs to avoid sleeplessness
• For obesity only if patient is on weight reduction program, includ-

F

ing dietary changes, exercise; patient will develop tolerance and weight loss won't occur without additional methods, give 1 hr before meals
• Gum, hard candy, frequent sips of water for dry mouth
Perform/provide:
• Check to see PO medication has been swallowed
Evaluate:
• Therapeutic response: decreased weight
• Mental status: mood, sensorium, affect, stimulation, insomnia, aggressiveness may occur
• Physical dependency: should not be used for extended time; dose should be discontinued gradually, drug tolerance will occur after long-term use
• Withdrawal symptoms: headache, nausea, vomiting, muscle pain, weakness
Teach patient/family:
• Not to take more frequently than prescribed
• To decrease caffeine consumption (coffee, tea, cola, chocolate); may increase irritability, stimulation
• Avoid OTC preparations unless approved by physician
• To taper off drug over several weeks, or depression, increased sleeping, lethargy may ensue
• To avoid alcohol ingestion
• To avoid hazardous activities until patient is stabilized on medication
• To get needed rest; patients will feel more tired at end of day
Treatment of overdose: Administer fluids, gastric lavage, hemodialysis or peritoneal dialysis; antihypertensive for increased B/P; ammonium Cl for increased excretion

fenoprofen calcium
(fen-oh-proe'fen)
Nalfon
Func. class.: Nonsteroidal antiinflammatory
Chem. class.: Propionic acid derivative

Action: May inhibit prostaglandin synthesis by decreasing enzyme needed for biosynthesis; possesses analgesic, antiinflammatory, antipyretic properties
Uses: Mild to moderate pain, osteoarthritis, rheumatoid arthritis, acute gout, arthritis, ankylosing spondylitis, inflammation, dysmenorrhea
Dosage and routes:
Pain
• *Adult:* PO 200 mg q4-6h as needed
Arthritis
• *Adult:* PO 300-600 mg qid, not to exceed 3.2 g/day
Available forms include: Caps 200, 300 mg; tabs 600 mg
Side effects/adverse reactions:
GI: Nausea, anorexia, vomiting, diarrhea, jaundice, ***cholestatic hepatitis,*** constipation, flatulence, cramps, dry mouth, peptic ulcer
CNS: Dizziness, headache, drowsiness, fatigue, tremors, confusion, insomnia, anxiety, depression
CV: Tachycardia, peripheral edema, palpitations, dysrhythmias
INTEG: Purpura, rash, pruritus, sweating
GU: ***Nephrotoxicity: dysuria, hematuria, oliguria, azotemia***
HEMA: ***Blood dyscrasias***
EENT: Tinnitus, hearing loss, blurred vision
Contraindications: Hypersensitivity, asthma, severe renal disease, severe hepatic disease

* Available in Canada only

Precautions: Pregnancy, (B) 1st and 2nd trimester, lactation, children, bleeding disorders, GI disorders, cardiac disorders, hypersensitivity to other antiinflammatory agents

Pharmacokinetics:

PO: Peak 2 hr, half-life 3-3½ hr, metabolized in liver, excreted in urine (metabolites), breast milk, 99% plasma protein binding

Interactions/incompatibilities:

- May increase the action of: coumarin, sulfonamides, salicyates
- May decrease effects of fenoprofen: phenobarbital, probenecid

NURSING CONSIDERATIONS

Assess:

- Renal, liver, blood studies: BUN, creatinine, AST, ALT, Hgb, before treatment, periodically thereafter
- Audiometric, ophthalmic examination before, during, after treatment

Administer:

- With food to decrease GI symptoms; however, best to take on empty stomach to facilitate absorption

Perform/provide:

- Storage at room temperature

Evaluate:

- Therapeutic response: decreased pain, stiffness in joints, decreased swelling in joints, ability to move more easily
- For eye, ear problems: blurred vision, tinnitus; may indicate toxicity

Teach patient/family:

- To report blurred vision, ringing, roaring in ears; may indicate toxicity
- To avoid driving, other hazardous activities if dizziness, drowsiness occurs
- To report change in urine pattern, increased weight, edema, increased pain in joints, fever, blood in urine; indicates nephrotoxicity
- That therapeutic effects may take up to 1 mo
- To take with a full glass of water to enhance absorption

fentanyl citrate

(fen'ta-nill)

Sublimaze

Func. class.: Narcotic analgesics

Chem. class.: Opiate, synthetic phenylpiperidine derivative

Controlled Substance Schedule II

Action: Inhibits ascending pain pathways in CNS, increases pain threshold, alters pain perception

Uses: Preoperatively, postoperatively; adjunct to general anesthetic, when combined with droperidol

Dosage and routes:

Anesthetic

- *Adult:* IV 0.05-0.1 mg q2-3min prn

Preoperatively

- *Adult:* IM 0.05-0.1 mg q30-60 min before surgery

Postoperatively

- *Adult:* IM 0.05-0.1 mg ql-2h prn
- *Child:* IM 0.02-0.03 mg/9 kg

Available forms include: Inj IM, IV 0.05 mg/ml

Side effects/adverse reactions:

CNS: Dizziness, delirium, euphoria

GI: Nausea, vomiting

MS: Muscle rigidity

EENT: Blurred vision, miosis

CV: ***Bradycardia, arrest,*** hypotension or hypertension

RESP: ***Respiratory depression, arrest, laryngospasm***

Contraindications: Hypersensitivity to opiates, myasthenia gravis

Precautions: Elderly, respiratory depression, increased intracranial pressure, seizure disorders, severe respiratory disorders, cardiac dysrhythmias, pregnancy (C)

Pharmacokinetics:

IM: Onset 7-15 min, peak 30 min, duration 1-2 hr

IV: Onset immediate, peak 3-5 min, duration ½-1 hr; metabolized by liver, excreted by kidneys, crosses placenta, excreted in breast milk, half-life 2½-4 hr, 80% bound to plasma proteins

Interactions/incompatibilities:

- Effects may be increased with other CNS depressants: alcohol, narcotics, sedative/hypnotics, antipsychotics, skeletal muscle relaxants

NURSING CONSIDERATIONS

Assess:

- VS after parenteral route, note muscle rigidity

Administer:

- By injection (IM, IV), give slowly to prevent rigidity
- Only with resuscitative equipment available
- IV; may be diluted with compatible sol and given as an infusion

Perform/provide:

- Storage in light-resistant area at room temperature
- Coughing, turning, deep breathing for postoperative patients
- Safety measures: siderails, night light, call bell within reach

Evaluate:

- Therapeutic response: induction of anesthesia
- CNS changes: dizziness, drowsiness, hallucinations, euphoria, LOC, pupil reaction
- Allergic reactions: rash, urticaria
- Respiratory dysfunction: respiratory depression, character, rate, rhythm; notify physician if respirations are <10/min

fentanyl citrate/droperidol combination

(fen'ta-nil) (droe-per'i-dole)

Innovar

Func. class.: General anesthetic/narcotic analgesic

Chem. class.: Phenylpiperone derivative

Controlled Substance Schedule II

Action: Action at subcortical levels to reduce motor activity, produces analgesia

Uses: Premedication, adjunct to general anesthesia, maintenance of anesthesia

Dosage and routes:

Induction

- *Adult:* IV 1 ml/20-25 lb
- *Child:* IV 0.5 ml/20 lb

Premedication

- *Adult:* IM 0.5-2 ml 45-60 min before surgery or procedure
- *Child:* IM 0.25 ml/20 lb 45-60 min before surgery or procedure

Available forms include: Inj IM, IV 0.05 mg fentanyl, 2.5 mg droperidol/ml

Side effects/adverse reactions:

RESP: ***Laryngospasm, bronchospasm, respiratory arrest***

CNS: Dystonia, akathisia, flexion of arms, fine tremors, dizziness, anxiety, drowsiness, restlessness, hallucination, depression

CV: Tachycardia, hypotension, circulatory depression

EENT: Upward rotation of eyes, oculogyric crisis, blurred vision

INTEG: Chills, facial sweating, shivering, diaphoresis

GI: Nausea, vomiting

Contraindications: Hypersensitivity, child < 2 yr, myasthenia gravis

Precautions: Elderly, increased intracranial pressure, cardiovascular

* Available in Canada only

disease (bradydysrhythmias), renal disease, liver disease, Parkinson's disease, COPD, pregnancy (C)

Pharmacokinetics:

IV: Onset 20 sec, peak 2-10 min, duration ½-2 hr; tranquilizing effect may last up to 12h

IM: Onset 7 min, duration 1-2 hr, metabolized in liver, excreted in urine metabolites (90%)

Interactions/incompatibilities:

- Increased CNS depression: alcohol, narcotics, barbiturates, antipsychotics or other CNS depressants
- Decreased effects of: amphetamines, anticonvulsants, anticoagulants
- Increased intraocular pressure: anticholinergics, antiparkinson drugs
- Increased side effects of: lithium
- Do not mix with barbiturates in solution

NURSING CONSIDERATIONS

Assess:

- VS q10min during IV administration, q30min after IM dose

Administer:

- Anticholinergics (benztropine, diphenhydramine) for extrapyramidal reaction
- Only with crash cart, resuscitative equipment nearby; narcotic antagonist for severe respiratory depression
- IV slowly only

Perform/provide:

- Slow movement of patient to avoid orthostatic hypotension

Evaluate:

- Therapeutic response: decreased anxiety, absence of vomiting, maintenance of anesthesia
- Rigidity of skeletal muscles
- Extrapyramidal reactions: dystonia, akathisia
- Increasing heart rate or decreasing B/P, notify physician at once; do not place patient in Trendelenburg position or sympathetic blockade may occur causing respiratory arrest

Teach patient/family:

- To use deep breathing, turning, coughing after surgery to prevent increased secretions in lungs

---

fentanyl transdermal

Duragesic

Func. class.: Narcotic analgesic
Chem. class.: Opiate, synthetic phenylpiperidine

Controlled Substance Schedule II

Action: Inhibits ascending pain pathways in CNS, increases pain threshold, alters pain perception

Uses: Management of chronic pains for those requiring opioid analgesia

Dosage and routes:

Adult: 25 μg/hr; may increase until pain relief occurs; apply patch to flat surface on upper torso and wear for 72 hr; apply new patch on different site for continued relief

Available forms include: Patch 2.5, 5, 7.5, 10 mg

Side effects/adverse reactions:

CNS: Dizziness, delirium, euphoria, light-headedness, sedation, dysphoria, agitation, anxiety

GI: Nausea, vomiting, diarrhea, cramps

EENT: Blurred vision, miosis

CV: Bradycardia, ***cardiac arrest,*** hypotension or hypertension, facial flushing, chills

RESP: ***Respiratory depression, laryngospasm, bronchospasm***

Contraindications: Hypersensitivity to opiates, myasthenia gravis

Precautions: Elderly, respiratory

depression, increased intracranial pressure, seizure disorders, severe respiratory disorders, cardiac dysrhythmias, pregnancy (C)

Interactions/incompatibilities:

• Effects may be increased with other CNS depressants: alcohol, narcotics, sedative/hypnotics, antipsychotics, skeletal muscle relaxants

NURSING CONSIDERATIONS

Assess:

• Pain contol; check for duration, site, character of pain

Administer:

• q72h for continuous pain relief

Perform/provide:

• Safety measures: siderails, night light, call bell within reach

Evaluate:

• Therapeutic response: decreased pain

• CNS changes: dizziness, drowsiness, hallucinations, euphoria, LOC, pupil reaction

• Allergic reactions: rash, urticaria

• Respiratory dysfunction: respiratory depression, character, rate, rhythm; notify physician if respirations are <10/min

---

ferrous fumarate/ferrous gluconate/ferrous sulfate

Eldofe, Farbegen, Fecot, Femiron, Feostat, Ferranol,* Fersamal, Fumasorb, Fumerin, Hemocyte, Ircon, Laud-Iron, Maniron, Neofer, Novofumar,* Palafer,* Palmiron/Fergon, Ferralet, Fertinic,* Novoferrogluc*, Simiron/Fer-in-Sol, Feosol, Fero-Grad,* Fero-Gradumet, Ferolix, Ferospace, Fesofor,* Irospan, Mol-Iron, Novoferrosulfa,* Slow-Fe, Telefon

Func. class.: Hematinic
Chem. class.: Iron preparation

Action: Replaces iron stores needed for red blood cell development, energy and O_2 transport, utilization; fumarate contains 33% elemental iron; gluconate, 12%; sulfate, 20%; iron, 30%; ferrous sulfate exsiccated

Uses:

Iron deficiency anemia, prophylaxis for iron deficiency in pregnancy

Dosage and routes:

Fumarate

• *Adult:* PO 200 mg tid-qid

• *Child:* 2-12 yr: PO 3 mg/kg/day (elemental iron) tid-qid

• *Child 6 mo-2 yr:* PO up to 6 mg/kg/day (elemental iron) tid-qid

• *Infants:* PO 10-25 mg/day (elemental iron) tid-qid

Gluconate

• *Adult:* PO 200-600 mg tid

• *Child 6-12 yr:* 300-900 mg qd

• *Child <6 yr:* 100-300 mg qd

Sulfate

• *Adult:* PO 0.750-1.5 g/day in divided doses tid

• *Child 6-12 yr:* 600 mg/day in divided doses

Pregnancy

• *Adult:* PO 300-600 mg/day in divided doses

Available forms include:

Fumarate

Tabs 63, 195, 200, 324, 325 mg; tabs chewable 100 mg; tabs controlled-release 300 mg; oral susp 100 mg/5 ml, 45 mg/0.6 ml

Gluconate

Tabs 300, 320, 325 mg; caps 86, 325, 435 mg; tabs film-coated 300 mg; elix 300 mg/5 ml

Sulfate

Tabs, 195, 300, 325 mg; tabs enteric-coated 325 mg; tabs extended-release, time-release caps, 525 mg

Side effects/adverse reactions:

GI: Nausea, constipation, epigas-

---

* Available in Canada only

tric pain, black and red tarry stools, vomiting, diarrhea

INTEG: Temporarily discolored tooth enamel and eyes

Contraindications: Hypersensitivity, ulcerative colitis/regional enteritis, hemosiderosis/hemochromatosis, peptic ulcer disease, hemolytic anemia, cirrhosis

Precautions: Anemia (long-term), pregnancy (A)

Pharmacokinetics:

PO: Excreted in feces, urine, skin, breast milk, enters bloodstream, bound to transferrin, crosses placenta

Interactions/incompatibilities:

• Decreased absorption of: penicillamine

• Decreased absorption of iron preparations: chloramphenicol, antacids, tetracycline, vitamin E

• Increased absorption of iron preparation: ascorbic acid

NURSING CONSIDERATIONS

Assess:

• Blood studies: Hct, Hgb, reticulocytes, bilirubin before treatment, at least monthly

Administer:

• Only with vitamin E supplements to infants or hemolytic anemia may occur

• Between meals for best absorption, may give with juice; do not give with antacids or milk, delay at least 1 hr; if GI symptoms occur, give PC even if absorption is decreased; eggs, milk products, chocolate, caffeine interfere with absorption

• Through plastic straw to avoid discoloration of tooth enamel; dilute thoroughly

• At least 1 hr before hs since corrosion may occur in stomach

• For <6 months for anemia

Perform/provide:

• Storage in tight, light-resistant container

Evaluate:

• Therapeutic response: improvement in Hct, Hgb, reticulocytes, decreased fatigue, weakness

• Toxicity: nausea, vomiting, diarrhea (green then tarry stools), hematemesis, pallor, cyanosis, shock, coma

• Elimination; if constipation occurs, increase water, bulk, activity

• Nutrition: amount of iron in diet (meat, dark green leafy vegetables, dried beans, dried fruits, eggs)

• Cause of iron loss or anemia, including salicylates, sulfonamides, antimalarials, quinidine

Teach patient/family:

• That iron will change stools black or dark green

• That iron poisoning may occur if increased beyond recommended level

• Not to crush; swallow tablet whole

• To keep out of reach of children

• Do not substitute one iron salt for another; elemental iron content differs (e.g., 300 mg ferrous fumarate contains about 100 mg elemental iron, whereas 300 mg ferrous gluconate contains only about 30 mg elemental iron)

• To avoid reclining position for 15-30 min after taking drug to avoid esophageal corrosion

• To follow diet high in iron

Lab test interferences:

False-positive: Occult blood

Treatment of overdose: Induce vomiting; give eggs, milk until lavage can be done

F

fibrinolysin/desoxyribonuclease

(fye-bri-noe-lye'sin)

Elase

Func. class.: Enzyme
Chem. class.: Proteolytic-bovine

Action: Dissolves fibrin in clots, attacks DNA in areas of disintegrating cells

Uses: Debridement of wounds, intravaginally; irrigating wounds, topically

Dosage and routes:

Debridement/intravaginally

• *Adult:* OINT 5 g

Irrigating

• *Adult:* IRIG dilution depends on type of wound

Available forms include: Fibrinolysin with desoxyribonuclease 666.6 U/g; top sol fibrinolysin 25 U/desoxyribonuclease 15,000 U

Side effects/adverse reactions:

INTEG: Hyperemia

Contraindications: Hypersensitivity to bovine or mercury products, hematoma

Precautions: Pregnancy (C)

NURSING CONSIDERATIONS

Assess:

• For signs of irritation and inflammation; drug should be discontinued

Administer:

• After reconstituting with 10 ml sterile NaCl solution, use only fresh solution

• After removing necrotic debris, dry eschar

• Wet dressing by mixing 1 vial elase/10-50 ml saline solution, saturate gauze with solution, pack area, remove in 6-8 hr, repeat tid-qid

Perform/provide:

• Cleaning of wound using aseptic technique, cover with drug then dressing, change at least qid

Evaluate:

• Therapeutic response: decrease in wound scarring, tissue necrosis

• Wound: drainage, color, odor, size, depth

filgrastim (G-CSF)

(fill-grass'stim)

Neupogen

Func. class.: Biologic modifier
Chem. class.: Granulocyte colony stimulating factor

Action: Stimulates proliferation and differentiation of neutrophils

Uses: To decrease chance of infection in patients receiving antineoplastics that are myelosuppressive

Dosage and routes:

• *Adult:* IV/SC 5 μg/kg/day in a single dose, may increase by 5 μg/kg in each chemotherapy cycle; give qd for up to 2 wk until the absolute neutrophil count (ANC) has reached 10,000/mm^3

Available forms include: Inj 300 μg/ml

Side effects/adverse reactions:

CNS: Fever

HEMA: ***Thrombocytopenia***

INTEG: Alopecia, exacerbation of skin conditions

MS: Osteoporosis, skeletal pain

GI: Nausea, vomiting, diarrhea, mucositis, anorexia

Contraindications: Hypersensitivity to proteins of *E. coli*

Precautions: Pregnancy (C), lactation, cardiac conditions

Pharmacokinetics: Metabolism, excretion, distribution is not known

Interactions/incompatibilities:

• Do not use this drug concomitantly with antineoplastics

* Available in Canada only

NURSING CONSIDERATIONS

Assess:

• Blood studies: CBC, platelet count before treatment and twice weekly; neutrophil counts may be increased for 2 days after therapy

Administer:

• Using single-use vials; after dose is withdrawn, do not reenter vial

• For 2 wk or until ANC is 10,000/ mm^3 after the expected chemotherapy neutrophil nadir

Perform/provide:

• Storage in refrigerator; do not freeze, may store at room temperature for up to 6 hr

• Avoid shaking

Evaluate:

• Therapeutic response: absence of infection

Teach patient/family:

• Technique for self-administration: dose, side effects, disposal of containers and needles; provide instruction sheet

Lab test interferences:

Increase: Uric acid, lactate dehydrogenase, alk, phosphatase

flavoxate HCl

(fla-vox'ate)

Urispas

Func. class.: Spasmolytic
Chem. class.: Flavone derivative

Action: Relaxes smooth muscles in urinary tract

Uses: Relief of nocturia, incontinence, suprapubic pain, dysuria, frequency associated with urologic conditions (symptomatic only)

Dosage and routes:

• *Adult and child >12 yr:* PO 100-200 mg tid-qid

Available forms include: Tabs 100 mg

Side effects/adverse reactions:

HEMA: ***Leukopenia, eosinophilia***

CNS: Anxiety, restlessness, dizziness, ***convulsions,*** headache, drowsiness, confusion, decreased concentration

CV: Palpitations, sinus tachycardia, hypotension

GI: Nausea, vomiting, anorexia, abdominal pain, constipation

GU: Dysuria

INTEG: Urticaria, dermatitis

EENT: Blurred vision, increased intraocular tension, dry mouth, throat

Contraindications: Hypersensitivity, GI obstruction, GI hemorrhage, GU obstruction

Precautions: Pregnancy (B), lactation, suspected glaucoma, children <12 yr

Pharmacokinetics: Excreted in urine

NURSING CONSIDERATIONS

Evaluate:

• Therapeutic response: decreased dysuria

• Urinary status: dysuria, frequency, nocturia, incontinence

• Allergic reactions: rash, urticaria; if these occur, drug should be discontinued

Teach patient/family

• To avoid hazardous activities; dizziness may occur

flecainide acetate

(fle-kay'nide)

Tambocor

Func. class.: Antidysrhythmic (Class IC)

Action: Decreases conduction in all parts of the heart, with greatest effect on His-Purkinje system, which stabilizes cardiac membrane

Uses: Life-threatening ventricular

F

dysrhythmias, sustained ventricular tachycardia

Dosage and routes:

• *Adult:* PO 100 mg q12h, may increase q4d by 50 mg q12h to desired response, not to exceed 400 mg/day

Available forms include: Tabs 50, 100, 150 mg

Side effects/adverse reactions:

CNS: Headache, dizziness, involuntary movement, confusion, psychosis, restlessness, irritability, paresthesias, ataxia, flushing, somnolence, depression, anxiety, malaise

EENT: Tinnitus, *blurred vision,* hearing loss

GI: Nausea, vomiting, anorexia, constipation, abdominal pain, flatulence, change in taste

CV: Hypotension, bradycardia, angina, PVCs, ***heart block, cardiovascular collapse, arrest,*** *dysrhythmias,* ***CHF, fatal ventricular tachycardia***

RESP: Dyspnea, ***respiratory depression***

INTEG: Rash, urticaria, edema, swelling

HEMA: Leukopenia, thrombocytopenia

GU: Impotence, decreased libido, polyuria, urinary retention

Contraindications: Hypersensitivity, severe heart block, cardiogenic shock, nonsustained ventricular dysrhythmias, frequent PVCs, nonlife-threatening dysrhythmias

Precautions: Pregnancy (C), lactation, children, renal disease, liver disease, CHF, respiratory depression, myasthenia gravis

Pharmacokinetics:

PO: Peak 3 hr; half-life 12-27 hr; metabolized by liver, excreted unchanged by kidneys (10%), excreted in breast milk

Interactions/incompatibilities:

• Increased levels of both drugs: propranolol

• Increased level of flecainide: amiodarone, cimetidine

• Increased negative inotropic effects: disopyramide, verapamil

• Increased digoxin level: digoxin

NURSING CONSIDERATIONS

Assess:

• For hypokalemia, hyperkalemia before administration; correct electrolytes

• Blood levels: trough (0.2-1 μg/ml)

• B/P, ECG continuously for fluctuations

Administer:

• Reduced dosage as soon as dysrhythmia is controlled

Evaluate:

• Therapeutic response: decreased dysrhythmias

• Malignant hyperthermia: tachypnea, tachycardia, changes in B/P, increased temperature

• Cardiac rate, respiration: rate, rhythm, character, continuously

• Respiratory status: rate, rhythm, lung fields for rales

• CNS effects: dizziness, confusion, psychosis, paresthesias, convulsions; drug should be discontinued

• Increased respiration, increased pulse; drug should be discontinued

Lab test interferences:

Increase: CPK

Treatment of overdose: O_2, artificial ventilation, ECG, administer dopamine for circulatory depression, administer diazepam or thiopental for convulsions, treat ventricular dysrhythmias

floxuridine

(flox-yoor'i-deen)
FUDR

Func. class.: Antineoplastic, antimetabolite
Chem. class.: Pyrimidine antagonist

Action: Inhibits DNA synthesis; interferes with cell replication by competitively inhibiting thymidylate synthesis

Uses: GI adenocarcinoma metastatic to liver, cancer of breast, head, neck, liver, brain, gallbladder, bile duct

Dosage and routes:

• *Adult:* INTRAARTERIAL 0.1-0.6 mg/kg/day × 1-6 wk; HEPATIC ARTERY INJ 0.4-0.6 mg/kg/day × 1-6 wk

Available forms include: Powder for inj (intraarterial, hepatic artery) 500 mg/5 ml vial

Side effects/adverse reactions:

HEMA: ***Thrombocytopenia, leukopenia, myelosuppression, anemia***
GI: Anorexia, diarrhea, nausea, vomiting, ***hemorrhage***
GU: ***Renal failure***
EENT: Epistaxis
INTEG: Rash, fever
CNS: Lethargy, malaise, weakness

Contraindications: Hypersensitivity, myelosuppression, pregnancy (D), poor nutritional states, serious infections

Precautions: Renal disease, hepatic disease, bone marrow depression

Pharmacokinetics: Half-life 10-20 min, 20 hr terminal, metabolized in liver, excreted in urine (active metabolite), crosses blood-brain barrier

Interactions/incompatibilities:

• Increased toxicity: radiation or other antineoplastics

NURSING CONSIDERATIONS

Assess:

• CBC, differential, platelet count weekly; withhold drug if WBC is <3500/mm^3 or platelet count is <100,000/mm^3; notify physician of these results; drug should be discontinued
• Renal function studies: BUN, serum uric acid, urine CrCl, electrolytes before, during therapy
• I&O ratio: report fall in urine output to <30 ml/hr
• Monitor temperature q4h; fever may indicate beginning infection
• Liver function tests before, during therapy: bilirubin, alk phosphatase, AST, ALT, LDH; as needed or monthly

Administer:

• By intraarterial infusion pump after diluting 5 ml drug/5 ml sterile H_2O for inj, dilute further with D_5W or normal saline to required dilution
• Antiemetic 30-60 min before giving drug to prevent vomiting and prn
• Antibiotics for prophylaxis of infection
• Topical or systemic analgesics for pain
• Transfusion for anemia
• Antispasmodic for diarrhea

Perform/provide:

• Wrapping solution, do not expose to light
• Strict medical asepsis and protective isolation if WBC levels are low
• Increased fluid intake to 2-3 L/day to prevent dehydration unless contraindicated
• Rinsing of mouth tid-qid with water, club soda, brushing of teeth bid-tid with soft brush or cotton-tipped applicators for stomatitis; use unwaxed dental floss
• Nutritious diet with iron, vitamin

F

supplements, low fiber, and no dairy products as ordered

Evaluate:

- Therapeutic response: decreased tumor size, spread of malignancy
- Bleeding: hematuria, guaiac, bruising or petechiae, mucosa or orifices q8h
- Food preferences; list likes, dislikes
- Inflammation of mucosa, breaks in skin
- Buccal cavity q8h for dryness, sores or ulceration, white patches, oral pain, bleeding, dysphagia
- Symptoms indicating severe allergic reaction: rash, urticaria, itching, flushing
- GI symptoms: frequency of stools, cramping; low-residue diet with elimination of milk products when used in conjunction with 5FUDR/radiation therapy
- Acidosis, signs of dehydration: rapid respirations, poor skin turgor, decreased urine output, dry skin, restlessness, weakness

Teach patient/family:

- Why protective isolation precautions are necessary
- To report signs of infection: increased temperature, sore throat, flu symptoms
- To report signs of anemia: fatigue, headache, faintness, shortness of breath, irritability
- To report bleeding: avoid use of razors, or commercial mouthwash
- To avoid use of aspirin products or ibuprofen
- To report stomatitis: any bleeding, white spots, ulcerations in mouth; tell patient to examine mouth qd, report symptoms

Lab test interferences:

Increase: Liver function studies

fluconazole

(floo-con'-a-zole)

Diflucan

Func. class.: Antifungal

Action: Inhibits ergosterol biosynthesis, causes direct damage to membrane phospholipids

Uses: Oropharyngeal candidiasis in AIDS patients, chronic mucocutaneous candidiasis, urinary candidiasis, cryptococcal meningitis

Dosage and routes:

Vaginal candidiasis

- *Adult:* PO 150 mg as a single dose

Serious fungal infections

- *Adult:* PO/IV 50-400 mg qd

Oropharyngeal candidiasis in AIDS patients:

- *Adult:* PO 50 mg qd

Available forms include: Tabs 50, 100, 200 mg, IV inj 200, 400 mg

Side effects/adverse reactions:

GI: Nausea, vomiting, diarrhea, cramping, flatus, increased AST, ALT

Contraindications: Hypersensitivity

Precautions: Renal disease, pregnancy (B)

Interactions/incompatibilities:

- Potentiation of anticoagulation: warfarin
- Increased renal dysfunction: cyclosporines

NURSING CONSIDERATIONS

Assess:

- VS q15-30min during first infusion, note changes in pulse, B/P
- I&O ratio; watch for decreasing urinary output, change in sp gr; discontinue drug to prevent renal damage
- Weigh weekly; if weight gain >2 lb/wk and edema is present, renal damage should be considered

Administer:
• After diluting according to package directions
• IV using an in-line filter, using distal veins; check for extravasation and necrosis q2h
• Drug only after C&S confirms organism, drug needed to treat condition
Perform/provide:
• Storage, protected from moisture and light, diluted solution is stable for 24 hr
Evaluate:
• Therapeutic response: decreasing oral candidiasis, fever, malaise, rash, negative C&S for infection organism
• Renal toxicity: increasing BUN, serum creatinine; if BUN is >40 mg/dl or if serum creatinine is >3 mg/dl, drug may be discontinued or dosage reduced
• For hepatotoxicity: increasing AST, ALT, alk phosphatase, bilirubin
Teach patient/family:
• That long-term therapy may be needed to clear infection

flucytosine

(floo-sye'toe-seen)
Ancobon, Ancotil*
Func. class.: Antifungal
Chem. class.: Pyrimidine (fluorinated)

Action: Converted to fluorouracil after entering fungi, which inhibits DNA synthesis
Uses: *Candida* infections (septicemia, endocarditis, pulmonary, urinary tract infections), *Cryptococcus* (meningitis, pulmonary, urinary tract infections)
Dosage and routes:
• *Adult and child >50 kg:* PO 50-150 mg/kg/day q6h
• *Adult and child <50 kg:* PO 1.5-4.5 g/m²/day in 4 divided doses
Available forms include: Caps 250, 500 mg
Side effects/adverse reactions:
INTEG: Rash
CNS: Headache, confusion, dizziness, sedation
GI: Nausea, vomiting, anorexia, diarrhea, cramps, enterocolitis, increased AST, ALT, alk phosphatase, ***bowel perforation*** (rare)
HEMA: ***Thrombocytopenia, agranulocytosis, anemia, leukopenia, pancytopenia***
GU: Increased BUN, creatinine
Contraindications: Hypersensitivity
Precautions: Renal disease, bone marrow depression, blood dyscrasias, radiation/chemotherapy, pregnancy (C)
Pharmacokinetics:
PO: Peak 2½-6 hr, half-life 3-6 hr, excreted in urine (unchanged), well-distributed to CSF, aqueous humor, joints
Interactions/incompatibilities:
• Synergisim: Amphotericin B

NURSING CONSIDERATIONS
Assess:
• VS q15-30min during first infusion, note changes in pulse and B/P
• Blood studies: CBC, including platelets
• Drug level during treatment (therapeutic level 25-100 μg/ml); if renal impairment is present level usually kept <100 μg/ml
Administer:
• Drug only after C&S confirms organism, drug needed to treat condition
• Few caps at a time to decrease nausea, vomiting over 15 min
Perform/provide:
• Symptomatic treatment as or-

dered for adverse reactions: aspirin, antihistamines, antiemetics, antispasmodics
• Storage in tight, light-resistant containers at room temperature

Evaluate:
• Therapeutic response: decreased fever, malaise, rash, negative C&S for infecting organism
• For renal toxicity: increasing BUN, serum creatinine; if serum creatinine >1.7 mg/100 dl, dosage may be reduced
• For hepatotoxicity: increasing AST, ALT, alk phosphatase
• For allergic reaction: dermatitis, rash; drug should be discontinued, antihistamines (mild reaction) or epinephrine (severe reaction) administered
• For blood dyscrasias, fatigue, bruising, malaise, dark urine

Teach patient/family:
• That long-term therapy may be needed to clear infection (1-2 mo depending on type of infection)
• To report symptoms of blood dyscrasias: fatigue, bruising, malaise, dark urine

Lab test interferences:
False-increase: Creatinine

fludarabine phosphate

(floo-dar'a-bine)
Fludara
Func. class.: Antineoplastic, antimetabolite
Chem. class.: Vidarabine derivative

Action: Competes with physiologic substrate that inhibits DNA synthesis

Uses: Chronic lymphocytic leukemia

Dosage and routes:
• *Adult:* IV 25 mg/m² over 30 min qd × 5 days, may repeat q28 days; reconstitute 2 ml of sterile water for inj; dissolution should occur in <15 sec

Available forms include: Lyophilized powder for reconstitution 50 mg

Side effects/adverse reactions:
SYST: Fever, chills, malaise, fatigue
META: Hyperuricemia, hyperphosphatemia, hypocalcemia, metabolic acidosis, hyperkalemia
HEMA: Thrombophlebitis, bleeding, ***thrombocytopenia, leukopenia, myelosuppression, anemia***
GI: Nausea, vomiting, anorexia, diarrhea, stomatitis, ***hepatotoxicity,*** abdominal pain, hematemesis, ***GI hemorrhage***
EENT: Visual disturbances, sinusitis
GU: Dysuria, infection
INTEG: Rash
RESP: ***Pneumonia,*** dyspnea, cough, interstitial pulmonary infiltrate
CV: Edema
CNS: Weakness, confusion, headache, depression, sleep disorder, impaired mentation, ***coma,*** peripheral neuropathy

Contraindications: Hypersensitivity, pregnancy (D)

Precautions: Renal disease, hepatic disease, infants

Pharmacokinetics: Rapidly converted to active metabolite; half-life of metabolite 10 hr; mean plasma clearance of metabolite 8.9 L/hr/m²; 23% excreted in urine as unchanged metabolite

Interactions/incompatibilities:
• Increased toxicity: radiation or other antineoplastics

NURSING CONSIDERATIONS

Assess:
• CBC (RBC, Hct, Hgb), differential, platelet count weekly; with-

*Available in Canada only

hold drug if CBC <4000/mm³, platelet count is <75,000/mm³, or RBC, Hct, Hgb are low; notify physician of these results

- Renal function studies: BUN, uric acid, urine creatinine clearance, electrolytes before and during therapy
- I&O ratio; report fall in urine output to <30 ml/hr
- Temperature q4h; fever may indicate beginning infection; no rectal temperature
- Liver function tests before, during therapy: bilirubin, ALT, AST, alk phosphatase, as needed or monthly
- Blood uric acid levels during therapy

Administer:

- Antiemetic 30 to 60 min before giving drug to prevent vomiting, and PRN
- Allopurinol or sodium bicarbonate to maintain uric acid levels and alkalinization or the urine; prevent hyperuricemia
- Antibiotics for prophylaxis of infection
- Topical or systemic analgesics for pain
- Transfusion for anemia
- Antispasmodic for GI symptoms

Perform/provide:

- Strict medical asepsis and protective isolation if WBC levels are low
- Increase fluid intake to 2-3 L/day to prevent urate deposits and calculi formation, unless contraindicated
- Diet low in purines: absence of organ meats (kidney, liver), dried beans, peas to prevent increased urate deposits
- Rinsing of mouth tid-qid with water, club soda; brushing of teeth bid-tid with soft brush or cotton-tipped applicators for stomatitis; use unwaxed dental floss
- HOB increased to facilitate breathing if dyspnea or pneumonia occurs
- Storage in refrigerator

Evaluate:

- Therapeutic response: decrease in tumor size, spread of malignancy
- Bleeding: hematuria, guaiac, bruising or petechiae, mucosa or orifices q8h
- Dyspnea, rales, unproductive cough, chest pain, tachypnea, fatigue, increased pulse, pallor, lethargy, personality changes with high doses
- Food preferences: list likes, dislikes
- Edema in feet, joint pain, stomach pain, shaking
- Inflammation of mucosa, breaks in skin
- Yellowing of skin, sclera, dark urine, clay-colored stools, itchy skin, abdominal pain, fever, diarrhea
- Buccal cavity q8h for dryness, sores or ulceration, white patches, oral pain, bleeding, dysphagia
- Local irritation, pain, burning, discoloration at injection site
- GI symptoms: frequency of stools, cramping
- Acidosis, signs of dehydration: rapid respirations, poor skin turgor, decreased urine output, dry skin, restlessness, weakness

Teach patient/family:

- Why protective isolation precautions are necessary
- To report any coughing, chest pain, or changes in breathing, which may indicate beginning pneumonia
- To avoid foods with citric acid, hot or rough texture if stomatitis is present
- To report stomatitis: any bleeding, white spots, ulcerations in

mouth; tell patient to examine mouth qd, report any symptoms
• To report signs of anemia: fatigue, headache, faintness, shortness of breath, irritability
• To report bleeding; avoid use of razors or commercial mouthwash
• To avoid use of aspirin products or ibuprofen

Overdose treatment: Discontinue drug, use supportive therapy

fludrocortisone acetate

(floo-droe-kor'ti-sone)
Florinef Acetate
Func. class.: Corticosteroid
Chem. class.: Mineralocorticoid

Action: Promotes increased reabsorption of sodium and loss of potassium from the renal tubules
Uses: Adrenal insufficiency, salt-losing adrenogenital syndrome
Dosage and routes:
• *Adult:* PO 0.1-0.2 mg qd
Available forms include: Tabs 0.1 mg
Side effects/adverse reactions:
CNS: Flushing, sweating, headache
CV: Hypertension, ***circulatory collapse, thrombophlebitis, embolism,*** tachycardia
MS: Fractures, osteoporosis, weakness
Contraindications: Hypersensitivity, acute glomerulonephritis, amebiasis
Precautions: Pregnancy (C), osteoporosis, CHF
Pharmacokinetics:
PO: Half-life 3.5 hr, metabolized by liver, excreted in urine
Interactions/incompatibilities:
• Decreased action of fludrocortisone: cholestyramine, colestipol, barbiturates, rifampin, ephedrine, phenytoin, theophylline
• Decreased effects of: diuretics, K-sparing diuretics, potassium supplements
• Increased side effects: sodium-containing food or medication, digitalis preparations

NURSING CONSIDERATIONS

Assess:
• Potassium, while on long-term therapy; hypokalemia
• Weight daily, notify physician of weekly gain >5 lb
• B/P q4h, pulse, notify physician if chest pain occurs
• I&O ratio; be alert for decreasing urinary output and increasing edema
Administer:
• Titrated dose, use lowest effective dose
• With food or milk to decrease GI symptoms
Perform/provide:
• Assistance with ambulation in patient with bone tissue disease to prevent fractures
Evaluate:
• Therapeutic response: correction of adrenal insufficiency
• Potassium depletion: paresthesias, fatigue, nausea, vomiting, depression, polyuria, dysrhythmias, weakness
• Edema, hypertension, cardiac symptoms
Teach patient/family:
• That ID as steroid user should be carried
• Not to discontinue this medication abruptly
Lab test interferences:
Increase: Potassium, sodium
Decrease: Hematocrit

* Available in Canada only

flumazenil

(floo-maz'een-ill)
Mazicon

Func. class.: Benzodiazepine receptor antagonist
Chem. class.: Imidazebenzodiazepine derivative

Action: Antagonizes the actions of benzodiazepines on the CNS, competitively inhibits the activity at the benzodiazepine recognition site on the GABA/benzodiazepine receptor complex

Uses: Reversal of the sedative effects of benzodiazepines

Dosage and routes:

Reversal of conscious sedation or in general anesthesia

• *Adult:* IV 0.2 mg (2 ml) given over 15 sec, wait 45 sec, then give 0.2 mg (2 ml) if consciousness does not occur; may be repeated at 60 sec intervals as needed, up to 4 additional times (max total dose 1 mg), dose is to be individualized

Management of suspected benzodiazepine overdose

• *Adult:* IV 0.2 mg (2 ml) given over 30 sec, wait 30 sec, then give 0.3 mg (3 ml) over 30 sec if consciousness does not occur; further doses of 0.5 mg (5 ml) can be given over 30 sec at intervals of 1 min up to cumulative dose of 3 mg

Available forms include: Inj 0.1 mg/ml

Side effects/adverse reactions:

EENT: Abnormal vision, blurred vision, tinnitus

CV: Hypertension, palpitations, cutaneous vasodilation, dysrhythmias, bradycardia, tachycardia, chest pain

GI: Nausea, vomiting, hiccups

CNS: Dizziness, agitation, emotional lability, confusion, ***convulsions,*** somnolence

SYST: Headache, injection site pain, increased sweating, fatigue, rigors

Contraindications: Hypersensitivity to this drug or benzodiazepines, serious cyclic antidepressant overdose, patients given benzodiazepine for control of life-threatening condition

Precautions: Pregnancy (C), lactation, children, elderly, renal disease, seizure disorders, head injury, labor and delivery, hepatic disease, hypoventilation, panic disorder, drug and alcohol dependency, ambulatory patients

Pharmacokinetics: Terminal half-life 41-79 min, metabolized in liver

Interactions/incompatibilities:

• Toxicity: mixed drug overdosage

NURSING CONSIDERATIONS

Assess:

• Assess cardiac status using continuous monitoring
• For seizures, protect patient from injury
• GI symptoms: nausea, vomiting, place in side-lying position to prevent aspiration

Administer:

• Over several minutes; check airway and IV access before administration

Evaluate:

• Therapeutic response: decreased sedation
• Allergic reactions: flushing, rash, urticaria, pruritus

Teach patient/family:

• That amnesia may continue
• Not to engage in hazardous activities for 18-24 hr after discharge
• Not to take any alcohol or nonprescription drugs for 18-24 hr

F

flunisolide

(floo-niss'oh-lide)

AeroBid,* Nasalide Nasal Solution, Rhinalar*

Func. class.: Steroid, intranasal
Chem. class.: Glucocorticoid

Action: Long-acting synthetic adrenocorticoid with antiinflammatory activity, minimal mineralocorticoid properties

Uses: Rhinitis (seasonal or perennial)

Dosage and routes:

- *Adult:* INSTILL 2 sprays in each nostril bid, then increase to tid if needed, not to exceed 8 sprays in each nostril/day
- *Child 6-14 yr:* INSTILL 1 spray in each nostril tid or 2 sprays bid, not to exceed 4 sprays in each nostril/day

Available forms include: Aerosol 25μg/spray

Side effects/adverse reactions:

EENT: Nasal irritation, dryness, rebound congestion, epistaxis, sneezing

INTEG: Urticaria

CNS: Headache, dizziness

SYST: ***CHF, convulsions,*** increased sodium, hypertension

Contraindications: Hypersensitivity, child <12 yr, fungal, bacterial infection of nose

Precautions: Lactation, pregnancy (C)

Pharmacokinetics:

AERO: Half-life 6 min, terminal half-life 1.8 hr, metabolized in liver, excreted in urine

NURSING CONSIDERATIONS

Administer:

- No more than q4h

Perform/provide:

- Storage in light-resistant container; discard open container after 3 mo

Evaluate:

- Therapeutic response: decreased congestion, runny nose
- Redness, swelling, pain in nasal passages

Teach patient/family:

- That stinging may occur for several applications; drying of mucosa may be decreased by environmental humidification
- To notify physician if irregular pulse, insomnia, dizziness, or tremors occur
- Proper administration to avoid systemic absorption
- To check with physician before using any other nasal medications

flunisolide

(floo-niss'oh-lide)

AeroBid, Nasalide

Func. class.: Corticosteroid
Chem. class.: Glucocorticoid

Action: Decreases inflammation by suppression of migration of polymorphonuclear leukocytes, fibroblasts, reversal of increased capillary permeability and lysosomal stabilization; does not depress hypothalamus

Uses: Rhinitis, allergies, nasal polyps

Dosage and routes:

- *Adult and child >6 yr:* SPRAY 2 puffs bid, not to exceed 4 puffs bid

Available forms include: Nasal sol 25 μg/metered dose (Nasalide), 250 μg/metered dose (AeroBid)

Side effects/adverse reactions:

CNS: Headache, nervousness, restlessness

EENT: Hoarseness, *Candida* infection of oral cavity, sore throat

GI: Nausea, vomiting, dry mouth

* Available in Canada only

Contraindications: Hypersensitivity, child <6 yr

Precautions: Nonasthmatic bronchial disease, bacterial, fungal, viral infections of mouth, throat, lungs, respiratory TB, untreated fungal, bacterial, or viral infections, pregnancy (C), glaucoma

Pharmacokinetics:

INH: Duration 1 hr

NURSING CONSIDERATIONS

Administer:

- Titrated dose, use lowest effective dose

Evaluate:

- Therapeutic response: ease of respirations, decreased inflammation
- Infection: increased temperature, WBC, even after withdrawal of medication; drug masks symptoms of infection

Teach patient/family:

- To use gum; rinse mouth after each dose
- That ID as steroid user should be carried
- To notify physician if therapeutic response decreases; dosage adjustment may be needed
- Proper administration technique, shake well before use
- Compliance to therapy
- Teach patient about cushingoid symptoms
- Symptoms of adrenal insufficiency: nausea, anorexia, fatigue, dizziness, dyspnea, weakness, joint pain

---

fluocinonide

(floo-oh-sin'oh-nide)

Lidex, Lidex-E, Lidemol*/Topsyn

Func. class.: Topical corticosteroid

Chem. class.: Synthetic fluorinated agent, group II potency

Action: Possesses antipruritic, antiinflammatory actions

Uses: Psoriasis, eczema, contact dermatitis, pruritus

Dosage and routes:

- *Adult and child:* Apply to affected area tid-qid

Available forms include: Oint 0.05%; cream 0.05%; sol 0.05%; gel 0.05%

Side effects/adverse reactions:

INTEG: Burning, dryness, itching, irritation, acne, folliculitis, hypertrichosis, perioral dermatitis, hypopigmentation, atrophy, striae, miliaria, allergic contact dermatitis, secondary infection

Contraindications: Hypersensitivity to corticosteroids, fungal infections

Precautions: Pregnancy (C), lactation, viral infections, bacterial infections

NURSING CONSIDERATIONS

Assess:

- Temperature: if fever develops, drug should be discontinued

Administer:

- Only to affected areas; do not get in eyes
- Medication, then cover with occlusive dressing (only if prescribed), seal to normal skin, change q12h; use occlusive dressings with extreme caution
- Only to dermatoses; do not use on weeping, denuded, or infected area

Perform/provide:

- Cleansing before application of drug
- Treatment for a few days after area has cleared
- Storage at room temperature

Evaluate:

- Therapeutic response: absence of severe itching, patches on skin, flaking

Teach patient/family:

- To avoid sunlight on affected area; burns may occur

fluorescein sodium

(flure'e-seen)

Fluorescite, Fluor-I-Strip, Ful-Glo, Funduscein Injections

Func. class.: Diagnostic agent, optic

Chem. class.: Fluorescent dye

Action: Allows breaks in the corneal tissue to absorb dye and show up as bright green under cobalt blue light

Uses: Diagnostic aid in identifying foreign bodies, fitting hard contact lenses, fundus photography, tonometry, identifying corneal abrasions, retinal angiography

Dosage and routes:

- *Adult:* INSTILL 1 gtt of 2% sol, irrigate or wet strip with sterile water and touch conjunctiva or fornix, flush eye with irrigating sol

Retinal angiography

- *Adult:* IV 5 ml 10% sol or 3 ml 25% sol injected in antecubital vein
- *Child:* IV 0.077 ml 10% sol or 0.044 ml 25% sol injected in antecubital vein

Available forms include: Inj IV 10%, 25%; sol 2%; strips 0.6, 9 mg

Side effects/adverse reactions:

CNS: Headache, dizziness, paresthesia, ***convulsions***

CV: Bradycardia, ***shock, cardiac arrest,*** hypertension

RESP: ***Dyspnea, acute pulmonary edema***

GI: Nausea, vomiting

EENT: Stinging, burning, conjunctival redness

Contraindications: Hypersensitivity

Precautions: Bronchial asthma, pregnancy (C), lactation

NURSING CONSIDERATIONS

Administer:

- Only after soft contact lens are removed
- Solution, have patient close eyelids for 1 min
- Only with resuscitative equipment nearby
- Test dose (IV) before angiography
- Epinephrine 1:1000 for IV, IM route; an antihistamine and O_2 should always be available

Perform/provide:

- Storage at room temperature

Evaluate:

- IV site for redness, inflammation, swelling
- Eye color after application: epithelial defects are green while normal precorneal tear film appears bright yellow
- For allergic reaction: rash, urticaria, pruritus, angioedema

Teach patient/family:

- To report stinging, burning, itching, lacrimation, puffiness
- That urine will be yellow after IV dose

fluorometholone

(flure-oh-meth'oh-lone)

FML Liquifilm Ophthalmic

Func. class.: Ophthalmic antiinflammatory

Action: Decreases inflammation, resulting in decreased pain, photophobia, hyperemia, cellular infiltration

Uses: Inflammation of eye, lids, conjunctiva, cornea, uveitis, iridocyclitis, allergic condition, burns, foreign bodies, postoperatively in cataract

Dosage and routes:

- *Adult and child:* Instill 1-2 gtts

* Available in Canada only

into conjunctival sac 1hr × 2 days, if needed, then bid-qid

Available forms include: Oint 0.1%; ophthalmic susp 0.1%, 0.25%

Side effects/adverse reactions:

EENT: ***Increased intraocular pressure,*** poor corneal wound healing, increased possibility of corneal infections, glaucoma exacerbation, ***optic nerve damage,*** decreased acuity, visual field

Contraindications: Hypersensitivity, acute superficial herpes simplex, fungal/viral diseases of the eye or conjunctiva, active diabetes mellitus, ocular TB, infections of the eye

Precautions: Corneal abrasions, glaucoma, pregnancy (C)

NURSING CONSIDERATIONS

Evaluate:

• Therapeutic response: absence of swelling, redness, exudate

Administer:

• After shaking

Perform/provide:

• Storage in tight, light-resistant container

Teach patient/family:

• Instillation method: pressure on lacrimal duct for 1 min

• Not to share eye medications with others

• Not to use if purulent drainage is present

• Not to discontinue steroids abruptly; they should be tapered over 1-2 wk

---

fluorouracil

(flure-oh-yoor'a-sil)

Efudex, Fluoroplex

Func. class.: Topical antineoplastic

Chem. class.: Antimetabolite

Action: Inhibits synthesis of DNA, RNA in susceptible cells

Uses: Keratosis (multiple/actinic), basal cell carcinoma

Dosage and routes:

• *Adult and child:* TOP apply to affected area bid

Available forms include: Sol 1%, 2%, 5%; cream 1%, 5%

Side effects/adverse reactions:

INTEG: Rash, irritation, pain, burning, contact dermatitis, scaling, swelling, soreness, hyperpigmentation, pruritus

Contraindications: Hypersensitivity, pregnancy (D)

NURSING CONSIDERATIONS

Assess:

• WBC, platelets at least monthly

Administer:

• Only 5% sol/cream for basal cell carcinoma

• Using gloves or applicator

• A low-residue diet with no dairy product where radiation is also used

Perform/provide:

• Covering of lesion with porous gauze dressing only

• Washing of hands after application if gloves or applicator is not used

• Storage at room temperature

Evaluate:

• Therapeutic response: decreased size of lesion

• Area of body involved for redness, swelling

• Check oral cavity qd for stomatitis; if present discontinue drug

Teach patient/family:

• To avoid application on normal skin or getting cream in eyes

• To discontinue use if rash or irritation occurs

• To avoid sunlight or use sunscreen; photosensitivity may occur

• To wash hands after application

• Not to change application and use exactly as prescribed

F

• That lesion will disappear in 1-2 mo

fluorouracil (5-fluorouracil)

(flure-oh-yoor'a-sil)

Adrucil, 5-FU

Func. class.: Antineoplastic, antimetabolite

Chem. class.: Pyrimidine antagonist

Action: Inhibits DNA synthesis; interferes with cell replication by competitively inhibiting thymidylate synthesis, a vesicant

Uses: Cancer of breast, colon, rectum, stomach, pancreas

Dosage and routes:

• *Adult:* IV 12 mg/kg/day × 4 days, not to exceed 800 mg/day; may repeat with 6 mg/kg on day 6, 8, 10, 12; maintenance is 10-15 mg/kg/wk as a single dose, not to exceed 1 g/wk

Available forms include: Inj IV 50 mg/ml

Side effects/adverse reactions:

CV: Myocardial ischemia, angina

HEMA: ***Thrombocytopenia, leukopenia, myelosuppression, anemia, agranulocytosis***

GI: Anorexia, stomatitis, diarrhea, nausea, vomiting, ***hemorrhage,*** *enteritis glossitis*

GU: ***Renal failure***

EENT: Epistaxis

INTEG: Rash, fever

CNS: Lethargy, malaise, weakness

Contraindications: Hypersensitivity, myelosuppression, pregnancy (D), poor nutritional states, serious infections

Precautions: Renal disease, hepatic disease, bone marrow depression, angina, lactation, children

Pharmacokinetics: Half-life 10-20 min, 20 hr terminal, metabolized in the liver, excreted in the urine, crosses blood-brain barrier

Interactions/incompatibilities:

• Increased toxicity: radiation or other antineoplastics

NURSING CONSIDERATIONS

Assess:

• CBC, differential, platelet count weekly; withhold drug if WBC is <3500/mm³ or platelet count is <100,000/mm³; notify physician of these results; drug should be discontinued

• Renal function studies: BUN, serum uric acid, urine CrCl, electrolytes before, during therapy

• I&O ratio; report fall in urine output to <30 ml/hr

• Temperature q4h; fever may indicate beginning infection

• Liver function tests before, during therapy: bilirubin, alk phosphatase, AST, ALT, LDH; as needed or monthly

Administer:

• IV undiluted, may inject through Y-tube or 3-way stopcock; give over 1-3 min

• Antiemetic 30-60 min before giving drug to prevent vomiting

• Antibiotics for prophylaxis of infection

• Topical or systemic analgesics for pain

• Transfusion for anemia

• Antispasmodic for diarrhea

Perform/provide:

• Protection from light

• Strict medical asepsis, protective isolation if WBC levels are low

• Increase fluid intake to 2-3 L/day to prevent dehydration, unless contraindicated

• Changing of IV site q48h

• Rinsing of mouth tid-qid with water, club soda; brushing of teeth bid-tid with soft brush or cotton-

tipped applicator for stomatitis; use unwaxed dental floss
• Nutritious diet with iron, vitamin supplements, low fiber, few dairy products especially when combined with radiotherapy as ordered

Evaluate:
• Therapeutic response: decreased tumor size, spread of malignancy
• Bleeding: hematuria, guaiac, bruising or petechiae, mucosa or orifices q8h
• Food preferences; list likes, dislikes
• Inflammation of mucosa, breaks in skin
• Buccal cavity q8h for dryness, sores or ulceration, white patches, oral pain, bleeding, dysphagia
• Symptoms indicating severe allergic reaction: rash, urticaria, itching, flushing
• GI symptoms: frequency of stools, cramping
• Acidosis, signs of dehydration: rapid respirations, poor skin turgor, decreased urine output, dry skin, restlessness, weakness

Teach patient/family:
• Why protective isolation precautions are necessary
• To avoid foods with citric acid, hot or rough texture if stomatitis is present; to drink adequate fluids
• To report stomatitis: any bleeding, white spots, ulcerations in mouth; tell patient to examine mouth qd, report symptoms
• To report signs of infection: increased temperature, sore throat, flu symptoms
• To report signs of anemia: fatigue, headache, faintness, shortness of breath, irritability
• To report bleeding: avoid use of razors, or commercial mouthwash
• To avoid use of aspirin products or ibuprofen
• To use contraception during therapy (men and women)

Lab test interferences:
Increase: Liver function studies, 6-HIAA
Decrease: Albumin

fluoxetine

(floo-ox'e-teen)
Prozac

Func. class.: Bicyclic antidepressant

Action: Inhibits CNS neuron uptake of serotonin, but not of norepinephrine

Uses: Major depressive disorder

Dosage and routes:
• *Adult:* PO 20 mg qd in AM; after 4 wk if no clinical improvement is noted, dose may be increased to 20 mg bid in AM, afternoon, not to exceed 80 mg/day

Available forms include: Pulvules 20 mg

Side effects/adverse reactions:
CNS: Headache, nervousness, insomnia, drowsiness, anxiety, tremor, dizziness, fatigue, sedation, poor concentration, abnormal dreams, agitation, ***convulsions,*** apathy, euphoria, hallucinations, delusions, psychosis
GI: Nausea, diarrhea, dry mouth, anorexia, dyspepsia, constipation, cramps, vomiting, taste changes, flatulence, decreased appetite
INTEG: Sweating, rash, pruritus, acne, alopecia, urticaria
RESP: Infection, pharyngitis, nasal congestion, sinus headache, sinusitus, cough, dyspnea, bronchitis, asthma, hyperventilation, pneumonia
CV: Hot flashes, palpitations, angina pectoris, ***hemorrhage,*** hypertension, tachycardia, first-degree

AV block, bradycardia, *MI*, thrombophlebitis
MS: Pain, arthritis, twitching
GU: Dysmenorrhea, decreased libido, urinary frequency, urinary tract infection, amenorrhea, cystitis, impotence
EENT: Visual changes, ear/eye pain, photophobia, tinnitus
SYST: Asthenia, viral infection, fever, allergy, chills

Contraindications: Hypersensitivity

Precautions: Pregnancy (B), lactation, children, elderly

Pharmacokinetics:
PO: Peak 6-8 hr; metabolized in liver, excreted in urine; half-life 2-7 days

Interactions/incompatibilities:
- Do not use with MAOIs
- Increased agitation: L-tryptophan
- Increased side effects: highly protein bound drugs (i.e., fluoxetine)
- Increased half-life of: diazepam

NURSING CONSIDERATIONS

Assess:
- Mental status: mood, sensorium, affect, suicidal tendencies, increase in psychiatric symptoms, depression, panic
- B/P (lying/standing), pulse q4h; if systolic B/P drops 20 mm Hg, hold drug, notify physician; take vital signs q4h in patients with cardiovascular disease
- Blood studies: CBC, leukocytes, differential, cardiac enzymes if patient is receiving long-term therapy
- Hepatic studies: AST, ALT, bilirubin, creatinine
- Weight qwk, appetite may decrease with drug
- ECG for flattening of T wave, bundle branch, AV block, dysrhythmias in cardiac patients

Administer:
- Increased fluids, bulk in diet if constipation, urinary retention occur
- With food or milk for GI symptoms
- Crushed if patient is unable to swallow medication whole
- Dosage hs if oversedation occurs during the day; may take entire dose hs; elderly may not tolerate once/day dosing
- Gum, hard candy, frequent sips of water for dry mouth

Perform/provide:
- Storage at room temperature, do not freeze
- Assistance with ambulation during therapy since drowsiness, dizziness occur
- Safety measures including side rails, primarily in elderly
- Checking to see PO medication swallowed

Evaluate:
- Therapeutic response: decreased depression
- EPS primarily in elderly, rigidity, dystonia, akathisia
- Urinary retention, constipation
- Withdrawal symptoms: headache, nausea, vomiting, muscle pain, weakness; do not usually occur unless drug was discontinued abruptly
- Alcohol consumption; if alcohol is consumed, hold dose until morning

Teach patient/family:
- That therapeutic effect may take 2-3 wk
- To use caution in driving or other activities requiring alertness because of drowsiness, dizziness, or blurred vision
- Not to discontinue medication quickly after long-term use, may cause nausea, headache, malaise
- To avoid alcohol ingestion or other CNS depressants

• To notify physician if pregnant or plan to become pregnant or breastfeed

Lab test interferences:
Increase: Serum bilirubin, blood glucose, alk phosphatase
Decrease: VMA, 5-HIAA
False increase: Urinary catecholamines

---

fluoxymesterone

(floo-ox-ee-mess'te-rone)
Android-F, Halotestin, Ora-Testryl
Func. class.: Androgenic anabolic steroid
Chem. class.: Halogenated testosterone derivative

Action: Increases weight by building body tissue, increases potassium, phosphorus, chloride, nitrogen levels, increases bone development

Uses: Impotence from testicular deficiency, hypogonadism, breast engorgement, palliative treatment of female breast cancer

Dosage and routes:

Hypogonadism/impotence
• *Adult:* PO 2-10 mg qd

Breast engorgement
• *Adult:* PO 2.5 mg qd, then 5-10 mg qd × 5 days

Breast cancer
• *Adult:* PO 15-30 mg qd in divided doses until therapeutic effect occurs, then dosage should be reduced

Available forms include: Tabs 2, 5, 10 mg

Side effects/adverse reactions:
INTEG: Rash, acneiform lesions, oily hair, skin, flushing, sweating, acne vulgaris, alopecia, hirsutism
CNS: Dizziness, headache, fatigue, tremors, paresthesias, flushing, sweating, anxiety, lability, insomnia
MS: Cramps, spasms
CV: Increased B/P
GU: ***Hematuria,*** amenorrhea, vaginitis, decreased libido, decreased breast size, clitoral hypertrophy, testicular atrophy
GI: Nausea, vomiting, constipation, weight gain, ***cholestatic jaundice***
EENT: Carpal tunnel syndrome, conjunctional edema, nasal congestion
ENDO: Abnormal GTT

Contraindications: Severe renal disease, severe cardiac disease, severe hepatic disease, hypersensitivity, pregnancy (X), lactation, genital bleeding (abnormal)

Precautions: Diabetes mellitus, CV disease, MI

Pharmacokinetics:
PO: Metabolized in liver, excreted in urine, crosses placenta, excreted in breast milk

Interactions/incompatibilities:
• Increased effects of: oral antidiabetics, oxyphenbutazone
• Increased PT: anticoagulants
• Edema: ACTH, adrenal steroids
• Decreased effects of: insulin

NURSING CONSIDERATIONS

Assess:
• Weight daily, notify physician if weekly weight gain is >5 lb
• B/P q4h
• I&O ratio; be alert for decreasing urinary output, increasing edema
• Growth rate in children since growth rate may be uneven (linear/bone growth) if used for extended periods of time
• Electrolytes: K, Na, Cl, cholesterol
• Liver function studies: ALT, AST, bilirubin

Administer:
• Titrated dose, use lowest effective dose
• With food or milk to decrease GI symptoms

Perform/provide:
• Diet with increased calories, protein; decrease sodium, if edema occurs

Evaluate:
• Therapeutic response: increased appetite, stamina
• Edema, hypertension, cardiac symptoms, jaundice
• Mental status: affect, mood, behavioral changes, aggression
• Signs of masculinization in female: increased libido, deepening of voice, breast tissue, enlarged clitoris, menstrual irregularities; male: gynecomastia, impotence, testicular atrophy
• Hypercalcemia: lethargy, polyuria, polydipsia, nausea, vomiting, constipation, drug may need to be decreased
• Hypoglycemia in diabetics, since oral anticoagulant action is decreased

Teach patient/family:
• That drug needs to be combined with complete health plan: diet, rest, exercise
• To notify physician if therapeutic response decreases
• Not to discontinue medication abruptly
• About change in sex characteristics
• Females to report menstrual irregularities
• That 1-3 mo course is necessary for response in breast cancer
• That steroids should not be used for body building

Lab test interferences:
Increase: Serum cholesterol, blood glucose, urine glucose
Decrease: Serum calcium, serum potassium, T_4, T_3, thyroid ^{131}I uptake test, urine 17-OHCS, 17-KS, PBI, BSP

---

fluphenazine decanoate/fluphenazine enanthate/fluphenazine HCl

(floo-fen´-a-zeen)

Modecate Decanoate,* Prolixin Decanoate/Moditen Enanthate,* Prolixin Enanthate/Moditen HCl,* Permitil HCl, Prolixin HCl

Func. class.: Antipsychotic/neuroleptic
Chem. class.: Phenothiazine, piperazine

Action: Depresses cerebral cortex, hypothalamus, limbic system, which control activity and aggression; blocks neurotransmission produced by dopamine at synapse; exhibits strong α-adrenergic and anticholinergic blocking action; mechanism for antipsychotic effects is unclear

Uses: Psychotic disorders, schizophrenia

Dosage and routes:

Enanthate, decanoate
• *Adult and child >12 yr:* SC 12.5-25 mg ql-3wk

HCl
• *Adult:* PO 2.5-10 mg, in divided doses q6-8h, not to exceed 20 mg qd; IM initially 1.25 mg then 2.5-10 mg in divided doses q6-8h

Available forms include: HCl tabs 1, 2.5, 5, 10 mg; elix 2.5 mg/5 ml; conc 5 mg/ml; inj IM 10 mg/ml, enanthate, decanoate, inj SC, IM 25 mg/ml

Side effects/adverse reactions:
RESP: ***Laryngospasm,*** dyspnea, ***respiratory depression***

---

* Available in Canada only

CNS: Extrapyramidal symptoms: pseudoparkinsonism, akathisia, dystonia, tardive dyskinesia, drowsiness, headache, seizures, ***neuroleptic malignant syndrome***

HEMA: Anemia, ***leukopenia, leukocytosis, agranulocytosis***

INTEG: Rash, photosensitivity, dermatitis

EENT: Blurred vision, glaucoma, dry eyes

GI: Dry mouth, nausea, vomiting, anorexia, constipation, diarrhea, jaundice, weight gain, ***paralytic ileus, hepatitis***

GU: Urinary retention, urinary frequency, enuresis, impotence, amenorrhea, gynecomastia

CV: Orthostatic hypotension, hypertension, ***cardiac arrest,*** ECG changes, ***tachycardia***

Contraindications: Hypersensitivity, circulatory collapse, liver damage, cerebral arteriosclerosis, coronary disease, severe hypertension/ hypotension, blood dyscrasias, coma, child <12 yr, brain damage, bone marrow depression, alcohol and barbiturate withdrawal states

Precautions: Pregnancy (C), lactation, seizure disorders, hypertension, hepatic disease, cardiac disease

Pharmacokinetics:

PO/IM (HCl): Onset 1 hr, peak 2-4 hr, duration 6-8 hr

SC (enanthate): Onset 1-2 days, peak 2-3 days, duration 1-3 wk, half-life 3.5-4 days; decanoate: onset 1-3 days, peak 1-2 days, duration over 4 wk, half-life (single dose) 6.8-9.6 days, (multiple dose) 14.3 days; metabolized by liver, excreted in urine (metabolites), crosses placenta, enters breast milk

Interactions/incompatibilities:

- Oversedation: other CNS depressants, alcohol, barbiturate anesthetics
- Toxicity: epinephrine
- Decreased effects of: levodopa, lithium
- Decreased effects of: fluphenazine: smoking, phenobarbital
- Increased effects of both drugs: β-adrenergic blockers, alcohol
- Increased anticholinergic effects anticholinergics

NURSING CONSIDERATIONS

Assess:

- Swallowing of PO medication; check for hoarding or giving of medication to other patients
- I&O ratio; palpate bladder if low urinary output occurs
- Bilirubin, CBC, liver function studies monthly
- Urinalysis is recommended before and during prolonged therapy

Administer:

- Concentrate with juice, milk, or uncaffeinated drinks
- Antiparkinsonian agent, to be used if extrapyramidal symptoms occur
- IM injection into large muscle mass, to minimize postural hypotension give injection and have patient remain seated or recumbent for ½ hr
- Use dry needle or solution will become cloudy; use No. 21 G or larger due to viscosity

Perform/provide:

- Decreased noise input by dimming lights, avoiding loud noises
- Supervised ambulation until stabilized on medication; do not involve in strenuous exercise program because fainting is possible; patient should not stand still for long periods of time

• Increased fluids to prevent constipation
• Sips of water, candy, gum for dry mouth
• Storage in tight, light-resistant container in cool environment

Evaluate:
• Therapeutic response: decrease in emotional excitement, hallucinations, delusions, paranoia, reorganization of patterns of thought, speech
• Affect, orientation, LOC, reflexes, gait, coordination, sleep pattern disturbances
• B/P standing and lying; take pulse and respirations q4h during initial treatment; establish baseline before starting treatment; report drops of 30 mm Hg
• Dizziness, faintness, palpitations, tachycardia on rising
• Extrapyramidal symptoms including akathisia (inability to sit still, no pattern to movements), tardive dyskinesia (bizarre movements of jaw, mouth, tongue, extremities), pseudoparkinsonism (rigidity, tremors, pill rolling, shuffling gait)
• Skin turgor daily
• Constipation, urinary retention daily; if these occur, increase bulk, water in diet

Teach patient/family:
• That orthostatic hypotension occurs often, to rise from sitting or lying position gradually; avoid hazardous activities until stabilized on medication
• To avoid hot tubs, hot showers, or tub baths since hypotension may occur
• To avoid abrupt withdrawal of this drug or extrapyramidal symptoms may result; drug should be withdrawn slowly
• To avoid OTC preparations (cough, hayfever, cold) unless approved by physician since serious drug interactions may occur; avoid use with alcohol or CNS depressants; increased drowsiness may occur
• To use a sunscreen during sun exposure to prevent burns
• Regarding compliance with drug regimen
• About extrapyramidal symptoms and necessity for meticulous oral hygiene since oral candidiasis may occur
• To report sore throat, malaise, fever, bleeding, mouth sores; if these occur, CBC should be drawn and drug discontinued
• That in hot weather heat stroke may occur; take extra precautions to stay cool
• That urine may turn pink to reddish-brown

Lab test interferences:
Increase: Liver function tests, cardiac enzymes, cholesterol, blood glucose, prolactin, bilirubin, PBI, cholinesterase, ^{131}I
Decrease: Hormones (blood and urine)
False positive: Pregnancy tests, PKU
False negative: Urinary steroids, 17-OHCS, pregnancy tests

Treatment of overdose: Lavage, if orally injested, provide an airway; *do not induce vomiting*

---

flurandrenolide

(flure-an-dren'oh-lide)
Cordran, Drenison 1/4,* Drenison Tape*

Func. class.: Topical corticosteroid
Chem. class.: Synthetic fluorinated agent

Action: Possesses antipruritic, antiinflammatory actions

* Available in Canada only

Uses: Corticosteroid-responsive dermatoses, pruritus

Dosage and routes:

• *Adult and child:* TOP apply to affected area tid-qid; apply tape q12-24h

Available forms include: Oint 0.025%, 0.05%; cream 0.025%, 0.05%; lotion 0.05%; tape 4 μg/cm^2

Side effects/adverse reactions:

INTEG: Burning, dryness, itching, irritation, acne, folliculitis, hypertrichosis, perioral dermatitis, hypopigmentation, atrophy, striae, miliaria, allergic contact dermatitis, secondary infection

Contraindications: Hypersensitivity to corticosteroids, fungal infections, viral infections

Precautions: Pregnancy (C), lactation, viral infections, bacterial infections

NURSING CONSIDERATIONS

Assess:

• Temperature, if fever develops drug should be discontinued

Administer:

• Only to affected areas, do not get in eyes

• Then cover with occlusive dressing if ordered, seal to normal skin, change q12h, systemic absorption may occur

• Only to dermatoses; do not use on weeping, denuded, or infected area

• Tape after cutting with scissors, apply only to clean dry wounds

Perform/provide:

• Cleansing before application of drug

• Treatment for a few days after area has cleared

• Storage at room temperature

Evaluate:

• Therapeutic response: absence of severe itching, patches on skin, flaking

• Systemic absorption: fever, infection, irritation

Teach patient/family:

• To avoid sunlight on affected area; burns may occur

---

flurazepam HCl

(flure-az'e-pam)

Dalmane, Durapam, Somnol*

Func. class.: Sedative-hypnotic

Chem. class.: Benzodiazepine derivative

Controlled Substance Schedule IV (USA), Schedule F (Canada)

Action: Produces CNS depression at the limbic, thalamic, hypothalamic levels of CNS; may be mediated by neurotransmitter γ-aminobutyric acid (GABA); results are sedation, hypnosis, skeletal muscle relaxation, anticonvulsant activity, anxiolytic action

Uses: Insomnia

Dosage and routes:

• *Adult:* PO 15-30 mg hs, may repeat dose once if needed

• *Geriatric:* PO 15 mg hs, may increase if needed

Available forms include: Caps 15, 30 mg

Side effects/adverse reactions:

HEMA: ***Leukopenia, granulocytopenia*** (rare)

CNS: Lethargy, drowsiness, daytime sedation, dizziness, confusion, light-headedness, headache, anxiety, irritability

GI: Nausea, vomiting, diarrhea, heartburn, abdominal pain, constipation

CV: Chest pain, pulse changes

Contraindications: Hypersensitivity to benzodiazepines, pregnancy,

lactation, intermittent porphyria, uncontrolled pain
Precautions: Anemia, hepatic disease, renal disease, suicidal individuals, drug abuse, elderly, psychosis, child <15 yr
Pharmacokinetics:
PO: Onset 15-45 min, duration 7-8 hr; metabolized by liver, excreted by kidneys (inactive/active metabolites), crosses placenta, excreted in breast milk; half-life 47-100 hr, additional 100 hr for active metabolites
Interactions/incompatibilities:
• Increased effects of flurazepam: cimetidine, disulfiram
• Increased action of both drugs: alcohol, CNS depressants
• Decreased effect of flurazepam: antacids

NURSING CONSIDERATIONS

Assess:
• Blood studies: Hct, Hgb, RBC (if on long-term therapy)
• Hepatic studies: AST, ALT, bilirubin
Administer:
• After removal of cigarettes, to prevent fires
• After trying conservative measures for insomnia
• ½-1 hr before hs for sleeplessness
• On empty stomach for fast onset, but may be taken with food if GI symptoms occur
Perform/provide:
• Assistance with ambulation after receiving dose
• Safety measure: siderails, night-light, call-bell within easy reach
• Checking to see PO medication has been swallowed
• Storage in tight container in cool environment
Evaluate:
• Therapeutic response: ability to sleep at night, decreased amount of early morning awakening if taking drug for insomnia
• Mental status: mood, sensorium, affect, memory (long, short)
• Blood dyscrasias: fever, sore throat, bruising, rash, jaundice, epistaxis (rare)
• Type of sleep problem: falling asleep, staying asleep
Teach patient/family:
• To avoid driving or other activities requiring alertness until drug is stabilized
• To avoid alcohol ingestion or CNS depressants; serious CNS depression may result
• That effects may take 2 nights for benefits to be noticed
• Alternate measures to improve sleep: reading, exercise several hours before hs, warm bath, warm milk, TV, self-hypnosis, deep breathing
• That hangover is common in elderly, but less common than with barbiturates
Lab test interferences:
Increase: AST/ALT, serum bilirubin
False increase: Urinary 17-OHCS
Decrease: RAI uptake
Treatment of overdose: Lavage, activated charcoal, monitor electrolytes, vital signs

---

flurbiprofen sodium

(flure-bi'proe-fen)
Ocufen
Func. class.: Nonsteroidal antiinflammatory ophthalmic
Chem. class.: Phenylalkanoic acid

Action: Inhibits enzyme system necessary for biosynthesis of prostaglandins; inhibits miosis
Uses: Inhibition of intraoperative miosis, corneal edema

* Available in Canada only

Dosage and routes:
• *Adult:* 1 gtt q½h 2 hr before surgery (4 gtt total)
Available forms include: Sol 0.03%
Side effects/adverse reactions:
EENT: Burning, stinging in the eye, irritation, bleeding or redness
Contraindications: Hypersensitivity, epithelial herpes simplex keratitis
Precautions: Pregnancy (C), lactation, child, aspirin or nonsteroidal antiinflammatory drug hypersensitivity, allergy, bleeding dis-

NURSING CONSIDERATIONS
Administer:
• Excess solution must be wiped away promptly to prevent its flow into lacrimal system, producing systemic symptoms
Perform/provide:
• Protect solution from sun
Teach patient/family:
• To report change in vision, blurring, or loss of sight during miosis
• Not to use for any other condition

---

flutamide
(floo′-ta-mide)
Eulexin
Func. class.: Antineoplastic-hormone
Chem. class.: Antiandrogen

Action: Interferes with testosterone at the cellular level. Inhibits androgen uptake by inhibiting nuclear binding or by interfering with androgen in target tissues. Prostatic carcinoma is androgen-sensitive, which results in arrested tumor growth
Uses: Metastatic prostatic carcinoma, stage D2 in combination with LHRH agonistic analogs (leuprolide)
Dosage and routes:
• *Adult:* PO 250 mg q8h tid, for a daily dosage of 750 mg
Available forms: cap 125 mg
Side effects/adverse reactions:
CNS: Hot flashes, drowsiness, confusion, depression, anxiety
GU: Decreased libido, impotence, gynecomastia
GI: Diarrhea, nausea, vomiting, increased liver function studies, ***hepatitis,*** anorexia
INTEG: Irritation at site, rash, photosensitivity
MISC: Edema, hematopoietic symptoms, neuromuscular and pulmonary symptoms, hypertension
Contraindications: Hypersensitivity, pregnancy (D)
Pharmacokinetics: Rapidly and completely absorbed; excreted in urine and feces as metabolites; half-life 6 hr, geriatric half-life 8 hr, 94% bound to plasma proteins

NURSING CONSIDERATIONS
Assess:
• Liver function studies: AST, ALT, alk phosphatase, which may be elevated
• For CNS symptoms: drowsiness, confusion, depression, anxiety
Evaluate:
• Therapeutic response: decrease in prostatic tumor size, decrease in spread of cancer
Teach patient/family:
• To report side effects of decreased libido, impotence, breast enlargement, hot flashes, diarrhea
• That this drug is taken with leuprolide
Treatment of overdose: Induce vomiting, provide supportive care

folic acid (vitamin B_9)

Apo-Folic, Folvite, Novofolacid*

Func. class.: Vitamin B complex group

Action: Needed for erythropoiesis; increases RBC, WBC, and platelet formation in megaloblastic anemias

Uses: Megaloblastic or macrocytic anemia caused by folic acid deficiency; liver disease, alcoholism, hemolysis, intestinal obstruction, pregnancy

Dosage and routes:

Supplement

• *Adult:* PO/IM/SC 0.1 mg qd

• *Child:* PO 0.05 mg qd

Megaloblastic/macrocytic anemia

• *Adult and child >4 yr:* PO/SC/IM 1 mg qd × 4-5 days

• *Child <4 yr:* PO/SC/IM 0.3 mg or less qd

• *Pregnancy/lactation:* PO/SC/IM 0.8 mg qd

Prevention of megaloblastic/macrocytic anemia

• *Pregnancy:* PO/SC/IM 1 mg qd

Available forms include: Tabs 0.1, 0.4, 0.8, 1 mg; inj SC, IM 5, 10 mg/ml

Side effects/adverse reactions:

RESP: ***Bronchospasm***

Contraindications: Hypersensitivity, anemias other than megaloblastic/macrocytic anemia, vitamin B_{12} deficiency anemia

Precautions: Pregnancy (A)

Pharmacokinetics:

PO: Peak ½-1 hr, bound to plasma proteins, excreted in breast milk, methylated in liver, excreted in urine (small amounts)

Interactions/incompatibilities:

• Decreased folate levels: chloramphenicol

• Increased metabolism of: phenobarbitol, hydantoins

• Do not use with methotrexate unless leucovorin rescue is available

NURSING CONSIDERATIONS

Assess:

• Folate levels: 6-15 μg/ml

Perform/provide:

• Storage in light-resistant container

Evaluate:

• Therapeutic response: increased weight, oriented well-being; absence of fatigue

• Nutritional status: bran, yeast, dried beans, nuts, fruits, fresh vegetables, asparagus

• Drugs currently taken: alcohol, oral contraceptives, hydantoins, trimethoprim, these drugs may cause increased folic acid use by body and contribute to a deficiency

Teach patient/family:

• To take drug exactly as prescribed

• To notify physician of side effects

foscarnet sodium

(foss-car'net)

Foscavir

Func. class.: Antiviral

Chem. class.: Inorganic pyrophosphate organic analog

Action: Antiviral activity is produced by selective inhibition at the pyrophosphate binding site on virus-specific DNA polymerases and reverse transcriptases at concentrations that do not affect cellular DNA polymerases

Uses: Treatment of CMV retinitis in AIDS

Dosage and routes:

• *Adult:* IV INF 60 mg/kg given over at least 1 hr, q8hr × 2-3 wk initially, then 90-120 mg/kg/day over 2 hr

* Available in Canada only

In renal abnormalities:

• *Adult:* IV Male:

$$\frac{140 - \text{age}}{\text{serum creatinine} \times 72} = \text{Ccr}$$

Female: 0.85 × above value

Dose based on table provided in package insert

Available forms include: Inj 24 mg/ml

Side effects/adverse reactions:

CNS: Fever, dizziness, headache, ***seizures,*** fatigue, neuropathy, tremor, ataxia, dementia, stupor, EEG abnormalities, vertigo, ***coma,*** abnormal gait, hypertonia, extrapyramidal disorders, hemiparesis, ***paralysis,*** hyperreflexia paraplegia, ***tetany,*** hyporeflexia, neuralgia, neuritis, cerebral edema, paresthesia, depression, confusion, anxiety, insomnia, somnolence, amnesia, hallucinations, agitation

GI: Nausea, vomiting, anorexia, abdominal pain, constipation, dysphagia, rectal hemorrhage, dry mouth, melena, flatulence, ulcerative stomatitis, pancreatitis, enteritis, enterocolitis, glossitis, proctitis, stomatitis, increased amylases, gastroenteritis, ***pseudomembranous colitis,*** duodenal ulcer, ***paralytic ileus, esophageal ulceration,*** abnormal A-G ratio, increased AST, ALT, cholecystitis, ***hepatitis,*** dyspepsia, tenesmus, hepatosplenomegaly, jaundice

INTEG: Rash, sweating, pruritus, skin ulceration, seborrhea, skin discoloration, alopecia, acne, dermatitis, pain/inflammation at injection site, facial edema, dry skin, urticaria

HEMA: Anemia, ***granulocytopenia, leukopenia, thrombocytopenia,*** platelet abnormalities, ***thrombosis, pulmonary embolism, coagulation disorders, decreased prothrombin, hypochromic anemia, pancytopenia, hemolysis, leukocytosis,*** lymphadenopathy, epistaxis, lymphopenia

SYST: Hypokalemia, hypocalcemia, hypomagnesemia, increased alk phosphatase, LDH, BUN, acidosis, hypophosphatemia, hyperphosphatemia, dehydration, glycosuria, increased creatine phosphokinase, hypervolemia, infection, ***sepsis, death, ascites,*** hyponatremia, hypochloremia, hypercalcemia

GU: ***Acute renal failure,*** decreased Ccr and increased serum creatinine, ***glomerulonephritis, toxic nephropathy, nephrosis, renal tubular disorders, pyelonephritis, uremia, hematuria, albuminuria,*** dysuria, polyuria

RESP: Coughing, dyspnea, pneumonia, sinusitis, pharyngitis, ***pulmonary infiltration,*** stridor, ***pneumothorax, hemoptysis, bronchospasm,*** bronchitis, ***respiratory depression, pleural effusion, pulmonary hemorrhage,*** rhinitis

EENT: Visual field defects, vocal cord paralysis, speech disorders, taste perversion, eye pain, conjunctivitis, tinnitus, otitis

CV: Hypertension, palpitations, ECG abnormalities, 1st degree AV block, nonspecific ST-T segment changes, hypotension, cerebrovascular disorder, cardiomyopathy, ***cardiac arrest,*** bradycardia, dysrhythmias

MS: Arthralgia, myalgia

Contraindications: Hypersensitivity

Precautions: Pregnancy (C), lactation, children, elderly, renal disease, seizure disorders, electrolyte/mineral imbalances, severe anemia

Pharmacokinetics: 14%-17%

plasma protein bound, half-life 2-8 hr in normal renal function

Interactions/incompatibilities:

- Nephrotoxicity: aminoglycosides, amphotericin B, IV pentamidine
- Hypocalcemia: pentamidine
- Increased anemia: zidovudine

NURSING CONSIDERATIONS

Assess:

- Kidney, liver function studies: BUN, creatinine, AST, ALT
- I&O ratio, urine pH
- Blood counts q2wk; watch for decreasing granulocytes, Hgb; if low, therapy may need to be discontinued and restarted after hematologic recovery; blood transfusions may be required
- GI symptoms: severe nausea, vomiting, diarrhea, severe symptoms may necessitate discontinuing drug
- Electrolytes and minerals: calcium, phosphorus, magnesium, sodium, potassium

Administer:

- Increased fluids before and during drug administration to induce diuresis and minimize renal toxicity
- Using infusion device, at no more than 1 mg/kg/min; do not give by rapid or bolus IV; give by CVP or peripheral vein; standard 24 mg/ml solution may be used without dilution if using by CVP; dilute the 24 mg/ml sol to 12 mg/ml with D_5W or normal saline if using peripheral vein

Perform/provide:

- Regular ophthalmologic exams
- Close monitoring during therapy, if tingling, numbness, paresthesias; if these occur stop infusion, obtain lab for electrolytes

Evaluate:

- Therapeutic response: improvement in CMV retinitis
- Blood dyscrasias (anemia, granulocytopenia); bruising, fatigue, bleeding, poor healing
- Allergic reactions: flushing, rash, urticaria, pruritus

Teach patient/family:

- To call physician if sore throat, swollen lymph nodes, malaise, fever occur since other infections may occur
- To report perioral tingling, numbness in extremities, and paresthesias
- That serious drug interactions may occur if OTC products are ingested; check first with physician
- That drug is not a cure, but will control symptoms

---

fosinopril

(foss-in-o'prel)

Monopril

Func. class.: Antihypertensive
Chem. class.: Angiotension-converting enzyme (ACE) inhibitor

Action: Selectively suppresses renin-angiotensin-aldosterone system; inhibits ACE; prevents conversion of angiotensin I to angiotensin II; results in dilation of arterial, venous vessels

Uses: Hypertension, alone or in combination with thiazide diuretics

Dosage and routes:

- *Adult:* PO 10 mg qd initially, then 20-40 mg/day divided bid or qd

Available forms include: Tabs 10, 20 mg

Side effects/adverse reactions:

CV: Hypotension, chest pain, palpitations, angina, orthostatic hypotension

GU: ***Proteinuria,*** Increased BUN, creatinine, decreased libido

HEMA: Decreased Hct, Hgb, ***eosinophilia, leukopenia, neutropenia***

* Available in Canada only

INTEG: ***Angioedema,*** rash, flushing, sweating, photosensitivity, pruritus
RESP: Cough, sinusitis, dyspnea, ***bronchospasm***
META: Hyperkalemia
GI: Nausea, constipation, vomiting, diarrhea
CNS: Insomnia, paresthesia, headache, dizziness, fatigue, memory disturbance, tremor, mood change
MS: Arthralgia, myalgia
Contraindications: Hypersensitivity to ACE inhibitors, pregnancy (D), lactation, children
Precautions: Impaired liver function, hypovolemia, blood dyscrasias, CHF, COPD, asthma, elderly
Pharmacokinetics:
PO: Peak 3 hr, serum protein binding 97%, half-life 12 hr, metabolized by liver (metabolites excreted in urine, feces)
Interactions/incompatibilities:
- Increased hypotension: diuretics, other antihypertensives, ganglionic blockers, adrenergic blockers
- Increased toxicity: vasodilators, hydralazine, prazosin, potassium-sparing diuretics, sympathomimetics
- Decreased absorption: antacids
- Decreased antihypertensive effect: indomethacin
- Increased serum levels of: digoxin, lithium
- Increased hypersensitivity: allopurinol

NURSING CONSIDERATIONS

Assess:
- Blood studies: neutrophils, decreased platelets
- B/P, orthostatic hypotension, syncope
- Renal studies: protein, BUN, creatinine; watch for increased levels that may indicate nephrotic syndrome
- Baselines in renal, liver function tests before therapy begins
- Potassium levels, although hyperkalemia rarely occurs
- Dipstick of urine for protein qd in first morning specimen; if protein is increased, a 24-hr urinary protein should be collected

Administer:
- IV infusion of 0.9% NaCl (as ordered) to expand fluid volume if severe hypotension occurs

Perform/provide:
- Storage in tight container at 30° C or less
- Supine or Trendelenburg position for severe hypotension

Evaluate:
- Therapeutic response: decrease in B/P
- Edema in feet, legs daily
- Allergic reactions: rash, fever, pruritus, urticaria; drugs should be discontinued if antihistamines fail to help
- Renal symptoms: polyuria, oliguria, frequency, dysuria

Teach patient/family:
- Not to discontinue drug abruptly
- Not to use OTC products (cough, cold, allergy) unless directed by physician; do not use salt substitutes containing potassium without consulting physician
- Importance of complying with dosage schedule, even if feeling better
- To rise slowly to sitting or standing position to minimize orthostatic hypotension
- To notify physician of: mouth sores, sore throat, fever, swelling of hands or feet, irregular heartbeat, chest pain
- To report excessive perspiration, dehydration, vomiting, diarrhea; may lead to fall in B/P
- That drug may cause dizziness,

F

fainting, light-headedness during 1st few days of therapy
• That drug may cause skin rash or impaired perspiration
• How to take B/P; normal readings for age group

Lab test interferences:
False positive: Urine acetone

Treatment of overdose: 0.9% NaCl IV INF, hemodialysis

---

furosemide

(fur-oh'se-mide)
Lasix, Novosemide,* Uritol*

Func. class.: Loop diuretic
Chem. class.: Sulfonamide derivative

Action: Acts on loop of Henle by increasing excretion of chloride, sodium

Uses: Pulmonary edema, edema in CHF, liver disease, nephrotic syndrome, ascites, hypertension

Dosage and routes:
• *Adult:* PO 20-80 mg/day in AM, may give another dose in 6 hr, up to 600 mg/day; IM/IV 20-40 mg, increased by 20 mg q2h until desired response
• *Child:* PO/IM/IV 2 mg/kg, may increase by 1-2 mg/kg/q6-8h up to 6 mg/kg

Pulmonary edema
• *Adult:* IV 40 mg given over several minutes, repeated in 1 hr; increase to 80 mg if needed

Available forms include: Tabs 20, 40, 80 mg; oral sol 10 mg/ml; inj IM, IV 10 mg/ml

Side effects/adverse reactions:
GU: Polyuria, ***renal failure,*** glycosuria
ELECT: Hypokalemia, hypochloremic alkalosis, hypomagnesemia, hyperuricemia, hypocalcemia, hyponatremia
CNS: Headache, fatigue, weakness, vertigo, paresthesias
GI: Nausea, diarrhea, dry mouth, vomiting, anorexia, cramps, oral, gastric irritations, pancreatitis
EENT: ***Loss of hearing,*** ear pain, tinnitus, blurred vision
INTEG: Rash, pruritus, purpura, ***Stevens-Johnson syndrome,*** sweating, photosensitivity, urticaria
MS: Cramps, arthritis, stiffness
ENDO: Hyperglycemia
HEMA: ***Thrombocytopenia, agranulocytosis, leukopenia, neutropenia, anemia***
CV: Orthostatic hypotension, chest pain, ECG changes, ***circulatory collapse***

Contraindications: Hypersensitivity to sulfonamides, anuria, hypovolemia, infants, lactation, electrolyte depletion

Precautions: Diabetes mellitus, dehydration, ascites, severe renal disease, pregnancy (C)

Pharmacokinetics:
PO: Onset 1 hr, peak 1-2 hr, duration 6-8 hr
IV: Onset 5 min, peak ½ hr, duration 2 hr
Excreted in urine, feces, crosses placenta, excreted in breast milk

Interactions/incompatibilities:
• Increased toxicity: lithium, nondepolarizing skeletal muscle relaxants, digitalis
• Increased action of: antihypertensives
• Increased ototoxicity: aminoglycosides, cisplatin, vancomycin
• Decreased antihypertensive effect of furosemide: indomethacin, metolazone

NURSING CONSIDERATIONS

Assess:
• Hearing when giving high doses
• Weight, I&O daily to determine

---

* Available in Canada only

fluid loss; effect of drug may be decreased if used qd
• Rate, depth, rhythm of respiration, effect of exertion
• B/P lying, standing; postural hypotension may occur
• Electrolytes: potassium, sodium, chloride; include BUN, blood sugar, CBC, serum creatinine, blood pH, ABGs, uric acid, calcium, magnesium
• Glucose in urine if patient is diabetic
• Hearing when giving high doses

Administer:
• IV undiluted may be given through Y-tube or 3-way stopcock; give 20 mg or less/min
• In AM to avoid interference with sleep if using drug as a diuretic
• Potassium replacement if potassium is less than 3.0
• With food, if nausea occurs, absorption may be decreased slightly

Evaluate:
• Therapeutic response: improvement in edema of feet, legs, sacral area daily if medication is being used in CHF
• Improvement in CVP q8h
• Signs of metabolic alkalosis: drowsiness, restlessness
• Signs of hypokalemia: postural hypotension, malaise, fatigue, tachycardia, leg cramps, weakness
• Rashes, temperature elevation qd
• Confusion, especially in elderly, take safety precautions if needed

Teach patient/family:
• To increase fluid intake 2-3 L/day unless contraindicated, to rise slowly from lying or sitting position
• Adverse reactions: muscle cramps, weakness, nausea, dizziness
• Take with food or milk for GI symptoms
• Take early in day to prevent nocturia

Lab test interferences:
Interfere: GTT

Treatment of overdose: Lavage if taken orally, monitor electrolytes, administer dextrose in saline, monitor hydration, CV, renal status

---

gallamine triethiodide

(gal'a-meen)
Flaxedil

Func. class.: Neuromuscular blocker (nondepolarizing)

Action: Inhibits transmission of nerve impulses by binding with cholinergic receptor sites, antagonizing action of acetylcholine

Uses: Facilitation of endotracheal intubation, skeletal muscle relaxation during mechanical ventilation, surgery, or general anesthesia

Dosage and routes:
• *Adult and child >1 mo:* IV 1 mg/kg, not to exceed 100 mg, then 0.5-1 mg/kg q30-40 min
• *Child <1 mo, >5 kg:* IV 0.25-0.75 mg/kg, then 0.01-0.05 mg/kg q30-40 min

Available forms include: Inj IV 20 mg/ml

Side effects/adverse reactions:
CV: Bradycardia, tachycardia, increased, decreased B/P
RESP: ***Prolonged apnea, bronchospasm, cyanosis, respiratory depression***
EENT: Increased secretions
INTEG: Rash, flushing, pruritus, urticaria
CNS: ***Malignant hyperthermia***
GI: Decreased motility

Contraindications: Hypersensitivity to iodides

Precautions: Pregnancy (C), thyroid disease, collagen disease, cardiac disease, lactation, children <2 yr, electrolyte imbalances, dehydration, neuromuscular disease (myasthenia gravis), respiratory disease

Pharmacokinetics:

IV: Onset 2 min, duration 20-60 min; half-life 2 min, 29 min (terminal), excreted in urine, feces (metabolites), crosses placenta

Interactions/incompatibilities:

• Increased neuromuscular blockade: aminoglycosides, clindamycin, lincomycin, quinidine, local anesthetics, polymyxin antibiotics, lithium, narcotic analgesics, thiazides, enflurane, isoflurane; used with cyclopropane, may provoke ventricular dysrhythmias
• Dysrhythmias: theophylline
• Do not mix with barbiturates in solution or syringe
• May be added to Pentothal, but not vice versa; do not use syringe previously used for Pentothal
• Do not use yellow-colored solutions of the drug

NURSING CONSIDERATIONS

Assess:

• For electrolyte imbalances (K, Mg); may lead to increased action of this drug
• Vital signs (B/P, pulse, respirations, airway) q15min until fully recovered; rate, depth, pattern of respirations, strength of hand grip
• I&O ratio; check for urinary retention, frequency, hesitancy

Administer:

• Using nerve stimulator by anesthesiologist to determine neuromuscular blockade
• Anticholinesterase to reverse neuromuscular blockade
• IV undiluted over 1-2 min (only by qualified person, usually an anesthesiologist)
• Only slight discolored solution

Perform/provide:

• Storage in light-resistant, cool area
• Reassurance if communication is difficult during recovery from neuromuscular blockade

Evaluate:

• Therapeutic response: paralysis of jaw, eyelid, head, neck, rest of body
• Recovery: decreased paralysis of face, diaphragm, leg, arm, rest of body
• Allergic reactions: rash, fever, respiratory distress, pruritus; drug should be discontinued

Treatment of overdose: Edrophonium or neostigmine, atropine, monitor VS; may require mechanical ventilation

gallium nitrate

(gal'ee-yum)

Ganite

Func. class.: Electrolyte modifier
Chem. class.: Hypocalcemic drug

Action: Lowers serum calcium levels by inhibiting calcium resorption from bone

Uses: To decrease hypercalcemia in cancer

Dosage and routes:

• *Adult:* IV 100-200 mg/m² qd × 5 days; infuse over 24 hr

Available forms: 25 mg/ml inj

Side effects/adverse reactions:

EENT: Blurred vision, optic neuritis, hearing loss

GU: ***Nephrotoxicity,*** increased BUN, creatinine

META: Hypophosphatemia, hypocalcemia

Contraindications: Hypersensitivity, severe renal disease

Precautions: Pregnancy (C), lactation, children, mild renal disease

Pharmacokinetics:
IV: Onset 12-24 hr, peak 5 days, duration 8 days
Interactions/incompatibilities:
• Increased toxicity: aminoglycosides, amphotericin B

NURSING CONSIDERATIONS

Assess:
• Renal status: BUN, creatinine, urine output
• Monitor calcium, phosphate, bicarbonate since all levels may be decreased and supplements of phosphate may be needed
• For hypercalcemia: nausea, vomiting, fatigue, weakness, thirst, dehydration, dysrhythmias, change in mental status
• For hypocalcemia: dysrhythmias; paresthesia; twitching; colic; laryngospasm; Trousseau's, Chvostek's sign; tremors
Administer:
• Adequate hydration with IV saline, 2000 mg/day during treatment
• After dilution of dose/1000 ml 0.9% NaCl or D_5W, run over 24 hr
Perform/provide:
• Storage of solution for 48 hr at room temperature or 1 wk in refrigerator
Evaluate:
• Therapeutic response: decreased serum calcium levels
Teach patient/family:
• To follow dietary guidelines given by physician, including adequate calcium (daily products, broccoli, canned) and vitamin D (fortified milk, grain products, fish oil)

gancyclovir (DHPG)

(gan-sy-clo-ver)
Cytovene
Func. class.: Antiviral
Chem. class.: Synthetic nucleoside analog

Action: Inhibits replication of herpes viruses in vitro; in vivo by selective inhibition of the human CMV DNA polymerase and by direct incorporation into viral DNA
Uses: Cytomegalovirus (CMV) retinitis in immunocompromised persons, including those with AIDS, after indirect ophthalmoscopy confirms diagnosis
Dosage and routes:
Induction treatment
• *Adult:* IV 5 mg/kg given over 1 hr, q12h × 2-3 wk
Maintenance treatment
• *Adult:* IV INF 5 mg/kg given over 1 hr, qd × 7 days/wk; or 6 mg/kg qd × 5 days/wk
• Dosage must be reduced in renal impairment
Available forms include: powder 500 mg/vial gancyclovir
Side effects/adverse reactions:
HEMA: ***Granulocytopenia, thrombocytopenia, irreversible neutropenia, anemia, eosinophilia***
GI: Abnormal LFTs, nausea, vomiting, anorexia, diarrhea, abdominal pain, ***hemorrhage***
INTEG: Rash, alopecia, pruritis, urticaria, pain at site, phlebitis
CNS: Fever, chills, ***coma***, confusion, abnormal thoughts, dizziness, bizarre dreams, headache, psychosis, tremors, somnolence, paresthesia
CV: Dysrhythmia, hypertension/hypotension
RESP: Dyspnea

EENT: Retinal detachment in CMV retinitis
GU: ***Hematuria,*** increased creatinine, BUN
Contraindications: Hypersensitivity to acyclovir or gancyclovir
Precautions: Preexisting cytopenias, renal function impairment, pregnancy (C), lactation, children <6 mo, elderly, platelet count <25,000/mm
Pharmacokinetics: Half-life 3-4½ hr, excreted by the kidneys (unchanged drug), crosses blood-brain barrier
Interactions/incompatibilities:
- Decreased renal clearance of gancyclovir: probenecid
- Increased toxicity: dapsone, pentamidine, flucytosine, vincristine, vinblastine, adriamycin, doxorubicin, amphotericin B, trimethoprim/sulfa combinations, or other nucleoside analogs
- Severe granulocytopenia: zidovudine; do not give together
- Increased seizures: imipenem-cilastatin

NURSING CONSIDERATIONS
Assess:
- For leukopenia/neutropenia/thrombocytopenia: WBCs, platelets q2d during twice a day dosing and q1wk thereafter
- For leukopenia with qd WBC count in patients with prior leukopenia with other nucleoside analogs or for whom leukopenia counts are <1,000 cells/mm^3 at start of treatment
- Serum creatinine or creatine clearance at least q2wk

Administer:
- IV after diluting 500 mg/10 ml sterile H_2O for injection, shake, further dilute in 100 ml compatible sol and run over 1 hr
- Slowly; do not give by bolus IV, IM, SC injection
- Using diluted solution within 24 hr

Evaluate:
- Therapeutic response: decreased symptoms of cytomegalovirus

Teach patient/family:
- That drug does not cure condition, that regular ophthalmologic examinations are necessary
- That major toxicities may necessitate discontinuing drug
- To use contraception during treatment and that infertility may occur; men should use barrier contraception for 90 days after treatment

Treatment of overdose: Discontinue drug, use hemodialysis, and increase hydration

---

gemfibrozil

(gem-fi'broe-zil)
Lopid
Func. class.: Antilipemic
Chem. class.: Aryloxisobutyric acid derivative

Action: Inhibits biosynthesis of VLDL, LDL, which are responsible for cholesterol development
Uses: Type III/IV, V hyperlipidemia
Dosage and routes:
- *Adult:* PO 1200 mg in divided doses bid 30 min before meals

Available forms include: Caps 300 mg
Side effects/adverse reactions:
GI: Nausea, vomiting, dyspepsia, diarrhea, abdominal pain
INTEG: Rash, urticaria, pruritus
HEMA: ***Leukopenia, anemia, eosinophilia***
CNS: Dizziness, blurred vision
Contraindications: Severe hepatic disease, preexisting gallbladder disease, severe renal disease, pri-

mary biliary cirrhosis, hypersensitivity

Precautions: Monitor hematologic and hepatic function, pregnancy (B), lactation

Pharmacokinetics:

PO: Peak 1-2 hr, plasma protein binding >90%, half-life 1.5 hr, excreted in urine, metabolized in liver

Interactions/incompatibilities:

- May increase anticoagulant properties: oral anticoagulants
- Increased risk of myositis, myalgia: lovastatin

NURSING CONSIDERATIONS

Assess:

- Renal, hepatic levels if patient is on long-term therapy

Administer:

- 30 min before morning and evening meals

Evaluate:

- Therapeutic response: decreased cholesterol levels
- Bowel pattern daily; increase bulk, water in diet if constipation develops, especially elderly

Teach patient/family:

- That compliance is needed since toxicity may result if doses are missed
- That risk factors should be decreased: high fat diet, smoking, alcohol consumption, absence of exercise
- Birth control should be practiced while on this drug

Lab test interferences:

Increase: Liver function studies, CPK, BSP, thymol turbidity, glucose

Decrease: Hgb, Hct, WBC

gentamicin sulfate

(jen-ta-mye'sin)

Alcomicin,* Apogen, Cidomycin,* Garamycin, Jenamicin, U-Gencin

Func. class.: Antibiotic

Chem. class.: Aminoglycoside

Action: Interferes with protein synthesis in bacterial cell by binding to ribosomal subunit, causing misreading of genetic code; inaccurate peptide sequence forms in protein chain, causing bacterial death

Uses: Severe systemic infections of CNS, respiratory, GI, urinary tract, bone, skin, soft tissues caused by susceptible strains of *P. aeruginosa, Proteus, Klebsiella, Serratia, E. coli, Enterobacter, Citrobacter, Staphylococcus, Shigella, Salmonella*

Dosage and routes:

Severe systemic infections

- *Adult:* IV INF 3-5 mg/kg/day in 3 divided doses q8h; dilute in 50-200 ml NS or D_5W given over 30 min-2 hr; IM 3 mg/kg/day in divided doses q8h
- *Adult:* INTRATHECAL 4-8 mg qd
- *Child:* IV/IM 2-2.5 mg/kg q8h
- *Neonates and infants:* IV/IM 2.5 mg/kg q8h
- *Neonates <1 wk:* 2.5 mg/kg q12h
- *Infants and child >3 months:* INTRATHECAL 1-2 mg qd

Dental/respiratory procedures/GI/GU surgery (prophylaxis endocarditis)

- *Adult:* IM 1.5 mg/kg ½-1 hr before procedure with ampicillin
- *Child:* IM 2.5 mg/kg ½-1 hr before procedure with ampicillin

Available forms include: Inj IM, IV 10, 40, 60, 80, 100 mg; intrathecal 2 mg/ml

Side effects/adverse reactions:
GU: ***Oliguria, hematuria, renal damage, azotemia, renal failure, nephrotoxicity***
CNS: Confusion, depression, numbness, tremors, ***convulsions,*** muscle twitching, ***neurotoxicity,*** dizziness, vertigo
EENT: ***Ototoxicity,*** *deafness,* visual disturbances, tinnitus
HEMA: ***Agranulocytosis, thrombocytopenia, leukopenia, eosinophilia,*** anemia
GI: Nausea, vomiting, anorexia, increased ALT, AST, bilirubin, hepatomegaly, ***hepatic necrosis,*** splenomegaly
CV: Hypotension, hypertension, palpitations
INTEG: Rash, burning, urticaria, dermatitis, alopecia

Contraindications: Severe renal disease, hypersensitivity

Precautions: Neonates, mild renal disease, pregnancy (C), hearing deficits, myasthenia gravis, lactation, elderly, Parkinson's disease

Pharmacokinetics:
IM: Onset rapid, peak 1-2 hr
IV: Onset immediate, peak 1-2 hr
Plasma half-life 1-2 hr; duration 6-8 hr, not metabolized, excreted unchanged in urine; crosses placental barrier

Interactions/incompatibilities:
- Increased ototoxicity, neurotoxicity, nephrotoxicity: other aminoglycosides, amphotericin B, polymyxin, vancomycin, ethacrynic acid, furosemide, mannitol, methoxyflurane, cisplatin, cephalosporins, bacitracin
- Do not mix in solution or syringe: carbenicillin, ticarcillin, amphotericin B, cephalothin, erythromycin, heparin
- Increased effects: nondepolarizing neuromuscular blockers

NURSING CONSIDERATIONS

Assess:
- Weight before treatment; calculation of dosage is usually done based on ideal body weight, but may be calculated on actual body weight
- I&O ratio, urinalysis daily for proteinuria, cells, casts; report sudden change in urine output, toxicity is increased in patients with decreased renal function if high doses are given
- VS during infusion, watch for hypotension, change in pulse
- IV site for thrombophlebitis including pain, redness, swelling q30min, change site if needed; apply warm compresses to discontinued site
- Serum peak, drawn at 30-60 min after IV infusion or 60 min after IM injection, and trough level drawn just before next dose; blood level should be 2-4 times bacteriostatic level
- Urine pH if drug is used for UTI; urine should be kept alkaline

Administer:
- IV after diluting in 50-200 ml of normal saline or D_5W, sol concentration should be 1 mg/ml or less, run over ½-1 hr (adults) or 2 hr (children)
- IM injection in large muscle mass, rotate injection sites
- Drug in evenly spaced doses to maintain blood level
- Bicarbonate to alkalinize urine if ordered for UTI, as drug is most active in alkaline environment

Perform/provide:
- Adequate fluids of 2-3 L/day unless contraindicated to prevent irritation of tubules
- Flush of IV line with NS or D_5W after infusion
- Supervised ambulation, other

* Available in Canada only

safety measures with vestibular dysfunction

Evaluate:

• Therapeutic response: absence of fever, draining wounds, negative C&S after treatment

• Renal impairment by securing urine for CrCl testing, BUN, serum creatinine; lower dosage should be given in renal impairment (CrCl <80 ml/min)

• Deafness by audiometric testing, ringing, roaring in ears, vertigo; assess hearing before, during, after treatment

• Dehydration: high sp gr, decrease in skin turgor, dry mucous membranes, dark urine

• Overgrowth of infection including increased temperature, malaise, redness, pain, swelling, perineal itching, diarrhea, stomatitis, change in cough or sputum

• C&S before starting treatment to identify infecting organism

• Vestibular dysfunction: nausea, vomiting, dizziness, headache; drug should be discontinued if severe

• Injection sites for redness, swelling, abscesses; use warm compresses at site

Teach patient/family:

• To report headache, dizziness, symptoms of overgrowth of infection, renal impairment

• To report loss of hearing, ringing, roaring in ears or feeling of fullness in head

Treatment of overdose: Hemodialysis, monitor serum levels of drug

gentamicin sulfate (ophthalmic)

(jen-ta-mye'sin)

Garamycin Ophthalmic, Genoptic

Func. class.: Antiinfective ophthalmic

Action: Inhibits bacterial protein synthesis

Uses: Infection of external eye

Dosage and routes:

• *Adult and child:* INSTILL 1 or 2 gtt q2-4h; TOP apply oint to conjunctival sac bid-qid

Available forms include: Oint, sol 3%

Side effects/adverse reactions:

EENT: Poor corneal wound healing, temporary visual haze, overgrowth of nonsusceptible organisms

Contraindications: Hypersensitivity

Precautions: Antibiotic hypersensitivity, pregnancy (C)

NURSING CONSIDERATIONS

Administer:

• After washing hands, cleanse crusts or discharge from eye before application

Perform/provide:

• Storage at room temperature

Evaluate:

• Therapeutic response: absence of redness, inflammation, tearing

• Allergy: itching, lacrimation, redness, swelling, photosensitivity

Teach patient/family:

• To use drug exactly as prescribed

• Not to use eye makeup, towels, washcloths, eye medication of others; reinfection may occur

• That drug container tip should not be touched to eye

• To report itching, increased redness, burning, stinging, swelling; drug should be discontinued

• That drug may cause blurred vision when ointment is applied

gentamicin sulfate (topical)

(jen-ta-mye'sin)

Garamycin

Func. class.: Local antiinfective
Chem. class.: Aminoglycoside

Action: Interferes with bacterial protein synthesis
Uses: Superficial skin infections
Dosage and routes:
• *Adult and child:* TOP rub into affected area tid-qid
Available forms include: Cream, oint 0.1%
Side effects/adverse reactions:
INTEG: Rash, urticaria, stinging, burning, photosensitivity, pruritus
Contraindications: Hypersensitivity
Precautions: Pregnancy (C), lactation

NURSING CONSIDERATIONS

Administer:
• Enough medication to completely cover lesions, may cover with gauze dressing
• After cleansing with soap, water before each application, dry well
Perform/provide:
• Storage at room temperature in dry place
Evaluate:
• Therapeutic response: decrease in size, number of lesions
• Allergic reaction: burning, stinging, swelling, redness, photosensitivity
Teach patient/family:
• To use medical asepsis (hand washing) before, after each application
• To apply with glove to prevent further infection
• To avoid use of OTC creams, ointments, lotions unless directed by physician
• To avoid sunlight or wear sunscreen to prevent burns
• Not to use in eyes or external ear if eardrum is perforated
• To notify physician if condition worsens

glipizide

(glip-i'zide)

Glucotrol

Func. class.: Antidiabetic
Chem. class.: Sulfonylurea (2nd generation)

Action: Causes functioning β-cells in pancreas to release insulin, leading to drop in blood glucose levels; may improve insulin binding to insulin receptors or increase the number of insulin receptors; not effective if patient lacks functioning β-cells
Uses: Stable adult-onset diabetes mellitus (Type II) NIDDM
Dosage and routes:
• *Adult:* PO 5 mg initially, then increased to desired response, do not exceed 15 mg once a day dose, 40 mg/day in divided doses
• *Elderly:* PO 2.5 mg initially, then increased to desired response, max 40 mg/day in divided doses or 15 mg once a day dose
Available forms include: Tabs 5, 10 mg
Side effects/adverse reactions:
CNS: Headache, weakness, dizziness, drowsiness, tinnitus, fatigue, vertigo
GI: ***Hepatotoxicity, cholestatic jaundice,*** nausea, vomiting, diarrhea, heartburn
HEMA: ***Leukopenia, thrombocytopenia, agranulocytosis, aplastic***

*Available in Canada only

anemia, increased AST, ALT, alk phosphatase, ***pancytopenia, hemolytic anemia***

INTEG: Rash, allergic reactions, pruritus, urticaria, eczema, photosensitivity, erythema

ENDO: ***Hypoglycemia***

Contraindications: Hypersensitivity to sulfonylureas, juvenile or brittle diabetes

Precautions: Pregnancy (C), elderly, cardiac disease, severe renal disease, severe hepatic disease, thyroid disease

Pharmacokinetics:

PO: Completely absorbed by GI route, onset 1-1½ hr, duration 10-24 hr, half-life 2-4 hr; metabolized in liver, excreted in urine, 90%-95% is plasma protein bound

Interactions/incompatibilities:

- Increased hypoglycemic effects: insulin, MAOIs, cimetidine, chloramphenicol, guanethidine, methyldopa, nonsteroidal antiinflammatories, salicylates, probenecid
- Decreased action of glipizide: calcium-channel blockers, corticosteroids, oral contraceptives, thiazide diuretics, thyroid preparations, estrogens, phenothiazines, phenytoin, rifampin, isoniazide, phenobarbital, sympathomimetics
- Disulfiram-like reaction: alcohol
- Decreased effects of both drugs: diazoxide

NURSING CONSIDERATIONS

Assess:

- Blood, urine glucose levels during treatment to determine diabetes control

Administer:

- Drug 30 min before meals

Perform/provide:

- Storage in tight light-resistant containers at room temperature

Evaluate:

- Therapeutic response: decrease in polyuria, polydipsia, polyphagia, clear sensorium, absence of dizziness, stable gait
- Hypo/hyperglycemic reaction that can occur soon after meals

Teach patient/family:

- Not to drink alcohol
- To check for symptoms of cholestatic jaundice: dark urine, pruritus, yellow sclera; if these occur physician should be notified
- To use a capillary blood glucose test while on this drug
- To test urine glucose levels with Chemstrip 3 × /day
- The symptoms of hypo/hyperglycemia, what to do about each
- That drug must be continued on daily basis; explain consequence of discontinuing drug abruptly
- To take drug in morning to prevent hypoglycemic reactions at night
- To avoid OTC medications unless prescribed by a physician
- That diabetes is a life-long illness; drug will not cure disease
- That all food included in diet plan must be eaten in order to prevent hypoglycemia
- To carry Medic-Alert ID for emergency purposes
- To test urine for glucose/ketones tid if this drug is replacing insulin
- To continue weight control, dietary restrictions, exercise, hygiene

Treatment of overdose: 10%-50% glucose solution or 1 mg glucagon

---

glutethimide

(gloo-teth'i-mide)

Doriden, Rolathimide

Func. class.: Sedative-hypnotic

Chem. class.: Piperidine derivative

Controlled Substance Schedule III (USA), Schedule F (Canada)

Action: Depresses activity in brain cells primarily in reticular activating system in brain stem, also selectively depresses neurons in posterior hypothalamus, limbic structures

Uses: Insomnia, labor (stage 1), preoperatively for relaxation

Dosage and routes:

Insomnia

• *Adult:* PO 250-500 mg hs, may repeat dose >4 hr before usual awakening, not to exceed 1 g

Preoperatively

• *Adult:* PO 500 mg hs the night before surgery, then 500 mg-1 g 1 hr before surgery

Labor

• *Adult:* PO 500 mg given at the onset of labor, may repeat

Available forms include: Tabs 250, 500 mg; caps 500 mg

Side effects/adverse reactions:

HEMA: ***Thrombocytopenia, aplastic anemia, leukopenia, megaloblastic anemia***

CNS: Residual sedation, dizziness, ataxia, stimulation, headache, hangover

GI: Nausea, vomiting, hiccups, diarrhea, jaundice

GU: Porphyria

INTEG: Rash, urticaria, purpura, ***exfoliative dermatitis*** *(rare)*

EENT: Dry mouth, blurred vision

Contraindications: Hypersensitivity to this drug or piperidine derivatives, severe pain, severe renal disease, porphyria

Precautions: Depression, suicidal individuals, drug abuse, cardiac dysrhythmias, narrow-angle glaucoma, prostatic hypertrophy, stenosed peptic ulcer, pyloroduodenal/bladder neck obstruction, pregnancy (C)

Pharmacokinetics:

PO: Onset 30 min, peak 1-2 hr, duration 4-8 hr; metabolized by liver, excreted by kidneys (metabolites), crosses placenta, excreted in breast milk; half-life 4 hr, 10-20 hr terminal

Interactions/incompatibilities:

• Decreased hypoprothrombinemic effect: oral anticoagulants

• Increased CNS depression: alcohol and other CNS depressants

• Increased anticholinergic effect: tricyclic antidepressants

NURSING CONSIDERATIONS

Assess:

• Blood studies: Hct, Hgb, RBCs (if on long-term therapy)

• Hepatic studies: AST, ALT, bilirubin

Administer:

• After removal of cigarettes, to prevent fires

• After trying conservative measures for insomnia

• ½-1 hr before hs for sleeplessness

• Several hours before patient is to arise (to avoid hangover)

Perform/provide:

• Assistance with ambulation after receiving dose

• Safety measures: siderails, nightlight, call bell within easy reach

• Checking to see PO medication has been swallowed

• Storage in tight container in cool environment

Evaluate:

• Therapeutic response: ability to sleep at night, decreased amount of early morning awakening if taking drug for insomnia

• Mental status: mood, sensorium, affect, memory (long, short)

• Blood dyscrasias: fever, sore throat, bruising, rash, jaundice, epistaxis (rare)

• Type of sleep problem: falling asleep, staying asleep

Teach patient/family:

• To avoid driving or other activities requiring alertness until drug is stabilized

• To avoid alcohol ingestion or CNS depressants; serious CNS depression may result

• Not to discontinue medication quickly after long-term use, drug should be tapered over 1-2 wk

• That effects may take 2 nights for benefits to be noticed

• Alternate measures to improve sleep: reading, exercise several hours before hs, warm bath, warm milk, TV, self-hypnosis, deep breathing

• That hangover is common in elderly, but less common than with barbiturates

• Symptoms of withdrawal: nausea, vomiting, anxiety, hallucinations, insomnia, tachycardia, fever, cramps, tremors, seizures

• Blood dyscrasias: fever, sore throat, bruising, rash, jaundice (rare)

• Allergic reaction: rash, discontinue drug if rash occurs

Lab test interferences:

Interferes: 17-OHCS

Treatment of overdose: Lavage, activated charcoal, monitor electrolytes, vital signs

glyburide

(glye'byoor-ide)

DiaBeta,* Micronase

Func. class.: Antidiabetic

Chem. class.: Sulfonylurea (2nd generation)

Action: Causes functioning β-cells in pancreas to release insulin, leading to drop in blood glucose levels; may improve insulin binding to insulin receptors and increase number of insulin receptors; not effective if patient lacks functioning β-cells

Uses: Stable adult-onset diabetes mellitus (type II) NIDDM

Dosage and routes:

• *Adult:* PO 2.5-5 mg initially, then increased to desired response

• *Elderly:* PO 1.25 mg initially, then increased to desired response; max 20 mg/day, maintenance 1.25-20 mg/qd

Available forms include: Tabs 1.25, 2.5, 5 mg

Side effects/adverse reactions:

CNS: Headache, weakness, paresthesia, tinnitus, fatigue, vertigo

GI: Nausea, fullness, heartburn, ***hepatotoxicity, cholestatic jaundice,*** vomiting, diarrhea

HEMA: ***Leukopenia, thrombocytopenia, agranulocytosis, aplastic anemia,*** increased AST, ALT, alk phosphatase

INTEG: Rash, allergic reactions, pruritus, urticaria, eczema, photosensitivity, erythema

ENDO: ***Hypoglycemia***

MS: Joint pains

Contraindications: Hypersensitivity to sulfonylureas, juvenile or brittle diabetes

Precautions: Pregnancy (B), elderly, cardiac disease, severe renal disease, severe hepatic disease, thyroid disease, severe hypoglycemic reactions

Pharmacokinetics:

PO: Completely absorbed by GI route, onset 2-4 hr, peak 2-8 hr, duration 24 hr; half-life 10 hr, metabolized in liver, excreted in urine, feces (metabolites), crosses placenta, 90%-95% is plasma protein bound

Interactions/incompatibilities:

• Both drugs effects may be decreased: diazoxide

• Decreased digoxin level: digoxin

G

• Increased hypoglycemic effects: insulin, MAOIs, cimetidine, oral anticoagulants, chloramphenicol, guanethidine, methyldopa, nonsteroidal antiinflammatories, salicylates, probenecid
• Decreased action of glyburide: calcium-channel blockers, corticosteroids, oral contraceptives, thiazide diuretics, thyroid preparations, estrogens, phenothiazines, phenytoin, rifampin, isoniazide, phenobarbital, sympathomimetics
• Disulfiram-like reaction: alcohol

NURSING CONSIDERATIONS

Administer:
• With breakfast

Perform/provide:
• Storage in tight container in cool environment

Evaluate:
• Therapeutic response: decrease in polyuria, polydipsia, polyphagia, clear sensorium, absence of dizziness, stable gait
• Hypo/hyperglycemic reaction that can occur soon after meals

Teach patient/family:
• Not to drink alcohol
• To check for symptoms of cholestatic jaundice: dark urine, pruritus, yellow sclera; if these occur a physician should be notified
• To use a capillary blood glucose test while on this drug
• To test urine glucose levels with Chemstrip 3 × /day
• The symptoms of hypo/hyperglycemia, what to do about each
• That drug must be continued on daily basis; explain consequence of discontinuing drug abruptly
• To take drug in morning to prevent hypoglycemic reactions at night
• To avoid OTC medications unless prescribed by a physician
• That diabetes is a life-long illness, drug will not cure disease
• That all food included in diet plan must be eaten to prevent hypoglycemia
• To carry a Medic-Alert ID for emergency purposes

Treatment of overdose: 10%-50% glucose solution or 1 mg glucagon

glycerin

(gli'ser-in)

Glycerol, Glyrol, Osmoglyn

Func. class.: Laxative, hyperosmotic

Chem. class.: Trihydric alcohol

Action: Increases osmotic pressure, draws fluid into colon

Uses: Constipation

Dosage and routes:
• *Adult and child >6 yr:* REC SUPP 3 g; ENEMA 5-15 ml
• *Child <6 yr:* REC SUPP 1-1.5 g; ENEMA 2-5 ml

Available forms include: Rec sol 4 ml/applicator; supp

Side effects/adverse reactions:

CNS: Headache, confusion, ***convulsions***

GI: Nausea, vomiting, diarrhea

META: Dehydration

Contraindications: Hypersensitivity

Precautions: Pregnancy (C)

NURSING CONSIDERATIONS

Administer:
• In morning or evening (oral dose)

Perform/provide:
• Storage in cool environment, do not freeze

Evaluate:
• Therapeutic response: decrease in constipation
• Cause of constipation; identify whether fluids, bulk, or exercise is missing from lifestyle
• Cramping, rectal bleeding, nau-

* Available in Canada only

sea, vomiting; if these symptoms occur, drug should be discontinued

Teach patient/family:

- Not to use laxatives for long-term therapy; bowel tone will be lost
- That normal bowel movements do not always occur daily
- Not to use in presence of abdominal pain, nausea, vomiting
- To notify physician if constipation unrelieved or if symptoms of electrolyte imbalance occur: muscle cramps, pain, weakness, dizziness, excessive thirst

glycerin, anhydrous

(gli'ser-in)

Ophthalgan

Func. class.: Ophthalmic
Chem. class.: Trihydric alcohol

Action: Reduces corneal edema by osmosis of water through corneal epithelium, which is semipermeable

Uses: Reduce corneal edema

Dosage and routes:

- *Adult:* INSTILL 1-2 gtts after local anesthetic

Available forms include: Sol

Side effects/adverse reactions:

EENT: Eye pain
CNS: Headache

Contraindications: Hypersensitivity

Precautions: Pregnancy (C)

Pharmacokinetics: Onset 10 min, peak 20 min, duration 6-8 hr

NURSING CONSIDERATIONS

Administer:

- Anesthetic (tetracaine or proparacaine) before instillation to decrease pain

Perform/provide:

- Storage in tight container

Evaluate:

- Therapeutic response: decreased corneal edema

Teach patient/family:

- Method of instillation, including pressure on lacrimal sac for 1 min, and not to touch dropper to eye

glycopyrrolate

(glye-koe-pye'roe-late)

Robinul, Robinul Forte

Func. class.: Cholinergic blocker
Chem. class.: Quaternary ammonium compound

Action: Inhibits acetylcholine at receptor sites in autonomic nervous system, which controls secretions, free acids in stomach

Uses: Decreased secretions before surgery, reversal of neuromuscular blockade, peptic ulcer disease, irritable bowel syndrome

Dosage and routes:

Preoperatively

- *Adult:* IM 0.002 mg/lb ½-1 hr before surgery
- *Child 2-12 yr:* IM 0.002-0.004 mg/lb
- *Child <2 yr:* IM 0.004 mg/lb

Reversal of neuromuscular blockage

- *Adult:* IV 0.2 mg for each 1 mg of neostigmine or 5 mg IV of pyridostigmine simultaneously

GI disorders

- *Adult:* PO 1-2 mg bid-tid; IM/IV 0.1-0.2 mg tid-qid, titrated to patient response

Available forms include: Tabs 1, 2 mg; inj 0.2 mg/ml

Side effects/adverse reactions:

INTEG: Urticaria, allergic reactions
MISC: Suppression of lactation, nasal congestion, decreased sweating
CNS: Confusion, anxiety, restlessness, irritability, delusions, hallucinations, headache, sedation, depression, incoherence, dizziness, lethargy, flushing, weakness

EENT: Blurred vision, photophobia, dilated pupils, difficulty swallowing, increased intraocular pressure, mydriasis, cycloplegia
CV: Palpitations, tachycardia, postural hypotension, paradoxical bradycardia
GI: Dryness of mouth, constipation, nausea, vomiting, abdominal distress, paralytic ileus, altered taste perception
GU: Hesitancy, retention, impotence

Contraindications: Hypersensitivity, narrow-angle glaucoma, myasthenia gravis, GI/GU obstruction, child <3 yr, tachycardia, myocardial ischemia, hepatic disease, ulcerative colitis, toxic megacolon

Precautions: Pregnancy (C), elderly, lactation, prostatic hypertrophy, renal disease, CHF, pulmonary disease, hyperthyroidism

Pharmacokinetics:
PO: Peak 1 hr, duration 6 hr
IM: Peak 30-45 min, duration 7 hr
IV: Peak 10-15 min, duration 4 hr
Excreted in urine, bile, feces (unchanged)

Interactions/incompatibilities:
- Increased anticholinergic effect: alcohol, antihistamines, phenothiazines, amantadine, tricyclics
- Do not mix with diazepam, chloramphenicol, pentobarbital, sodium bicarbonate, sodium chloride in syringe or solution

NURSING CONSIDERATIONS

Assess:
- I&O ratio; retention commonly causes decreased urinary output

Administer:
- IV undiluted, give through a Y-tube or 3-way stopcock; give 0.2 mg or less over 1-2 min
- Parenteral dose with patient recumbent to prevent postural hypotension
- With or after meals to prevent GI upset; may give with fluids other than water
- Parenteral dose slowly; keep in bed for at least 1 hr after dose, monitor vital signs
- After checking dose carefully, even slight overdose could lead to toxicity

Perform/provide:
- Storage at room temperature
- Hard candy, frequent drinks, sugarless gum to relieve dry mouth

Evaluate:
- Therapeutic response: decreased secretions
- Urinary hesitancy, retention: palpate bladder if retention occurs
- Constipation; increase fluids, bulk, exercise if this occurs
- For tolerance over long-term therapy; dose may need to be increased or changed
- Mental status: affect, mood, CNS depression, worsening of mental symptoms during early therapy

Teach patient/family:
- Not to discontinue this drug abruptly; to taper off over 1 wk
- To avoid driving or other hazardous activities; drowsiness may occur
- To avoid OTC medication: cough, cold preparations with alcohol, antihistamines unless directed by physician

---

gonadorelin acetate

Lutrepulse

Func. class.: Gonadotropin
Chem. class.: Synthetic endogenous gonadotropin-releasing hormone (GnRH)

Action: Induces ovulation in

women by release of LH in the anterior pituitary gland

Uses: Primary hypothalamic amenorrhea

Dosage and routes:

• IV Pump: 5 μg/min, × 21 days; after three treatment intervals, it may be necessary to raise the dose in a stepwise program

Available forms include: Powder for inj, IV 0.8, 3.2 mg

Side effects/adverse reactions:

INTEG: Inflammation at injection site, phlebitis, hematoma at catheter site

SYST: ***Anaphylaxis (bronchospasm, tachycardia, flushing, urticaria, induration of injection site)***

REPRO: Ovarian hyperstimulation, multiple pregnancy

Contraindications: Hypersensitivity; patients with ovarian cysts or hormonally dependent tumors; causes of anovulation other than those of hypothalamic origin

Precautions: Pregnancy (B)

Pharmacokinetics: Excreted by kidneys, half-life (initial) 2-10 min, (terminal 10-40 min)

Interaction/incompatibilities:

• Ovulation stimulators should not be used with this drug

NURSING CONSIDERATIONS

Assess:

• Effects by ovarian ultrasound—baseline, after 1 wk, after 2 wk, midluteal phase serum progesterone

Administer:

• Using Lutrepulse pump only; detailed instructions are given with pump

• After reconstituting 8 ml of diluent provided and transferring to plastic reservoir, withdraw 8 ml of diluent and inject into lyophile drug cake; shake, fill reservoir bag with reconstituted solution, and administer IV using pump provider

Perform/provide:

• Storage at room temperature; use prepared solution within 24 hr

Evaluate:

• Therapeutic response: absence of amenorrhea with drug use

---

gonadorelin HCl

(goe-nad-oh-rell'in)

Factrel

Func. class.: Gonadotropin

Chem. class.: Synthetic luteinizing hormone–releasing hormone

Action: Combination luteinizing hormone (releasing hormone) that acts on anterior pituitary

Uses: Evaluation of response of gonadotropic hormone

Dosage and routes:

• *Adult:* SC/IV 100 μg usually given between day 1-7 of menstrual cycle

• *Child:* SC/IV 2 μg/kg

Available forms include: Powder for inj SC, IV 100, 500 μg/vial

Side effects/adverse reactions:

CNS: Dizziness, headache, flushing

GI: Nausea

INTEG: Inflammation at injection site

Contraindications: Hypersensitivity

Precautions: Pregnancy (B)

Pharmacokinetics: Excreted by kidneys

Interactions/incompatibilities:

• Increased level of gonadorelin: levodopa, spironolactone

• Decreased level of gonadorelin: digoxin, oral contraceptives, phenothiazines, dopamine antagonists

• May produce false test results when used with androgens, glucocorticoids, estrogens, progestins

NURSING CONSIDERATIONS
Assess:
• Test result: pituitary/hypothalamus dysfunction (decreased LH); postmenopausal (increased LH)
Administer:
• After reconstituting with sterile diluent (1 ml)/100 μg enclosed in package; give over 30 sec
• Repeated doses may be necessary to elevate pituitary gonadotropin reserve
Perform/provide:
• Storage at room temperature; use prepared solution within 24 hr

goserelin acetate

(go'seh-rel-in)
Zoladex

Func. class.: Gonadotropin-releasing hormone
Chem. class.: Synthetic decapeptide analog of LHRH

Action: Inhibitor of pituitary gonadotropin secretion. Initially increases LH and FSH with increases in testosterone, and reduction in sex steroid levels
Uses: Advanced prostate cancer, premenopausal breast cancer
Dosage and routes:
• *Adult:* SC 3.6 mg q28d
Available forms include: Depot inj 3.6 mg
Side effects/adverse reactions:
CNS: Headaches, ***spinal cord compression,*** anxiety, depression
CV: ***Dysrhythmia, cerebrovascular accident,*** hypertension, ***MI,*** chest pain
ENDO: Gynecomastia, breast tenderness, hot flashes
GI: Nausea, vomiting, constipation, diarrhea, ulcer
GU: Spotting, breakthrough bleeding, decreased libido, renal insufficiency, urinary obstruction, urinary tract infection
INTEG: Rash, pain on injection
MS: Osteoneuralgia
Contraindications: Hypersensitivity, pregnancy
Pharmacokinetics: Peak serum concentrations in 12-15 days
NURSING CONSIDERATIONS
Assess:
• For relief of bone pain
Evaluate:
• Therapeutic response: more normal levels of prostate-specific antigen, acid phosphatase, alk phosphatase, testosterone level of <25 ng/dl
Teach patient/family:
• That gynecomastia and postmenopausal symptoms may occur, but will decrease after treatment is discontinued
Lab test interferences:
Increased: Alk phosphatase, estradiol, FSH, LH, testosterone levels
Decreased: Testosterone levels, progesterone

griseofulvin microsize/griseofulvin ultramicrosize

(gri-see-oh-ful'vin)
Fulvicin-U/F, Grifulvin-V, Grasactin, Grisovin-FP, Fulvicin P/G, Grisactin-Ultra, Gris-PEG

Func. class.: Antifungal
Chem. class.: Penicillium griseofulvum derivative

Action: Arrests fungal cell division at metaphase, binds to human keratin making it resistant to disease
Uses: Mycotic infections: tinea corporis, tinea pedis, tinea cruris, tinea barbae, tinea capitis, tinea unguium if caused by *Epidermophyton, Microsporum, Trichophyton*

Dosage and routes:

• *Adult:* PO 500-1000 mg qd in single or divided doses (microsize), 125-165 mg bid (ultramicrosize) or 250-330 mg qd; may need 500-660 mg in divided doses for severe infections

• *Child:* PO 10 mg/kg/day or 30 mg/m^2/day (microsize) or 5 mg/kg/day (ultramicrosize)

Available forms include: Microcaps 125, 250 mg; tabs 250, 500 mg; oral susp 125 mg/ml; ultratabs 125, 165, 250, 330 mg

Side effects/adverse reactions:

INTEG: Rash, urticaria, photosensitivity, lichen planus, angioedema

CNS: Headache, peripheral neuritis, paresthesias, confusion, dizziness, fatigue, insomnia, psychosis

EENT: Blurred vision, oral candidiasis, furry tongue, transient hearing loss

GU: Proteinuria, cylinduria, precipitate porphyria, increased thirst

GI: Nausea, vomiting, anorexia, diarrhea, cramps, dry mouth, flatulence

HEMA: ***Leukopenia, granulocytopenia, neutropenia, monocytosis***

Contraindications: Hypersensitivity, porphyria, hepatic disease, lupus erythematosus

Precautions: Penicillin sensitivity, pregnancy (C)

Pharmacokinetics:

PO: Peak 4 hr, half-life 9-24 hr, metabolized in liver, excreted in urine (inactive metabolites), feces, perspiration

Interactions/incompatibilities:

• Tachycardia: alcohol

• Decreased action of griseofulvin: barbiturates

• Decreased action of: warfarin, anticoagulants (oral)

NURSING CONSIDERATIONS

Assess:

• I&O ratio

• Liver studies qwk (ALT, AST, bilirubin, alk phosphatase)

• Renal studies: BUN, serum creatinine

• Blood studies: CBC, platelets, q2wk

• Drug level during treatment

Administer:

• Drug carefully, making sure there is no confusion with dosage form (microsize vs ultrasize)

• With meals to decrease GI symptoms

• Until 3 separate cultures are negative for infective organism

Perform/provide:

• Storage in tight, light-resistant containers at room temperature

Evaluate:

• Therapeutic response: decreased fever, malaise, rash, negative C&S for infecting organism

• For history of penicillin allergy; may be cross-sensitive to this drug

• For renal toxicity: increasing BUN, serum creatinine, proteinuria, cylinduria

• For hepatotoxicity: increasing ALT, AST, bilirubin, alk phosphatase

• For blood dyscrasias: fatigue, malaise, dark urine, bruising

Teach patient/family:

• That long-term therapy may be needed to clear infection (2 wk-6 mo depending on organism)

• Proper hygiene: handwashing technique, nail care, use of concomitant topical agents if prescribed

• Importance of compliance even after feeling better

• To avoid alcohol since nausea, vomiting, hypertension may occur

• To use sunscreen or avoid direct sunlight to prevent photosensitivity

• To notify physician of sore

G

throat, fever, skin rash, which may indicate overgrowth of organisms

guaifenesin

(gwye-fen'e-sin)

Anti-Tuss, Balminil,* Bowtussin, Breonesin, Colrex, Cosin-GG, Dilyn, Glycotuss, Gly-O-Tussin, Glytuss, G-Tussin, Hytuss, Malotuss, Nortussin Proco, Recsei-Tuss, Resyl,* Robitussin, Tursen, Wal-Tussin DM

Func. class.: Expectorant

Action: Acts as an expectorant by stimulating a gastric mucosal reflex to increase the production of lung mucus

Uses: Dry, nonproductive cough

Dosage and routes:

- *Adult:* PO 100-400 mg q4-6h, not to exceed 1.2 g/day
- *Child:* PO 12 mg/kg/day in 6 divided doses

Available forms include: Tabs 100, 200 mg; caps 200 mg; syr 100 mg/5 ml

Side effects/adverse reactions:

CNS: Drowsiness

GI: Nausea, anorexia, vomiting

Contraindications: Hypersensitivity, persistent cough

Precautions: Pregnancy (C)

NURSING CONSIDERATIONS

Perform/provide:

- Storage at room temperature
- Increased fluids, room humidification to liquefy secretions

Evaluate:

- Therapeutic response: absence of cough
- Cough: type, frequency, character including sputum

Teach patient/family:

- To avoid driving, other hazardous activities if drowsiness occurs (rare)
- To avoid smoking, smoke-filled room, perfumes, dust, environmental pollutants, cleansers

guanabenz acetate

(gwan'a-benz)

Wytensin

Func. class.: Antihypertensive

Chem. class.: Central α_2-adrenergic agonist

Action: Stimulates central α_2-adrenergic receptors resulting in decreased sympathetic outflow from brain

Uses: Hypertension

Dosage and routes:

- *Adult:* PO 4 mg bid, increasing in increments of 4-8 mg/day q1-2wk, not to exceed 32 mg bid

Available forms include: Tabs 4, 8, 16 mg

Side effects/adverse reactions:

CV: ***Severe rebound hypertension,*** chest pain, dysrhythmias, palpitations

CNS: Drowsiness, dizziness, sedation, headache, depression, weakness

EENT: Dry mouth, nasal congestion, blurred vision

GI: Nausea, diarrhea, constipation

GU: Impotence

Contraindications: Hypersensitivity to guanabenz

Precautions: Pregnancy (C), lactation, children <12 yr, severe coronary insufficiency, recent myocardial infarction, cerebrovascular disease, severe hepatic or renal failure

Pharmacokinetics:

PO: Peak 2-4 hr; half-life 6 hr, excreted in urine

Interactions/incompatibilities:

- Increased sedation: CNS depressants

*Available in Canada only

NURSING CONSIDERATIONS

Assess:

- Renal studies: protein, BUN, creatinine, watch for increased levels; may indicate nephrotic syndrome
- Baselines in renal, liver function tests before therapy begins
- K levels, although hyperkalemia rarely occurs
- Dipstick of urine for protein qd in first morning specimen, if protein is increased a 24 hr urinary protein should be collected
- B/P during beginning treatment, periodically thereafter

Evaluate:

- Therapeutic response: decrease in B/P
- Edema in feet and legs daily
- Allergic reaction: rash, fever, pruritus, urticaria; drug should be discontinued if antihistamines fail to help
- Renal symptoms: polyuria, oliguria, frequency

Teach patient/family:

- To avoid hazardous activities, sedation may occur
- Not to discontinue drug abruptly or withdrawal symptoms may occur: anxiety, increased B/P, headache, insomnia, increased pulse, tremors, nausea, sweating
- Not to use OTC (cough, cold, or allergy) products unless directed by physician
- Importance of complying with dosage schedule even if feeling better
- To notify physician of: swelling of hands or feet, irregular heartbeat, chest pain
- About excessive perspiration, dehydration, vomiting, diarrhea; may lead to fall in blood pressure—consult physician if these occur
- That drug may cause dizziness, fainting; light-headedness may occur during 1st few days of therapy
- That compliance is necessary, not to skip or stop drug unless directed by physician
- That drug may cause skin rash or impaired perspiration

Treatment of overdose: Administer vasopressor, discontinue drug, supine position

guanadrel sulfate

(gwahn'a-drel)

Hylorel

Func. class.: Antihypertensive
Chem. class.: Adrenergic blocker, peripheral guinidine derivative

Action: Inhibits sympathetic vasoconstriction by inhibiting release of norepinephrine, depletes norepinephrine stores in adrenergic nerve endings

Uses: Hypertension

Dosage and routes:

- *Adult:* PO 5 mg bid, adjusted to desired response, may need 20-75 mg/day in divided doses

Available forms include: Tabs 10, 25 mg

Side effects/adverse reactions:

CV: Orthostatic hypotension, bradycardia, ***CHF,*** palpitations, chest pain, tachycardia, dysrhythmias

CNS: Drowsiness, fatigue, weakness, feeling of faintness, insomnia, dizziness, mental changes, memory loss, hallucinations, *depression,* anxiety, *confusion, paresthesias, headache*

GI: Nausea, cramps, diarrhea, constipation, dry mouth, anorexia, indigestion

INTEG: Rash, purpura, alopecia

EENT: Nasal stuffiness, tinnitus, visual changes, sore throat, double vision, dry burning eyes

G

GU: Ejaculation failure, impotence, dysuria, nocturia, frequency
RESP: ***Bronchospasm,*** dyspnea, cough, rales, SOB
MS: Leg cramps, aching, pain, inflammation
Contraindications: Hypersensitivity, pregnancy (B), pheochromocytoma, lactation, CHF, child <18 yr
Precautions: Elderly, bronchial asthma, peptic ulcer, electrolyte imbalances, vascular disease
Pharmacokinetics:
PO: Onset 0.5-2 hr, peak 1½-2 hr, duration 4-14 hr; half-life 10-12 hr, excreted in urine (50% unchanged)
Interactions/incompatibilities:
- Increased hypotension: diuretics, other antihypertensives
- Do not use with MAOIs
- Increased orthostatic hypotension: alcohol, opioids
- Decreased hypotensive effect: tricyclic antidepressants, phenothiazines, ephedrine, phenylpropanolamine

NURSING CONSIDERATIONS

Assess:
- Renal function studies in renal impairment (BUN, creatinine)
- Bleeding time, check for ecchymosis, thrombocytopenia, purpura
- I&O in renal disease patient

Evaluate:
- Therapeutic response: decreased B/P
- Cardiac status: B/P lying and standing, pulse, watch for hypotension
- Edema in feet, legs daily; take weight daily
- Skin turgor, dryness of mucous membranes for hydration status
- Symptoms of CHF: edema, dyspnea, wet rales

Teach patient/family:
- To avoid driving, hazardous activities if drowsiness occurs
- Not to discontinue drug abruptly
- Not to use OTC products unless directed by physician: cough, cold preparations
- To report bradycardia, dizziness, confusion, depression, fever or sore throat
- That impotence, gynecomastia may occur but are reversible
- To rise slowly to sitting or standing position to minimize orthostatic hypotension
- That therapeutic effect may take 2-4 wk

guanethidine sulfate

(gwahn-eth'i-deen)
Ismelin
Func. class.: Antihypertensive
Chem. class.: Antiadrenergic agent, peripheral

Action: Inhibits norepinephrine release, depleting norepinephrine stores in adrenergic nerve endings
Uses: Moderate to severe hypertension
Dosage and routes:
- *Adult:* PO 10 mg qd, increase by 10 mg qwk at monthly intervals; may require 25-50 mg qd
- *Adult:* (Hospitalized) 25-50 mg; may increase by 25-50 mg/day or every other day
- *Child:* PO 200 μg/kg/day; increase q7-10d, not to exceed 3000 μg/kg/24 hr

Available forms include: Tabs 10, 25 mg
Side effects/adverse reactions:
CV: Orthostatic hypotension, dizziness, weakness, lassitude, bradycardia, ***CHF,*** fatigue, angina, heart block, chest paresthesia
CNS: Depression
GI: Nausea, vomiting, *diarrhea,*

* Available in Canada only

constipation, dry mouth, weight gain, anorexia
INTEG: Dermatitis, loss of scalp hair
HEMA: ***Thrombocytopenia, leukopenia***
EENT: Nasal congestion, ptosis, blurred vision
GU: Ejaculation failure, impotence, nocturia, edema, retention, increased BUN
RESP: Dyspnea
Contraindications: Hypersensitivity, pheochromocytoma, recent MI, CHF, cardiac failure, sinus bradycardia
Precautions: Pregnancy (B), lactation, peptic ulcer, asthma
Pharmacokinetics:
PO: Therapeutic level: 1-3 wk; half-life 5 days, metabolized by liver, excreted in urine (metabolites), breast milk
Interactions/incompatibilities:
- Increased hypotension: diuretics, other antihypertensives
- Do not use with MAOIs
- Increased orthostatic hypotension: alcohol
- Decreased hypotensive effect: tricyclic antidepressants, phenothiazines, ephedrine, phenylpropanolamine, oral contraceptives, thiothixine, doxepin, haloperidol, amphetamines

NURSING CONSIDERATIONS
Assess:
- Renal function studies in renal impairment (BUN, creatinine)
- Bleeding time, check for ecchymosis, thrombocytopenia, purpura
- I&O in renal disease patient

Evaluate:
- Therapeutic response: decreased B/P
- Cardiac status: B/P, pulse, watch for hypotension
- Edema in feet, legs daily; take weight daily
- Skin turgor, dryness of mucous membranes for hydration status
- Symptoms of CHF: edema, dyspnea, wet rales

Teach patient/family:
- To avoid driving, hazardous activities if drowsiness occurs
- Not to discontinue drug abruptly
- Not to use OTC products unless directed by physician: cough, cold preparations
- To report bradycardia, dizziness, confusion, depression, fever, sore throat
- That impotence, gynecomastia may occur, but are reversible
- To rise slowly to sitting or standing position to minimize orthostatic hypotension, more common in AM, hot weather, exercise or when using alcohol
- That therapeutic effect may take 2-4 wk
- Notify physicians of severe diarrhea

Lab test interferences:
Increase: BUN
Decrease: Blood glucose, VMA excretion, urinary norepinephrine
Treatment of overdose: Lavage, vasopressors given cautiously

---

guanfacine HCl

(gwahn'fa-seen)
Tenex
Func. class.: Antihypertensive
Chem. class.: α-2 Adrenergic receptor agonist

Action: Stimulates central α-adrenergic receptors resulting in decreased sympathetic outflow from brain
Uses: Hypertension in individual using a thiazide diuretic

G

Dosage and routes:
- *Adult:* PO 1 mg/day hs, may increase dose in 2-3 wk to 2-3 mg/day

Available forms include: Tabs 1 mg

Side effects/adverse reactions:
GI: Dry mouth, constipation, cramps, nausea, diarrhea
CNS: Somnolence, dizziness, headache, fatigue
GU: Impotence, urinary incontinence
EENT: Taste change, tinnitus, vision change, rhinitis
MS: Leg cramps
RESP: Dyspnea
INTEG: Dermatitis, pruritus, purpura
CV: Bradycardia, chest pain

Contraindications: Hypersensitivity

Precautions: Pregnancy (B), lactation, children <12 yr, severe coronary insufficiency, recent MI, renal or hepatic disease, CVA

Pharmacokinetics:
Peak 1-4 hr, 70% bound to plasma proteins, half-life 17 hr, eliminated via kidney unchanged and as metabolites

Interactions/incompatibilities:
- Increased sedation: CNS depressants, other antihypertensives

NURSING CONSIDERATIONS

Assess:
- Blood studies: neutrophils, decrease in platelets
- Renal studies: protein, BUN, creatinine; watch for increased levels that may indicate nephrotic syndrome
- Baselines in renal, liver function tests before therapy begins
- Potassium levels, although hyperkalemia rarely occurs
- Dipstick of urine for protein in first morning specimen, if protein is increased, a 24 hr urinary protein should be collected
- B/P before, during, after treatment; notify physician of significant changes

Perform/provide:
- Storage of tablets in tight containers

Evaluate:
- Therapeutic response: decreased B/P in hypertension
- Edema in feet, legs daily
- Allergic reaction: rash, fever, pruritus, urticaria; drug should be discontinued if antihistamines fail to help
- Symptoms of CHF: edema, dyspnea, wet rales, B/P
- Renal symptoms: polyuria, oliguria, frequency

Teach patient/family:
- To avoid hazardous activities
- Not to discontinue drug abruptly or withdrawal symptoms may occur: anxiety, increased B/P, headache, insomnia, increased pulse, tremors, nausea, sweating
- Not to use OTC (cough, cold, or allergy) products unless directed by physician
- To avoid sunlight or to wear sunscreen; photosensitivity may occur
- Importance of complying with dosage schedule even if feeling better

haemophilus b vaccines (polysaccharide, conjugate)

(hee-moef'ii-lus)

Hib-Imune, HibVAX (polysaccharide), b-Capsa 1, ProHIBIT (conjugate)

Func. class.: Vaccine
Chem. class.: Haemophilus influenzae capsular polysaccharide

Action: Stimulates antibody pro-

* Available in Canada only

duction to *Haemophilus influenzae b*

Uses: Polysaccharide immunization of children 2-6 yr against *H. influenzae b,* conjugate immunization of child 1½-5 yr against invasive disease of *H. influenzae b*

Dosage and routes:

- *Child:* SC 0.5 ml (polysaccharide), IM 0.5 mg (conjugate)

Available forms include: Polysaccharide powder for injection 25 μg/0.5 ml after reconstituting; conjugate powder for injection 25 μg polysaccharide and 18 μg conjugated diphtheria toxoid/0.5 ml

Side effects/adverse reactions:

INTEG: Redness, soreness at injection site, rash

SYST: Low-grade fever, acute febrile reactions

Contraindications: Hypersensitivity, febrile illness, active infection

Precautions: Pregnancy (C)

NURSING CONSIDERATIONS

Assess:

- For skin reactions: swelling, rash, urticaria

Administer:

- After diluting with 0.6 ml diluent, which will yield 10 doses of 0.5 ml
- Only with epinephrine 1:1000 on unit to treat laryngospasm
- Only by SC or IM route

Perform/provide:

- Storage in refrigerator
- Written record of immunization

Evaluate:

- For history of allergies, skin conditions (eczema, psoriasis, dermatitis), reactions to vaccinations
- For anaphylaxis: inability to breathe, bronchospasm

Teach patient/family:

- That usually one dose is required

Lab test interferences:

Interference: Latex agglutination, countercurrent immunoelectrophoresis

halazepam

(hal-az'e-pam)

Paxipam

Func. class.: Antianxiety

Chem. class.: Benzodiazepine

Controlled Substance Schedule IV

Action: Depresses subcortical levels of CNS, including limbic system, reticular formation

Uses: Anxiety

Dosage and routes:

- *Adult:* PO 20-40 mg tid-qid
- *Geriatric:* PO 20 mg qd-bid

Available forms include: Tabs 20, 40 mg

Side effects/adverse reactions:

CNS: Dizziness, drowsiness, confusion, headache, anxiety, tremors, stimulation, fatigue, depression, insomnia, hallucinations

GI: Constipation, dry mouth, nausea, vomiting, anorexia, diarrhea

INTEG: Rash, dermatitis, itching

CV: Orthostatic hypotension, ***ECG changes, tachycardia,*** hypotension

EENT: Blurred vision, tinnitus, mydriasis

Contraindications: Hypersensitivity to benzodiazepines, narrow-angle glaucoma, psychosis, pregnancy (D), child <18 yr

Precautions: Elderly, debilitated, hepatic disease, renal disease

Pharmacokinetics:

PO: Peak 1-3 hr, duration 3-6 hr; metabolized by liver, excreted by kidneys, crosses placenta, breast milk, half-life 14 hr

Interactions/incompatibilities:
• Decreased effects of halazepam: oral contraceptives, valproic acid
• Increased effects of halazepam: CNS depressants, alcohol, disulfiram, oral contraceptives

NURSING CONSIDERATIONS

Assess:
• B/P (lying, standing), pulse; if systolic B/P drops 20 mm Hg, hold drug, notify physician, respirations q5-15min if given IV
• Blood studies: CBC during long-term therapy, blood dyscrasias have occurred rarely
• Hepatic studies: AST, ALT, bilirubin, creatinine, LDH, alk phosphatase

Administer:
• With food or milk for GI symptoms
• Crushed if patient is unable to swallow medication whole
• Sugarless gum, hard candy, frequent sips of water for dry mouth

Perform/provide:
• Assistance with ambulation during beginning therapy, since drowsiness/dizziness occurs
• Safety measures, including siderails
• Check to see PO medication has been swallowed

Evaluate:
• Therapeutic response: decreased anxiety, restlessness, sleeplessness
• Mental status: mood, sensorium, affect, sleeping pattern, drowsiness, dizziness
• Physical dependency, withdrawal symptoms: headache, nausea, vomiting, muscle pain, weakness after long-term use
• Suicidal tendencies

Teach patient/family:
• That drug may be taken with food
• Not to be used for everyday stress or used longer than 4 mo, unless directed by physician, not to take more than prescribed amount, may be habit forming
• To avoid OTC preparations (hay fever, cough, cold) unless approved by physician
• To avoid driving or other activities that require alertness; drowsiness may occur
• To avoid alcohol ingestion or other psychotropic medications, unless prescribed by physician
• Not to discontinue medication abruptly after long-term use
• To rise slowly or fainting may occur
• That drowsiness might worsen at beginning of treatment

Lab test interferences:
Increase: AST/ALT, serum bilirubin
False increase: 17-OHCS
Decrease: RAIU

Treatment of overdose: Lavage, VS, supportive care

halcinonide

(hal-sin'oo-nide)
Halciderm, Halog

Func. class.: Corticosteroid, synthetic
Chem. class.: Fluorinated corticosteroid

Action: Antiinflammatory, antipruritic, vasoconstrictor actions

Uses: Inflammation of corticosteroid-responsive dermatoses

Dosage and routes:
• *Adult:* TOP apply to affected area bid-tid

Available forms include: Cream 0.025%, 0.1%; oint 0.1%; sol 0.1%

Side effects/adverse reactions:
INTEG: Acne, atrophy, epidermal thinning, purpura, striae

Contraindications: Hypersensitivity, viral infections, fungal infections

Precautions: Pregnancy (C)

NURSING CONSIDERATIONS

Administer:

• Using an occlusive dressing, systemic absorption may occur

• For 3-5 days after lesions are gone

Perform/provide:

• Washing of skin before application

• Dressing change qd; check area for redness, rash, inflammation, discoloration; do not leave dressing in place over 16 hr

Evaluate:

• Therapeutic response: decreased inflammation

• Infection: increased temperature, WBC, even after withdrawal of medication; keep in mind these may be systemically absorbed

Teach patient/family:

• Not to get drug in eyes or mucous membranes

---

haloperidol/haloperidol decanoate

(ha-loe-per'idole)

Haldol, Peridol/Haloperidol Decanoate

Func. class.: Antipsychotic/neuroleptic

Chem. class.: Butyrophenone

Action: Depresses cerebral cortex, hypothalamus, limbic system, which control activity and aggression; blocks neurotransmission produced by dopamine at synapse; exhibits strong α-adrenergic, anticholinergic blocking action; mechanism for antipsychotic effects is unclear.

Uses: Psychotic disorders, control of tics, vocal utterances in Gilles de la Tourette syndrome, short-term treatment of hyperactive children showing excessive motor activity, prolonged parenteral therapy in chronic schizophrenia

Dosage and routes:

Psychosis

• *Adult:* PO 0.5-5 mg bid or tid initially depending on severity of condition; dose is increased to desired dose, max 100 mg/day; IM 2-5 mg q1-8h

• *Child 3-12 yr:* PO/IM 0.05-0.15 mg/kg/day

• *Decanoate:* Initial dose IM is 10-15 x daily oral dose at 4 wk interval; do not administer IV, not to exceed 100 mg

Chronic schizophrenia

• *Adult:* IM 10-15 times the PO dose q4 wk (decanoate)

• *Child 3-12 yr:* PO/IM 0.05-0.15 mg/kg/day

Tics/vocal utterances

• *Adult:* PO 0.5-5 mg bid or tid increased until desired response occurs

• *Child 3-12 yr:* PO 0.05-0.075 mg/kg/day

Hyperactive children

• *Child 3-12 yr:* PO 0.05-0.075 mg/kg/day

Available forms include: Tabs 0.5, 1, 2, 5, 10, 20 mg; conc 2 mg/ml; inj IM 5 mg/ml

Side effects/adverse reactions:

RESP: ***Laryngospasm,*** dyspnea, ***respiratory depression***

CNS: Extrapyramidal symptoms: pseudoparkinsonism, akathisia, dystonia, tardive dyskinesia, drowsiness, headache, ***seizures neuroleptic malignant syndrome,*** confusion

INTEG: Rash, photosensitivity, dermatitis

EENT: Blurred vision, glaucoma, dry eyes
GI: Dry mouth, nausea, vomiting, anorexia, constipation, diarrhea, jaundice, weight gain, ***ileus, hepatitis***
GU: Urinary retention, urinary frequency, enuresis, impotence, amenorrhea, gynecomastia
CV: Orthostatic hypotension, hypertension, ***cardiac arrest,*** ECG changes, ***tachycardia***
Contraindications: Hypersensitivity, blood dyscrasias, coma, child <3 yr, brain damage, bone marrow depression, alcohol and barbiturate withdrawal states, Parkinson's disease, angina, epilepsy, urinary retention, narrow-angle glaucoma
Precautions: Pregnancy (C), lactation, seizure disorders, hypertension, hepatic disease, cardiac disease
Pharmacokinetics:
PO: Onset erratic, peak 2-6 hr, half-life 24 hr
IM: Onset 15-30 min, peak 15-20 min, half-life 21 hr
IM (Decanoate): Peak 4-11 days, half-life 3 wk
Metabolized by liver, excreted in urine, bile, crosses placenta, enters breast milk
Interactions/incompatibilities:
• Oversedation: other CNS depressants, alcohol, barbiturate anesthetics
• Toxicity: epinephrine
• Toxicity: with lithium, neurotoxicity and brain damage possible
• Decreased effects of: lithium, levodopa
• Increased effects of both drugs: β-adrenergic blockers, alcohol
• Increased anticholinergic effects: anticholinergics
• Decreased effects of: haloperidol; phenobarbital

NURSING CONSIDERATIONS
Assess:
• Swallowing of PO medication; check for hoarding or giving of medication to other patients
• I&O ratio; palpate bladder if low urinary output occurs
• Bilirubin, CBC, liver function studies monthly
• Urinalysis is recommended before and during prolonged therapy
Administer:
• Reduced dose to elderly
• Antiparkinsonian agent, to be used if extrapyramidal symptoms occur
• IM injection into large muscle mass, use No. 21G, 2″ needle; give no more than 3 ml/injection site; patient should remain recumbent for ½ hr
• Oral liquid use calibrated dropper, do not mix in coffee or tea
• PO with food or milk
Perform/provide:
• Decreased noise input by dimming lights, avoiding loud noises
• Supervised ambulation until stabilized on medication; do not involve in strenuous exercise program because fainting is possible; patient should not stand still for long periods of time
• Increased fluids to prevent constipation
• Sips of water, candy, gum for dry mouth
• Storage in tight, light-resistant container
Evaluate:
• Therapeutic response: decrease in emotional excitement, hallucinations, delusions, paranoia, reorganization of patterns of thought, speech
• For depression in bipolar patients; rapid mood swings may occur with this drug

* Available in Canada only

• Affect, orientation, LOC, reflexes, gait, coordination, sleep pattern disturbances
• B/P standing and lying; take pulse and respirations q4h during initial treatment; establish baseline before starting treatment; report drops of 30 mm Hg
• Dizziness, faintness, palpitations, tachycardia on rising
• Extrapyramidal symptoms including akathisia (inability to sit still, no pattern to movements), tardive dyskinesia (bizarre movements of jaw, mouth, tongue, extremities), pseudoparkinsonism (rigidity, tremors, pill rolling, shuffling gait)
• Skin turgor daily
• For neuroleptic malignant syndrome: hyperthermia, muscle rigidity, altered mental status, increased CPK
• Constipation, urinary retention daily; if these occur, increase bulk, water in diet

Teach patient/family:
• That orthostatic hypotension occurs often, and to rise from sitting or lying position gradually to avoid hazardous activities until stabilized on medication
• To remain lying down after IM injection for at least 30 min
• To avoid hot tubs, hot showers, or tub baths since hypotension may occur
• To avoid abrupt withdrawal of this drug or extrapyramidal symptoms may result; drug should be withdrawn slowly
• To avoid OTC preparations (cough, hayfever, cold) unless approved by physician since serious drug interactions may occur; avoid use with alcohol or CNS depressants, increased drowsiness may occur
• To use a sunscreen during sun exposure to prevent burns
• Regarding compliance with drug regimen
• About EPS and necessity for meticulous oral hygiene since oral candidiasis may occur
• To report impaired vision, jaundice, tremors, muscle twitching
• That in hot weather, heat stroke may occur; take extra precautions to stay cool

Lab test interferences:
Increase: Liver function tests, cardiac enzymes, cholesterol, blood glucose, prolactin, bilirubin, PBI, cholinesterase, ^{131}I
Decrease: Hormones (blood, urine)
False positive: Pregnancy tests, PKU
False negative: Urinary steroids

Treatment of overdose: Induce emesis, activated charcoal lavage, if orally injested, provide an airway; *do not induce vomiting*

haloprogin (topical)

(ha-loe-proe'jin)
Halotex

Func. class.: Local antiinfective, antifungal
Chem. class.: Iodinated phenolic ester

Action: Interferes with fungal cell membrane permeability

Uses: Tinea pedis, tinea cruris, tinea corporis, tinea manus, tinea versicolor

Dosage and routes:
• *Adult and child:* TOP apply to affected area bid × 14-21 days

Available forms include: Cream, sol 1%

Side effects/adverse reactions:
INTEG: Rash, urticaria, stinging,

burning, vesiculation, pruritus, erythema, scaling, folliculitis sensitization
Contraindications: Hypersensitivity
Precautions: Pregnancy (B), lactation, children

NURSING CONSIDERATIONS

Administer:
- Enough medication to completely cover lesions
- After cleansing with soap, water before each application, dry well

Perform/provide:
- Storage at room temperature in dry place

Evaluate:
- Therapeutic response: decrease in size, number of lesions
- Allergic reaction: burning, stinging, swelling, redness, vesiculation, scaling

Teach patient/family:
- To use medical asepsis (hand washing) before, after each application
- To apply with glove to prevent further infection
- To avoid use of OTC creams, ointments, lotions unless directed by physician
- To avoid contact with eyes
- To continue even though condition improves
- To use for full duration even if condition subsides, or irritation increases; if condition does not improve after 4 wk another treatment should be considered

heparin calcium/heparin sodium

(hep'a-rin)
Calciparine,* Calcilean,* Liquaemin/Hepalean,* Hep Lock
Func. class.: Anticoagulant

Action: Prevents conversion of fibrinogen to fibrin, and prothrombin to thrombin by enhancing inhibitory effects of antithrombin III
Uses: Deep vein thrombosis, pulmonary emboli, myocardial infarction, open heart surgery, disseminated intravascular clotting syndrome, atrial fibrillation with embolization, as an anticoagulant in transfusion and dialysis procedures

Dosage and routes:

Deep vein thrombosis/MI
- *Adult:* IV PUSH 5000-7000 U q4h then titrated to PTT or ACT level, IV BOL 5000-7500 U, then IV INF; IV INF After bolus dose, then 1000 U/hr titrated to PTT or ACT level
- *Child:* IV INF 50 U/kg, maintenance 100 U/kg q4h or 20,000 U/m^2 qd

Pulmonary embolism
- *Adult:* IV PUSH 7500-10,000 q4h then titrated to PTT or ACT level; IV BOL 7500-10,000, then IV INF; IV INF After bolus dose, then 1000 U/hr titrated to PTT or ACT level
- *Child:* IV INF 50 U/kg, maintenance 100 U/kg q4h or 20,000 U/m^2 qd

Open heart surgery
- *Adult:* IV INF 150-300 U/kg

Available forms include: (Heparin sodium) inj 1000, 2500, 5000, 7500, 10,000, 15,000, 20,000, 40,000 U/ml; (Heparin calcium) inj 5000, 12,500, 20,000 U/dose

Side effects/adverse reactions:
GI: Diarrhea, nausea, vomiting, anorexia, stomatitis, abdominal cramps, ***hepatitis***
GU: ***Hematuria***
INTEG: Rash, dermatitis, urticaria, alopecia, pruritus
CNS: Fever, chills

* Available in Canada only

HEMA: ***Hemorrhage, thrombocytopenia***

Contraindications: Hypersensitivity, hemophilia, leukemia with bleeding, peptic ulcer disease, thrombocytopenic purpura, hepatic disease (severe), renal disease (severe), blood dyscrasias, pregnancy, severe hypertension, subacute bacterial endocarditis, acute nephritis

Precautions: Alcoholism, elderly, pregnancy (C)

Pharmacokinetics:

IV: Peak 5 min, duration 2-6 hr

SC: Onset 20-60 min, duration 8-12 hr

Half-life 1½ hr, excreted in urine, 95% bound to plasma proteins

Interactions/incompatibilities:

- Decreased action of: corticosteroids
- Increased action of: diazepam
- Decreased action of heparin: digitalis, tetracyclines, antihistamines
- Increased action of heparin: oral anticoagulants, salicylates, dextran, steroids, nonsteroidal antiinflammatories

NURSING CONSIDERATIONS

Assess:

- Blood studies (Hct, platelets, occult blood in stools) q3mo
- Partial prothrombin time, which should be 1½-2 × control, PTT; often done qd, APTT, ACT
- B/P, watch for increasing signs of hypertension

Administer:

- IV undiluted or diluted in compatible sol and given by direct, intermittent, or continuous infusion; give 1000 U or less over 1 min; then 5000 U or less over 1 min; infusion may run from 4-24 hr
- At same time each day to maintain steady blood levels
- Do not massage area or aspirate when giving SC injection, give in abdomen between pelvic bone, rotate sites; do not pull back on plunger, leave in for 10 sec; apply gentle pressure for 1 min
- Changing needles is not recommended
- Avoiding all IM injections that may cause bleeding

Perform/provide:

- Storage in tight container

Evaluate:

- Therapeutic response: decrease of deep vein thrombosis
- Bleeding gums, petecchiae, ecchymosis, black tarry stools, hematuria
- Fever, skin rash, urticaria
- Needed dosage change q1-2wk

Teach patient/family:

- To avoid OTC preparations that may cause serious drug interactions unless directed by physician
- That drug may be held during active bleeding (menstruation), depending on condition
- To use soft-bristle toothbrush to avoid bleeding gums, avoid contact sports, use electric razor
- To carry a Medic-Alert ID identifying drug taken
- To report any signs of bleeding: gums, under skin, urine, stools

Lab test interferences:

Increase: T_3 uptake

Decrease: Uric acid

Treatment of overdose:

Protamine SO_4 1:1 solution

hepatitis B vaccine

Heptavax-B

Func. class.: Vaccine

Action: Provides active immunity to hepatitis B

Uses: Prevention of hepatitis B virus

Dosage and routes:

• *Adult and child >10 yr:* IM 1 ml, then 1 ml after 1 mo, then 1 ml 6 mo after initial dose

• *Child 3 mo-10 yr:* IM 0.5 ml, then 0.5 ml after 1 mo, then 0.5 ml 6 mo after initial dose

• *Patients with decreased immunity:* IM 2 ml, then 2 ml after 1 mo, then 2 ml 6 mo after initial dose

Available forms include: Inj IM 10 mg/0.5 ml, 20 μg/ml

Side effects/adverse reactions:

INTEG: Soreness at injection site, urticaria, erythema, swelling

SYST: Induration

CNS: Headache, dizziness, fever

GI: Nausea, vomiting

Contraindications: Hypersensitivity

Precautions: Pregnancy, elderly, lactation, children; active infection, compromised cardiac or pulmonary status

NURSING CONSIDERATIONS

Assess:

• For skin reactions: rash, induration, urticaria

Administer:

• After rotating vial, do not shake

• Only with epinephrine 1:1000 on unit to treat laryngospasm

• In deltoid for better protection, give 2 ml dose in two different sites

Perform/provide:

• Written record of immunization

• Comfort measures

Evaluate:

• For history of allergies, skin conditions (eczema, psoriasis, dermatitis), reactions to vaccinations

• For anaphylaxis: inability to breathe, bronchospasm

hetastarch

(het'a-starch)

Hespan, HES, Volex

Func. class.: Plasma expander

Chem. class.: Synthetic polymer

Action: Similar to human albumin, which expands plasma volume by colloidal osmotic pressure

Uses: Plasma volume expander, leukapheresis

Dosage and routes:

• *Adult:* IV INF 500-1000 ml, total dose not to exceed 1500 ml/day, not to exceed 20 ml/kg/hr (hemorrhagic shock)

Leukapheresis

• *Adult:* IV INF 250-700 ml infused at 1:8 ratio with whole blood, may be repeated 2/wk up to 10 treatments

Available forms include: 6% hetastarch/0.9% NaCl

Side effects/adverse reactions:

HEMA: Decreased hematocrit, platelet function, increased bleeding/coagulation times, increased sed rate

INTEG: Rash, urticaria, pruritus, angioedema, chills, fever, flushing, peripheral edema

RESP: Wheezing, dyspnea, ***bronchospasm, pulmonary edema***

GI: Nausea, vomiting

SYST: ***Anaphylaxis***

CNS: Headache

Contraindications: Hypersensitivity, severe bleeding disorders, renal failure, CHF (severe)

Precautions: Pregnancy (C), liver disease

Pharmacokinetics:

IV: Expands blood volume 1-2 × amount infused, excreted in urine

NURSING CONSIDERATIONS

Assess:

• VS q5min × 30 min

• CVP during infusion (5-10 cm H_2O normal range)
• Urine output q1h, watch for increase in urinary output, which is common; if output does not increase, infusion should be decreased or discontinued
• I&O ratio and specific gravity, urine osmolarity; if specific gravity is very low, renal clearance is low, drug should be discontinued

Administer:
• IV, run at 20 ml/kg/hr; reduced rate in septic shock, burns

Perform/provide:
• Storage at room temperature; discard unused portions, do not freeze, do not use if turbid, deep brown, or precipitate forms

Evaluate:
• Therapeutic response: increased plasma volume
• Allergy: rash, urticaria, pruritus, wheezing, dyspnea, bronchospasm, drug should be discontinued immediately
• For circulatory overload: increased pulse, respirations, SOB, wheezing, chest tightness, chest pain
• For dehydration after infusion: decreased output, increased temperature, poor skin turgor, increased specific gravity, dry skin

Lab test interferences:
False increase: bilirubin

---

hexamethylmelamine

Hexalen

Func. class.: Antineoplastic, alkylating agent

Action: Responsible for inhibition of cell DNA and RNA synthesis, cell death; rapidly degraded; cell-cycle nonspecific

Uses: Resistant or recurrent ovarian cancer; may be used alone or in combination

Dosage and routes:
Adult: PO 260 mg/m²; average dose 400 qd × 14 days, then rest for 14 days; cycle should continue until patient no longer responds

Available forms include: Caps 50 mg

Side effects/adverse reactions:
EENT: Tinnitus, hearing loss
HEMA: ***Thrombocytopenia, leukopenia***
GI: Nausea, vomiting, diarrhea, stomatitis, weight loss, colitis, hepatotoxicity, anorexia
CNS: Headache, dizziness, drowsiness, paresthesia, peripheral neuropathy, coma, hyporeflexia, muscle weakness
INTEG: Alopecia, pruritus, herpes zoster

Contraindications: Lactation, pregnancy (first trimester) (D), myelosuppression, acute herpes zoster, hypersensitivity

Precautions: Radiation therapy, leukopenia, thrombocytopenia

Pharmacokinetics: Metabolized in liver, excreted in urine

Interactions/incompatibilities:
• Increased toxicity: antineoplastics, radiation
• Reduced efficiency: influenza vaccine, pneumococcal vaccine

NURSING CONSIDERATIONS

Assess:
• CBC, differential, platelet count weekly; withhold drug if WBC is <4000 or platelet count is 75,000; notify physician of these results
• Renal function studies: BUN, serum uric acid, urine CrCl before, during therapy
• I&O ratio; report fall in urine output to <30 ml/hr
• Monitor temperature q4h; fever

H

may indicate beginning infection, no rectal temperatures
• Liver function tests before, during therapy: (bilirubin, AST, ALT, LDH) as needed or monthly

Administer:
• As divided daily doses 1-2 hr pc and hs
• Antiemetic 30-60 min before giving drug to prevent vomiting and prn
• Topical or systemic analgesics for pain
• Local or systemic drugs for infection

Perform/provide:
• Storage at room temperature in dry form
• Strict medical asepsis, protective isolation if WBC levels are low
• Special skin care
• Increase fluid intake to 2-3 L/day to prevent urate deposits, calculi information
• Diet low in purines: organ meats (kidney, liver), dried beans, peas to maintain alkaline urine
• Rinsing of mouth tid-qid with water, club soda; brushing of teeth bid-tid with soft brush or cotton-tipped applicators for stomatitis; use unwaxed dental floss

Evaluate:
• Therapeutic response: decreased tumor size, decreased spread of malignancy
• Bleeding: hematuria, guaiac, bruising, or petechiae, mucosa or orifices q8h
• Food preferences: list likes, dislikes
• Yellowing of skin, sclera, dark urine, clay-colored stools, itchy skin, abdominal pain, fever, diarrhea
• Effects of alopecia on body image; discuss feelings about body changes
• Inflammation of mucosa, breaks in skin
• Buccal cavity q8h for dryness, sores, or ulceration, white patches, oral pain, bleeding, dysphagia
• Symptoms indicating severe allergic reaction: rash, pruritus, urticaria, purpuric skin lesions, itching, flushing

Teach patient/family:
• About protective isolation precautions
• That sterility, amenorrhea can occur; reversible after discontinuing treatment
• That hair may be lost during treatment; a wig or hairpiece may make patient feel better; new hair may be different in color, texture
• To avoid foods with citric acid, hot or rough texture
• To report any bleeding, white spots, or ulcerations in mouth to physician; tell patient to examine mouth qd
• To report signs of infection: increased temperature, sore throat, flu symptoms
• To report signs of anemia: fatigue, headache, faintness, shortness of breath, irritability

---

hexocyclium methylsulfate

(hex-oh-sye'klee-um)

Tral

Func. class.: Gastrointestinal anticholinergic
Chem. class.: Synthetic quaternary ammonium compound

Action: Inhibits muscarinic actions of acetylcholine at postganglionic parasympathetic neuroeffector sites
Uses: Treatment of peptic ulcer disease in combination with other drugs; other GI disorders

* Available in Canada only

Dosage and routes:
• *Adult:* PO 25 mg qid ac, hs
Available forms include: Tabs 25 mg

Side effects/adverse reactions:
CNS: Confusion, stimulation in elderly, headache, insomnia, dizziness, drowsiness, anxiety, weakness, hallucination
GI: Dry mouth, constipation, ***paralytic ileus,*** heartburn, nausea, vomiting, dysphagia, absence of taste
GU: Hesitancy, retention, impotence
CV: Palpitations, tachycardia
EENT: Blurred vision, photophobia, mydriasis, cycloplegia, increased ocular tension
INTEG: Urticaria, rash, pruritus, anhidrosis, fever, allergic reactions

Contraindications: Hypersensitivity to anticholinergics, narrow-angle glaucoma, GI obstruction, myasthenia gravis, paralytic ileus, GI atony, toxic megacolon

Precautions: Hyperthyroidism, coronary artery disease, dysrhythmias, CHF, ulcerative colitis, hypertension, hiatal hernia, hepatic disease, renal disease, pregnancy (C), urinary retention, prostatic hypertrophy, elderly

Pharmacokinetics:
PO: Onset 1 hr, duration 3-4 hr; metabolized by liver, excreted in urine

Interactions/incompatibilities:
• Increased anticholinergic effect: amantadine, tricyclic antidepressants, MAOIs
• Decreased effect of: phenothiazines, levodopa, ketoconazole

NURSING CONSIDERATIONS

Assess:
• VS, cardiac status: checking for dysrhythmias, increased rate, palpitations
• I&O ratio; check for urinary retention or hesitancy

Administer:
• ½-1 hr ac for better absorption
• Decreased dose to elderly patients; their metabolism may be slowed
• Gum, hard candy, frequent rinsing of mouth for dryness of oral cavity

Perform/provide:
• Storage in tight container protected from light
• Increased fluids, bulk, exercise to patient's lifestyle to decrease constipation

Evaluate:
• Therapeutic response: absence of epigastric pain, bleeding, nausea, vomiting
• GI complaints: pain, bleeding (frank or occult), nausea, vomiting, anorexia

Teach patient/family:
• To avoid driving or other hazardous activities until stabilized on medication
• To avoid alcohol or other CNS depressants; will enhance sedating properties of drug
• To avoid hot environments, stroke may occur, drug suppresses perspiration
• To use sunglasses when outside to prevent photophobia, may cause blurred vision
• To drink plenty of fluids
• To report dysphagia

homatropine hydrobromide (optic)

(hoe'ma-troe-peen)
Homatrocel, Isopto Homatropine, Murrocoll Homatropine

Func. class.: Mydriatic
Chem. class.: Synthetic alkaloid

Action: Blocks response of iris

sphincter muscle, muscle of accommodation of ciliary body to cholinergic stimulation, resulting in dilation, paralysis of accommodation

Uses: Uveitis, iritis

Dosage and routes:

• *Adult and child:* INSTILL 1-2 gtts repeat in 5-10 min for refraction or q3-4h for uveitis

Available forms include: Sol 2%, 5%

Side effects/adverse reactions:

CV: Tachycardia

CNS: Confusion, somnolence, flushing, fever

EENT: Blurred vision, photophobia, increased intraocular pressure, irritation, edema

Contraindications: Hypersensitivity, children <6 yr, narrow-angle glaucoma, increased intraocular pressure, infants

Precautions: Children, elderly, hypertension, hyperthyroidism, diabetes, pregnancy (C)

Pharmacokinetics:

INSTILL: Peak ½-1 hr, duration 1-3 days

NURSING CONSIDERATIONS

Evaluate:

• Therapeutic response: decrease in inflammation or cycloplegic refraction

• Eye pain, discontinue use

Teach patient/family:

• To report change in vision, blurring or loss of sight, trouble breathing, sweating, flushing

• Method of instillation: pressure on lacrimal sac for 1 min, do not touch dropper to eye

• That blurred vision will decrease with repeated use of drug

• Not to engage in hazardous activities until able to see

• To wait 5 min to use other drops

• Not to blink more than usual

hyaluronidase

(hye-l-yoor-on'i-dase)

Wydase

Func. class.: Enzyme

Action: Hydrolyzes hyaluronic within areas filled with exudates

Uses: Hypodermoclysis, subcutaneous urography, adjunct to dispersion of other drugs

Dosage and routes:

Adjunct

• *Adult and child:* INJ 150 U with other drug

Urography

• *Adult and child:* SC 75 U over scapula, then contrast medium is injected at same site

Hypodermoclysis

• *Adult and child >3 yr:* SC 150 U/L of clysis sol for 1000 ml of clysis sol

Available forms include: Inj powder 150, 1500 U; inj sol 150 U/ml

Side effects/adverse reactions:

INTEG: Rash, urticaria, itching

OTHER: Overhydration (hyperdermoclysis)

Contraindications: Hypersensitivity to bovine products, CHF, hypoproteinemia

Precautions: Pregnancy (C)

NURSING CONSIDERATIONS

Assess:

• Site before administration (hypodermoclysis)

Administer:

• After test dose: 0.02 ml of 150 u/ml solution is injected if wheal develops, itching test is positive

• Right after mixing since solution is unstable

• To child <3 yr, not exceeding 200 ml; in neonates not exceeding 2 ml/min

Evaluate:

• Therapeutic response: absence of

swelling, pain after hypodermoclysis
• For overhydration in child <3 yr

hydralazine HCl

(hye'dral'a-zeen)

Apresoline, Hydralyn, Rolazine

Func. class.: Antihypertensive, direct-acting peripheral vasodilator
Chem. class.: Phthalazine

Action: Vasodilates arteriolar smooth muscle by direct relaxation; reduction in blood pressure with reflex increases in cardiac function
Uses: Essential hypertension; *parenteral:* severe essential hypertension
Dosage and routes:
• *Adult:* PO 10 mg qid 2-4 days, then 25 mg for rest of 1st wk, then 50 mg qid individualized to desired response, not to exceed 300 mg; IV/IM BOL 20-40 mg q4-6h, administer PO as soon as possible; IM 20-40 mg q4-6h
• *Child:* PO 0.75 mg/kg qd 0.75-3 mg/kg/day in 4 divided doses; max 7.5 mg/kg/24 hr; IV BOL 0.1-0.2 mg/kg q4-6h; IM 0.1-0.2 mg/kg q4-6h
Available forms include: Inj IV, IM 20 mg/ml; tabs 10, 25, 50, 100 mg
Side effects/adverse reactions:
MISC: Nasal congestion, muscle cramps, *lupuslike symptoms*
CV: Palpitations, reflex tachycardia, angina, ***shock,*** edema, rebound hypertension
CNS: Headache, tremors, dizziness, anxiety, peripheral neuritis, depression
GI: Nausea, vomiting, anorexia, diarrhea, constipation
INTEG: Rash, pruritus
HEMA: ***Leukopenia, agranulocytosis,*** anemia
GU: Impotence, urinary retention, sodium, water retention
Contraindications: Hypersensitivity to hydralazines, coronary artery disease, mitral valvular rheumatic heart disease, rheumatic heart disease
Precautions: Pregnancy (C), CVA, advanced renal disease
Pharmacokinetics:
PO: Onset 20-30 min, peak 1 hr, duration 2-4 hr
IM: Onset 5-10 min, peak 1 hr, duration 2-4 hr
IV: Onset 5-20 min, peak 10-80 min, duration 2-6 hr; half-life 2-8 hr, metabolized by liver, less than 10% present in urine
Interactions/incompatibilities:
• Increased tachycardia, angina: sympathomimetics (epinephrine, norepinephrine)
• Increased effects of: β-blockers
• Use MAOIs with caution in patients receiving hydralazine
• Do not mix with any drug in syringe or solution

NURSING CONSIDERATIONS

Assess:
• B/P q5min × 2 hr, then q1h × 2 hr, then q4h
• Pulse, jugular venous distention q4h
• Electrolytes, blood studies: potassium, sodium, chloride, CO_2, CBC, serum glucose
• Weight daily, I&O
• LE prep, ANA titer before starting therapy
Administer:
• IV undiluted; give through Y-tube or 3-way stopcock each 10 mg or less/min
• To patient in recumbent position, keep in that position for 1 hr after administration
Evaluate:
• Therapeutic response: decreased B/P

- Edema in feet, legs daily
- Skin turgor, dryness of mucous membranes for hydration status
- Rales, dyspnea, orthopnea
- IV site for extravasation, rate
- Fever, joint pain, tachycardia, palpitations, headache, nausea
- Mental status: affect, mood, behavior, anxiety; check for personality changes

Teach patient/family:
- To take with food to increase bioavailability
- To avoid OTC preparations unless directed by physician
- To notify physician if chest pain, severe fatigue, fever, muscle or joint pain occurs

Treatment of overdose: Administer vasopressors, volume expanders for shock; if PO lavage or give activated charcoal, digitalization

---

hydrochlorothiazide

(hye-droe-klor-oh-thye'a-zide)

Chlorzide, Diaqua, Diu-Scrip, Diuchlor H,* Esidrix, Hydrodiuril, Hydromal, Hydroz-50, Hydrozide,* Hyperetic, Neo-Codema,* Novohydrazide,* Oretic, Urozide*

Func. class.: Thiazide diuretic
Chem. class.: Sulfonamide derivative

Action: Acts on distal tubule by increasing excretion of water, sodium, chloride, potassium

Uses: Edema, hypertension, diuresis, CHF

Dosage and routes:
- *Adult:* PO 25-100 mg/day
- *Child >6 mo:* PO 2.2 mg/kg/day in divided doses
- *Child <6 mo:* PO up to 3.3 mg/kg/day in divided doses

Available forms include: Tabs 25, 50, 100 mg; sol 50 mg/5 ml, 100 mg/ml

Side effects/adverse reactions:
GU: Frequency, polyuria, ***uremia, glucosuria***
CNS: Drowsiness, paresthesia, anxiety, depression, headache, *dizziness, fatigue, weakness*
GI: Nausea, vomiting, anorexia, constipation, diarrhea, cramps, pancreatitis, GI irritation, ***hepatitis***
EENT: Blurred vision
INTEG: Rash, urticaria, purpura, photosensitivity, fever
META: Hyperglycemia, hyperuricemia, increased creatinine, BUN
HEMA: ***Aplastic anemia, hemolytic anemia, leukopenia, agranulocytosis, thrombocytopenia, neutropenia***
CV: Irregular pulse, orthostatic hypotension, palpitations, volume depletion
ELECT: Hypokalemia, hypercalcemia, hyponatremia, hypochloremia, hypomagnesemia

Contraindications: Hypersensitivity to thiazides or sulfonamides, anuria, renal decompensation, hypomagnesemia

Precautions: Hypokalemia, renal disease, pregnancy (D), hepatic disease, gout, COPD, lupus erythematosus, diabetes mellitus

Pharmacokinetics:
PO: Onset 2 hr, peak 4 hr, duration 6-12 hr; excreted unchanged by kidneys, crosses placenta, enters breast milk

Interactions/incompatibilities:
- Increased toxicity of: lithium, nondepolarizing skeletal muscle relaxants, digitalis
- Decreased effects of: antidiabetics
- Decreased absorption of thiazides: cholestyramine, colestipol

---

* Available in Canada only

• Decreased hypotensive response: indomethacin
• Hyperglycemia, hyperuricemia, hypotension: diazoxide

NURSING CONSIDERATIONS
Assess:
• Weight, I&O daily to determine fluid loss; effect of drug may be decreased if used qd
• Rate, depth, rhythm of respiration, effect of exertion
• B/P lying, standing; postural hypotension may occur
• Electrolytes: potassium, magnesium, sodium chloride; include BUN, blood sugar, CBC, serum creatinine, blood pH, ABGs, uric acid, calcium
• Glucose in urine if patient is diabetic
Administer:
• In AM to avoid interference with sleep if using drug as a diuretic
• Potassium replacement if potassium is less than 3.0
• With food, if nausea occurs, absorption may be decreased slightly
Evaluate:
• Therapeutic response: improvement in edema of feet, legs, sacral area daily if medication is being used in CHF
• Improvement in CVP q8h
• Signs of metabolic alkalosis: drowsiness, restlessness
• Signs of hypokalemia: postural hypotension, malaise, fatigue, tachycardia, leg cramps, weakness, dehydration
• Rashes, temperature elevation qd
• Confusion, especially in elderly; take safety precautions if needed
Teach patient/family:
• To increase fluid intake 2-3 L/day unless contraindicated; to rise slowly from lying or sitting position
• To notify physician of muscle weakness, cramps, nausea, dizziness
• That drug may be taken with food or milk
• That blood sugar may be increased in diabetics
• To take early in day to avoid nocturia
Lab test interferences:
Increase: BSP retention, amylase, parathyroid test
Decrease: PBI, PSP
Treatment of overdose: Lavage if taken orally, monitor electrolytes, administer dextrose in saline, monitor hydration, CV, renal status

hydrocodone bitartrate
(hye-droe-koe'done)
Dihydrocodeinone bitartrate, Hycodan,* Robidone*
Func. class.: Narcotic analgesic
Chem. class.: Opiate

Controlled Substance III
Action: Acts directly on cough center in medulla to suppress cough
Uses: Hyperactive and nonproductive cough, mild pain
Dosages and routes:
• *Adults:* PO 5 mg q4h prn or 10 mg q12h (long-acting)
• *Child:* PO, 2-12 mg 1.25-5 mg q4h prn
Available forms include: Caps 5 mg, susp 5 mg/ml, tabs 5 mg, 10 mg (long-acting)
Side effects/adverse reactions:
CNS: Drowsiness, dizziness, lightheadedness, confusion, headache, sedation, euphoria, dysphoria, weakness, hallucinations, disorientation, ***convulsions***
GI: Nausea, vomiting, anorexia, constipation, cramps, dry mouth
GU: Increased urinary output, dysuria, urinary retention

INTEG: Rash, urticaria, flushing, pruritus
EENT: Tinnitus, blurred vision, miosis, diplopia
CV: Palpitations, tachycardia, bradycardia, change in B/P, ***circulatory depression,*** syncope
RESP: ***Respiratory depression***
Contraindications: Hypersensitivity, addiction (narcotic)
Precautions: Addictive personality, pregnancy (C), lactation, increased intracranial pressure, MI (acute), severe heart disease, respiratory depression, hepatic disease, renal disease, child <18 yr
Pharmacokinetics: Onset 10-20 min, duration 3-6 hr, half-life 3-4 hr; metabolized in liver, excreted in urine, crosses placenta
Interactions/incompatibilities:
• Increased CNS depression: alcohol, narcotics, sedative/hypnotics, phenothiazines, skeletal muscle relaxants, general anesthetics, tricyclic antidepressants

NURSING CONSIDERATIONS
Assess:
• I&O ratio; check for decreasing output; may indicate urinary retention
Administer:
• With antiemetic after meals if nausea or vomiting occur
Perform/provide:
• Storage in light-resistant area at room temperature
• Assistance with ambulation
• Safety measures: siderails, night light, call bell within easy reach
Evaluate:
• Therapeutic response: decrease in pain or cough
• CNS changes: dizziness, drowsiness, hallucinations, euphoria, LOC, pupil reaction
• Allergic reactions: rash, urticaria
• Respiratory dysfunction: respiratory depression, character, rate, rhythm; notify physician if respirations are <10/min
• Need for pain medication, physical dependence
Teach patient/family:
• To report any symptoms of CNS changes, allergic reactions
• That physical dependency may result when used for extended periods of time
• Withdrawal symptoms may occur: nausea, vomiting, cramps, fever, faintness, anorexia
Lab test interferences:
Increase: Amylase, lipase
Treatment of overdose: Narcan 0.2-0.8 IV, O_2, IV fluids, vasopressors

hydrocortisone/hydrocortisone acetate

(hye-droe-kor'ti-sone)
Cortamed,* Otall
Func. class.: Otic
Chem. class.: Synthetic steroid

Action: Antiinflammatory, antipruritic
Uses: Ear canal inflammation
Dosage and routes:
• *Adult and child:* INSTILL 3-4 gtt bid-qid
Available forms include: Otic sol 0.25%, 0.5%, 1%
Side effects/adverse reactions:
EENT: Itching, irritation in ear
INTEG: Rash, urticaria
Contraindications: Hypersensitivity, perforated eardrum
Precautions: Pregnancy (C)

NURSING CONSIDERATIONS
Administer:
• After removing impacted cerumen by irrigation
• After cleaning stopper with alcohol

* Available in Canada only

• After restraining child if necessary
• Warming solution to body temperature

Evaluate:
• Therapeutic response: decreased ear pain, inflammation
• For redness, swelling, fever, pain in ear, which indicates infection

Teach patient/family:
• Method of instillation using aseptic technique, including not touching dropper to ear
• That dizziness may occur after instillation

hydrocortisone/hydrocortisone acetate/hydrocortisone valerate

(hye-droe-kor'ti-sone)

Acticort, Aeroseb-HC, Carmol HC, Cetacort, Cort-Dome, Delacort, Dermicort, Dermolate, Proctocort, Cortaid, Cortef, Cortifoam, Epifoam, My-Cort, Proctofoam-HC, Westcort Cream

Func. class.: Topical corticosteroid
Chem. class.: Natural nonfluorinated, group IV potency (Valerate), group VI potency (acetate and plain)

Action: Possesses antipruritic, antiinflammatory actions

Uses: Psoriasis, eczema, contact dermatitis, pruritus

Dosage and routes:
• *Adult and child >2 yr:* Apply to affected area qd-qid

Available forms include: *Hydrocortisone*—oint 0.5%, 1%, 2.5%; cream 0.25%, 0.5%, 1%, 2.5%; lotion 0.25%, 0.5%, 1%, 2%, 2.5%; gel 1%; sol 1%; aerosol/pump spray 0.5%; *acetate*—oint 0.5%, 1%, 2.5%; cream 0.5%; lotion 0.05%; aerosol 1%; *valerate*—oint 0.2%; cream 0.2% (many others)

Side effects/adverse reactions:
INTEG: Burning, dryness, itching, irritation, acne, folliculitis, hypertrichosis, perioral dermatitis, hypopigmentation, atrophy, striae, miliaria, allergic contact dermatitis, secondary infection

Contraindications: Hypersensitivity to corticosteroids, fungal infections

Precautions: Pregnancy (C), lactation, viral infections, bacterial infections

NURSING CONSIDERATIONS

Assess:
• Temperature; if fever develops, drug should be discontinued

Administer:
• Only to affected areas; do not get in eyes
• Medication, then cover with occlusive dressing (only if prescribed), seal to intact skin, change q12h; systemic absorption may occur, use gloves
• Only to dermatoses; do not use on weeping, denuded, or infected area
• Apply aerosol at distance 15 cm for 1-2 sec

Perform/provide:
• Cleansing before application of drug
• Treatment for a few days after area has cleared
• Storage at room temperature

Evaluate:
• Therapeutic response: absence of severe itching, patches on skin, flaking
• For systemic absorption: increased temperature, inflammation, irritation

Teach patient/family:
• To avoid sunlight on affected area; burns may occur

• Not to use other OTC products unless approved by physician

hydrocortisone/hydrocortisone acetate/hydrocortisone sodium phosphate/hydrocortisone sodium succinate

(hye-dro-kor'ti-sone)

Cortef, Hydrocortone/ Cortef Acetate, Hydrocortone Acetate/Hydrocortone Phosphate/A-Hydrocort, Solu-Cortef, Cortenema

Func. class.: Corticosteroid
Chem. class.: Glucocorticoid, short-acting

Action: Decreases inflammation by suppression of migration of polymorphonuclear leukocytes, fibroblasts, reversal of increased capillary permeability and lysosomal stabilization

Uses: Severe inflammation, shock, adrenal insufficiency, ulcerative colitis, collagen disorders

Dosage and routes:

Adrenal insufficiency/inflammation

• *Adult:* PO 5-30 mg bid-qid; IM/IV 100-250 mg (succinate), then 50-100 mg IM as needed; IM/IV 15-240 mg q12h (phosphate)

Shock

• *Adult:* 500 mg-2 g q2-6h, (succinate)

• *Child:* IM/IV 0.16-1 mg/kg bid-tid (succinate)

Colitis

• *Adult:* ENEMA 100 mg nightly for 21 days

Available forms include: Retention enema 100 mg/60 ml; tabs 5, 10, 20 mg; inj 25, 50 mg/ml; inj 50 mg/ml; phosphate inj 100, 250, 500, 1000 mg/vial; succinate inj 25, 50 mg/ml

Side effects/adverse reactions:

INTEG: Acne, poor wound healing, ecchymosis, petechiae

CNS: Depression, flushing, sweating, headache, mood changes

CV: Hypertension, ***circulatory collapse, thrombophlebitis, embolism***, tachycardia, edema

HEMA: ***Thrombocytopenia***

MS: Fractures, osteoporosis, weakness

GI: Diarrhea, nausea, abdominal distention, ***GI hemorrhage***, increased appetite, ***pancreatitis***

EENT: Fungal infections, increased intraocular pressure, blurred vision

Contraindications: Psychosis, hypersensitivity, idiopathic thrombocytopenia, acute glomerulonephritis, amebiasis, fungal infections, nonasthmatic bronchial disease, child <2 yr, AIDS, TB

Precautions: Pregnancy (C), diabetes mellitus, glaucoma, osteoporosis, seizure disorders, ulcerative colitis, CHF, myasthenia gravis, renal disease, esophagitis, peptic ulcer

Pharmacokinetics:

PO: Onset 1-2 hr, peak 1 hr, duration 1-1½ days

IM/IV: Onset 20 min, peak 4-8 hr, duration 1-1½ days

REC: Onset 3-5 days

Metabolized by liver, excreted in urine (17-OHCS, 17-KS), crosses placenta

Interactions/incompatibilities:

• Decreased action of hydrocortisone: cholestyramine, colestipol, barbiturates, rifampin, ephedrine, phenytoin, theophylline

• Decreased effects of: anticoagulants, anticonvulsants, antidiabetics, ambenonium, neostigmine, isoniazid, toxoids, vaccines, anticholinesterases, salicylates, somatrem

• Increased side effects: alcohol, salicylates, indomethacin, amphotericin B, digitalis, cyclosporine, diuretics
• Increased action of hydrocortisone: salicylates, estrogens, indomethacin, oral contraceptives, ketoconazole, macrolide antibiotics

NURSING CONSIDERATIONS

Assess:
• Potassium, blood sugar, urine glucose while on long-term therapy; hypokalemia and hyperglycemia
• Weight daily, notify physician of weekly gain >5 lb
• B/P q4h, pulse, notify physician if chest pain occurs
• I&O ratio; be alert for decreasing urinary output and increasing edema
• Plasma cortisol levels during long-term therapy (normal level: 138-635 nmol/L SI units when drawn at 8 AM)

Administer:
• IV undiluted or added to dextrose or saline inj and given by infusion; give 25 mg or less/min
• After shaking suspension (parenteral)
• Titrated dose, use lowest effective dose
• IM inj deeply in large mass, rotate sites, avoid deltoid, use 21G needle
• In one dose in AM to prevent adrenal suppression, avoid SC administration, damage may be done to tissue
• With food or milk to decrease GI symptoms

Perform/provide:
• Assistance with ambulation in patient with bone tissue disease to prevent fractures

Evaluate:
• Therapeutic response: ease of respirations, decreased inflammation
• Infection: increased temperature, WBC, even after withdrawal of medication; drug masks symptoms of infection
• Potassium depletion: paresthesias, fatigue, nausea, vomiting, depression, polyuria, dysrhythmias, weakness
• Edema, hypertension, cardiac symptoms
• Mental status: affect, mood, behavioral changes, aggression

Teach patient/family:
• That ID as steroid user should be carried
• To notify physician if therapeutic response decreases; dosage adjustment may be needed
• Not to discontinue this medication abruptly or adrenal crisis can result
• To avoid OTC products: salicylates, alcohol in cough products, cold preparations unless directed by physician
• About cushingoid symptoms
• Symptoms of adrenal insufficiency: nausea, anorexia, fatigue, dizziness, dyspnea, weakness, joint pain

Lab test interferences:
Increase: Cholesterol, sodium, blood glucose, uric acid, calcium, urine glucose
Decrease: Calcium, potassium, T_4, T_3, thyroid ^{131}I uptake test, urine 17-OHCS, 17-KS, PBI
False negative: Skin allergy tests

---

hydrogen peroxide

(per-ox'ide)

Func. class.: Disinfectant
Chem. class.: Oxidizing drug

Action: Destroys bacteria (primarily anaerobic) by mechanical action

Uses: Douche, cleansing wounds, mouthwash for Vincent's stomatitis, removal of ear wax

Dosage and routes:

• *Adult and child:* SOL Use as needed

Available forms include: Top sol 1.5%, 3%

Side effects/adverse reactions:

CV: ***Oxygen emboli***

INTEG: Irritation

EENT: Black hairy tongue, decalcification of tooth enamel

Contraindications: Hypersensitivity to this drug, closed wounds

Precautions: 3rd degree burns, deep wounds

Pharmacokinetics:

TOP: Duration to end of bubbling

NURSING CONSIDERATIONS

Administer:

• To ear canal to facilitate removal of cerumen

• As mouthwash for Vincent's stomatitis; do not use everyday as mouthwash

• After dilution with water or salt water solution

• Only when oxygen can flow in and out of wound; emboli may result

Evaluate:

• Therapeutic response: cleansing of area

• Area of body involved: irritation, rash, breaks, dryness, scales

hydromorphone HCl

(hye-droe-mor'fone)

Dilaudid

Func. class.: Narcotic analgesics

Chem. class.: Opiate, semisynthetic phenanthrene

Controlled Substance Schedule II

Action: Inhibits ascending pain pathways in CNS, increases pain threshold, alters pain perception

Uses: Moderate to severe pain

Dosage and routes:

• *Adult:* PO 1-6 mg q4-6h prn; IM/SC/IV 2-4 mg q4-6h; REC 3 mg hs prn

Available forms include: Inj IM, IV 1, 2, 3, 4 mg/ml; tabs 1, 2, 3, 4 mg; rec supp 3 mg

Side effects/adverse reactions:

CNS: Drowsiness, dizziness, confusion, headache, sedation, euphoria

GI: Nausea, vomiting, anorexia, constipation, cramps

GU: Increased urinary output, dysuria, urinary retention

INTEG: Rash, urticaria, bruising, flushing, diaphoresis, pruritus

EENT: Tinnitus, blurred vision, miosis, diplopia

CV: Palpitations, bradycardia, change in B/P

RESP: ***Respiratory depression***

Contraindications: Hypersensitivity, addiction (narcotic)

Precautions: Addictive personality, pregnancy (C), lactation, increased intracranial pressure, MI (acute), severe heart disease, respiratory depression, hepatic disease, renal disease, child <18 yr

Pharmacokinetics:

Onset 15-30 min, peak ½-1½ hr, duration 4-5 hr; metabolized by liver, excreted by kidneys, crosses placenta, excreted in breast milk

Interactions/incompatibilities:

• Effects may be increased with other CNS depressants: alcohol, narcotics, sedative/hypnotics, antipsychotics, skeletal muscle relaxants

NURSING CONSIDERATIONS

Assess:

• I&O ratio; check for decreasing

output; may indicate urinary retention
• Need for drug

Administer:
• IV diluted with 5 ml of sterile H_2O or normal saline; give through Y-tube, or 3-way stopcock; give 2 mg or less/5 min
• With antiemetic if nausea, vomiting occur
• When pain is beginning to return; determine dosage interval by patient response

Perform/provide:
• Storage in light-resistant area at room temperature
• Assistance with ambulation
• Safety measures: siderails, night light, call bell within easy reach

Evaluate:
• Therapeutic response: decrease in pain
• CNS changes: dizziness, drowsiness, hallucinations, euphoria, LOC, pupil reaction
• Allergic reactions: rash, urticaria
• Respiratory dysfunction: respiratory depression, character, rate, rhythm; notify physician if respirations are <10/min
• Need for pain medication, physical dependence

Teach patient/family:
• To report any symptoms of CNS changes, allergic reactions
• That physical dependency may result when used for extended periods of time
• Withdrawal symptoms may occur: nausea, vomiting, cramps, fever, faintness, anorexia

Lab test interferences:
Increase: Amylase

Treatment of overdose: Narcan 0.2-0.8 IV, O_2, IV fluids, vasopressors

hydromorphone HCl

(hye-droe-mor'fone)
Dilaudid Cough Syrup

Func. class.: Antitussive, narcotic
Chem. class.: Phenanthrene derivative, guaifenesin

Controlled Substance Schedule II

Action: Increases respiratory tract fluid by decreasing surface tension, adhesiveness, which increases removal of mucus; possesses analgesic, antitussive properties

Uses: Cough

Dosage and routes:
• *Adult:* PO 1 mg q3-4h prn
• *Child 6-12 yr:* PO 0.5 mg q3-4h prn

Available forms include: Syr 1 mg/5 ml

Side effects/adverse reactions:
CNS: Dizziness, drowsiness
GI: Nausea, constipation, vomiting, anorexia
CV: Hypotension
INTEG: Urticaria, rash
RESP: ***Respiratory depression***

Contraindications: Hypersensitivity, increased intracranial pressure, status asthmaticus

Precautions: Hypothyroidism, Addison's disease, CNS depression, brain tumor, asthma, hepatic disease, renal disease, COPD, psychosis, alcoholism, convulsive disorders, pregnancy (C)

Pharmacokinetics: Metabolized by liver, half-life 2-4 hr

Interactions/incompatibilities:
• Enhanced CNS depression: barbiturates, narcotics, antipsychotics, antidepressants

NURSING CONSIDERATIONS

• VS, cardiac status including hypotension
• Respiratory rate, depth

Administer:
• Decreased dose to elderly patients; their metabolism may be slowed
Perform/provide:
• Storage at room temperature
• Increased fluids, bulk, exercise to patient's lifestyle to decrease constipation
Evaluate:
• Therapeutic response: absence of cough
• Cough: type, frequency, character including sputum
Teach patient/family:
• To avoid driving, other hazardous activities until patient is stabilized on this medication if drowsiness occurs
• To avoid alcohol, other CNS depressants; will enhance sedating properties of this drug

hydroquinone

(hye'droe-kwin-one)

Derma-Blanch, Eldopaque, Eldoquin, Esoterica Medicated Cream, Melanex, Quinnone, Porcelana, Solaquin

Func. class.: Depigmentating agent
Chem. class.: Enzyme inhibitor

Action: Inhibits production of tyrosine, which is needed in formation of melanin
Uses: Bleaching skin, including age spots, freckles, lentigo, chloasma
Dosage and routes:
• *Adult and child:* TOP apply to affected area qd-bid
Available forms include: Top cream 2%, 4%; top lotion 2%; gel 4%; sol 3%
Side effects/adverse reactions:
INTEG: Rash, dryness, fissures, stinging, contact dermatitis, erythema, irritation
Contraindications: Hypersensitivity, inflamed skin, prickly heat, sunburn
Precautions: Pregnancy (C), lactation, child <1 yr

NURSING CONSIDERATIONS

Administer:
• Topical corticosteroid for irritation
• Test dose to be applied to area 25 mm in diameter, check site after 24 hr; if itching or excessive inflammation occurs, drug should not be used
Perform/provide:
• Storage at room temperature in tight container
Evaluate:
• Therapeutic response: fading of spots over time
• Area of body involved, including time involved, what helps or aggravates condition
Teach patient/family:
• To avoid application on normal skin or getting cream in eyes
• To use opaque sunscreen during day on exposed areas or bleaching effect may be reversed
• That minor redness is not a contraindication
• To continue to use sunscreen after bleaching is complete

hydroxocobalamin (vitamin B_{12})

Acti-B_{12},* Alpha Redisol, Alpha-Ruvite, Codrozomin, Droxomin, Neo-Betalin 12, Rubesol-LA

Func. class.: Vitamin
Chem. class.: B_{12}—water-soluble vitamin

Action: Needed for adequate nerve functioning, protein and carbohy-

* Available in Canada only

drate metabolism, normal growth, RBC development

Uses: Vitamin B_{12} deficiency, pernicious anemia, vitamin B_{12} malabsorption syndrome, Schilling test

Dosage and routes:

• *Adult:* IM 30-100 μg qd × 5-10 days, maintenance 100-200 mg IM qmo

• *Child:* IM 1-30 μg qd × 5-10 days, maintenance 60 μg IM qmo or more often

Pernicious anemia/malabsorption syndrome

• *Adult:* IM 100-1000 μg qd × 2 wk, then 100-1000 μg IM qmo

• *Child:* IM 1000-5000 μg × 2 wk or more given in 100-500 μg doses, then 60 μg IM/SC mo

Schilling test

• *Adult and child:* IM 1000μg in one dose

Available forms include: Inj IM 100, 120, 1000 μg/ml

Side effects/adverse reactions:

CNS: Flushing, optic nerve atrophy

GI: Diarrhea

CV: ***CHF,*** peripheral vascular thrombosis, ***pulmonary edema***

INTEG: Itching, rash

Contraindications: Hypersensitivity, optic nerve atrophy

Precautions: Pregnancy (A), lactation, children

Pharmacokinetics: Stored in liver, kidneys, stomach; 50%-90% excreted in urine, crosses placenta, breast milk

Interactions/incompatibilities:

• Decreased absorption of hydroxocobalamin: aminoglycosides, anticonvulsants, colchicine, chloramphenicol, aminosalicylic acid, potassium preparations

• Increased absorption of this drug: prednisone

NURSING CONSIDERATIONS

Assess:

• Potassium levels during beginning treatment

• CBC for increased reticulocyte count during 1st week of therapy, followed by increase in RBC and hemoglobin

Administer:

• With fruit juice to disguise taste

• With meals if possible for better absorption

• By IM inj for pernicious anemia unless contraindicated

Evaluate:

• Therapeutic response: decreased anorexia, dyspnea on excretion, palpitations, paresthesias, psychosis, visual disturbances

• Nutritional status: egg yolks, fish, organ meats, dairy products, clams, oysters, which are good sources for vitamin B_{12}

• For pulmonary edema, or worsening of CHF in cardiac patients

Teach patient/family

• That treatment must continue for life if diagnosed as having pernicious anemia

• Importance of well-balanced diet

• To avoid persons with infections

Lab test interferences:

False positive: Intrinsic factor

---

hydroxychloroquine sulfate

(hye-drox-ee-klor'oh-kwin)

Plaquenil Sulfate

Func. class.: Antimalarial

Chem. class.: 4-aminoquinoline derivative

Action: Inhibits parasite replications, transcription of DNA to RNA by forming complexes with DNA of parasite

Uses: Malaria caused by *P. vivax,*

P. malariae, P. ovale, P. falciparum (some strains): lupus erythematosus, rheumatoid arthritis

Dosage and routes:

Malaria

• *Adult and child:* PO 5 mg/kg/wk on same day of week, not to exceed 400 mg; treatment should begin 2 wk before entering endemic area, continue 8 wk after leaving; if treatment begins after exposure, 800 mg for adult, 10 mg/kg for children in 2 divided doses 6 hr apart

Lupus erythematosus

• *Adult:* PO 400 mg qd-bid, length depends on patient response; maintenance 200-400 mg qd

Rheumatoid arthritis

• *Adult:* PO 400-600 mg qd, then 200-300 mg qd after good response

Available forms include: Tabs 200 mg

Side effects/adverse reactions:

CV: Hypotension, heart block, ***asystole with syncope***

INTEG: Pruritus, pigmentation changes, skin eruptions, lichen planuslike eruptions, eczema, ***exfoliative dermatitis,*** alopecia

CNS: Headache, stimulation, fatigue, irritability, ***convulsion,*** bad dreams, dizziness, confusion, psychosis, decreased reflexes

EENT: Blurred vision, corneal changes, retinal changes, difficulty focusing, tinnitus, vertigo, deafness, photophobia, corneal edema

GI: Nausea, vomiting, anorexia, diarrhea, cramps

HEMA: ***Thrombocytopenia, agranulocytosis, hemolytic anemia, leukopenia***

Contraindications: Hypersensitivity, retinal field changes, prophyria, children (long-term)

Precautions: Blood dyscrasias, severe GI disease, neurologic disease, alcoholism, hepatic disease, G-6-PD deficiency, psoriasis, eczema, pregnancy (C)

Pharmacokinetics:

PO: Peak 1-2 hr, half-life 3-5 days, metabolized in liver, excreted in urine, feces, breast milk, crosses placenta

Interactions/incompatibilities:

• Decreased action of hydroxychloroquine: magnesium or aluminum compounds

• Increased levels of: digoxin

NURSING CONSIDERATIONS

Assess:

• Ophthalmic test if long-term treatment or drug dosage >150 mg/day

• Liver studies qwk: AST, ALT, bilirubin

• Blood studies: CBC, since blood dyscrasias occur

• For decreased reflexes: knee, ankle

• ECG during therapy

• Watch for depression of T waves, widening of QRS complex

Administer:

• Before or after meals at same time each day to maintain drug level

• IM after aspirating to avoid injection into blood system, which may cause hypotension, asystole, heart block; rotate injection sites

Perform/provide:

• Storage in tight, light-resistant containers at room temperature; injection should be kept in cool environment

Evaluate:

• Therapeutic response: decreased symptoms of malaria

• Allergic reactions: pruritus, rash, urticaria

• Blood dyscrasias: malaise, fever, bruising, bleeding (rare)

• For ototoxicity (tinnitus, vertigo, change in hearing); audiometric testing should be done before, after treatment

• For toxicity: blurring vision, difficulty focusing, headache, dizziness, knee, ankle reflexes; drug should be discontinued immediately

Teach patient/family:

• To use sunglasses in bright sunlight to decrease photophobia

• That urine may turn rust or brown color

• To report hearing, visual problems, fever, fatigue, bruising, bleeding, which may indicate blood dyscrasias

Treatment of overdose: Induce vomiting, gastric lavage, administer barbiturate (ultrashort-acting), vasopressin, ammonium chloride; tracheostomy may be necessary

---

hydroxyprogesterone caproate

(hye-drox-ee-proe-jess'te-rone)
Delalutin, Dura-lutin

Func. class.: Progestogen, hormone

Action: Inhibits secretion of pituitary gonadotropins, which prevents follicular maturation, ovulation, stimulates growth of mammary tissue, antineoplastic action against endometrial cancer

Uses: Uterine cancer, menstrual disorders

Dosage and routes:

• *Adult:* IM 125-375 mg q4wk, discontinue after 4 cycles

Uterine cancer

• *Adult:* IM 1-5 g/wk

Available forms include: Inj IM 125, 250 mg/ml

Side effects/adverse reactions:

CNS: Dizziness, headache, migraines, depression, fatigue

CV: Hypotension, thrombophlebitis, edema, ***thromboembolism, stroke, pulmonary embolism, myocardial infarction***

GI: Nausea, vomiting, anorexia, cramps, increased weight, ***cholestatic jaundice***

EENT: Diplopia

GU: Amenorrhea, cervical erosion, breakthrough bleeding, dysmenorrhea, vaginal candidiasis, breast changes, *gynecomastia, testicular atrophy, impotence,* endometriosis, ***spontaneous abortion***

INTEG: Rash, urticaria, acne, hirsutism, alopecia, oily skin, seborrhea, purpura, melasma, photosensitivity

META: Hyperglycemia

Contraindications: Breast cancer, hypersensitivity, thromboembolic disorders, reproductive cancer, genital bleeding (abnormal, undiagnosed), pregnancy (X)

Precautions: Lactation, hypertension, asthma, blood dyscrasias, gallbladder disease, HF, diabetes mellitus, bone disease, depression, migraine headache, convulsive disorders, hepatic disease, renal disease, family history of breast or reproductive tract cancer

Pharmacokinetics:

IM: Half-life 5 min, duration 24 hr, excreted in urine, feces, metabolized in liver

NURSING CONSIDERATIONS

Assess:

• Weight daily, notify physician of weekly weight gain >5 lb

• B/P at beginning of treatment and periodically

• I&O ratio; be alert for decreasing urinary output, increasing edema

• Liver function studies: ALT, AST, bilirubin, periodically during long-term therapy

Administer:
• Titrated dose, use lowest effective dose
• Oil solution deeply in large muscle mass (IM), rotate sites
• In one dose in AM
• With food or milk to decrease GI symptoms
• After warming to dissolve crystals

Perform/provide:
• Storage in dark area

Evaluate:
• Therapeutic response: decreased abnormal uterine bleeding, absence of amenorrhea
• Edema, hypertension, cardiac symptoms, jaundice
• Mental status: affect, mood, behavioral changes, depression
• Hypercalcemia

Teach patient/family:
• To avoid sunlight or use sunscreen; photosensitivity can occur
• About cushingoid symptoms
• To report breast lumps, vaginal bleeding, edema, jaundice, dark urine, clay-colored stools, dyspnea, headache, blurred vision, abdominal pain, numbness or stiffness in legs, chest pain; male to report impotence or gynecomastia
• To report suspected pregnancy

Lab test interferences:
Increase: Alk phosphatase, nitrogen (urine), pregnanediol, amino acids
Decrease: GTT, HDL

---

hydroxyurea

(hye-drox'ee-yoo-ree-ah)
Hydrea
Func. class.: Antineoplastic-antimetabolite
Chem. class.: Synthetic urea analog

Action: Acts by inhibiting DNA synthesis without interfering with RNA or protein synthesis; incorporates thymidine into DNA, causing direct damage to DNA strands

Uses: Melanoma, chronic myelocytic leukemia, recurrent or metastatic ovarian cancer, squamous cell carcinoma of the head and neck

Dosage and routes:
Solid tumors
• *Adult:* PO 80 mg/kg as a single dose q3 days or 20-30 mg/kg as a single dose qd
In combination with radiation
• *Adult:* PO 80 mg/kg as a single dose q3d
Resistant chronic myelocytic leukemia
• *Adult:* PO 20-30 mg/kg/day as a single daily dose
Available forms include: Caps 500 mg

Side effects/adverse reactions:
HEMA: ***Leukopenia, anemia, thrombocytopenia***
GI: Nausea, vomiting, anorexia, diarrhea, stomatitis, constipation
GU: Increased BUN, uric acid, creatinine, temporary renal function impairment
INTEG: *Rash,* urticaria, pruritus, dry skin
CV: Angina, ischemia
CNS: Headache, confusion, hallucinations, dizziness, ***convulsions***

Contraindications: Hypersensitivity, leukopenia (<2500/mm^3), thrombocytopenia (<100,000/mm^3), anemia (severe), pregnancy (D)

Precautions: Renal disease (severe)

Pharmacokinetics: Readily absorbed when taken orally, peak level in 2 hr, degraded in liver, excreted in urine, almost totally eliminated in 24 hr; readily crosses blood-brain barrier

---

* Available in Canada only

Interactions/incompatibilities:
- Increased toxicity: radiation or other antineoplastics

NURSING CONSIDERATIONS

Assess:
- CBC, differential, platelet count weekly; withhold drug if WBC is <3500/mm^3 or platelet count is <100,000/mm^3; notify physician of these results; drug should be discontinued
- Renal function studies: BUN, serum uric acid, urine CrCl, electrolytes before, during therapy
- I&O ratio; report fall in urine output to <30 ml/hr
- Monitor temperature q4h; fever may indicate beginning infection
- Liver function tests before, during therapy: bilirubin, alk phosphatase, AST, ALT, LDH; as needed or monthly
- B/P q3-4h; check for chest pain; angina, ischemia may occur

Administer:
- Allopurinol or $NaHCO_3$ concurrently to prevent high uric acid levels; extra fluids
- Antiemetic 30-60 min before giving drug to prevent vomiting and prn
- Antibiotics for prophylaxis of infection
- Transfusion for anemia

Perform/provide:
- Rinsing of mouth tid-qid with water, club soda; brushing of teeth bid-tid with soft brush or cotton-tipped applicators for stomatitis; use unwaxed dental floss
- Nutritious diet with iron, vitamin supplements as ordered

Evaluate:
- Therapeutic response: decreased tumor size, spread of malignancy
- Bleeding: hematuria, guaiac, bruising or petechiae, mucosa or orifices q8h
- Food preferences; list likes, dislikes
- Inflammation of mucosa, breaks in skin
- Buccal cavity q8h for dryness, sores or ulceration, white patches, oral pain, bleeding, dysphagia
- Symptoms indicating severe allergic reaction: rash, urticaria, itching, flushing
- Neurotoxicity: headaches, hallucinations, convulsions, dizziness

Teach patient/family:
- To report signs of infection: increased temperature, sore throat, flu symptoms
- To report signs of anemia: fatigue, headache, faintness, shortness of breath, irritability
- To report bleeding: avoid use of razors, or commercial mouthwash
- To avoid use of aspirin products or ibuprofen
- To avoid foods with citric acid, hot or rough texture if stomatitis is present
- To report stomatitis: any bleeding, white spots, ulcerations in the mouth; tell patient to examine mouth qd, report symptoms
- That contraceptive measures are recommended during therapy
- To drink 10-12 (8 oz) glasses of fluid/day
- To notify physician of fever, chills, sore throat, nausea, vomiting, anorexia, diarrhea, bleeding, bruising; may indicate blood dyscrasias

Lab test interferences:
Increase: Renal function studies

H

hydroxyzine HCl/ hydroxyzine pamoate

(hye-drox'i-zeen)

Atarax, Durrax, Orgatrax, Quiess, Vistaril/Vistaril IM

Func. class.: Antianxiety
Chem. class.: Piperazine derivative

Action: Depresses subcortical levels of CNS, including limbic system, reticular formation

Uses: Anxiety, preoperatively, postoperatively to prevent nausea, vomiting, to potentiate narcotic analgesics, sedation, pruritus

Dosage and routes:

- *Adult:* PO 25-100 mg tid-qid
- *Child >6 yr:* 50-100 mg/day in divided doses
- *Child <6 yr:* 50 mg/day in divided doses

Preoperatively/postoperatively

- *Adult:* IM 25-100 mg q4-6h
- *Child:* IM 1.1 mg/kg q4-6h

Available forms include: Tabs 10, 25, 50, 100 mg; caps 25, 50, 100 mg; syrup 10 mg/5 ml; oral susp 25 mg/5 ml; IM inj

Side effects/adverse reactions:

CNS: Dizziness, drowsiness, confusion, headache, tremors, fatigue, depression, convulsions

GI: Dry mouth

Contraindications: Hypersensitivity, pregnancy (C)

Precautions: Elderly, debilitated, hepatic disease, renal disease

Pharmacokinetics:

PO: Onset 15-30 min, duration 4-6 hr, half-life 3 hr

Interactions/incompatibilities:

- Increased CNS depressant effect: barbiturates, narcotics, analgesics, alcohol

NURSING CONSIDERATIONS

Assess:

- B/P (lying, standing), pulse; if systolic B/P drops 20 mm Hg, hold drug, notify physician
- Blood studies: CBC
- Hepatic studies: AST, ALT, bilirubin, creatinine

Administer:

- By Z-track injection in large muscle for IM to decrease pain, chance of necrosis
- With food or milk for GI symptoms
- Crushed if patient is unable to swallow medication whole
- Gum, hard candy, frequent sips of water for dry mouth

Perform/provide:

- Assistance with ambulation during beginning therapy, since drowsiness/dizziness occurs
- Safety measures, including siderails
- Checking to see PO medication has been swallowed

Evaluate:

- Therapeutic response: decreased anxiety
- Mental status: mood, sensorium, affect
- Increased sedation

Teach patient/family:

- Not to be used for everyday stress or used longer than 4 mo
- Avoid OTC preparations (cold, cough, hay fever) unless approved by physician
- To avoid driving, activities that require alertness
- To avoid alcohol ingestion, or other psychotropic medications
- Not to discontinue medication quickly after long-term use
- To rise slowly or fainting may occur

Lab test interferences:

False increase: 17-OHCS

Treatment of overdose: Lavage if orally ingested; VS, supportive care; IV norepinephrine for hypotension

hyoscyamine sulfate

(hye-oh-sye'a-meen)

Anaspaz, Levsin, Levsinex

Func. class.: Gastrointestinal anticholinergic

Chem. class.: Belladonna alkaloid

Action: Inhibits muscarinic actions of acetylcholine at postganglionic parasympathetic neuroeffector sites

Uses: Treatment of peptic ulcer disease in combination with other drugs; other GI disorders, other spastic disorders

Dosage and routes:

- *Adult:* PO/SL 0.125-0.25 mg tid-qid ac, hs; TIME REL 0.375 q12h; IM/SC/IV 0.25-0.5 mg q6h
- *Child 2-10 yr:* ½ adult dose
- *Child <2 yr:* ¼ adult dose

Available forms include: Tabs 0.125, 0.13, 0.15 mg; caps time rel 0.375 mg; sol 0.125 mg/ml; elix 0.125 mg/5 ml; inj IM, IV, SC 0.5 mg/ml

Side effects/adverse reactions:

CNS: Confusion, stimulation in elderly, headache, insomnia, dizziness, drowsiness, anxiety, weakness, hallucination

GI: Dry mouth, constipation, paralytic ileus, heartburn, nausea, vomiting, dysphagia, absence of taste

GU: Hesitancy, retention, impotence

CV: Palpitations, tachycardia

EENT: Blurred vision, photophobia, mydriasis, cycloplegia, increased ocular tension

INTEG: Urticaria, rash, pruritus, anhidrosis, fever, allergic reactions

Contraindications: Hypersensitivity to anticholinergics, narrow-angle glaucoma, GI obstruction, myasthenia gravis, paralytic ileus, GI atony, toxic megacolon, prostatic hypertrophy

Precautions: Hyperthyroidism, coronary artery disease, dysrhythmias, CHF, ulcerative colitis, hypertension, hiatal hernia, hepatic disease, renal disease, pregnancy (C), urinary retention

Pharmacokinetics:

PO: Duration 4-6 hr; metabolized by liver, excreted in urine, half-life 3.5 hr

Interactions/incompatibilities:

- Decreased effect of hyoscyamine: antacids
- Increased anticholinergic effect: amantadine, tricyclic antidepressants, MAOIs, H_1 antihistamines
- Decreased effect of: phenothiazines, levodopa, ketoconazole

NURSING CONSIDERATIONS

Assess:

- VS, cardiac status: checking for dysrhythmias, increased rate, palpitations
- I&O ratio; check for urinary retention or hesitancy

Administer:

- ½ hr ac for better absorption
- Decreased dose to elderly patients; their metabolism may be slowed
- Gum, hard candy, frequent rinsing of mouth for dryness of oral cavity

Perform/provide:

- Storage is tight container protected from light
- Increased fluids, bulk, exercise to patient's lifestyle to decrease constipation

Evaluate:

- Therapeutic response: absence of epigastric pain, bleeding, nausea, vomiting
- GI complaints: pain, bleeding

H

(frank or occult), nausea, vomiting, anorexia

Teach patient/family:

- To avoid driving or other hazardous activities until stabilized on medication
- To avoid alcohol or other CNS depressants; will enhance sedating properties of this drug
- To avoid hot environments, stroke may occur, drug suppresses perspiration
- To use sunglasses when outside to prevent photophobia, may cause blurred vision

ibuprofen

(eye-byoo'proe-fen)

Amersol, Motrin, Rufen

Func. class.: Nonsteroidal antiinflammatory

Chem. class.: Propionic acid derivative

Action: Inhibits prostaglandin synthesis by decreasing enzyme needed for biosynthesis; possesses analgesic, antiinflammatory, antipyretic properties

Uses: Rheumatoid arthritis, osteoarthritis, primary dysmenorrhea, gout, dental pain, musculoskeletal disorders

Dosage and routes:

- *Adult:* PO 200-800 mg qid, not to exceed 3.2 g/day

Available forms include: Tabs 200, 300, 400, 600, 800 mg

Side effects/adverse reactions:

GI: Nausea, anorexia, vomiting, diarrhea, jaundice, ***cholestatic hepatitis,*** constipation, flatulence, cramps, dry mouth, peptic ulcer

CNS: Dizziness, drowsiness, fatigue, tremors, confusion, insomnia, anxiety, depression

CV: Tachycardia, peripheral edema, palpitations, dysrhythmias

INTEG: Purpura, rash, pruritus, sweating

GU: ***Nephrotoxicity: dysuria, hematuria, oliguria, azotemia***

HEMA: ***Blood dyscrasias***

EENT: Tinnitus, hearing loss, blurred vision

Contraindications: Hypersensitivity, asthma, severe renal disease, severe hepatic disease

Precautions: Pregnancy (B) 1st and 2nd trimester, lactation, children, bleeding disorders, GI disorders, cardiac disorders, hypersensitivity to other antiinflammatory agents

Pharmacokinetics:

PO: Peak 1-2 hr, half-life 2-4 hr, metabolized in liver (inactive metabolites), excreted in urine (inactive metabolites), 90%-99% plasma protein binding

Interactions/incompatibilities:

- May increase action of: coumarin, phenytoin, sulfonamides
- Decreased action of ibuprofen: salicylates

NURSING CONSIDERATIONS

Assess:

- Renal, liver, blood studies: BUN, creatinine, AST, ALT, Hgb, before treatment, periodically thereafter
- Audiometric, ophthalmic examination before, during, after treatment
- Cardiac status: edema (peripheral), tachycardia, palpitations; monitor B/P, pulse for character, quality, rhythm
- For past history of peptic ulcer disorder

Administer:

- With food to decrease GI symptoms; however, best to take on empty stomach to facilitate absorption

Perform/provide:
• Storage at room temperature
Evaluate:
• Therapeutic response: decreased pain, stiffness in joints, decreased swelling in joints, ability to move more easily
• For eye, ear problems: blurred vision, tinnitus; may indicate toxicity
Teach patient/family:
• To report blurred vision, ringing, roaring in ears; may indicate toxicity
• To avoid driving, other hazardous activities if dizziness, drowsiness occurs
• To report change in urine pattern, increased weight, edema, increased pain in joints, fever, blood in urine; indicate nephrotoxicity
• That therapeutic inflammatory effects may take up to 1 mo
• To avoid alcohol, salicylates; bleeding may occur
• To avoid sun or sunlamp exposure

---

idarubicin HCl

(eye-dah-roob'ih-sin)
Idamycin

Func. class.: Antineoplastic, antibiotic
Chem. class.: Anthracycline glycoside

Action: Inhibits DNS synthesis derived from daunorubicin by binding to DNA, which causes strand splitting; cell cycle specific (S phase); a vesicant
Uses: Used in combination with other antineoplastics for acute myelocytic leukemia in adults
Dosage and routes:
Adult: IV 12 $mg/m^2/day \times 3$ days in combination with cytosine arabinoside, or 25 mg/m^2 IV bolus followed by 200 $mg/m^2/day \times 5$ days by continuous INF
Available forms include: inj IV 5, 10 mg
Side effects/adverse reactions:
HEMA: ***Thrombocytopenia, leukopenia, anemia***
GI: Nausea, vomiting, abdominal pain, mucositis, diarrhea, ***hepatoxicity***
INTEG: Rash, extravasation, dermatitis, reversible alopecia, urticaria, thrombophlebitis at injection site
CV: ***Dysrhythmias, CHF, pericarditis, myocarditis,*** peripheral edema
CNS: Fever, chills, headache
Contraindications: Hypersensitivity, pregnancy (D)
Precautions: Renal and hepatic disease, gout, bone marrow depression, children
Pharmacokinetics: Half-life 22 hr, metabolized by liver, crosses placenta, excreted in bile, urine (primarily as metabolites)
Interactions/incompatibilities:
• Increased toxicity: other antineoplastics or radiation
• Do not mix with other drugs in solution or syringe

NURSING CONSIDERATIONS

Assess:
• CBC, differential, platelet count weekly; withhold drug if WBC is 4000/mm^3 or platelet count is 75,000/mm^3; notify physician of these results
• Blood, urine, uric acid levels
• Renal function studies: BUN, serum uric acid, urine CrCl, electrolytes before, during therapy
• I&O ratio; report fall in urine output to <30 ml/hr
• Monitor temperature q4h; fever may indicate beginning infection
• Liver function tests before, dur-

ing therapy: bilirubin, AST, ALT, alk phosphatase as needed or monthly
• ECG: watch for ST-T wave changes, low QRS and T, possible dysrhythmias (sinus tachycardia, heart block, PVCs)

Administer:
• Antiemetic 30-60 min before giving drug and 6-10 hr after treatment to prevent vomiting
• After reconstituting 5 mg vial with 5 ml 0.9% NaCl (1 mg/1 ml), give over 10-15 min
• Antibiotics for prophylaxis of infection
• Allopurinol or sodium bicarbonate to reduce uric acid levels, alkalinization, or urine
• Transfusion for anemia
• Hydrocortisone for extravasation; apply ice compress after stopping infusion

Perform/provide:
• Strict handwashing technique, gloves, protective clothing
• Liquid diet: carbonated beverages, gelatin may be added if patient is not nauseated or vomiting
• Increase fluid intake to 2-3 L/day to prevent urate and calculi formation
• Diet low in purines: absence of organ meats (kidney, liver), dried beans, peas to reduce uric acid level
• Rinsing of mouth tid-qid with water, club soda; brushing of teeth tid-qid with soft brush or cotton-tipped applicators for stomatitis; use unwaxed dental floss
• Storage at room temperature for 3 days after reconstituting or 7 days refrigerated

Evaluate:
• Therapeutic response: decreased tumor size, spread of malignancy
• Bleeding: hematuria, guaiac stools, bruising or petechiae, mucosa or orifices q8h
• Food preferences: list likes, dislikes
• Effects of alopecia on body image; discuss feelings about body changes
• Inflammation of mucosa, breaks in skin
• Yellowing of skin, sclera, dark urine, clay-colored stools, itchy skin, abdominal pain, fever, diarrhea
• Buccal cavity q8h for dryness, sores, or ulceration, white patches, oral pain, bleeding, dysphagia
• Local irritation, pain, burning at injection site
• GI symptoms: frequency of stools, cramping
• Acidosis, signs of dehydration: rapid respirations, poor skin turgor, decreased urine output, dry skin, restlessness, weakness
• Cardiac status: B/P, pulse, character, rhythm, rate

Teach patient/family:
• To report any complaints, side effects to nurse or physician
• That hair may be lost during treatment and wig or hairpiece may make patient feel better; tell patient that new hair may be different in color, texture
• To avoid foods with citric acid, hot or rough texture
• To report any bleeding, white spots, ulcerations in mouth; tell patient to examine mouth qd
• That urine may be red-orange for 48 hr

Lab test interferences:
Increase: Uric acid

idoxuridine-IDU (ophthalmic)

(eye-dox-your'ih-deen)
Dendrid Herplex, IDU Stoxil
Func. class.: Antiviral
Chem. class.: Pyrimidine nucleoside

Action: Inhibits viral replication by interfering with viral DNA synthesis
Uses: Herpes simplex keratitis, cytomegalovirus, varicella-zoster alone or with corticosteroids
Dosage and routes:
• *Adult and child:* INSTILL 1 gtt q1h during day and 2 hr during night; TOP apply oint q4h × 1 wk, if no response, discontinue
Available forms include: Oint 0.5%, sol 0.1%
Side effects/adverse reactions:
EENT: Poor corneal wound healing, temporary visual haze, overgrowth of nonsusceptible organisms
Contraindications: Hypersensitivity
Precautions: Antibiotic hypersensitivity, pregnancy (C)
Interactions/incompatibilities:
• Do not use boric acid with this drug

NURSING CONSIDERATIONS
Administer:
• After washing hands, cleanse crusts or discharge from eye before application
Perform/provide:
• Storage in refrigerator, in light-resistant container until used
Evaluate:
• Therapeutic response: absence of redness, inflammation, tearing, photophobia
• Allergy: itching, lacrimation, redness, swelling
Teach patient/family:
• To use drug exactly as prescribed
• Not to use eye makeup, towels, washcloths, eye medication of others; reinfection may occur
• That drug container tip should not be touched to eye
• To report itching, increased redness, burning, stinging, swelling; drug should be discontinued
• That drug may cause blurred vision when ointment is applied

ifosfamide

(i-foss'fa-mid)
Ifex
Func. class.: Antineoplastic alkylating agent
Chem. class.: Nitrogen mustard

Action: Alkylates DNA, RNA, inhibits enzymes that allow synthesis of amino acids in proteins; also responsible for cross-linking DNA strands
Uses: Testicular cancer
Dosage and routes:
• *Adult:* IV 1.2 g/m^2/day × 5 days, repeat course q3wk
Available forms include: Inj 1, 3 g
Side effects/adverse reactions:
CNS: Facial paresthesia, fever, malaise, somnolence, confusion, depression, hallucinations, dizziness, disorientation, ***seizures, coma***
GI: Nausea, vomiting, anorexia, ***hepatotoxicity,*** stomatitis, constipation
INTEG: Dermatitis, alopecia, pain at injection site
GU: ***Hematuria, nephrotoxicity, hemorrhagic cystitis,*** dysuria, urinary frequency
HEMA: ***Thrombocytopenia, leukopenia, anemia***

Contraindications: Hypersensitivity, bone marrow suppression

Precautions: Renal disease, pregnancy (D), lactation, children

Pharmacokinetics: Metabolized by liver, saturation occurs at high doses, excreted in urine, half-life 7-15 hr

NURSING CONSIDERATIONS

Assess:

• Liver function studies before, during therapy (bilirubin, AST, ALT, LDH) as needed or monthly

• CBC, differential, platelet count weekly; withhold drug if WBC is <4000 or platelet count is <75,000; notify physician of results

• Monitor temperature q4h (may indicate beginning infection)

Administer:

• Antiemetic 30-60 min before giving drug to prevent vomiting

• Antibiotics for prophylaxis of infection

• Slow IV infusion using 21-, 23-, 25-gauge needle; watch for extravasation

Perform/provide:

• Storage of powder at room temperature

• Strict medical asepsis, protective isolation if WBC levels are low

• Increase fluid intake to 2-3 L/day to prevent urate deposits, calculi formation

• Warm compresses at injection site for inflammation

Evaluate:

• Therapeutic response: decrease in size and spread of tumor

• Blood dyscrasias (anemia, granulocytopenia); bruising, fatigue, bleeding, poor healing

• Allergic reactions: dermatitis, exfoliative dermatitis, pruritus, urticaria

• Bleeding: hematuria, guaiac, bruising or petechiae, mucosa or orifices q8h

• Food preferences; list likes, dislikes

• Effects of alopecia on body image, discuss feelings about body changes

• Yellowing of skin, sclera, dark urine, clay-colored stools, itchy skin, abdominal pain, fever, diarrhea

• Inflammation of mucosa, breaks in skin

Teach patient/family:

• To call physician if sore throat, swollen lymph nodes, malaise, fever occur since other infections may occur

• About protective isolation precautions

• That hair may be lost during treatment; a wig or hairpiece may make the patient feel better; new hair may be different in color, texture

• To report signs of anemia: fatigue, headache, faintness, shortness of breath, irritability

• To report bleeding; avoid use of razors or commercial mouthwash

• To avoid use of aspirin products or ibuprofen

• To use contraceptive measures during therapy

---

imipenem/cilastatin

i-me-pen′em sye-la-stat′in

Primaxin

Func. class.: Antiinfective-misc penicillin

Action: Interferes with cell wall replication of susceptible organisms; osmotically unstable cell wall swells, bursts from osmotic pressure; addition of cilastatin prevents renal inactivation that occurs with high urinary concentrations of imipenem

Uses: Serious infections caused by gram-positive: *S. pneumoniae*, group A beta-hemolytic streptococci, *S. aureus*, enterococcus; gram-negative: *Klebsiella, Proteus, E. coli, Acinetobacter, Serratia, P. aeruginosa; Salmonella, Shigella*

Dosage and routes:

• *Adult:* IV 250-500 mg q6h; severe infections may require 1 g q6h; may give IM (total daily IM dosage >1500 mg not recommended)

Available forms include: Inj 250, 500, 750 mg vials

Side effects/adverse reactions:

CNS: Fever, somnolence, ***seizures,*** dizziness, weakness

GI: Diarrhea, nausea, vomiting, ***pseudomembranous colitis, hepatitis,*** glossitis

CV: Hypotension, palpitations

HEMA: ***Eosinophilia, neutropenia,*** decreased HGb, HtC

INTEG: Rash, urticaria, pruritus, pain at injection site, phlebitis, erythema at injection site

SYST: ***Anaphylaxis***

RESP: Chest discomfort, dyspnea, hyperventilation

Contraindications: Hypersensitivity, IM hypersensitivity to local anesthetics of the amide type

Precautions: Pregnancy (C), lactation, elderly, hypersensitivity to penicillins, seizure disorders, renal disease, children

Pharmacokinetics:

IV: Onset immediate, peak ½-1 hr, half-life 1 hr

Interactions/incompatibilities:

• Increased imipenem plasma levels: probenecid

• Do not mix or physically add to other antibiotics

NURSING CONSIDERATIONS

Assess:

• Sensitivity to penicillin or other cephalosporins

• Renal disease: lower dose may be required

• Bowel pattern qd; if severe diarrhea occurs, drug should be discontinued; may indicate pseudomembranous colitis

Administer:

• After reconstitution of 250 or 500 mg with 10 ml of diluent and shake; add to at least 100 ml of diluent; place contents in infusion bottle with 100 ml of compatible diluent, shake

• 250-500 mg over 20-30 min; 1 g over 40-60 min; do not give by IV bolus or cloudy solutions

• After C&S is taken

Evaluate:

• Therapeutic response: negative C&S

• Allergic reactions: rash, urticaria, pruritus; may occur few days after therapy begins

• Overgrowth of infection: perineal itching, fever, malaise, redness, pain, swelling, drainage, rash, diarrhea, change in cough, sputum

Teach patient/family:

• To report severe diarrhea; may indicate pseudomembranous colitis

• To report sore throat, bruising, bleeding, joint pain; may indicate blood dyscrasias (rare)

Lab test interferences:

Increase: AST, ALT, LDH, BUN, alk phosphatase, bilirubin, creatinine

False positive: Direct Coombs' test

Treatment of overdose: Epinephrine, antihistamines; resuscitate if needed (anaphylaxis)

imipramine HCl

(im-ip'ra-meen)

Impril,* Janimine, Novopramine,* Presamine, Ropramine, Tipramine, Tofranil

Func. class.: Antidepressant—tricyclic

Chem. class.: Dibenzazepine—tertiary amine

Action: Blocks reuptake of norepinephrine, serotonin into nerve endings, increasing action of norepinephrine, serotonin in nerve cells

Uses: Depression, enuresis in children

Dosage and routes:

- *Adult:* PO/IM 75-100 mg/day in divided doses, may increase by 25-50 mg to 200 mg, not to exceed 300 mg/day; may give daily dose hs
- *Child:* PO 25-75 mg/day

Available forms include: Tabs 10, 25, 50 mg; inj IM 25 mg/2 ml

Side effects/adverse reactions:

HEMA: ***Agranulocytosis, thrombocytopenia, eosinophilia, leukopenia***

CNS: Dizziness, drowsiness, confusion, headache, anxiety, tremors, stimulation, weakness, insomnia, nightmares, EPS (elderly), increased psychiatric symptoms, paresthesia

GI: Diarrhea, dry mouth, nausea, vomiting, ***paralytic ileus,*** increased appetite, cramps, epigastric distress, jaundice, ***hepatitis,*** stomatitis

GU: Retention, ***acute renal failure***

INTEG: Rash, urticaria, sweating, pruritus, photosensitivity

CV: Orthostatic hypotension, ECG changes, tachycardia, ***hypertension,*** palpitations

EENT: Blurred vision, tinnitus, mydriasis

Contraindications: Hypersensitivity to tricyclic antidepressants, recovery phase of myocardial infarction, convulsive disorders, prostatic hypertrophy

Precautions: Suicidal patients, severe depression, increased intraocular pressure, narrow-angle glaucoma, urinary retention, cardiac disease, hepatic disease, hyperthyroidism, electroshock therapy, elective surgery, elderly, pregnancy (C)

Pharmacokinetics:

PO: Steady state 2-5 days; metabolized by liver, excreted by kidneys, feces, crosses placenta, excreted in breast milk, half-life 6-20 hr

Interactions/incompatibilities:

- Decreased effects of: guanethidine, clonidine, indirect acting sympathomimetics (ephedrine)
- Increased effects of: direct acting sympathomimetics (epinephrine), alcohol, barbiturates, benzodiazepines, CNS depressants
- Hyperpyretic crisis, convulsions, hypertensive episode: MAOI (pargyline [Eutonyl])

NURSING CONSIDERATIONS

Assess:

- B/P (lying, standing), pulse q4h; if systolic B/P drops 20 mm Hg hold drug, notify physician; take vital signs q4h in patients with cardiovascular disease
- Blood studies: CBC, leukocytes, differential, cardiac enzymes if patient is receiving long-term therapy
- Hepatic studies: AST, ALT, bilirubin, creatinine
- Weight qwk, appetite may increase with drug
- ECG for flattening of T wave,

*Available in Canada only

bundle branch block, AV block, dysrhythmias in cardiac patients

Administer:

• Increased fluids, bulk in diet if constipation, urinary retention occur

• With food or milk for GI symptoms

• Dosage hs if oversedation occurs during day; may take entire dose hs; elderly may not tolerate once/day dosing

• Gum, hard candy, or frequent sips of water for dry mouth

Perform/provide:

• Storage in tight container at room temperature, do not freeze

• Assistance with ambulation during beginning therapy since drowsiness/dizziness occurs

• Safety measures including side rails primarily in elderly

• Checking to see PO medication swallowed

Evaluate:

• Therapeutic response: decreased depression, enuresis

• EPS primarily in elderly: rigidity, dystonia, akathisia

• Mental status: mood, sensorium, affect, suicidal tendencies, increase in psychiatric symptoms: depression, panic

• Urinary retention, constipation; constipation is more likely to occur in children, elderly

• Withdrawal symptoms: headache, nausea, vomiting, muscle pain, weakness; do not usually occur unless drug was discontinued abruptly

• Alcohol consumption; if alcohol is consumed, hold dose until morning

Teach patient/family:

• That therapeutic effects may take 2-3 wk

• To use caution in driving or other activities requiring alertness because of drowsiness, dizziness, blurred vision

• To avoid alcohol ingestion, other CNS depressants

• Not to discontinue medication quickly after long-term use, may cause nausea, headache, malaise

• To wear sunscreen or large hat since photosensitivity occurs

Lab test interferences:

Increase: Serum bilirubin, alk phosphatase, blood glucose

Decrease: 5-HIAA, VMA, urinary catecholamines

Treatment of overdose: ECG monitoring, induce emesis, lavage, activated charcoal, administer anticonvulsant

---

immune globulin

Gamastan, Gamimune, Gammar, Immuglobin, Sandoglobulin

Func. class.: Immune serum
Chem. class.: IgG

Action: Provides passive immunity to hepatitis A, measles, varicella, rubella, immune globulin deficiency

Uses: Agammaglobulinemia, hepatitis A exposure, measles exposure, measles vaccine complications, purpura, rubella exposure, chickenpox exposure

Dosage and routes:

• *Adult:* IM 30-50 ml q mo; IV 100 mg/kg qmo, 0.01-0.02 ml/kg/min × ½ hr (Gamimune); IV 200 mg/kg q, 0.05-1 ml/min × 15-30 min, then increase to 1.5-2.5 ml/min (Sandoglobulin)

• *Child:* IM 20-40 ml qmo

Hepatitis A exposure

• *Child and adult:* IM 0.02-0.04 ml/kg or 0.1 mg/kg if treatment is delayed

Hepatitis B exposure
• *Adult and child:* IM 0.06 ml/kg within 1 wk, qmo
Measles
• *Child:* IM 0.25 ml/kg within 6 days
Immunoglobulin deficiency
• *Child:* IM 1.3 ml/kg, then 0.66 ml/kg after 2-4 wk and q2-4wk thereafter
Idiopathic thrombocytopenia purpura
• *Adult:* IV 0.4 g/kg × 5 days
Available forms include: IV, IM inj 2, 10 ml/vial
Side effects/adverse reactions:
INTEG: Pain at injection site, rash, pruritus, chills, chest pain
MS: Arthralgia
SYST: Lymphadenopathy, ***anaphylaxis***
CNS: Headache, fatigue, malaise
GI: Abdominal pain
Contraindications: Hypersensitivity
Precautions: Pregnancy (C)
Interactions/incompatibilities:
• Do not administer live virus vaccines within 3 mo of this drug

NURSING CONSIDERATIONS
Administer:
• Gamimune: IV undiluted or dilute with D_5; give 0.01 ml/kg/ min; may increase to 0.02-0.04 ml/kg/ min
• Sandoglobulin: IV diluted with provided diluent; give 0.5-1 ml/ min × 15-30 min; may increase to 1.5-2.5 ml/min
• IM ≤3ml in one site, use large muscle mass
• Only after epinephrine 1:1000, resuscitative equipment are available
• Only within 2 wk of exposure to hepatitis A
Perform/provide:
• Storage at 2°-8° C
Teach patient/family:
• Passive immunity is temporary

indapamide

(in-dap'a-mide)
Lozol, Lozide*
Func. class.: Diuretic—thiazide-like
Chem. class.: Indoline

Action: Acts on proximal section of distal renal tubule by inhibiting reabsorption of sodium; may act by direct vasodilation caused by blocking of calcium channel
Uses: Edema, hypertension, diuresis
Dosage and routes:
• *Adult:* PO 2.5 mg qd in AM, may be increased to 5 mg qd if needed
Available forms include: Tabs 2.5 mg
Side effects/adverse reactions:
GU: Polyuria, dysuria, frequency
ELECT: Hypochloremic alkalosis, hypomagnesemia, hyperuricemia, hypercalcemia, hyponatremia, hypokalemia, hyperglycemia
CNS: Headache, dizziness, fatigue, weakness, paresthesias, depression
GI: Nausea, diarrhea, dry mouth, vomiting, anorexia, cramps, constipation, pancreatitis, abdominal pain, jaundice, hepatitis
EENT: Loss of hearing, tinnitus, blurred vision, nasal congestion, increased intraocular pressure
INTEG: Rash, pruritus, photosensitivity, alopecia, urticaria
MS: Cramps
HEMA: ***Thrombocytopenia, agranulocytosis, leukopenia, neutropenia, anemia***
CV: Orthostatic hypotension, volume depletion, palpitations
Contraindications: Hypersensitivity, anuria

*Available in Canada only

Precautions: Hypokalemia, dehydration, ascites, hepatic disease, severe renal disease, pregnancy (B)
Pharmacokinetics:
PO: Onset 1-2 hr, peak 2 hr, duration up to 36 hr; excreted in urine, feces, half-life 14-18 hr
Interactions/incompatibilities:
• Hyperglycemia, hyperuricemia, hypotension: diazoxide
• Muscle relaxants, steroids, lithium, digitalis
• Decreased potassium: steroids
• Decreased effects: antidiabetics
• Decreased absorption: cholestyramine, colestipol
• Decreased hypotensive effect: indomethacin

NURSING CONSIDERATIONS
Assess:
• Weight daily, I&O daily to determine fluid loss; effect of drug may be decreased if used qd
• Rate, depth, rhythm of respiration, effect of exertion
• B/P lying, standing; postural hypotension may occur
• Electrolytes: potassium, magnesium, sodium chloride; include BUN, CBC, serum creatinine, blood pH, ABGs, uric acid, calcium, glucose
Administer:
• In AM to avoid interference with sleep
• With food, if nausea occurs, absorption may be decreased slightly
Evaluate:
• Therapeutic response: improvement in edema of feet, legs, sacral area daily if medication is being used in CHF
• Improvement in CVP q8h
• Signs of metabolic alkalosis
• Signs of hypokalemia
• Rashes, temperature elevation qd
• Confusion, especially in elderly; take safety precautions if needed
• Hydration: skin turgor, thirst, dry mucous membranes
Teach patient/family:
• To increase fluid intake 2-3 L/day unless contraindicated; to rise slowly from lying or sitting position
• Adverse reactions: muscle cramps, weakness, nausea, dizziness
• To take with food or milk for GI symptoms
• To take early in day to prevent nocturia
Lab test interferences:
Increase: Calcium, parathyroid test
Treatment of overdose: Lavage if taken orally, monitor electrolytes, administer IV fluids, monitor hydration, CV, renal status

indecainide HCl
(in-de-kane'ide)
Decabid
Func. class.: Antidysrhythmic, (Class Ic)

Action: Unknown; able to slow conduction, reduce membrane responsiveness, inhibits automaticity, increases ratio of effective refractory period to action potential duration
Uses: Life-threatening dysrhythmias, sustained ventricular tachycardia
Dosage and routes:
• *Adult:* PO 100-200 mg/day in divided dose q12h; 50 mg q12h initially, then increase dose by 25 mg increments q4d, max 400 mg/day
Available forms include: Ext Rel tabs 50, 75, 100 mg
Side effects/adverse reactions:
CV: ***Dysrhythmias, CHF***
CNS: Headache, dizziness, lightheadedness
GI: Constipation, nausea

GU: Impotence
EENT: Blurred vision, diplopia
Contraindications: 2nd or 3rd degree AV block, right bundle branch block, cardiogenic shock, hypersensitivity
Precautions: Severe CHF, hypokalemia, hyperkalemia, sick-sinus syndrome, pregnancy (B), lactation, children, impaired hepatic or renal disease
Pharmacokinetics:
Half-life 9-10 hr metabolized by the liver; 63% of drug recovered in urine
Interactions/incompatibilities:
- Increased effect of indecainide: cimetidine
- Increased serum concentrations of: digoxin

NURSING CONSIDERATIONS
Assess:
- GI status: bowel pattern, number of stools
- Cardiac status: rate, rhythm, quality
- Chest x-ray, pulmonary function test during treatment
- I&O ratio; check for decreasing output
- B/P for fluctuations
- Lung fields; bilateral rales may occur in CHF patient
- Increased respiration, increased pulse; drug should be discontinued

Evaluate:
- Therapeutic response: absence of dysrhythmias
- Cardiac rate: respiration, rate, rhythm, character continuously

Lab test interferences:
Increase: CPK
Treatment of overdose: O_2, artificial ventilation, ECG, administer dopamine for circulatory depression, administer diazepam or thiopental for convulsions

indomethacin/ indomethacin sodium trihydrate

(in-doe-meth'a-sin)
Indocid, Indocin, Indocin SR, Indomed/Indocin IV
Func. class.: Nonsteroidal
Chem. class.: Propionic acid derivative

Action: Inhibits prostaglandin synthesis by decreasing enzyme needed for biosynthesis; possesses analgesic, antiinflammatory, antipyretic properties
Uses: Rheumatoid arthritis, ankylosing rheumatoid spondylitis, acute gouty arthritis, closure of patent ductus arteriosus in premature infants
Dosage and routes:
Arthritis
- *Adult:* PO/REC 25 mg bid-tid, may increase by 25 mg/day qwk, not to exceed 200 mg/day; SUS REL 75 mg qd, may increase to 75 mg bid

Acute arthritis
- *Adult:* PO/REC 50 mg tid; use only for acute attack, then reduce dose

Patent ductus arteriosus
- *Infant <2 days:* IV 0.2 mg/kg, then 0.1 mg/kg q12-24 hr
- *Infant 2-7 days:* IV 0.2 mg/kg, then 0.2 mg × 2 doses after 12, 24 hr
- *Infant >7 days:* IV 0.2 mg/kg, then 0.25 mg/kg × 2 doses after 12, 24 hr

Available forms include: Caps 25, 50 mg; caps ext rel 75 mg; susp 25 mg/5 ml; rec supp 50 mg
Side effects/adverse reactions:
GI: Nausea, anorexia, vomiting, diarrhea, jaundice, ***cholestatic hep-***

*Available in Canada only

atitis, constipation, flatulence, cramps, dry mouth, peptic ulcer
CNS: Dizziness, drowsiness, fatigue, tremors, confusion, insomnia, anxiety, depression
CV: Tachycardia, peripheral edema, palpitations, dysrhythmias
INTEG: Purpura, rash, pruritus, sweating
GU: ***Nephrotoxicity: dysuria, hematuria, oliguria, azotemia***
HEMA: ***Blood dyscrasias***
EENT: Tinnitus, hearing loss, blurred vision
Contraindications: Hypersensitivity, asthma, severe renal disease, severe hepatic disease
Precautions: Pregnancy, lactation, children, bleeding disorders, GI disorders, cardiac disorders, hypersensitivity to other antiinflammatory agents, pregnancy (B) 1st and 2nd trimesters, depression
Pharmacokinetics:
PO: Onset 1-2 hr, peak 3 hr, duration 4-6 hr; metabolized in liver, kidneys, excreted in urine, bile, feces, crosses placenta, excreted in breast milk, 99% plasma protein binding
Interactions/incompatibilities:
- Increased action of: coumarin, phenytoin, sulfonamides
- Toxicity: lithium, methotrexate
- Decreased action of: triamterene
- Do not give with antacids

NURSING CONSIDERATIONS
Assess:
- Renal, liver, blood studies: BUN, creatinine, AST, ALT, Hgb, before treatment, periodically thereafter
- Audiometric, ophthalmic exam before, during, after treatment

Administer:
- IV after diluting 1 mg/ml or more normal saline or sterile H_2O for inj without preservative; give over 5-10 sec
- With food to decrease GI symptoms; however, best to take on empty stomach to facilitate absorption

Perform/provide:
- Storage at room temperature

Evaluate:
- Therapeutic response: decreased pain, stiffness in joints, decreased swelling in joints, ability to move more easily
- For eye, ear problems: blurred vision, tinnitus; may indicate toxicity
- For confusion, mood changes, hallucinations

Teach patient/family:
- To report blurred vision, ringing, roaring in ears; may indicate toxicity
- To avoid driving, other hazardous activities if dizziness, drowsiness occurs
- To report change in urine pattern, increased weight, edema, increased pain in joints, fever, blood in urine; indicate nephrotoxicity; to report mood changes: anxiety, depression
- That therapeutic antiinflammatory effects may take up to 1 mo
- To avoid alcohol, salicylates; bleeding may occur

influenza virus vaccine, trivalent A & B (whole virus/split virus)

Fluzone, Fluogen, Fluviral*
Func. class.: Vaccine

Action: Produces antibodies to influenza virus by production of antibodies; split virus vaccine causes less adverse reactions
Uses: Prevention of Russian, Chile, Philippine influenza
Dosage and routes:
- *Adult and child >12 yr:* IM 0.5 ml in 1 dose

• *Child 3-12 yr:* IM 0.5 ml, repeat in 1 mo (split) unless 1978-1985 vaccine was given
• *Child 6 mo to 3 yr:* IM 0.25 ml, repeat in 1 mo (split) unless 1978-1985 vaccine was given
Available forms include: Inj IM 100 μg/ml
Side effects/adverse reactions:
CNS: Fever, Guillain-Barré syndrome
INTEG: Urticaria, induration, erythema
SYST: ***Anaphylaxis,*** malaise
MS: Myalgia
Contraindications: Hypersensitivity, active infection, chicken, egg allergy, Guillain-Barré syndrome
Precautions: Elderly, immunosuppression, pregnancy

NURSING CONSIDERATIONS
Assess:
• For skin reactions: rash, induration, erythema
Administer:
• Only with epinephrine 1:1000 on unit to treat laryngospasm
• Only IM
Perform/provide:
• Written record of immunization
• At least 2 mo after measles virus vaccine; do not administer at same time as DPT
Evaluate:
• For history of allergies, skin conditions (eczema, psoriasis, dermatitis), reactions to vaccinations
• For anaphylaxis: inability to breathe, bronchospasm

insulin, isophane suspension (NPH)

Beef NPH Iletin II, Humulin N, Iletin NPH,* Insulatard NPH, NPH Iletin I, Pork NPH Iletin II, Protaphane NPH, Novolin N,* NPH Insulin, NPH Purified Pork

Func. class.: Antidiabetic
Chem. class.: Exogenous unmodified insulin

Action: Decreases blood sugar, and indirectly increases blood pyruvate, lactate, decreases phosphate, potassium
Uses: Ketoacidosis, Type I (IDDM), Type II (NIDDM) diabetes mellitus, hyperkalemia
Dosage and routes:
• *Adult:* SC dosage individualized by blood, urine glucose, usual dose 7-26 U, may increase by 2-10 U/day if needed
Available forms include: SC 40, 100 U/ml
Side effects/adverse reactions:
CNS: Headache, lethargy, tremors, weakness, fatigue, delirium, sweating
CV: Tachycardia, palpitations
EENT: Blurred vision, dry mouth
GI: Hunger, nausea
META: Hypoglycemia
INTEG: Flushing, rash, urticaria, warmth, lipodystrophy, lipohypertrophy
SYST: ***Anaphylaxis***
Contraindications: Hypersensitivity to protamine
Precautions: Pregnancy (B)
Interactions/incompatibilities:
• Increased hypoglycemia: salicylate, alcohol, β-blockers, anabolic steroids, fenfluramine, phenylbutazone, sulfinpyrazone, guanethidine, oral hypoglycemics, MAOIs, tetracycline

*Available in Canada only

• Decreased hypoglycemia: thiazides, thyroid hormones, oral contraceptives, corticosteroids, estrogens, dobutamine, epinephrine

Pharmacokinetics:

SC: Onset 1-2 hr, peak 4-12 hr, duration 18-24 hr

Metabolized by liver, muscle, kidneys; excreted in urine

NURSING CONSIDERATIONS

Assess:

• Fasting blood glucose, 2 hr PP (80-150 mg/dl normal fasting level) (70-130 mg/dl-normal 2 hr level)

• Urine ketones during times of illness; insulin requirements may increase during times of stress, illness

Administer:

• After warming to room temperature by rotating in palms to prevent injecting cold insulin

• Increased doses if tolerance occurs

• Human insulin to those allergic to beef or pork

Perform/provide:

• Storage at room temperature for <1 mo, keep away from heat and sunlight, refrigerate all other supply, do not use if discolored; do not freeze

• Rotation of injection sites within one area: abdomen, upper back, thighs, upper arm, buttocks; keep record of sites

Evaluate:

• Therapeutic response: decrease in polyuria, polydipsia, polyphagia, clear sensorium, absence of dizziness, stable gait

• Hypoglycemic reaction that can occur during peak time

Teach patient/family:

• That blurred vision occurs, not to change corrective lens until vision is stabilized 1-2 mo

• To keep insulin, equipment available at all times

• That drug does not cure diabetes, but controls symptoms

• To carry Medic Alert ID as diabetic

• Hypoglycemia reaction: headache, tremors, fatigue, weakness

• Dosage, route, mixing instructions, if any diet restrictions, disease process

• To carry candy or lump sugar to treat hypoglycemia

• Symptoms of ketoacidosis: nausea, thirst, polyuria, dry mouth, decreased B/P, dry, flushed skin, acetone breath, drowsiness, Kussmaul respirations

• That a plan is necessary for diet, exercise; all food on diet should be eaten, exercise routine should not vary

• About urine glucose testing; make sure patient is able to determine glucose, acetone levels

• To use glucose oxidase reagents

• To avoid OTC drugs unless directed by physician

Lab test interferences:

Increase: VMA

Decrease: Potassium, calcium

Interference: Liver function studies, thyroid function studies

Treatment of overdose: 10%-50% glucose PO if conscious or IV if comatose or 1 mg glucagon

---

insulin, isophane suspension and regular insulin

Humulin 70/30, Mixtard, Novolin 70/30

Func. class.: Antidiabetic
Chem. class.: Exogenous unmodified insulin

Action: Decreases blood sugar, indirectly increases blood pyruvate, lactate, decreases phosphate, potassium

Uses: Ketoacidosis, Type I (IDDM), Type II (NIDDM) diabetes mellitus, hyperkalemia

Dosage and routes:

• *Adult:* SC individualized dose

Available forms include: 70 U/ml isophane insulin with 30 U/ml regular insulin = 100 U/ml

Side effects/adverse reactions:

CNS: Headache, lethargy, tremors, weakness, fatigue, delirium, sweating

CV: Tachycardia, palpitations

EENT: Blurred vision, dry mouth

GI: Hunger, nausea

META: Hypoglycemia

INTEG: Flushing, rash, urticaria, warmth, lipodystrophy, lipohypertrophy

SYST: ***Anaphylaxis***

Contraindications: Hypersensitivity to protamine

Precautions: Pregnancy (B)

Interactions/incompatibilities:

• Increased hypoglycemia: salicylate, alcohol, β-blockers, anabolic steroids, fenfluramine, guanethidine, sulfinpyrazone, oral hypoglycemics, MAOIs, tetracycline

• Decreased hypoglycemia: thiazides, thyroid hormones, oral contraceptives, corticosteroids, estrogens, dobutamine, epinephrine, smoking, levothyroxine

Pharmacokinetics:

SC: Onset 30 min, peak 4-8 hr, duration 12-24 hr

Metabolized by liver, muscle, kidneys; excreted in urine

NURSING CONSIDERATIONS

Assess:

• Fasting blood glucose, 2 hr PP (80-150 mg/dl normal fasting level) (70-130 mg/dl-normal 2 hr level)

• Urine ketones during times of illness; insulin requirement increases during times of stress; illness

Administer:

• After warming to room temperature by rotating in palms to prevent injecting cold insulin

• Increased doses if tolerance occurs

• Human insulin to those allergic to beef or pork

Perform/provide:

• Storage at room temperature for <1 mo, keep cool and away from heat, refrigerate all other supply, do not use if discolored

• Rotation of injection sites within one area: abdomen, upper back, thighs, upper arm, buttocks; keep record of sites

Evaluate:

• Therapeutic response: decrease in polyuria, polydipsia, polyphagia, clear sensorium, absence of dizziness, stable gait

• Hypoglycemic reaction that can occur during peak time

Teach patient/family:

• That blurred vision occurs, not to change corrective lens until vision is stabilized 1-2 mo

• To keep insulin, equipment available at all times

• That drug does not cure diabetes, but controls symptoms

• To carry Medic Alert ID as diabetic

• Hypoglycemia reaction: headache, tremors, fatigue, weakness

• Dosage, route, mixing instructions, if any diet restrictions, disease process

• To carry candy or lump sugar to treat hypoglycemia

• Symptoms of ketoacidosis: nausea, thirst, polyuria, dry mouth, decreased B/P, dry, flushed skin, ace-

* Available in Canada only

tone breath, drowsiness, Kussmaul respirations
• That a plan is necessary for diet, exercise; all food on diet should be eaten, exercise routine should not vary
• About urine glucose testing; make sure patient is able to determine glucose, acetone levels
• That pregnant patient should use glucose oxidase reagents
• To avoid OTC drugs unless directed by physician

Lab test interferences:
Increase: VMA
Decrease: Potassium, calcium
Interference: Liver function studies, thyroid function studies
Treatment of overdose: 10%-50% glucose PO if conscious or IV if comatose or glucogon 1 mg

insulin, regular

Beef Regular Iletin II, Humulin BR, Humulin R, Iletin Regular,* Novolin R, Pork Regular Iletin II, Regular Iletin I, Regular Pork Insulin, Regular purified Pork, Novolin R PenFill, Velosulin

Func. class.: Antidiabetic
Chem. class.: Exogenous unmodified insulin

Action: Decreases blood sugar, indirectly increases blood pyruvate, lactate, decreases phosphate, potassium
Uses: Adult-onset diabetes, juvenile diabetes, ketoacidosis, Type I, II, NIDDM, IDDM, hyperkalemia
Dosage and routes:
Ketoacidosis
• *Adult:* IV/IM 5-10 U, then 5-10 U/hr until desired response, then switch to SC dose; IV/INF 2-12 U (50 U/500 ml of normal saline)
• *Child:* IV/IM 0.1 U/kg
Replacement
• *Adult:* SC dosage individualized by blood, urine glucose levels, up to qid given ½ hr before meals
Available forms include: IV/IM/SC inj U 40, U 100/ml
Side effects/adverse reactions:
CNS: Headache, lethargy, tremors, weakness, fatigue, delirium, sweating
CV: Tachycardia, palpitations
EENT: Blurred vision, dry mouth
GI: Hunger, nausea
META: Hypoglycemia
INTEG: Flushing, rash, urticaria, warmth, lipodystrophy, lipohypertrophy
SYST: ***Anaphylaxis***
Contraindications: Hypersensitivity
Precautions: Pregnancy (B)
Interactions/incompatibilities:
• Increased hypoglycemia: salicylate, alcohol, β-blockers, anabolic steroids, fenfluramine, guanethidine, oral hypoglycemics, MAOIs, tetracycline, sulfinpyrazone
• Decrease hypoglycemia: thiazides, thyroid hormones, oral contraceptives, corticosteroids, estrogens, dobutamine, epinephrine, dextrothyroxine, smoking
• Mask signs/symptoms of hypoglycemia: β-blocker
Pharmacokinetics:
SC: Onset 30-60 min, peak 2-3 hr, duration 5-7 hr
IV: Onset 10-30 min, peak 30-60 min, duration 1-2 hr, half-life 3-5 min; metabolized by liver, muscle, kidneys, excreted in urine

NURSING CONSIDERATIONS

Assess:
• Fasting blood glucose, 2 hr PP (60-100 mg/dl normal fasting level) (70-130 mg/dl-normal 2 hr level)

• Urine ketones during illness; insulin requirements increase during times of stress, illness

Administer:

• After warming to room temperature by rotating in palms, to prevent lipodystrophy (from injecting cold insulin)

• ½ hr ac, so peak action coincides with peak sugar level

• Increased doses if tolerance occurs

• Human insulin to those allergic to beef or pork

• IV undiluted through Y-tube or 3-way stopcock, give 50 U or less/min; may be diluted in 0.9% NS or 0.45% saline for INF; run at rate ordered

Perform/provide:

• Storage at room temperature for <1 month, keep in cool area, refrigerate all other supply, do not use discolored, or cloudy solution

• Rotation of injection sites: abdomen, upper back, thighs, upper arm, buttocks; keep record of sites

Evaluate:

• Therapeutic response: decrease in polyuria, polydipsia, polyphagia, clear sensorium, absence of dizziness, stable gait

• Hypoglycemic/hyperglycemic reaction that can occur soon after meals

Teach patient/family:

• That blurred vision occurs, not to change corrective lens until vision is stabilized 1-2 mo

• To keep insulin, equipment available at all times

• That drug does not cure diabetes, but controls symptoms

• To carry Medic Alert ID as diabetic

• Hypoglycemia reaction: headache, tremors, fatigue, weakness, sweating

• Dosage, route, mixing instructions if any diet restrictions, disease process

• To carry candy or lump sugar to treat hypoglycemia

• Symptoms of ketoacidosis: nausea, thirst, polyuria, dry mouth, decrease B/P, dry, flushed skin, acetone breath, drowsiness, Kussmaul respirations

• That a plan is necessary for diet, exercise; all food on diet should be eaten, exercise routine should not vary

• About urine glucose testing; make sure patient is able to determine glucose, acetone levels, also home blood glucose monitoring

• That pregnant patients should use glucose oxidase reagents

• To avoid OTC drugs unless directed by physician

Lab test interferences:

Increase: VMA

Decrease: Potassium, calcium

Interference: Liver function studies, thyroid function studies

Treatment of overdose: 10%-50% glucose PO if conscious or IV if comatose or 1 mg glucagon

---

insulin, regular concentrated

Regular (concentrated) Iletin II U-500

Func. class.: Antidiabetic
Chem. class.: Exogenous unmodified insulin

Action: Decreases blood sugar, indirectly increases blood pyruvate, lactate, decreases phosphate, potassium

Uses: Treatment of diabetic patients with marked insulin resistance (>200 U/day)

Dosage and routes:
• *Adult:* SC/IM dosage individualized by blood, urine glucose qd-tid
Available forms include: Inj SC, IM 500 U/ml
Side effects/adverse reactions:
CNS: Headache, lethargy, tremors, weakness, fatigue, delirium, sweating
CV: Tachycardia, palpitations
EENT: Blurred vision
GI: Hunger, nausea, dry mouth
META: Hypoglycemia
INTEG: Flushing, rash, urticaria, warmth, lipodystrophy, lipohypertrophy
SYST: ***Anaphylaxis***
MISC: Thirst, leg pain, increased urination
Contraindications: Hypersensitivity
Precautions: Pregnancy (B)
Pharmacokinetics:
SC: Onset 30-60 min, peak 2-5 hr, duration 5-7 hr
Metabolized by liver, muscle, kidneys, excreted in urine
Interactions/incompatibilities:
• Increased hypoglycemia: salicylate, alcohol, β-blockers, anabolic steroids, fenfluramine, guanethidine, oral hypoglycemics, MAOIs, tetracycline, sulfinpyrazone
• Decreased hypoglycemia: thiazides, thyroid hormones, oral contraceptives, corticosteroids, estrogens, smoking, dextrothyroxine, dobutamine, epinephrine

NURSING CONSIDERATIONS

Assess:
• Fasting blood glucose, 2 hr PP (60-100 mg/dl normal fasting level) (70-130 mg/dl-normal 2 hr level)
• Urine ketones during times of illness; insulin requirements increase during stress, illness

Administer:
• After warming to room temperature by rotating in palms, to prevent lipodystrophy from injecting cold insulin
• ½ hr ac, so peak action coincides with peak sugar level
• Increased doses if tolerance occurs

Perform/provide:
• Storage in refrigerator, do not freeze, do not use discolored, or cloudy solution
• Rotation of injection sites: abdomen, upper back, thighs, upper arms, buttocks; keep record of sites

Evaluate:
• Therapeutic response: decrease in polyuria, polydipsia, polyphagia, clear sensorium, absence of dizziness, stable gait
• Hypoglycemic/hyperglycemic reaction that can occur soon after meals or suddenly while on therapy

Teach patient/family:
• That blurred vision occurs, not to change corrective lens until vision is stabilized 1-2 mo
• To keep insulin, equipment available at all times
• That drug does not cure diabetes, but controls symptoms
• To carry Medic Alert ID as diabetic
• Hypoglycemia reaction: headache, tremors, fatigue, weakness
• Dosage, route, mixing instructions if any diet restrictions, disease process
• To carry candy or lump sugar to treat hypoglycemia
• Symptoms of ketoacidosis: nausea, thirst, polyuria, dry mouth, decrease B/P, dry, flushed skin, acetone breath, drowsiness, Kussmaul respirations
• That a plan is necessary for diet, exercise; all food on diet should be

eaten, exercise routine should not vary
- About urine glucose testing, make sure patient is able to determine glucose, acetone levels
- That pregnant patients should use glucose oxidase reagents
- To avoid OTC drugs unless directed by physician

Lab test interferences:
Increase: VMA
Decrease: Potassium, calcium
Interference: Liver function studies, thyroid function studies
Treatment of overdose: 10%-50% glucose PO if conscious or IV if comatose or 1 mg glucagon

insulin, zinc suspension (Lente)

Beef Lente Iletin II, Lente Iletin I, Lente Insulin, Pork Lente Iletin II, Lentard Monotard,* Novolin L, Humulin L, Lente Purified Pork Insulin

Func. class.: Antidiabetic
Chem. class.: Exogenous unmodified insulin

Action: Decreases blood sugar, indirectly increases blood pyruvate, lactate, decreases phosphate, potassium
Uses: Ketoacidosis, Type I (IDDM), Type II (NIDDM) diabetes mellitus, hyperkalemia
Dosage and routes:
- *Adult:* SC individualized

Available forms include: SC 40, 100 U/ml
Side effects/adverse reactions:
CNS: Headache, lethargy, tremors, weakness, fatigue, delirium, sweating
CV: Tachycardia, palpitations
EENT: Blurred vision, dry mouth
GI: Hunger, nausea
META: ***Hypoglycemia***
INTEG: Flushing, rash, urticaria, warmth, lipodystrophy, lipohypertrophy
SYST: ***Anaphylaxis***
Contraindications: Hypersensitivity to protamine
Precautions: Pregnancy (B)
Pharmacokinetics:
SC: Onset 1-2½ hr, peak 7-15 hr, duration 12-24 hr
Metabolized by liver, muscle, kidneys; excreted in urine
Interactions/incompatibilities:
- Increased hypoglycemia: salicylate, alcohol, β-blockers, anabolic steroids, fenfluramine, guanethidine, oral hypoglycemics, MAOIs, tetracycline, sulfinpyrazone
- Hyperglycemia: thiazides, thyroid hormones, oral contraceptives, corticosteroids, estrogens, dobutamine, epinephrine, smoking, levothyroxine

NURSING CONSIDERATIONS
Assess:
- Fasting blood glucose, 2 hr PP (80-150 mg/dl normal fasting level) (70-130 mg/dl-normal 2 hr level)
- Urine ketones during times of illness; insulin requirements increase during times of illness, stress

Administer:
- After warming to room temperature by rotating in palms to prevent injecting cold insulin
- Increased doses if tolerance occurs
- Human insulin to those allergic to beef or pork

Perform/provide:
- Storage at room temperature for <1 mo, keep in cool area, refrigerate all other supply, do not use if discolored
- Rotation of injection sites within one area: abdomen, upper back,

*Available in Canada only

thighs, upper arm, buttocks; keep record of sites

Evaluate:

• Therapeutic response: decrease in polyuria, polydipsia, polyphagia, clear sensorium, absence of dizziness, stable gait

• Hypoglycemic reaction that can occur during peak time

Teach patient/family:

• That blurred vision occurs, not to change corrective lens until vision is stabilized 1-2 mo

• To keep insulin, equipment available at all times

• That drug does not cure diabetes, but controls symptoms

• To carry Medic Alert ID as diabetic

• About hypoglycemia reaction: headache, tremors, fatigue, weakness

• Dosage, route, mixing instructions, if any diet restrictions, disease process

• To carry candy or lump sugar to treat hypoglycemia

• Symptoms of ketoacidosis: nausea, thirst, polyuria, dry mouth, decreased B/P, dry, flushed skin, acetone breath, drowsiness, Kussmaul respirations

• That a plan is necessary for diet, exercise; all food on diet should be eaten, exercise routine should not vary

• About urine glucose testing, make sure patient is able to determine glucose, acetone levels

• That pregnant patients should use glucose oxidase reagents

• To avoid OTC drugs unless directed by physician

Lab test interferences:

Increase: VMA

Decrease: Potassium, calcium

Interference: Liver function studies, thyroid function studies

Treatment of overdose: 10%-50% glucose PO if conscious or IV if comatose or 1 mg glucagon

---

insulin, zinc suspension extended (Ultralente)

Iletin Ultralente,* Ultralente,* Ultralente Iletin I, Ultralente Insulin, Ultralente Purified Beef

Func. class.: Antidiabetic
Chem. class.: Exogenous unmodified insulin

Action: Decreases blood sugar, indirectly increases blood pyruvate, lactate, decreases phosphate, potassium

Uses: Ketoacidosis, Type I (IDDM), Type II (NIDDM) diabetes mellitus, hyperkalemia

Dosage and routes:

• *Adult:* SC individualized

Available forms include: SC 40, 100 U/ml

Side effects/adverse reactions:

CNS: Headache, lethargy, tremors, weakness, fatigue, delirium, sweating

CV: Tachycardia, palpitations

EENT: Blurred vision, dry mouth

GI: Hunger, nausea

META: Hypoglycemia

INTEG: Flushing, rash, urticaria, warmth, lipodystrophy, lipohypertrophy

SYST: ***Anaphylaxis***

Contraindications: Hypersensitivity to protamine

Precautions: Pregnancy (C)

Pharmacokinetics:

SC: Onset 4-8 hr, peak 10-30 hr, duration 7-36 hr

Metabolized by liver, muscle, kidneys, excreted in urine

Interactions/incompatibilities:

• Increased hypoglycemia: salicylate, alcohol, β-blockers, anabolic

steroids, fenfluramine, guanethidine, oral hypoglycemics, MAOIs, tetracycline, sulfinpyrazone
• Decreased hypoglycemia: thiazides, thyroid hormones, oral contraceptives, corticosteroids, estrogens, dobutamine, epinephrine, smoking, levothyroxine

NURSING CONSIDERATIONS

Assess:
• Fasting blood glucose, 2 hr PP (80-150 mg/dl normal fasting level) (70-130 mg/dl-normal 2 hr level)
• Urine ketones during illness; insulin requirements increase during times of stress, illness

Administer:
• After warming to room temperature by rotating in palms to prevent injecting cold insulin
• Increased doses if tolerance occurs

Perform/provide:
• Storage at room temperature for <1 mo, refrigerate all other supply, do not use if discolored
• Rotation of injection sites within one area: abdomen, upper back, thighs, upper arm, buttocks; keep record of sites

Evaluate:
• Therapeutic response: decrease in polyuria, polydipsia, polyphagia, clear sensorium, absence of dizziness, stable gait
• Hypoglycemic reaction that can occur during peak time

Teach patient/family:
• That blurred vision occurs, not to change corrective lens until vision is stabilized 1-2 mo
• To keep insulin, equipment available at all times
• That drug does not cure diabetes, but controls symptoms
• To carry Medic Alert ID as diabetic
• Hypoglycemia reaction: headache, tremors, fatigue, weakness
• Dosage, route, mixing instructions, if any diet restrictions, disease process
• To carry candy or lump sugar to treat hypoglycemia
• Symptoms of ketoacidosis: nausea, thirst, polyuria, dry mouth, decreased B/P, dry, flushed skin, acetone breath, drowsiness, Kussmaul respirations
• That a plan is necessary for diet, exercise; all food on diet should be eaten, exercise routine should not vary
• About urine glucose testing, make sure patient is able to determine glucose, acetone levels
• That pregnant patients should use glucose oxidase reagents
• To avoid OTC drugs unless directed by physician

Lab test interferences:
Increase: VMA
Decrease: Potassium, calcium
Interference: Liver function studies, thyroid function studies

Treatment of overdose: 10%-50% glucose PO if conscious or IV if comatose or 1 mg glucagon

---

insulin, zinc suspension, prompt (semilente)

Semilente Iletin I, Semilente Insulin, Semilente Purified Pork

Func. class.: Antidiabetic
Chem. class.: Exogenous unmodified insulin

Action: Decreases blood sugar, indirectly increases blood pyruvate, lactate, decreases phosphate, potassium

Uses: Ketoacidosis, Type I (IDDM), Type II (NIDDM) diabetes mellitus, hyperkalemia

---

* Available in Canada only

Dosage and routes:
• *Adult:* SC dosage individualized by blood, urine glucose qd-tid
Available forms include: SC 40, 100 U/ml
Side effects/adverse reactions:
CNS: Headache, lethargy, tremors, weakness, fatigue, delirium, sweating
CV: Tachycardia, palpitations
EENT: Blurred vision, dry mouth
GI: Hunger, nausea
META: *Hypoglycemia*
INTEG: Flushing, rash, urticaria, warmth, lipodystrophy, lipohypertrophy
SYST: ***Anaphylaxis***
Contraindications: Hypersensitivity to protamine
Precautions: Pregnancy (B)
Pharmacokinetics:
SC: Onset 1-1½ hr, peak 5-10 hr, duration 12-16 hr
Metabolized by liver, muscle, kidneys; excreted in urine
Interactions/incompatibilities:
• Increased hypoglycemia: salicylate, alcohol, β-blockers, anabolic steroids, fenfluramine, guanethidine, oral hypoglycemics, MAOIs, tetracycline, sulfinpyrazone
• Hyperglycemia: thiazides, thyroid hormones, oral contraceptives, corticosteroids, estrogens, dobutamine, epinephrine, smoking, levothyroxine

NURSING CONSIDERATIONS

Assess:
• Fasting blood glucose, 2 hr PP (80-150 mg/dl normal fasting level) (70-130 mg/dl-normal 2 hr level)
• Urine ketones during illness; insulin requirements increase during times of stress, illness
Administer:
• After warming to room temperature by rotating in palms, to prevent injecting cold insulin
• Increased doses if tolerance occurs
Perform/provide:
• Storage at room temperature for <1 mo in cool area, refrigerate all other supply, do not use if discolored
• Rotation of injection sites within one area: abdomen, upper back, thighs, upper arm, buttocks; keep record of sites
Evaluate:
• Therapeutic response: decrease in polyuria, polydipsia, polyphagia, clear sensorium, absence of dizziness, stable gait
• Hypoglycemic reaction that can occur during peak time
Teach patient/family:
• That blurred vision occurs, not to change corrective lens until vision is stabilized 1-2 mo
• To keep insulin, equipment available at all times
• That drug does not cure diabetes, but controls symptoms
• To carry Medic Alert ID as diabetic
• Hypoglycemia reaction: headache, tremors, fatigue, weakness
• Dosage, route, mixing instructions, if any diet restrictions, disease process
• To carry candy or lump sugar to treat hypoglycemia
• Symptoms of ketoacidosis: nausea, thirst, polyuria, dry mouth, decreased B/P, dry, flushed skin, acetone breath, drowsiness, Kussmaul respirations
• That a plan is necessary for diet, exercise; all food on diet should be eaten, exercise routine should not vary
• Urine glucose testing, make sure

patient is able to determine glucose, acetone levels
• That pregnant patients should use glucose oxidase reagents
• To avoid OTC drugs unless directed by physician
Lab test interferences:
Increase: VMA
Decrease: Potassium, calcium
Interference: Liver function studies, thyroid function studies
Treatment of overdose: 10%-50% glucose PO if conscious or IV if comatose or 1 mg glucagon

interferon alfa-2a/interferon alfa-2b

(in-ter-ferón)
Roferon-a/Intron-a
Func. class.: Miscellaneous antineoplastic
Chem. class.: Protein product

Action: Antiviral action inhibits viral replication by reprogramming virus; antitumor action suppresses cell proliferation; immunomodulating action phagocytizes target cells
Uses: Hairy cell leukemia in persons >18 yr, condylomata acuminata, metastatic melanoma, AIDS
Dosage and routes:
• *Adult:* SC/IM (interferon alfa-2a) 3,000,000 IU × 16-24 wk, then 3,000,000 IU 3 × wk maintenance; SC/IM (interferon alfa-2b) 2,000,000 IU/m^2 3 × wk; if severe adverse reactions occur, dose should be skipped or reduced by ½
Available forms include: alfa-2a inj 3, 18 million IU/vial; alfa-2b inj 3, 5, 10, 25 million IU/vial
Side effects/adverse reactions:
CNS: Dizziness, confusion, numbness, paresthesias, hallucinations, ***convulsions, coma,*** amnesia, anxiety, mood changes
CV: Edema, hypotension, hypertension, chest pain, palpitations, dysrhythmias, ***CHF, MI, CVA***
INTEG: Rash, dry skin, itching, alopecia, flushing
GI: Weight loss, taste changes
GU: Impotence
MISC: Flulike syndrome; fever, fatigue, myalgias, headache, chills
Contraindications: Hypersensitivity
Precautions: Severe hypotension, dysrhythmia, tachycardia, pregnancy (C), lactation, children, severe renal or hepatic disease, convulsion disorder
Pharmacokinetics:
Half-life (interferon alfa-2a) 3.7-8.5 hr, peak 3-4 hr; half-life (interferon alfa-2b) 2-7 hr, peak 6-8 hr

NURSING CONSIDERATIONS

Assess:
• For symptoms of infection, may be masked by drug fever
• CNS reaction: LOC, mental status, dizziness, confusion
Administer:
• At hs for minimizing side effects
• Acetaminophen as ordered to alleviate fever and headache
Perform/provide:
• Storage of reconstituted solution for 1 mo in refrigerator
• Increased fluid intake to 2-3 L/day
Evaluate:
• Therapeutic response: decrease in tumor size, increase in ease of breathing
Teach patient/family:
• To avoid hazardous tasks, since confusion, dizziness may occur
• That brands of this drug should not be changed; each form is different with different doses

• That fatigue is common, activity may need to be altered
• Not to become pregnant while taking drug; possible mutagenic effects
• To report signs of infection: sore throat, fever, diarrhea, vomiting
• That impotence may occur during treatment, but is temporary

Lab test interferences:
Interference: AST, ALT, LDH, alk phosphatase, WBC, platelets, granulocytes, creatinine

Interferon alfa-n 3

(in-ter-feer'on)
Alferon N

Func. class.: Antineoplastic
Chem. class.: Human interferon alfa protein

Action: Binds interferon to membrane receptors on cell surface with high specificity; this produces protein synthesis, inhibition of virus replication, suppression of cell proliferide, and increased phagocytosis

Uses: Condylomata acuminata (veneral/genital warts)

Dosages and routes:
• *Adult:* 0.05 ml (250,000 IU) per wart, given 2 ×/wk × 8 wk; not to exceed 0.5 ml (2.5 million IU); inject into base of wart

Available forms include: Inj 5 m IU/1 ml vial with 3.3 mg/ml phenol and 1 mg/ml human albumin

Side effects/adverse reactions:
CNS: Fever, headache, sweating, vasovagal reaction, chills, fatigue, dizziness, insomnia, sleepiness, depression
GI: Nausea, vomiting, heartburn, diarrhea, constipation, anorexia, stomatitis, dry mouth
MS: Myalgias, arthralgia, back pain
INTEG: Pain at injection site, pruritis
CV: Chest pain, hypotension

Contraindications: Hypersensitivity to this product, egg protein, IgG, neomycin

Precautions: Pregnancy (C), lactation, children, CHF, angina (unstable), COPD, diabetes mellitus with ketoacidosis, hemophilia, pulmonary embolism, thrombophlebitis, bone marrow depression, convulsive disorder

Pharmacokinetics: Unable to detect

NURSING CONSIDERATIONS

Assess:
• For symptoms of infection, may be masked by drug fever
• CNS reaction: LOC, mental status, dizziness, confusion
• For body image disturbance

Administer:
• Acetaminophen to alleviate fever and headache

Perform/provide:
• Storage of reconstituted solution for 1 mo in refrigerator
• Increased fluid intake to 2-3 L/day

Evaluate:
• Therapeutic response: decrease in wart size

Teach patient/family:
• To avoid hazardous tasks, since confusion, dizziness may occur
• That brands of this drug should not be changed; each form is different with different doses
• That fatigue is common, activity may need to be altered
• Not to become pregnant while taking drug; possible mutagenic effects
• To report signs of infection: sore throat, fever, diarrhea, vomiting

• Signs of hypersensitivity: liver, urticaria, wheezing, dyspnea; notify physician immediately

Lab test interferences:
Interferences: AST, ALT, LDH, alk phosphatase, WBC, platelets, granulocytes, creatinine

---

interferon gamma-1b

(in-ter-fer'on)
Actimmune
Func. class.: Biologic response modifier
Chem. class.: Lymphokine, interleukin type

Action: Species-specific protein synthesized in response to viruses, potent phagocyte-activating effects, capable of mediating the killing of *S. aureus, T. gondii, L. donovani, L. monocytogenes, M. avium-intracellulare;* enhances oxidative metabolism of macrophages, enhances antibody-dependent cellular cytotoxicity

Uses: Serious infections associated with chronic granulomatous disease

Dosage and routes:
• *Adult:* SC 50 μg/m^2 (1.5 million U/m^2) for patients with a surface area of >0.5 m^2; 1.5 μg/kg/dose for patient with a surface area of <0.5/m^2; give on Monday, Wednesday, Friday for 3 × /wk dosing

Available forms include: Inj 100 μg (3 million U) single-dose vial

Side effects/adverse reactions:
GI: Nausea, anorexia, abdominal pain, weight loss, diarrhea, vomiting
CNS: Headache, fatigue, depression, fever, chills
INTEG: Rash, pain at injection site
MS: Myalgia, arthralgia

Contraindications: Hypersensitivity to interferon gamma, *E. coli*–derived products

Precautions: Pregnancy (C), cardiac disease, seizure disorders, CNS disorders, myelosuppression, lactation, children

Pharmacokinetics:
SC: Dose absorbed 89%, elimination half-life 5.9 hr, peak 7 hr

Interactions/incompatibilities:
• Increased myelosuppression: other myelosuppressive agents

NURSING CONSIDERATIONS

Assess:
• Blood, renal, hepatic studies: CBC, differential, platelet counts, BUN, creatinine ALT, urinalysis
• CNS symptoms: headache, fatigue, depression

Administer:
• At HS to minimize adverse reactions; administer acetaminophen for fever, headache
• 50% of the dose if severe reactions occur or discontinue treatment until reactions subside
• Using sterilized glass or plastic disposable syringes
• In right and left deltoid and anterior thigh
• Warm to room temperature before use; do not leave at room temperature over 12 hr (unopened vial)

Perform/provide:
• Storage in refrigerator upon receipt; do not freeze, do not shake

Evaluate:
• Therapeutic response: decreased serious infections, improve existing infections and inflammatory conditions

Teach patient/family:
• Method of administration if family members will be giving medication

---

• To provide patient or family member with written, detailed information about the drug

iodinated glycerol

Organidin, Isophen Elixir

Func. class.: Expectorant

Chem. class.: Iodopropylidene glycerol isom

Action: Increases respiratory tract fluid by decreasing surface tension, adhesiveness, which increases removal of mucus

Uses: Bronchial asthma, emphysema, bronchitis

Dosage and routes:

• *Adult:* PO 60 mg qid; SOL 20 gtts qid; ELIX 5 ml qid

• *Child:* PO up to half adult dose, depending on weight

Available forms include: Tabs 30 mg; sol 50 mg/ml, 60 mg/5 ml

Side effects/adverse reactions:

EENT: Burning mouth, throat, eye irritation, swelling of eyelids

GI: Gastric irritation

ENDO: Iodism, goiter, myxedema

RESP: Pulmonary edema

INTEG: ***Angioedema,*** rash

CNS: Frontal headache, ***CNS depression,*** fever, parkinsonism

Contraindications: Hypersensitivity to iodides, pulmonary TB, pregnancy (X), hyperthyroidism, hyperkalemia, newborns, lactation, acute bronchitis

Precautions: Hypothyroidism, cystic fibrosis, lactation

Pharmacokinetics: Excreted in urine

Interactions/incompatibilities:

• Increased hypothyroid effects: lithium, antithyroid drugs

• Dysrhythmias, hyperkalemia: potassium-sparing diuretics, potassium-containing medication

NURSING CONSIDERATIONS

Administer:

• Orally in solution or tablet form

Perform/provide:

• Increased fluids to liquefy secretions

Evaluate:

• Therapeutic response: absence of cough

• Cough: type, frequency, character including sputum

Teach patient/family:

• Not to use if pregnant or if any potential for pregnancy

• Symptoms of iodism: eruptions, burning of oral cavity, eye irritation

• Symptoms of hyperthyroidism: CNS depression, fever, glomerulonephritis

iodoquinol

(eye-oh-do-kwin'ole)

Diodoquin,* Yodoxin, Amebaquine

Func. class.: Amebicide

Chem. class.: Dihalogenated derivative of 8-hydroxyquinoline

Action: Direct-acting amebicide; action occurs in intestinal lumen

Uses: Intestinal amebiasis

Dosage and routes:

• *Adult:* PO 630-650 mg tid × 20 days, not to exceed 2 g/day

• *Child:* PO 30-40 mg/kg/day in 2-3 divided doses × 20 days; do not repeat treatment before 2-3 wk

Available forms include: Tabs 210, 650 mg; powder

Side effects/adverse reactions:

HEMA: ***Agranulocytosis*** (rare)

INTEG: Rash, pruritus, discolored skin, alopecia

CNS: Headache, dizziness, ataxia

EENT: Blurred vision, sore throat,

retinal edema, subacute myelo-optic neuropathy
GI: Nausea, vomiting, diarrhea, epigastric distress, anorexia, gastritis, constipation, abdominal cramps, rectal irritation, itching
Contraindications: Hypersensitivity to this drug or iodine, renal disease, hepatic disease, severe thyroid disease, preexisting optic neuropathy
Precautions: Pregnancy (C)

NURSING CONSIDERATIONS

Assess:
- Stools during entire treatment; should be clear at end of therapy, stools should be free of parasites for 1 yr before patient is considered cured
- I&O, stools for number, frequency, character

Administer:
- PO after meals to avoid GI symptoms

Perform/provide:
- Storage in tight container

Evaluate:
- Therapeutic response: decreased diarrhea, symptoms in amebiasis
- Iodism: skin eruption, urticaria, discoloring of hair, nails
- Allergic reaction: fever, rash, itching, chills; drug should be discontinued if these occur
- Blurred vision
- Superimposed infection, fever, monilial growth, fatigue, malaise
- Diarrhea for 2-3 days

Teach patient/family:
- Proper hygiene after BM: handwashing technique
- To avoid contact of drug with eyes, mouth, nose, other mucous membranes
- About need for compliance with dosage schedule, duration of treatment

Lab test interferences:
False positive: PKU
Increase: PBI
Decrease: ^{131}I uptake test

ipecac syrup

(ip'e-kak)

Func. class.: Emetic
Chem. class.: Cephaelis ipecacuanha derivative

Action: Acts on chemoreceptor trigger zone to induce vomiting, irritates gastric mucosa
Uses: In poisoning to induce vomiting
Dosage and routes:
- *Adult:* PO 15 ml, then 200-300 ml water
- *Child >1 yr:* PO 15 ml, then 200-300 ml water
- *Child <1 yr:* PO 5-10 ml, then 100-200 ml water; may repeat dose if needed

Available forms include: Liq
Side effects/adverse reactions:
CNS: ***Depression, convulsions, coma***
GI: Nausea, vomiting, bloody diarrhea
CV: ***Circulatory failure, atrial fibrillation, fatal myocarditis, dysrhythmias***
Contraindications: Hypersensitivity, unconscious/semiconscious, depressed gag reflex, poisoning with petroleum products or caustic substances, convulsions
Precautions: Lactation, pregnancy (C)
Pharmacokinetics:
PO: Onset 15-30 min
Interactions/incompatibilities:
- Do not administer with activated charcoal; effect will be decreased

NURSING CONSIDERATIONS

Assess:

• VS, B/P; check patients with cardiac disease more often

Administer:

• **Ipecac *syrup* not ipecac,** which is 14 times stronger; death may occur

• Then bounce child to increase emetic effect

• Activated charcoal if this drug doesn't work; may begin lavage after 10-15 min

Evaluate:

• Therapeutic response: vomiting

• Type of poisoning; do not administer if petroleum products or caustic substances have been ingested: kerosene, gasoline, lye, Drano

• Respiratory status before, during, after administration of emetic; check rate, rhythm, character; respiratory depression can occur rapidly with elderly or debilitated patients

---

ipratropium bromide

(eye-pra-troep'ee-um)

Atrovent

Func. class.: Anticholinergic

Chem. class.: Synthetic quaternary ammonium compound

Action: Inhibits interaction of acetylcholine at receptor sites on the bronchial smooth muscle, resulting in bronchodilation

Uses: Bronchodilation during bronchospasm in those with COPD

Dosage and routes:

• *Adult:* 2 INH 4 × day, not to exceed 12 INH/24 hr

Available forms include: Aerosol 18 μg/actuation

Side effects/adverse reactions:

GI: Nausea, vomiting, cramps

EENT: Dry mouth, blurred vision

CNS: Anxiety, dizziness, headache

RESP: Cough, worsening of symptoms

INTEG: Rash

CV: Palpitation

Contraindications: Hypersensitivity to this drug or atropine

Precautions: Pregnancy (B), lactation, children <12 yr, narrow-angle glaucoma, prostatic hypertrophy, bladder neck obstruction

Pharmacokinetics:

Half-life 2 hr, does not cross blood-brain barrier

NURSING CONSIDERATIONS

Assess:

• For palpitations; if severe, drug may need to be changed

Perform/provide:

• Storage at room temperature

• Hard candy, frequent drinks, sugarless gum to relieve dry mouth

Evaluate:

• Therapeutic response: ability to breathe adequately

• For tolerance over long-term therapy; dose may need to be increased or changed

Teach patient/family:

• That compliance is necessary with number of inhalations/24 hr, or overdose may occur

• To shake before using

• Correct method of inhalation

---

iron dextran

Dextraron, Feostat, Hematran, Hydextran, Imferon, Irodex, K-Feron, Proferdex, Rocyte, Nor-Feran

Func. class.: Hematinic

Chem. class.: Ferric hydroxide complexed with dextran

Action: Iron is carried by transferrin to the bone marrow where it is incorporated into hemoglobin

Uses: Iron deficiency anemia

Dosage and routes:

- *Adult and child:* IM 0.5 ml as a test dose by Z-track, then no more than the following per day
- *Adult <50 kg:* IM 100 mg
- *Adult >50 kg:* IM 250 mg
- *Infant <5 kg:* IM 25 mg
- *Child <9 kg:* IM 50 mg
- *Adult:* IV 0.5 ml test dose then 100 mg qd after 2-3 days; IV 250/1000 ml of NaCl, give 25 mg test dose, wait 5 min, then infuse over 6-12 hr or follow equation

$$\frac{0.3 \times \text{wt (lb)} \times 100\text{-Hgb (g/dl)} \times 100}{14.8} = \text{mg iron}$$

<30 lb should be given 80% of above formula dose

Available forms include: Inj IM/IV 50 mg/ml, inj IM only 50 mg/ml

Side effects/adverse reactions:

CNS: Headache, paresthesia, dizziness, shivering, weakness, ***seizures***

GI: Nausea, vomiting, metallic taste, abdominal pain

INTEG: Rash, pruritus, urticaria, fever, sweating, chills, brown skin discoloration, pain at injection site, necrosis, sterile abscesses, phlebitis

CV: Chest pain, ***shock,*** hypotension, tachycardia

RESP: Dyspnea

HEMA: ***Leukocytosis***

Other: ***Anaphylaxis***

Contraindications: Hypersensitivity, all anemias excluding iron deficiency anemia, hepatic disease

Precautions: Acute renal disease, children, asthma, lactation, rheumatoid arthritis (IV), infants <4 mo, pregnancy (C)

Pharmacokinetics:

IM: Excreted in feces, urine, bile, breast milk, crosses placenta, most absorbed through lymphatics, can be gradually absorbed over weeks/months from fixed locations

Interactions/incompatibilities:

- Not to mix with other drugs in syringe or D_5W
- Decreased reticulocyte response: chloramphenicol
- Increased toxicity: oral iron—do not use

NURSING CONSIDERATIONS

Assess:

- Blood studies: Hct, Hgb, reticulocytes, bilirubin before treatment, at least monthly

Administer:

- D/c oral iron before parenteral; only after test dose of 25 mg by preferred route; wait at least 1 hr before giving remaining portion
- IM deeply in large muscle mass, use Z-track method and a 19-20 G 2-3 inch needle; ensure needle is long enough to place drug deep in muscle
- IV, after flushing with 10 ml of NS; give undiluted; may be diluted in 50-250 normal saline for infusion
- IV injection requires single dose vial without preservative; verify on label IV use is approved
- Only with epinephrine available in case of anaphylactic reaction during dose

Perform/provide:

- Storage at room temperature in cool environment
- Recumbent position 30 min after IV injection to prevent orthostatic hypotension

Evaluate:

- Therapeutic response: increased serum iron levels
- Allergy: ***anaphylaxis***, rash, pruritus, fever, chills
- Cardiac status: anginal pain, hypotension, tachycardia
- Nutrition: amount of iron in diet

(meat, dark green leafy vegetables, dried beans, dried fruits, eggs)
• Cause of iron loss or anemia including salicylates, sulfonamides

Teach patient/family:
• That iron poisoning may occur if increased beyond recommended level
• That delayed reaction may occur 1-2 days after administration and last 3-4 days (IV) 3-7 days (IM); report fever, chills, malaise, muscle, joint aches, nausea, vomiting, backache

Lab test interferences:
False increase: Serum bilirubin
False decrease: Serum calcium
False positive: ^{99m}Tc diphosphate bone scan, iron test (large doses >2 ml)

---

isocarboxazid

(eye-soe-kar-box'a-zid)
Marplan

Func. class.: Antidepressant—MAOI
Chem. class.: Hydrazine

Action: Increases concentrations of endogenous epinephrine, norepinephrine, serotonin, dopamine in storage sites in CNS by inhibition of MAO; increased concentration reduces depression

Uses: Depression, when uncontrolled by other means

Dosage and routes:
• *Adult:* PO 30 mg/day in divided doses, reduce dose to lowest effective dose when condition improves

Available forms include: Tabs 10 mg

Side effects/adverse reactions:
HEMA: Anemia
CNS: Dizziness, drowsiness, confusion, headache, anxiety, tremors, stimulation, weakness, hyperreflexia, mania, insomnia, fatigue, weight gain
GI: Constipation, dry mouth, nausea, vomiting, *anorexia,* diarrhea, weight gain
GU: Change in libido, frequency
INTEG: Rash, flushing, increased perspiration, jaundice
CV: Orthostatic hypotension, hypertension, dysrhythmias, hypertensive crisis
EENT: Blurred vision
ENDO: ***SIADH-like syndrome***

Contraindications: Hypersensitivity to MAOIs, elderly, hypertension, CHF, severe hepatic disease, pheochromocytoma, severe renal disease, severe cardiac disease

Precautions: Suicidal patients, convulsive disorders, severe depression, schizophrenia, hyperactivity, diabetes mellitus, pregnancy (C)

Pharmacokinetics:
PO: Duration up to 2 wk; metabolized by liver, excreted by kidneys

Interactions/incompatibilities:
• Increased pressor effects: guanethidine, clonidine, indirect acting sympathomimetics (ephedrine)
• Increased effects of: direct acting sympathomimetics (epinephrine), alcohol, barbiturates, benzodiazepines, CNS depressants, levodopa
• Hyperpyretic crisis, convulsions, hypertensive episode: tricyclic antidepressants, meperidine
• Hypoglycemic effect: increased insulin

NURSING CONSIDERATIONS

Assess:
• B/P (lying, standing), pulse; if systolic B/P drops 20 mm Hg hold drug, notify physician
• Blood studies: CBC, leukocytes, cardiac enzymes if patient is receiving long-term therapy
• Hepatic studies: ALT, AST, bili-

rubin, creatinine, hepatotoxicity may occur

Administer:

• Increased fluids, bulk in diet if constipation, urinary retention occur

• With food or milk for GI symptoms

• Crushed if patient is unable to swallow medication whole

• Dosage hs if oversedation occurs during day

• Gum, hard candy, or frequent sips of water for dry mouth

• Phentolamine for severe hypertension

Perform/provide:

• Storage in tight container in cool environment, away from children

• Assistance with ambulation during beginning therapy since drowsiness/dizziness occurs

• Safety measures including siderails

• Checking to see PO medication swallowed

Evaluate:

• Therapeutic response: decreased depression

• Toxicity: increased headache, palpitation; discontinue drug immediately; prodromal signs of hypertensive crisis

• Mental status: mood, sensorium, affect, memory (long, short), increase in psychiatric symptoms

• Urinary retention, constipation, edema, take weight weekly

• Withdrawal symptoms: headache, nausea, vomiting, muscle pain, weakness

Teach patient/family:

• That therapeutic effects may take 1-4 wk

• To avoid driving or other activities requiring alertness; hypotension may be increased in the elderly

• To avoid alcohol ingestion, CNS depressants or OTC medications: cold, weight, hay fever, cough syrup

• Not to discontinue medication quickly after long-term use

• To avoid high tyramine foods: cheese (aged), sour cream, beer, wine, pickled products, liver, raisins, bananas, figs, avocados, meat tenderizers, chocolate, yogurt; increase caffeine

• Report headache, palpitation, neck stiffness

Treatment of overdose: Lavage, activated charcoal, monitor electrolytes, vital signs, diazepam IV, $NaHCO_3$

isoetharine HCl/ isoetharine mesylate

(eye-soe-eth'a-reen)

Beta-Z solution, Bronkosol/Bronkometer

Func. class.: Adrenergic β_2-agonist

Action: Causes bronchodilation by β_2 stimulation, resulting in increased levels of cAMP, causing relaxation of bronchial smooth muscle with very little effect on heart rate

Uses: Bronchospasm, asthma

Dosage and routes:

• *Adult:* INH 3-7 puffs undiluted, IPPB 0.5 ml diluted 1:3 with NS

Available forms include: Sol for nebulization 0.06%, 0.08%, 0.1%, 0.125%, 0.17%, 0.2%, 0.25%, 0.5%, 10%

Side effects/adverse reactions:

CNS: Tremors, anxiety, insomnia, headache, dizziness, stimulation

CV: Palpitations, tachycardia, hypertension, ***cardiac arrest,*** dysrhythmias

GI: Nausea

* Available in Canada only

• *META:* Hyperglycemia
Contraindications: Hypersensitivity to sympathomimetics, narrow-angle glaucoma
Precautions: Pregnancy (C), cardiac disorders, hyperthyroidism, diabetes mellitus, prostatic hypertrophy
Pharmacokinetics:
INH: Onset immediate, peak 5-15 min, duration 1-4 hr, metabolized in liver, GI tract, lungs, excreted in urine
Interactions/incompatibilities:
• Increased effects of both drugs: other sympathomimetics
• Decreased action when used with other β-blockers
• Hypertensive crisis: MAOIs

NURSING CONSIDERATIONS
Assess:
• Respiratory function: vital capacity, forced expiratory volume, ABGs, pulse, B/P
Administer:
• 2 hr before hs to avoid sleeplessness
Perform/provide:
• Storage at room temperature. Do not use solution if brown or contains a precipitate
Evaluate:
• Therapeutic response: ease of breathing
• Paresthesias and coldness of extremities, peripheral blood flow may decrease
Teach patient/family:
• Not to use OTC medications, extra stimulation may occur
• Use of inhaler, review package insert with patient
• To avoid getting aerosol in eyes
• To wash inhaler in warm water and dry qd
• About all aspects of drug; avoid smoking, smoke-filled rooms, persons with respiratory infections

isoflurophate

(eye-soe-flure'oh-fate)
Floropryl, Diisopropyl Fluorophosphate, Diflupyl
Func. class.: Miotic
Chem. class.: Cholinesterase inhibitor, irreversible

Action: Prevents breakdown of neurotransmitter acetylcholine, which then accumulates, causing enhancement, prolongation of its physiologic effects
Uses: Open-angle glaucoma, accommodative esotropia, conditions obstructing aqueous outflow
Dosage and routes:
• *Adult and child:* INSTILL ¼ in strip of 0.25% oint in conjunctival sac q8-72 hr for glaucoma or qhs × 2 wk for esotropia
Available forms include: Only as ophthalmic ointment 0.25%
Side effects/adverse reactions:
CNS: Headache
CV: Hypotension, bradycardia, paradoxic tachycardia
RESP: ***Bronchospasm,*** dyspnea, bronchoconstriction, wheezing
EENT: Blurred vision, lacrimation, conjunctival congestion
GU: Urinary incontinence
GI: Abdominal cramps, diarrhea, increased salivation, nausea, vomiting
Contraindications: Hypersensitivity, uveal inflammation
Precautions: History of retinal detachment

NURSING CONSIDERATIONS
Administer:
• Ointment to conjunctival sac with patient supine
Evaluate:
• Therapeutic response: decreased aqueous outflow

Teach patient/family:

- That top of tube must not come in contact with moisture; keep tube closed, dry, away from tears or cornea; to wash hands after application of ointment
- To report change in vision, blurring or loss of sight, trouble breathing, sweating, flushing
- That long-term therapy may be required
- That blurred vision will decrease with repeated use of drug
- To minimize effects of blurred vision, application should take place at bedtime
- To observe for signs/symptoms of systemic absorption (i.e., diarrhea, weakness)
- To observe eyes for irritation
- To monitor for cardiac, respiratory, or GI problems

isoniazid (INH)

(eye-soe-nye'a-zid)

Hyzyd, Isotamine,* Laniazid, Nydrazid, PMS-Isoniazid,* Rolazid, Teebaconin

Func. class.: Antitubercular
Chem. class.: Isonicotinic acid hydrazide

Action: Bactericidal interference with lipid, nucleic acid biosynthesis

Uses: Treatment, prevention of tuberculosis

Dosage and routes:

Treatment

- *Adult:* PO/IM 5 mg/kg qd as single dose for 9 mo to 2 yr, not to exceed 300 mg/day
- *Child and infants:* PO/IM 10-20 mg/kg qd as single dose for 18-24 mo, not to exceed 300 mg/day

Prevention

- *Adult* PO 300 mg qd as single dose × 12 mo
- *Child and infants:* PO/IM 10 mg/kg qd as single dose for 12 mo, not to exceed 300 mg/day

Available forms include: Tabs 50, 100, 300 mg; inj 100 mg/ml; powder, syrup 50 mg/5 ml

Side effects/adverse reactions:
Hypersensitivity: fever, skin eruptions, lymphadenopathy, vasculitis
CNS: Peripheral neuropathy, memory impairment, ***toxic encephalopathy, convulsions,*** psychosis
EENT: Blurred vision, optic neuritis
HEMA: ***Agranulocytosis, hemolytic, aplastic anemia, thrombocytopenia, eosinophilia, methemoglobinemia***
MISC: Dyspnea, B_6-deficiency, pellegra, hyperglycemia, metabolic acidosis, gynecomastia, rheumatic syndrome, SLE-like syndrome
GI: Nausea, vomiting, epigastric distress, ***jaundice, fatal hepatitis***

Contraindications: Hypersensitivity, optic neuritis

Precautions: Pregnancy (C), renal disease, diabetic retinopathy, cataracts, ocular defects, hepatic disease, child <13 yr

Pharmacokinetics:
PO: Peak 1-2 hr, duration 6-8 hr
IM: Peak 45-60 min
Metabolized in liver, excreted in urine (metabolites), crosses placenta, excreted in breast milk

Interactions/incompatibilities:

- Increased toxicity: alcohol, cycloserine, ethionamide, rifampin, carbamazepine
- Decreased absorption: aluminum antacids

NURSING CONSIDERATIONS

Assess:

- Liver studies qwk: ALT, AST, bilirubin

*Available in Canada only

• Renal status: before, qmo: BUN, creatinine, output, sp gr, urinalysis

Administer:

• With meals to decrease GI symptoms; better to take on empty stomach 1 hr ac or 2 hr pc

• Antiemetic if vomiting occurs

• After C&S is completed; qmo to detect resistance

Evaluate:

• Therapeutic response: decreased symptoms of TB

• Mental status often: affect, mood, behavioral changes; psychosis may occur

• Hepatic status: decreased appetite, jaundice, dark urine, fatigue

Teach patient/family:

• That compliance with dosage schedule, duration is necessary

• That scheduled appointments must be kept or relapse may occur

• To avoid alcohol while taking drug

• That, if diabetic, use Clinitest to obtain correct result

• To report weakness, fatigue, loss of appetite, nausea, vomiting, yellowing of skin or eyes, tingling/numbness of hands/feet

---

isoproterenol HCl/isoproterenol sulfate

(eye-soe-proe-ter'e-nole)

Isuprel, Proternol, Norisodrine, Vapo-Iso/Iso-Autohaler, Luf-Iso Inhalation, Medihaler-Iso, Norisodrine

Func. class.: Adrenergic
Chem. class.: Catecholamine

Action: Has β_1 and β_2 action. Relaxes bronchial smooth muscle and dilates the trachea and main bronchi, by increasing levels of cAMP, which relaxes smooth muscles; causes increased contractility and heart rate by acting on β-receptors in heart

Uses: Bronchospasm, asthma, heart block, ventricular dysrhythmias, shock

Dosage and routes:

Asthma, bronchospasm

• *Adult:* SL 10-20 mg q6-8h HCl; INH 1 puff, may repeat in 2-5 min, maintenance 1-2 puffs 4-6 × per day

• *Child:* SL 5-10 mg q6-8 HCl; INH 1 puff, may repeat in 2-5 min, maintenance 1-2 puffs 4-6 × per day

Heart block/ventricular dysrhythmias

• *Adult:* IV 0.02-0.06, then 0.01-0.2 mg or 5 μg/min HCl; IM 0.2 mg, then 0.02-1 mg as needed HCl

• *Child:* IV/IM ½ of beginning adult dose

Shock

• *Adult and child:* IV INF 0.5-5 μg/min 1 mg/500 ml D_5W, titrate to B/P, CVP, and hourly urine output

Available forms include: Sol for nebulization 1:400 (0.25%), 1:200 (0.5%), 1:100 (1%); aerosol 0.25%, 0.2%; powd for INH 0.1 mg/cart; inj 1:5000 (0.2 mg/ml) IV, IM; glossets (SL) 10 mg

Side effects/adverse reactions:

CNS: Tremors, anxiety, insomnia, headache, dizziness, stimulation

CV: Palpitations, tachycardia, hypertension, ***cardiac arrest***

GI: Nausea, vomiting

RESP: Bronchial irritation, edema, dryness of oropharynx

META: Hyperglycemia

Contraindications: Hypersensitivity to sympathomimetics, narrow-angle glaucoma

Precautions: Pregnancy (C), cardiac disorders, hyperthyroidism, diabetes mellitus, prostatic hypertrophy

Pharmacokinetics:

INH/SL: Onset 1-2 hr

SC: Onset 2 hr

REC: Onset 2-4 hr; metabolized in liver, lungs, GI tract

Interactions/incompatibilities:

• Increased effects of both drugs: other sympathomimetics

• Decreased action when used with β-blockers

NURSING CONSIDERATIONS

Assess:

• Resp. function: B/P, pulse, lung sounds

• Blood studies (CBC, WBC, differential) since blood dyscrasias may occur (rare)

• I&O ratio; check for urinary retention, frequency, hesitancy

Administer:

• IV; dilute 0.2 mg/10 ml normal saline (1:50,000 sol); give over 1 min; 2 mg/500 ml of D_5W; run each 1 ml (1:250,000) sol/min; may be increased

• With meals for GI symptoms

Perform/provide:

• Storage at room temperature, do not use discolored solutions

Evaluate:

• Therapeutic response: increased B/P with stabilization, ease of breathing

• For paresthesias and coldness of extremities, peripheral blood flow may decrease

• Injection site: tissue sloughing; if this occurs administer phentolamine mixed with NS

Teach patient/family:

• To rinse mouth after use

• Use of inhaler, review package insert with patient

• To avoid getting aerosol in eyes

• To wash inhaler in warm water and dry qd

• About all aspects of drug; avoid smoking, smoke-filled rooms, persons with respiratory infections

Treatment of overdose: Administer a β-blocker

---

isosorbide

(eye-soe-sor'bide)

Ismotic

Func. class.: Miscellaneous ophthalmic agent

Action: Increases osmotic gradient between plasma and ocular fluids, which decreases intraocular pressure

Uses: Intraocular pressure from glaucoma and cataract

Dosage and routes:

• *Adult:* PO 1.5 g/kg, then increase to 1-3 g/kg bid-qid

Available forms include: Sol 45%

Side effects/adverse reactions:

CNS: Headache, light-headedness, irritability, lethargy, syncope

GI: Nausea, vomiting, anorexia, diarrhea, cramps, thirst

INTEG: Rash

META: Hypernatremia, hyperosmolarity

Contraindications: Hypersensitivity, anuria, severe renal disease, pulmonary edema, hemorrhagic glaucoma, dehydration

Precautions: Pregnancy (C), patients on sodium restricted diet

NURSING CONSIDERATIONS

Assess:

• I&O; report decrease urinary output

• Electrolytes during treatment

Administer:

• After pouring over ice (oral)

Evaluate:

• Therapeutic response: decreased intraocular pressure

---

isosorbide dinitrate

(eye-soe-sor'bide)

Iso-Bid, Isotrate, Isonate, Dilatrate-SR, Coronex,* Isordil, Sorbitrate

Func. class.: Antianginal
Chem. class.: Nitrate

Action: Decreases preload, afterload, which is responsible for decreasing left ventricular end-diastolic pressure, systemic vascular resistance

Uses: Chronic stable angina pectoris, prophylaxis of angina pain

Dosage and routes:

• *Adult:* PO 5-40 mg qid; SL 2.5-10 mg, may repeat q2-3h; CHEW TAB 5-10 mg prn or q2-3h as prophylaxis, sus rel 40-80 mg q8-12 h

Available forms include: Caps ext rel 40 mg; caps 40; tabs 5, 10, 20, 30, 40 mg; chew tabs 5, 10 mg; tabs ext rel 40 mg; SL tabs 2.5, 5, 10 mg

Side effects/adverse reactions:

MISC: Twitching, hemolytic anemia, ***methemoglobinemia***

CV: Postural hypotension, tachycardia, ***collapse,*** syncope

GI: Nausea, vomiting

INTEG: Pallor, sweating, rash

CNS: Vascular headache, flushing, dizziness, weakness, faintness

Contraindications: Hypersensitivity to this drug or nitrites, severe anemia, increased intracranial pressure, cerebral hemorrhage, acute MI

Precautions: Postural hypotension, pregnancy (C), lactation, children

Pharmacokinetics:

SUS ACTION: Duration 6-8 hr

PO: Onset 15-30 min, duration 4-6 hr

SL: Onset 2-5 min, duration 1-4 hr

CHEW TAB: Onset 3 min, duration ½-3 hr; metabolized by liver, excreted in urine as metabolites (80%-100%)

Interactions/incompatibilities:

• Increased effects: β-blockers, diuretics, antihypertensives, alcohol

NURSING CONSIDERATIONS

Assess:

• B/P, pulse, respirations during beginning therapy

Administer:

• After checking expiration date

• With 8 oz of water on empty stomach (oral tablet)

Evaluate:

• Therapeutic response: decrease or prevention of anginal pain

• Pain: duration, time started, activity being performed, character

• Tolerance if taken over long period of time

• Headache, light-headedness, decreased B/P; may indicate a need for decreased dosage

Teach patient/family:

• To leave tabs in original container

• If 3 SL tabs in 15 min does not relieve pain, activate EMS

• To avoid alcohol

• That drug may cause headache, but tolerance usually develops, taking with meals may reduce or eliminate headache

• That drug may be taken before stressful activity (exercise, sexual activity)

• That SL may sting when drug comes in contact with mucous membranes

• To avoid hazardous activities if dizziness occurs

• Importance of complying with complete medical regimen

• To make position changes slowly to prevent fainting

• Not to crush, chew SL or sus rel tabs

isosorbide mononitrate

(eye-soe-sor'bide)
ISMO

Func. class.: Antianginal
Chem. class.: Nitrate

Action: Decreases preload, afterload, resulting in decreased left ventricular end-diastolic pressure, systemic vascular resistance
Uses: Prevention of angina pectoris due to coronary artery disease
Dosage and routes:
• *Adult:* PO 20 mg bid, 7 hr apart
Available forms include: Tabs 20 mg
Side effects/adverse reactions:
MISC: Twitching, hemolytic anemia, methemoglobinemia
CV: Postural hypotension, tachycardia, ***collapse,*** syncope
GI: Nausea, vomiting
INTEG: Pallor, sweating, rash
CNS: Vascular headache, flushing, dizziness, weakness, faintness
Contraindications: Hypersensitivity to nitrites, severe anemia, increased intracranial pressure, cerebral hemorrhage, acute MI, closed-angle glaucoma
Precautions: Postural hypotension, pregnancy (C), lactation, children, glaucoma
Pharmacokinetics: Metabolized by the liver, excreted in urine as metabolites (80%-100%)
Interactions/incompatibilities:
• Increased effects: β-blockers, diuretics, antihypertensives, alcohol, calcium-channel blockers

NURSING CONSIDERATIONS

Assess
• B/P, pulse, respirations during beginning therapy
Administer:
• With 8 oz of water on empty stomach (oral tablet)
Evaluate:
• Therapeutic response: absence of anginal pain
• Headache, light-headedness, decreased B/P; may indicate a need for decreased dosage
Teach patient/family:
• That drug may cause headache, but tolerance usually develops; taking with meals may reduce or eliminate headache
• To avoid hazardous activities if dizziness occurs
• To make position changes slowly to prevent fainting

isotretinoin

(eye-soe-tret'i-noyn)
Accutane

Func. class.: Dermatologic
Chem. class.: Retinoic acid isomer, vitamin A derivative

Action: Decreases sebum secretion; improves cystic acne
Uses: Severe recalcitrant cystic acne
Dosage and routes:
• *Adult:* PO 0.5-2 mg/kg/day in 2 divided doses × 15-20 wk
Available forms include: Caps 10, 20, 40 mg
Side effects/adverse reactions:
INTEG: Dry skin, pruritus, cheilosis, joint muscle pain, hair loss, photosensitivity, urticaria, bruising, hirsutism, petechiae, hypo/hyperpigmentation, nail brittleness
MS: Hyperosiosis, arthralgia, bone, joint, muscle pain
CV: Chest pain
GI: Nausea, vomiting, anorexia, increased liver enzymes, regional ileus, abdominal pain, weight loss
EENT: Eye irritation, conjunctivitis, epistaxis, dry nose, mouth,

* Available in Canada only

contact lens intolerance, optic neuritis
GU: ***Hematuria, proteinuria,*** hypouricemia
HEMA: ***Thrombocytopenia,*** decreased H&H, WBC, reticulocyte count
CNS: Lethargy, fatigue, headache, depression, ***pseudotumor cerebri***
Contraindications: Hypersensitivity, inflamed skin, pregnancy (X)
Precautions: Lactation, diabetes, photosensitivity, hepatic disease
Pharmacokinetics:
PO: Peak 2.9-3.2 hr, half-life 10-20 hr; metabolized in liver, excreted in urine, feces
Interactions/incompatibilities:
- Additive toxic effects: vitamin A, do not use together
- Pseudotumor cerebri: minocycline or tetracycline
- Increased triglyceride levels: alcohol

NURSING CONSIDERATIONS
Assess:
- Triglyceride levels, AST, ALT, alk phosphatase; before, during treatment
- Urinalysis qwk for protein, blood
- Blood glucose in diabetics periodically

Administer:
- Whole, do not crush; give with meals
- Second course of treatment if needed after waiting 2 mo

Perform/provide:
- Storage in tight, light-resistant container

Evaluate:
- Therapeutic response: decrease in size and number of lesions
- Area of body involved, including time involved, what helps or aggravates condition
- Pseudotumor cerebri: headache, vomiting, nausea, visual disturbance; discontinue drug

Teach patient/family:
- To avoid sunlight or wear sunscreen since photosensitivity may occur
- That an increase in acne may occur during initial treatment; decrease in 4-6 wk
- Not to become pregnant while taking drug
- Not to take vitamin A supplements, to take drug with meals
- Not to crush
- To minimize or eliminate alcohol consumption

Lab test interferences:
Increase: Sedimentation rate, triglyceride, liver function studies
Decrease: RBC/WBC count

isoxsuprine HCl
(eye-sox'syoo-preen)
Vasodilan, Voxsuprine
Func. class.: Peripheral vasodilator
Chem. class.: Nylidrin-related agent

Action: α-Adrenoreceptor antagonist with β-adrenoreceptor stimulate properties; may also act directly on vascular smooth muscle; causes cardiac stimulation, uterine relaxation
Uses: Symptoms of cerebrovascular insufficiency, peripheral vascular disease including arteriosclerosis obliterans, thromboangiitis obliterans, Raynaud's disease
Dosage and routes:
- *Adult:* PO 10-20 mg tid or qid

Available forms include: Tabs 10, 20 mg
Side effects/adverse reactions:
CV: Hypotension, ***tachycardia,*** palpitations, chest pain

CNS: Dizziness, weakness, tremors, anxiety
GI: Nausea, vomiting, abdominal pain, distention
INTEG: Severe rash, flushing
Contraindications: Hypersensitivity, postpartum, arterial bleeding
Precautions: Pregnancy (C), tachycardia
Pharmacokinetics:
PO: Peak 1 hr, duration 3 hr, half-life 1¼ hr; excreted in urine, crosses placenta

NURSING CONSIDERATIONS

Assess:
- B/P, pulse during treatment until stable; take B/P lying, standing; orthostatic hypotension is common

Administer:
- With meals to reduce GI upset

Perform/provide:
- Storage at room temperature

Evaluate:
- Therapeutic response: ability to walk without pain, increased pulse volume, increased temperature in extremities, orientation, long- and short-term memory

Teach patient/family:
- That medication is not cure, may need to be taken continuously depending on condition; therapeutic response may not be evident for 2-3 mo
- That it is necessary to quit smoking to prevent excessive vasoconstriction
- To avoid hazardous activities until stabilized on medication; dizziness may occur
- To make position changes slowly, or fainting will occur
- To discontinue drug, notify physician if rash develops
- To report palpitations, flushing if severe
- To avoid changes in temperature; extremities should be kept warm to promote better circulation

isradipine

DynaCirc
Func. class.: Calcium channel blocker
Chem. class.: Dihydropyridine

Action: Inhibits calcium ion influx across cell membrane during cardiac depolarization; produces relaxation of coronary vascular smooth muscle, peripheral vascular smooth muscle; dilates coronary vascular arteries; increases myocardial oxygen delivery in patients with vasospastic angina
Uses: Essential hypertension, angina
Dosage and routes:
Hypertension:
Adult: PO 1.25 mg bid, increase at 3-4 wk intervals up to 10 mg bid
Angina
Adult: PO 2.5-7.5 mg tid
Available forms include: Tabs 1.25 mg
Side effects/adverse reactions:
HEMA: ***Thrombocytopenia, leukopenia, anemia***
CV: Peripheral edema, tachycardia, hypotension, chest pain
GI: Nausea, vomiting, diarrhea, gastric upset, constipation, hepatitis
GU: Nocturia, polyuria, ***acute renal failure***
INTEG: Rash, pruritus, urticaria, photosensitivity, hair loss
CNS: Headache, fatigue, dizziness, fainting, sleep disturbances
MISC: Flushing
Contraindications: Sick sinus syndrome, 2nd or 3rd degree heart block, hypotension less than 90 mm Hg systolic, hypersensitivity

Precautions: CHF, hypotension, hepatic disease, pregnancy (C), lactation, children, renal disease, elderly

Pharmacokinetics: Metabolized in liver; metabolites are excreted in urine and feces; secreted in breast milk, peak plasma levels at 2-3 hr

Interactions/incompatibilities:

• Increased effects of: digitalis, neuromuscular blocking agents, cyclosporine

• Increased effects of isradipine: cimetidine, carbamazepine

NURSING CONSIDERATIONS

Assess:

• B/P, pulse rate, chest pain; monitor ECG periodically during therapy

Evaluate:

• Therapeutic response: decreased anginal pain, decreased B/P

• Cardiac status: B/P, pulse, respiration, ECG

Teach patient/family:

• To avoid hazardous activities until stabilized on drug, dizziness is no longer a problem

• To limit caffeine consumption

• To avoid OTC drugs unless directed by physician

• Importance of compliance in all areas of medical regimen: diet, exercise, stress reduction, drug therapy

• To notify physician of: irregular heartbeat, shortness of breath, swelling of feet and hands, pronounced dizziness, constipation, nausea, hypotension

Treatment of overdose: Defibrillation, β-agonists, IV calcium inotropic agents, diuretics, atropine for AV block, vasopressor for hypotension

kanamycin sulfate

(kan-a-mye'sin)

Anamid,* Kantrex, Klebcil

Func. class.: Antibiotic

Chem. class.: Aminoglycoside

Action: Interferes with protein synthesis in bacterial cell by binding to ribosomal subunit, causing inaccurate peptide sequence to form in protein chain, causing bacterial death

Uses: Severe systemic infections of CNS, respiratory, GI, urinary tract, bone, skin, soft tissues caused by *E. coli, Enterobacter, Acinetobacter, Proteus, N. gonorrhoeae, H. influenzae, Shigella, K. pneumoniae, S. marcescens, Staphylococcus;* also used as adjunct in hepatic coma, peritonitis, preoperatively to sterilize bowel

Dosage and routes:

Severe systemic infections

• *Adult and child:* IV INF 15 mg/kg/day in divided doses q8-12h; diluted 500 mg/200 ml of NS or D_5W given over 30-60 min, not to exceed 1.5 g/day; IM 15 mg/kg/day in divided doses q8-12h, not to exceed 1.5 g/day, irrigation not to exceed 1.5 g/day

Hepatic coma

• *Adult:* PO 8-12 g/day in divided doses

Preoperative bowel sterilization

• *Adult:* PO 1 g qh × 4 doses, then q6h × 36-72 hr

Available forms include: Inj IM, IV 75, 500 mg/2ml, 1 g/3 ml; cap 500 mg

Side effects/adverse reactions:

GU: ***Oliguria, hematuria, renal damage, azotemia, renal failure, nephrotoxicity***

CNS: Confusion, depression,

K

numbness, tremors, ***convulsions,*** muscle twitching, ***neurotoxicity***
EENT: ***Ototoxicity,*** deafness, visual disturbances, dizziness, vertigo, tinnitus
HEMA: ***Agranulocytosis, thrombocytopenia, leukopenia, eosinophilia, anemia***
GI: Nausea, vomiting, anorexia, increased ALT, AST, bilirubin, hepatomegaly, ***hepatic necrosis,*** splenomegaly
CV: Hypotension
INTEG: Rash, burning, urticaria, dermatitis, alopecia
Contraindications: Bowel obstruction, severe renal disease, hypersensitivity
Precautions: Neonates, myasthenia gravis, hearing deficits, mild renal disease, pregnancy (D), lactation, Parkinson's disease
Pharmacokinetics:
IM: Onset rapid, peak 1-2 hr
IV: Onset immediate, peak 1-2 hr
Plasma half-life 2-3 hr; not metabolized, excreted unchanged in urine, crosses placental barrier
Interactions/incompatibilities:
• Increased ototoxicity, neurotoxicity, nephrotoxicity: other aminoglycosides, amphotericin B, polymyxin, vancomycin, ethacrynic acid, furosemide, mannitol, methoxyflurane, cisplatin, cephalosporins, bacitracin
• Do not mix in solution or syringe: carbenicillin, ticarcillin, amphotericin B, cephalothin, erythromycin, heparin
• Increased effects: nondepolarizing muscle relaxants, succinylcholine
• Decreased effects of: oral anticoagulants

NURSING CONSIDERATIONS

Assess:
• Weight before treatment; calculation of dosage is usually done based on ideal body weight, but may be calculated on actual body weight
• I&O ratio, urinalysis daily for proteinuria, cells, casts; report sudden change in urine output
• VS during infusion, watch for hypotension, change in pulse
• IV site for thrombophlebitis including pain, redness, swelling q30min, change site if needed; apply warm compresses to discontinued site
• Serum peak, drawn at 30-60 min after IV infusion or 60 min after IM injection; trough level drawn just before next dose; blood level should be 2-4 times bacteriostatic level
• Urine pH if drug is used for UTI; urine should be kept alkaline
Administer:
• IV after diluting 500 mg/100 ml of D_5W, D_5/NaCl normal saline or more, give 3-4 ml/min
• IM injection in large muscle mass, rotate injection sites
• Drug in evenly spaced doses to maintain blood level
• Bicarbonate to alkalinize urine if ordered in treating UTI, as drug is most active in alkaline environment
Perform/provide:
• Adequate fluids of 2-3 L/day unless contraindicated to prevent irritation of tubules
• Flush of IV line with NS or D_5W after infusion
• Supervised ambulation, other safety measures with vestibular dysfunction
Evaluate:
• Therapeutic effect: absence of fever, draining wounds, negative C&S after treatment
• Renal impairment by securing urine for CrCl testing, BUN, serum

* Available in Canada only

creatinine; lower dosage should be given in renal impairment (CrCl <80 ml/min)

- Deafness by audiometric testing, ringing, roaring in ears, vertigo; assess hearing before, during, after treatment
- Dehydration: high sp gr, decrease in skin turgor, dry mucous membranes, dark urine
- Overgrowth of infection: increased temperature, malaise, redness, pain, swelling, perineal itching, diarrhea, stomatitis, change in cough, sputum
- C&S before starting treatment to identify infecting organism
- Vestibular dysfunction: nausea, vomiting, dizziness, headache; drug should be discontinued if severe
- Injection sites for redness, swelling, abscesses; use warm compresses at site

Teach patient/family:

- To report headache, dizziness, symptoms of overgrowth of infection, renal impairment
- To report loss of hearing, ringing, roaring in ears or feeling of fullness in head

Treatment of overdose: Hemodialysis, monitor serum levels of drug

---

kaolin, pectin

(kay'o-lynn)

Baropectin, Kaoparin, Kaopectate, Kapectin, Keotin, Pectokay

Func. class.: Antidiarrheal
Chem. class.: Hydrous magnesium aluminum silicate

Action: Decreases gastric motility, H_2O content of stool, adsorbent, demulcent

Uses: Diarrhea (cause undetermined)

Dosage and routes:

- *Adult:* PO 60-120 ml (45-90 ml conc) after each loose bowel movement
- *Child >12 yr:* PO 60 ml after each loose bowel movement
- *Child 6-12 yr:* PO 30-60 ml 30 ml conc after each loose bowel movement
- *Child 3-6 yr:* PO 15-30 ml 15 ml conc after each loose bowel movement

Available forms include: Susp Kaolin 0.87 g/5ml, pectin 43 mg/5 ml; Kaolin 0.98 g/5 ml, pectin 21.7 mg/5 ml

Side effects/adverse reactions:

GI: Constipation (chronic use)

Precautions: Pregnancy (C)

Interactions/incompatibilities:

- Decreased action of: all other drugs

NURSING CONSIDERATIONS

Administer:

- For 48 hr only

Evaluate:

- Therapeutic response: decreased diarrhea
- Bowel pattern before; for rebound constipation
- Dehydration in children

Teach patient/family:

- Not to exceed recommended dose
- To shake well before administration

---

ketamine HCl

(keet'a-meen)

Ketalar

Func. class.: General anesthetic
Chem. class.: Phencyclidine derivative

Action: Acts on limbic system, cortex to provide anesthesia

Uses: Short anesthesia for diagnostic/surgical procedures

K

Dosage and routes:
- *Adult and child:* IV 1-4.5 mg/kg over 1 min
- *Adult and child:* IM 6.5-13 mg/kg

Available forms include: Inj IM, IV 10, 50, 100 mg/ml vial
Side effects/adverse reactions:
CNS: Hallucinations, confusion, delirium, tremors, polyneuropathy, fasciculations, pseudoconvulsions
CV: Increased BP, hypotension, bradycardia
EENT: Diplopia, salivation, small increase in intraocular pressure
INTEG: Rash, pain at injection site
Contraindications: Hypersensitivity, CVA, increased intracranial pressure, severe hypertension, cardiac decompensation, child <2 yr
Precautions: Pregnancy (C), seizure disorders, elderly, psychiatric disorders
Pharmacokinetics:
IV: Peak 40 sec, duration 10 min
IM: Peak 3-8 min, duration 25 min
Interactions/incompatibilities:
- Increased action of ketamine: narcotics or atropine
- Respiratory depression: antihypertensives with CNS depressant effects
- Hypertension, tachycardia: thyroid hormones
- Increased action of: tubocurarine
- Do not mix with barbiturates in solution or syringe

NURSING CONSIDERATIONS
Assess:
- VS q10min during IV administration, q30min after IM dose

Administer:
- IV after diluting 100 mg/ml with equal parts of compatible sol; give over 1 min; may be diluted 10 ml (50 mg/ml)/500 ml of normal saline or D_5W; run at 1-2 mg/min
- Anticholinergic preoperatively to decrease solution
- Only with crash cart, resuscitative equipment nearby
- Narcotic, or diazepam to control recovery symptoms

Perform/provide:
- Quiet environment for recovery to decrease psychotic symptoms

Evaluate:
- Therapeutic response: maintenance of anesthesia
- Hallucinations, delusions, separation from environment
- Extrapyramidal reactions: dystonia, akathisia
- Increasing heart rate or decreasing B/P, notify physician at once

ketoconazole
(ke-to-con'a-zol)
Nizoral
Func. class.: Antifungal
Chem. class.: Imidazole derivative

Action: Alters cell membranes and inhibits several fungal enzymes
Uses: Systemic candidiasis, chronic mucocandidiasis, oral thrush, candiduria, coccidioidomycosis, histoplasmosis, chromomycosis, paracoccidioidomycosis
Dosage and routes:
- *Adult and child >40 kg:* PO 200 mg qd, may increase to 400 mg qd if needed
- *Child 20-40 kg:* PO 100 mg qd
- *Child <20 kg:* PO 50 mg qd

Available forms include: Tabs 200 mg; susp 100 mg/5 ml
Side effects/adverse reactions:
GU: Gynecomastia, impotence
INTEG: Pruritus, fever, chills, photophobia, rash, dermatitis, purpura, urticaria
CNS: Headache, dizziness, lethargy, anxiety, insomnia, dreams, paresthesia
SYST: ***Anaphylaxis***

* Available in Canada only

GI: Nausea, vomiting, anorexia, diarrhea, cramps, abdominal pain, constipation, flatulence, GI bleeding, ***hepatotoxicity***

Contraindications: Hypersensitivity, pregnancy (C), lactation, meningitis

Precautions: Renal disease, hepatic disease, achlorhydria (drug-induced)

Pharmacokinetics:

PO: Peak 1-2 hr, half-life 2 hr, terminal 8 hr, metabolized in liver, excreted in bile, feces, requires acid pH for absorption, distributed poorly to CSF, highly protein bound

Interactions/incompatibilities:

- Hepatotoxicity: other hepatotoxic drugs
- Increased action of ketoconazole: cyclosporine
- Decreased action of: antacids, H_2-receptor antagonists, isoniazid, rifampin
- Increased anticoagulant effect, coumarin anticoagulants
- Severe hypoglycemia; oral hypoglycemics
- Disulfuram reaction: alcohol

NURSING CONSIDERATIONS

Assess:

- I&O ratio
- Liver studies (ALT, AST, bilirubin) if on long-term therapy

Administer:

- In the presence of acid products only; do not use alkaline products or antacids within 2 hr of drug; may give coffee, tea, acidic fruit juices
- With food to decrease GI symptoms
- With hydrochloric acid if achlorhydria is present

Perform/provide:

- Storage in tight containers at room temperature

Evaluate:

- Therapeutic response: decreased fever, malaise, rash, negative C&S for infecting organism
- For allergic reaction: rash, photosensitivity, urticaria, dermatitis
- For hepatotoxicity: nausea, vomiting, jaundice, clay-colored stools, fatigue

Teach patient/family:

- That long-term therapy may be needed to clear infection (1 wk-6 mo depending on infection)
- To avoid hazardous activities if dizziness occurs
- To take 2 hr ac administration of other drugs that increase gastric pH (antacids, H_2-blockers, anticholinergics
- Importance of compliance with drug regimen
- To notify physician if GI symptoms, signs of liver dysfunction (fatigue, nausea, anorexia, vomiting, dark urine, pale stools)

ketoprofen

(ke-to-proe'fen)

Orudis

Func. class.: Nonsteroidal

Chem. class.: Propionic acid derivative

Action: Inhibits prostaglandin synthesis by decreasing enzyme needed for biosynthesis; possesses analgesic, antiinflammatory, antipyretic properties

Uses: Mild to moderate pain, osteoarthritis, rheumatoid arthritis, dysmenorrhea

Dosage and routes:

- *Adult:* PO 150-300 mg in divided doses tid-qid, not to exceed 300 mg/day

Available forms include: Caps 50, 75 mg

Side effects/adverse reactions:
GI: Nausea, anorexia, vomiting, diarrhea, jaundice, ***cholestatic hepatitis,*** constipation, flatulence, cramps, dry mouth, peptic ulcer
CNS: Dizziness, drowsiness, fatigue, tremors, confusion, insomnia, anxiety, depression
CV: Tachycardia, peripheral edema, palpitations, dysrhythmias
INTEG: Purpura, rash, pruritus, sweating
GU: ***Nephrotoxicity: dysuria, hematuria, oliguria, azotemia***
HEMA: ***Blood dyscrasias***
EENT: Tinnitus, hearing loss, blurred vision
Contraindications: Hypersensitivity, asthma, severe renal disease, severe hepatic disease
Precautions: Pregnancy (B), lactation, children, bleeding disorders, GI disorders, cardiac disorders, hypersensitivity to other antiinflammatory agents, elderly
Pharmacokinetics:
PO: Peak 2 hr, half-life 3-3½ hr, metabolized in liver, excreted in urine (metabolites), excreted in breast milk, 99% plasma protein binding
Interactions/incompatibilities:
- Increased action of: coumarin, streptokinase, probenecid

NURSING CONSIDERATIONS

Assess:
- Renal, liver, blood studies: BUN, creatinine, AST, ALT, Hgb, before treatment, periodically thereafter
- Audiometric, ophthalmic examination before, during, after treatment

Administer:
- With food to decrease GI symptoms; however, best to take on empty stomach to facilitate absorption

Perform/provide:
- Storage at room temperature

Evaluate:
- Therapeutic response: decreased pain, stiffness in joints, decreased swelling in joints, ability to move more easily
- For eye, ear problems: blurred vision, tinnitus; may indicate toxicity

Teach patient/family:
- To report blurred vision, ringing, roaring in ears; may indicate toxicity
- To avoid driving, other hazardous activities if dizziness, drowsiness occurs, especially elderly
- To report change in urine pattern, increased weight, edema, increased pain in joints, fever, blood in urine; indicate nephrotoxicity
- That therapeutic effects may take up to 1 mo

---

ketorolac

(kec'toe-role-ak)
Toradol
Func. class.: Nonsteroidal antiinflammatory
Chem. class.: Pyrrole acetic acid derivative

Action: Inhibits prostaglandin synthesis by decreasing an enzyme needed for biosynthesis; possesses analgesic, antiinflammatory, antipyretic properties
Uses: Mild to moderate pain, osteoarthritis, rheumatoid arthritis
Dosage and routes:
- *Adult:* IM 30-60 mg loading dose, then 15-30 mg q6h

Available forms include: inj 15, 30, 60 mg (prefilled syringes)
Side effects/adverse reactions:
GI: Nausea, anorexia, vomiting, diarrhea, jaundice, ***cholestatic hepatitis,*** constipation, flatulence,

cramps, dry mouth, peptic ulcer
CNS: Dizziness, drowsiness, fatigue, tremors, confusion, insomnia, anxiety, depression
CV: Tachycardia, peripheral edema, palpitations, dysrhythmias
INTEG: Purpura, rash, pruritus, sweating
GU: ***Nephrotoxicity: dysuria, hematuria, oliguria, azotemia***
HEMA: ***Blood dyscrasias***
EENT: Tinnitus, hearing loss, blurred vision
Contraindications: Hypersensitivity, asthma, severe renal disease, severe hepatic disease
Precautions: Pregnancy (B), lactation, children, bleeding disorders, GI disorders, cardiac disorders, hypersensitivity to other antiinflammatory agents
Pharmacokinetics:
IM: Peak 50 min, half-life 6 hr
Interactions/incompatibilities:
• Increased action of ketorolac: phenytoin, sulfonamides

NURSING CONSIDERATIONS

Assess:
• Renal, liver, blood studies: BUN, creatinine, AST, ALT, Hgb before treatment, periodically thereafter
• Audiometric, ophthalmic exam before, during, after treatment
Administer:
• With food to decrease GI symptoms; best to take on empty stomach to facilitate absorption
Perform/provide:
• Storage at room temperature
Evaluate:
• Therapeutic response: decreased pain, stiffness, swelling in joints, ability to move more easily
• For eye, ear problems: blurred vision, tinnitus (may indicate toxicity)
Teach patient/family:
• To report blurred vision or ringing, roaring in ears (may indicate toxicity)
• To avoid driving or other hazardous activities if dizziness or drowsiness occurs
• To report change in urine pattern, weight increase, edema, pain increase in joints, fever, blood in urine (indicates nephrotoxicity)
• That therapeutic effects may take up to 1 mo
• To take with a full glass of water

---

labetalol

(la-bet'a-lole)
Normodyne, Trandate
Func. class.: Antihypertensive
Chem. class.: Nonselective β-blocker

Action: Produces falls in B/P without reflex tachycardia or significant reduction in heart rate through mixture of α-blocking, β-blocking effects; elevated plasma renins are reduced
Uses: Mild to moderate hypertension
Dosage and routes:
Hypertension
• *Adult:* PO 100 mg bid, may be given with a diuretic, may increase to 200 mg bid after 2 days, may continue to increase q1-3 days; max 400 mg bid
Hypertensive crisis
• *Adult:* IV INF 200 mg/160 ml D_5W, run at 2 ml/min; stop infusion after desired response obtained, repeat q6-8h as needed; IV BOL 20 mg over 2 min, may repeat 40-80 mg q10min, not to exceed 300 mg
Available forms include: Tabs 100, 200, 300 mg, inj 5 mg/ml in 20 ml amps

Side effects/adverse reactions:
CV: Orthostatic hypotension, bradycardia, ***CHF,*** chest pain, ***ventricular dysrhythmias***, AV block
CNS: Dizziness, mental changes, drowsiness, fatigue, headache, catatonia, depression, anxiety, nightmares, paresthesias, lethargy
GI: Nausea, vomiting, diarrhea
INTEG: Rash, alopecia, urticaria, pruritus, fever
HEMA: ***Agranulocytosis, thrombocytopenia, purpura*** (rare)
EENT: Tinnitus, visual changes, sore throat, double vision, dry burning eyes
GU: Impotence, dysuria, ejaculatory failure
RESP: ***Bronchospasm,*** dyspnea, wheezing
Contraindications: Hypersensitivity to β-blockers, cardiogenic shock, heart block (2nd or 3rd degree), sinus bradycardia, CHF, bronchial asthma
Precautions: Major surgery, pregnancy (C), lactation, diabetes mellitus, renal disease, thyroid disease, COPD, well compensated heart failure, CAD, nonallergic bronchospasm
Pharmacokinetics:
PO: Onset 1-2 hr, peak 2-4 hr, duration 8-12 hr
IV: Peak 5 min
Half-life 6-8 hr, metabolized by liver (metabolites inactive), excreted in urine, bile, crosses placenta, excreted in breast milk
Interactions/incompatibilities:
• Increased bronchodilation: β-adrenergic agonists
• Increased hypotension: diuretics, other antihypertensives, halothane, cimetidine, nitroglycerin
• Decreased effects: sympathomimetics, lidocaine, indomethacin, theophylline, cimetidine
• Increased hypoglycemia: insulin

NURSING CONSIDERATIONS

Assess:
• I&O, weight daily
• B/P during beginning treatment, periodically thereafter, pulse q4h; note rate, rhythm, quality
• Apical/radial pulse before administration; notify physician of any significant changes
• Baselines in renal, liver function tests before therapy begins
Administer:
• IV undiluted or diluted in compatible sol; give undiluted 20 mg or less/2 min; infusion is titrated to patient response
• PO ac, hs, tablet may be crushed or swallowed whole
• Reduced dosage in renal dysfunction
• IV, keep patient recumbent for 3 hr
Perform/provide:
• Storage in dry area at room temperature, do not freeze
Evaluate:
• Therapeutic response: decreased B/P after 1-2 wk
• Edema in feet, legs daily
• Skin turgor, dryness of mucous membranes for hydration status
Teach patient/family:
• Not to discontinue drug abruptly, taper over 2 wk, may cause precipitate angina
• Not to use OTC products containing α-adrenergic stimulants (nasal decongestants, OTC cold preparations) unless directed by physician
• To report bradycardia, dizziness, confusion, depression, fever
• To take pulse at home, advise when to notify physician

• To avoid alcohol, smoking, sodium intake
• To comply with weight control, dietary adjustments, modified exercise program
• To carry Medic Alert ID to identify drug you are taking, allergies
• To avoid hazardous activities if dizziness is present
• To report symptoms of CHF: difficult breathing, especially on exertion or when lying down, night cough, swelling of extremities
• To take medication at bedtime to prevent effect of orthostatic hypotension
• To wear support hose to minimize effects of orthostatic hypotension

Lab test interferences:
False increase: Urinary catecholamines

Treatment of overdose: Lavage, IV atropine for bradycardia, IV theophylline for bronchospasm, digitalis, O_2, diuretic for cardiac failure; hemodialysis is useful for removal, hypotension; administer vasopressor (norepinephrine)

---

lactulose

(lak'tyoo-lose)

Cephulac, Chronulac

Func. class.: Ammonia detoxicant
Chem. class.: Lactose synthetic derivative

Action: Prevents absorption of ammonia in colon

Uses: Constipation, portal-systemic encephalopathy in patients with hepatic disease

Dosage and routes:
Constipation
• *Adult:* PO 15-60 ml qd
Encephalopathy
• *Adult:* PO 20-30 g tid or qid until stools are soft; RET ENEMA 30-45 ml in 100 ml of fluid

Available forms include: Oral sol, rec sol 3.33 g/5 ml

Side effects/adverse reactions:
GI: Nausea, vomiting, anorexia, cramps, diarrhea, flatulence

Contraindications: Hypersensitivity, low galactose diet

Precautions: Pregnancy (C), lactation, diabetes mellitus

Pharmacokinetics: Metabolized in intestine, excreted by kidneys

Interactions/incompatibilities:
• Decreased effects of lactulose: neomycin, other oral antiinfectives

NURSING CONSIDERATIONS

Assess:
• Blood ammonia level (30-70 mg/100 ml)
• Blood, urine electrolytes if drug is used often by patient
• I&O ratio to identify fluid loss

Administer:
• With fruit juice, water, milk to increase palatability of oral form
• Retention enema by diluting 300 ml lactose/700 ml of water; administer by rectal balloon catheter
• Increase fluids to 2 L/day, do not give with other laxatives; if diarrhea occurs, reduce dosage

Evaluate:
• Therapeutic response: decreased constipation, decreased blood ammonia level
• Cause of constipation; identify whether fluids, bulk, or exercise is missing from lifestyle
• Cramping, rectal bleeding, nausea, vomiting; if these symptoms occur, drug should be discontinued
• Clearing of confusion, lethargy, restlessness, irritability

Teach patient/family:
• Not to use laxatives for long-term therapy; bowel tone will be lost

L

leucovorin calcium (citrovorum factor/folinic acid)

(loo-koe-vor'in)

Calcium Folinate, Wellcovorin

Func. class.: Vitamin/folic acid antagonist antidote

Chem. class.: Tetrahydrofolic acid derivative

Action: Needed for normal growth patterns, prevents toxicity during antineoplastic therapy by protecting normal cells

Uses: Megaloblastic or macrocytic anemia caused by folic acid deficiency, overdose of folic acid antagonist, methotrexate toxicity, toxicity caused by pyrimethamine or trimethoprim, pneumocystosis, toxoplasmosis

Dosage and routes:

Megaloblastic anemia caused by enzyme deficiency

• *Adult and child:* IM 3-6 mg qd, then 1 mg PO for life

Megaloblastic anemia caused by deficiency of folate

• *Adult and child:* IM 1 mg or less qd, continued until adequate response

Methotrexate toxicity

• *Adult and child:* Given 6-36 hr after dose of methotrexate

Pyrimethamine toxicity

• *Adult and child:* PO/IM 5 mg qd

Trimethoprim toxicity

• *Adult and child:* PO IM 400 μg qd

Available forms include: Tabs 5, 25 mg; inj IM 3, 5 mg/ml; powder for inj 10 mg/ml

Side effects/adverse reactions:

RESP: Wheezing

INTEG: Rash, pruritus, erythema

Contraindications: Hypersensitivity, anemias other than megaloblastic not associated with B_{12}-deficiency

Precautions: Pregnancy (C)

Interactions/incompatibilities:

• Decreased folate levels: chloramphenicol

• Increased metabolism of: phenobarbitol, hydantoins

NURSING CONSIDERATIONS

Assess:

• CrCl before leucovorin rescue and qd to detect nephrotoxicity

• I&O; watch for nausea and vomiting

Administer:

• Within 1 hr of folic acid antagonist

• After reconstituting with bacteriostatic water for inj

Perform/provide:

• Increase fluid intake if used to treat folic acid inhibitor overdose

• Protection from light and heat

Evaluate:

• Therapeutic response: increased weight, oriented, well-being, absence of fatigue

• Nutritional status: bran, yeast, dried beans, nuts, fruits, fresh vegetables, asparagus

• Drugs currently taken: alcohol, hydantoins, trimethoprim may cause increased folic acid use by body

Teach patient/family:

• To take drug exactly as prescribed

• To notify physician of side effects

leuprolide acetate

(loo-proe'-lide)

Lupron

Func. class.: Antineoplastic hormone

Chem. class.: Gonadotropin-releasing hormone

Action: Causes initial increase

* Available in Canada only

in circulating levels of LH, FSH; continuous administration results in decreased LH, FSH. In males, testosterone is reduced to castrate levels; in premenopausal females, estrogen is reduced to menopausal levels
Uses: Metastatic prostate cancer, management of endometriosis
Dosage and routes:
• *Adult:* SC 1 mg/day
Available forms include: Inj IM 3.75 mg, 7.5 mg single dose, multiple dose vials
Side effects/adverse reactions:
GU: Edema, hot flashes, impotence, decreased libido, amenorrhea, vaginal dryness, gynecomastia
Contraindications: Hypersensitivity to GnRH or analogs, thromboembolic disorders, pregnancy (X), lactation, undiagnosed vaginal bleeding
Precautions: Edema, hepatic disease, CVA, MI, seizures, hypertension, diabetes mellitus

NURSING CONSIDERATIONS

Assess:
• Liver function tests before, during therapy (bilirubin, AST, ALT, LDH) as needed or monthly
• Pituitary gonadotropic and gonadal function during therapy and 4-8 wk after therapy is decreased
• Increased worsening of signs and symptoms is normal during beginning therapy
Perform/provide:
• Nutritious diet with iron, vitamin supplements as ordered
• Storage in tight container at room temperature
Evaluate:
• Therapeutic response: decreased tumor size. spread of malignancy
• Fatigue, increased pulse, pallor, lethargy
• Food preferences; list likes, dislikes
• Edema in feet, joint, stomach pain, shaking
• Symptoms indicating severe allergic reaction: rash, pruritus, urticaria, purpuric skin lesions, itching, flushing
Teach patient/family:
• To notify physician if menstruation continues; menstruation should stop
• To use a nonhormoral method of contraception during therapy
• That bone pain will disappear after 1 wk
• To report any complaints, side effects to nurse or physician
• How to prepare, give and rotate sites for SC injections
• To keep accurate records of dose
• That tumor flare may occur: increase in size of tumor, increased bone pain, and will subside rapidly, may take analgesics for pain; premenopausal women need to use mechanical birth control because ovulation may be induced.

levamisole HCl

(lee-vam'i-sol)
Ergamisol
Func. class.: Immunomodulator

Action: May increase the action of macrophages, monocytes, and T cells, which will restore immune function; complete action is unknown
Uses: Treatment of Dukes' stage C colon cancer given with fluorouracil after surgical resection
Dosage and routes:
• *Adult:* PO 50 mg q8h × 3 days, begin treatment at least 1 wk but no more than 4 wk after resection; given with fluorouracil 450 mg/m^2/

L

day; IV given daily × 5 days beginning 21-34 days after resection, maintenance is 50 mg q8h × 3 days q2wk × 1 yr; given with fluorouracil 45 mg/m^2/day by IV push qwk starting 28 days after the initial 5-day course × 1 yr
Available forms include: Tab 50 mg (base)
Side effects/adverse reactions:
CNS: Dizziness, headache, paresthesia, somnolence, depression, anxiety, fatigue, fever, mental changes, ataxia, insomnia
GI: Nausea, vomiting, anorexia, diarrhea, stomatitis, constipation, flatulence, dyspepsia, abdominal pain
INTEG: Rash, pruritus, alopecia, dermatitis, urticaria
HEMA: ***Granulocytopenia, leukopenia, thrombocytopenia***
CV: Chest pain, edema
META: Hyperbilirubinemia
EENT: Blurred vision, conjunctivitis
OTHER: Rigors, infection, altered sense of smell, arthralgia, myalgia
Contraindications: Hypersensitivity
Precautions: Pregnancy (C), lactation, children, blood dyscrasias
Pharmacokinetics: Peak 1.5-2 hr, elimination half-life 3-4 hr, metabolized by the liver
Interactions/incompatibilities:
• Increased plasma levels: phenytoin
• Disulfiram-like reaction: alcohol

NURSING CONSIDERATIONS

Assess:
• Kidney, liver function studies: BUN, creatinine, AST, ALT, alk phosphatase, bilirubin
• Baseline blood counts with differential, platelets, electrolyte, repeat q3mo for 1 yr; if platelets are <100,000/mm^3 therapy, should be discontinued and restarted after recovery; fluorouracil should not be given if WBC is 2500-3500/mm^3; after WBC is >3500/mm^3, dose should be reduced by 20%; if WBC <2500/mm^3 for 10 days, discontinue levamisole
• Stomatitis or GI symptoms, drug may need to be discontinued, then start fluorouracil 28 days after the start of 1st course
Administer:
• 7-20 days after surgery, start fluorouracil with 2nd course of levamisole; begin no sooner than 21 days and no later than 35 days after surgery; if levamisole therapy begins 21-30 days after resection, fluorouracil should be given with 1st course
Evaluate:
• Therapeutic response: decrease in size and spread of tumor
• Blood dyscrasias (anemia, granulocytopenia); bruising, fatigue, bleeding, poor healing
• Allergic reactions: dermatitis, exfoliative dermatitis, pruritus, urticaria
Teach patient/family:
• To call physician if sore throat, swollen lymph nodes, malaise, fever occur since other infections may occur

---

levodopa

(lee-voe-doe'pa)
Dopar, Larodopa, Levopa, Parda, Rio-Dopa
Func. class.: Antiparkinson agent
Chem. class.: Catecholamine

Action: Decarboxylation to dopamine, which increases dopamine levels in brain
Uses: Parkinsonism, carbon mon-

* Available in Canada only

oxide, chronic manganese intoxication, cerebral arteriosclerosis

Dosage and routes:

• *Adult:* PO 0.5-1 g qd divided bid-qid with meals, may increase by up to 0.75 g q3-7 days, not to exceed 8 g/day unless closely supervised

Available forms include: Caps 100, 250, 500 mg; tabs 100, 250, 500 mg

Side effects/adverse reactions:

HEMA: ***Hemolytic anemia, leukopenia, agranulocytosis***

CNS: Involuntary choreiform movements, hand tremors, fatigue, headache, anxiety, twitching, numbness, weakness, confusion, agitation, insomnia, nightmares, psychosis, hallucination, hypomania, severe depression, dizziness

GI: Nausea, vomiting, anorexia, abdominal distress, dry mouth, flatulence, dysphagia, bitter taste, diarrhea, constipation

INTEG: Rash, sweating, alopecia

CV: Orthostatic hypotension, tachycardia, hypertension, palpitation

EENT: Blurred vision, diplopia, dilated pupils

MISC: Urinary retention incontinence, weight change, dark urine

Contraindications: Hypersensitivity, narrow-angle glaucoma, undiagnosed skin lesions

Precautions: Renal disease, cardiac disease, hepatic disease, respiratory disease, MI with dysrhythmias, convulsions, peptic ulcer, pregnancy (C), asthma, endocrine disease, affective disorders, psychosis, lactation, children <12 yrs

Pharmacokinetics:

PO: Peak 1-3 hr, excreted in urine (metabolites)

Interactions/incompatibilities:

• Hypertensive crisis: MAOIs, furazolidone

• Decreased effects of levodopa: anticholinergics, hydantoins, methionine, papaverine, pyridoxine, tricyclics

• Increased effects of levodopa: antacids, metoclopramide

NURSING CONSIDERATIONS

Assess:

• B/P, respiration

Administer:

• Drug up until NPO before surgery

• Adjust dosage depending on patient response

• With meals; limit protein taken with drug

• Only after MAOIs have been discontinued for 2 wk

Perform/provide:

• Assistance with ambulation, during beginning therapy

• Testing for diabetes mellitus, acromegaly if on long-term therapy

Evaluate:

• Therapeutic response: decrease in akathisia, increased mood

• Mental status: affect, mood, behavioral changes, depression, complete suicide assessment

Teach patient/family:

• To change positions slowly to prevent orthostatic hypotension

• To report side effects: twitching, eye spasms; indicate overdose

• To use drug exactly as prescribed; if drug is discontinued abruptly, parkinsonian crisis may occur

• That urine, sweat may darken

• To avoid vitamin B_6-preparations, vitamin-fortified foods containing B_6; these foods can reverse effects of levodopa

Lab test interferences:

False positive: Urine ketones, urine glucose

False negative: Urine glucose (glucose oxidase)

L

False increase: Uric acid, urine protein
Decrease: VMA

levodopa-carbidopa

(lee-voe-doe'pa) (kar-bi-doe'pa)
Sinemet
Func. class.: Antiparkinson agent
Chem. class.: Catecholamine

Action: Decarboxylation of levodopa to periphery is inhibited by carbidopa; more levodopa is made available for transport to brain and conversion to dopamine in the brain
Uses: Parkinsonism resulting from carbon monoxide, chronic manganese intoxication, cerebral arteriosclerosis
Dosage and routes:
• *Adult:* PO 3-6 tabs of 25 mg carbidopa/250 mg levodopa qd in divided doses, not to exceed 8 tabs/day
Available forms include: Tabs 10/100, 25/100, 25 mg carbidopa/250 mg levodopa
Side effects/adverse reactions:
HEMA: ***Hemolytic anemia, leukopenia, agranulocytosis***
CNS: Involuntary choreiform movements, hand tremors, fatigue, headache, anxiety, twitching, numbness, weakness, confusion, agitation, insomnia, nightmares, psychosis, hallucination, hypomania, severe depression, dizziness
GI: Nausea, vomiting, anorexia, abdominal distress, dry mouth, flatulence, dysphagia, bitter taste, diarrhea, constipation
INTEG: Rash, sweating, alopecia
CV: Orthostatic hypotension, tachycardia, hypertension, palpitation
EENT: Blurred vision, diplopia, dilated pupils
MISC: Urinary retention, incontinence, weight change, dark urine
Contraindications: Hypersensitivity, narrow-angle glaucoma, undiagnosed skin lesions
Precautions: Renal disease, cardiac disease, hepatic disease, respiratory disease, MI with dysrhythmias, convulsions, peptic ulcer, pregnancy (C)
Pharmacokinetics:
PO: Peak 1-3 hr, excreted in urine (metabolites)
Interactions/incompatibilities:
• Hypertensive crisis: MAOIs, furazolidone
• Decreased effects of levodopa: anticholinergics, hydantoins, methionine, papaverine, pyridoxine, tricyclics
• Increased effects of levodopa: antacids, metoclopramide

NURSING CONSIDERATIONS

Assess:
• B/P, respiration
Administer:
• Drug up until NPO before surgery
• Adjust dosage depending on patient response
• With meals; limit protein taken with drug
• Only after MAOIs have been discontinued for 2 wk; if previously on levodopa, discontinue for at least 8 hr before change to levodopa-carbidopa
Perform/provide:
• Assistance with ambulation during beginning therapy
• Testing for diabetes mellitus, acromegaly if on long-term therapy
Evaluate:
• Therapeutic response: decrease in akathisia, increased mood
• Mental status: affect, mood, be-

havioral changes, depression, complete suicide assessment

Teach patient/family:

• To change positions slowly to prevent orthostatic hypotension

• To report side effects: twitching, eye spasms; indicate overdose

• To use drug exactly as prescribed; if drug is discontinued abruptly, parkinsonian crisis may occur; physician may recommend drug-free holidays

• That urine, sweat may darken

• To use physical activities to maintain mobility and lessen spasms

• That improvement may not occur for 3-4 months

Lab test interferences:

False positive: Urine ketones

False negative: Urine glucose

False increase: Uric acid, urine protein

Decrease: VMA, BUN, creatinine

---

levonorgestrel implant

(lee-voe-nor-jess'trel)

Norplant

Func. class.: Contraceptive system

Chem. class.: Synthetic progestin

Action: As a progestin it transforms proliferative endometrium into secretory endometrium; inhibits secretion of pituitary gonadotropins, which prevents follicular maturation and ovulation

Uses: Prevention of pregnancy for 5 yr

Dosage and routes:

• *Adult:* 6 caps subdermally implanted in the upper arm during 1st 7 days of onset of menses

Available forms include: Kit of 6 cap, 36 mg/cap

Side effects/adverse reactions:

CNS: Dizziness, headache, nervousness

GU: Amenorrhea, cervical erosion, breakthrough bleeding, dysmenorrhea, vaginal candidiasis, breast changes, vaginitis

GI: Nausea, abdominal discomfort

INTEG: Alopecia, dermatitis, hirsutism, acne, hypertrichosis, infection at site, pain/itching at site

OTHER: Change in appetite, weight gain

Contraindications: Hypersensitivity, pregnancy (X), thrombophlebitis, undiagnosed genital bleeding, liver tumors, breast carcinoma, liver disease

Precautions: Depression, psychosis, lactation, fluid retention, contact lens wearers

Pharmacokinetics: Max concentration at 24 hr

Interactions/incompatibilities:

• Decreased contraception: phenytoin, carbamazepine

NURSING CONSIDERATIONS

Assess:

• Blood studies: cholesterol, triglycerides; may be increased or decreased; sex hormone-binding globulin, thyroxine, T_3 uptake

• Menstrual irregularities: spotting, prolonged bleeding, amenorrhea; usually diminish

• For jaundice, thrombophlebitis, implants should be removed

• For acne, dermatitis, hirsutism, alopecia

Administer:

• 8 cm above the crease of the elbow; implantation should be during first 7 days of the onset of menses; implantation should be fanlike, 15 degrees apart

Evaluate:

• Therapeutic response: absence of pregnancy

Teach patient/family:

• That if vision problems occur, an ophthalmologist should be seen

• That physical examinations are necessary

levorphanol tartrate

(lee-vor'fa-nole)

Levo-Dromoran

Func. class.: Narcotic analgesics
Chem. class.: Opiate, synthetic morphine derivative

Controlled Substance Schedule II
Action: Depresses pain impulse transmission at the spinal cord level by interacting with opioid receptors
Uses: Moderate to severe pain
Dosage and routes:
• *Adult:* PO/SC/IV 2-3 mg q6-8h prn
Available forms include: Inj SC/IV 2 mg/ml; tabs 2 mg
Side effects/adverse reactions:
CNS: Drowsiness, dizziness, confusion, headache, sedation, euphoria
GI: Nausea, vomiting, anorexia, constipation, cramps
GU: Increased urinary output, dysuria
INTEG: Rash, urticaria, bruising, flushing, diaphoresis, pruritus
EENT: Tinnitus, blurred vision, miosis, diplopia
CV: Palpitations, bradycardia, change in B/P
RESP: ***Respiratory depression***
Contraindications: Hypersensitivity, addiction (narcotic)
Precautions: Addictive personality, pregnancy (B), lactation, increase intracranial pressure, MI (acute), severe heart disease, respiratory depression, hepatic disease, renal disease, child <18 yr
Pharmacokinetics:
SC: Peak 1-½ hr, duration 6-8 hr
IV: Peak 20 min, duration 6-8 hr; metabolized by liver, excreted by kidneys, crosses placenta, excreted in breast milk, half-life 11 hr
Interactions/incompatibilities:
• Effects may be increased with other CNS depressants: alcohol, narcotics, sedative/hypnotics, antipsychotics, skeletal muscle relaxants

NURSING CONSIDERATIONS
Assess:
• I&O ratio; check for decreasing output; may indicate urinary retention
Administer:
• With antiemetic if nausea, vomiting occur
• When pain is beginning to return; determine dosage interval by patient response
• IV directly over 5 min
Perform/provide:
• Storage in light-resistant area at room temperature
• Assistance with ambulation
• Safety measures: siderails, night light, call bell within easy reach
Evaluate:
• Therapeutic response: decrease in pain
• CNS changes: dizziness, drowsiness, hallucinations, euphoria, LOC, pupil reaction
• Allergic reactions: rash, urticaria
• Respiratory dysfunction: respiratory depression, character, rate, rhythm; notify physician if respirations are <10/min
• Need for pain medication, physical dependence
Teach patient/family:
• To report any symptoms of CNS changes, allergic reactions
• That physical dependency may result when used for extended periods of time
• Withdrawal symptoms may occur: nausea, vomiting, cramps, fever, faintness, anorexia

Lab test interferences:
Increase: Amylase
Treatment of overdose: Narcan 0.2-0.8 IV, O_2, IV fluids, vasopressors

levothyroxine sodium (T_4, L-thyroxine sodium)

(lee-voe-thye-rox'een)

Eltroxin, Levoid, Levothroid, Noroxine, Synthroid, Syroxine, Synthrox

Func. class.: Thyroid hormone
Chem. class.: Levoisomer of thyroxine

Action: Increases metabolic rates, increases cardiac output, O_2 consumption, body temperature, blood volume, growth, development at cellular level
Uses: Hypothyroidism, myxedema coma, thyroid hormone replacement, cretinism, euthyroid states, thyrotoxicosis
Dosage and routes:
- *Adult:* PO 0.025-0.1 mg qd, increased by 0.05-0.1 mg q1-4 wk until desired response, maintenance dose 0.1-0.4 mg qd
- *Child:* PO 0.01-0.05 qd, may increase 0.025-0.05 mg q1-4 wk until desired response

Cretinism
- *Child:* IV 0.025-0.05 mg qd, may increase by 0.05-0.1 mg PO q2-3wk

Myxedema coma
- *Adult:* IV 0.2-0.5 mg, may increase by 0.1-0.3 mg after 24 hr; place on oral medication as soon as possible

Available forms include: Inj IV 200, 500 μg/vial; tabs 0.025, 0.05, 0.075, 0.1, 0.125, 0.15, 0.175, 0.2, 0.3 mg

Side effects/adverse reactions:
CNS: Anxiety, insomnia, tremors, headache, ***thyroid storm***
CV: Tachycardia, palpitations, angina, dysrhythmias, hypertension, ***cardiac arrest***
GI: Nausea, diarrhea, increased or decreased appetite, cramps
MISC: Menstrual irregularities, weight loss, sweating, heat intolerance, fever
Contraindications: Adrenal insufficiency, myocardial infarction, thyrotoxicosis
Precautions: Elderly, angina pectoris, hypertension, ischemia, cardiac disease, pregnancy (A), lactation
Pharmacokinetics:
IV/PO: Peak 12-48 hr, half-life 6-7 days; distributed throughout body tissues
Interactions/incompatibilities:
- Decreased absorption of levothyroxine: cholestyramine
- Increased effects of: anticoagulants, sympathomimetics, tricyclic antidepressants
- Decreased effects of: digitalis drugs, insulin, hypoglycemics
- Decreased effects of levothyroxine: estrogens

NURSING CONSIDERATIONS

Assess:
- B/P, pulse before each dose
- I&O ratio
- Weight qd in same clothing, using same scale, at same time of day
- Height, growth rate if given to a child
- T_3, T_4, FTIs which are decreased, radioimmunoassay of TSH, which is increased, radio uptake, which is decreased if patient is on too low a dose of medication
- Pro-time may require decreased anticoagulant, check for bleeding, bruising

Administer:
• IV after diluting with provided diluent 0.5 mg/5 ml; shake; give through Y-tube or 3-way stopcock; give 0.1 mg or less over 1 min
• In AM if possible as a single dose to decrease sleeplessness
• At same time each day, to maintain drug level
• Only for hormone imbalances, not to be used for obesity, male infertility, menstrual conditions, lethargy
• Lowest dose that relieves symptoms

Perform/provide:
• Storage in tight, light-resistant container; solutions should be discarded if not used immediately
• Removal of medication 4 wk before RAIU test

Evaluate:
• Therapeutic response: absence of depression, increased weight loss, diuresis, pulse, appetite, absence of constipation, peripheral edema, cold intolerance, pale, cool dry skin, brittle nails, alopecia, coarse hair, menorrhagia, night blindness, paresthesias, syncope, stupor, coma, rosy cheeks
• Increased nervousness, excitability, irritability, which may indicate too high dose of medication, usually after 1-3 wk of treatment
• Cardiac status: angina, palpitation, chest pain, change in VS

Teach patient/family:
• That hair loss will occur in child, is temporary
• To report excitability, irritability, anxiety, which indicate overdose
• Not to switch brands unless approved by physician
• That drug may be discontinued after birth, thyroid panel evaluated after 1-2 mo
• That hypothyroid child will show almost immediate behavior/personality change
• That treatment drug is not to be taken to reduce weight
• To avoid OTC preparations with iodine, read labels
• To avoid iodine food, salt-iodinized, soy beans, tofu, turnips, some seafood, some bread

Lab test interferences:
Increase: CPK, LDH, AST, PBI, blood glucose
Decrease: TSH, ^{131}I uptake test, uric acid, triglycerides

---

lidocaine/lidocaine HCl (topical)

(lye'-doe-kane)
Stanacaine, Xylocaine
Func. class.: Topical anesthetic
Chem. class.: Aminoacylamide

Action: Inhibits nerve impulses from sensory nerves, which produces anesthesia
Uses: Pruritus, sunburn, toothache, sore throat, cold sores, oral pain

Dosage and routes:
• *Adult and child:* TOP apply q3-4h to affected area; INSTILL 15 ml (male) or 5 ml (female) into urethra

Available forms include: Top sol

Side effects/adverse reactions:
INTEG: Rash, irritation, sensitization

Contraindications: Hypersensitivity, application to large areas
Precautions: Sepsis, pregnancy (B), denuded skin

NURSING CONSIDERATIONS

Administer:
• After cleansing and drying of affected area

Evaluate:
• Therapeutic response: absence of pain, itching of affected area

• Allergy: rash, irritation, reddening, swelling
• Infection: if affected area is infected, do not apply

Teach patient/family:
• To report rash, irritation, redness, swelling
• How to apply ointment

lidocaine HCl

(lye-doe-kane)
Lido Pen Auto-Injector, Xylocaine
Func. class.: Antidysrhythmic (Class IB)
Chem. class.: Aminoacyl amide

Action: Increases electrical stimulation threshold of ventricle, His Purkinje system, which stabilizes cardiac membrane, decreases automaticity

Uses: Ventricular tachycardia, ventricular dysrhythmias during cardiac surgery, myocardial infarction, digitalis toxicity, cardiac catheterization

Dosage and routes:
• *Adult:* IV BOL 50-100 mg over 2-3 min, repeat q3-5 min, not to exceed 300 mg in 1 hr; begin IV INF; IV INF 20-50 μg/kg/min; IM 200-300 mg in deltoid muscle
• *Elderly, CHF reduced liver function:* IV BOL give ½ adult dose
• *Child:* IV BOL 1 mg/kg, then IV INF 30 μg/kg/min

Available forms include: IV INF 0.2%, 0.4%, 0.8%; IV Ad 4%, 10%, 20%; IV Dir 1%, 2%; IM 300 mg/ml, 10%

Side effects/adverse reactions:
CNS: Headache, dizziness, involuntary movement, confusion, tremor, drowsiness, euphoria, ***convulsions***
EENT: Tinnitus, blurred vision
GI: Nausea, vomiting, anorexia
CV: Hypotension, bradycardia, ***heart block, cardiovascular collapse, arrest***
RESP: Dyspnea, ***respiratory depression***
INTEG: Rash, urticaria, edema, swelling
MISC: Febrile response, phlebitis at injection site

Contraindications: Hypersensitivity to amides, severe heart block, supraventricular dysrhythmias, Adams-Stokes syndrome, Wolff-Parkinson-White syndrome

Precautions: Pregnancy (B), lactation, children, renal disease, liver disease, CHF, respiratory depression, malignant hyperthermia

Pharmacokinetics:
IV: Onset 2 min, duration 20 min
IM: Onset 5-15 min, duration 1½ hr; half-life 8 min, 1-2 hr (terminal), metabolized in liver excreted in urine, crosses placenta

Interactions/incompatibilities:
• Increased neuromuscular blockade of: neuromuscular blockers, tubocurarine
• Increased effects of lidocaine: cimetidine, phenytoin, propranolol, metoprolol
• Decreased effects of lidocaine: barbiturates

NURSING CONSIDERATIONS

Assess:
• ECG continuously to determine increased PR or QRS segments; if these develop, discontinue or reduce rate; watch for increased ventricular ectopic beats, may need to rebolus
• IV infusion rate using infusion pump, run at less than 4 mg/min
• Blood levels (therapeutic level: 1.5-6 μg/ml)
• B/P continuously for fluctuations
• I&O ratio, electrolytes (K, Na, Cl)

Administer:

• IV bolus undiluted; give 50 mg or less over 1 min or dilute 1 g/ 250-500 ml of D_5W; titrate to patient response

• IM injection in deltoid; aspirate to avoid intravascular administration; check site daily for infiltration or extravasation

Evaluate:

• Therapeutic response: decreased dysrhythmias

• Malignant hyperthermia: tachypnea, tachycardia, changes in B/ P, increased temperature

• Cardiac rate, respiration: rate, rhythm, character, continuously

• Respiratory status: rate, rhythm, lung fields for rales, watch for respiratory depression

• CNS effects: dizziness, confusion, psychosis, paresthesias, convulsions; drug should be discontinued

• Lung fields, bilateral rales may occur in CHF patient

• Increased respiration, increased pulse; drug should be discontinued

Teach patient/family:

• Use of automatic lidocaine injection device if ordered

Lab test interferences:

Increase: CPK

Treatment of overdose: O_2, artificial ventilation, ECG, administer dopamine for circulatory depression, administer diazepam or thiopental for convulsions, decrease drug if needed

---

lidocaine HCl (local)

(lye'doe-kane)

Ardecaine, Dilocaine, Dolicaine, Nervocaine, Norocaine, Rocaine, Stanacaine, Ultracaine, Xylocaine

Func. class.: Local anesthetic
Chem. class.: Amide

Action: Competes with calcium for sites in nerve membrane that control sodium transport across cell membrane; decreases rise of depolarization phase of action potential

Uses: Peripheral nerve block, caudal anesthesia, epidural, spinal, surgical anesthesia

Dosage and routes:

Varies depending on route of anesthesia

Available forms include: Inj 0.5%, 1%, 1.5%, 2%, 4%, 5%; inj with epinephrine 0.5%, 1%, 1.5%, 2%

Side effects/adverse reactions:

CNS: Anxiety, restlessness, ***convulsions, loss of consciousness,*** drowsiness, disorientation, tremors, shivering

CV: ***Myocardial depression, cardiac arrest, dysrhythmias,*** bradycardia, hypotension, hypertension, fetal bradycardia

GI: Nausea, vomiting

EENT: Blurred vision, tinnitus, pupil constriction

INTEG: Rash, urticaria, allergic reactions, edema, burning, skin discoloration at injection site, tissue necrosis

RESP: ***Status asthmaticus, respiratory arrest, anaphylaxis***

Contraindications: Hypersensitivity, child <12 yr, elderly, severe liver disease

Precautions: Elderly, severe drug allergies, pregnancy (C)

Pharmacokinetics:

Onset 4-17 min, duration 3-6 hr; metabolized by liver, excreted in urine (metabolites)

Interactions/incompatibilities:

• Dysrhythmias: epinephrine, halothane, enflurane

• Hypertension: MAOIs, tricyclic antidepressants, phenothiazines

• Decreased action of lidocaine: chloroprocaine

---

*Available in Canada only

NURSING CONSIDERATIONS
Assess:
• B/P, pulse, respiration during treatment
• Fetal heart tones if drug is used during labor
Administer:
• Only with crash cart, resuscitative equipment nearby
• Only drugs without preservatives for epidural or caudal anesthesia
Perform/provide:
• Use of new solution, discard unused portions
Evaluate:
• Therapeutic response: anesthesia necessary for procedure
• For allergic reactions: rash, urticaria, itching
• Cardiac status: ECG for dysrhythmias, pulse, B/P during anesthesia
Treatment of overdose: Airway, O_2, vasopressor, IV fluids, anticonvulsants for seizures

lincomycin HCl

(lin-koe-mye'sin)
Lincocin
Func. class.: Antibacterial
Chem. class.: Lincomycin derivative

Action: Binds to 50S subunit of bacterial ribsomes, suppresses protein synthesis
Uses: Infections caused by group A β-hemolytic streptococci, pneumococci, staphylococci (respiratory tract, skin, soft tissue, urinary tract infections, osteomyelitis, septicemia)
Dosage and routes:
• *Adult:* PO 500 mg q6-8h, not to exceed 8 g/day; IM 600 mg/day or q12h; IV 600 mg-1 g q8-12h, dilute in 100 ml IV sol, infuse over 1 hr, not to exceed 8 g/day
• *Child >1 mo:* PO 30-60 mg/kg/day in divided doses q6-8h; IM 10 mg/kg/day q12h; IV 10-20 mg/kg/day in divided doses q8-12h; dilute to 100 ml IV sol, infuse over 1 hr
Available forms include: Caps 500 mg; caps pediatric 250 mg; inj IM, IV 300 mg/ml
Side effects/adverse reactions:
HEMA: ***Leukopenia, eosinophilia, agranulocytosis, thrombocytopenia***
GI: Nausea, vomiting, abdominal pain, tenesmus, diarrhea, ***pseudomembranous colitis***
GU: Increased AST, ALT, bilirubin, alk phosphatase, jaundice, *vaginitis,* urinary frequency
EENT: Rash, urticaria, pruritus, erythema, pain, abscess at injection site
Contraindications: Hypersensitivity, ulcerative colitis/enteritis, infants <1 mo
Precautions: Renal disease, liver disease, GI disease, elderly, pregnancy (C), lactation
Pharmacokinetics:
PO: Peak 2-4 hr, duration 6 hr
IM: Peak 30 min, duration 8-12 hr
Half-life 4-6 hr, metabolized in liver, excreted in urine, bile, feces as active, inactive metabolites, crosses placenta, excreted in breast milk
Interactions/incompatibilities:
• Increased neuromuscular blockage: nondepolarizing muscle relaxants
• Decreased absorption of lincomycin: kaolin
• Decreased action of: chloramphenicol, erythromycin
NURSING CONSIDERATIONS
Assess:
• Signs of infection

L

• Any patient with compromised renal system; drug is excreted slowly in poor renal system function; toxicity may occur rapidly
• Liver studies: AST, ALT
• Blood studies: WBC, RBC, Hct, Hgb, platelets, serum iron, reticulocytes; drug should be discontinued if bone marrow depression occurs
• Renal studies: urinalysis, protein, blood, BUN, creatinine
• C&S before drug therapy; drug may be taken as soon as culture is taken
• Drug level in impaired hepatic, renal systems
• B/P, pulse in patient receiving drug parenterally

Administer:
• IV by infusion only; do not administer bolus dose; dilute 1g or less/100 ml or more D_5W, NS, not to exceed 100 ml/hr
• IM deep injection; rotate sites
• Orally with at least 8 oz water on empty stomach

Perform/provide:
• Storage at room temperature (capsules) and up to 2 wk (reconstituted solution)
• Adrenalin, suction, tracheostomy set, endotracheal intubation equipment on unit
• Adequate intake of fluids (2000 ml) during diarrhea episodes

Evaluate:
• Therapeutic response: decreased temperature, negative C&S
• Bowel pattern before, during treatment
• Skin eruptions, itching, dermatitis
• Respiratory status: rate, character, wheezing, tightness in chest
• Allergies before treatment, reaction of each medication; place allergies on chart, Kardex in bright red letters; notify all people giving drugs

Teach patient/family:
• To take oral drug with full glass of water; may give with food if GI symptoms occur
• Aspects of drug therapy: need to complete entire course of medication to ensure organism death (10-14 days); culture may be taken after completed course of medication
• To report sore throat, fever, fatigue; could indicate superimposed infection
• That drug must be taken in equal intervals around clock to maintain blood levels
• To notify nurse of diarrhea

Lab test interferences:
Increase: Alk phosphatase, bilirubin, CPK, AST/ALT

Treatment of hypersensitivity: Withdraw drug, maintain airway, administer epinephrine, aminophylline, O_2, IV corticosteroids

lindane (gamma benzene hexachloride)

(lin-dane)

gBh,* Kwell, Kwellada,* Kwildane, Scabene, G-Well

Func. class.: Scabicide
Chem. class.: Chlorinated hydrocarbon (synthetic)

Action: Stimulates nervous system of arthropods, resulting in seizures, death of organism

Uses: Scabies, lice (head/pubic), nits

Dosage and routes:
• *Adult and child:* CREAM/LOTION wash area with soap, water, remove visible crusts, apply to skin surfaces, remove with soap, water in 8-12 hr, may reapply in 1 wk if needed; shampoo using 30 ml

* Available in Canada only

work into lather, rub for 5 min, rinse, dry with towel; comb with fine-toothed comb to remove nits
Available forms include: Lotion, shampoo, cream (1%)
Side effects/adverse reactions:
INTEG: Pruritus, rash, irritation, contact dermatitis
GI: Nausea, vomiting, diarrhea, liver damage (inhalation of vapors)
HEMA: ***Aplastic anemia*** (chronic inhalation of vapors)
CV: ***Ventricular fibrillation*** (chronic inhalation of vapors)
GU: ***Kidney damage*** (chronic inhalation of vapors)
CNS: Tremors, ***convulsions,*** stimulation, dizziness (chronic inhalation of vapors)
Contraindications: Hypersensitivity, premature neonate, patients with known seizure disorders, inflammation of skin, abrasions, or breaks in skin
Precautions: Pregnancy (B), avoid contact with eyes, children <10 yr, infants, lactation
Pharmacokinetics:
Stored in body fat, metabolized in liver, excreted in urine, feces
Interactions/incompatibilities:
• Oils may enhance absorption; if an oil-based hair dressing is used, shampoo, rinse, dry hair before applying lindane shampoo

NURSING CONSIDERATIONS
Administer:
• To body areas, scalp only; do not apply to face, lips, mouth, eyes, any mucous membrane, anus, or meatus
• Topical corticosteroids as ordered to decrease contact dermatitis
• Lotions of menthol or phenol to control itching
• Topical antibiotics for infection
Perform/provide:
• Isolation until areas on skin, scalp have cleared and treatment is completed
• Removal of nits by using a fine-toothed comb rinsed in vinegar after treatment; use gloves
Evaluate:
• Therapeutic response: decreased crusts, nits, brownish trails on skin, itching papules in skin folds
Teach patient/family:
• To wash all inhabitants' clothing, using insecticide; preventive treatment may be required of all persons living in same house, using lotion or shampoo to decrease spread of infection; use rubber gloves when applying drug
• That itching may continue for 4-6 wk
• That drug must be reapplied if accidently washed off or treatment will be ineffective
• Not to apply to face; if accidental contact with eyes occurs, flush with water
• To treat sexual contacts simultaneously
Treatment of ingestion: Gastric lavage, saline laxatives, IV valium for convulsions

---

liothyronine sodium (T_3)

(lye-oh-thye'roe-neen)
Cytomel, Cyronine
Func. class.: Thyroid hormone
Chem. class.: Synthetic T_3

Action: Increases metabolic rates, increases cardiac output, O_2 consumption, body temperature, blood volume, growth, development at cellular level
Uses: Hypothyroidism, myxedema coma, thyroid hormone replacement, cretinism, nontoxic goiter, T_3 suppression test

L

Dosage and routes:

• *Adult:* PO 25 μg qd, increased by 12.5-25 μg q1-2 wk until desired response, maintenance dose 25-75 μg qd

Cretinism

• *Child >3 yr:* PO 50-100 μg qd

• *Child <3 yr:* PO 5 μg qd, increased by 5 μg q3-4 days titrated to response

Myxedema

• *Adult:* PO 5 μg qd, may increase by 5-10 μg q1-2 wk, maintenance dose 50-100 μg qd

Nontoxic goiter

• *Adult:* PO 5 μg qd, increased by 12.5-25 μg q1-2 wk, maintenance dose 75 μg qd

Suppression test

• *Adult:* PO 75-100 μg qd × 1 wk

Available forms include: Tabs 5, 25, 50 μg

Side effects/adverse reactions:

CNS: Insomnia, tremors, headache, ***thyroid storm***

CV: Tachycardia, palpitations, angina, dysrhythmias, hypertension, cardiac arrest

GI: Nausea, diarrhea, increased or decreased appetite, cramps

MISC: Menstrual irregularities, weight loss, sweating, heat intolerance, fever

Contraindications: Adrenal insufficiency, myocardial infarction, thyrotoxicosis

Precautions: Elderly, angina pectoris, hypertension, ischemia, cardiac disease, pregnancy (A), lactation

Pharmacokinetics:

PO: Peak 12-48 hr, half-life 6-7 days

Interactions/incompatibilities:

• Decreased absorption of liothyronine: cholestyramine

• Increased effects of: anticoagulants, sympathomimetics, tricyclic antidepressants

• Decreased effects of: digitalis drugs, insulin, hypoglycemics

• Decreased effects of liothyronine: estrogens

NURSING CONSIDERATIONS

Assess:

• B/P, pulse before each dose

• I&O ratio

• Weight qd in same clothing, using same scale, at same time of day

• Height, growth rate if given to a child

• T_3, T_4, which are decreased, radioimmunoassay of TSH, which is increased, radio uptake, which is decreased if patient is on too low a dose of medication

• Pro-time may require decreased anticoagulant, check for bleeding, bruising

Administer:

• In AM if possible as a single dose to decrease sleeplessness

• At same time each day to maintain drug level

• Only for hormone imbalances; not to be used for obesity, male infertility, menstrual conditions, lethargy

• Lowest dose that relieves symptoms

Perform/provide:

• Removal of medication 4 wk before RAIU test

Evaluate:

• Therapeutic response: absence of depression, increased weight loss, diuresis, pulse, appetite, absence of constipation, peripheral edema, cold intolerance, pale, cool dry skin, brittle nails, alopecia, coarse hair, menorrhagia, night blindness, paresthesia, snycope, stupor, coma, rosy cheeks

• Increased nervousness, excitability, irritability, which may indicate

* Available in Canada only

too high dose of medication usually after 1-3 wk of treatment
• Cardiac status: angina, palpitation, chest pain, change in VS

Teach patient/family:
• That hair loss will occur in child but is temporary
• To report excitability, irritability, anxiety, which indicates overdose
• Not to switch brands unless approved by physician
• That hypothyroid child will show almost immediate behavior/personality change
• That treatment drug is not to be taken to reduce weight
• To avoid OTC preparations with iodine, read labels
• To avoid iodine food, salt-iodinized, soy beans, tofu, turnips, some seafood, some bread

Lab test interferences:
Increase: CPK, LDH, AST, PBI, blood glucose
Decrease: TSH, ^{131}I uptake test, uric acid, triglycerides

---

liotrix

(lye'oh-trix)
Euthroid, Thyrolar

Func. class.: Thyroid hormone
Chem. class.: Levothyroxine/liothyronine (synthetic T_4, T_3)

Action: Increases metabolic rates, increases cardiac output, O_2 consumption, body temperature, blood volume, growth, development at cellular level

Uses: Hypothyroidism, thyroid hormone replacement

Dosage and routes:
• *Adult and child:* PO 15-30 mg qd, increased by 15-30 mg q1-2wk until desired response, may increase by 15-30 mg q2wk in child
• *Geriatric:* PO 15-30 mg, double dose q6-8wk until desired response

Available forms include: Tabs 15, 30, 60, 120, 180 mg as thyroid equivalent

Side effects/adverse reactions:
CNS: Insomnia, tremors, headache, thyroid storm
CV: Tachycardia, palpitations, angina, dysrhythmias, hypertension, cardiac arrest
GI: Nausea, diarrhea, increased or decreased appetite, cramps
MISC: Menstrual irregularities, weight loss, sweating, heat intolerance, fever

Contraindications: Adrenal insufficiency, myocardial infarction, thyrotoxicosis

Precautions: Elderly, angina pectoris, hypertension, ischemia, cardiac disease, pregnancy (A), lactation

Pharmacokinetics:
PO: Peak 12-48 hr, half-life 6-7 days

Interactions/incompatibilities:
• Decreased absorption of liotrix: cholestyramine
• Increased effects of: anticoagulants, sympathomimetics, tricyclic antidepressants, catecholamines
• Decreased effects of: digitalis drugs, insulin, hypoglycemics
• Decreased effects of liotrix: estrogens

NURSING CONSIDERATIONS

Assess:
• B/P, pulse before each dose
• I&O ratio
• Weight qd in same clothing, using same scale, at same time of day
• Height, growth rate if given to a child
• T_3, T_4 FTIs that are decreased, radioimmunoassay of TSH, which is increased, radio uptake, which is decreased if patient is on too low a dose of medication

• Pro-time may require decreased anticoagulant, check for bleeding, bruising

Administer:
• In AM if possible as a single dose to decrease sleeplessness
• At same time each day to maintain drug level
• Only for hormone imbalances, not to be used for obesity, male infertility, menstrual conditions, lethargy
• Lowest dose that relieves symptoms

Perform/provide:
• Removal of medication 4 wk before RAIU test

Evaluate:
• Therapeutic response: absence of depression, increased weight loss, diuresis, pulse, appetite, absence of constipation, peripheral edema, cold intolerance, pale, cool dry skin, brittle nails, coarse hair, menorrhagia, night blindness, paresthesias, syncope, stupor, coma, rosy cheeks
• Increased nervousness, excitability, irritability, which may indicate too high dose of medication usually after 1-3 wk of treatment
• Cardiac status: angina, palpitation, chest pain, change in VS

Teach patient/family:
• That hair loss will occur in child, is temporary
• To report excitability, irritability, anxiety, which indicate overdose
• Not to switch brands unless approved by physician
• That hypothyroid child will show almost immediate behavior/personality change
• That treatment drug is not to be taken to reduce weight
• To avoid OTC preparations with iodine, read labels
• To avoid iodine food, salt-iodinized, soy beans, tofu, turnips, some seafood, some bread

Lab test interferences:
Increase: CPK, LDH, AST, PBI, blood glucose
Decrease: TSH, ^{131}I uptake test, uric acid, triglycerides

lisinopril

(lyse-in'oh-pril)
Prinivil, Zestril

Func. class.: Angiotensin converting enzyme (ACE) inhibitor
Chem. class.: Enalaprilat lysine analog

Action: Selectively suppresses renin-angiotensin-aldosterone system; inhibits ACE preventing conversion of angiotensin I to angiotensin II

Uses: Mild to moderate hypertension

Dosage and routes:
• *Adult:* PO 10-40 mg qd, may increase to 80 mg qd if required

Available forms include: Tabs 5, 10, 20 mg

Side effects/adverse reactions:
GI: Nausea, vomiting, anorexia, constipation, flatulence, GI irritation
GU: ***Proteinuria, renal insufficiency,*** sexual dysfunction, impotence
INTEG: Rash, pruritus
CNS: Vertigo, depression, stroke, insomnia, paresthesias, headache, fatigue, asthenia
EENT: Blurred vision, nasal congestion
RESP: Cough, dyspnea

Contraindications: Hypersensitivity

Precautions: Pregnancy (C), lactation, renal disease, hyperkalemia

Pharmacokinetics:

* Available in Canada only

Peak 6-8 hr, excreted unchanged in urine

Interactions/incompatibilities:

• Increased hypotensive effect: diuretics, other hypertensives, probenecid

• Decreased effects of lisinopril: aspirin, indomethacin

• Increased potassium levels: potassium salt substitutes, potassium-sparing diuretics, potassium supplements

• Increased effects of: antihypertensives, reserpine, diuretics

• Increased hypersensitivity reactions: allopurinol

NURSING CONSIDERATIONS

Assess:

• B/P, pulse q4h; note rates rhythm, quality

• Electrolytes: potassium, sodium, chloride

• Apical/pedal pulse before administration; notify physician of any significant changes

• Baselines in renal, liver function tests before therapy begins

Evaluate:

• Therapeutic response: decreased B/P

• Edema in feet, legs daily

• Skin turgor, dryness of mucous membranes for hydration status

• Symptoms of CHF: edema, dyspnea, wet rales

Teach patient/family:

• Not to discontinue drug abruptly

• To rise slowly to sitting or standing position to minimize orthostatic hypotension

Lab test interferences:

Interfere: Glucose/insulin tolerance tests

Treatment of overdose: Lavage, IV atropine for bradycardia, IV theophylline for bronchospasm, digitalis, O_2, diuretic for cardiac failure, hemodialysis

lithium carbonate

(li'thee-um)

Carbolith,* Lithane, Eskalith, Lithonate, Lithotabs, Lithobid, Lithium Citrate, Lithonate-S

Func. class.: Antimanic
Chem. class.: Alkali metal ion salt

Action: May alter sodium, potassium ion transport across cell membrane in nerve, muscle cells; may balance biogenic amines of norepinephrine, serotonin in CNS areas involved in emotional responses

Uses: Manic-depressive illness (manic phase), prevention of bipolar manic depressive psychosis

Dosage and routes:

• *Adult:* PO 600 mg tid, maintenance 300 mg tid or qid; slow rel tabs 300 mg bid, dose should be individualized to maintain blood levels at 0.5-1.5 mEq/L

Available forms include: Caps 150, 300 mg; tabs 300 mg; tabs ext rel 300, 450 mg; oral sol 8 mEq/5 ml

Side effects/adverse reactions:

CNS: Headache, drowsiness, dizziness, tremors, twitching, ataxia, seizure, slurred speech, restlessness, confusion, stupor, memory loss, clonic movements

GI: Dry mouth, anorexia, nausea, vomiting, diarrhea, incontinence, abdominal pain, metallic taste

GU: ***Polyuria, glycosuria, proteinuria, albuminuria,*** urinary incontinence, polydipsia, edema

CV: Hypotension, ECG changes, dysrhythmias, ***circulatory collapse, edema***

INTEG: Drying of hair, alopecia, rash, pruritus, hyperkeratosis

HEMA: ***Leukocytosis***

EENT: Tinnitus, blurred vision

ENDO: Hyponatremia

L

MS: Muscle weakness

Contraindications: Hepatic disease, renal disease, brain trauma, OBS, pregnancy (D), lactation, children <12 yr, schizophrenia, severe cardiac disease, severe renal disease, severe dehydration

Precautions: Elderly, thyroid disease, seizure disorders, diabetes mellitus, systemic infection, urinary retention

Pharmacokinetics:

PO: Onset rapid, peak ½-4 hr, half-life 18-36 hr depending on age; crosses blood-brain barrier, 80% of filtered lithium is reabsorbed by the renal tubules, excreted in urine, crosses placenta, enters breast milk, well absorbed by oral method

Interactions/incompatibilities:

- Increased hypothyroid effects: antithyroid effects, calcium iodide, potassium iodide, iodinated glycerol
- Brain damage: haloperidol
- Increased effects of: neuromuscular blocking agents, phenothiazines
- Increased renal clearance: sodium bicarbonate, acetazolamide, mannitol, aminophylline
- Increased toxicity: indomethacin, diuretics, nonsteroidal antiinflammatories
- Decreased effects of lithium: theophyllines, urea, urinary alkalinizers

NURSING CONSIDERATIONS

Assess:

- Weight daily, check for edema in legs, ankles, wrists; report if present
- Sodium intake; decreased sodium intake with decreased fluid intake may lead to lithium retention; increased sodium and fluids may decrease lithium retention
- Skin turgor at least daily
- Urine for albuminuria, glycosuria, uric acid during beginning treatment, q2mo thereafter
- Neuro status: LOC, gait, motor reflexes, hand tremors
- Serum lithium levels weekly initially, then q2mo (therapeutic level: 0.5-1.5 mEq/L)

Administer:

- Reduced dose to elderly
- With meals to avoid GI upset
- Adequate fluids (2-3 L/day) to prevent dehydration during initial treatment, 1-2 L/day during maintenance

Evaluate:

- Therapeutic response: decrease in excitement, manic phase

Teach patient/family:

- Symptoms of minor toxicity: vomiting, diarrhea, poor coordination, fine motor tremors, weakness, lassitude; major toxicity: coarse tremors, severe thirst, tinnitus, dilute urine
- To monitor urine specific gravity, emphasize need for follow-up care to determine lithium levels
- That contraception is necessary since lithium may harm fetus
- Not to operate machinery until lithium levels are stable
- Provide a list of drugs that interact with lithium, and discuss need for adequate salt and fluid intake

Lab test interferences:

Increase: Potassium excretion, urine glucose, blood glucose, protein, BUN

Decrease: VMA, T_3, T_4, PBI, ^{131}I

Treatment of overdose: Induce emesis or lavage, maintain airway, respiratory function; dialysis for severe intoxication

* Available in Canada only

lomefloxacin HCl

(lome-flock'a-sin)

Maxaquin

Func. class.: Antiinfective
Chem. class.: Fluoroquinolone

Action: Interferes with conversion of intermediate DNA fragments into high-molecular-weight DNA in bacteria

Uses: Treatment of lower respiratory tract infections (pneumonia, bronchitis), genitourinary infections (prostatitis, UTIs), preoperatively to reduce urinary tract infections in transurethral surgical procedures

Dosage and routes:

- *Adult:* PO 400 mg/day 7-14 days depending on type of infection

In renal impairment

- *Adult:* PO 200 mg/dose

Prophylaxis of UTI

- *Adult:* PO 400 mg 2-6 hr before surgery

Available forms include: Tabs 400

Side effects/adverse reactions:

CNS: Dizziness, headache, somnolence, depression, insomnia, nervousness, confusion, agitation

GI: Diarrhea, nausea, vomiting, anorexia, flatulence, heartburn, dry mouth, increased AST, ALT, constipation, abdominal pain, oral thrush, glossitis, stomatitis

INTEG: Rash, pruritus, urticaria

EENT: Visual disturbances

Contraindications: Hypersensitivity to quinolones

Precautions: Pregnancy (C), lactation, children, elderly, renal disease, seizure disorders, excessive sunlight

Pharmacokinetics:

PO: Peak 1-2 hr, half-life 6-8 hr; excreted in urine as active drug, metabolites

Interactions/incompatibilities:

- Decreased effects of lomefloxacin: antacids, nitrofurantoin, sucralfate, iron salts, zinc salts
- Increased lomefloxacin levels: probenecid, cimetidine
- Increased levels of: cyclosporine, warfarin

NURSING CONSIDERATIONS

Assess:

- Kidney, liver function studies: BUN, creatinine, AST, ALT
- I&O ratio, urine pH; <5.5 is ideal

Administer:

- After clean-catch urine is obtained for C&S

Perform/provide:

- Limited intake of alkaline foods, drugs; milk, dairy products, peanuts, vegetables, alkaline actacids, sodium bicarbonate

Evaluate:

- Therapeutic response: negative C&S
- CNS symptoms: insomnia, vertigo, headache, agitation, confusion
- Allergic reactions: rash, flushing, urticaria, pruritus

Teach patient/family:

- That fluids must be increased to 3L/day to avoid crystallization in kidneys
- That if dizziness or light-headedness occurs, to ambulate, perform activities with assistance
- To complete full course of drug therapy
- To contact physician if adverse reactions occur
- To avoid iron- or mineral-containing supplements within 2 hr before and after dosing

L

lomustine (CCNU)

(loe-mus'teen)
CeeNU, CCNU
Func. class.: Antineoplastic alkylating agent
Chem. class.: Nitrosourea

Action: Responsible for cross-linking DNA strands, which leads to cell death
Uses: Hodgkin's disease, lymphomas, melanomas, multiple myeloma; brain, lung, bladder, kidney, colon cancer
Dosage and routes:
• *Adult:* PO 130 mg/m^2 as a single dose q6wk; titrate dose to WBC level; do not give repeat dose unless WBCs are >4000/mm^3, platelet count >100,000/mm^3
Available forms include: Cap 10, 40, 100 mg
Side effects/adverse reactions:
HEMA: ***Thrombocytopenia, leukopenia, myelosuppression, anemia***
GI: Nausea, vomiting, anorexia, stomatitis, ***hepatotoxicity***
GU: ***Azotemia, renal failure***
INTEG: Burning at injection site
RESP: ***Fibrosis, pulmonary infiltrate***
Contraindications: Hypersensitivity, leukopenia, thrombocytopenia, pregnancy (D)
Precautions: Radiation therapy
Pharmacokinetics:
Metabolized in liver, excreted in urine; half-life 16-48 hr, 50% protein bound, crosses blood-brain barrier, appears in breast milk
Interactions/incompatibilities:
• Increased toxicity: barbiturates, phenytoin, chloral hydrate
• Increased metabolism of lomustine: phenobarbital
• Potentiation of lomustine: succinylcholine
• Increased bone marrow depression: allopurinol

NURSING CONSIDERATIONS
Assess:
• CBC, differential, platelet count weekly; withhold drug if WBC is <4000 or platelet count is <75,000; notify physician of results
• Pulmonary function tests, chest x-ray films before, during therapy; chest film should be obtained q2wk during treatment
• Renal function studies: BUN, serum uric acid, urine CrCl before, during therapy
• I&O ratio; report fall in urine output of 30 ml/hr
• Monitor temperature q4h (may indicate beginning infection); no rectal temperatures
• Liver function tests before, during therapy (bilirubin, AST, ALT, LDH) as needed or monthly
Administer:
• Antiemetic 30-60 min before giving drug to prevent vomiting
• Antibiotics for prophylaxis of infection
• Topical or systemic analgesics for pain
• Local or systemic drugs for infection
Perform/provide:
• Storage in tight container at room temperature
• Strict medical asepsis, protective isolation if WBC levels are low
• Special skin care
• Deep breathing exercises with patient tid-qid; place in semi-Fowler's position
• Increase fluid intake to 2-3 L/day to prevent urate deposits, calculi formation
• Rinsing of mouth tid-qid with water, club soda; brushing of teeth bid-tid with soft brush or cotton-

tipped applicators for stomatitis; use unwaxed dental floss

Evaluate:

- Therapeutic response: decreased tumor size, spread of malignancy
- Bleeding: hematuria, guaiac, bruising or petechiae, mucosa or orifices q8h
- Dyspnea, rales, unproductive cough, chest pain, tachypnea
- Food preferences; list likes, dislikes
- Yellowing of skin, sclera, dark urine, clay-colored stools, itchy skin, abdominal pain, fever, diarrhea
- Inflammation of mucosa, breaks in skin
- Buccal cavity q8h for dryness, sores or ulceration, white patches, oral pain, bleeding, dysphagia
- Local irritation, pain, burning, discoloration at injection site
- Symptoms indicating severe allergic reaction: rash, pruritus, urticaria, purpuric skin lesions, itching, flushing

Teach patient/family:

- Of protective isolation precautions
- To report any changes in breathing or coughing
- To avoid foods with citric acid, hot or rough texture if buccal inflammation is present
- To report any bleeding, white spots or ulcerations in mouth to physician; tell patient to examine mouth qd
- To report signs of infection: increased temperature, sore throat, flu symptoms
- To report signs of anemia: fatigue, headache, faintness, shortness of breath, irritability
- To avoid use of razors or commercial mouthwash
- To avoid use of aspirin products or ibuprofen

---

loperamide HCl

(loe-per'a-mide)

Imodium

Func. class.: Antidiarrheal
Chem. class.: Piperidine derivative

Action: Direct action on intestinal muscles to decrease GI peristalsis

Uses: Diarrhea (cause undetermined), chronic diarrhea, ileostomy discharge

Dosage and routes:

- *Adult:* PO 4 mg, then 2 mg after each loose stool, not to exceed 16 mg/day
- *Child 2-5 yr:* PO 1 mg then 1, 0.1 mg/kg after each loose stool
- *Child 5-8 yr:* PO 2 mg bid on day 1, then 0.1 mg/kg after each loose stool
- *Child 8-12 yr:* PO 2 mg tid on day 1, then 0.1 mg/kg after each loose stool

Available forms include: Caps 2 mg; liq 1 mg/5 ml

Side effects/adverse reactions:

CNS: Dizziness, drowsiness, fatigue, fever

GI: Nausea, dry mouth, vomiting, constipation, abdominal pain, anorexia, ***toxic megacolon***

INTEG: Rash

RESP: ***Respiratory depression***

Contraindications: Hypersensitivity, severe ulcerative colitis, pseudomembranous colitis

Precautions: Pregnancy (B), lactation, children <2 yr, liver disease, dehydration, bacterial disease

Pharmacokinetics:

PO: Onset ½-1 hr, duration 4-5 hr, half-life 7-14 hr; metabolized in liver, excreted in feces as un-

L

changed drug, small amount in urine

Interactions/incompatibilities:

• Do not mix oral solution with other solutions

NURSING CONSIDERATIONS

Assess:

• Electrolytes (K, Na, Cl) if on long-term therapy

• Skin turgor q8h if dehydration is suspected

Administer:

• For 48 hr only, cont INF

Perform/provide:

• Storage in tight containers

Evaluate:

• Therapeutic response: decreased diarrhea

• Bowel pattern before; for rebound constipation

• Response after 48 hr; if no response, drug should be discontinued

• Dehydration in children

• Abdominal distention, toxic megacolon; may occur in ulcerative colitis

Teach patient/family:

• To avoid OTC products unless directed by physician

• That ostomy patient may take this drug for extended time

---

loracarbef

(lor-a-kar'bef)

Lorabid

Func. class.: Antibiotic
Chem. class.: Carbacephem

Action: Inhibits bacterial cell wall synthesis, which renders cell wall osmotically unstable

Uses: Gram-negative: *H. influenzae, E. coli, P. mirabilis, Klebsiella;* gram-positive: *S. pneumoniae, S. pyogenes, S. aureus;* upper and lower respiratory tract, urinary tract, skin infections, otitis media

Dosage and routes:

• *Adult:* PO UTI 200 mg qd × 7 days

• *Child:* PO Acute otitis media 15 mg/kg bid × 7 days

Available forms include: Caps 200 mg; 100, 200 mg/5 ml suspension

Side effects/adverse reactions:

CNS: Dizziness, headache, fatigue, paresthesia, fever, chills, confusion

GI: Diarrhea, nausea, vomiting, anorexia, dysgeusia, glossitis, bleeding, increased AST, ALT, bilirubin, LDH, alk phosphatase, abdominal pain, loose stools, flatulence, heartburn, stomach cramps, colitis, jaundice

INTEG: Rash, urticaria, dermatitis, ***anaphylaxis***

GU: Vaginitis, pruritus, candidiasis, increased BUN, ***nephrotoxicity, renal failure,*** pyuria, dysuria, reversible interstitial nephritis

HEMA: ***Leukopenia, thrombocytopenia, agranulocytosis,*** anemia, ***neutropenia, lymphocytosis, eosinophilia, pancytopenia, hemolytic anemia, leukocytosis, granulocytopenia***

RESP: Dyspenia

Contraindications: Hypersensitivity to cephalosporins or related antibiotics

Precautions: Pregnancy (B), lactation, children, renal disease

Pharmacokinetics:

PO: Peak 1 hr, half-life 1 hr; excreted in urine as unchanged drug

Interactions/incompatibilities:

• Decreased effects: tetracyclines, erythromycins

• Increased effect/toxicity: aminoglycosides, furosemide, probenecid, ethacrynic acid, vancomycin

NURSING CONSIDERATIONS

Assess:

---

* Available in Canada only

• Nephrotoxicity: increased BUN, creatinine
• I&O ratio
• Blood studies: AST, ALT, CBC, Hct, bilirubin, LDH, alk phosphatase, Coombs' test monthly if patient is on long-term therapy
• Electrolytes: potassium, sodium, chloride monthly if patient is on long-term therapy
• Bowel pattern qd; if severe diarrhea occurs, drug should be discontinued; may indicate pseudomembranous colitis

Administer:
• One hour before or 2 hr after a meal
• After C&S is completed
• For 7 days to ensure organism death, prevent superimposed infection

Evaluate:
• Therapeutic response: negative C&S
• Urine output; if decreasing, notify physician (may indicate nephrotoxicity)
• Allergic reactions: rash, flushing, urticaria, pruritus
• Bleeding: ecchymosis, bleeding gums, hematuria, stool guaiac daily
• Overgrowth of infection: perineal itching, fever, malaise, redness, pain, swelling, drainage, rash, diarrhea, change in cough sputum

Teach patient/family:
• If diabetic, to use Clinistix or Ketodiastix
• Not to drink alcohol or take meds with alcohol or reaction may occur
• Complete full course of drug therapy
• Take on an empty stomach, 1 hr before or 2 hr after a meal
• Notify physician if breastfeeding or of any side effects

Lab test interferences:
Increase (false): Creatinine (serum urine), urinary 17-KS
False positive: Urinary protein, direct Coombs' test, urine glucose
Interference: Cross-matching

Treatment of overdose: Epinephrine, antihistamines; resuscitate if needed (anaphylaxis)

---

loratidine

(loer-at-i-deen)
Claritin

Func. class.: Antihistamine
Chem. class.: Selective histamine-l (Hl) receptor antagonist

Action: Binds to peripheral histamine receptors, which provides antihistamine action without sedation

Uses: Seasonal rhinitis

Dosage and routes:
• *Adult:* PO 10-40 mg qd

Available forms include: Tabs 10 mg

Side effects/adverse reactions:
CNS: Sedation (more common with increased doses)

Contraindications: Hypersensitivity, acute asthma attacks, lower respiratory tract disease

Precautions: Pregnancy (B), increased intraocular pressure, bronchial asthma

Pharmacokinetics:
Peak 1½ hr, elimination half-life 14½ hr; metabolized in liver to active metabolites, excreted in urine

NURSING CONSIDERATIONS

Perform/provide:
• Storage in tight container at room temperature

Evaluate:
• Therapeutic response: absence of running or congested nose

Teach patient/family:

- To avoid driving or other hazardous activities if drowsiness occurs

lorazepam

(lor-a'ze-pam)

Ativan, Novolorazem*

Func. class.: Antianxiety

Chem. class.: Benzodiazepine

Controlled Substance Schedule IV

Action: Depresses subcortical levels of CNS, including limbic system and reticular formation

Uses: Anxiety, irritability in psychiatric or organic disorders, preoperatively, insomnia, acute alcohol withdrawal symptoms, anticonvulsant, adjunct in endoscopic procedures

Dosage and routes:

Anxiety

- Adult: PO 2-6 mg/day in divided doses, not to exceed 10 mg/day

Insomnia

- Adult: PO 2-4 mg hs; only minimally effective after 2 wk continuous therapy

Preoperatively

- Adult: IM/IV 2-4 mg

Available forms include: Tabs 0.5, 1, 2 mg; IM/IV inj 2, 4 mg/ml

Side effects/adverse reactions:

CNS: Dizziness, drowsiness, confusion, headache, anxiety, tremors, stimulation, fatigue, depression, insomnia, hallucinations, weakness, unsteadiness

GI: Constipation, dry mouth, nausea, vomiting, anorexia, diarrhea

INTEG: Rash, dermatitis, itching

CV: Orthostatic hypotension, ***ECG changes, tachycardia,*** hypotension

EENT: Blurred vision, tinnitus, mydriasis

Contraindications: Hypersensitivity to benzodiazepines, narrow-angle glaucoma, psychosis, pregnancy (D), child <12 yr, history of drug abuse, COPD

Precautions: Elderly, debilitated, hepatic disease, renal disease

Pharmacokinetics:

PO: Peak 1-3 hr, duration 3-6 hr, metabolized by liver, excreted by kidneys, crosses placenta, breast milk, half-life 14 hr

Interactions/incompatibilities:

- Decreased effects of lorazepam: oral contraceptives, valproic acid
- Increased effects of lorazepam: CNS depressants, alcohol, disulfiram, oral contraceptives

NURSING CONSIDERATIONS

Assess:

- B/P (lying, standing), pulse; if systolic B/P drops 20 mm Hg, hold drug, notify physician; respirations q5-15 min if given IV
- Blood studies: CBC during long-term therapy, blood dyscrasias have occurred rarely
- Hepatic studies: AST, ALT, bilirubin, creatinine, LDH, alk phosphatase

Administer:

- With food or milk for GI symptoms
- Crushed if patient is unable to swallow medication whole
- Sugarless gum, hard candy, frequent sips of water for dry mouth
- IV after diluting in an equal volume of compatible sol; give through Y-tube or 3-way stopcock; give at 2 mg or less over 1 min
- Deep into large muscle mass (IM inj)

Perform/provide:

- Assistance with ambulation during beginning therapy since drowsiness/dizziness occurs

* Available in Canada only

• Safety measures, including siderails
• Check to see whether PO medication has been swallowed

Evaluate:
• Therapeutic response: decreased anxiety, restlessness, insomnia
• Mental status: mood, sensorium, affect, sleeping pattern, drowsiness, dizziness
• Physical dependency, withdrawal symptoms: headache, nausea, vomiting, muscle pain, weakness, tremors, convulsions, after long-term, excessive use
• Suicidal tendencies

Teach patient/family:
• That drug may be taken with food
• Not to be used for everyday stress or used longer than 4 mo unless directed by physician
• Not to take more than prescribed amount, may be habit forming
• To avoid OTC preparations (cough, cold, hay fever) unless approved by physician
• To avoid driving, activities that require alertness, since drowsiness may occur
• To avoid alcohol ingestion or other psychotropic medications, unless prescribed by physician
• Not to discontinue medication abruptly after long-term use
• To rise slowly or fainting may occur, especially elderly
• That drowsiness might worsen at beginning of treatment
• To use birth-control if child-bearing age

Lab test interferences:
Increase: AST/ALT, serum bilirubin
Decrease: RAIU
False increase: 17-OHCS

Treatment of overdose: Lavage, VS, supportive care

lovastatin

(lo'va-sta-tin)
Mevacor

Func. class.: Cholesterol-lowering agent
Chem. class.: Aspergillus terreus strain derivative

Action: Inhibits HMG-COA reductase enzyme, which reduces cholesterol synthesis

Uses: As an adjunct in primary hypercholesterolemia (types IIa, IIb), mixed hyperlipidemia

Dosage and routes:
(Patient should first be placed on a cholesterol-lowering diet)
• *Adult:* PO 20 mg qd with evening meal, may increase to 20-80 mg/day in single or divided doses, not to exceed 80 mg/day; dosage adjustments should be made qm

Available forms include: Tabs 20 mg

Side effects/adverse reactions:
GI: Nausea, constipation, diarrhea, dyspepsia, flatus, abdominal pain, heartburn, ***liver dysfunction***
MS: Muscle cramps, myalgia, ***myositis, rhabdomyolysis***
CNS: Dizziness, headache
INTEG: Rash, pruritus
EENT: Blurred vision, dysgeusia, lens opacities

Contraindications: Pregnancy (X), lactation, active liver disease

Precautions: Past liver disease, alcoholics, severe acute infections, trauma, hypotension, uncontrolled seizure disorders, severe metabolic disorders, electrolyte imbalances

Pharmacokinetics:
PO: Peak 2-4 hr, metabolized in liver (metabolites), highly protein bound, excreted in urine, feces, crosses placenta, excreted in breast milk

Interactions/incompatibilities:
• Increased effects: bile acid sequestrants, coumadin
• Increased myalgia, myositis: cyclosporine, gemfibrozil, niacin

NURSING CONSIDERATIONS

Assess:
• Cholesterol levels periodically during treatment
• Liver function studies q1-2mo during the first 1½ yr of treatment; AST, ALT, liver function tests may increase
• Renal function in patients with compromised renal system: BUN, creatinine, I&O ratio
• Eyes with slit lamp before, 1 mo after treatment begins, anually, lens opacities may occur

Administer:
• In evening with meal; if dose is increased, take with breakfast and evening meal

Perform/provide:
• Storage in cool environment in tight container protected from light

Evaluate:
• Therapeutic response: decrease in cholesterol to desired level after 8 wk

Teach patient/family:
• That treatment will be ongoing for several years
• That blood work and eye exam will be necessary during treatment
• To report blurred vision, severe GI symptoms, dizziness, headache
• That previously prescribed regimen will continue: low-cholesterol diet, exercise program

Lab test interferences:
Increase: CPK, liver function tests

loxapine succinate/ loxapine HCl

(lox'a'peen)

Loxapax,* Loxitane, Loxitane-C

Func. class.: Antipsychotic/neuroleptic

Chem. class.: Dibenzoxazepine

Action: Depresses cerebral cortex, hypothalamus, limbic system, which control activity and aggression; blocks neurotransmission produced by dopamine at synapse; exhibits strong α-adrenergic, anticholinergic blocking action; mechanism for antipsychotic effects is unclear

Uses: Psychotic disorders

Dosage and routes:
• *Adult:* PO 10 mg bid-qid initially, may be rapidly increased depending on severity of condition, maintenance 60-100 mg/day; IM 12.5-50 mg q4-6hr or more until desired response, then start PO form

Available forms include: Caps 5, 10, 25, 50 mg; conc 25 mg/ml; inj IM 50 mg/ml

Side effects/adverse reactions:

RESP: ***Laryngospasm,*** dyspnea, ***respiratory depression***

CNS: Extrapyramidal symptoms: pseudoparkinsonism, akathisia, dystonia, tardive dyskinesia, drowsiness, headache, ***seizures,*** confusion

HEMA: ***Anemia, leukopenia, leukocytosis, agranulocytosis***

INTEG: Rash, photosensitivity, dermatitis

EENT: Blurred vision, glaucoma

GI: Dry mouth, nausea, vomiting, anorexia, constipation, diarrhea, jaundice, weight gain

GU: Urinary retention, urinary frequency, enuresis, impotence, amenorrhea, gynecomastia

*Available in Canada only

CV: Orthostatic hypotension, ***cardiac arrest,*** ECG changes, tachycardia

Contraindications: Hypersensitivity, blood dyscrasias, coma, child, brain damage, bone marrow depression, alcohol and barbiturate withdrawal states

Precautions: Pregnancy (C), lactation, seizure disorders, hepatic disease, cardiac disease, prostatic hypertrophy, cardiac conditions child <16 yr

Pharmacokinetics:

PO: Onset 20-30 min, peak 2-4 hr, duration 12 hr

IM: Onset 15-30 min, peak 15-20 min, duration 12 hr

Metabolized by liver, excreted in urine, crosses placenta, enters breast milk, initial half-life 5 hr, terminal half-life 19 hr

Interactions/incompatibilities:

- Toxicity: epinephrine
- Increased extrapyramidal effect: other antipsychotics
- Decreased effects: guanadrel, guanethidine
- Increased CNS depression: MAOIs, antidepressants

NURSING CONSIDERATIONS

Assess:

- Mental status before initial administration
- Swallowing of PO medication; check for hoarding or giving of medication to other patients
- I&O ratio; palpate bladder if low urinary output occurs
- Bilirubin, CBC, liver function studies monthly
- Urinalysis is recommended before and during prolonged therapy

Administer:

- Reduced dose to elderly
- Antiparkinsonian agent, to be used if extrapyramidal symptoms occur
- IM injection into large muscle mass
- Concentrate mixed in orange or grapefruit juice

Perform/provide:

- Decreased noise input by dimming lights, avoiding loud noises
- Supervised ambulation until stabilized on medication; do not involve in strenuous exercise program because fainting is possible; patient should not stand still for long periods of time
- Increased fluids to prevent constipation
- Sips of water, candy, gum for dry mouth
- Storage in tight, light-resistant container

Evaluate:

- Therapeutic response: decrease in emotional excitement, hallucinations, delusions, paranoia; reorganization of patterns of thought, speech
- Affect, orientation, LOC, reflexes, gait, coordination, sleep pattern disturbances
- B/P standing and lying; take pulse and respirations q4h during initial treatment; establish baseline before starting treatment; report drops of 30 mm Hg
- Dizziness, faintness, palpitations, tachycardia on rising
- Extrapyramidal symptoms including akathisia (inability to sit still, no pattern to movements), tardive dyskinesia (bizarre movements of the jaw, mouth, tongue, extremities), pseudoparkinsonism (rigidity, tremors, pill rolling, shuffling gait)
- Skin turgor daily
- For neuroleptic malignant syndrome: muscle rigidity, increased CPK, altered mental status, hyperthermia

• Constipation, urinary retention daily; if these occur, increase bulk, water in diet

Teach patient/family:

• That orthostatic hypotension may occur and to rise from sitting or lying position gradually
• To remain lying down after IM injection for at least 30 min
• To avoid hot tubs, hot showers, or tub baths since hypotension may occur
• To avoid abrupt withdrawal of this drug or EPS may result; drug should be withdrawn slowly
• To avoid OTC preparations (cough, hayfever, cold) unless approved by physician since serious drug interactions may occur; avoid use with alcohol or CNS depressants, increased drowsiness may occur
• To avoid hazardous activities until stabilized on medication
• To use a sunscreen during sun exposure to prevent burns
• Regarding compliance with drug regimen; warn patient about avoiding OTC preparation
• About necessity for meticulous oral hygiene since oral candidiasis may occur
• To report impaired vision, jaundice, tremors, muscle twitching
• That in hot weather heat stroke may occur; take extra precautions to stay cool

Treatment of overdose: Lavage if orally ingested, provide an airway

---

lypressin

(lye-press'in)

Diapid

Func. class.: Pituitary hormone
Chem. class.: Lysine vasopressin

Action: Promotes reabsorption of water by action on renal tubular epithelium

Uses: Nonnephrogenic diabetes insipidus

Dosage and routes:

• *Adult:* Intranasal 1-2 sprays in one or both nostrils qid, an extra dose hs if needed

Available forms include: Intranasal 0.185 mg/ml

Side effects/adverse reactions:

EENT: Nasal irritation, congestion, rhinitis, conjunctivitis, rhinorrhea
CNS: Headache
GI: Nausea, heartburn, cramps
MISC: Chest tightness, cough, dyspnea

Precautions: CAD, pregnancy (B)

Pharmacokinetics:

NASAL: Onset 1 hr, duration 3-8 hr, half-life 15 min; metabolized in liver, kidneys, excreted in urine

NURSING CONSIDERATIONS

Assess:

• I&O ratio; weight daily, check for edema in extremities, if water retention is severe, diuretic may be prescribed

Perform/provide:

• Storage at room temperature

Evaluate:

• Therapeutic response: absence of severe thirst, decreased urine output, osmolality
• Water intoxication: lethargy, behavioral changes, disorientation, neuromuscular excitability

Teach patient/family:

• To clear nasal passages before using drug, not to inhale spray
• To carry drug at all times

---

* Available in Canada only

mafenide acetate (topical)

(ma'fe-nide)

Sulfamylon

Func. class.: Local antiinfective
Chem. class.: Sulfonamide

Action: Interferes with bacterial cell wall synthesis
Uses: Burns (2nd, 3rd degree)
Dosage and routes:
• *Adult and child:* TOP apply 1/16 in to affected area qd-bid, reapply as needed
Available forms include: Cream 85 mg/g as acetate
Side effects/adverse reactions:
INTEG: Rash, urticaria, stinging, burning, bleeding, excoriation of new skin, super infections, pruritus, blisters, facial edema, hives, erythema
OTHER: Metabolic acidosis, tachypnea, ***bone marrow suppression, fatal hemolytic anemia, eosinophilia***
Contraindications: Hypersensitivity, inhalation injury
Precautions: Pregnancy (C), impaired pulmonary function, lactation, impaired renal function

NURSING CONSIDERATIONS
Administer:
• Analgesic before application if needed
• Enough medication to completely cover burns; they must be covered at all times
• After cleansing debris from burn before each application
• Using aseptic technique to debrided areas
Perform/provide:
• Storage at room temperature in dry place
Evaluate:
• Therapeutic response: appearance of granulation tissue
• Allergic reaction: burning, stinging, swelling, redness
• Fluid loss: decreased urinary output
Teach patient/family:
• That therapy will continue until area is ready for grafting
• About signs of superimposed infection
• About changes in respiratory activity

magaldrate (aluminum magnesium complex)

(mag' al-drate)

Hydromagnesium, Lowsium, Riopan, Riopan Plus

Func. class.: Antacid
Chem. class.: Aluminum/magnesium hydroxide

Action: Neutralizes gastric acidity
Uses: Antacid
Dosage and routes:
• *Adult:* PO 1-2 (480-1080 mg) between meals, hs, not to exceed 20 tabs/day; chew tab 1-2 (480-960 mg) between meals, hs, not to exceed 20 tabs/day; susp 5-10 ml (400-800 mg) with water between meals, hs, not to exceed 100 ml/day
Available forms include: Tabs 480 mg; chew tabs 480 mg; susp 540 mg/5 ml, 480 mg/5 ml, 1080 mg/5 ml
Side effects/adverse reactions:
GI: Constipation, diarrhea
META: Hypermagnesium
Contraindications: Hypersensitivity to this drug or aluminum products
Precautions: Elderly, fluid restriction, decreased GI motility, GI obstruction, dehydration, renal disease, sodium-restricted diets, pregnancy (C)

Pharmacokinetics:
PO: Duration 60 min
Interactions/incompatibilities:
• Decreased effectiveness of: tetracyclines, ketoconazole
• Decreased absorption of: anticholinergics, chlordiazepoxide, cimetidine, corticosteroids, iron salts, phenothiazines, phenytoin, salicylates
NURSING CONSIDERATIONS
Assess:
• Serum Mg^{++} levels with impaired renal function
Administer:
• Laxatives or stool softeners if constipation occurs
• After shaking, give between meals and hs
• To separate enteric-coated drugs and antacid by 1 hr
Evaluate:
• Therapeutic response: absence of pain, decreased acidity
• Constipation: increase bulk in diet if needed

magnesium carbonate

Func. class.: Antacid
Chem. class.: Magnesium product

Action: Neutralizes gastric acidity
Uses: Antacid, constipation
Dosage and routes:
• *Adult:* PO 0.5-2 g between meals with water
Laxative
• *Adult:* PO 8 g with water hs
Available forms include: Powder
Side effects/adverse reactions:
GI: Diarrhea, flatulence, cramps, belching, nausea, vomiting, impaction, ***obstruction,*** pain
META: Hypermagnesia: *weakness, lethargy, depression, decreased B/P, increased pulse,* ***respiratory depression, coma***
Contraindications: Hypersensitivity
Precautions: Severe renal disease, GI bleeding, diarrhea, intestinal obstruction, pregnancy (C)
Pharmacokinetics:
PO: Excreted in urine
Interactions/incompatibilities:
• Decreased effectiveness of: tetracyclines
• Decreased absorption of: anticholinergics, chlordiazepoxide, cimetidine, corticosteroids, iron salts
NURSING CONSIDERATIONS
Administer:
• After mixing with water
Evaluate:
• Therapeutic response: absence of pain, decreased acidity
Teach patient/family:
• Not to change antacids unless directed by physician
• To store in tightly covered container
Lab test interferences:
Increase: Urinary pH, gastrin
Decrease: K^{+}

magnesium oxide

Mag-Ox, Maox, Par-Mag, Uro-Mag
Func. class.: Antacid
Chem. class.: Magnesium product

Action: Neutralizes gastric acidity
Uses: Constipation, hypomagnesemia, antacid
Dosage and routes:
• *Adult:* PO 250 mg-1 g pc, hs with 4-8 oz water
Laxative
• *Adult:* PO 2-4 g with water hs
Hypomagnesemia
• *Adult:* PO 650-1.3 g qd
Available forms include: Caps 140; tabs 400, 420 mg

Side effects/adverse reactions:
GU: Renal stones
GI: Diarrhea, flatulence, cramps, belching, nausea, vomiting
META: Hypermagnesemia: *weakness, lethargy, depression, decreased B/P, increased pulse,* ***respiratory depression, coma***
Contraindications: Hypersensitivity
Precautions: Severe renal disease, GI bleeding, diarrhea, intestinal obstruction, pregnancy (C)
Pharmacokinetics:
PO: Excreted in urine
Interactions/incompatibilities:
• Decreased effectiveness of: tetracyclines, ketoconazole
• Decreased absorption of: anticholinergics, chlordiazepoxide, cimetidine, corticosteroids, iron salts, phenothiazines, phenytoin

NURSING CONSIDERATIONS

Perform/provide:
• Storage in airtight container
Evaluate:
• Therapeutic response: absence of pain, decreased acidity
• Decreased constipation, characteristics of stools
Teach patient/family:
• Not to change antacids unless directed by physician
Lab test interferences:
Increase: Urinary pH, gastrin
Decrease: K+

magnesium salicylate

Analate, Arthrin, Doan's pills, Efficin, Magan, Mobidin
Func. class.: Nonnarcotic analgesic
Chem. class.: Salicylate

Action: Blocks pain impulses in CNS that occur in response to inhibition of prostaglandin synthesis; antipyretic action results from inhibition of hypothalamic heat-regulating center to produce vasodilation to allow heat dissipation
Uses: Mild to moderate pain or fever including arthritis, juvenile rheumatoid arthritis
Dosage and routes:
Arthritis
• *Adult:* PO not to exceed 4.8 g/day in divided doses
Pain/fever
• *Adult:* PO 600 mg tid or qid
Available forms include: Tabs 325, 545, 600 mg
Side effects/adverse reactions:
HEMA: ***Thrombocytopenia, agranulocytosis, leukopenia, neutropenia, hemolytic anemia,*** increased pro-time
CNS: Stimulation, drowsiness, dizziness, confusion, ***convulsion,*** headache, flushing, hallucinations, coma
GI: Nausea, vomiting, GI bleeding, diarrhea, heartburn, anorexia, ***hepatitis***
INTEG: Rash, urticaria, bruising
EENT: Tinnitus, hearing loss
CV: Rapid pulse, ***pulmonary edema***
RESP: Wheezing, hyperpnea
ENDO: Hypoglycemia, hyponatremia, hypokalemia
Contraindications: Hypersensitivity to salicylates, GI bleeding, bleeding disorders, children < 3 yr, vitamin K deficiency
Precautions: Anemia, hepatic disease, renal disease, Hodgkin's disease, pregnancy (C), lactation
Pharmacokinetics:
PO: Onset 15-30 min, peak 1-2 hr, duration 4-6 hr, metabolized by liver, excreted by kidneys, crosses placenta, excreted in breast milk, half-life 1-3½ hr

Interactions/incompatibilities:

- Decreased effects of magnesium salicylate: antacids, steroids, urinary alkalizers
- Increased blood loss: alcohol, heparin
- Increased effects of: anticoagulants, insulin, methotrexate
- Decreased effects of: probenecid, spironolactone, sulfinpyrazone, sulfonylmides
- Toxic effects: PABA
- Decreased blood sugar levels: salicylates

NURSING CONSIDERATIONS

Assess:

- Liver function studies: AST, ALT, bilirubin, creatinine if patient is on long-term therapy
- Renal function studies: BUN, urine creatinine if patient is on long-term therapy
- Blood studies: CBC, Hct, Hgb, pro-time if patient is on long-term therapy
- I&O ratio; decreasing output may indicate renal failure (long-term therapy)

Administer:

- To patient crushed or whole; chewable tablets may be chewed
- With food or milk to decrease gastric symptoms; give 30 min before or 2 hr after meals
- With full glass of water

Evaluate:

- Therapeutic response: decreased pain, fever
- Hepatotoxicity: dark urine, clay-colored stools, yellowing of skin, sclera, itching, abdominal pain, fever, diarrhea if patient is on long-term therapy
- Allergic reactions: rash, urticaria; if these occur, drug may need to be discontinued
- Renal dysfunction: decreased urine output
- Ototoxicity: tinnitus, ringing, roaring in ears; audiometric testing is needed before, after long-term therapy
- Visual changes: blurring, halos, corneal and retinal damage
- Edema in feet, ankles, legs
- Prior drug history; there are many drug interactions

Teach patient/family:

- To report any symptoms of hepatotoxicity, renal toxicity, visual changes, ototoxicity, allergic reactions, bleeding (long-term therapy)
- Not to exceed recommended dosage; acute poisoning may result
- To read label on other OTC drugs; many contain aspirin
- That therapeutic response takes 2 wk (arthritis)
- To avoid alcohol ingestion; GI bleeding may occur
- That if anticoagulants are given, this drug should be discontinued 2 wks before surgery

Lab test interferences:

Increase: Coagulation studies, liver function studies, serum uric acid, amylase, CO_2, urinary protein
Decrease: Serum potassium, PBI, cholesterol, blood glucose
Interfere: Urine catecholamines, pregnancy test

Treatment of overdose: Lavage, activated charcoal, monitor electrolytes, VS

---

magnesium salts

Magnesium Citrate, Magnesium Sulfate, Milk of Magnesia (MOM), Mint-O-Mag

Func. class.: Laxative, saline

Action: Increases osmotic pressure, draws fluid into colon

Uses: Constipation, bowel prepa-

* Available in Canada only

ration before surgery or examination

Dosage and routes:

• *Adult:* PO 30-60 ml hs (Milk of Magnesia), 300 mg

• *Adult and child >6 yr:* PO 15 g in 8 oz of water (magnesium sulfate); PO 10-20 ml (concentrated Milk of Magnesia); PO 5-10 oz hs (Magnesium Citrate)

• *Child 2-6 yr:* 5-15 ml (Milk of Magnesia)

Available forms include: Oral sol, susp 77.5 mg/g; tabs 300, 600 mg

Side effects/adverse reactions:

CNS: Muscle weakness, flushing, sweating, confusion, sedation, depressed reflexes, ***flaccid, paralysis,*** hypothermia

GI: Nausea, vomiting, anorexia, cramps

CV: Hypotension, heart block, ***circulatory collapse***

META: Electrolyte, fluid imbalances

Contraindications: Hypersensitivity, renal diseases, abdominal pain, nausea/vomiting, obstruction, acute surgical abdomen, rectal bleeding

Precautions: Pregnancy (B)

Pharmacokinetics:

PO: Peak 1-2 hr; excreted in feces

Interactions/incompatibilities:

• Increased CNS depression: CNS depressants, barbiturates, narcotics, anesthetics

NURSING CONSIDERATIONS

Assess:

• I&O ratio; check for decrease in urinary output

Administer:

• With 8 oz of water

Evaluate:

• Therapeutic response: decreased constipation

• Cause of constipation; identify whether fluids, bulk, or exercise is missing from lifestyle

• Cramping, rectal bleeding, nausea, vomiting; if these symptoms occur, drug should be discontinued

• Magnesium toxicity: thirst, confusion, decrease in reflexes

Teach patient/family:

• Not to use laxatives for long-term therapy; bowel tone will be lost

• Chilling helps the taste of Magnesium Citrate

magnesium sulfate

Func. class.: Anticonvulsant

Chem. class.: Magnesium product

Action: Decreases acetylcholine in motor nerve terminals, which is responsible for anticonvulsant properties; osmotically retains fluid, which increases amount of water in feces when used as laxative; reduces SA node impulse formation, prolongs conduction time in myocardium

Uses: Hypomagnesemic seizures, control of seizures in pregnancy-induced hypertension, seizures in acute nephritis

Dosage and routes:

Hypomagnesemic seizures

• *Adult:* IV 1-2 g over 15 min, then 1 g IM q4-6h, depending on response

Nephritis

• *Child:* IM 20-40 mg/kg in 20% sol, repeat as needed

Preeclampsia/eclampsia

• *Adult:* IV 4 g/250 ml D_5W and 4 g IM, then 4 g IM q4h prn; or 4 g IV loading dose, then 1-4 g IV inf hourly, not to exceed 3 ml/min

Available forms include: Inj IV, IM 10%, 50%, 12.5%, 25%; granules,

Side effects/adverse reactions:

CNS: Sweating, depressed reflexes,

flushing, drowsiness, flaccid paralysis, hypothermia, weakness, sedation
RESP: ***Paralysis***
CV: Hypotension, ***circulatory collapse, heart block,*** decreased cardiac function
Contraindications: Hypersensitivity, myocardial infarction, renal disease
Precaution: Pregnancy (C)
Pharmacokinetics:
IV: Onset 1-5 min, duration 30 min
IM: Onset 1 hr, duration 3-4 hr
Excreted by kidneys
Interactions/incompatibilities:
- Increased CNS depression: barbiturates, general anesthetics, narcotics, antipsychotics
- Increased effects of: neuromuscular blockers

NURSING CONSIDERATIONS
Assess:
- VS q15min after IV dose; do not exceed 150 mg/min
- Cardiac function: monitoring, magnesium levels
- Timing of contractions, determine intensity, monitor fetal heart rate, reactivity, may decrease with this drug if using during labor
- I&O: should remain at 30 ml/hr or more; if less than this, notify physician

Administer:
- Only after calcium gluconate is available for magnesium toxicity
- IV undiluted 1.5 ml of 10% sol over 1 min; may dilute to 20% sol, infuse over 3 hr
- IV at less than 150 mg/min; circulatory collapse may occur

Perform/provide:
- Seizure precautions: placing in dark room with decreased stimuli, padded siderails

Evaluate:
- Therapeutic response absence of seizures
- Urine output before each dose, output should be 100 ml/4 hr or more
- Mental status: mood, sensorium, affect, memory (long, short)
- Respiratory dysfunction: respiratory depression, character, rate, rhythm; hold drug if respirations are <16/min
- Hypermagnesemia: depressed patellar reflex, flushing, polydipsia, confusion, weakness, flaccid paralysis, hypothermia, dyspnea begin to appear at blood levels of 4 mEq/L
- Respiratory rate, rhythm of newborn if drug was given 24 hr before delivery or less; check reflexes of newborn whose mother received this drug before delivery
- Reflexes: knee jerk, patellar; decrease signals Mg^{++} toxicity

Teach patient/family:
- Symptoms of hypermagnesemia

Treatment of overdose: Stop drug, administer calcium gluconate, monitor reflexes, magnesium levels

magnesium trisilicate

Trisomin

Func. class.: Antacid
Chem. class.: Magnesium product

Action: Neutralizes gastric acidity
Uses: Constipation, hypomagnesemia
Dosage and routes:
- *Adult:* PO 1-4 g qid with 4 oz of water

Available forms include: Powder, tabs 488 mg
Side effects/adverse reactions:
GI: Diarrhea, flatulence, cramps, belching, nausea, vomiting
META: Hypermagnesemia: *weakness, lethargy, depression, de-*

creased B/P, increased pulse, ***respiratory depression, coma***
Contraindications: Hypersensitivity to this drug
Precautions: Severe renal disease, pregnancy (C)
Pharmacokinetics:
PO: Excreted in urine
Interactions/incompatibilities:
• Decreased effectiveness of: tetracyclines, ketoconazole
• Decreased absorption of: anticholinergics, chlordiazepoxide, cimetidine, corticosteroids, iron salts, phenothiazines, phenytoin

NURSING CONSIDERATIONS
Administer:
• After mixing with water
Evaluate:
• Therapeutic response: absence of pain, decreased acidity
• Decreased constipation, characteristics of stools
Teach patient/family:
• Not to change antacids unless directed by physician
• That tabs must be chewed before swallowing
• That drug has a delayed reaction
• To separate doses of other drugs by 1 hr
Lab test interferences:
Increase: Urinary pH, gastrin
Decrease: K+

---

mannitol

(man'i-tole)
Osmitrol, Resectial

Func. class.: Osmotic diuretic
Chem. class.: Hexahydric alcohol

Action: Acts by increasing osmolarity of glomerular filtrate, which raises osmotic pressure of fluid in renal tubules; there is a decrease in reabsorption of water, increase in urinary output, sodium, chloride excretion
Uses: Edema, promote systemic diuresis in cerebral edema, decrease intraocular pressure, improve renal function in acute renal failure, chemical poisoning
Dosage and routes:
Oliguria, prevention
• *Adult:* IV 50-100 g of a 5%-25% sol
Oliguria, treatment
• *Adult:* IV 300-400 mg/kg of a 20%-25% sol up to 100 g of a 15%-20% sol
Intraocular pressure/intracranial pressure
• *Adult:* IV 1.5-2 g/kg of a 15%-25% sol over ½-1 hr
Renal failure
• *Adult:* IV 50-200 g/24 hr, adjusted to maintain output of 30-50 mg/hr
Diuresis in drug intoxication
• *Adult and child >12 yr:* 5%-10% sol continuously up to 200 g IV, while maintaining 100-500 ml output/hr
Available forms include: Inj IV 5%, 10%, 15%, 20%, 25%
Side effects/adverse reactions:
GU: Marked diuresis, urinary retention, thirst
CNS: Dizziness, headache, ***convulsions,*** rebound increased ICP
GI: Nausea, vomiting, dry mouth, diarrhea
CV: Edema, thrombophlebitis, hypotension, hypertension, tachycardia, angina-like chest pains, fever, chills
RESP: Pulmonary congestion
ELECT: Fluid, electrolyte imbalances, acidosis, electrolyte loss, dehydration
EENT: Loss of hearing, blurred vision, nasal congestion, decreased intraocular pressure

Contraindications: Active intracranial bleeding, hypersensitivity, anuria, severe pulmonary congestion, edema, severe dehydration
Precautions: Dehydration, pregnancy (C), severe renal disease, CHF, lactation
Pharmacokinetics:
IV: Onset 30-60 min for diuresis, ½-1 hr for intraocular pressure, 25 min for cerebrospinal fluid; duration 4-6 hr for intraocular pressure, 3-8 hr for cerebrospinal fluid; excreted in urine
Interactions/incompatibilities:
• Decreased effect: lithium
• Increased effects of: EDTA
• Incompatible with whole blood, in solution or syringe with any other drug or solution

NURSING CONSIDERATIONS
Assess:
• Weight, I&O daily to determine fluid loss; effect of drug may be decreased if used qd
• Rate, depth, rhythm of respiration, effect of exertion
• B/P lying, standing, postural hypotension may occur
• Electrolytes: potassium, sodium, chloride; include BUN, CBC, serum creatinine, blood pH, ABGs
Administer:
• IV in 15%-25% solutions with filter; give over ½-1½ hr, rapid infusion may worsen CHF
• Test dose in severe oliguria, 0.2 g/kg over 3-5 min, if no urine increase, give 2nd test dose; if no response, reassess patient
Evaluate:
• Therapeutic response: improvement in edema of feet, legs, sacral area daily if medication is being used in CHF
• Improvement in CVP q8h
• Signs of metabolic acidosis: drowsiness, restlessness
• Signs of hypokalemia: postural hypotension, malaise, fatigue, tachycardia, leg cramps, weakness
• Rashes, temperature elevation qd
• Confusion, especially in elderly; take safety precautions if needed
• Hydration including skin turgor, thirst, dry mucous membranes
Teach patient/family:
• To increase fluid intake 2-3 L/day unless contraindicated; to rise slowly from lying or sitting position
Lab test interferences:
Interference: Inorganic phosphorus, ethylene glycol
Treatment of overdose: Discontinue infusion, correct fluid, electrolyte imbalances, hemodialysis, monitor hydration, CV, renal function

---

maprotiline HCl
(ma-proe'ti-leen)
Ludiomil
Func. class.: Antidepressant
Chem. class.: Tetracyclic

Action: Blocks reuptake of norepinephrine, serotonin into nerve endings, increasing action of norepinephrine, serotonin in nerve cells
Uses: Depression, dysthymic disorder, manic depressive—depressed, agitated depression
Dosage and routes:
• *Adult:* PO 75 mg/day in moderate depression, may increase to 150 mg/day; not to exceed 225 mg in hospitalized patients, severely depressed patients that are hospitalized may be given 300 mg/day
• *Elderly:* 50-75 mg/day
Available forms include: Tabs 25, 50, 75 mg
Side effects/adverse reactions:
HEMA: ***Agranulocytosis, throm-***

*Available in Canada only

bocytopenia, eosinophilia, leukopenia

CNS: Dizziness, drowsiness, confusion, headache, anxiety, tremors, stimulation, weakness, insomnia, nightmares, EPS (elderly), increased psychiatric symptoms, ***seizures***

GI: Diarrhea, dry mouth, nausea, vomiting, ***paralytic ileus,*** increased appetite, cramps, epigastric distress, jaundice, ***hepatitis,*** stomatitis

GU: Retention, ***acute renal failure***

INTEG: Rash, urticaria, sweating, pruritus, photosensitivity

CV: Orthostatic hypotension, ECG changes, tachycardia, ***hypertension,*** palpitations

EENT: Blurred vision, tinnitus, mydriasis

Contraindications: Hypersensitivity to tricyclic antidepressants, recovery phase of myocardial infarction, convulsive disorders, prostatic hypertrophy

Precautions: Suicidal patients, severe depression, increased intraocular pressure, narrow-angle glaucoma, urinary retention, cardiac disease, hepatic disease, hypothyroidism, hyperthyroidism, electroshock therapy, elective surgery, elderly, pregnancy (B)

Pharmacokinetics:

PO: Onset 15-30 min, peak 12 hr, duration up to 3 wk, steady state 6-10 days; metabolized by liver, excreted by kidneys, feces, crosses placenta, half-life 21-25 hr

Interactions/incompatibilities:

- Decreased effects of: guanethidine, clonidine, indirect acting sympathomimetics (ephedrine)
- Increased effects of: direct acting sympathomimetics (epinephrine), alcohol, barbiturates, benzodiazepines, CNS depressants
- Hyperpyretic crisis, convulsions, hypertensive episode: MAOI (pargyline [Eutonyl])

NURSING CONSIDERATIONS

Assess:

- B/P (lying, standing), pulse q4h; if systolic B/P drops 20 mm Hg hold drug, notify physician; take vital signs q4h in patients with cardiovascular disease
- Blood studies: CBC, leukocytes, differential, cardiac enzymes if patient is receiving long-term therapy
- Hepatic studies: AST, ALT, bilirubin, creatinine
- Weight qwk, appetite may increase with drug
- ECG for flattening of T wave, bundle branch block, AV block, dysrhythmias in cardiac patients

Administer:

- Increased fluids, bulk in diet if constipation, urinary retention occur, especially elderly
- With food or milk for GI symptoms
- Dosage hs if oversedation occurs during day; may take entire dose hs; elderly may not tolerate once/day dosing
- Gum, hard candy, or frequent sips of water for dry mouth
- Concentrate with fruit juice, water, or milk to disguise taste

Perform/provide:

- Storage in tight container at room temperature, do not freeze
- Assistance with ambulation during beginning therapy since drowsiness/dizziness occurs
- Safety measures including siderails primarily in elderly
- Checking to see PO medication swallowed

Evaluate:

- Therapeutic response: decreased depression

M

• EPS primarily in elderly: rigidity, dystonia, akathisia
• Mental status: mood, sensorium, affect, suicidal tendencies, increase in psychiatric symptoms: depression, panic
• Urinary retention, constipation; constipation is more likely to occur in children
• Withdrawal symptoms: headache, nausea, vomiting, muscle pain, weakness; do not usually occur unless drug was discontinued abruptly
• Alcohol consumption; if alcohol is consumed, hold dose until morning

Teach patient/family:
• That therapeutic effects may take 2-3 wk
• Use of caution in driving or other activities requiring alertness because of drowsiness, dizziness, blurred vision
• To avoid alcohol ingestion, other CNS depressants
• Not to discontinue medication quickly after long-term use; may cause nausea, headache, malaise
• To wear sunscreen or large hat since photosensitivity occurs

Lab test interferences:
Increase: Serum bilirubin, blood glucose, alk phosphatase
False increase: Urinary catecholamines
Decrease: VMA, 5-HIAA

Treatment of overdose: ECG monitoring, induce emesis, lavage, activated charcoal, administer anticonvulsant

mazindol

(may'zin-dole)
Mazanor, Sanorex
Func. class.: Anorexiant
Chem. class.: Imidazoisoindole derivative

Controlled Substance Schedule IV

Action: Acts on central adrenergic and dopaminergic pathways to stimulate satiety center in hypothalamic, limbic regions

Uses: Exogenous obesity

Dosage and routes:
• *Adult:* PO 1 mg ac, or 2 mg 1 hr ac lunch

Available forms include: Tabs 1, 2 mg

Side effects/adverse reactions:
HEMA: ***Bone marrow depression, leukopenia, agranulocytosis***
EENT: Mydriasis, blurred vision, eye irritation
MISC: Hair loss, muscle pain, flushing, fever
CNS: *Hyperactivity, insomnia, restlessness,* dizziness, headache, stimulation, irritability, drowsiness, weakness, tremor
GI: Nausea, anorexia, dry mouth, diarrhea, constipation
GU: Impotence, change in libido, difficulty urinating
CV: Palpitations, tachycardia
INTEG: Urticaria, rash, pallor, shivering, sweating

Contraindications: Hypersensitivity to sympathomimetic amine, glaucoma, drug abuse, cardiovascular disease, children <12 yr, hypertension, hypotension, severe arteriosclerosis, agitated states

Precautions: Diabetes mellitus, pregnancy (C), lactation

Pharmacokinetics:
PO: Onset ½-1 hr, duration 8-15 hr,

metabolized by liver, excreted by kidneys

Interactions/incompatibilities:

• Hypertensive crisis: MAOIs or within 14 days of MAOIs

• Increased effect of mazindol: acetazolamide, antacids, sodium bicarbonate

• Decreased effects of mazindol: tricyclics, ascorbic acid, ammonium chloride

• Decreased effects of: guanethidine, other antihypertensives

• Increased effects of: insulin

NURSING CONSIDERATIONS

Assess:

• VS, B/P since this drug may reverse antihypertensives; check patients with cardiac disease more often

• CBC, urinalysis, in diabetes: blood sugar, urine sugar; insulin changes may need to be made since eating will decrease

• Height, growth rate in children; growth rate may be decreased

Administer:

• At least 6 hr before hs to avoid sleeplessness, 1 hr ac meals

• For obesity only if patient is on weight reduction program including dietary changes, exercise; patient will develop tolerance, and weight loss won't occur without additional methods

• Gum, hard candy, frequent sips of water for dry mouth

Evaluate:

• Therapeutic response: decreased weight

• Mental status: mood, sensorium, affect, stimulation, insomnia, aggressiveness

• Physical dependency: should not be used for extended time; dose should be discontinued gradually, tolerance will occur after long-term use

• Withdrawal symptoms: headache, nausea, vomiting, muscle pain, weakness

Teach patient/family:

• To take with meals to avoid GI symptoms

• To decrease caffeine consumption (coffee, tea, cola, chocolate), which may increase irritability, stimulation

• To avoid OTC preparations unless approved by physician

• To taper off drug over several weeks, or depression, increased sleeping, lethargy may ensue

• To avoid alcohol ingestion

• To avoid hazardous activities until patient is stabilized on medication

• To get needed rest; patients will feel more tired at end of day

Treatment of overdose: Administer fluids, chlorpromazine 1 mg/kg; antihypertensive for increased B/P; ammonium Cl for increased excretion

measles, mumps, and rubella virus vaccine, live

M-M-R-II

Func. class.: Vaccine

Action: Produces antibodies to measles, mumps, rubella

Uses: Prevention of measles, mumps, rubella

Dosage and routes:

• *Child 1-13 yr:* SC 1000 U

Available forms include: Inj SC measles 1000 $TCID_{50}$, mumps 5000 $TCID_{50}$, rubella 1000 $TCID_{50}$

Side effects/adverse reactions:

CNS: Fever, ***subacute sclerosing panencephalitis and blindness associated with optic neuritis,*** paresthesias

INTEG: Urticaria, erythema, burning, stinging at injection site
SYST: Lymphadenitis, ***anaphylaxis,*** malaise, sore throat, headache
MS: Osteomyelitis, arthralgia, arthritis
Contraindications: Hypersensitivity, blood dyscrasias, anemia, active infection, immunosuppression, egg, chicken allergy, pregnancy, febrile illness, neomycin allergy, neoplasms
Interactions/incompatibilities:
- Decreased response to: TB skin test
- Other live virus vaccines

NURSING CONSIDERATIONS
Assess:
- For skin reactions: rash, induration, erythema

Administer:
- Only with epinephrine 1 : 1000 on unit to treat laryngospasm
- Only SC

Perform/provide:
- Storage at 39° F (4° C), protect from heat and light; do not give within 1 month of other live virus vaccines
- Written record of immunization

Evaluate:
- For history of allergies, skin conditions (eczema, psoriasis, dermatitis), reactions to vaccinations
- For anaphylaxis: inability to breathe, bronchospasm

Teach patient/family:
- That fever may occur between the 5-12th day after vaccine given
- That joint pains, tingling in extremities may occur 5-12 days after vaccine given
- That pain and inflammation may occur
- To take acetaminophen for fever

mebendazole

(me-ben'da-zole)
Vermox
Func. class.: Anthelmintic
Chem. class.: Carbamate

Action: Inhibits glucose uptake, degeneration of cytoplasmic microtubules in the cell; interferes with absorption, secretory function
Uses: Pinworms, roundworms, hookworms, whipworms, threadworms, pork tapeworms, dwarf tapeworms, beef tapeworms, hydatid cyst
Dosage and routes:
- *Adult and child >2 yr:* PO 100 mg as a single dose or bid × 3 days, depending on type of infection; course may be repeated in 3 wk if needed

Available forms include: Tabs, chewable 100 mg
Side effects/adverse reactions:
CNS: Dizziness, fever
GI: Transient diarrhea, abdominal pain
Contraindications: Hypersensitivity
Precautions: Child <2 yr, lactation, pregnancy (1st trimester) (C)
Pharmacokinetics:
PO: Peak ½-7 hr, excreted in feces primarily (metabolites), small amount in urine (unchanged), highly bound to plasma proteins

NURSING CONSIDERATIONS
Assess:
- Stools during entire treatment; specimens must be sent to lab while still warm

Administer:
- May be crushed, chewed if unable to swallow whole
- PO after meals to avoid GI symptoms since absorption is not altered by food

• Second course after 3 wk if needed; usually recommended

Perform/provide:

• Storage in tight container

Evaluate:

• Therapeutic response: expulsion of worms and 3 negative stool cultures after completion of treatment

• For allergic reaction: rash (rare)

• For diarrhea during expulsion of worms; avoid self-contamination with patient's feces

• For infection in other family members since infection from person to person is common

Teach patient/family:

• Proper hygiene after BM including handwashing technique; tell patient to avoid putting fingers in mouth

• That infected person should sleep alone; do not shake bed linen, change bed linen qd, wash in hot water

• To clean toilet qd with disinfectant (green soap solution)

• Need for compliance with dosage schedule, duration of treatment

• To wear shoes, wash all fruits and vegetables well before eating

---

mecamylamine HCl

(mek-a-mill'a-meen)

Inversine

Func. class.: Antihypertensive
Chem. class.: Ganglionic blocker

Action: Occupies receptor site, prevents acetylcholine from attaching to postsynaptic nerve ending in sympathetic ganglia

Uses: Moderate to severe hypertension, malignant hypertension

Dosage and routes:

• *Adult:* PO 2.5 mg bid, may increase in increments of 2.5 mg × 2 days until desired response, maintenance 25 mg/day in 3 divided doses

Available forms include: Tabs 2.5 mg

Side effects/adverse reactions:

CV: Postural hypotension, irregular heart rate, ***CHF***

CNS: *Drowsiness, sedation,* headache, tremors, weakness, syncope, paresthesia, dizziness, ***convulsions***

EENT: *Blurred vision,* nasal congestion, dry mouth, dilated pupils

GU: Impotence, urinary retention, decreased libido

GI: Anorexia, glossitis, nausea, vomiting, constipation, ***paralytic ileus***

Contraindications: Hypersensitivity, myocardial infarction, coronary insufficiency, renal disease, glaucoma, organic pyloric stenosis, uremia, uncooperative patients, mild/labile hypertension

Precautions: CVA, prostatic hypertrophy, bladder neck obstruction, urethral stricture, renal dysfunction (elevated BUN), cerebral dysfunction, pregnancy (C)

Pharmacokinetics:

PO: Onset ½-2 hr, duration 6-12 hr; excreted in urine, feces, breast milk; crosses placenta

Interactions/incompatibilities:

• Increased effects: thiazide diuretics, antihypertensives, CNS depressants (alcohol, anesthetics, MAOIs), bethanechol

NURSING CONSIDERATIONS

Assess:

• B/P lying and standing, other VS throughout treatment

• Weight daily, I&O

Administer:

• Whole, do not chew or crush tablets

• After meals for better absorption;

M

give larger dose at noon and evening, smaller dose in AM
• Gum, frequent rinsing of mouth, hard candy for dry mouth

Evaluate:
• Therapeutic response: decreased B/P
• Edema in feet, legs daily
• Skin turgor, dryness of mucous membranes for hydration status
• Tolerance to drug that occurs with prolonged use
• Constipation: number of stools, consistency, give stool softener as ordered or increase bulk in diet

Teach patient/family:
• To notify physician if tremor, seizure, or signs of paralytic ileus occur
• To avoid OTC preparations unless directed by physician
• To rise slowly from sitting or lying position, orthostatic hypotension may occur
• That impotence may occur, but is reversible after discontinuing drug

Treatment of overdose: Administer gastric lavage, discontinue drug, administer small doses of pressor amines for hypotension

mechlorethamine HCl (nitrogen mustard)

(me-klor-eth'a-meen)

Mustargen

Func. class.: Antineoplastic alkylating agent
Chem. class.: Nitrogen mustard

Action: Responsible for cross-linking DNA strands leading to cell death; rapidly degraded, a vesicant

Uses: Hodgkin's disease, lymphomas, lymphosarcoma; ovarian, breast, lung cancer; neoplastic effusions

Dosage and routes:
• *Adult:* IV 0.4 mg/kg or 10 mg/m^2 as 1 dose or divided doses

Neoplastic effusions
• *Adult:* Intracavity 10-20 mg

Available forms include: Inj IV, intracavity 10 mg; powder for inj

Side effects/adverse reactions:
EENT: Tinnitus, hearing loss
HEMA: ***Thrombocytopenia, leukopenia, agranulocytosis,*** anemia
GI: Nausea, vomiting, diarrhea, stomatitis, weight loss, colitis, ***hepatotoxicity***
CNS: Headache, dizziness, drowsiness, paresthesia, peripheral neuropathy, ***coma***
INTEG: Alopecia, pruritus, herpes zoster

Contraindications: Lactation, pregnancy (1st trimester) (D), myelosuppression, acute herpes zoster

Precautions: Radiation therapy, chronic lymphocytic leukopenia

Pharmacokinetics:
Metabolized in liver, excreted in urine

Interactions/incompatibilities:
• Increased toxicity: antineoplastics, radiation

NURSING CONSIDERATIONS

Assess:
• CBC, differential, platelet count weekly; withhold drug if WBC is <4000 or platelet count is <75,000; notify physician of results
• Renal function studies: BUN, serum uric acid, urine CrCl before, during therapy
• I&O ratio; report fall in urine output of 30 ml/hr
• Monitor temperature q4h (may indicate beginning infection), no rectal temperatures
• Liver function tests before, during therapy (bilirubin, AST, ALT, LDH) as needed or monthly

* Available in Canada only

Administer:

- After using guidelines for preparation of cytotoxic drugs
- Antiemetic 30-60 min before giving drug to prevent vomiting and prn
- Antibiotics for prophylaxis of infection
- IV after diluting 10 mg/10 ml sterile H_2O or NaCl; leave needle in vial, shake, withdraw dose, give through Y-tube or 3-way stopcock or directly
- Slow IV infusion using 21-, 23-, 25-gauge needle, watch for infiltration. If infiltration occurs, infiltrate area with isotonic sodium thiosulfate or 1% lidocaine. Apply ice for 6-12 hr
- Topical or systemic analgesics for pain
- Local or systemic drugs for infection

Perform/provide:

- Storage at room temperature in dry form
- Strict medical asepsis, protective isolation if WBC levels are low
- Special skin care
- Increase fluid intake to 2-3 L/day to prevent urate deposits, calculi formation
- Diet low in purines: organ meats (kidney, liver), dried beans, peas to maintain alkaline urine
- Preparation under hood using gloves and mask
- Rinsing of mouth tid-qid with water, club soda; brushing of teeth bid-tid with soft brush or cotton-tipped applicators for stomatitis; use unwaxed dental floss
- Warm compresses at injection site for inflammation

Evaluate:

- Therapeutic response: decreased tumor size, spread of malignancy
- Bleeding: hematuria, guaiac, bruising or petechiae, mucosa or orifices q8h
- Food preferences; list likes, dislikes
- Yellowing of skin, sclera, dark urine, clay-colored stools, itchy skin, abdominal pain, fever, diarrhea
- Effects of alopecia on body image; discuss feelings about body changes
- Inflammation of mucosa, breaks in skin
- Buccal cavity q8h for dryness, sores, ulceration, white patches, oral pain, bleeding, dysphagia
- Local irritation, pain, burning, discoloration at injection site
- Symptoms indicating severe allergic reaction: rash, pruritus, urticaria, purpuric skin lesions, itching, flushing

Teach patient/family:

- About protective isolation precautions
- That sterility, amenorrhea can occur; reversible after discontinuing treatment
- That hair may be lost during treatment; a wig or hairpiece may make patient feel better; new hair may be different in color, texture
- To avoid foods with citric acid, hot or rough texture
- To report any bleeding, white spots, or ulcerations in mouth to physician; tell patient to examine mouth qd
- To report signs of infection: increased temperature, sore throat, flu symptoms
- To report signs of anemia: fatigue, headache, faintness, shortness of breath, irritability
- To avoid use of razors or commercial mouthwash
- To avoid use of aspirin products or ibuprofen

meclizine HCl

(mek'li-zeen)

Antivert, Bonamine,* Bonine, Lamine, Roclizine, Vertol

Func. class.: Antiemetic, antihistamine, anticholinergic

Chem. class.: H_1-receptor antagonist, piperazine derivative

Action: Acts centrally by blocking chemoreceptor trigger zone, which in turn acts on vomiting center

Uses: Dizziness, motion sickness

Dosage and routes:

• *Adult:* PO 25-100 mg qd in divided doses or 1 hr before traveling

Available forms include: Tabs 12.5, 25, 50 mg; chew tabs 25 mg; tabs film coated 25 mg

Side effects/adverse reactions:

CNS: Drowsiness, dizziness, fatigue, restlessness, headache, insomnia

GI: Nausea, anorexia

EENT: Dry mouth, blurred vision

Contraindications: Hypersensitivity to cyclizines, shock, lactation, pregnancy

Precautions: Children, narrow-angle glaucoma, glaucoma, urinary retention, lactation, prostatic hypertrophy, elderly, pregnancy (B)

Pharmacokinetics:

PO: Duration 8-24 hr, half-life 6 hr

Interactions/incompatibilities:

• Increased effect of: alcohol, tranquilizers, narcotics

NURSING CONSIDERATIONS

Assess:

• VS, B/P

Administer:

• Tablets may be swallowed whole, chewed, or allowed to dissolve

Evaluate:

• Therapeutic response: absence of dizziness, vomiting

• Signs of toxicity of other drugs or masking of symptoms of disease: brain tumor, intestinal obstruction

• Observe for drowsiness, dizziness, LOC

Teach patient/family:

• That a false-negative result may occur with skin testing; these procedures should not be scheduled for 4 days after discontinuing use

• To avoid hazardous activities, activities requiring alertness; dizziness may occur; instruct patient to request assistance with ambulation

• To avoid alcohol, other depressants

Lab test interferences:

False negative: Allergy skin testing

meclofenamate

(me-kloe-fen-am'ate)

Meclomen

Func. class.: Nonsteroidal antiinflammatory

Chem. class.: Anthranilic acid derivative

Action: Inhibits prostaglandin synthesis by decreasing an enzyme needed for biosynthesis; possesses analgesic, antiinflammatory, antipyretic properties

Uses: Mild to moderate pain, osteoarthritis, rheumatoid arthritis

Dosage and routes:

• *Adult:* PO 200-400 mg/day in divided doses tid-qid

Available forms include: Caps 50, 100 mg

Side effects/adverse reactions:

GI: Nausea, anorexia, vomiting, diarrhea, jaundice, ***cholestatic hepatitis,*** constipation, flatulence, cramps, dry mouth, peptic ulcer

CNS: Dizziness, drowsiness, fatigue, tremors, confusion, insomnia, anxiety, depression

CV: Tachycardia, peripheral

* Available in Canada only

edema, palpitations, dysrhythmias
INTEG: Purpura, rash, pruritus, sweating
GU: ***Nephrotoxicity: dysuria, hematuria, oliguria, azotemia***
HEMA: ***Blood dyscrasias***
EENT: Tinnitus, hearing loss, blurred vision
Contraindications: Hypersensitivity, asthma, severe renal disease, severe hepatic disease
Precautions: Pregnancy (B), lactation, children, bleeding disorders, GI disorders, cardiac disorders, hypersensitivity to other antiinflammatory agents
Pharmacokinetics:
PO: Peak 2 hr, half-life 3-3½ hr; metabolized in liver, excreted in urine (metabolites), excreted in breast milk
Interactions/incompatibilities:
• Increased action of: coumarin, phenytoin, sulfonamides

NURSING CONSIDERATIONS
Assess:
• Renal, liver, blood studies: BUN, creatinine, AST, ALT, Hgb, Hct before treatment, periodically thereafter
• Audiometric and ophthalmic exam before, during, after treatment
• For history of peptic ulcer disease
Administer:
• With food to decrease GI symptoms; best to take on empty stomach to facilitate absorption
Perform/provide:
• Storage at room temperature
Evaluate:
• Therapeutic response: decreased pain, stiffness, swelling in joints, ability to move more easily
• For eye, ear problems: blurred vision, tinnitus (may indicate toxicity)
Teach patient/family:
• To report increased GI symptoms; dose may need to be reduced
• To report blurred vision, ringing, roaring in ears (may indicate toxicity)
• To avoid driving or other hazardous activities if dizziness or drowsiness occurs
• To report change in urine pattern, weight increase, edema, pain increase in joints, fever, blood in urine (indicates nephrotoxicity)
• That therapeutic effects may take up to 1 mo

medium-chain triglycerides

MCT Oil
Func. class.: Caloric

Action: Needed for energy in body; more rapidly hydrolyzed than fat
Uses: Inadequate dietary fat intake or absorption
Dosage and routes:
• *Adult:* PO 15 ml tid-qid, not to exceed 100 ml/day
Available forms include: Oil (115 calories/15 ml)
Side effects/adverse reactions:
CNS: Loss of consciousness (reversible)
GI: Nausea, vomiting, anorexia, cramps, diarrhea, distention
Contraindications: Hypersensitivity, severe hepatic disease, lipoproteinemia
Precautions: Portacaval shunts, pregnancy (C), pancreatitis, hyperlipemia

NURSING CONSIDERATIONS
Assess:
• Triglycerides, free-fatty-acid levels, platelet counts daily to prevent fat overload, thrombocytopenia
• Liver function: AST, ALT

Evaluate:
• Therapeutic response: increased weight
• Nutritional status: calorie count by dietitian

Teach patient/family:
• Reason for use of lipids
• Methods of incorporating drug in food or beverages (salad dressings, chilled fruit juices)

---

medroxyprogesterone acetate

(me-drox'ee-proe-jess'te-rone)
Amen, Curretab, Depo-Provera, Provera

Func. class.: Progestogen
Chem. class.: Progesterone derivative

Action: Inhibits secretion of pituitary gonadotropins, which prevents follicular maturation and ovulation, stimulates growth of mammary tissue, antineoplastic action against endometrial cancer

Uses: Uterine bleeding (abnormal), secondary amenorrhea, endometrial cancer, renal cancer

Dosage and routes:

Secondary amenorrhea
• *Adult:* PO 5-10 mg qd × 5-10 days

Endometrial/renal cancer
• *Adult:* IM 400-1000 mg/wk

Uterine bleeding
• *Adult:* PO 5-10 mg qd × 5-10 days starting on 16th day of menstrual cycle

Available forms include: Tabs 2.5, 10 mg; inj susp 100, 400 mg/ml

Side effects/adverse reactions:
CNS: Dizziness, headache, migraines, depression, fatigue
CV: Hypotension, thrombophlebitis, edema, ***thromboembolism, stroke, pulmonary embolism, myocardial infarction***
GI: Nausea, vomiting, anorexia, cramps, increased weight, ***cholestatic jaundice***
EENT: Diplopia
GU: Amenorrhea, cervical erosion, breakthrough bleeding, dysmenorrhea, vaginal candidiasis, breast changes, *gynecomastia, testicular atrophy, impotence,* endometriosis, ***spontaneous abortion***
INTEG: Rash, urticaria, acne, hirsutism, alopecia, oily skin, seborrhea, purpura, melasma, photosensitivity
META: Hyperglycemia

Contraindications: Breast cancer, hypersensitivity, thromboembolic disorders, reproductive cancer, genital bleeding (abnormal, undiagnosed), pregnancy (X)

Precautions: Lactation, hypertension, asthma, blood dyscrasias, gallbladder disease, CHF, diabetes mellitus, bone disease, depression, migraine headache, convulsive disorders, hepatic disease, renal disease, family history of cancer of breast or reproductive tract

Pharmacokinetics:
PO: Duration 24 hr, excreted in urine and feces, metabolized in liver

NURSING CONSIDERATIONS

Assess:
• Weight daily, notify physician of weekly weight gain >5 lb
• B/P at beginning of treatment and periodically
• I&O ratio; be alert for decreasing urinary output, increasing edema
• Liver function studies: ALT, AST, bilirubin, periodically during long-term therapy

Administer:
• Titrated dose, use lowest effective dose

- Oil solution deeply in large muscle mass (IM), rotate sites
- In one dose in AM
- With food or milk to decrease GI symptoms
- After warming to dissolve crystals

Perform/provide:
- Storage in dark area

Evaluate:
- Therapeutic response: decreased abnormal uterine bleeding, absence of amenorrhea
- Edema, hypertension, cardiac symptoms, jaundice
- Mental status: affect, mood, behavioral changes, depression
- Hypercalcemia

Teach patient/family:
- To avoid sunlight or use sunscreen; photosensitivity can occur
- About cushingoid symptoms
- To report breast lumps, vaginal bleeding, edema, jaundice, dark urine, clay-colored stools, dyspnea, headache, blurred vision, abdominal pain, numbness or stiffness in legs, chest pain; male to report impotence or gynecomastia
- To report suspected pregnancy

Lab test interferences:
Increase: Alk phosphatase, nitrogen (urine), pregnanediol, amino acids
Decrease: GTT, HDL

mefenamic acid

(me-fe-nam′-ik)
Ponstan, Ponstel

Func. class.: Nonsteroidal antiinflammatory
Chem. class.: Anthranilic acid derivative

Action: Inhibits prostaglandin synthesis by decreasing an enzyme needed for biosynthesis and interferes with prostaglandins at receptor sites; possesses analgesic, antiinflammatory, antipyretic properties

Uses: Mild to moderate pain, dysmenorrhea, inflammatory disease

Dosage and routes:
- *Adult and child >14 yr:* PO 500 mg, then 250 mg q4h, use not to exceed 1 wk

Available forms include: Caps 250 mg

Side effects/adverse reactions:
GI: Nausea, anorexia, vomiting, diarrhea, jaundice, ***cholestatic hepatitis,*** constipation, flatulence, cramps, dry mouth, peptic ulcer
CNS: Dizziness, drowsiness, fatigue, tremors, confusion, insomnia, anxiety, depression
CV: Tachycardia, peripheral edema, palpitations, dysrhythmias
INTEG: Purpura, rash, pruritus, sweating
GU: ***Nephrotoxicity: dysuria, hematuria, oliguria, azotemia***
HEMA: ***Blood dyscrasias***
EENT: Tinnitus, hearing loss, blurred vision

Contraindications: Hypersensitivity, asthma, severe renal disease, severe hepatic disease

Precautions: Pregnancy (C), lactation, children, bleeding disorders, GI disorders, cardiac disorders, hypersensitivity to other antiinflammatory agents

Pharmacokinetics:
PO: Peak 2 hr, half-life 3-3½ hr; metabolized in liver, excreted in urine (metabolites), excreted in breast milk, extensive protein binding

Interactions/incompatibilities:
- Increased action of: coumarin, phenytoin, sulfonamides

NURSING CONSIDERATIONS

Assess:
- Renal, liver, blood studies: BUN,

M

creatinine, AST, ALT, Hgb before treatment, periodically thereafter
• Audiometric, ophthalmic exam before, during, after treatment
Administer:
• With food to decrease GI symptoms; take on empty stomach to facilitate absorption
Perform/provide:
• Storage at room temperature
Evaluate:
• Therapeutic response: decreased pain, stiffness, swelling in joints, ability to move more easily
• For eye, ear problems: blurred vision, tinnitus (may indicate toxicity)
Teach patient/family:
• To report blurred vision, or ringing, roaring in ears (may indicate toxicity)
• To avoid driving or other hazardous activities if dizziness or drowsiness occurs
• To report change in urine pattern, weight increase, edema, pain increase in joints, fever, blood in urine (indicates nephrotoxicity)
• That therapeutic effects may take up to 1 mo
• To report diarrhea or skin rash: drug may be discontinued
• To take with full glass of water

---

mefloquine HCl

(me-flow′quine)
Lariam
Func. class.: Antimalarial
Chem. class.: Analog of quinine

Action: Exact mechanism not known; blood schizonticide
Uses: Treatment and prevention of *Plasmodium falciparum* malaria, *P. vivax*
Dosage and routes:
• *Adult:* PO 1250 mg as a single dose (treatment); 250 mg qwk × 4 wk, then 250 mg q other wk (prevention)
Available forms include: Tabs 250 mg
Side effects/adverse reactions:
CV: Bradycardia, extrasystole
CNS: Dizziness, headache, syncope, *neuropsychiatric disturbances: disorientation, hallucinations,* ***coma, convulsions***
GI: Nausea, vomiting, loss of appetite, diarrhea, abdominal pain
INTEG: Itching, rash
MISC: Myalgia
Contraindications: Hypersensitivity, pregnancy (C)
Precautions: Cardiac dysrhythmias, neurologic disease, lactation, children
Pharmacokinetics:
Protein binding 98%, excreted in breast milk and urine, half-life 21 days (adults)
Interactions/incompatibilities:
• Increased ECG abnormalities, possible cardiac arrest: β-blockers, quinine, quinidine
• Increased potential for convulsions: chloroquine, valproic acids

NURSING CONSIDERATIONS

Assess:
• B/P, pulse, watch for bradycardia
• Neuropsychiatric symptoms: disorientation, hallucinations; drug should be discontinued
• Liver studies weekly: ALT, AST, bilirubin
Administer:
• On empty stomach with at least 8 oz of water
Perform/provide:
• Storage in tight, light-resistant container
Evaluate:
• Therapeutic response: decreased symptoms of malaria

---

* Available in Canada only

Teach patient/family:
- To take drug on an empty stomach with full glass of water

---

megestrol acetate

(me-jess'trole)

Megace, Pallace

Func. class.: Antineoplastic
Chem. class.: Hormone, progestin

Action: Affects endometrium by antiluteinizing effect; this is thought to bring about cell death

Uses: Breast, endometrial cancer, renal cell cancer

Dosage and routes:
- *Adult:* PO 40-320 mg/day in divided doses

Available forms include: Tabs 20, 40 mg

Side effects/adverse reactions:

GI: Nausea, vomiting, anorexia, diarrhea, abdominal cramps

GU: Gynecomastia, fluid retention, ***hypercalcemia***

CV: ***Thrombophlebitis***

INTEG: Alopecia, rash, pruritus, purpura, itching

CNS: Mood swings

Contraindications: Hypersensitivity, pregnancy (X)

Pharmacokinetics:

PO: Duration 1-3 days, half-life 60 min, metabolized in liver, excreted in feces, breast milk

NURSING CONSIDERATIONS

Assess:
- I&O ratio; weights
- Serum Ca levels
- Homan's sign

Administer:
- Antispasmodic
- Diuretics for increased fluids

Perform/provide:
- Increase fluid intake to 2-3 L/day to prevent dehydration and maintain normal Ca
- Nutritious diet with iron, vitamin supplements as ordered
- Limitation of calcium (dairy products)
- Storage in tight container at room temperature

Evaluate:
- Therapeutic response: decreased tumor size, spread of malignancy
- Food preferences; list likes, dislikes
- Effects of alopecia on body image; discuss feelings about body changes
- Symptoms indicating severe allergic reaction: rash, pruritus, urticaria, purpuric skin lesions, itching, flushing
- Frequency of stools, characteristics: cramping, acidosis, signs of dehydration (rapid respirations, poor skin turgor, decreased urine output, dry skin, restlessness, weakness)
- Mood swings
- Anorexia, nausea, vomiting, constipation, weakness, loss of muscle tone

Teach patient/family:
- To report any complaints or side effects to nurse or physician
- That gynecomastia can occur; reversible after discontinuing treatment
- To recognize and report signs of fluid retention, thromboemboli, hepatotoxicity

Lab test interferences:

Increase: Alk phosphatase, urinary nitrogen, urinary pregnanediol, plasma amino acids

False positive: Urine glucose

Decrease: HDL, glucose tolerance test

M

melphalan

(mel'fa-lan)

Alkeran

Func. class.: Antineoplastic alkylating agent

Chem. class.: Nitrogen mustard

Action: Responsible for cross-linking DNA strands leading to cell death

Uses: Multiple myeloma, breast cancer, reticulum cell sarcoma, testicular seminoma, malignant melanoma, advanced ovarian cancer

Dosage and routes:

• *Adult:* PO 6 mg qd × 2-3 wk, stop drug for 4 wk or until WBC level begins to rise; do not administer if WBC <3000/mm^3 or platelets <100,000/mm^3; may be given 0.15 mg/kg/day × 7 days; wait until platelets and WBCs rise, then 0.05 mg/kg/day

Available forms include: Tabs 2 mg

Side effects/adverse reactions:

HEMA: ***Thrombocytopenia, neutropenia, myelosuppression,*** anemia

GI: Nausea, vomiting, stomatitis

GU: Amenorrhea, hyperuricemia

INTEG: Rash, urticaria

RESP: ***Fibrosis, dysplasia***

Contraindications: Lactation, pregnancy (D)

Precautions: Radiation therapy, bone marrow depression

Pharmacokinetics:

Metabolized in liver, excreted in urine, half-life 1½ hr

Interactions/incompatibilities:

• Increased toxicity: antineoplastics, radiation

NURSING CONSIDERATIONS

Assess:

• CBC, differential, platelet count weekly; withhold drug if WBC is <4000 or platelet count is <75,000; notify physician of results

• Renal function studies: BUN, serum uric acid, urine CrCl before, during therapy

• I&O ratio; report fall in urine output of 30 ml/hr

• Monitor temperature q4h (may indicate beginning infection), no rectal temperatures

• Liver function tests before, during therapy (bilirubin, AST, ALT, LDH) as needed or monthly

Administer:

• Antiemetic 30-60 min before giving drug to prevent vomiting

• Antibiotics for prophylaxis of infection

• Topical or systemic analgesics for pain

• Local or systemic drugs for infection

Perform/provide:

• Storage in tight, light-resistant container

• Strict medical asepsis, protective isolation if WBC levels are low

• Special skin care

• Increase fluid intake to 2-3 L/day to prevent urate deposits, calculi formation

• Diet low in purines: organ meats (kidney, liver), dried beans, peas to maintain alkaline urine

• Rinsing of mouth tid-qid with water, club soda; brushing of teeth bid-tid with soft brush or cotton-tipped applicators for stomatitis; use unwaxed dental floss

• Warm compresses at injection site for inflammation

Evaluate:

• Therapeutic response: decreased tumor size, spread of malignancy

• Bleeding: hematuria, guaiac, bruising or petechiae, mucosa or orifices q8h

• Food preferences; list likes, dislikes
• Yellowing of skin, sclera, dark urine, clay-colored stools, itchy skin, abdominal pain, fever, diarrhea
• Inflammation of mucosa, breaks in skin
• Buccal cavity q8h for dryness, sores, ulceration, white patches, oral pain, bleeding, dysphagia
• Local irritation, pain, burning, discoloration at injection site
• Symptoms indicating severe allergic reaction: rash, pruritus, urticaria, purpuric skin lesions, itching, flushing

Teach patient/family:
• Of protective isolation precautions
• That sterility, amenorrhea can occur; reversible after discontinuing treatment
• To avoid foods with citric acid, hot or rough texture
• To report any bleeding, white spots, or ulcerations in mouth to physician; tell patient to examine mouth qd
• To report signs of infection: increased temperature, sore throat, flu symptoms
• To report signs of anemia: fatigue, headache, faintness, shortness of breath, irritability
• To avoid use of razors or commercial mouthwash
• To avoid use of aspirin products or ibuprofen

menadione/menadiol sodium diphosphate (vitamin K_3)

(men-a-dye'one)
Synkavite,* Synkayvite
Func. class.: Vitamin, fat soluble

Action: Needed for adequate blood clotting (factors II, VII, IX, X)
Uses: Vitamin K malabsorption, hypoprothrombinemia
Dosage and routes:
• *Adult:* PO 2-10 mg (menadione)
• *Adult:* PO/IM 5-15 mg (menadiol sodium diphosphate)
Available forms include: Tabs 5 mg; inj 5, 10, 37.5 mg/ml
Side effects/adverse reactions:
CNS: Headache, ***brain damage*** (large doses)
GI: Nausea, decreased liver function tests
HEMA: ***Hemolytic anemia, hemoglobinuria, hyperbilirubinemia***
INTEG: Rash, urticaria
Contraindications: Hypersensitivity, severe hepatic disease, last few weeks of pregnancy (X)
Precautions: Neonates
Pharmacokinetics: Metabolized, crosses placenta
Interactions/incompatibilities:
• Decreased action of menadione: oral antibiotics, cholestyramine, mineral oil
• Decreased action of: oral anticoagulants

NURSING CONSIDERATIONS

Assess:
• Pro-time during treatment (2 sec deviation from control time, bleeding time, and clotting time)
Administer:
• Deep IM, IV slowly over 7 min
Evaluate:
• Therapeutic response: decreased bleeding tendencies, decreased pro-time, decreased clotting time
• Nutritional status: liver (beef), spinach, tomatoes, coffee, asparagus, broccoli, cabbage, lettuce, greens
Teach patient/family:
• Not to take other supplements, unless directed by physician

M

- Necessary foods to be included in diet
- To avoid use of mineral oil

menotropins

(men-oh-troe'pin)

Pergonal

Func. class.: Gonadotropin

Chem. class.: Exogenous gonadotropin

Action: In women, increases follicular growth, maturation; in men, when given with HCG, stimulates spermatogenesis

Uses: Infertility, anovulation

Dosage and routes:

Infertility

- *Adult (men):* IM 1 amp 3 × wk with HCG 2000 U 2 × wk × 4 mo
- *Adult (women):* IM 75 IU of FSH, LH qd × 9-12 days, then 10,000 U HCG 1 day after these drugs; repeat × 2 menstrual cycles, then increase to 150 IU of FSH, LH qd × 9-12 days, then 10,000 U HCG 1 day after these drugs × 2 menstrual cycles

Anovulation

- *Adult (women):* IM 75 IU FSH, LH qd × 9-12 days, then 10,000 U HCG 1 day after last dose of these drugs; repeat × 1-3 menstrual cycles

Available forms include: Powder for inj 17 IU/amp

Side effects/adverse reactions:

CNS: Fever

CV: Hypovolemia

GI: Nausea, vomiting, diarrhea, anorexia

GU: Ovarian enlargement, abdominal distention/pain, multiple births, ovarian hyperstimulation: sudden ovarian enlargement, ascites with or without pain, pleural effusion

HEMA: ***Hemoperitoneum***

Contraindications: Primary anovulation, thyroid/adrenal dysfunction, organic intracranial lesion, ovarian cysts, primary testicular failure

Precautions: Pregnancy (C)

NURSING CONSIDERATIONS

Assess:

- Weight qd; notify physician if weight gain increases rapidly
- Estrogen excretion level; if >100 μg/24 hr, drug is withheld, hyperstimulation syndrome may occur
- I&O ratio; be alert for decreasing urinary output

Administer:

- After reconstituting with 1-2 ml sterile saline injection; use immediately

Evaluate:

- Therapeutic response: ovulation, pregnancy
- Ovarian enlargement, abdominal distention/pain; report symptoms immediately

Teach patient/family:

- That multiple births are possible. If pregnancy occurs, it usually occurs in 4-6 wk after start of treatment
- To keep appointment during treatment qd × 2 wk
- That daily intercourse is necessary from day preceding administration of gonadotropin until ovulation occurs

mepenzolate bromide

(me-pen'zoe'late)

Cantil

Func. class.: Gastrointestinal anticholinergic

Chem. class.: Synthetic quaternary ammonium antimuscarinic

Action: Inhibits muscarinic actions

of acetylcholine at postganglionic parasympathetic neuroeffector sites
Uses: Treatment of peptic ulcer disease, irritable bowel syndrome in combination with other drugs; for other GI disorders
Dosage and routes:
• *Adult:* PO 25-50 mg qid with meals, hs, titrate to patient response
Available forms include: Tabs 25 mg
Side effects/adverse reactions:
CNS: Confusion, stimulation in elderly, headache, insomnia, dizziness, drowsiness, anxiety, weakness, hallucination
GI: Dry mouth, constipation, ***paralytic ileus,*** heartburn, nausea, vomiting, dysphagia, absence of taste
GU: Hesitancy, retention, impotence
CV: Palpitations, tachycardia
EENT: Blurred vision, photophobia, mydriasis, cycloplegia, increased ocular tension
INTEG: Urticaria, rash, pruritus, anhidrosis, fever, allergic reactions
Contraindications: Hypersensitivity to anticholinergics, narrow-angle glaucoma, GI obstruction, myasthenia gravis, paralytic ileus, GI atony, toxic megacolon
Precautions: Hyperthyroidism, coronary artery disease, dysrhythmias, CHF, ulcerative colitis, hypertension, hiatal hernia, hepatic disease, renal disease, pregnancy (C), elderly, urinary retention, prostatic hypertrophy
Pharmacokinetics:
PO: Onset 1 hr, duration 3-4 hr; metabolized by liver, excreted in urine
Interactions/incompatibilities:
• Increased anticholinergic effect: amantadine, tricyclic antidepressants, MAOIs
• Decreased effect of: phenothiazines, levodopa, ketoconazole

NURSING CONSIDERATIONS

Assess:
• VS, cardiac status: checking for dysrhythmias, increased rate, palpitations
• I&O ratio; check for urinary retention or hesitancy
Administer:
• ½-1 hr ac for better absorption
• Decreased dose to elderly patients; their metabolism may be slowed
• Gum, hard candy, frequent rinsing of mouth for dryness of oral cavity
Perform/provide:
• Storage in tight container protected from light
• Increased fluids, bulk, exercise to patient's lifestyle to decrease constipation
Evaluate:
• Therapeutic response: absence of epigastric pain, bleeding, nausea, vomiting
• GI complaints: pain, bleeding (frank or occult), nausea, vomiting, anorexia
Teach patient/family:
• Avoid driving or other hazardous activities until stabilized on medication
• Avoid alcohol or other CNS depressants; will enhance sedating properties of this drug
• To avoid hot environments, stroke may occur, drug suppresses perspiration
• Use sunglasses when outside to prevent photophobia, may cause blurred vision
• To drink plenty of fluids
• To report dysphagia

meperidine HCl

(me-per'i-deen)

Demerol

Func. class.: Narcotic analgesic
Chem. class.: Opiate, phenylpiperidine derivative

Controlled Substance Schedule II

Action: Depresses pain impulse transmission at the spinal cord level by interacting with opioid receptors

Uses: Moderate to severe pain, preoperatively

Dosage and routes:

Pain

• *Adult:* PO/SC/IM 50-150 mg q3-4h prn, dose should be decreased if given IV

• *Child:* PO/SC/IM 1 mg/kg q4-6h prn, not to exceed 100 mg q4h

Preoperatively

• *Adult:* IM/SC 50-100 mg q30-90 min before surgery, dose should be reduced if given IV

• *Child:* IM/SC 1-2.2 mg/kg 30-90 min before surgery

Available forms include: Inj SC, IM, IV 25, 50, 75, 100 mg/ml; tabs 50, 100 mg; syr 50 mg/5 ml

Side effects/adverse reactions:

CNS: Drowsiness, dizziness, confusion, headache, sedation, euphoria, ***increased intracranial pressure***

GI: Nausea, vomiting, anorexia, constipation, cramps

GU: Increased urinary output, dysuria, urinary retention

INTEG: Rash, urticaria, bruising, flushing, diaphoresis, pruritus

EENT: Tinnitus, blurred vision, miosis, diplopia, depressed corneal reflex

CV: Palpitations, bradycardia, change in B/P, tachycardia (IV)

RESP: ***Respiratory depression***

Contraindications: Hypersensitivity, addiction (narcotic)

Precautions: Addictive personality, pregnancy (B), lactation, increased intracranial pressure, MI (acute), severe heart disease, respiratory depression, hepatic disease, renal disease, child <18 yr

Pharmacokinetics:

PO: Onset 15 min, peak 1 hr, duration 4-5 hr

SC/IM: Onset 10 min, peak 1 hr, duration 2-4 hr

IV: Onset 5 min, duration 2 hr

Metabolized by liver (to active/inactive metabolites), excreted by kidneys, crosses placenta, excreted in breast milk, half-life 3-4 hr; a toxic by-product can result from regular use

Interactions/incompatibilities:

• Increased effects with other CNS depressants: alcohol, narcotics, sedative/hypnotics, antipsychotics, skeletal muscle relaxants, MAO inhibitors, chlorpromazine

NURSING CONSIDERATIONS

Assess:

• I&O ratio; check for decreasing output; may indicate urinary retention

• Need for drug

Administer:

• IV after diluting with 5 ml or more sterile H_2O or NS, give directly over 4-5 min; may be further diluted in solutions to 1 mg/ml during anesthesia

• With antiemetic if nausea, vomiting occur

• When pain is beginning to return; determine dosage interval by patient response

Perform/provide:

• Storage in light-resistant area at room temperature

• Assistance with ambulation

* Available in Canada only

• Safety measures: siderails, night light, call bell within easy reach

Evaluate:

• Therapeutic response: decrease in pain

• CNS changes: dizziness, drowsiness, hallucinations, euphoria, LOC, pupil reaction

• Allergic reactions: rash, urticaria

• Respiratory dysfunction: respiratory depression, character, rate, rhythm; notify physician if respirations are <12/min

• Need for pain medication, physical dependence

Teach patient/family:

• To report any symptoms of CNS changes, allergic reactions

• That physical dependency may result when used for extended periods of time

• Withdrawal symptoms may occur: nausea, vomiting, cramps, fever, faintness, anorexia

Lab test interferences:

Increase: Amylase

Treatment of overdose: Narcan 0.2-0.8 IV, O_2, IV fluids, vasopressors

mephentermine sulfate

(me-fen'ter-meen)

Wyamine

Func. class.: Adrenergic, direct and indirect acting

Chem. class.: Substituted phenylethylamine

Action: Causes increased contractility and heart rate by acting on β-receptors in heart; also, acts on α-receptors, causing vasoconstriction in blood vessels, cardiac output is elevated and systolic and diastolic pressures are increased

Uses: Shock and hypotension following variety of procedures

Dosage and routes:

Hypotension

• *Adult:* IV 15-45 mg depending on procedure

Hypotension/shock

• *Adult:* IV 0.5 mg/kg

• *Child:* IV 0.4 mg/kg

Available forms include: Inj IV 15, 30 mg/ml

Side effects/adverse reactions:

CV: Palpitations, tachycardia, hypertension

CNS: Tremors, drowsiness, confusion, incoherence

Contraindications: Hypersensitivity to sympathomimetics

Precautions: Pregnancy (B), cardiac disorders, hyperthyroidism, diabetes mellitus, prostatic hypertrophy

Pharmacokinetics:

IV: Onset immediate, duration ½-1 hr; metabolized in liver, excreted in urine

Interactions/incompatibilities:

• Do not use with MAOIs or tricyclic antidepressants; hypertensive crisis may occur

• Decreased effect of mephentermine: methyldopa, urinary acidifiers, rauwolfia alkaloids

• Increased effect of mephentermine: urinary alkalizers

• Dysrhythmias: halothane, cyclopropaine, digitalis

NURSING CONSIDERATIONS

Assess:

• I&O ratio; notify MD if output is < 30 cc/hr

• ECG during administration continuously; if B/P increases, drug is decreased

• B/P, pulse q5min after parenteral route

• CVP or PWP during infusion if possible

Administer:

• Plasma expanders for hypovolemia

• IV undiluted 30 mg or less/1 min, or diluted 600 mg/500 ml D_5W, titrate to patient response, check site for extravasation; use an infusion pump

Perform/provide:

• Storage of reconstituted solution if refrigerated for no longer than 24 hr

• Do not use discolored solutions

Evaluate:

• Therapeutic response: increased B/P with stabilization

Teach patient/family:

• Reason for drug administration

---

mephenytoin

(me-fen′i-toyn)

Mesantoin

Func. class.: Anticonvulsant
Chem. class.: Hydantoin derivative

Action: Reduces electrical discharges in motor cortex, reducing seizures; increases AV conduction velocity, prolongs refractory period

Uses: Generalized tonic-clonic, complex-partial seizures

Dosage and routes:

• *Adult:* PO 50-100 mg/day, may increase by 50-100 mg q7d, up to 200 mg tid

• *Child:* PO 50-100 mg/day or 100-450 mg/m^2/day in 3 divided doses, initially; then increase 50-100 mg q7d, up to 200 mg tid in divided doses q8h

Available forms include: Tabs 100 mg

Side effects/adverse reactions:

HEMA: ***Agranulocytosis, leukopenia, neutropenia, pancytopenia, eosinophilia, lymphadenopathy***

CNS: Drowsiness, dizziness, fatigue, irritability, tremors, insomnia, depression

GI: Nausea, vomiting

INTEG: Rash, exfoliative dermatitis

EENT: Photophobia, conjunctivitis, nystagmus, diplopia

RESP: ***Pulmonary fibrosis***

Contraindications: Hypersensitivity to hydantoins, sinus bradycardia, heart block, Adams-Stokes syndrome

Precautions: Alcoholism, hepatic disease, renal disease, blood dyscrasias, CHF, elderly, pregnancy (C), respiratory depression, diabetes mellitus

Pharmacokinetics:

PO: Onset 30 min, duration 24-48 hr, metabolized by liver, excreted by kidneys, half-life 144 hr

Interactions/incompatibilities:

• Decreased effects: rifampin, chronic alcohol use, barbiturates, antihistamines, antacids, other anticonvulsants antineoplastics, calcium products, folic acid, oxacillin

• Increased effects: benzodiazepines, cimetidine, salicylates, sulfonamide, pyrazolones, phenothiazines, estrogens, disulfiram, chloramphenicol, anticoagulants

• Seizures: valproic acid

• Myocardial depression: lidocaine, propanolol, sympathomimetics

NURSING CONSIDERATIONS

Assess:

• Blood studies: CBC, platelets q2 wk until stabilized, then qmo × 12, then q3mo; discontinue drug if neutrophils are $<1600/mm^3$, liver function tests with long-term use

• Drug level: therapeutic level 25-40 μg/ml

Evaluate:

• Therapeutic response: decreased seizure activity

• Mental status: mood, sensorium, affect, behavioral changes; if mental status changes, notify physician

---

• Eye problems: need for ophthalmic examinations before, during, after treatment (slit lamp, fundoscopy, tonometry)
• Allergic reaction: red raised rash; if this occurs, drug should be discontinued
• Blood dyscrasias: fever, sore throat, bruising, rash, jaundice
• Toxicity: bone marrow depression, nausea, vomiting, ataxia, diplopia, cardiovascular collapse, Stevens-Johnson syndrome

Teach patient/family:
• Not to discontinue drug quickly; should be tapered
• To avoid activities that require alertness if drowsiness or dizziness occur
• That use of alcohol may decrease effects of drug

mephobarbital

(me-foe-bar'bi-tal)
Mebaral, Mentabal, Mephoral
Func. class.: Anticonvulsant
Chem. class.: Barbiturate

Controlled Substance Schedule IV
Action: Depresses sensory cortex, motor activity; inhibits ascending conduction in reticular formation of thalamus
Uses: Generalized tonic-clonic (grand mal), absence (petit mal) seizures
Dosage and routes:
• *Adult:* PO 400-600 mg/day or in divided doses
• *Child:* PO 6-12 mg/kg/day in divided doses q6-8h
Available forms include: Tabs 32, 50, 100, 200 mg
Side effects/adverse reactions:
HEMA: ***Thrombocytopenia, agranulocytosis, megaloblastic anemia***
CNS: Dizziness, headache, hangover, paradoxic stimulation, drowsiness, increased pain
GI: Nausea, vomiting, epigastric pain
INTEG: Rash, urticaria, purpura, erythema multiforme, facial edema
EENT: Tinnitus, hearing loss
CV: Hypotension, bradycardia
RESP: Wheezing, hyperpnea
ENDO: Hypoglycemia, hyponatremia, hypokalemia
Contraindications: Hypersensitivity to barbiturates, pregnancy (D)
Precautions: Hepatic disease, renal disease, lactation, alcoholism, drug abuse, hyperthyroidism
Pharmacokinetics:
PO: Onset 20-60 min, duration 6-8 hr
REC: Onset slow, duration 4-6 hr; metabolized by liver, excreted by kidneys, half-life 34 hr
Interactions/incompatibilities:
• Increased effects: CNS depressants, chloramphenicol, valproic acid, disulfiram, nondepolarizing skeletal muscle relaxants, sulfonamides
• Increased orthostatic hypotension: furosemide

NURSING CONSIDERATIONS

Assess:
• Drug level, CBC, BUN, creatinine
Perform/provide:
• Storage in light-resistant container
Evaluate:
• Therapeutic response: decreased seizure activity
• Mental status: mood, sensorium, affect, memory (long, short)
• Respiratory depression: respiration <10/min, shallow
• Blood dyscrasias: fever, sore throat, bruising, rash, jaundice

M

Teach patient/family:

• Never to withdraw drug abruptly; notify physician if side effects occur

• To avoid hazardous activities until stabilized on drug

• That dreaming may increase when drug is discontinued

Treatment of overdose: Administer calcium gluconate IV

mepivacaine HCl

(meep-ee-va-kane)

Carbocaine, Cavacaine, Isocaine

Func. class.: Local anesthetic
Chem. class.: Amide

Action: Competes with calcium for sites in nerve membrane that control sodium transport across cell membrane; decreases rise of depolarization phase of action potential

Uses: Nerve block, caudal anesthesia, epidural, pain relief, paracervical block, transvaginal block or infiltration

Dosage and routes:

Varies depending on route of anesthesia

Available forms include: Inj 1%, 1.5%, 2%, 3%

Side effects/adverse reactions:

CNS: Anxiety, restlessness, ***convulsions, loss of consciousness,*** drowsiness, disorientation, tremors, shivering

CV: ***Myocardial depression, cardiac arrest, dysrhythmias,*** bradycardia, hypotension, hypertension, fetal bradycardia

GI: Nausea, vomiting

EENT: Blurred vision, tinnitus, pupil constriction

INTEG: Rash, urticaria, allergic reactions, edema, burning, skin discoloration at injection site, tissue necrosis

RESP: ***Status asthmaticus, respiratory arrest, anaphylaxis***

Contraindications: Hypersensitivity, child <12 yr, elderly, severe liver disease

Precautions: Elderly, severe drug allergies, pregnancy (C)

Pharmacokinetics:

Onset 15 min, duration 3 hr; metabolized by liver, excreted in urine (metabolites)

Interactions/incompatibilities:

• Dysrhythmias: epinephrine, halothane, enflurane

• Hypertension: MAOIs, tricyclic antidepressants, phenothiazines

• Decreased action of mepivacaine: chloroprocaine

NURSING CONSIDERATIONS

Assess:

• B/P, pulse, respiration during treatment

• Fetal heart tones if drug is used during labor

Administer:

• Only with crash cart, resuscitative equipment nearby

• Only drugs without preservatives for epidural or caudal anesthesia

Perform/provide:

• Use of new solution, discard unused portions

Evaluate:

• Therapeutic response: anesthesia necessary for procedure

• Allergic reactions: rash, urticaria, itching

• Cardiac status: ECG for dysrhythmias, pulse, B/P during anesthesia

Treatment of overdose: Airway, O_2, vasopressor, IV fluids, anticonvulsants for seizures

meprobamate

(me-proe-ba'mate)

Arcoban, Equanil, Kalmm, Meditran,* Meprocon, Meprotabs, Meribam, Miltown, Neo-Tran,* Novomepro,* Saronil, Tranmep

Func. class.: Sedative/hypnotic
Chem. class.: Propanediol carbamate derivative

Controlled Substance Schedule IV

Action: Blocks impulses from cortex to thalamus in CNS

Uses: Anxiety

Dosage and routes:

- *Adult:* PO 1.2-1.6 g in 2-3 divided doses, not to exceed 2.4 g/day
- *Child 6-12 yr:* PO 100-200 mg bid-tid

Available forms include: Tabs 200, 400, 600 mg; caps 400 mg sust rel caps 200, 400 mg

Side effects/adverse reactions:

HEMA: ***Thrombocytopenia, leukopenia, eosinophilia***

CNS: Dizziness, drowsiness, headache, ***convulsions***

GI: Nausea, vomiting, anorexia, diarrhea, stomatitis

INTEG: Urticaria, pruritus, maculopapular rash

CV: Hypotension, tachycardia, palpitations, ***hyperthermia***

EENT: Blurred vision, tinnitus, mydriasis, slurred speech

Contraindications: Hypersensitivity, renal failure, porphyria, pregnancy (D), history of drug abuse or dependence

Precautions: Suicidal patients, severe depression, renal disease, hepatic disease, elderly

Pharmacokinetics:

PO: Onset 1 hr, metabolized by liver, excreted by kidneys, in feces, crosses placenta, breast milk, half-life 6-16 hr

Interactions/incompatibilities:

- Increased effects of meprobamate: CNS depressants, alcohol, tricyclic antidepressants

NURSING CONSIDERATIONS

Assess:

- B/P (lying, standing), pulse; if systolic B/P drops 20 mm Hg, hold drug, notify physician; respirations q5-15min if given IV
- Blood studies: CBC during long-term therapy, blood dyscrasias have occurred rarely
- Hepatic studies: AST, ALT, bilirubin, creatinine, LDH, alk phosphatase

Administer:

- With food or milk for GI symptoms
- Crushed tabs if patient is unable to swallow medication whole
- Sugarless gum, hard candy, frequent sips of water for dry mouth

Perform/provide

- Assistance with ambulation during beginning therapy since drowsiness/dizziness occurs
- Safety measures, including siderails
- Check to see PO medication has been swallowed

Evaluate:

- Therapeutic response: decreased anxiety, restlessness, insomnia
- Mental status: mood, sensorium, affect, sleeping pattern, drowsiness, dizziness
- Physical dependency, withdrawal symptoms: headache, nausea, vomiting, muscle pain, weakness, hyperthermia, death, convulsions after long-term use
- Suicidal tendencies

Teach patient/family:

- That drug may be taken with food

• Not to be used for everyday stress or used longer than 4 months, unless directed by physician, not to take more than prescribed amount, may be habit forming
• To avoid OTC preparations (alcohol, cold, hay fever) unless approved by physician
• To avoid driving, activities that require alertness, since drowsiness may occur
• To avoid alcohol ingestion or other psychotropic medications, unless prescribed by physician
• Not to discontinue medication abruptly after long-term use
• To rise slowly or fainting may occur, especially elderly
• That drowsiness might worsen at beginning of treatment

Lab test interferences:
False increase: 17-OHCS
False positive: Phentolamine test

Treatment of overdose: Lavage, VS, supportive care

mercaptopurine (6-MP)

(mer-kap-toe-pyoor'een)
Purinethol

Func. class.: Antineoplastic-antimetabolite
Chem. class.: Purine analog

Action: Inhibits purine metabolism at multiple sites, which inhibits DNA and RNA synthesis

Uses: Chronic myelocytic leukemia, acute lymphoblastic leukemia in children, acute myelogenous leukemia

Dosage and routes:
• *Adult and child:* PO 2.5 mg/kg/day, not to exceed 5 mg/kg/day; maintenance 1.5-2.5 mg/kg/day
• *Child:* 70 mg/m²/day

Available forms include: Tabs 50 mg

Side effects/adverse reactions:
CNS: Fever, headache, weakness
HEMA: ***Thrombocytopenia, leukopenia, myelosuppression, anemia***
GI: Nausea, vomiting, anorexia, diarrhea, stomatitis, ***hepatotoxicity*** (with high doses), jaundice, gastritis
GU: ***Renal failure,*** hyperuricemia, ***oliguria,*** crystalluria, ***hematuria***
INTEG: Rash, dry skin, urticaria

Contraindications: Patients with prior drug resistance, leukopenia (<2500/mm³), thrombocytopenia (<100,000/mm³), anemia, pregnancy (D)

Precautions: Renal disease

Pharmacokinetics: Incompletely absorbed when taken orally, metabolized in liver, excreted in urine

Interactions/incompatibilities:
• Increased toxicity: radiation or other antineoplastics
• Increased bone marrow depression: allopurinol
• Reversal of neuromuscular blockade: nondepolarizing muscle relaxants

NURSING CONSIDERATIONS

Assess:
• CBC, differential, platelet count weekly; withhold drug if WBC is <3500 or platelet count is <100,000; notify physician of these results; drug should be discontinued
• Renal function studies: BUN, serum uric acid, urine CrCl, electrolytes before, during therapy
• I&O ratio; report fall in urine output to <30 ml/hr
• Monitor temperature q4h; fever may indicate beginning infection; no rectal temperatures
• Liver function tests before, during therapy: bilirubin, alk phosphatase, AST, ALT, qwk during beginning therapy

Administer:
- Antacid before oral agent; give drug after evening meal before bedtime
- Allopurinol or sodium bicarbonate to maintain uric acid levels, alkalinization of urine
- Antibiotics for prophylaxis of infection
- Topical or systemic analgesics for pain
- Transfusion for anemia

Perform/provide:
- Strict medical asepsis, protective isolation if WBC levels are low
- Increase fluid intake to 2-3 L/day to prevent urate deposits, calculi formation, unless contraindicated
- Diet low in purines: absence of organ meats (kidney, liver), dried beans, peas to maintain alkaline urine
- Rinsing of mouth tid-qid with water, club soda; brushing of teeth bid-tid with soft brush or cotton-tipped applicators for stomatitis; use unwaxed dental floss
- Nutritious diet with iron, vitamin supplements as ordered
- Storage in tightly closed container in cool environment

Evaluate:
- Therapeutic response: decreased size of tumor, spread of malignancy
- Bleeding: hematuria, guaiac, bruising, petechiae, mucosa or orifices q8h
- Food preferences; list likes, dislikes
- Inflammation of mucosa, breaks in skin
- Buccal cavity q8h for dryness, sores, ulceration, white patches, oral pain, bleeding, dysphagia
- Symptoms indicating severe allergic reaction: rash, urticaria, itching, flushing

Teach patient/family:
- To avoid foods with citric acid, hot or rough texture if stomatitis is present
- To report stomatitis: any bleeding, white spots, ulcerations in mouth; tell patient to examine mouth qd, report symptoms
- Contraceptive measures are recommended during therapy
- To drink 10-12 (8 oz) glasses of fluid/day
- Notify physician of fever, chills, sore throat, nausea, vomiting, anorexia, diarrhea, bleeding, bruising, which may indicate blood dyscrasias
- To report signs of infection: increased temperature, sore throat, flu symptoms
- To report signs of anemia: fatigue, headache, faintness, shortness of breath, irritability
- To report bleeding: avoid use of razors or commercial mouthwash
- To avoid use of aspirin products or ibuprofen

---

mesalamine

(mez-al'a-meen)

Rowasa

Func. class.: GI antiinflammatory
Chem. class.: 5-aminosalicylic acid

Action: May diminish inflammation by blocking cyclooxygenase, inhibiting prostaglandin production in colon

Uses: Mild to moderate active distal ulcerative colitis, proctosigmoiditis, proctitis

Dosage and routes:
- *Adult:* REC 60 ml (4 g) hs, retained for 8 hr × 3-6 wk

Available forms include: Rec susp 4 g/60 ml

Side effects/adverse reactions:
GI: Cramps, gas, nausea, diarrhea, rectal pain, constipation
CNS: Headache, fever, dizziness, insomnia, asthenia, weakness, fatigue
INTEG: Rash, itching, alopecia
SYST: Flu, malaise, back pain, peripheral edema, leg and joint pain, urinary tract infection
EENT: Sore throat
Contraindications: Hypersensitivity
Precautions: Renal disease, pregnancy (B), lactation, children, sulfite sensitivity
Pharmacokinetics:
REC: Primarily excreted in feces but some in urine as metabolite; half-life 1 hr, metabolite half-life 5-10 hr

NURSING CONSIDERATIONS

Assess:
- GI symptoms: cramps, gas, nausea, diarrhea, rectal pain; if severe the drug should be discontinued

Administer:
- Rectally only, drug should be given hs, retained until morning

Perform/provide:
- Storage at room temperature

Evaluate:
- Therapeutic response: absence of pain, bleeding from GI tract, decrease in number of diarrhea stools

Teach patient/family:
- That usual course of therapy is 3-6 wk
- To shake bottle well
- Method of rectal administration
- To inform physician of GI symptoms

mesoridazine besylate

(mez-oh-rid'a-zeen)
Serentil
Func. class.: Antipsychotic/neuroleptic
Chem. class.: Phenothiazine, piperidine

Action: Depresses cerebral cortex, hypothalamus, limbic system, which control activity, aggression; blocks neurotransmission produced by dopamine at synapse; exhibits strong α-adrenergic, anticholinergic blocking action; mechanism for antipsychotic effects is unclear
Uses: Psychotic disorders, schizophrenia, anxiety, alcoholism, behavioral problems in mental deficiency, chronic brain syndrome
Dosage and routes:
Schizophrenia
- *Adult:* PO 50 mg tid, optimum dose 100-400 mg/day; IM 25 mg may repeat ½-1 hr; dosage range 25-200 mg/day

Behavior problems
- *Adult:* PO 25 mg tid; optimum dose 75-300 mg/day;

Alcoholism
- *Adult:* PO 25 mg bid; optimum dose 50-200 mg/day

Schizoaffective disorders
- *Adult:* PO 10 mg tid; optimum dose 30-150 mg/day

Available forms include: Tabs 10, 25, 50, 100 mg; conc 25 mg/ml; inj IM 25 mg/ml
Side effects/adverse reactions:
RESP: ***Laryngospasm,*** dyspnea, ***respiratory depression***
CNS: Extrapyramidal symptoms: pseudoparkinsonism, akathisia, dystonia, tardive dyskinesia, drowsiness, headache,
HEMA: ***Anemia, leukopenia, leukocytosis, agranulocytosis***

* Available in Canada only

INTEG: Rash, photosensitivity, dermatitis
EENT: Blurred vision, glaucoma
GI: Dry mouth, nausea, vomiting, anorexia, constipation, diarrhea, jaundice, weight gain
GU: Urinary retention, urinary frequency, enuresis, impotence, amenorrhea, gynecomastia
CV: Orthostatic hypotension, hypertension, ***cardiac arrest,*** ECG changes, tachycardia
Contraindications: Hypersensitivity, circulatory collapse, liver damage, cerebral arteriosclerosis, coronary disease, severe hypertension/hypotension, blood dyscrasias, coma, brain damage, bone marrow depression, narrow-angle glaucoma
Precautions: Pregnancy (C), lactation, seizure disorders, hypertension, hepatic disease, cardiac disease, prostatic hypertrophy, intestinal obstruction, respiratory conditions
Pharmacokinetics:
PO: Onset erratic, peak 2 hr, duration 4-6 hr
IM: Onset 15-30 min, peak 30 min, duration 6-8 hr; metabolized by liver, excreted in urine, crosses placenta, enters breast milk
Interactions/incompatibilities:
• Oversedation: other CNS depressants, alcohol, barbiturate anesthetics
• Toxicity: epinephrine
• Decreased absorption: aluminum hydroxide or magnesium hydroxide antacids
• Decreased effects of: lithium, levodopa
• Increased effects of both drugs: β-adrenergic blockers, alcohol
• Increased anticholinergic effects: anticholinergics

NURSING CONSIDERATIONS
Assess:
• Mental status before initial administration
• Swallowing of PO medication; check for hoarding or giving of medication to other patients
• I&O ratio; palpate bladder if low urinary output occurs
• Bilirubin, CBC, liver function studies monthly
• Urinalysis is recommended before, during prolonged therapy
Administer:
• Antiparkinsonian agent, after securing order from physician to be used if extrapyramidal symptoms occur
• Concentrate mixed in distilled water, orange, grape juice; do not prepare, store bulk dilutions
• IM injection into large muscle mass; do not use if precipitate present
Perform/provide:
• Decreased noise input by dimming lights, avoiding loud noises
• Supervised ambulation until stabilized on medication; do not involve in strenuous exercise program because fainting is possible; patient should not stand still for long periods of time
• Increased fluids to prevent constipation
• Sips of water, candy, gum for dry mouth
• Storage in tight, light-resistant container
Evaluate:
• Therapeutic response: decrease in emotional excitement, hallucinations, delusions, paranoia, and reorganization of patterns of thought, speech
• Affect, orientation, LOC, reflexes, gait, coordination, sleep pattern disturbances

• B/P standing and lying; also include pulse and respirations; take these q4h during initial treatment; establish baseline before starting treatment; report drops of 30 mm Hg
• Dizziness, faintness, palpitations, tachycardia on rising
• Extrapyramidal symptoms including akathisia (inability to sit still, no pattern to movements), tardive dyskinesia (bizarre movements of jaw, mouth, tongue, extremities), pseudoparkinsonism (rigidity, tremors, pill rolling, shuffling gait)
• For neuroleptic malignant syndrome: hyperthermia, altered mental status, muscle rigidity, increased CPK
• Skin turgor daily
• Constipation, urinary retention daily; if these occur increase bulk, water in diet

Teach patient/family:
• That orthostatic hypotension occurs frequently, and to rise from sitting or lying position gradually; to avoid hazardous activities until stabilized on medication
• To remain lying down after IM injection for at least 30 min
• To avoid hot tubs, hot showers, or tub baths since hypotension may occur
• To avoid abrupt withdrawal of mesoridazine or extrapypramidal symptoms may result; drugs should be withdrawn slowly
• To avoid OTC preparations (cough, hayfever, cold) unless approved by physician since serious drug interactions may occur; to avoid use with alcohol or CNS depressants, increased drowsiness may occur
• To use sunscreen during sun exposure to prevent burns
• Regarding compliance with drug regimen
• About necessity for meticulous oral hygiene since oral candidiasis may occur
• To report sore throat, malaise, fever, bleeding, mouth sores; if these occur, a CBC should be drawn and drug discontinued
• That in hot weather heat stroke may occur; take extra precautions to stay cool

Lab test interferences:
Increase: Liver function tests, cardiac enzymes, cholesterol, blood glucose, prolactin, bilirubin, PBI, cholinesterase, ^{131}I
Decrease: Hormones (blood, urine)
False positive: Pregnancy tests, PKU
False negative: Urinary steroids, 17-OHCS

Treatment of overdose: Lavage if orally injested, provide an airway; *do not induce vomiting*

---

metaproterenol sulfate

(met-a-proe-ter'e-nole)
Alupent, Metaprel
Func. class.: Selective β_2-agonist

Action: Relaxes bronchial smooth muscle by direct action on β_2-adrenergic receptors

Uses: Bronchial asthma, bronchospasm

Dosage and routes:
• *Adult and child>12 yr:* INH 2-3 puffs, may repeat q 3-4h, not to exceed 12 puffs/day

Asthma/bronchospasm
• *Adult:* PO 20 mg q6-8h
• *Child >9 yr or >27 kg:* PO 20 mg q6-8h or 0.4-0.9 mg/kg/dose tid
• *Child 6-9 yr or <27 kg:* PO 10

* Available in Canada only

mg q6-8h or 0.4-0.9 mg/kg/dose tid
Available forms include: Tabs 10, 20 mg; aerosol 0.65 mg/dose; syrup 10 mg/5 ml; sol nebulizer 0.6%, 5%
Side effects/adverse reactions:
CNS: Tremors, anxiety, insomnia, headache, dizziness, stimulation
CV: Palpitations, tachycardia, hypertension, ***cardiac arrest***
GI: Nausea
RESP: Dyspnea
Contraindications: Hypersensitivity to sympathomimetics, narrow-angle glaucoma
Precautions: Pregnancy (C), cardiac disorders, hyperthyroidism, diabetes mellitus, prostatic hypertrophy
Pharmacokinetics:
PO: Onset 15-30 min, peak 1 hr, duration 4 hr, excreted in urine as metabolites
Interactions/incompatibilities:
• Increased effects of both drugs: other sympathomimetics
• Decreased action of: β-blockers

NURSING CONSIDERATIONS

Assess:
• Respiratory function: vital capacity, forced expiratory volume, ABGs
Administer:
• 2 hr before hs to avoid sleeplessness
Perform/provide:
• Storage at room temperature, do not use discolored solutions
Evaluate:
• Therapeutic response: absence of dyspnea, wheezing
• Tolerance over long-term therapy, dose may need to be increased or changed
Teach patient/family:
• Not to use OTC medications, extra stimulation may occur
• Use of inhaler, review package insert with patient
• To avoid getting aerosol in eyes
• To wash inhaler in warm water and dry qd
• On all aspects of drug; avoid smoking, smoke-filled rooms, persons with respiratory infections

---

methadone HCl

(meth'a-done)
Dolophine, Methadone HCl Oral Solution
Func. class.: Narcotic analgesics
Chem. class.: Opiate, synthetic diphenylheptane derivative

Controlled Substance Schedule II
Action: Depresses pain impulse transmission at the spinal cord level by interacting with opioid receptors
Uses: Severe pain, narcotic withdrawal
Dosage and routes:
Pain
• *Adult:* PO/SC/IM 2.5-10 mg q4-12h prn
Narcotic withdrawal
• *Adult:* PO 15-40 mg/day individualized initially, then 20-120 mg/day titrated to patient response
Available forms include: Inj SC, IM 10 mg/ml; tabs 5, 10 mg; oral sol 5, 10 mg/5 ml; dispersible tabs 40 mg
Side effects/adverse reactions:
CNS: Drowsiness, dizziness, confusion, headache, sedation, euphoria
GI: Nausea, vomiting, anorexia, constipation, cramps, biliary tract spasm
GU: Increased urinary output, dysuria, urinary retention
INTEG: Rash, urticaria, bruising, flushing, diaphoresis, pruritus

M

EENT: Tinnitus, blurred vision, miosis, diplopia
CV: Palpitations, bradycardia, change in B/P
RESP: ***Respiratory depression***
Contraindications: Hypersensitivity, addiction (narcotic)
Precautions: Addictive personality, pregnancy (B), lactation, increased intracranial pressure, MI (acute), severe heart disease, respiratory depression, hepatic disease, renal disease, child <18 yr
Pharmacokinetics:
PO: Onset 30-60 min, duration 6-8 hr, cumulative 22-48 hr
SC/IM: Onset 10-20 min, peak 1 hr, duration 6-8 hr, cumulative 22-48 hr
Metabolized by liver, excreted by kidneys, crosses placenta, excreted in breast milk, half-life 1-1½ days, 90% bound to plasma proteins
Interactions/incompatibilities:
• Increased effects with other CNS depressants: alcohol, narcotics, sedative/hypnotics, antipsychotics, skeletal muscle relaxants, rifampin, phenytoin

NURSING CONSIDERATIONS

Assess:
• I&O ratio; check for decreasing output; may indicate urinary retention
Administer:
• With antiemetic if nausea, vomiting occurs
• When pain is beginning to return; determine dosage interval by patient response
• Rotating injection sites
Perform/provide:
• Storage in light-resistant area at room temperature
• Assistance with ambulation
• Safety measures: siderails, night light, call bell within easy reach
Evaluate:
• Therapeutic response: decrease in pain
• CNS changes: dizziness, drowsiness, hallucinations, euphoria, LOC, pupil reaction
• Allergic reactions: rash, urticaria
• Respiratory dysfunction: respiratory depression, character, rate, rhythm; notify physician if respirations are <10/min
• Need for pain medication, physical dependence
Teach patient/family:
• To report any symptoms of CNS changes, allergic reactions
• That physical dependency may result when used for extended periods of time
• Withdrawal symptoms may occur: nausea, vomiting, cramps, fever, faintness, anorexia
Lab test interferences:
Increase: Amylase
Treatment of overdose: Narcan 0.2-0.8 IV, O_2, IV fluids, vasopressors

---

methamphetamine HCl

(meth-am-fet'a-meen)
Desoxyn Gradumey
Func. class.: Cerebral stimulants
Chem. class.: Amphetamine

Controlled Substance Schedule II
Action: Increases release of norepinephrine and dopamine in cerebral cortex to reticular activating system
Uses: Exogenous obesity, minimal brain dysfunction, attention deficit disorder with hyperactivity
Dosage and routes:
Attention deficit disorder
• *Child >6 yr:* 2.5-5 mg qd or bid increasing by 5 mg/wk
Obesity

• *Adult:* PO 2.5-5 mg, 30 min ac or 10-15 mg long-acting tab qd in AM

Available forms include: Tabs 5; tabs long-acting 5, 10, 15 mg

Side effects/adverse reactions:

CNS: Hyperactivity, insomnia, restlessness, talkativeness, dizziness, headache, chills, stimulation, dysphoria, irritability, aggressiveness, tremor

GI: Anorexia, dry mouth, diarrhea, constipation, weight loss, metallic taste, cramps

GU: Impotence, change in libido

CV: Palpitations, tachycardia, hypertension, decreased heart rate, dysrhythmia

INTEG: Urticaria

Contraindications: Hypersensitivity to sympathomimetic amines, hyperthyroidism, hypertension, glaucoma hypertrophy, severe arteriosclerosis, drug abuse, cardiovascular disease, anxiety

Precautions: Gilles de la Tourette's disorder, pregnancy (C), lactation, child <3 years

Pharmacokinetics:

PO: Duration 3-6 hr, metabolized by liver, excreted by kidneys, crosses blood-brain barrier

Interactions/incompatibilities:

• Hypertensive crisis: MAOIs or within 14 days of MAOIs

• Increased effect of methamphetamine: acetazolamide, antacids, sodium bicarbonate

• Decreased effects of methamphetamine: barbiturates, tricyclics, ascorbic acid, ammonium chloride

• Decreased effects of: guanethidine

NURSING CONSIDERATIONS

Assess:

• VS, B/P since this drug may reverse antihypertensives; check patients with cardiac disease more often

• CBC, urinalysis, in diabetes: blood sugar, urine sugar; insulin changes may need to be made since eating will decrease

• Height, growth rate in children; growth rate may be decreased

Administer:

• At least 6 hr before hs to avoid sleeplessness

• For obesity only if patient is on weight reduction program including dietary changes, exercise; patient will develop tolerance, loss of weight won't occur without additional methods give 2 hr before meals

• Gum, hard candy or frequent sips of water for dry mouth

Evaluate:

• Therapeutic response: decreased weight, decreased hyperactivity

• Mental status: mood, sensorium, affect, stimulation, insomnia, aggressiveness

• Physical dependency: should not be used for extended time; dose should be discontinued gradually, tolerance will occur after long-term use

• Withdrawal symptoms: headache, nausea, vomiting, muscle pain, weakness

Teach patient/family:

• To decrease caffeine consumption (coffee, tea, cola, chocolate), which may increase irritability, stimulation

• To avoid OTC preparations unless approved by physician

• To taper off drug over several weeks, or depression, increased sleeping, lethargy may ensue

• To avoid alcohol ingestion

• To avoid hazardous activities until patient is stabilized on medication

• To get needed rest; patients will feel more tired at end of day
• Not to chew or crush sus rel forms

Treatment of overdose: Administer fluids, hemodialysis or peritoneal dialysis; antihypertensive for increased B/P; ammonium Cl for increased excretion.

---

methantheline bromide

(meth-an'tha-leen)

Banthine

Func. class.: Gastrointestinal anticholinergic

Chem. class.: Synthetic quaternary ammonium antimuscarinic

Action: Inhibits muscarinic actions of acetylcholine at postganglionic parasympathetic neuroeffector sites

Uses: Treatment of peptic ulcer disease, irritable bowel syndrome, pancreatitis, gastritis, biliary dyskinesia, pylorospasm, reflex neurogenic bladder in children

Dosage and routes:
• *Adult:* PO 50-100 mg q6h
• *Child >1 yr:* PO 12.5-50 mg qid
• *Child <1 yr:* PO 12.5-25 mg qid
• *Neonate:* PO 12.5 mg bid-tid

Available forms include: Tabs 50 mg

Side effects/adverse reactions:

CNS: Confusion, stimulation in elderly, headache, insomnia, dizziness, drowsiness, anxiety, weakness, hallucination

GI: Dry mouth, constipation, paralytic ileus, heartburn, nausea, vomiting, dysphagia, absence of taste

GU: Hesitancy, retention, impotence

CV: Palpitations, tachycardia

EENT: Blurred vision, photophobia, mydriasis, cycloplegia, increased ocular tension

INTEG: Urticaria, rash, pruritus, anhidrosis, fever, allergic reactions

Contraindications: Hypersensitivity to anticholinergics, narrow-angle glaucoma, GI obstruction, myasthenia gravis, paralytic ileus, GI atony, toxic megacolon

Precautions: Hyperthyroidism, coronary artery disease, dysrhythmias, CHF, ulcerative colitis, hypertension, hiatal hernia, hepatic disease, renal disease, pregnancy (C), urinary retention, prostatic hypertrophy

Pharmacokinetics:

PO: Onset 30-45 min, duration 4-6 hr; metabolized by liver, excreted in urine, bile

Interactions/incompatibilities:
• Increased anticholinergic effect: amantadine, tricyclic antidepressants, MAOIs, H_1 antihistamines
• Increased effect of: nitrofurantoin
• Decreased effect of: phenothiazines, levodopa

NURSING CONSIDERATIONS

Assess:
• VS, cardiac status: checking for dysrhythmias, increased rate, palpitations
• I&O ratio; check for urinary retention, hesitancy

Administer:
• ½-1 hr ac for better absorption
• Decreased dose to elderly patients; their metabolism may be slowed
• Gum, hard candy, frequent rinsing of mouth for dryness of oral cavity

Perform/provide:
• Storage in tight container protected from light
• Increased fluids, bulk, exercise to patient's lifestyle to decrease constipation

Evaluate:
• Therapeutic response: absence of

---

* Available in Canada only

epigastric pain, bleeding, nausea, vomiting

- GI complaints: pain, bleeding (frank or occult), nausea, vomiting, anorexia

Teach patient/family:

- To avoid driving or other hazardous activities until stabilized on medication
- To avoid alcohol or other CNS depressants; will enhance sedating properties of this drug
- That drug may cause blurred vision

---

methazolamide

(meth-a-zoe'la-mide)

Neptazane

Func. class.: Carbonic anhydrase inhibitor diuretic

Chem. class.: Sulfonamide derivative

Action: Decreases production of aqueous humor in eye, which lowers intraocular pressure

Uses: Open-angle glaucoma or preoperatively in narrow-angle glaucoma, can be used with miotic, osmotic agents

Dosage and routes:

- *Adult:* PO 50-100 mg bid or tid

Available forms include: Tabs 50 mg

Side effects/adverse reactions:

GU: Frequency, hypokalemia, polyuria, uremia, ***glucosuria, hematuria,*** dysuria

CNS: Drowsiness, paresthesia, anxiety, depression, headache, dizziness, confusion, stimulation, fatigue, ***convulsions***, sedation, nervousness

GI: Nausea, vomiting, anorexia, constipation, diarrhea, melena, weight loss, hepatic insufficiency

EENT: Myopia, tinnitus

INTEG: Rash, pruritus, urticaria, fever, photosensitivity, Stevens-Johnson syndrome

ENDO: Hyperglycemia

HEMA: ***Aplastic anemia, hemolytic anemia, leukopenia, agranulocytosis, thrombocytopenia, purpura, pancytopenia***

Contraindications: Hypersensitivity to sulfonamides, severe renal disease, severe hepatic disease, electrolyte imbalances (hyponatremia, hypokalemia), hyperchloremic acidosis, Addison's disease, COPD

Precautions: Hypercalciuria, pregnancy (C)

Pharmacokinetics:

PO: Onset 2-4 hr, peak 6-8 hr, duration 10-18 hr; excreted in urine, crosses placenta

Interactions/incompatibilities:

- Increased action of: amphetamines, procainamide, quinidine, flecainide, ephedrine, pseudoephedrine
- Hypokalemia: with other diuretics, corticosteroids, amphotericin B
- Toxicity: salicylates

NURSING CONSIDERATIONS

Assess:

- Weight, I&O daily to determine fluid loss; effect of drug may be decreased if used qd
- Rate, depth, rhythm of respiration, effect of exertion
- B/P lying, standing; postural hypotension may occur
- Electrolytes: potassium, sodium, chloride; include BUN, blood sugar, CBC, serum creatinine, blood pH, ABGs, liver function tests

Administer:

- In AM to avoid interference with sleep

• Potassium replacement if potassium is less than 3.0
• With food, if nausea occurs, absorption may be decreased slightly

Evaluate:
• Therapeutic response: decrease in aqueous humor
• Signs of metabolic acidosis: drowsiness, restlessness
• Signs of hypokalemia: postural hypotension, malaise, fatigue, tachycardia, leg cramps, weakness
• Rashes, temperature elevation qd
• Confusion, especially in elderly; take safety precautions if needed

Teach patient/family:
• To increase fluid intake 2-3 L/day unless contraindicated; to rise slowly from lying or sitting position
• To notify physician if sore throat, unusual bleeding, bruising, paresthesias, tremors, flank pain, or skin rash occurs
• To avoid hazardous activities if drowsiness occurs

Lab test interferences:
False positive: Urinary protein

Treatment of overdose: Lavage if taken orally, monitor electrolytes, administer dextrose in saline, monitor hydration, CV, renal status

---

methenamine hippurate/methenamine mandelate

(meth-en'a-meen) (hip'yoo-rate)
Hiprex, Hip-Rex,* Urex/Mandelamine

Func. class.: Urinary antiinfective
Chem. class.: Methenamine, mandelic acid

Action: In acid urine, it is hydrolyzed to ammonia, formaldehyde, which are bactericidal

Uses: Urinary tract infections caused by *E. coli, Klebsiella, Enterobacter, P. mirabilis, P. morganii, Serratia, Citrobacter*

Dosage and routes:
• *Adult and child >12 yr:* PO 1 g q12h, maximum: 4 g/24 hr
• *Child 6-12 yr:* PO 500 mg-1g q12h

Neurogenic bladder
• *Adult:* PO 1 g qid pc
• *Child 6-12 yr:* PO 500 mg qid pc
• *Child <6 yr:* PO 50 mg/kg in 4 divided doses pc

Available forms include: Tabs 500 mg, 1 g; oral sol 500 mg, 1 g; susp 250, 500 mg/5 ml; tabs, enteric-coated 250, 500 mg, g; tabs, film-coated 500 mg, 1g

Side effects/adverse reactions:
CNS: Headache
INTEG: Pruritus, rash, urticaria
GI: Nausea, vomiting, anorexia, abdominal pain, increase AST, ALT
GU: Dysuria, bladder irritation, ***albuminuria, hematuria,*** crystalluria
EENT: Tinnitus, stomatitis

Contraindications: Hypersensitivity, severe dehydration, renal insufficiency

Precautions: Renal disease, pregnancy (C), lactation

Pharmacokinetics:
PO: Excreted in urine, half-life 4 hr

Interactions/incompatibilities:
• Insoluble precipitate in urine: sulfonamides
• Do not use with silver, iron, mercury salts

NURSING CONSIDERATIONS

Assess:
• I&O ratio; urine pH <5.5 is ideal; monitor for hematuria indicating crystalluria
• Periodic liver function test: AST, ALT, alk phosphatase

---

* Available in Canada only

• C&S before treatment, after completion

Administer:

• After clean-catch urine is obtained for C&S
• Two daily doses if urine output is high or if patient has diabetes
• Up to 12 g of Vitamin C if needed to acidify urine; cranberry, prune juice may be used

Perform/provide:

• Storage protected from high temperature
• Limited intake of alkaline foods or drugs: milk, dairy products, peanuts, vegetables, alkaline antacids, sodium bicarbonate

Evaluate:

• Therapeutic response: decreased pain, frequency, urgency, negative C&S, absence of infection
• Allergy: fever, flushing, rash, urticaria, pruritus

Teach patient/family:

• To keep urine acidic by eating food that acidifies urine (meats, eggs, fish, gelatin products, prunes, plums, cranberries)
• That fluids must be increased to 3 L/day to avoid crystallization in kidneys
• To complete full course of drug therapy; to take drug at evenly spaced intervals around clock for best results

Lab test interferences:

Interfere: VMA, urinary catecholamines
False decrease: Urine estriol, 5HIAA
False increase: 17-OHCS

methicillin sodium

(meth-i-sill'in)
Celbenin, Staphcillin
Func. class.: Broad-spectrum antibiotic
Chem. class.: Penicillinase-resistant penicillin

Action: Interferes with cell wall replication of susceptible organisms; osmotically unstable cell wall swells, bursts from osmotic pressure

Uses: Effective for gram-positive cocci *(S. aureus, S. pyogenes, S. viridans, S. faecalis, S. bovis, S. pneumoniae)*, infections caused by penicillinase-producing *Staphylococcus*

Dosage and routes:

• *Adult:* IM/IV 4-12 g/day in divided doses q4-6h
• *Child:* IM/IV 50-300 mg/kg/day in divided doses q4-12h

Available forms include: Powder for inj IM, IV 1, 4, 6, 10 g; IV INF only 1 g

Side effects/adverse reactions:

HEMA: Anemia, increased bleeding time, ***bone marrow depression, granulocytopenia***
GI: Nausea, vomiting, diarrhea, increased AST, ALT, abdominal pain, glossitis, colitis
GU: Oliguria, ***proteinuria, hematuria,*** *vaginitis, moniliasis,* ***glomerulonephritis***
CNS: Lethargy, hallucinations, anxiety, depression, twitching, ***coma, convulsions***

Contraindications: Hypersensitivity to penicillins

Precautions: Pregnancy (B), hypersensitivity to cephalosporins, neonates

Pharmacokinetics:

IM: Peak ½-1 hr, duration 4 hr

M

IV: Peak 15 min, duration 2 hr; metabolized in liver, excreted in urine, bile, breast milk, crosses placenta

Interactions/incompatibilities:
• Decreased antimicrobial effectiveness of methicillin: tetracyclines, erythromycins
• Increased methicillin concentrations: aspirin, probenecid

NURSING CONSIDERATIONS

Assess:
• I&O ratio; report hematuria, oliguria since penicillin in high doses is nephrotoxic
• Any patient with compromised renal system since drug is excreted slowly in poor renal system function; toxicity may occur rapidly
• Liver studies: AST, ALT
• Blood studies: WBC, RBC, H&H, bleeding time
• Renal studies: urinalysis, protein, blood
• C&S before drug therapy; drug may be taken as soon as culture is taken

Administer:
• IV after diluting 1 g/1.8 ml sterile H_2O, further dilute each 500 mg/25 ml or more NaCl; give directly over 1 min or more or by inf over ½-8 hr
• Drug after C&S has been completed

Perform/provide:
• Adrenalin, suction, tracheostomy set, endotracheal intubation equipment
• Adequate fluid intake (2000 ml) during diarrhea episodes
• Scratch test to assess allergy after securing order from physician; usually done when penicillin is only drug of choice
• Storage at room temperature; reconstituted solution is stable for 8 hr

Evaluate:
• Therapeutic response: absence of fever, draining wounds
• Bowel pattern before, during treatment
• Skin eruptions after administration of penicillin to 1 wk after discontinuing drug
• Respiratory status: rate, character, wheezing, tightness in chest
• Allergies before initiation of treatment, reaction of each medication; highlight allergies on chart, Kardex

Teach patient/family:
• That culture may be taken after completed course of medication
• To report sore throat, fever, fatigue (could indicate superimposed infection)
• To wear or carry Medic Alert ID if allergic to penicillins
• To notify nurse of diarrhea

Lab test interferences:
False positive: Urine glucose, urine protein

Treatment of overdose: Withdraw drug, maintain airway, administer epinephrine, aminophylline, O_2, IV corticosteroids for anaphylaxis

methimazole

(meth-im'a-zole)

Tapazole

Func. class.: Antithyroid hormone
Chem. class.: Thioamide

Action: Inhibits synthesis of thyroid hormones by decreasing iodine use in manufacture of thyroglobin and iodothyronine; does not affect already formed hormones

Uses: Hyperthyroidism, preparation for thyroidectomy, thyrotoxic crisis, thyroid storm

Dosage and routes:
Hyperthyroidism

• *Adult:* PO 5-20 mg tid depending on severity of condition, continue until euthyroid, maintenance dose 5 mg qd-tid, maximal dose 150 mg qd
• *Child:* PO 0.4 mg/kg/day in divided doses q8h, continue until euthyroid maintenance dose 0.2 mg/kg/day in divided doses q8h

Preparation for thyroidectomy
• *Adult and child:* PO same as above; iodine may be added × 10 days before surgery

Thyrotoxic crisis
• *Adult and child:* PO same as hyperthyroidism with iodine and propranolol

Available forms include: Tabs 5, 10 mg

Side effects/adverse reactions:
ENDO: Enlarged thyroid
INTEG: Rash, urticaria, pruritus, alopecia, hyperpigmentation, lupuslike syndrome
GU: ***Nephritis***
CNS: Drowsiness, headache, vertigo, fever, paresthesias, neuritis
HEMA: ***Agranulocytosis, leukopenia, thrombocytopenia, hypothrombinemia, lymphadenopathy,*** bleeding, vasculitis
GI: Nausea, diarrhea, vomiting, ***jaundice, hepatitis,*** loss of taste
MS: Myalgia, arthralgia, nocturnal muscle cramps

Contraindications: Hypersensitivity, pregnancy (3rd trimester) (D), lactation

Precautions: Infection, bone marrow depression, hepatic disease, pregnancy (1st, 2nd trimester)

Pharmacokinetics:
PO: Onset 30-40 min, duration 2-4 hr, half-life 1-2 hr, excreted in urine, bile, breast milk, crosses placenta

NURSING CONSIDERATIONS

Assess:
• Pulse, B/P, temperature
• I&O ratio, check for edema: puffy hands, feet, periorbits; indicate hypothyroidism
• Weight qd; same clothing, scale, time of day
• T_3, T_4, which are increased; serum TSH, which is decreased; free thyroxine index, which is increased if dosage is too low; discontinue drug 3-4 wk before RAIU
• Blood work: CBC for blood dyscrasias: leukopenia, thrombocytopenia, agranulocytosis; LFTs

Administer:
• With meals to decrease GI upset
• At same time each day, to maintain drug level
• Lowest dose that relieves symptoms, discontinue before RAI

Perform/provide:
• Storage in light-resistant container
• Fluids to 3-4 L/day, unless contraindicated

Evaluate:
• Therapeutic response: weight gain, decreased pulse, decreased T_4, B/P
• Overdose: peripheral edema, heat intolerance, diaphoresis, palpitations, dysrhythmias, severe tachycardia, increased temperature, delirium, CNS irritability
• Hypersensitivity: rash, enlarged cervical lymph nodes; drug may need to be discontinued
• Hypoprothrombinemia: bleeding, petechiae, ecchymosis
• Clinical response: after 3 wk should include increased weight, pulse; decreased T_4
• Bone marrow depression: sore throat, fever, fatigue

Teach patient/family:
• To abstain from breast feeding after delivery
• To take pulse daily
• To report redness, swelling, sore

M

throat, mouth lesions, which indicate blood dyscrasias
• To keep graph of weight, pulse, mood
• Avoid OTC products that contain iodine
• That seafood, other iodine products may be restricted
• Not to discontinue this medication abruptly; thyroid crisis may occur; stress patient response
• That response may take several months if thyroid is large
• Symptoms/signs of overdose: periorbital edema, cold intolerance, mental depression
• Symptoms of inadequate dose: tachycardia, diarrhea, fever, irritability

Lab test interferences:
Increase: Pro-time, AST/ALT, alk phosphatase

---

methocarbamol

(meth-oh-kar'ba-mole)
Delaxin, Forbaxin, Robamol, Robaxin, Romethocarb, Spenaxin, Tresortil*

Func. class.: Skeletal muscle relaxant
Chem. class.: Carbamate derivative

Action: Depresses multisynaptic pathways in the spinal cord
Uses: Adjunct for relief of spasm and pain in musculoskeletal conditions, tetanus management
Dosage and routes:
Pain
• *Adult:* PO 1.5 g × 2-3 days, then 1 g qid; IM 500 mg in each gluteal region, may repeat q8h; IV BOL 1-3 g/day at 3 ml/min; IV INF 1 gm/250 ml D_5W or NS, not to exceed 3 g/day

Tetanus
• *Adult:* IV INF 1-3 g/L of solution q6h; IV BOL 1-2 g injected into running IV
• *Child:* IV 15 mg/kg q6h

Available forms include: Tabs 500, 750 mg; inj IM, IV 100 mg/ml
Side effects/adverse reactions:
CNS: Dizziness, weakness, drowsiness, headache, tremor, depression, insomnia, ***seizures***
HEMA: Hemolysis, increased hemoglobin (IV only)
EENT: Diplopia, temporary loss of vision, blurred vision, nystagmus
CV: Postural hypotension, bradycardia
GI: Nausea, vomiting, hiccups, anorexia, metallic taste
GU: Brown, black, green urine
INTEG: Rash, pruritus, fever, facial flushing, urticaria
Contraindications: Hypersensitivity, child <12 yr, intermittent porphyria
Precautions: Renal disease, hepatic disease, addictive personalities, pregnancy (C), myasthenia gravis, epilepsy
Pharmacokinetics:
PO: Onset ½ hr, peak 1-2 hr, half-life 1-2 hr, metabolized in liver, excreted in urine (unchanged), crosses placenta
Interactions/incompatibilities:
• Increased CNS depression: alcohol, tricyclic antidepressants, narcotics, barbiturates, sedatives, hypnotics

NURSING CONSIDERATIONS

Assess:
• Blood studies: CBC, WBC, differential; blood dyscrasias may occur
• During and after injection: CNS effects, rash, conjunctivitis, and nasal congestion may occur
• Liver function studies: AST,

---

* Available in Canada only

ALT, alk phosphatase; hepatitis may occur
- ECG in epileptic patients; poor seizure control has occurred with patients taking this drug

Administer:
- With meals for GI symptoms
- IV undiluted over 1 min or more, give 300 mg or less/1 min or longer; may be diluted in 250 ml or less compatible sol
- By slow IV to prevent phlebitis; keep recumbent for 15 min to prevent orthostatic hypotension; check for extravasation
- IM deeply in large muscle mass; rotate sites

Perform/provide:
- Storage in tight container at room temperature
- Assistance with ambulation if dizziness, drowsiness occurs

Evaluate:
- Therapeutic response: decreased pain, spasticity
- Allergic reactions: rash, fever, respiratory distress
- Severe weakness, numbness in extremities
- Psychologic dependency: increased need for medication, more frequent requests for medication, increased pain
- CNS depression: dizziness, drowsiness, psychiatric symptoms

Teach patient/family:
- Not to discontinue medication quickly; insomnia, nausea, headache, spasticity, tachycardia will occur; drug should be tapered off over 1-2 wk
- That urine may turn green, black or brown
- Not to take with alcohol, other CNS depressants
- To avoid altering activities while taking this drug
- To avoid hazardous activities if drowsiness, dizziness occurs
- To avoid using OTC medication: cough preparations, antihistamines, unless directed by physician

Lab test interferences:
False increase: VMA, urinary 5-HIAA

Treatment of overdose: Induce emesis of conscious patient, lavage, dialysis; have epinephrine, antihistamines, and corticosteroids available

---

methohexital sodium

(meth-oh-hex′i-tal)

Brevital Sodium, Brietal Sodium*

Func. class.: General anesthetic
Chem. class.: Barbiturate

Controlled Substance Schedule IV

Action: Acts in reticular-activating system to produce anesthesia

Uses: General anesthesia, for electroshock therapy, reduction of fractures

Dosage and routes:
- *Adult and child:* IV 50-100 mg given 1 ml/5 sec

Maintenance
- *Adult and child:* IV 20-40 mg q4-7 min of a 0.1% solution; cont IV 1 gtt/sec of a 0.2% solution

Available forms include: Inj IV 500 mg, 2.5, 5g

Side effects/adverse reactions:
RESP: ***Respiratory depression, bronchospasm***
CNS: Retrograde amnesia, prolonged somnolence
CV: Tachycardia, hypotension, ***myocardial depression, dysrhythmias***
EENT: Sneezing, coughing
INTEG: Chills, *shivering,* necrosis, pain at injection site

M

MS: Muscle irritability

Contraindications: Hypersensitivity, status asthmaticus, hepatic/intermittent porphyrias, pregnancy (D)

Precautions: Severe cardiovascular disease, renal disease, hypotension, liver disease, myxedema, myasthenia gravis, asthma, increased intracranial pressure

Pharmacokinetics:

IV: Onset 30-40 sec; half-life 11.5 hr, crosses placenta

Interactions/incompatibilities:

• Increased action: CNS depressants

• Do not mix with atropine or silicone in solution or syringe

NURSING CONSIDERATIONS

Assess:

• VS q3-5 min during IV administration, after dose, q4 hr postoperatively

Administer:

• After preparation with sterile water 0.9%, NaCl or 5% dextrose

• Only with crash cart, resuscitative equipment nearby

• IV slowly only by qualified persons

Evaluate:

• Therapeutic response: induction of anesthesia

• Extravasation, if it occurs use chloroprocaine to decrease pain, increase circulation

• Dysrhythmias or myocardial depression

methotrexate/methotrexate sodium (amethopterin, MTX)

(meth-oh-trex'ate)

Folex, Mexate

Func. class.: Antineoplastic-antimetabolite

Chem. class.: Folic acid antagonist

Action: Inhibits an enzyme that reduces folic acid, which is needed for nucleic acid synthesis in all cells

Uses: Acute lymphocytic leukemia, in combination for breast, lung, head, neck cancer, lymphosarcoma, psoriasis, gestational choriocarcinoma, hydatidiform mole

Dosage and routes:

Leukemia

• *Adult and child:* PO 3.3 mg/m^2/day, maintenance 30 mg/m^2/day 2×/wk; IV 2.5 mg/kg q2wk

Choriocarcinoma

• *Adult and child:* PO 15-30 mg/m^2 qd × 5 days, then off 1 wk; may repeat

Available forms include: Tabs, 2.5 mg; inj IV 25 mg/ml; powder for inj IV 20, 25, 50, 100, 250 mg; sodium inj IV 2.5, 25 mg/ml

Side effects/adverse reactions:

HEMA: ***Leukopenia, thrombocytopenia, myelosuppression, anemia***

GI: Nausea, vomiting, anorexia, diarrhea, stomatitis, ***hepatotoxicity,*** cramps, ulcer, gastritis, ***GI hemorrhage,*** abdominal pain, hematemesis

GU: Urinary retention, ***renal failure,*** menstrual irregularities, defective spermatogenesis, ***hematuria, azotemia, uric acid nephropathy***

INTEG: Rash, alopecia, dry skin, urticaria, photosensitivity, folliculitis, vasculitis, petechiae, ecchymosis, acne, alopecia

CNS: Dizziness, ***convulsions,*** headache, confusion, hemiparesis, malaise, fatigue, chills, fever

Contraindications: Hypersensitivity, leukopenia (<2500/mm^3), thrombocytopenia (<100,000/mm^3), anemia, psoriatic patients with severe renal/hepatic disease, pregnancy (D)

Precautions: Renal disease, lactation

* Available in Canada only

Pharmacokinetics:
PO: Readily absorbed when taken orally, peak 1-4 hr
IV/IM: Peak ½-2 hr
Not metabolized, excreted in urine (unchanged), crosses placenta, blood-brain barrier, 50% plasma protein bound

Interactions/incompatibilities:
- Increased toxicity: aspirin, sulfa drugs, other antineoplastics, radiation, alcohol, probenecid, phenytoin, phenylbutazone, pyrimethamine
- Decreased effect of: oral digoxin
- Increased hypoprothrombinemia: oral anticoagulants
- Decreased effect of methotrexate: folic acid supplements
- Possible fatal interactions: nonsteroidal antiinflammatory drugs

NURSING CONSIDERATIONS

Assess:
- CBC, differential, platelet count weekly; withhold drug if WBC is <3500/mm³ or platelet count is <100,000/mm³; notify physician of these results; drug should be discontinued
- Renal function studies: BUN, serum uric acid, urine CrCl, electrolytes before, during therapy
- I&O ratio; report fall in urine output to <30 ml/hr
- Monitor temperature q4h; fever may indicate beginning infection, no rectal temperatures
- Liver function tests before and during therapy: bilirubin, alk phosphatase, AST, ALT; liver biopsy should be done before start of therapy (psoriasis patients)
- Bleeding time, coagulation time during treatment

Administer:
- IV after diluting 5 mg/2 ml of sterile H_2O for inj; give through Y-tube or 3-way stopcock at 10 mg or less/min
- Antacid before oral agent; give drug after evening meal before bedtime
- Antiemetic 30-60 min before giving drug to prevent vomiting
- Allopurinol or sodium bicarbonate to maintain uric acid levels, alkalinization of urine, adequate fluids
- Leucovorin calcium within 12 hr of this drug to prevent tissue damage, check agency policy
- Antibiotics for prophylaxis of infection
- Topical or systemic analgesics for pain
- Transfusion for anemia

Perform/provide:
- Strict medical asepsis and protective isolation if WBC levels are low
- Liquid diet: carbonated beverage, Jell-O; dry toast, crackers may be added when patient is not nauseated or vomiting
- Increased fluid intake to 2-3 L/day to prevent urate deposits, calculi formation, unless contraindicated
- Diet low in purines: absence of organ meats (kidney, liver), dried beans, peas to maintain alkaline urine
- Rinsing of mouth tid-qid with water, club soda; brushing of teeth bid-tid with soft brush or cotton-tipped applicators for stomatitis; use unwaxed dental floss
- Nutritious diet with iron, vitamin supplements
- Storage in tightly closed container in cool environment; store injection, powder for injection in dark, dry area

Evaluate:
- Therapeutic response: decreased tumor size, spread of malignancy

M

• Bleeding: hematuria, guaiac, bruising or petechiae, mucosa or orifices q8h
• Food preferences; list likes, dislikes
• Effects of alopecia on body image; discuss feelings about body changes
• Hepatotoxicity: yellowing of skin, sclera, dark urine, clay-colored stools, pruritus, abdominal pain, fever, diarrhea
• Buccal cavity q8h for dryness, sores, ulceration, white patches, oral pain, bleeding, dysphagia
• Symptoms indicating severe allergic reaction: rash, urticaria, itching, flushing

Teach patient/family:
• Why protective isolation precautions are needed
• To report any complaints, side effects to nurse or physician: black tarry stools, chills, fever, sore throat, bleeding, bruising, cough, shortness of breath, dark or bloody urine
• That hair may be lost during treatment; wig or hairpiece may make patient feel better; tell patient that new hair may be different in color, texture (alopecia is rare)
• To avoid foods with citric acid, hot or rough texture if stomatitis is present
• To report stomatitis: any bleeding, white spots, ulcerations in mouth to physician; tell patient to examine mouth qd, report symptoms to nurse
• That contraceptive measures are recommended during therapy for at least 8 wk following cessation of therapy
• To drink 10-12 glasses of fluid/day
• To avoid alcohol, salicylates
• To avoid use of razors or commercial mouthwash

methotrimeprazine HCl

(meth-oh-trye-mep'ra-zeen)
Levoprome, Nozinan*
Func. class.: Analgesic
Chem. class.: Aliphatic (propylamine-phenothiazine derivative)

Action: Depresses cerebral cortex, hypothalamus, limbic system; blocks neurotransmission produced by dopamine at synapse; exhibits strong α-adrenergic, anticholinergic blocking action, antihistamine

Uses: Sedation, analgesia, preoperative and postoperative analgesia, obstetric analgesia

Dosage and routes:
Analgesia/sedation
• *Adult and child >12 yr:* IM 10-20 mg q4-6h prn
• *Elderly:* IM 5-10 mg q4-6h

Preoperative medication
• *Adult and child >12 yr:* IM 2-20 mg 45 min to 3 hr before surgery

Postoperative medication
• *Adult and child >12 yr:* IM 2.5-7.5 mg q4-6h titrated to patient's needs

Available forms include: Inj IM 20 mg/ml

Side effects/adverse reactions:
HEMA: ***Thrombocytopenia, agranulocytosis, leukopenia, neutropenia, hemolytic anemia*** (long-term, high dose)
CNS: Weakness, dizziness, drowsiness, confusion, delirium, euphoria, headache, sedation, EPS
GI: Nausea, vomiting, abdominal pain, dry mouth, jaundice (long-term use)
GU: ***Hematuria,*** dysuria, hesitancy, retention, uterine inertia (rare)

* Available in Canada only

INTEG: Pain, edema at injection site, fever, chills
EENT: Nasal congestion, blurred vision, slurred speech
CV: Orthostatic hypotension, palpitations, tachycardia, bradycardia
Contraindications: Hypersensitivity to this drug, phenothiazines, bisulfite; seizures; severe hepatic disease; severe renal disease; severe cardiac disease; coma
Precautions: Elderly, pregnancy (C)
Pharmacokinetics:
IM: Onset 20-30 min, peak 1-2 hr, duration 4 hr; metabolized by liver, excreted by kidneys and in feces, crosses placenta, excreted in breast milk
Interactions/incompatibilities:
• Mix only with scopolamine or atropine; not to be mixed in syringe or solution with any other drugs
• Increased sedation: CNS depressants, alcohol, barbiturates, reserpine, narcotics, general anesthetics, meprobamate

NURSING CONSIDERATIONS

Assess:
• Blood studies: CBC, ALT, AST, bilirubin
• VS q10min for 30 min; watch for decreasing B/P with increased pulse that may occur 10-30 min after injection; continue to closely monitor for 6-12 hr after several injections
• Effect on uterine contractions, fetal heart tones if using for labor
Administer:
• After removal of cigarettes, to prevent fires
• IM injection in deep large muscle mass to prevent tissue sloughing, rotate sites
• Lowest dose, then gradually increase; lower doses are required after general anesthesia
Perform/provide:
• Bed rest for several hours after injection if orthostatic hypotension occurs
• Safety measure: siderails, nightlight, call bell within easy reach
• Storage in darkness, expires after 5 yr
• Assistance with ambulation for 6 hr after injection
Evaluate:
• Therapeutic response: decrease in pain, grimacing, absence of change in VS, ability to cough and breathe deep after surgery
Teach patient/family:
• To avoid ambulation without assistance for 6 hr after drug is given
Treatment of overdose: Lavage, activated charcoal, monitor electrolytes, vital signs

methoxsalen

(meth-ox'a-len)
Oxsoralen, Oxsoralen-Ultra 8-MOP, UltraMOP
Func. class.: Pigmenting agent
Chem. class.: Psoralen derivative

Action: Decreases cell turnover by combining with epidermal cell DNA, causing photo damage when used with ultraviolet rays
Uses: Vitiligo, psoriasis
Dosage and routes:
Vitiligo
• *Adult and child >12 yr:* PO 20 mg qd 2-4 hr before exposure to therapeutic ultraviolet rays; administer on alternate days; TOP apply 1-2 hr before exposure to UVA light; treatment intervals regulated by erythema response
Psoriasis
Adult PO: Dosage individualized according to weight; taken 2 hr be-

fore exposure to therapeutic ultraviolet rays

Available forms include: Lotion 1%; hard caps 10 mg; soft caps 10 mg; contains tartrazine

Side effects/adverse reactions:

CNS: Headache, depression, restlessness, anxiety, nervousness, vertigo, insomnia, malaise

GI: Nausea

INTEG: Rash, pruritus, burning, peeling, erythema, edema, urticaria, hypopigmentation

MISC: Leg cramps, hypotension, herpes simplex

Contraindications: Hypersensitivity, melanoma, LE, albinism, sunburn, cataracts, squamous cell cancer, child ≤12 yr, diseases associated with photosensitivity

Precautions: Hepatic disease, cardiac disease, children, lactation, pregnancy (C); contains tartrazine (FD & C #5), photosensitizing agents

Pharmacokinetics:

PO: Duration 8 hr, half-life 2 hr, metabolized in liver, excreted in urine

Interactions/incompatibilities:

• Increased effects of methoxsalen: other photosensitizing agents, phenothiazines, thiazides, tetracyclines, griseofulvin, halogenated salicylanides, sulfonamides, coal tar derivatives, nalidixic acid

NURSING CONSIDERATIONS

Assess:

• Hepatic test (AST, ALT, bilirubin), renal test (BUN, protein), antinuclear antibodies during treatment

Administer:

• With food or milk to prevent GI upset

• To prevent extensive phototoxicity, qod

• Lotion to small areas, use systemic treatment for large areas

Perform/provide:

• Protection to eyes, lips during treatment

• Use of finger cot or gloves to apply lotion

Evaluate:

• Therapeutic response: increased pigmentation in vitiligo, decreased psoriatic areas

Teach patient/family:

• To avoid UVA exposure for at least 24 hr after topical application, and 8 hr after PO dose

• That sunscreen may be used if exposure to sunlight occurs after treatment

• That repigmentation may require 6-9 mo

methscopolamine bromide

(meth-skoe-pol'a-meen)

Pamine

Func. class.: Gastrointestinal anticholinergic

Chem. class.: Synthetic quaternary ammonium antimuscarinic

Action: Inhibits muscarinic actions of acetylcholine at postganglionic parasympathetic neuroeffector sites

Uses: Treatment of peptic ulcer disease

Dosage and routes:

• *Adult:* PO 2.5-5 mg ½ hr ac, hs

Available forms include: Tabs 2.5 mg

Side effects/adverse reactions:

CNS: Confusion, stimulation in elderly, headache, insomnia, dizziness, drowsiness, anxiety, weakness, hallucination

GI: Dry mouth, constipation, ***paralytic ileus,*** heartburn, nausea,

vomiting, dysphagia, absence of taste
GU: Hesitancy, retention, impotence
CV: Palpitations, tachycardia
EENT: Blurred vision, photophobia, mydriasis, cycloplegia, increased ocular tension
INTEG: Urticaria, rash, pruritus, anhidrosis, fever, allergic reactions
Contraindications: Hypersensitivity to anticholinergics, narrow-angle glaucoma, GI obstruction, myasthenia gravis, paralytic ileus, GI atony, toxic megacolon
Precautions: Hyperthyroidism, coronary artery disease, dysrhythmias, CHF, ulcerative colitis, hypertension, hiatal hernia, hepatic disease, renal disease, pregnancy (C), urinary retention, prostatic hypertrophy
Pharmacokinetics:
PO: Onset 1 hr, duration 6-8 hr; metabolized by liver, excreted in urine
Interactions/incompatibilities:
• Increased anticholinergic effect: amantadine, tricyclic antidepressants, MAOIs, H_1 antihistamines
• Decreased effect of: phenothiazines, levodopa, ketoconazole

NURSING CONSIDERATIONS

Assess:
• VS, cardiac status: checking for dysrhythmias, increased rate, palpitations
• I&O ratio; check for urinary retention or hesitancy
Administer:
• ½-1 hr ac for better absorption
• Decreased dose to elderly patients; their metabolism may be slowed
• Gum, hard candy, frequent rinsing of mouth for dryness of oral cavity
Perform/provide:
• Storage in tight container protected from light
• Increased fluids, bulk, exercise to patient's lifestyle to decrease constipation
Evaluate:
• Therapeutic response: absence of epigastric pain, bleeding, nausea, vomiting
• GI complaints: pain, bleeding (frank or occult), nausea, vomiting, anorexia
Teach patient/family:
• To avoid driving or other hazardous activities until stabilized on medication
• To avoid alcohol or other CNS depressants; will enhance sedating properties of this drug
• To drink plenty of fluids
• To report dysphagia
• That drug may cause blurred vision

---

methsuximide

(meth-sux'i-mide)
Celontin
Func. class.: Anticonvulsant
Chem. class.: Succinimide

Action: Inhibits spike, wave formation in absence seizures (petit mal), decreases amplitude, frequency, duration, spread of discharge in minor motor seizures
Uses: Refractory absence seizures (petit mal)
Dosage and routes:
• *Adult and child:* PO 300 mg/day; may increase by 300 mg/wk, not to exceed 1.2 g/day in divided doses
Available forms include: Caps, half-strength 150 mg; caps 300 mg
Side effects/adverse reactions:
HEMA: ***Agranulocytosis, aplastic anemia, thrombocytopenia, leukocytosis, eosinophilia, pancytopenia***

CNS: Drowsiness, dizziness, fatigue, euphoria, lethargy, irritability, depression, insomnia, anxiety, aggressiveness, ataxia, headache, confusion

GI: Nausea, vomiting, heartburn, anorexia, diarrhea, abdominal pain, cramps, constipation, gum hypertrophy, tongue swelling

GU: Vaginal bleeding, ***hematuria, renal damage***

INTEG: Urticaria, pruritic erythema, hirsutism, ***Stevens-Johnson syndrome***

EENT: Myopia, blurred vision

Contraindications: Hypersensitivity to succinimide derivatives

Precautions: Hepatic disease, renal disease, pregnancy (C), lactation

Pharmacokinetics:

PO: Onset 15-30 min, peak 1-2 hr, duration 4-6 hr

REC: Onset slow, duration 4-6 hr; metabolized by liver, excreted by kidneys, half-life 2⅗-4 hr

Interactions/incompatibilities:

• Antagonist effect: tricyclic antidepressants

• Decreased effects of: estrogens, oral contraceptives

NURSING CONSIDERATIONS

Assess:

• Renal studies: urinalysis, BUN, urine creatinine

• Blood studies: CBC, Hct, Hgb, reticulocyte counts qwk for 4 wk then qmo

• Hepatic studies: ALT, AST, bilirubin, creatinine

• Drug levels during initial treatment, therapeutic range (40-80 μg/ml)

Administer:

• With food, milk to decrease GI symptoms

Perform/provide:

• Hard candy, frequent rinsing of mouth, gum for dry mouth

• Assistance with ambulation during early part of treatment; dizziness occurs

Evaluate:

• Therapeutic response: decreased seizure activity, document on patient's chart

• Mental status: mood, sensorium, affect, behavioral changes; if mental status changes notify physician

• Eye problems; need for ophthalmic exams before, during, after treatment (slit lamp, fundoscopy, tonometry)

• Allergic reaction: red raised rash; if this occurs, drug should be discontinued

• Blood dyscrasias: fever, sore throat, bruising, rash, jaundice

• Toxicity: bone marrow depression, nausea, vomiting, ataxia, diplopia

Teach patient/family:

• To avoid driving, other activities that require alertness

• To avoid alcohol ingestion, CNS depressants; increased sedation may occur

• Not to discontinue medication quickly after long-term use

• To call physician promptly if lupuslike syndrome occurs (enlarged lymph nodes, fever, bruising, sore throat)

• That drug may change urine to pink or brown

Lab test interferences:

Increase: Coombs' test

Treatment of overdose: Lavage, activated charcoal, monitor electrolytes, VS

methylcellulose

(meth-ill-sell'yoo-lose)

Cellothyl, Citrucel, Cologel, Hydrolose, Syncelose,

Func. class.: Laxative, bulk
Chem. class.: Hydrophilic semisynthetic cellulose derivative

Action: Attracts water, expands in intestine to increase peristalsis; also absorbs excess water in stool; decreases diarrhea
Uses: Constipation
Dosage and routes:
• *Adult:* PO 5-20 ml tid with 8 oz of water
• *Child:* PO 5-10 ml qd or bid with water or 500 mg tid with 8 oz of water
Available forms include: Powder 105 mg/g; sol 450 mg/5 ml; tab 500 mg
Side effects/adverse reactions:
GI: ***Obstruction,*** abdominal distention
Contraindications: Hypersensitivity, GI obstruction, hepatitis
Pharmacokinetics:
PO: Onset 12-24 hr, peak 1-3 days
Interactions/incompatibilities:
• Decreased absorption: antibiotics, digitalis, nitrofurantoin, salicylates, tetracyclines, oral anticoagulants

NURSING CONSIDERATIONS
Assess:
• Blood, urine electrolytes if drug is used often by patient
• I&O ratio to identify fluid loss
Administer:
• Alone for better absorption; do not take within 1 hr of other drugs
• In morning or evening (oral dose)
Evaluate:
• Therapeutic response: decrease in constipation
• Cause of constipation; identify whether fluids, bulk, or exercise is missing from lifestyle
• Cramping, rectal bleeding, nausea, vomiting; if these symptoms occur, drug should be discontinued
Teach patient/family:
• To swallow tabs whole; do not chew, increase fluid intake
• That normal bowel movements do not always occur daily
• Not to use in presence of abdominal pain, nausea, vomiting
• To notify physician if constipation unrelieved or if symptoms of electrolyte imbalance occur: muscle cramps, pain, weakness, dizziness, excessive thirst

methyldopa/methyldopate

(meth-ill-doe'pa)

Aldomet, Dopamet,* Medimet,* Novomedopa*

Func. class.: Antihypertensive
Chem. class.: Centrally-acting adrenergic inhibitor

Action: Stimulates central inhibitory α-adrenergic receptors or acts as false transmitter, resulting in reduction of arterial pressure
Uses: Hypertension
Dosage and routes:
• *Adult:* PO 250 mg bid or tid, then adjusted q2d as needed, 0.5-3 g qd in 2-4 divided doses (maintenance), not to exceed 3 g/day; IV 250 mg-500 mg in 100 ml D_5W q6h, run over 30-60 min, not to exceed 1 g q6h
• *Child:* PO 10 mg/kg/day in 2-4 divided doses, not to exceed 65 mg/kg or 3 g/day, whichever is less; IV 20-40 mg/kg/day in 4 divided doses, not to exceed 65 mg/kg
Available forms include: Tabs 125,

250, 500 mg; oral susp 250 mg/5ml; inj IV 50 mg/ml

Side effects/adverse reactions:
GI: Nausea, vomiting, diarrhea, constipation, hepatic dysfunction
CV: Bradycardia, myocarditis, orthostatic hypotension, angina, edema, weight gain
CNS: Drowsiness, weakness, dizziness, sedation, headache, depression, psychosis
EENT: Nasal congestion, eczema
HEMA: ***Leukopenia, thrombocytopenia,*** anemia, positive Coombs' test
INTEG: Lupuslike syndrome
GU: Impotence, failure to ejaculate

Contraindications: Active hepatic disease, hypersensitivity, blood dyscrasias

Precautions: Pregnancy (C), liver disease, eclampsia, severe cardiac disease

Pharmacokinetics:
PO: Peak 2-4 hr, duration 12-24 hr
IV: Peak 2 hr, duration 10-16 hr; metabolized by liver, excreted in urine

Interactions/incompatibilities:
- Increased hypoglycemia: talbutal
- Increased pressor effect: sympathomimetic amines (norepinephrine, phenylpropanolamine)
- Increased hypotension: levodopa
- Increased sedation: haloperidol
- Increased action of: anesthetics

NURSING CONSIDERATIONS

Assess:
- Blood studies: neutrophils, decreased platelets
- Renal studies: protein, BUN, creatinine, watch for increased levels, may indicate nephrotic syndrome
- Baselines in renal, liver function tests before therapy begins
- K levels, although hyperkalemia rarely occurs
- B/P during beginning treatment, periodically thereafter

Administer:
- IV after diluting with 100 mg of compatible sol run over ½-1 hr

Perform/provide:
- Storage of tablets in tight containers

Evaluate:
- Therapeutic response: decrease in B/P in hypertension
- Allergic reaction: rash, fever, pruritus, urticaria; drug should be discontinued if antihistamines fail to help
- Symptoms of CHF: edema, dyspnea, wet rales, B/P
- Renal symptoms: polyuria, oliguria, frequency

Teach patient/family:
- To avoid hazardous activities
- To administer 1 hr before meals
- Not to discontinue drug abruptly or withdrawal symptoms may occur: anxiety, increased B/P, headache, insomnia, increased pulse, tremors, nausea, sweating
- Not to use OTC (cough, cold, allergy) products unless directed by physician
- To avoid sunlight or wear sunscreen if in sunlight, photosensitivity may occur
- To comply with dosage schedule even if feeling better
- To rise slowly to sitting or standing position to minimize orthostatic hypotension
- To notify physician of: mouth sores, sore throat, fever, swelling of hands or feet, irregular heartbeat, chest pain, signs of angioedema
- That excessive perspiration, dehydration, vomiting, diarrhea may lead to fall in blood pressure; consult physician if these occur
- That dizziness, fainting, light-

headedness may occur during 1st few days of therapy

- That compliance is necessary; not to skip or stop drug unless directed by physician
- That drug may cause skin rash or impaired perspiration

methylene blue

(meth'i-leen)

MG-Blue, Urolene Blue, Wright's Stain

Func. class.: Urinary tract antiseptic

Chem. class.: Antiseptic dye

Action: Oxidation-reduction; has opposite action on hemoglobin depending on concentration; with increased concentration, converts ferrous ion of reduced hemoglobin to ferric form, methemoglobin is thus produced; prolonged administration accelerates destruction of erythrocytes

Uses: Oxalate urinary tract calculi; urinary tract infections caused by *E. coli, Klebsiella, Enterobacter, P. mirabilis, P. vulgaris, P. morganii, Serratia, Citrobacter*

Dosage and routes:

- *Adult:* PO 65-130 mg pc with full glass of water

Cyanide poisoning/methemoglobinemia

- *Adult and child:* IV 1-2 mg/kg of 1% sol, inject slowly over 5 min or more

Available forms include: Tabs 65 mg, inj 10 mg/ml

Side effects/adverse reactions:

CV: Cyanosis, CV abnormalities

INTEG: Pruritus, rash, urticaria, photosensitivity, profuse sweating

CNS: Dizziness, headache, drowsiness, mental confusion, fever with large doses

GI: Nausea, vomiting, abdominal pain, diarrhea

GU: Bladder irritation

Contraindications: Hypersensitivity to this drug, renal insufficiency

Precautions: Anemia, renal disease, hepatic disease, G-6-PD deficiency, pregnancy (C)

Pharmacokinetics:

PO/IV: Excreted in urine, bile, feces

NURSING CONSIDERATIONS

Assess:

- For cyanosis
- I&O ratio; urine pH <5.5 is ideal
- Hct, Hgb

Administer:

- After clean-catch urine is obtained for C&S
- Two daily doses if urine output is high or if patient has diabetes

Perform/provide:

- Limited intake of alkaline foods, drugs: milk, dairy products, peanuts, vegetables, alkaline antacids, sodium bicarbonate

Evaluate:

- Therapeutic response: decreased pain, frequency, urgency, C&S absence of infection
- CNS symptoms: insomnia, headache, drowsiness, confusion
- Allergic reactions: fever, flushing, rash, urticaria, pruritus

Teach patient/family:

- That anemia may result with continued administration
- That drug turns urine, sometimes stool, blue green
- To notify physician if symptoms do not improve, or become worse
- To notify physician of any sign/symptoms of side effects or adverse reactions

M

methylergonovine maleate

(meth-ill-er-goe-noe′veen)

Methergine, Methylergobasine*

Func. class.: Oxytocic

Chem. class.: Ergot alkaloid

Action: Stimulates uterine contractions, decreases bleeding

Uses: Treatment of hemorrhage associated with postpartum or postabortion

Dosage and routes:

• *Adult:* IM 0.2 mg q2-5h, not to exceed 5 doses; IV 0.2 mg given over 1 min; PO 0.2-0.4 mg q6-12h × 2-7 days after initial IM or IV dose

Available forms include: Inj IM, IV 0.2 mg/ml; tabs 0.2 mg

Side effects/adverse reactions:

CNS: Headache, dizziness

GI: Nausea, vomiting

CV: Chest pain, palpitation, hypertension

EENT: Tinnitus

INTEG: Sweating, rash

Contraindications: Hypersensitivity to ergot preparations, indication of labor, before delivery of placenta, hypertension, pelvic inflammatory disease (PID), respiratory disease, cardiac disease, peripheral vascular disease

Precautions: Pregnancy (C), severe hepatic disease, severe renal disease, jaundice, diabetes mellitus, convulsive disorders

Pharmacokinetics:

PO: Onset 5-25 min, duration 3 hr

IM: Onset 2-5 min, duration 3 hr

IV: Onset immediate, duration 45 min

Metabolized in liver, excreted in urine

NURSING CONSIDERATIONS

Assess:

• B/P, pulse, character and amount of vaginal bleeding; watch for changes that may indicate hemorrhage

• Respiratory rate, rhythm, depth; notify physician of abnormalities

Administer:

• IV undiluted through Y-tube or 3-way stopcock; give 0.2 mg or less/min

• Only during fourth stage of labor, not to be used to augment labor

• IM in deep muscle mass; rotate injection sites if additional doses are given

• After having crash cart available on unit, IV route used only in emergencies

Evaluate:

• Therapeutic response: absence of postpartum, post abortion hemorrhage

• For uterine relaxation, observe for severe cramping

• Ergot toxicity: tinnitus, hypertension, palpitations, chest pain

Teach patient/family:

• To report increased blood loss, severe abdominal cramps, increased temperature or foul-smelling lochia

methylphenidate HCl

(meth-ill-fen′i-date)

Methidate, Ritalin, Ritalin SR

Func. class.: Cerebral stimulant

Chem. class.: Piperidine derivative

Controlled Substance Schedule II

Action: Increases release of norepinephrine, dopamine in cerebral cortex to reticular activating system; exact action not known

Uses: Attention deficit disorder with hyperactivity, narcolepsy

Dosage and routes:

Attention deficit disorder

• *Child >6 yr:* 5 mg before break-

*Available in Canada only

fast and lunch, increasing by 5-10 mg/wk, not to exceed 60 mg/day

Narcolepsy

• *Adult:* PO 10 mg bid-tid, 30-45 min before meals, may increase up to 40-50 mg/day

Available forms include: Tabs 5, 10, 20 mg; tabs sus rel 20 mg

Side effects/adverse reactions:

CNS: Hyperactivity, insomnia, restlessness, talkativeness, dizziness, headache, akathisia, dyskinesia, Gilles de la Tourette's syndrome

GI: Nausea, anorexia, dry mouth, diarrhea, constipation, weight loss, abdominal pain

CV: Palpitations, tachycardia, B/P changes, angina, dysrhythmias

INTEG: ***Exfoliative dermatitis,*** urticaria, rash, erythema-multiforme

ENDO: Growth retardation

GU: ***Uremia***

HEMA: ***Thrombocytopenia***

Contraindications: Hypersensitivity, anxiety, history of Gilles de la Tourette's syndrome; with history of seizures

Precautions: Hypertension, depression, pregnancy (C), seizures, lactation, drug abuse

Pharmacokinetics:

PO: Onset ½-1 hr, duration 4-6 hr, metabolized by liver, excreted by kidneys

Interactions/incompatibilities:

• Hypertensive crisis: MAOIs or within 14 days of MAOIs, vasopressors

• Decreased effects of: guanethidine, other antihypertensives

• Increased effects: oral anticoagulants, tricyclics, anticonvulsants, caffeine

NURSING CONSIDERATIONS

Assess:

• VS, B/P since this drug may reverse antihypertensives; check patients with cardiac disease more often

• CBC, urinalysis, in diabetes: blood sugar, urine sugar; insulin changes may need to be made since eating will decrease

• Height, growth rate in children; growth rate may be decreased

Administer:

• At least 6 hr before hs to avoid sleeplessness

• For obesity only if patient is on weight reduction program including dietary changes, exercise; patient will develop tolerance, and weight loss won't occur without additional methods, give 30-45 min before meals

• Gum, hard candy, frequent sips of water for dry mouth

Evaluate:

• Therapeutic response: decreased hyperactivity or ability to stay awake

• Mental status: mood, sensorium, affect, stimulation, insomnia, aggressiveness

• Physical dependency: should not be used for extended time; dose should be discontinued gradually, tolerance occurs after long-term use

• Withdrawal symptoms: headache, nausea, vomiting, muscle pain, weakness

Teach patient/family:

• To decrease caffeine consumption (coffee, tea, cola, chocolate); may increase irritability, stimulation

• To avoid OTC preparations unless approved by physician

• To taper off drug over several weeks, or depression, increased sleeping, lethargy will ensue

• To avoid alcohol ingestion

• To avoid hazardous activities until patient is stabilized on medication

M

• To get needed rest; patients will feel more tired at end of day
Treatment of overdose: Administer fluids, hemodialysis or peritoneal dialysis; antihypertensive for increased B/P, administer short-acting barbiturate before lavage

methylprednisolone/methylprednisolone acetate/methylprednisolone sodium succinate

(meth-ill-pred-niss'oh-lone)
Medrol/Depo-Medrol, Duralone, Medralone, Rep-Pred/A-Methapred, Solu-Medrol

Func. class.: Corticosteroid
Chem. class.: Glucocorticoid, immediate acting

Action: Decreases inflammation by suppression of migration of polymorphonuclear leukocytes, fibroblasts, reversal of increased capillary permeability and lysosomal stabilization
Uses: Severe inflammation, shock, adrenal insufficiency, collagen disorders
Dosage and routes:
Adrenal insufficiency/inflammation
• *Adult:* PO 2-60 mg in 4 divided doses; IM 40-80 mg (acetate); IM/IV 10-250 mg (succinate); intra-articular: 4-30 mg (acetate)
• *Child:* IV 117 μg-1.66 mg/kg in 3-4 divided doses (succinate)
Shock
• *Adult:* IV 100-250 mg q2-6h, (succinate)
Available forms include: Tabs 2, 4, 6, 8, 16, 24, 32 mg; inj 20, 40, 80 mg/ml acetate; inj 40, 125, 500, 1000 mg/vial succinate
Side effects/adverse reactions:
INTEG: Acne, poor wound healing, ecchymosis, petechiae
CNS: Depression, flushing, sweating, headache, mood changes
CV: Hypertension, ***circulatory collapse, thrombophlebitis, embolism***, tachycardia
HEMA: ***Thrombocytopenia***
MS: Fractures, osteoporosis, weakness
GI: Diarrhea, nausea, abdominal distention, ***GI hemorrhage,*** *increased appetite,* ***pancreatitis***
EENT: Fungal infections, increased intraocular pressure, blurred vision
Contraindications: Psychosis, hypersensitivity, idiopathic thrombocytopenia, acute glomerulonephritis, amebiasis, fungal infections, nonasthmatic bronchial disease, child <2 yr, *AIDS*, TB
Precautions: Pregnancy (C), diabetes mellitus, glaucoma, osteoporosis, seizure disorders, ulcerative colitis, CHF, myasthenia gravis, renal disease, esophagitis, peptic ulcer
Pharmacokinetics:
PO: Peak 1-2 hr, duration 1½ day
IM: Peak 4-8 days, duration 1-4 wk
INTRAARTICULAR: Peak 1 wk
Half-life >3½ hr
Interactions/incompatibilities:
• Decreased action of methylprednisolone: cholestyramine, colestipol, barbiturates, rifampin, ephedrine, phenytoin, theophylline
• Decreased effects of: anticoagulants, anticonvulsants, antidiabetics, ambenonium, neostigmine, isoniazid, toxoids, vaccines, anticholinesterases, salicylates, somatrem
• Increased side effects: alcohol, salicylates, indomethacin, amphotericin B, digitalis, cyclosporine, diuretics
• Increased action of methylprednisolone: salicylates, estrogens, in-

domethacin, oral contraceptive, ketoconazole, macrolide antibiotics

NURSING CONSIDERATIONS

Assess:

• Potassium, blood sugar, urine glucose while on long-term therapy; hypokalemia and hyperglycemia
• Weight daily, notify physician of weekly gain >5 lb
• B/P q4h, pulse, notify physician if chest pain occurs
• I&O ratio; be alert for decreasing urinary output and increasing edema
• Plasma cortisol levels during long-term therapy (normal level: 138-635 nmol/L SI units when drawn at 8 AM)

Administer:

• IV after diluting with diluent provided, agitate slowly, give 500 mg or less/1 min or longer; may be given as IV infusion
• After shaking suspension (parenteral)
• Titrated dose, use lowest effective dose
• IM inj deeply in large mass, rotate sites, avoid deltoid, use 21G needle
• In one dose in AM to prevent adrenal suppression, avoid SC administration, damage may be done to tissue
• With food or milk to decrease GI symptoms

Perform/provide:

• Assistance with ambulation in patient with bone tissue disease to prevent fractures

Evaluate:

• Therapeutic response: ease of respirations, decreased inflammation
• Infection: increased temperature, WBC, even after withdrawal of medication; drug masks symptoms of infection
• Potassium depletion: paresthesias, fatigue, nausea, vomiting, depression, polyuria, dysrhythmias, weakness
• Edema, hypertension, cardiac symptoms
• Mental status: affect, mood, behavioral changes, aggression

Teach patient/family:

• That ID as steroid user should be carried
• To notify physician if therapeutic response decreases; dosage adjustment may be needed
• Not to discontinue this medication abruptly or adrenal crisis can result
• To avoid OTC products: salicylates, alcohol in cough products, cold preparations unless directed by physician
• About cushingoid symptoms
• Symptoms of adrenal insufficiency: nausea, anorexia, fatigue, dizziness, dyspnea, weakness, joint pain

Lab test interferences:

Increase: Cholesterol, sodium, blood glucose, uric acid, calcium, urine glucose
Decrease: Calcium, potassium, T_4, T_3, thyroid ^{131}I uptake test, urine 17-OHCS, 17-KS, PBI
False negative: Skin allergy tests

methylprednisolone acetate

(meth-ill-pred-niss'oh-lone)
Medrol

Func. class.: Topical corticosteroid
Chem. class.: Synthetic nonfluorinated agent, group VI potency

Action: Possesses antipruritic, antiinflammatory actions
Uses: Psoriasis, eczema, contact dermatitis, pruritus

Dosage and routes:
- *Adult and child:* Apply to affected area qd-qid

Available forms include: Oint 0.25%, 1%

Side effects/adverse reactions:
INTEG: Burning, dryness, itching, irritation, acne, folliculitis, hypertrichosis, perioral dermatitis, hypopigmentation, atrophy, striae, miliaria, allergic contact dermatitis, secondary infection

Contraindications: Hypersensitivity to corticosteroids, fungal infections

Precautions: Pregnancy (C), lactation, viral or bacterial infections

NURSING CONSIDERATIONS

Assess:
- Temperature: if fever develops, drug should be discontinued

Administer:
- Only to affected areas; do not get in eyes
- Medication, then cover with occlusive dressing (only if prescribed), seal to normal skin, change q12h; systemic absorption may occur, use gloves for application
- Only to dermatoses; do not use on weeping, denuded, or infected area

Perform/provide:
- Cleansing before application of drug
- Treatment for a few days after area has cleared
- Storage at room temperature

Evaluate:
- Therapeutic response: absence of severe itching, patches on skin, flaking
- For systemic absorption: increased temperature, inflammation, irritation

Teach patient/family:
- To avoid sunlight on affected area, burns may occur

methyprylon

(meth-i-prye'lon)

Noludar

Func. class.: Sedative-hypnotic
Chem. class.: Piperidine derivative

Controlled Substance Schedule III (USA), Schedule F (Canada)

Action: Acts at level of thalamus to produce CNS mood alterations by interfering with nerve impulse transmission in sensory cortex by increasing threshold of arousal centers

Uses: Insomnia

Dosage and routes:
- *Adult:* PO 200-400 mg 15-30 min before hs
- *Child >12 yrs:* PO 50 mg hs, may increase to 200 mg

Available forms include: Caps 300 mg, tabs 50, 200 mg

Side effects/adverse reactions:
CNS: Residual sedation, dizziness, ataxia, stimulation, headache, pyrexia, nightmares, depression
GI: Nausea, vomiting, diarrhea, esophagitis, constipation
INTEG: Rash, pruritus

Contraindications: Hypersensitivity to piperidine derivatives, severe pain, severe renal or hepatic disease, porphyria

Precautions: Depression, suicidal individuals, drug abuse, cardiac dysrhythmias, narrow-angle glaucoma, prostatic hypertrophy, stenosed peptic ulcer, pyloroduodenal/bladder neck obstruction, pregnancy (B)

Pharmacokinetics:
PO: Onset 45 min, peak 1-2 hr, duration 5-8 hr; metabolized by the liver, excreted by the kidneys, crosses placenta, excreted in breast milk; half-life 3-6 hr

* Available in Canada only

Interactions/incompatibilities:
• Increased CNS depression: alcohol, barbiturates, narcotics and other CNS depressants

NURSING CONSIDERATIONS

Assess:
• Blood studies: Hct, Hgb, RBCs (long-term therapy)
• Hepatic studies: AST, ALT, bilirubin (long-term therapy)

Administer:
• After removal of cigarettes to prevent fires
• After trying conservative measures for insomnia
• ½-1 hr before hs for sleeplessness
• On empty stomach for fast onset, but may be taken with food if GI symptoms occur
• Overdosing symptoms: respiratory depression, hypotension, confusion, coma, constricted pupils

Perform/provide:
• Assistance with ambulation after receiving dose
• Safety measures: siderails, nightlight, call bell within easy reach
• Checking to see PO medication has been swallowed, watch depressed, drug-dependent patients for hoarding, self-overdosing
• Storage in tight, light-resistant container in cool environment

Evaluate:
• Therapeutic response: ability to sleep at night, decreased amount of early morning awakening if taking drug for insomnia
• Mental status: mood, sensorium, affect, memory (long, short)
• Type of sleep problem: falling asleep, staying asleep
• Physical dependency including more frequent requests for medication, shakes, anxiety
• Withdrawal: nausea, vomiting, anxiety, hallucinations, insomnia, tachycardia, fever, cramps, tremors, seizures
• Allergic reaction: rash; discontinue drug if rash occurs

Teach patient/family:
• To avoid driving or other activities requiring alertness until drug stabilizes
• To avoid alcohol ingestion or CNS depressants; serious CNS depression may result
• Not to discontinue medication quickly after long-term use; drug should be tapered over 1-2 wk
• That effects may take 2 nights for benefits to be noticed
• Alternate measures to improve sleep: reading, exercise several hours before hs, warm bath, warm milk, TV, self-hypnosis, deep breathing
• That hangover is common in elderly, but less common than with barbiturates

Treatment of overdose: Lavage, activated charcoal, monitor electrolytes, vital signs

---

methysergide maleate

(meth-i-ser'jide)

Sansert

Func. class.: Serotonin antagonist
Chem. class.: Ergot derivative

Action: Competitively blocks serotonin HT receptors in CNS and periphery; potent vasoconstrictor

Uses: Prophylaxsis for migraine and other vascular headaches

Dosage and routes:
• *Adult:* PO 2 mg bid with meals

Available forms include: Tabs 2 mg

Side effects/adverse reactions:
CNS: Tremors, anxiety, insomnia, headache, dizziness, euphoria, confusion, depersonalization, hal-

lucination, paresthesias, drowsiness
CV: ***Retroperitoneal fibrosis,*** valvular thickening, palpitations, tachycardia, postural hypertension, angina, thrombophlebitis, ECG changes, ***cardiac fibrosis***
GI: Nausea, vomiting, weight gain
MS: Arthralgia, myalgia
INTEG: Flushing, rash, alopecia
HEMA: ***Blood dyscrasias***
Contraindications: Hypersensitivity to ergot, tartrazine, pregnancy, occlusion (peripheral, vascular), CAD, hepatic disease, renal disease, peptic ulcer, hypertension, connective tissue disease, fibrotic pulmonary disease
Precautions: Pregnancy (C), lactation, children
Pharmacokinetics:
PO: Half-life 10 hr, metabolized by liver, excreted in urine (metabolites/unchanged drug)
Interactions/incompatibilities:
• Increased vasoconstriction: β-blockers
• Decreased effect of: narcotic analgesics

NURSING CONSIDERATIONS
Assess:
• Weight daily, check for peripheral edema in feet, legs, B/P
Administer:
• At beginning of headache, dose must be titrated to patient response
• Give with or after meals to avoid GI symptoms
• Only to women who are not pregnant, harm to fetus may occur
Perform/provide:
• Storage in dark area
• Quiet, calm environment with decreased stimulation for noise, bright light, or excessive talking
Evaluate:
• Therapeutic response: decrease in frequency, severity of headache
• For stress level, activity, recreation, coping mechanisms of patient
• Neurologic status: LOC, blurring vision, nausea, vomiting, tingling in extremities that occur preceding headache
• Ingestion of tyramine foods (pickled products, beer, wine, aged cheese), food additives, preservatives, colorings, artificial sweeteners, chocolate, caffeine may precipitate these types of headaches
Teach patient/family:
• Not to use OTC medications; serious drug interactions may occur
• To maintain dose at approved level, not to increase even if drug does not relieve headache
• To report side effects: increased vasoconstriction starting with cold extremities, then paresthesia, weakness
• That an increase in headaches may occur when this drug is discontinued after long-term use
• To keep drug out of reach of children, death may occur
• To report at once: dyspnea, paresthesias, urinary problems, pain in abdomen, chest, back, legs
• To use drug for less than 6 months
• That drug may cause drowsiness

metipranolol HCl

(met-ee-pran'oh-lole)
Betamet
Func. class.: I-isomer

Action: Reduces production of aqueous humor by unknown mechanism
Uses: Ocular hypertension, chronic open-angle glaucoma, secondary glaucoma, aphakic glaucoma
Dosage and routes:
• *Adult:* Instill bid
Available forms include: Sol 0.6%

Side effects/adverse reactions:
CNS: Weakness, fatigue, depression, anxiety, headache, confusion
GI: Nausea, anorexia, dyspepsia
EENT: Eye irritation, conjunctivitis, keratitis
INTEG: Rash, urticaria
Contraindications: Hypersensitivity, asthma, 2nd or 3rd degree heart block, right ventricular failure, congenital glaucoma (infants)
Pharmacokinetics:
INSTILL: Onset 15-30 min, peak 1-2 hr, duration 24 hr
Interactions/incompatibilities:
• Increased effect: propranolol, metoprolol

NURSING CONSIDERATIONS

Evaluate:
• Therapeutic response: decreased intraocular pressure

Teach patient/family:
• To report change in vision (blurring or loss of sight), trouble breathing, sweating, flushing
• Method of instillation, including pressure on lacrimal sac for 1 min, and not to touch dropper to eye
• That long-term therapy may be required
• That blurred vision will decrease with continued use of drug

---

metoclopramide HCl

(met-oh-kloe-pra' mide)
Maxeran,* Reglan

Func. class.: Cholinergic
Chem. class.: Central dopamine receptor antagonist

Action: Enhances response to acetylcholine of tissue in upper GI tract, which causes contraction of gastric muscle, relaxes pyloric, duodenal segments, increases peristalsis without stimulating secretions

Uses: Prevention of nausea, vomiting induced by chemotherapy, radiation, delayed gastric emptying, gastroesophageal reflux

Dosage and routes:

Nausea/vomiting
• *Adult:* IV 2 mg/kg q2h × 5 doses 30 min before administration of chemotherapy

Delayed gastric emptying
• *Adult:* PO 10 mg 30 min ac, hs × 2-8 wk

Gastroesophageal reflux
• *Adult:* PO 10-15 mg qid 30 min ac

Available forms include: Tabs 5, 10 mg; syr 5 mg/5 ml; inj IV 5 mg/ml

Side effects/adverse reactions:
CNS: Sedation, fatigue, restlessness, headache, sleeplessness, dystonia, dizziness, drowsiness
GI: Dry mouth, constipation, nausea, anorexia, vomiting
GU: Decreased libido, prolactin secretion, amenorrhea, galactorrhea
CV: Hypotension, supraventricular tachycardia
INTEG: Urticaria, rash

Contraindications: Hypersensitivity to this drug or procaine or procainamide, seizure disorder, pheochromocytoma, breast cancer, GI obstruction

Precautions: Pregnancy (B), lactation, GI hemorrhage, CHF

Pharmacokinetics:
IV: Onset 1-3 min, duration 1-2 hr
PO: Onset ½-1 hr, duration 1-2 hr
IM: Onset 10-15 min, duration 1-2 hr
Metabolized by liver, excreted in urine, half-life 4 hr

Interactions/incompatibilities:
• Decreased action of metoclopramide: anticholinergics, opiates
• Increased sedation: alcohol, other CNS depressants

M

NURSING CONSIDERATIONS

Administer:

- IV undiluted if dose is <10 mg; give over 2 min; 10 mg or more may be diluted in 50 ml or more compatible sol and given over 15 min or more
- ½-1 hr before meals for better absorption
- Gum, hard candy, frequent rinsing of mouth for dryness of oral cavity

Perform/provide:

- Protect from light with aluminum foil during infusion
- Discard open ampules

Evaluate:

- Therapeutic response: absence of nausea, vomiting, anorexia, fullness
- GI complaints: nausea, vomiting, anorexia, constipation

Teach patient/family:

- To avoid driving or other hazardous activities until patient is stabilized on this medication
- To avoid alcohol or other CNS depressants that will enhance sedating properties of this drug

Lab test interferences:

Increase: Prolactin, aldosterone, thyrotropin

---

metocurine iodide

(met-oh-kyoo'reen)

Metubine Iodide

Func. class.: Neuromuscular blocker (nondepolarizing)

Chem. class.: Methyl analog of tubocurarine

Action: Inhibits transmission of nerve impulses by binding with cholinergic receptor sites, antagonizing action of acetylcholine

Uses: Facilitation of endotracheal intubation, skeletal muscle relaxation during mechanical ventilation, surgery, or general anesthesia, reduction of fractures/dislocations

Dosage and routes:

- *Adult:* IV 2-4 mg if given cyclopropane as an anesthetic; 1.5-3 mg if given ether as an anesthetic; 4-7 mg if given nitrous oxide

Available forms include: Inj IV 2 mg/ml

Side effects/adverse reactions:

CV: Bradycardia, tachycardia, increased, decreased B/P

RESP: ***Prolonged apnea, bronchospasm, cyanosis, respiratory depression***

EENT: Increased secretions

INTEG: Rash, flushing, pruritus, urticaria

Contraindications: Hypersensitivity to iodides

Precautions: Pregnancy (C), cardiac disease, hepatic disease, renal disease, lactation, children <2 yr, electrolyte imbalances, dehydration, neuromuscular disease (myasthenia gravis), respiratory disease, or when histamine release is a definite hazard (e.g., asthma)

Pharmacokinetics:

IV: Peak 3-5 min, duration 35-90 min; half-life 3½ hr, excreted in urine, bile (½ unchanged), crosses placenta

Interactions/incompatibilities:

- Increased neuromuscular blockade: aminoglycosides, clindamycin, lincomycin, quinidine, local anesthetics, polymyxin antibiotics, lithium, narcotic analgesics, thiazides, enflurane, isoflurane
- Dysrhythmias: theophylline
- Do not mix with barbiturates in solution or syringe

NURSING CONSIDERATIONS

Assess:

- For electrolyte imbalances (K,

* Available in Canada only

Mg), may lead to increased action of this drug
• Vital signs (B/P, pulse, respirations, airway) until fully recovered; rate, depth, pattern of respirations (keep airway clear), strength of hand grip
• I&O ratio; check for urinary retention, frequency, hesitancy

Administer:
• Using nerve stimulator by anesthesiologist to determine neuromuscular blockade
• Anticholinesterase to reverse neuromuscular blockade
• By slow IV over 1-2 min (only by qualified person, usually an anesthesiologist)
• Only slightly discolored solution

Perform/provide:
• Storage in light-resistant, cool area
• Reassurance if communication is difficult during recovery from neuromuscular blockade

Evaluate:
• Therapeutic response: paralysis of jaw, eyelid, head, neck, rest of body
• Recovery: decreased paralysis of face, diaphragm, leg, arm, rest of body
• Allergic reactions: rash, fever, respiratory distress, pruritus; drug should be discontinued

Treatment of overdose: Edrophonium or neostigmine, atropine, monitor VS; may require mechanical ventilation

Teach patient/family: That postoperative stiffness is normal and will subside

metolazone

(me-tole'a-zone)
Diulo, Zaroxolyn

Func. class.: Diuretic
Chem. class.: Thiazide-like; quinazoline derivative

Action: Acts on distal tubule by increasing excretion of water, sodium, chloride, potassium

Uses: Edema, hypertension, CHF

Dosage and routes:

Edema
• *Adult:* PO 5-20 mg/day

Hypertension
• *Adult:* PO 2.5-5 mg/day

Available forms include: Tabs 0.5, 2.5, 5, 10 mg

Side effects/adverse reactions:

GU: Frequency, polyuria, ***uremia, glucosuria***

CNS: Drowsiness, paresthesia, anxiety, depression, headache, *dizziness, fatigue, weakness*

GI: Nausea, vomiting, anorexia, constipation, diarrhea, cramps, pancreatitis, GI irration, ***hepatitis***

EENT: Blurred vision

INTEG: Rash, urticaria, purpura, photosensitivity, fever

META: Hyperglycemia, hyperuricemia, increased creatinine, BUN

HEMA: ***Aplastic anemia, hemolytic anemia, leukopenia, agranulocytosis, thrombocytopenia,*** neutropenia

CV: Irregular pulse, orthostatic hypotension, palpitations, volume depletion

ELECT: Hypokalemia, hypomagnesemia, hypercalcemia, hyponatremia, hypochloremia

Contraindications: Hypersensitivity to thiazides or sulfonamides, anuria, pregnancy (D)

Precautions: Hypokalemia, renal

disease, hepatic disease, gout, COPD, lupus erythematosus, diabetes mellitus

Pharmacokinetics:

PO: Onset 1 hr, peak 2 hr, duration 12-24 hr; excreted unchanged by kidneys, crosses placenta, enters breast milk, half-life 8 hr

Interactions/incompatibilities:

• Synergism: furosemide
• Increased toxicity of: lithium, nondepolarizing skeletal muscle relaxants
• Decreased effects of: antidiabetics
• Decreased absorption of: thiazides, cholestyramine, colestipol
• Decreased hypotensive response: indomethacin
• Hyperglycemia, hyperuricemia, hypotension: diazoxide

NURSING CONSIDERATIONS

Assess:

• Weight, I&O daily to determine fluid loss; effect of drug may be decreased if used qd
• Rate, depth, rhythm of respiration, effect of exertion
• B/P lying, standing, postural hypotension may occur
• Electrolytes: potassium, magnesium, sodium, chloride; include BUN, blood sugar, CBC, serum creatinine, blood pH, ABGs, uric acid, calcium
• Glucose in urine if patient is diabetic

Administer:

• In AM to avoid interference with sleep if using drug as a diuretic
• Potassium replacement if potassium is less than 3.0
• With food, if nausea occurs, absorption may be decreased slightly

Evaluate:

• Therapeutic response: decreased edema, B/P
• Improvement in edema of feet, legs, sacral area daily if medication is being used in CHF
• Improvement in CVP q8h
• Signs of metabolic alkalosis: drowsiness, restlessness
• Signs of hypokalemia: postural hypotension, malaise, fatigue, tachycardia, leg cramps, weakness
• Rashes, temperature elevation qd
• Confusion, especially in elderly; take safety precautions if needed

Teach patient/family:

• To increase fluid intake 2-3 L/day unless contraindicated, to rise slowly from lying or sitting position
• To notify physician of muscle weakness, cramps, nausea, dizziness
• That drug may be taken with food or milk
• That blood sugar may be increased in diabetics
• To take early in day to avoid nocturia

Lab test interferences:

Increase: BSP retention, calcium, amylase, parathyroid test
Decrease: PBI, PSP

Treatment of overdose: Lavage if taken orally, monitor electrolytes, administer dextrose in saline, monitor hydration, CV, renal status

---

metoprolol tartrate

(met-oh'proe-lole)
Betaloc,* Lopresor,* Lopressor
Func. class.: Antihypertensive
Chem. class.: β_1-blocker

Action: Produces falls in B/P without reflex tachycardia or significant reduction in heart rate through β-blocking effects; elevated plasma renins are reduced; blocks β_2-adrenergic receptors in bronchial, vascular smooth muscle only at

* Available in Canada only

high doses (decreases rate of SA node)

Uses: Mild to moderate hypertension, acute myocardial infarction to reduce cardiovascular mortality, angina pectoris

Dosage and routes:

Hypertension

• *Adult:* PO 50 mg bid, or 100 mg qd, may give up to 200-450 mg in divided doses

Myocardial infarction

• *Adult:* (early treatment) IV bol 5 mg q2min × 3, then 50 mg PO 15 min after last dose and q6h × 48 hr; (late treatment) PO maintenance 100 mg bid for 3 mo

Available forms include: Tabs 50, 100 mg; inj IV 1 mg/ml

Side effects/adverse reactions:

CV: Hypotension, *bradycardia, CHF: Palpitations,* dysrhythmias, ***cardiac arrest, AV block***

CNS: Insomnia, dizziness, mental changes, hallucinations, ***depression,*** anxiety, headaches, nightmares, confusion, fatigue

GI: Nausea, vomiting, colitis, cramps, ***diarrhea,*** constipation, flatulence, dry mouth, ***hiccups***

INTEG: Rash, purpura, alopecia, dry skin, urticaria, pruritus

HEMA: ***Agranulocytosis, eosinophilia, thrombocytopenia, purpura***

EENT: Sore throat, dry burning eyes

GU: Impotence

RESP: ***Bronchospasm,*** dyspnea, wheezing

Contraindications: Hypersensitivity to β-blockers, cardiogenic shock, heart block (2nd, 3rd degree), sinus bradycardia, CHF, bronchial asthma

Precautions: Major surgery, pregnancy (C), lactation, diabetes mellitus, renal disease, thyroid disease, COPD, heart failure, CAD, nonallergic bronchospasm, hepatic disease

Pharmacokinetics:

PO: Peak 2-4 hr, duration 13-19 hr; half-life 3-4 hr, metabolized in liver (metabolites), excreted in urine, crosses placenta, enters breast milk

Interactions/incompatibilities:

• Increased hypotension, bradycardia: reserpine, hydralazine, methyldopa, prazosin, anticholinergics

• Decreased antihypertensive effects: indomethacin, sympathomimetics

• Increased hypoglycemic effects: insulin

• Decreased bronchodilation: theophyllines

NURSING CONSIDERATIONS

Assess:

• ECG, directly when giving IV during initial treatment

• I&O, weight daily

• B/P during initial treatment, periodically thereafter; pulse q4h; note rate, rhythm, quality

• Apical/radial pulse before administration; notify physician of any significant changes

• Baselines in renal, liver function tests before therapy begins

Administer:

• PO ac, hs, tablet may be crushed or swallowed whole

• Reduced dosage in renal dysfunction

• IV, undiluted, give over 1 min, keep patient recumbent for 3 hr

Perform/provide:

• Storage in dry area at room temperature, do not freeze

Evaluate:

• Therapeutic response: decreased B/P after 1-2 wk

• Edema in feet, legs daily

• Skin turgor, dryness of mucous membranes for hydration status

M

Teach patient/family:

• To take with or immediately after meals

• Not to discontinue drug abruptly, taper over 2 wk, may cause precipitate angina

• Not to use OTC products containing α-adrenergic stimulants (nasal decongestants, OTC cold preparations) unless directed by physician

• To report bradycardia, dizziness, confusion, depression, fever, sore throat, shortness of breath to physician

• To take pulse at home, advise when to notify physician

• To avoid alcohol, smoking, sodium intake

• To comply with weight control, dietary adjustments, modified exercise program

• To carry Medic Alert ID to identify drug you are taking, allergies

• To avoid hazardous activities if dizziness is present

• To report symptoms of CHF: difficult breathing, especially on exertion or when lying down, night cough, swelling of extremities

• To take medication hs to prevent effect of orthostatic hypotension

• To wear support hose to minimize effects of orthostatic hypotension

Lab test interferences:

Increase: Liver function tests, renal function tests

Treatment of overdose: Lavage, IV atropine for bradycardia, IV theophylline for bronchospasm, digitalis, O_2, diuretic for cardiac failure, hemodialysis, hypotension administer vasopressor (norepinephrine)

metronidazole/metronidazole HCl

(me-troe-ni'da-zole)

Apo-Metronidazole,* Flagyl, Metryl, Neo-Tric,* Novonidazole,* PMS-Metronidazole,* Satric, Trikacide,* Flagyl IV, Flagyl IV RTU, Metro IV, Femazole, Metizol, Metronid, Protostat

Func. class.: Trichomonacide, amebicide

Chem. class.: Nitroimidazole derivative

Action: Direct-acting amebicide/trichomonacide binds, degrades DNA in organism

Uses: Intestinal amebiasis, amebic abscess, trichomoniasis, refractory trichomoniasis, bacterial anaerobic infections, giardiasis

Dosage and routes:

Trichomoniasis

• *Adult:* PO 250 mg tid × 7 days, or 2 g in single dose; do not repeat treatment for 2-3 wk

Refractory trichomoniasis

• *Adult:* PO 250 mg bid × 10 days

Amebic abscess

• *Adult:* PO 500-750 mg tid × 5-10 days

• *Child:* PO 35-50 mg/kg/day in 3 divided doses × 10 days

Intestinal amebiasis

• *Adult:* PO 750 mg tid × 5-10 days

• *Child:* PO 35-50 mg/kg/day in 3 divided doses × 10 days; then give oral iodoquinol

Anerobic bacterial infections

• *Adult:* IV INF 15 mg/kg over 1 hr, then 7.5 mg/kg IV or PO q6h, not to exceed 4 g/day

Giardiasis

• *Adult:* PO 250 mg tid × 5 days

• *Child:* PO 5 mg/kg tid × 5 days

* Available in Canada only

Available forms include: Tabs 250, 500 mg; film-coated tabs 250, 1500 mg; inj IV 5 mg/vial; HCl inj IV 500 mg

Side effects/adverse reactions:

CV: Flat T waves

HEMA: ***Leukopenia, bone marrow aplasia***

INTEG: Rash, pruritus, urticaria, flushing

CNS: Headache, dizziness, confusion, depression, fatigue, drowsiness, insomnia, paresthesia, peripheal neuropathy, ***convulsions,*** incoordination, depression

EENT: Blurred vision, sore throat, retinal edema, dry mouth, bitter taste, furry tongue, glossitis, stomatitis

GI: Nausea, vomiting, diarrhea, epigastric distress, anorexia, constipation, abdominal cramps, metallic taste, ***pseudomembranous colitis***

GU: Polyuria, ***albuminuria,*** dysuria, cystitis, decreased libido, ***nephrotoxicity,*** incontinence, dyspareunia

Contraindications: Hypersensitivity to this drug, renal disease, hepatic disease, contracted visual or color fields, blood dyscrasias, pregnancy (1st trimester), lactation, CNS disorders

Precautions: *Candida* infections, pregnancy (2nd, 3rd trimesters) (B)

Pharmacokinetics:

IV/PO: Peak 1-2 hr, half-life 6⅕-11½ hr, crosses placenta, excreted in feces

Interactions/incompatibilities:

- Disulfiram reaction: alcohol
- May increase action of: warfarin
- Psychosis: disulfiram
- Decreased action of metronidazole: phenobarbital

NURSING CONSIDERATIONS

Assess:

- Stools during entire treatment; should be clear at end of therapy, stools should be free of parasites for 1 yr before patient is considered cured (amebiasis)
- Vision by ophthalmic exam during, after therapy; vision problems occur often
- I&O, stools for number, frequency, character

Administer:

- IV is prediluted, Flagyl IV; dilute with 4.4 ml sterile H_2O or 0.9% sodium chloride; must be diluted further with 8 mg/ml or more compatible sol, must neutralize with 5 mEq of Na_2CO_3/500 mg; may need to vent, run over 1 hr; primary IV must be discontinued; may be given as continuous infusion
- PO after meals to avoid GI symptoms, metallic taste

Perform/provide:

- Storage in light-resistant container

Evaluate:

- Therapeutic response: decreased symptoms of infection
- Neurotoxicity: peripheral neuropathy, seizures, dizziness, incoordination, pruritus, joint pains; may be discontinued
- Allergic reaction: fever, rash, itching, chills; drug should be discontinued if these occur
- Superimposed infection: fever, monilial growth, fatigue, malaise
- Renal and reproductive dysfunction: dysuria, polyuria, impotence, dyspareunia, decreased libido

Teach patient family:

- That urine may turn dark reddish brown
- Proper hygiene after BM: handwashing technique
- Need for compliance with dosage schedule, duration of treatment
- To use condoms if treatment for

trichomoniasis or cross contamination may occur
• That treatment of both partners is necessary
• Not to drink alcohol
Lab test interferences:
Decrease: AST, ALT

metyrosine

(me-tye'roe-seen)
Demser

Func. class.: Antihypertensive
Chem. class.: Adrenergic blocker

Action: Inhibits enzyme tyrosine hydroxylase, resulting in decreased levels of catecholamines
Uses: Pheochromocytoma
Dosage and routes:
• *Adult and child >12 yr:* PO 250 mg qid, may increase by 250-500 mg qd to a max of 4 g/day in divided doses
Available forms include: Caps 250 mg
Side effects/adverse reactions:
CNS: Sedation, drowsiness, dizziness, headache, depression, EPS, hallucinations, psychosis, agitation
INTEG: Rash, urticaria
EENT: Dry mouth
GU: Dysuria, ***oliguria, hematuria,*** enuresis, impotence
GI: Nausea, vomiting, anorexia, diarrhea, abdominal pain
MISC: Breast swelling, nasal stuffiness
Contraindications: Hypersensitivity, essential hypertension, children <12 yr
Precautions: Pregnancy (C), lactation, hepatic disease, renal disease
Pharmacokinetics:
PO: Onset 2 days, duration 3-4 days; half-life 3.4-3.7 hr, excreted in urine
Interactions/incompatibilities:
• Increased sedation: CNS depressants: alcohol, barbiturates, antipsychotics
• Decreased effects of: levodopa
• Extrapyramidal effects: phenothiazines, haloperidol

NURSING CONSIDERATIONS

Assess:
• Electrolytes: K, Na, Cl, CO_2
• Renal function studies: catecholamines, BUN, creatinine
• Hepatic function studies: AST, ALT, alk phosphatase
• ECG, BMR
• B/P, other VS throughout treatment
• Weight daily, I&O
Administer:
• Antiemetic or antidiarrheals for vomiting, diarrhea
Perform/provide:
• Fluids to 2 L/day to prevent crystallization by kidneys
Evaluate:
• Therapeutic response: decreased B/P, decreased levels of catecholamines
• Change in behavior or personality: psychosis, anxiety, hallucinations, EPS
• Nausea, vomiting, diarrhea
• Edema in feet, legs daily
• Skin turgor, dryness of mucous membranes for hydration status
Teach patient/family:
• To take each dose with a full glass of water; maintain sufficient daily intake
• Not to drive or perform hazardous tasks if behavioral changes, dizziness, or drowsiness occurs
• To avoid alcohol or other CNS depressants
• To notify physician if any of following occur: jaw stiffness, drooling, speech difficulty, tremors, dis-

orientation, diarrhea, painful urination
Lab test interferences:
False increase: Urinary catecholamines
Treatment of overdose: Administer vasopressors, discontinue drug

mexiletine HCl

(mex-il'e-teen)
Mexitil
Func. class.: Antidysrhythmic (Class IB)
Chem. class.: Lidocaine analog

Action: Increases electrical stimulation threshold of ventricle, His-Purkinje system, which stabilizes cardiac membrane
Uses: Ventricular tachycardia, ventricular dysrhythmias during cardiac surgery, myocardial infarction
Dosage and routes:
• *Adult:* PO 200-400 mg q8h
Available forms include: Caps 150, 200, 250 mg
Side effects/adverse reactions:
CNS: Headache, dizziness, confusion, ***convulsions,*** tremors, psychosis, nervousness, paresthesias, weakness, fatigue, coordination difficulties, change in sleep habits
EENT: Blurred vision, hearing loss, tinnitus
GI: Nausea, vomiting, anorexia, diarrhea, abdominal pain, ***hepatitis,*** dry mouth, peptic ulcer, altered taste, GI bleeding
CV: Hypotension, bradycardia, angina, PVCs, ***heart block, cardiovascular collapse, arrest,*** sinus node slowing, ***left ventricular failure***, syncope, ***cardiogenic shock***
RESP: Dyspnea, ***fibrosis, embolism,*** pneumonia
INTEG: Rash, alopecia, dry skin
HEMA: ***Thrombocytopenia, leukopenia, agranulocytosis, hypoplastic anemia,*** systemic lupus erythematosus syndrome
GU: Urinary hesitancy, decreased libido
MISC: Edema, arthralgia, fever
Contraindications: Hypersensitivity to amides, cardiogenic shock, blood dyscrasias, severe heart block
Precautions: Pregnancy (C), lactation, children, renal disease, liver disease, CHF, respiratory depression, myasthenia gravis
Pharmacokinetics:
PO: Peak 2-3 hr; half-life 12 hr, metabolized by liver, excreted unchanged by kidneys (10%), excreted in breast milk
Interactions/incompatibilities:
• Increased effects: cimetidine
• Decreased levels of mexiletine: phenytoin, phenobarbital, rifampin

NURSING CONSIDERATIONS

Assess:
• ECG continuously to determine increased PR or QRS segments; if these develop, discontinue or reduce rate; watch for increased ventricular ectopic beats, may need to rebolus
• Blood levels (therapeutic level 0.5-2 μg/ml)
• B/P continuously for fluctuations
• I&O ratio, electrolytes (K, Na, Cl), liver enzymes
Evaluate:
• Therapeutic response: decreased dysrhythmias
• Malignant hyperthermia: tachypnea, tachycardia, changes in B/P, increased temperature
• Cardiac rate, respiration: rate, rhythm, character
• Respiratory status: rate, rhythm,

M

lung fields for rales, watch for respiratory depression

• CNS effects: dizziness, confusion, psychosis, paresthesias, convulsions; drug should be discontinued

• Lung fields, bilateral rales may occur in CHF patient

• Increased respiration, increased pulse, drug should be discontinued

Lab test interferences:

Increase: CPK

Treatment of overdose: O_2, artificial ventilation, ECG, administer dopamine for circulatory depression, administer diazepam or thiopental for convulsions, acidify urine

mezlocillin sodium

(mez-loe-sill'in)

Mezlin

Func. class.: Broad-spectrum antibiotic

Chem. class.: Extended-spectrum penicillin

Action: Interferes with cell wall replication of susceptible organisms; osmotically unstable cell wall swells, bursts from osmotic pressure

Uses: Effective for gram-positive cocci (*S. aureus, S. viridans, S. faecalis, S. pneumoniae),* gram-negative cocci *(N. gonorrhoeae),* gram-positive bacilli, *C. perfringens, C. tetani,* gram-negative bacilli (*Bacteroides, E. coli, H. influenzae, Klebsiella, P. mirabilis, Peptococcus, Peptostreptococcus, M. morganii, Enterobacter, Serratia, Pseudomonas, P. vulgaris, P. rettgeri, Shigella, Citrobacter, Veillonella)*

Dosage and routes:

• *Adult:* IM/IV 200-300 mg/kg/day in divided doses q4-6h, may give up to 24 g/day for severe infections

• *Child:* IM/IV 50 mg/kg q4-6h

• *Infants >8 days; >*2000 g: 75 mg/kg q6h; <2000 g: 75 mg/kg q8h

• *Infants <8 days:* 75 mg/kg q12h

Available forms include: Powder for inj IM, IV 1, 2, 3, 4 g; IV INF 2, 3, 4 g

Side effects/adverse reactions:

HEMA: Anemia, increased bleeding time, ***bone marrow depression, granulocytopenia***

GI: Nausea, vomiting, diarrhea, increased AST, ALT, abdominal pain, glossitis, colitis

GU: Oliguria, proteinuria, hematuria, (vaginitis, moniliasis), ***glomerulonephritis***

CNS: Lethargy, hallucinations, anxiety, depression, twitching, ***coma, convulsions***

META: Hyperkalemia, hypokalemia, alkalosis, hypernatremia

Contraindications: Hypersensitivity to penicillins

Precautions: Pregnancy (B), hypersensitivity to cephalosporins, neonates

Pharmacokinetics:

IM: Peak 45 min

IV: Peak 5 min

Half-life 50-55 min, partially metabolized in liver, excreted in urine, bile, breast milk (small amount), crosses placenta

Interactions/incompatibilities:

• Decreased effectiveness of: aminoglycosides

• Decreased antimicrobial effectiveness of mezlocillin: tetracyclines, erythromycins

• Increased mezlocillin concentrations: aspirin, probenecid

NURSING CONSIDERATIONS

Assess:

• I&O ratio; report hematuria, oli-

* Available in Canada only

guria since penicillin in high doses is nephrotoxic

- Any patient with compromised renal system since drug is excreted slowly in poor renal system function; toxicity may occur rapidly
- Liver studies: AST, ALT
- Blood studies: WBC, RBC, H&H, bleeding time
- Renal studies: urinalysis, protein, blood
- C&S before drug therapy; drug may be taken as soon as culture is taken

Administer:

- IV after diluting 1g or less/10 ml of sterile H_2O, D_5, or 0.9% NaCl for inj, shake, dilute further with D_5W or 0.45 NaCl and give over 3-5 min; may be given by intermittent INF over ½ hr
- Drug after C&S has been completed

Perform/provide:

- Adrenalin, suction, tracheostomy set, endotracheal intubation equipment
- Adequate fluid intake (2000 ml) during diarrhea episodes
- Scratch test to assess allergy, after securing order from physician; usually done when penicillin is only drug of choice
- Storage at room temperature; reconstituted solution is stable for 24 hr refrigerated

Evaluate:

- Therapeutic response: absence of fever, draining wounds
- Bowel pattern before and during treatment
- Skin eruptions after administration of penicillin to 1 wk after discontinuing drug
- Respiratory status: rate, character, wheezing, and tightness in chest
- Allergies before initiation of treatment, and reaction of each medication; highlight allergies on chart, Kardex

Teach patient/family:

- That culture may be taken after completed course of medication
- To report sore throat, fever, fatigue (could indicate superimposed infection)
- To wear or carry Medic Alert ID if allergic to penicillins
- To notify nurse of diarrhea

Lab test interferences:
False positive: Urine glucose, urine protein

Treatment of overdose: Withdraw drug, maintain airway, administer epinephrine, aminophylline, O_2, IV corticosteroids for anaphylaxis

miconazole

(mi-kon'a-zole)
Monistat, Monistat IV
Func. class.: Antifungal
Chem. class.: Imidazole

Action: Alters cell membranes and inhibits fungal enzymes

Uses: Coccidioidomycosis, candidiasis, cryptococcosis, paracoccidioidomycosis, chronic mucocutaneous candidiasis, fungal meningitis; IV used for severe infections only

Dosage and routes:

- *Adult:* IV INF 200-3600 mg/day; may be divided in 3 infusions 200-1200 mg/infusion; may need to repeat course; intrathecal 20 mg given simultaneously with IV for fungal meningitis q3-7d
- *Adult:* TOP apply to affected areas bid; vag cream apply × 1 wk qhs or × 3 days (Monistat 3 vs Monistat 7)
- *Child:* IV 20-40 mg/kg/day, not to exceed 15 mg/kg/inf

Available forms include: Inj IV 10 mg/ml; aerosol 2%; cream, lotion, powder, vaginal cream (2%); supp, vaginal 100, 200 mg

Side effects/adverse reactions:

CV: Tachycardia, dysrhythmias (rapid IV)

INTEG: Pruritus, rash, fever, flushing, ***anaphylaxis,*** hives

CNS: Drowsiness, headache

GU: Vulvovaginal burning, itching, hyponatremia, pelvic cramps (topical forms)

GI: Nausea, vomiting, anorexia, diarrhea, cramps

HEMA: Decreased Hct, ***thrombocytopenia,*** hyperlipidemia

Contraindications: Hypersensitivity

Precautions: Renal disease, hepatic disease, pregnancy (B)

Pharmacokinetics:

IV: Half-life triphasic 0.4, 2.1, 24.1 hr, metabolized in liver, excreted in feces, urine (inactive metabolites), >90% protein binding

Interactions/incompatibilities:

• Increased action of: anticoagulants

• Decreased action of both drugs: amphotericin

NURSING CONSIDERATIONS

Assess:

• Cardiac system: B/P, pulse, ECG; watch for increasing pulse, cardiac dysrhythmias; drug should be discontinued if these occur

• Blood studies: Hct, Ca, cholesterol, triglycerides, platelets, sodium

Administer:

• After C&S is obtained to identify causative organism

• Antiemetic for nausea and vomiting as ordered

• After test dose of 200 mg is given by physician; watch for allergic reactions

• IV over ½-1 hr, dilute in 200 ml isotonic saline or D_5W

• IV after diluting with NS if hyponatremia has occurred

• Topical by rubbing into affected area

Evaluate:

• Therapeutic response: decreased fever, malaise, rash, negative C&S for infecting organism

• For phlebitis, pruritus; may need benadryl IV, continue unless reaction is severe

• Allergic reaction after test dose; have epinephrine available

Perform/provide:

• Storage of diluted preparations at room temperature for 24 hr

Teach patient/family:

• That long-term therapy may be needed to clear infection (1 wk-1 mo)

• Proper hygiene: handwashing techniques, nail care

• To report vaginitis; use light-day pad for vaginal dose

• To avoid contact with eyes, nose

• To avoid sexual contact during treatment; reinfection may occur

• To avoid use of occlusive dressings

miconazole nitrate (topical)

(mi-kon'a-zole)

Micatin, Monistat-Derm, Monistat

Func. class.: Local antiinfective

Chem. class.: Antifungal

Action: Interferes with fungal cell membrane, which increases permeability, leaking of nutrients

Uses: Tinea pedis, tinea cruris, tinea corporis, tinea versicolor, vaginal or vulvae *Candida albicans*

Dosage and routes:

• *Adult and child:* TOP apply to affected area bid × 2-4 wk

* Available in Canada only

• *Adult:* Intra vag give 1 applicator or suppository ×7 days hs
Available forms include: Cream, lotion, powder, spray 2%; vag cream 2%; vag supp 100, 200 mg
Side effects/adverse reactions:
GU: Vulvovaginal burning, itching, pelvic cramps
INTEG: Rash, urticaria, stinging, burning, contact dermatitis
Contraindications: Hypersensitivity
Precautions: Child <2 yr, pregnancy (B), lactation

NURSING CONSIDERATIONS

Administer:
• Enough medication to completely cover lesions
• After cleansing with soap, water before each application, dry well
Perform/provide:
• Storage at room temperature in dry place
Evaluate:
• Therapeutic response: decrease in size, number of lesions
• Allergic reaction: burning, stinging, swelling, redness
Teach patient/family:
• To use medical asepsis (hand washing) before, after each application
• To apply with glove to prevent further infection
• To avoid use of OTC creams, ointments, lotions unless directed by physician
• To avoid contact with eyes
• To avoid use of occlusive dressings
• To notify physician if no improvement in condition in 4 wk

microfibrillar collagen hemostat

Avitene, MCH

Func. class.: Hemostatic
Chem. class.: Purified cattle collagen

Action: Platelets adhere to hemostat, cause aggregation to and formation of thrombi
Uses: For hemostasis in surgery when ligature is ineffective/impractical
Dosage and routes:
• *Adult and child:* TOP apply to bleeding area after drying with sponge, compress for 1-5 min, may reapply if needed
• ***Available forms include:*** Fibrous form, non-woven web form
Side effects/adverse reactions:
INTEG: Rash, abscess, allergic reactions, infection, wound dehiscence
HEMA: Hematoma
Contraindications: Hypersensitivity, closure of skin incision
Precautions: Pregnancy (C)

NURSING CONSIDERATIONS

Administer:
• Dry, do not moisten
• Using gloves with forceps; area must be dry for drug to work
• Only new product; do not resterilize
Evaluate:
• Therapeutic response: decreased bleeding in surgery
• Possible infection: hematoma, abscess
• Allergy: rash, itching

M

midazolam HCl

(mid′-az-zoe-lam)

Versed

Func. class.: General anesthetic
Chem. class.: Benzodiazepine, short-acting

Controlled Substance Schedule IV

Action: Depresses subcortical levels in CNS; may act on limbic system, reticular formation; may potentiate γ-aminobenzoic acid (GABA) by binding to specific benzodiazepine receptors

Uses: Preoperative sedation, general anesthesia induction, sedation for diagnostic endoscopic procedures, intubation

Dosage and routes:

Preoperative sedation

Adult: IM 0.07-0.08 mg/kg ½-1 hr before general anesthesia

Induction of general anesthesia

Adult: IV (unpremedicated patients) 0.3-0.35 mg/kg over 30 sec, wait 2 min, follow with 25% of initial dose if needed; (premedicated patients) 0.15-0.35 mg/kg over 20-30 sec, allow 2 min for effect

Available forms include: Inj 1, 5 mg/ml

Side effects/adverse reactions:

CNS: Retrograde amnesia, euphoria, confusion, headache, anxiety, insomnia, slurred speech, paresthesia, tremors, weakness, chills

RESP: Coughing, ***apnea, bronchospasm, laryngospasm,*** dyspnea

CV: Hypotension, PVCs, tachycardia, bigeminy, nodal rhythm

EENT: Blurred vision, nystagmus, diplopia, blocked ears, loss of balance

GI: Nausea, vomiting, increased salivation, hiccups

INTEG: Urticaria, pain, swelling at injection site, rash, pruritus

Contraindications: Pregnancy (D), hypersensitivity to benzodiazepines, shock, coma, alcohol intoxication, acute narrow-angle glaucoma

Precautions: COPD, CHF, chronic renal failure, chills, elderly, debilitated

Pharmacokinetics:

IM: Onset: 15 min, peak ½-1 hr

IV: Onset: 3-5 min, onset of anesthesia 1½-2½ min, protein binding 97%, half-life 1.2-12.3 hr, metabolized in liver, metabolites excreted in urine, crosses placenta, blood-brain barrier

Interactions/incompatibilities:

- Prolonged respiratory depression: other CNS depressants, alcohol, barbiturates
- Increased hypnotic effect: fentanyl, narcotic agonists, analgesics, droperidol

NURSING CONSIDERATIONS

Assess:

- Injection site for redness, pain, swelling
- Degree of amnesia in elderly; may be increased

Administer:

- IV after diluting with D_5W or 0.9% NaCl to a concentration of 0.25 mg/ml; give over 2 min (conscious sedation) or over 30 sec (anesthesia induction)
- IM deep into large muscle mass

Perform/provide:

- Assistance with ambulation until drowsy period relieved
- Storage at room temperature

Evaluate:

- Therapeutic response: induction of sedation, general anesthesia
- Anterograde amnesia
- Vital signs for recovery period in

obese patient, since half-life may be extended

Teach patient/family:
- To avoid hazardous activities until drowsiness, weakness subsides
- That amnesia occurs, events may not be remembered

Treatment of overdose: O_2, vasopressors, physostigmine, resuscitation

mineral oil

Agoral Plain, Fleet Mineral Oil Enema, Kondremul, Milkinol, Neo-Cultol, Petrogalar Plain, Zymenol

Func. class.: Laxative
Chem. class.: Petroleum hydrocarbon

Action: Eases passage of stool by decreasing water absorption from feces, acts as lubricant

Uses: Constipation, preparation for bowel surgery or examination

Dosage and routes:
- *Adult:* PO 15-30 ml hs; enema 4 oz
- *Child:* PO 5-15 ml hs; enema 1-2 oz

Available forms include: Oil, enema; jelly 55%; susp 1.4, 2.5, 2.75 mg/5 ml

Side effects/adverse reactions:
CNS: Muscle weakness
GI: Nausea, vomiting, anorexia, diarrhea, pruritus ani, hepatic infiltration
META: ***Hypoprothrombinemia***
RESP: Lipoid pneumonia

Contraindications: Hypersensitivity, intestinal obstruction, abdominal pain, nausea/vomiting

Precautions: Pregnancy (C)

Pharmacokinetics: Excreted in feces

Interactions/incompatibilities:
- Increased effect of: oral anticoagulants
- Decreased absorption: fat-soluble vitamins (A, D, E, K) if used for prolonged time

NURSING CONSIDERATIONS

Assess:
- Blood, urine electrolytes if drug is used often by patient
- I&O ratio to identify fluid loss

Administer:
- Alone for better absorption
- In morning or evening (oral dose)
- Cautiously in elderly to prevent aspiration

Evaluate:
- Therapeutic response: decrease in constipation
- Cause of constipation; identify whether fluids, bulk, or exercise is missing from lifestyle
- Cramping, rectal bleeding, nausea, vomiting; if these symptoms occur, drug should be discontinued

Teach patient/family:
- Not to use laxatives for long-term therapy; bowel tone will be lost
- That normal bowel movements do not always occur daily
- Not to use in presence of abdominal pain, nausea, vomiting
- To notify physician if constipation unrelieved or if symptoms of electrolyte imbalance occur: muscle cramps, pain, weakness, dizziness, excessive thirst

minocycline HCl

(mi-noe-sye'kleen)

Minocin, Vectrin, Minocin IV

Func. class.: Broad-spectrum antibiotic
Chem. class.: Tetracycline

Action: Inhibits protein synthesis, phosphorylation in microorganisms by binding to 30S ribosomal subunits, reversibly binding to 50S ribosomal subunits, bacteriostatic

M

Uses: Syphilis, chlamydia trachomatis, gonorrhea, lymphogranuloma venereum, rickettsial infections, inflammatory acne, *Mycobacterium marinum, Neisseria* meningitis carriers

Dosage and routes:

• *Adult:* PO/IV 200 mg, then 100 mg q12h or 50 mg q6h, not to exceed 400 mg/24h IV

• *Child >8 yr:* PO/IV 4 mg/kg then 4 mg/kg/day PO in divided doses q12h

Gonorrhea

• *Adult:* PO 200 mg, then 100 mg q12h × 4 days

Chlamydia trachomatis

• *Adult:* PO 100 mg bid × 7 days

Syphilis

• *Adult:* PO 200 mg, then 100 mg q12h × 10-15 days

Available forms include: Tabs 50, 100 mg; caps 50, 100 mg oral susp 50 mg/5 ml; powder for inj IV 100 mg/vial

Side effects/adverse reactions:

CNS: Dizziness, fever, lightheadedness, vertigo

HEMA: ***Eosinophilia, neutropenia, thrombocytopenia, hemolytic anemia***

EENT: Dysphagia, glossitis, decreased calcification of deciduous teeth, oral candidiasis

GI: Nausea, abdominal pain, *vomiting, diarrhea,* anorexia, enterocolitis, ***hepatotoxicity,*** flatulence, abdominal cramps, epigastric burning, stomatitis

CV: Pericarditis

GU: Increased BUN, polyuria, polydipsia, ***renal failure, nephrotoxicity***

INTEG: Rash, urticaria, photosensitivity, increased pigmentation, ***exfoliative dermatitis,*** pruritus, angioedema, blue-gray color of skin, mucous membranes

Contraindications: Hypersensitivity to tetracyclines, children <8 yr, pregnancy (D)

Precautions: Hepatic disease, lactation

Pharmacokinetics:

PO: Peak 2-3 hr half-life 11-17 hr; excreted in urine, feces, crosses placenta, excreted in breast milk, 55%-88% protein bound

Interactions/incompatibilities:

• Decreased effect of minocycline: antacids, $NaHCO_3$, alkali products, iron, kaolin/pectin, cimetidine

• Increased effect of: anticoagulants

• Decreased effect of: penicillins, oral contraceptives

• Nephrotoxicity: methoxyflurane

• Do not mix with other drugs

NURSING CONSIDERATIONS

Assess:

• I&O ratio

• Blood studies: PT, CBC, AST, ALT, BUN, creatinine

• Signs of anemia: Hct, Hgb, fatigue

Administer:

• IV after diluting 100 mg/5 ml sterile H_2O for inj; further dilute in 500-1000 ml of compatible sol; run 100 mg/6 hr

• After C&S obtained

• 2 hr before or after laxative or ferrous products; 3 hr after antacid or kaolin-pectin product

Perform/provide:

• Storage in tight, light-resistant container at room temperature

Evaluate:

• Therapeutic response: decreased temperature, absence of lesions, negative C&S

• Allergic reactions: rash, itching, pruritus, angioedema

• Nausea, vomiting, diarrhea; administer antiemetic, antacids as ordered

• Overgrowth of infection: increased temperature, malaise, redness, pain, swelling, drainage, perineal itching, diarrhea, changes in cough or sputum

Teach patient/family:

• To avoid sun exposure since burns may occur; sunscreen does not seem to decrease photosensitivity

• That diabetics should avoid use of Clinistix, Diastix, or Tes-Tape for urine glucose testing

• That all prescribed medication must be taken to prevent superimposed infection

• To take with a full glass of water; may take with food or milk if GI symptoms occur

Lab test interferences:

False negative: Urine glucose with Clinistix or Tes-Tape

minoxidil

(mi-nox-i-dill)

Loniten, Minodyl, Rogaine

Func. class.: Antihypertensive
Chem. class.: Vasodilator—peripheral

Action: Directly relaxes arteriolar smooth muscle, causing vasodilation

Uses: Severe hypertension not responsive to other therapy (use with diuretic) topically to treat alopecia

Dosage and routes:

• *Adult:* PO 5 mg/day not to exceed 100 mg daily, usual range 10-40 mg/day in single doses

• *Child <12 yr:* (initial) 0.2 mg/kg/day; (effective range) 0.25-1 mg/kg/day; (max) 50 mg/day

Alopecia

• *Adult:* Apply topically, rub into scalp daily

Available forms include: Tabs 2.5, 10 mg, top 20 mg/ml

Side effects/adverse reactions:

CV: Severe rebound hypertension, tachycardia, angina, increased T wave, ***CHF, pulmonary edema, pericardial effusion,*** edema, sodium, water retention

CNS: Drowsiness, dizziness, sedation, headache, depression, fatigue

GI: Nausea, vomiting

GU: Gynecomastia, breast tenderness

INTEG: Pruritus, ***Stevens-Johnson syndrome,*** rash, hirsutism

HEMA: Hct, Hgb, erythrocyte count may decrease initially

Contraindications: Acute myocardial infarction, dissecting aortic aneurysm, hypersensitivity, pheochromocytoma

Precautions: Pregnancy (C), lactation, children, renal disease, CAD, CHF

M

Pharmacokinetics:

PO: Onset 30 min, peak 2-3 hr, duration 75 hr; half-life 4.2 hr, metabolized in liver, metabolites, excreted in urine, feces

Interactions/incompatibilities:

• Orthostatic hypotension: guanethidine

NURSING CONSIDERATIONS

Monitor:

• Electrolytes: K, Na, Cl, CO_2

• Renal function studies: catecholamines, BUN, creatinine

• Hepatic function studies: AST, ALT, alk phosphatase

• B/P, pulse

• Weight daily, I&O

Administer:

• With meals for better absorption, to decrease GI symptoms

• With β-blocker and/or diuretic

Evaluate:

• Therapeutic response: decreased B/P or increased hair growth

• Nausea, edema in feet, legs daily
• Skin turgor, dryness of mucous membranes for hydration status
• Rales, dyspnea, orthopnea

Teach patient/family:
• That body hair will increase but is reversible after discontinuing treatment
• Not to discontinue drug abruptly
• To report pitting edema, dizziness, weight gain >5 lb, shortness of breath, bruising or bleeding, heart rate >20 beats/min over normal, severe indigestion, dizziness, light-headedness, panting, new or aggravated symptoms of angina
• To take drug exactly as prescribed or serious side effects may occur

Lab test interferences:
Increase: Renal function studies
Decrease: Hgb/Hct/RBC

Treatment of overdose: Administer normal saline IV, phenylephrine, angiotensin II, vasopressor, dopamine may reverse hypotension

misoprostol

(mye-soe-prost′ ole)

Cytotec

Func. class.: Gastric mucosa protectant

Chem. class.: Prostaglandin E_1 analog

Action: Inhibits gastric acid secretion, may protect gastric mucosa; can increase bicarbonate, mucus production

Uses: Prevention of nonsteroidal antiinflammatory drug-induced gastric ulcers

Dosage and routes:
• *Adult:* PO 200 μg qid with food for duration of nonsteroidal antiinflammatory therapy; if 200 μg is not tolerated, 100 μg may be given

Available forms include: Tabs 200 μg

Side effects/adverse reactions:
GI: Diarrhea, nausea, vomiting, flatulence, constipation, dyspepsia, abdominal pain
GU: Spotting, cramps, hypermenorrhea, menstrual disorders

Contraindications: Hypersensitivity, pregnancy (X)

Precautions: Lactation, children, elderly, renal disease

Pharmacokinetics:
PO: Peak 12 min, plasma steady state achieved within 2 days, excreted in urine

NURSING CONSIDERATIONS

Assess:
• Gastric pH (>5 should be maintained)
• I&O ratio, BUN, creatinine

Perform/provide:
• Storage at room temperature

Evaluate:
• Therapeutic response: absence of pain or GI complaints

Teach patient/family:
• To take only as directed
• Not to take if pregnant (can cause miscarriage) and do not become pregnant while taking this medication; if pregnancy occurs during therapy, discontinue drug, notify physician
• Not to give drug to anyone else or take for more than 4 wk unless directed by physician

mitomycin

(mye-toe-mye′sin)

Mutamycin

Func. class.: Antineoplastic, antibiotic

Action: Inhibits DNA synthesis, primarily; derived from *Streptomyces caespitosus;* appears to cause cross-linking of DNA, a vesicant

Uses: Pancreas, stomach cancer, head and neck or breast cancer

Dosage and routes:

• *Adult:* IV 2 mg/m²/day × 5 days, stop drug for 2 days, then repeat cycle; or 10-20 mg/m² as a single dose, repeat cycle in 6-8 wk; stop drug if platelets are <75,000/mm³ or WBC is <3000/mm³

Available forms include: Inj IV

Side effects/adverse reactions:

HEMA: ***Thrombocytopenia, leukopenia, anemia***

GI: Nausea, vomiting, anorexia, stomatitis, ***hepatotoxicity,*** diarrhea

GU: Urinary retention, ***renal failure,*** edema

INTEG: Rash, alopecia, ***extravasation***

RESP: ***Fibrosis, pulmonary infiltrate,*** dyspnea

CNS: Fever, headache, confusion, drowsiness, syncope, fatigue

EENT: Blurred vision, drowsiness, syncope

Contraindications: Hypersensitivity, pregnancy (1st trimester) (D), as a single agent, thrombocytopenia, coagulation disorders

Precautions: Renal disease, bone marrow depression

Pharmacokinetics: Half-life 17 min, metabolized in liver, 10% excreted in urine (unchanged)

Interactions/incompatibilities:

• Increased toxicity: other antineoplastics (vinca alkaloids) or radiation

NURSING CONSIDERATIONS

Assess:

• CBC, differential, platelet count weekly; withhold drug if WBC is <4000/mm³ or platelet count is <75,000/mm³; notify physician of these results

• Pulmonary function tests, chest x-ray before, during therapy; chest x-ray should be obtained q2wk during treatment

• Renal function studies: BUN, serum uric acid, urine CrCl, electrolytes before, during therapy

• I&O ratio; report fall in urine output to <30 ml/hr

• Monitor temperature q4h; fever may indicate beginning infection

• Liver function tests before, during therapy: bilirubin, AST, ALT, alk phosphatase as needed or monthly

Administer:

• Sodium thiosulfate for extravasation, apply ice compress

• Antiemetic 30-60 min before giving drug to prevent vomiting

• IV after diluting 5 mg/10 ml sterile H_2O for inj; allow to stand, give through Y-tube or 3-way stopcock; give over 5-10 min

• Transfusion for anemia

• Antispasmodic for GI symptoms

Perform/provide:

• Liquid diet: carbonated beverages, gelatin may be added if patient is not nauseated or vomiting

• Rinsing of mouth tid-qid with water; brushing of teeth with baking soda bid-tid with soft brush or cotton-tipped applicators for stomatitis; use unwaxed dental floss

• Storage at room temperature for 1 wk after reconstituting or 2 wk refrigerated

Evaluate:

• Therapeutic response: decreased tumor size, spread of malignancy

• Alkalosis if severe vomiting is present

• Bleeding: hematuria, guaiac, bruising, petechiae, mucosa or orifices q8h

• Dyspnea, rales, unproductive cough, chest pain, tachypnea, fa-

tigue, increased pulse, pallor, lethargy
• Food preferences; list likes, dislikes
• Effects of alopecia on body image; discuss feelings about body changes
• Inflammation of mucosa, breaks in skin
• Yellowing of skin, sclera, dark urine, clay-colored stools, itchy skin, abdominal pain, fever, diarrhea
• Buccal cavity q8h for dryness, sores, ulceration, white patches, oral pain, bleeding, dysphagia
• Local irritation, pain, burning at injection site
• GI symptoms: frequency of stools, cramping
• Acidosis, signs of dehydration: rapid respirations, poor skin turgor, decreased urine output, dry skin, restlessness, weakness

Teach patient/family:
• To report any complaints, side effects to nurse or physician
• That hair may be lost during treatment and wig or hairpiece may make the patient feel better; tell patient that new hair may be different in color, texture
• To avoid foods with citric acid, hot or rough texture
• To report any bleeding, white spots, ulcerations in mouth; tell patient to examine mouth qd
• To avoid crowds, people with infections if granulocyte count is low

mitotane

(mye'toe-tane)

Lysodren

Func. class.: Antineoplastic
Chem. class.: Hormone, adrenal cytotoxic agent

Action: Acts on adrenal cortex to suppress activity; a cytotoxic agent that suppresses activity and causes cell death

Uses: Adrenocortical carcinoma

Dosage and routes:
• *Adult:* PO 9-10 g/day in divided doses tid or qid; may need to decrease dose if severe reactions occur

Available forms include: Tabs 500 mg

Side effects/adverse reactions:
GI: Nausea, vomiting, anorexia, diarrhea
GU: ***Proteinuria, hematuria***
INTEG: Rash
RESP: ***Fibrosis, pulmonary infiltrate***
CV: Hypertension, orthostatic hypotension
CNS: Light-headedness, flushing, sedation, vertigo
EENT: Lethargy, blurring, retinopathy

Contraindications: Hypersensitivity

Precautions: Lactation, hepatic disease, pregnancy (C)

Pharmacokinetics: Adequately absorbed orally (40%), excreted in urine, bile

Interactions/incompatibilities:
• Decreased effects of: corticosteroids

NURSING CONSIDERATIONS

Assess:
• Adrenal insufficiency: fatigue, orthostatic hypotension, weight loss, weakness, nausea, vomiting, diarrhea
• Pulmonary function tests, chest x-ray films before, during therapy; chest film should be obtained q2wk during treatment
• Renal function studies: BUN, serum uric acid, urine CrCl electrolytes before, during therapy
• I&O ratio

• Urinary 17-OHCS before, during treatment

Administer:

• Antacid before oral agent, give drug after evening meal, before bedtime

• Antiemetic 30-60 min before giving drug to prevent vomiting

• Antispasmodic

Perform/provide:

• Increase fluid intake to 2-3 L/day to prevent dehydration

• HOB raised to facilitate breathing

• Increased fluid intake to 2000 ml/day if not contraindicated

• Nutritious diet with iron, vitamin supplements as ordered

• Storage in tight, light-resistant container

Evaluate:

• Therapeutic response: decreased tumor size, spread of malignancy

• Dyspnea, chest pain, tachypnea, fatigue, increased pulse, pallor, lethargy

• Food preferences; list likes, dislikes

• Muscular weakness, fatigue, oliguria, hypoglycemia

• Frequency of stools, characteristics: cramping, acidosis, signs of dehydration (rapid respirations, poor skin turgor, decreased urine output, dry skin, restlessness, weakness)

• Symptoms indicating severe allergic reactions: rash, pruritus, itching, flushing

• Signs of infection: increased temperature, cough, fatigue, malaise

Teach patient/family:

• To report any complaints, side effects to nurse or physician

• To report any changes in breathing, coughing

• To avoid driving or other activities requiring alertness

Lab test interferences:

Decrease: PBI, urinary 17-OHCS

---

mitoxantrone HCl

(mye-toe-zan'trone)

Novantrone

Func. class.: Antineoplastic

Chem. class.: Synthetic anthraquinone

Action: DNA reactive agent, cytocidal effect on both proliferating and nonproliferating cells suggesting lack of cell cycle phase specificity

Uses: Acute nonlymphocytic leukemia (adult)

Dosage and routes:

• *Adult:* IV inf 12 mg/m^2/day on days 1-3, and 100 mg/m^2 cytosine arabinoside × 7 days

Available forms include: Inj 2 mg/ml

M

Side effects/adverse reactions:

GI: Nausea, vomiting, diarrhea, anorexia, mucositis, ***hepatotoxicity***

HEMA: ***Thrombocytopenia, leukopenia, myelosuppression, anemia***

INTEG: Rash, necrosis at injection site, dermatitis, thrombophlebitis at injection site, alopecia

CV: ***CHF, cardiopathy, dysrhythmias***

MISC: Fever

RESP: Cough, dyspnea

Contraindications: Hypersensitivity

Precautions: Myelosuppression, lactation, cardiac disease, children, pregnancy (D), renal, hepatic disease, gout

Pharmacokinetics:

Highly bound to plasma proteins, metabolized in liver, excreted via renal, hepatobiliary systems; half-life 24-72 hr

Interactions/incompatibilities:
• Do not mix with heparin, precipitate will form

NURSING CONSIDERATIONS

Assess:
• CBC, differential, platelet count weekly, withhold drug if WBC is <4000/mm³ or platelet count is <75,000/mm³, notify physician of these results
• Liver function test before, during therapy: bilirubin, AST, ALT, alk phosphatase prn or monthly
• Renal function studies: BUN, serum uric acid, urine CrCl, electrolytes before, during therapy

Administer:
• Medications by oral route if possible, avoid IM, SC, IV routes to prevent infections
• Antiemetic 30-60 min before giving drug to prevent vomiting
• IV after diluting with 50 ml or more normal saline or D_5W; give over 3-5 min running IV of D_5W or NS; may be diluted further in compatible sol and run over 15-30 min; check for extravasation

Perform/provide:
• Liquid diet: carbonated beverages, Jell-O; dry toast, crackers may be added if patient is not nauseated or vomiting
• Rinsing of mouth tid-qid with water, club soda, brushing of teeth bid-qid with soft brush or cotton-tipped applicators for stomatitis; use unwaxed dental floss

Evaluate:
• Therapeutic response: decreased tumor size, spread of malignancy
• Bleeding, hematuria, guaiac, bruising or petechiae, mucosa or orifices q8h
• Food preferences; list likes, dislikes
• Yellowing of skin, sclera, dark urine, clay-colored stools, itchy skin, abdominal pain, fever, diarrhea
• Acidosis, signs of dehydration: rapid respirations, poor skin turgor, decreased urine output, dry skin, restlessness, weakness

Teach patient/family:
• To report side effects to nurse or physician
• To avoid foods with citric acid, rough texture, or hot
• To report any bleeding, white spots, ulcerations in mouth; tell patient to examine mouth daily

---

mivacurium chloride

(miv-a-kure'ee-um)

Mivacron

Func. class.: Nondepolarizing neuromuscular blocker

Action: Inhibits transmission of nerve impulses by binding competitively with cholinergic receptor sites, antagonizing the action of acetylcholine

Uses: Facilitation of endotracheal intubation, skeletal muscle relaxation during mechanical ventilation, surgery, or general anesthesia

Dosage and routes:
• *Adult:* IV 0.15 mg/kg; maintenance q15min
• *Child:* 2-12 IV 0.2 mg/kg for a 10 min block

Available forms include: 5, 10 ml single-use vial (2 mg/ml); premixed infusion in D_5W 50 ml flex container

Side effects/adverse reactions:
CV: Decreased B/P, bradycardia, tachycardia
RESP: ***Prolonged apnea, bronchospasm, wheezing, respiratory depression***
EENT: Diplopia

* Available in Canada only

MS: Weakness, prolonged skeletal muscle relaxation, ***paralysis***
INTEG: Rash, urticaria
Contraindications: Hypersensitivity
Precautions: Pregnancy (C), renal, hepatic disease, lactation, children <3 mo, fluid and electrolyte imbalances, neuromuscular disease, respiratory disease, obesity, elderly
Pharmacokinetics: Rapidly hydrolyzed by plasma cholinesterases, peak 2-3 min, reversal within 15-30 min
Interactions/incompatibilities:
- Increased neuromuscular blockade: aminoglycosides, quinidine, local anesthetics, polymyxin antibiotics, enflurane, isoflurane, tetracyclines, halothane, magnesium, colistin, procainamide, bacitracin, lincomycin, clindamycin, lithium

NURSING CONSIDERATIONS
Assess
- For electrolyte imbalances (K, Mg); may lead to increased action of this drug
- Vital signs (B/P, pulse, respirations, airway) until fully recovered; rate, depth, pattern of respirations, strength of hand grip
- I&O ratio; check for urinary retention, frequency, hesitancy

Administer:
- Using nerve stimulator by anesthesiologist to determine neuromuscular blockade
- Anticholinesterase to reverse neuromuscular blockade
- By slow IV over 1-2 min (only by qualified persons, usually an anesthesiologist)
- Only fresh solution

Perform/provide:
- Storage at room temperature; do not freeze
- Reassurance if communication is difficult during recovery from neuromuscular blockade
- Frequent (q2h) instillation of artificial tears and covering eyes to prevent drying of cornea

Evaluate:
- Therapeutic response: paralysis of jaw, eyelid, head, neck, rest of body
- Recovery: decreased paralysis of face, diaphragm, leg, arm, rest of body
- Allergic reactions: rash, fever, respiratory distress, pruritus; drug should be discontinued

Treatment of overdose: Neostigmine, monitor VS; may require mechanical ventilation

---

molindone HCl
(moe-lin'done)
Moban
Func. class.: Antipsychotic/neuroleptic
Chem. class.: Dihydroindolone

Action: Depresses cerebral cortex, hypothalamus, limbic system, which control activity, aggression; blocks neurotransmission produced by dopamine at synapse; exhibits strong α-adrenergic, anticholinergic blocking action; mechanism for antipsychotic effects is unclear
Uses: Psychotic disorders
Dosage and routes:
- *Adult:* PO 50-75 mg/day increasing to 225 mg/day if needed

Available forms include: Tabs 5, 10, 25, 50, 100 mg; conc 20 mg/ml
Side effects/adverse reactions:
RESP: ***Laryngospasm,*** dyspnea, ***respiratory depression***
CNS: Extrapyramidal symptoms: pseudoparkinsonism, akathisia,

M

dystonia, tardive dyskinesia, drowsiness, headache, seizures
HEMA: ***Anemia, leukopenia, leukocytosis, agranulocytosis***
INTEG: Rash, photosensitivity, dermatitis
EENT: Blurred vision, glaucoma
GI: Dry mouth, nausea, vomiting, anorexia, constipation, diarrhea, jaundice, weight gain
GU: Urinary retention, urinary frequency, enuresis, impotence, amenorrhea, gynecomastia
CV: Orthostatic hypotension, hypertension, ***cardiac arrest,*** ECG changes, ***tachycardia***

Contraindications: Hypersensitivity, coma, child

Precautions: Pregnancy (C), lactation, hypertension, hepatic disease, cardiac disease, Parkinson's disease, brain tumor, glaucoma, urinary retention, diabetes mellitus, respiratory disease, prostatic hypertrophy

Pharmacokinetics:
PO: Onset erratic, peak 1½ hr, duration 24-36 hr; metabolized by liver, excreted in urine and feces, may cross placenta, enters breast milk, half-life 1½ hr

Interactions/incompatibilities:
• Increased sedation: other CNS depressants
• Increased EPS: other antipsychotics, lithium

NURSING CONSIDERATIONS

Assess:
• Mental status before initial administration
• Swallowing of PO medication; check for hoarding or giving of medication to other patients
• I&O ratio; palpate bladder if low urinary output occurs
• Bilirubin, CBC, liver function studies monthly
• Urinalysis is recommended before, during prolonged therapy

Administer:
• Reduced dose in elderly
• Antiparkinsonian agent, after securing order from physician, to be used if extrapyramidal symptoms occur
• IM injection into large muscle mass
• Concentrate mixed in orange or grapefruit juice

Perform/provide:
• Decreased noise input by dimming lights, avoiding loud noises
• Supervised ambulation until stabilized on medication; do not involve in strenuous exercise program because fainting is possible; patient should not stand still for a long time
• Increased fluids to prevent constipation
• Sips of water, candy, gum for dry mouth
• Storage in tight, light-resistant container

Evaluate:
• Therapeutic response: decrease in emotional excitement, hallucinations, delusions, paranoia, reorganization of patterns of thought, speech
• Affect, orientation, LOC, reflexes, gait, coordination, sleep pattern disturbances
• B/P standing and lying; also include pulse, respirations; take these q4h during initial treatment; establish baseline before starting treatment; report drops of 30 mm Hg, watch for ECG changes
• Dizziness, faintness, palpitations, tachycardia on rising
• Extrapyramidal symptoms including akathisia (inability to sit still, no pattern to movements), tardive dyskinesia (bizarre move-

ments of the jaw, mouth, tongue, extremities), pseudoparkinsonism (rigidity, tremors, pill rolling, shuffling gait)
- For neuroleptic malignant syndrome: hyperthermia, increased CPK, altered mental status, muscle rigidity
- Skin turgor daily
- Constipation, urinary retention daily; if these occur, increase bulk and water in diet

Teach patient/family:
- That orthostatic hypotension may occur and to rise from sitting or lying position gradually
- To avoid hot tubs, hot showers, or tub baths since hypotension may occur
- To avoid abrupt withdrawal of this drug or EPS may result; drugs should be withdrawn slowly
- To avoid OTC preparations (cough, hayfever, cold) unless approved by physician since serious drug interactions may occur; avoid use with alcohol or CNS depressants, increased drowsiness may occur
- To avoid hazardous activities if drowsiness or dizziness occurs
- To use sunscreen during sun exposure to prevent burns
- Regarding compliance with drug regimen
- About necessity for meticulous oral hygiene since oral candidiasis may occur
- To report impaired vision, jaundice, tremors, muscle twitching
- In hot weather, that heat stroke may occur; take extra precautions to stay cool

Lab test interferences:
Alterations in: BUN, RBC, serum glucose, WBC
Increase: Serum prolactin levels

Treatment of overdose: Lavage if orally injested, provide an airway; *do not induce vomiting*

moricizine

(mor iss' i-zeen)
Ethmozine

Func. class.: Antidysrhythmic, type I
Chem. class.: Phenothiazine

Action: Decreased rate of rise of action potential, prolonging refractory period and shortening the action potential duration; depression of inward influx if sodium mediates the effects; drug may slow atrial and AV nodal conduction

Uses: Symptomatic vertricular and life-threatening dysrhythmias

Dosage and routes:
Adult: PO 10-15 mg/kg/day in 2-3 divided doses

Available forms include: Film-coated tabs 200, 250, 300 mg

Side effects/adverse reactions:
GI: Nausea, abdominal pain, vomiting, diarrhea
CNS: (Dizziness, headache, fatigue, perioral numbness, euphoria) nervousness, sleep disorders, depression, tinnitus, fatigue
RESP: Dyspnea, hyperventilation, ***apnea,*** asthma, pharyngitis, cough
GU: Sexual dysfunction, difficult urination, dysuria, incontinence
CV: Palpitations, chest pain, ***CHF,*** hypertension, syncope, dysrythmias, bradycardia, ***MI,*** thrombophlebitis
MISC: Sweating, musculoskeletal pain

Contraindications: 2-3 degree AV block, right bundle branch block, cardiogenic shock, hypersensitivity

Precautions: CHF, hypokalemia, hyperkalemia, sick sinus syndrome, pregnancy (B), lactation,

children, impaired hepatic and renal function, cardiac dysfunction
Pharmacokinetics: Half-life 1.5-3.5 hr; peak 0.5-2.2 hr; metabolized by the liver; metabolites are excreted in feces and urine, protein binding >90%
Interactions/incompatibilities:
• Increased plasma levels of moricizine: ametadine
• Digoxin or propranolol may enhance some of cardiac effects of moricizine; moricizine may decrease effects of theophylline

NURSING CONSIDERATIONS

Assess:
• GI status: bowel pattern, number of stools
• Cardiac status: rate, rhythm, quality
• Chest x-ray, pulmonary function test during treatment
• I&O ratio; check for decreasing output
• B/P for fluctuations
• Lung fields: bilateral rales may occur in CHF patient
• Increased respiration, increased pulse; drug should be discontinued
Evaluate:
• Therapeutic response: absence of dysrhythmias
• Toxicity: fine tremors, dizziness
• Cardiac rate: respiration, rate, rhythm, character continuously
Lab test interferences:
Increase: CPK
Treatment of overdose: O_2 artificial ventilitation, ECG, administer dopamine for circulatory depression, administer diazepam or thiopental for convulsions

morphine sulfate

(mor'feen)
Duramorph PF, MS Contin, RMS, Roxanol, Roxanol SR, M.O.S.*
Func. class.: Narcotic analgesics
Chem. class.: Opiate

Controlled Substance Schedule II
Action: Depresses pain impulse transmission at the spinal cord level by interacting with opioid receptors
Uses: Severe pain
Dosage and routes:
• *Adult:* SC/IM 4-15 mg q4h prn; PO 10-30 mg q4h prn; EXT REL q8-12h; REC 10-20 mg q4h prn; IV 4-10 mg diluted in 4-5 ml of water for injection, over 5 min
• *Child:* SC 0.1-0.2 mg/kg, not to exceed 15 mg
Available forms include: Inj SC, IM, IV 2, 4, 5, 8, 10, 15 mg/ml; sol tabs 10, 15, 30 mg; oral sol 10, 20 mg/5 ml, 20 mg/10 ml, 20 mg/ml; oral tabs 15, 30 mg; rec supp 5, 10, 20 mg; ext rel tabs 300 mg
Side effects/adverse reactions:
CNS: Drowsiness, dizziness, confusion, headache, sedation, euphoria
GI: Nausea, vomiting, anorexia, constipation, cramps, biliary tract pressure
GU: Increased urinary output, dysuria, urinary retention
INTEG: Rash, urticaria, bruising, flushing, diaphoresis, pruritus
EENT: Tinnitus, blurred vision, miosis, diplopia
CV: Palpitations, bradycardia, change in B/P
RESP: ***Respiratory depression***
Contraindications: Hypersensitivity, addiction (narcotic), hemorrhage, bronchial asthma, increased intracranial pressure

* Available in Canada only

Precautions: Addictive personality, pregnancy (B), lactation, MI (acute), severe heart disease, elderly, respiratory depression, hepatic disease, renal disease, child <18 yr

Pharmacokinetics:

PO: Onset variable, peak variable, duration variable

SC: Onset 15-30 min, peak 50-90 min, duration 3-5 hr

IV: Peak 20 min; metabolized by liver, excreted by kidneys, crosses placenta, excreted in breast milk, half-life 2½-3 hr

Interactions/incompatibilities:

- Increased effects with other CNS depressants: alcohol, narcotics, sedative/hypnotics, antipsychotics, skeletal muscle relaxants

NURSING CONSIDERATIONS

Assess:

- I&O ratio; check for decreasing output; may indicate urinary retention

Administer:

- IV after diluting with 5 ml of compatible sol; give 15 mg or less over 4-5 min; give through Y-tube or 3-way stopcock; may be added to IV sol
- With antiemetic if nausea, vomiting occur
- When pain is beginning to return; determine dosage interval by patient response

Perform/provide:

- Storage in light-resistant area at room temperature
- Assistance with ambulation
- Safety measures: siderails, night light, call bell within easy reach

Evaluate:

- Therapeutic response: decrease in pain
- CNS changes: dizziness, drowsiness, hallucinations, euphoria, LOC, pupil reaction
- Allergic reactions: rash, urticaria
- Respiratory dysfunction: respiratory depression, character, rate, rhythm; notify physician if respirations are <10/min
- Need for pain medication, physical dependence

Teach patient/family:

- To report any symptoms of CNS changes, allergic reactions
- That physical dependency may result when used for extended periods of time
- That withdrawal symptoms may occur: nausea, vomiting, cramps, fever, faintness, anorexia

Lab test interferences:

Increase: Amylase

Treatment of overdose: Narcan 0.2-0.8 IV, O_2, IV fluids, vasopressors

---

moxalactam disodium

(mox'a-lak-tam)

Moxam

Func. class.: Antibiotic, broad-spectrum

Chem. class.: Cephalosporin (3rd generation)

Action: Inhibits bacterial cell wall synthesis, rendering cell wall osmotically unstable

Uses: Gram-negative organisms: *H. influenzae, E. coli, P. mirabilis, Klebsiella, Citrobacter, Salmonella, Shigella, Serratia;* gram-positive organisms: *S. pneumoniae, S. pyogenes, S. aureus;* serious lower respiratory tract, urinary tract, skin, bone infections, septicemia, meningitis, intraabdominal infections

Dosage and routes:

- *Adult:* IM/IV 2-4 g q8-12h

Mild infections

• *Adult:* IM/IV 250-500 mg q8-12h

Severe infections

• *Adult:* IM/IV 2-6 g q8h

• *Child:* IM/IV 50 mg/kg q6-8h

• Dosage reduction indicated even for mild renal impairment (CrCl < 80 ml/min)

Available forms include: Powder for inj IM, IV 1, 2, 10 g

Side effects/adverse reactions:

CNS: Headache, dizziness, weakness, paresthesia, fever, chills

GI: Nausea, vomiting, diarrhea, anorexia, pain, glossitis, bleeding, increased AST, ALT, bilirubin, LDH, alk phosphatase, abdominal pain

GU: ***Proteinuria,*** vaginitis, pruritus, candidiasis, increased BUN, ***nephrotoxicity, renal failure***

HEMA: ***Leukopenia, thrombocytopenia, agranulocytosis, anemia, neutropenia, lymphocytosis, eosinophilia, pancytopenia, hemolytic anemia, bleeding, hypoprothrombinemia***

INTEG: Rash, urticaria, dermatitis, ***anaphylaxis***

RESP: Dyspnea

Contraindications: Hypersensitivity to cephalosporins

Precautions: Hypersensitivity to penicillins, pregnancy (C), lactation, renal disease

Pharmacokinetics:

IV: Peak 5 min

IM: Peak ½-2 hr

Half-life 1½-2½ hr, 25% bound by plasma proteins, 60%-97% eliminated unchanged in urine in 24 hr, crosses placenta, blood-brain barrier, excreted in breast milk, not metabolized

Interactions/incompatibilities:

• Do not mix with tetracyclines, erythromycins, aminoglycosides in same parenteral fluid

• Decreased effects of: tetracyclines, erythromycins

• Increased toxicity: aminoglycosides, furosemide, probenecid, sulfinpyrazone, colistin, ethacrynic acid, vancomycin, agents affecting platelet function

• Disulfiram reaction: ethanol

NURSING CONSIDERATIONS

Assess:

• Nephrotoxicity: increased BUN, creatinine

• I&O daily

• Blood studies: AST, ALT, CBC, Hct, bilirubin, LDH, alk phosphatase, Coombs' test pro-time monthly if patient is on long-term therapy

• Electrolytes: potassium, sodium, chloride monthly if patient is on long-term therapy

• Bowel pattern qd; if severe diarrhea occurs, drug should be discontinued; may indicate pseudomembranous colitis

• IV site for extravasation, phlebitis; change site q72h

Administer:

• For 10-14 days to ensure organism death, prevent superimposed infection

• IV after diluting 1 g/10 ml sterile H_2O, D_5, 0.9% NaCl; give through Y-tube over 3-5 min; may be further diluted 1 g/20 ml in compatible sol, give over ½ hr; may be added 500-1000, give over 6-24 hr

• Vitamin K for bleeding (10 mg/wk)

• After C&S

Evaluate:

• Therapeutic response: decreased fever, malaise, chills

• Urine output: if decreasing, notify physician; may indicate nephrotoxicity

• Allergic reactions: rash, urticaria, pruritus, chills, fever, joint

* Available in Canada only

pain, angioedema; may occur few days after therapy begins
• Bleeding: ecchymosis, bleeding gums, hematuria, stool guaiac daily
• Overgrowth of infection: perineal itching, fever, malaise, redness, pain, swelling, drainage, rash, diarrhea, change in cough, sputum
Teach patient/family:
• To report sore throat, bruising, bleeding, joint pain; may indicate blood dyscrasias (rare)
• Not to drink alcohol while taking this drug
Lab test interferences:
Increase (false): Urinary 17-KS
False positive: Urinary protein, direct Coombs', urine glucose
Interference: Cross-matching
Treatment of overdose: Epinephrine, antihistamines, resuscitate if needed (anaphylaxis)

multivitamins

Many brands
Func. class.: Vitamin

Action: Needed for adequate metabolism
Uses: Prevention and treatment of vitamin deficiencies
Dosage and routes:
• *Adult and child:* PO depends on brand
Available forms include: Many forms available
Side effects/adverse reactions: None known
Precautions: Pregnancy (A)
Interactions/incompatibilities:
• Check each vitamin for specific interactions
NURSING CONSIDERATIONS
Evaluate:
• Therapeutic response: check each individual vitamin for guidelines
• Vitamin deficiency: usually more than one vitamin is deficient
Teach patient/family:
• That adequate nutrition must be maintained to prevent further deficiencies
• Drug interaction that should be avoided
• To comply with regimen
• To avoid using flavored multivitamins as candy; child may overdose
• To store out of children's reach

mupirocin

(meew-per'-o-sen)
Bactroban
Func. class.: Topical antiinfective
Chem. class.: Pseudomonic acid A

Action: Inhibits bacterial protein synthesis, shows no cross resistance to most antibiotics
Uses: Impetigo caused by *S. aureus,* β-hemolytic *Streptococcus, S. pyogenes*
Dosage and routes:
Apply small amount to affected area tid
Available forms include: Oint 2% (20 mg/g)
Side effects/adverse reactions:
INTEG: Burning, stinging, itching, rash, dry skin, swelling, contact dermatitis, erythema, tenderness, increased exudate
Contraindications: Hypersensitivity
Precautions: Pregnancy (B), lactation
NURSING CONSIDERATIONS
Assess:
• Affected area for continuing infection: increased size, amount of lesions
Administer:
• Then cover with 2 × 2 in gauze if needed

Perform/provide:
- Storage at room temperature
- Isolation (wound) for hospitalized child (2-5 days)
- Washing of hands after applying ointment

Evaluate:
- Therapeutic response: reduction in size, amount of lesions

Teach patient/family:
- To wash hands after applying ointment
- To trim fingernails to prevent scratching
- To report irritation, worsening of rash, itching, pain at site; if no improvement within 3-5 days report to physician

---

muromonab-CD3

(mur-oo-mone'ab)
Orthoclone OKT3

Func. class.: Immunosuppressive
Chem. class.: Murine monoclonal antibody

Action: Reverses graft rejection by blocking T-cell function
Uses: Acute allograft rejection in renal transplant patients
Dosage and routes:
- *Adult:* IV BOL 5 mg/day × 10-14 days; usually methylprednisolone sodium succinate, 1 mg/kg IV is given before muromonab-CD3, 100 mg IV hydrocortisone sodium succinate is given ½ hr after muromonab-CD3

Available forms include: Inj 5 mg/5 ml
Side effects/adverse reactions:
CNS: Pyrexia, chills, tremors
RESP: Dyspnea, wheezing, ***pulmonary edema***
CV: Chest pain
GI: Vomiting, nausea, diarrhea
MISC: Infection

Contraindications: Hypersensitivity to murine origin, fluid overload
Precautions: Pregnancy (C), child <2 yr, fever
Pharmacokinetics:
Trough level steady state 3-14 days

NURSING CONSIDERATIONS

Assess:
- Blood studies: Hgb, WBC, platelets during treatment monthly; if leukocytes are <3000/mm³ drug should be discontinued
- Liver function studies: alk phosphatase, AST, ALT, bilirubin

Administer:
- IV undiluted, withdraw with a 0.2-0.22 low protein-binding micron filter, discard and use new needle for administration; give over 1 min
- For several days before transplant surgery
- All medications PO if possible, avoid IM injection since infection may occur

Evaluate:
- Therapeutic response: decreased tumor size, spread of malignancy
- Hepatotoxicity: dark urine, jaundice, itching, light-colored stools; drug should be discontinued

Teach patient/family:
- To report fever, chills, sore throat, fatigue since serious infection may occur
- To use contraceptive measures during treatment, for 12 wk after ending therapy; possible mutagenic effects

---

* Available in Canada only

nabumetone

(nay-bume'tone)

Relafen

Func. class.: Nonsteroidal antiinflammatory

Chem. class.: Acetic acid derivative

Action: May inhibit prostaglandin synthesis by decreasing enzyme needed for biosynthesis; possesses analgesic, antiinflammatory, antipyretic properties

Uses: Osteoarthritis, rheumatoid arthritis, acute or chronic treatment

Dosage and routes:

• *Adult:* PO 1000 mg as a single dose; may increase to 1500-2000 mg/day if needed; may give qd or bid

Available forms include: Tabs 500, 750 mg

Side effects/adverse reactions:

CNS: Dizziness, headache, drowsiness, fatigue, tremors, confusion, insomnia, anxiety, depression, nervousness

GU: ***Nephrotoxicity, dysuria, hematuria, oliguria, azotemia,*** cystitis

GI: Nausea, anorexia, vomiting, diarrhea, jaundice, ***cholestatic hepatitis,*** constipation, flatulence, cramps, dry mouth, peptic ulcer, gastritis

CV: Tachycardia, peripheral edema, palpitations, dysrhythmias, CHF

INTEG: Purpura, rash, pruritus, sweating, photosensitivity

HEMA: ***Blood dyscrasias***

EENT: Tinnitus, hearing loss, blurred vision

RESP: Dyspnea, pharyngitis, ***bronchospasm***

Contraindications: Hypersensitivity to this drug or aspirin, iodides, NSAIDs, asthma, severe renal disease, severe

Precautions: Pregnancy (B) 1st and 2nd trimester, lactation, children, bleeding disorders, GI disorders, cardiac disorders, renal disorders, hepatic dysfunction, elderly

Pharmacokinetics:

PO: Peak 2½-4 hr, plasma protein binding >90%, half-life 22-30 hr; metabolized in liver to active metabolite, excreted in urine (metabolites), breast milk

Interactions/incompatibilities:

• May increase the action or increased toxicity of: coumarin, cyclosporine, phenytoin, methotrexate, probenecid

• May decrease effects of nabumetone: salicylates

NURSING CONSIDERATIONS

Assess:

• Renal, liver, blood studies: BUN, creatinine, AST, ALT, Hgb, before treatment, periodically thereafter

• Audiometric, ophthalmic exam before, during, after treatment

Administer:

• With food to decrease GI symptoms

• Avoid alcoholic beverages and aspirin

Perform/provide:

• Storage at room temperature

Evaluate:

• Therapeutic response: decreased pain and stiffness in joints

• For eye, ear problems: blurred vision, tinnitus; may indicate toxicity

Teach patient/family:

• To report blurred vision, ringing, roaring in ears; may indicate toxicity

• To avoid driving, other hazardous activities if dizziness, drowsiness occur

• To report change in urine pattern,

N

increased weight, edema, increased pains in joints, fever, blood in urine; indicates nephrotoxicity
• That therapeutic effects may take up to 1 mo
• To take with a full glass of water to enhance absorption
• To report dark stools; may indicate GI bleeding

nadolol

(nay-doe'-lole)
Corgard
Func. class.: Antihypertensive, antianginal
Chem. class.: β-adrenergic receptor blocker

Action: Long-acting, nonselective β-adrenergic receptor blocking agent; mechanism is similar to propranolol
Uses: Chronic stable angina pectoris, mild to moderate hypertension
Dosage and routes:
• *Adult:* PO 40 mg qd, increase by 40-80 mg q3-7d; maintenance 40-240 mg/day for angina, 40-320 mg/day for hypertension
Available forms include: Oral tabs 20, 40, 80, 120, 160 mg
Side effects/adverse reactions:
RESP: Dyspnea, respiratory dysfunction, ***bronchospasm,*** cough, wheezing, nasal stuffiness, pharyngitis, ***laryngospasm***
CV: Bradycardia, hypotension, ***CHF,*** palpitations, AV block
HEMA: ***Agranulocytosis, thrombocytopenia,*** chest pain, peripheral ischemia, flushing, edema, vasodilation, conduction disturbances
GI: Nausea, vomiting, diarrhea, colitis, constipation, cramps, dry mouth, flatulence, hepatomegaly, pancreatitis, taste distortion
INTEG: Rash, pruritus, fever
CNS: Depression, hallucinations, dizziness, fatigue, lethargy, paresthesias, headache
EENT: Sore throat
Contraindications: Hypersensitivity to this drug, cardiac failure, cardiogenic shock, 2nd or 3rd degree heart block, bronchospastic disease, sinus bradycardia, CHF, COPD
Precautions: Diabetes mellitus, pregnancy (C), renal disease, lactation, hyperthyroidism, peripheral vascular disease, myasthenia gravis
Pharmacokinetics:
PO: Onset variable, peak 3-4 hr, duration 17-24 hr; half-life 16-20 hr, not metabolized, excreted in urine (unchanged), bile, breast milk
Interactions/incompatibilities:
• Increased effects of: reserpine, digitalis, ergots, neuromuscular blocking agents, calcium channel blockers
• Decreased effects of: norepinephrine, xanthines, isoproterenol, thyroid, nonsteroidals, salicylates

NURSING CONSIDERATIONS

Assess:
• B/P, pulse, respirations during beginning therapy
• Weight qd, report gain of 5 lb
• I&O ratio, CrCl if kidney damage is diagnosed
• qd, note need to be administered more often
Administer:
• With 8 oz water
Evaluate:
• Therapeutic response: decreased B/P, symptoms of angina
• Pain: duration, time started, activity being performed, character
• Tolerance if taken over long time
• Headache, light-headedness, decreased B/P; may indicate a need for decreased dosage

Teach patient/family:

- That drug may mask signs of hypoglycemia or alter blood glucose in diabetics
- Not to discontinue abruptly
- To avoid OTC drugs unless physician approves
- To avoid hazardous activities if dizziness occurs
- To comply with complete medical regimen

Lab test interferences:

Increase: Serum potassium, serum uric acid, ALT/AST, alk phosphatase, LDH

Decrease: Blood glucose

---

nafarelin acetate

Synarel

Func. class.: Gonadotropin

Chem. class.: Analog of gonadotropin-releasing hormone

Action: Stimulates the release of LH and FSH, which increases ovarian steroid production; repeated dosing prevents stimulation of the pituitary gland

Uses: Endometriosis

Doses and routes: 400 μg/day as one spray (200 μg) into one nostril in morning and one spray into other nostril in evening; start treatment between days 2 and 4 of menstrual cycle; may increase to 800 μg/day (one spray into each nostril twice a day); recommended duration of treatment is 6 months

Available forms include: Nasal sol 2 mg/ml

Side effects/adverse reactions:

GU: Decreased libido, vaginal dryness, breast tenderness

CNS: Headache, flushing, depression, insomnia, emotional lability, hot flashes

INTEG: Nasal irritation, acne

Contraindications: Hypersensitivity, pregnancy (X), lactation, undiagnosed abnormal vaginal bleeding

Precautions: Children

Pharmacokinetics: Rapidly absorbed, peak 10-40 min, half-life 3 hr, 80% bound to plasma proteins

NURSING CONSIDERATIONS

Assess:

- Test results: pituitary/hypothalamus dysfunction (decreased LH); postmenopausal (increased LH)

Administer:

- Repeated doses may be necessary to elevate pituitary gonadotropin reserve

Perform/provide:

- Storage at room temperature; protect from light

Evaluate:

- Therapeutic response: decreased symptoms of endometriosis

---

nafcillin sodium

(naf-sill'-in)

Nafcil, Nallpen, Unipen

Func. class.: Broad-spectrum antibiotic

Chem. class.: Penicillinase-resistant penicillin

Action: Interferes with cell wall replication of susceptible organisms; osmotically unstable cell wall swells, bursts from osmotic pressure

Uses: Effective for gram-positive cocci *(S. aureus, S. viridans, S. pneumoniae)*, infections caused by penicillinase-producing *Staphylococcus*

Dosage and routes:

- *Adult:* IM/IV 2-6 g/day in divided doses q4-6h; PO 2-6 g/day in divided doses q4-6h
- *Child:* IM 25 mg/kg q12h; PO

25-50 mg/kg/day in divided doses q6h
• *Neonates* IM 10 mg/kg bid
Available forms include: Caps 250 mg; tabs 500 mg; powder for oral susp 250 mg/5 ml; powder for inj IM, IV 500 mg, 1, 2, 10 g; IV 1, 1.5, 2, 4 g
Side effects/adverse reactions:
HEMA: Anemia, increased bleeding time, ***bone marrow depression, granulocytopenia***
GI: Nausea, vomiting, diarrhea, increased AST, ALT, abdominal pain, glossitis, colitis
GU: Oliguria, ***proteinuria, hematuria,*** *vaginitis, moniliasis,* ***glomerulonephritis***
CNS: Lethargy, hallucinations, anxiety, depression, twitching, ***coma, convulsions***
Contraindications: Hypersensitivity to penicillins
Precautions: Pregnancy (B), hypersensitivity to cephalosporins, neonates
Pharmacokinetics:
IM/PO: Peak 30-60 min, duration 4-6 hr, half-life 1 hr, metabolized by the liver, excreted in bile, urine
Interactions/incompatibilities:
• Decreased antimicrobial effectiveness of nafcillin: tetracyclines, erythromycins
• Increased nafcillin concentrations: aspirin, probenecid

NURSING CONSIDERATIONS

Assess:
• I&O ratio; report hematuria, oliguria since penicillin in high doses is nephrotoxic
• Any patient with compromised renal system since drug is excreted slowly in poor renal system function; toxicity may occur rapidly
• Liver studies: AST, ALT
• Blood studies: WBC, RBC, H&H, bleeding time
• Renal studies: urinalysis, protein, blood
• C&S before drug therapy; drug may be taken as soon as culture is taken
Administer:
• IV after diluting 500 mg/1.7 ml of sterile H_2O for inj; further dilute each 500 mg/15-30 ml of compatible sol; give through Y-tube or stopcock 500 mg or less/5-10 min; may be further diluted and run over 24 hr
• Drug after C&S has been completed
• Divided oral doses on empty stomach before meals
Perform/provide:
• Adrenalin, suction, tracheostomy set, endotracheal intubation equipment
• Adequate fluid intake (2000 ml) during diarrhea episodes
• Scratch test to assess allergy, after securing order from physician; usually done when penicillin is only drug of choice
• Storage in tight container; refrigerate reconstituted solution
Evaluate:
• Therapeutic response: absence of fever, draining wounds
• Bowel pattern before and during treatment
• Skin eruptions after administration of penicillin to 1 wk after discontinuing drug
• Respiratory status: rate, character, wheezing, and tightness in chest
• Allergies before initiation of treatment, and reaction of each medication; highlight allergies on chart, Kardex
Teach patient/family:
• Aspects of drug therapy, including need to complete course of medication to ensure organism

* Available in Canada only

death (10-14 days); culture may be taken after completed course

• To report sore throat, fever, fatigue (could indicate superimposed infection)

• To wear or carry Medic Alert ID if allergic to penicillins

• To notify nurse of diarrhea

Lab test interferences:

False positive: Urine glucose, urine protein

Treatment of overdose: Withdraw drug, maintain airway, administer epinephrine, aminophylline, O_2, IV corticosteroids for anaphylaxis

naftifine HCl

(naf-tee-fin)

Naftin

Func. class.: Topical antifungal

Chem. class.: Synthetic allylamine derivative

Action: Interferes with cell membrane permeability in fungi such as *T. rubrum, T. mentagrophytes, T. tonsurans, E. floccosum, M. canis, M. audouinii, M. gypseum, Candida,* broad-spectrum antifungal

Uses: Tinea cruris, tinea corporis

Dosage and routes:

Massage into affected area, surrounding area bid, continue for 7-14 days

Available forms include: Cream 1%

Side effects/adverse reactions:

INTEG: Burning, stinging, dryness, itching, local irritation

Contraindications: Hypersensitivity

Precautions: Pregnancy (B), lactation, children

NURSING CONSIDERATIONS

Assess:

• For continuing infection: increased size, amount of lesions

Administer:

• To affected area, surrounding area; do not cover with occlusive dressings

Perform/provide:

• Storage below 30° C (86° F)

Evaluate:

• Therapeutic response: decrease in size, amount of lesions

Teach patient/family:

• To wear cotton clothing

• To use clean towel, dry well

• To avoid contact with mucous membranes

• Not to cover areas unless directed to by physician

• To report excessive itching, burning

• How to apply; massage cream into affected area and surrounding skin in AM, PM; effects observed within 1 wk, continue 1-2 wk after symptoms decrease

nalbuphine HCl

(nal'byoo-feen)

Nubain

Func. class.: Nonnarcotic analgesics

Chem. class.: Synthetic opiate

Controlled Substance Schedule II

Action: Depresses pain impulse transmission at the spinal cord level by interacting with opioid receptors

Uses: Moderate to severe pain

Dosage and routes:

• *Adult:* SC/IM/IV 10-20 mg q3-6h prn, not to exceed 160 mg/day

Available forms include: Inj SC, IM, IV 10, 20 mg/ml

Side effects/adverse reactions:

CNS: Drowsiness, dizziness, confusion, headache, sedation, euphoria, dysphoria (high doses)

GI: Nausea, vomiting, anorexia, constipation, cramps

GU: Increased urinary output, dysuria, urinary retention
INTEG: ***Rash,*** urticaria, bruising, flushing, diaphoresis, pruritus
EENT: Tinnitus, blurred vision, miosis, diplopia
CV: Palpitations, bradycardia, change in B/P
RESP: ***Respiratory depression***
Contraindications: Hypersensitivity, addiction (narcotic)
Precautions: Addictive personality, pregnancy (B), lactation, increased intracranial pressure, MI (acute), severe heart disease, respiratory depression, hepatic disease, renal disease
Pharmacokinetics:
SC/IM/IV: Duration 3-6 hr; metabolized by liver, excreted by kidneys, half-life 5 hr
Interactions/incompatibilities:
• Increased effects with other CNS depressants: alcohol, narcotics, sedative/hypnotics, antipsychotics, skeletal muscle relaxants

NURSING CONSIDERATIONS

Assess:
• I&O ratio; check for decreasing output; may indicate urinary retention
• For withdrawal reactions in narcotic-dependent individuals: pulmonary embolus, vascular occlusion; abscesses, ulcerations, nausea, vomiting, convulsions
Administer:
• IV undiluted 10 mg or less over 3-5 min
• With antiemetic if nausea, vomiting occur
• When pain is beginning to return; determine dosage interval by patient response
Perform/provide:
• Storage in light-resistant area at room temperature
• Assistance with ambulation
• Safety measures: siderails, night light, call bell within easy reach
Evaluate:
• Therapeutic response: decrease in pain
• CNS changes: dizziness, drowsiness, hallucinations, euphoria, LOC, pupil reaction
• Allergic reactions: rash, urticaria
• Respiratory dysfunction: respiratory depression, character, rate, rhythm; notify physician if respirations are <10/min
• Need for pain medication, physical dependence
Teach patient/family:
• To report any symptoms of CNS changes, allergic reactions
• That physical dependency may result when used for extended periods of time
• Withdrawal symptoms may occur: nausea, vomiting, cramps, fever, faintness, anorexia
Lab test interferences:
Increase: Amylase
Treatment of overdose: Narcan 0.2-0.8 IV, O_2, IV fluids, vasopressors

---

nalidixic acid

(nal-i-dix'ik)
NegGram, Nogram, Cybis, Wintomylon
Func. class.: Urinary tract anti-infective
Chem. class.: Synthetic naphthyridine derivative

Action: Appears to inhibit DNA polymerization, primary target being single-stranded DNA precursors in late stages of chromosomal replication
Uses: Urinary tract infections (acute/chronic) caused by *E. coli,*

---

* Available in Canada only

Klebsiella, Enterobacter, P. mirabilis, P. vulgaris, P. morganii

Dosage and routes:

• *Adult:* PO 1 g qid × 1-2 wk, 2 g/day for long-term treatment

• *Child >3 mo:* PO 55 mg/kg/day in 4 divided doses for 1-2 wk; 33 mg/kg/day in 4 divided doses for long-term treatment

Available forms include: Tabs 100, 250, 500 mg, 1 g susp 250 mg/5 ml

Side effects/adverse reactions:

INTEG: Pruritus, rash, urticaria, photosensitivity

CNS: Dizziness, headache, drowsiness, insomnia, ***convulsions***

GI: Nausea, vomiting, abdominal pain, diarrhea

EENT: Sensitivity to light, blurred vision, change in color perception

Contraindications: Hypersensitivity, CNS damage, liver disease, liver failure, infants <3 months

Precautions: Elderly, renal disease, hepatic disease, pregnancy (B)

Pharmacokinetics:

PO: Peak 1-2 hr, metabolized in liver, excreted in urine (unchange/conjugates), crosses placenta, enters breast milk

Interactions/incompatibilities:

• Increased effects of: oral coagulants

• Decreased effects of: antacids

NURSING CONSIDERATIONS

Assess:

• Blood count for patients on chronic therapy

• I&O ratio, urine pH <5.5 is ideal

• Renal, hepatic function

• Photosensitivity: if present, drug should be discontinued

Administer:

• After clean-catch urine is obtained for C&S

• Two daily doses if urine output is high or if patient has diabetes

Perform/provide:

• Limited intake of alkaline foods, drugs: milk, dairy products, peanuts, vegetables, alkaline antacids, sodium bicarbonate

• Protection from freezing

Evaluate:

• Therapeutic response: decreased dysuria, negative culture

• CNS symptoms: insomnia, vertigo, headache, drowsiness, convulsions

• Allergy: fever, flushing, rash, urticaria, pruritus

Teach patient/family:

• That photosensitivity occurs; that patient should avoid sunlight or use sunscreen to prevent burns

• To take medication with food or milk to decrease GI irritation

• To protect suspension from freezing, shake well before taking

• That drug may cause drowsiness; instruct client to seek aid in walking, other activities; advise client not to drive or operate machinery while on medication

• That diabetics should use ketodiastix to measure blood glucose level

Lab test interferences:

False positive: Urinary glucose

False increase: 17-OHCS, VMA

naloxone HCl

Narcan

Func. class.: Narcotic antagonist

Chem. class.: Thebaine derivative

Action: Competes with narcotics at narcotic receptor sites

Uses: Respiratory depression induced by narcotics, pentazocine, propoxyphene

Dosage and routes:
Narcotic-induced respiratory depression
• *Adult:* IV/SC/IM 0.4-2 mg; repeat q2-3 min, if needed
Postoperative respiratory depression
• *Adult:* IV 0.1-0.2 mg q2-3min prn
• *Child:* IV/IM/SC 0.01 mg/kg q2-3min prn
Asphyxia neonatorum
• *Neonates:* IV 0.01 mg/kg given into umbilical vein after delivery, may repeat in q2-3min × 3 doses
Available forms include: Inj IV, IM, SC 0.02, 0.4, 1 mg/ml
Side effects/adverse reactions:
CNS: Drowsiness, nervousness
GI: Nausea, vomiting
CV: Rapid pulse, increased systolic B/P high doses
RESP: Hyperpnea
Contraindications: Hypersensitivity, respiratory depression
Precautions: Pregnancy (B), children
Pharmacokinetics:
Metabolized by liver, excreted by kidneys, crosses placenta, excreted in breast milk, half-life 1 hr, onset 1-2 min (IV)

NURSING CONSIDERATIONS

Assess:
• VS q3-5min
• ABGs including PO_2, PCO_2
Administer:
• IV undiluted, diluted with sterile H_2O for inj, may be further diluted with NS or D_5 and given as an inf; give 0.4 mg or less over 15 sec or titrate inf to response
• Only if resuscitative equipment is nearby
• Only solutions prepared within 24 hr
Perform/provide:
• Storage at room temperature in darkness
Evaluate:
• Therapeutic response: reversal of respiratory depression
• Signs of withdrawal in drug-dependent individuals
• Cardiac status: tachycardia, hypertension
• Respiratory dysfunction: respiratory depression, character, rate, rhythm; if respirations are <10/min, administer Narcan, it is probably due to narcotic overdose not Narcan
Lab test interferences:
Interfere: Urine VMA, 5-HIAA, urine glucose

---

naltrexone HCl

(nal-trex'one)
Trexan

Func. class.: Narcotic antagonist
Chem. class.: Thebaine derivative

Action: Competes with narcotics at narcotic receptor sites
Uses: Blockage of opioid analgesics, used in treatment of opiate addiction
Dosage and routes:
• *Adult:* PO 25 mg, may give 25 mg after 1 hr if there are no withdrawal symptoms; 50-150 mg may be given qd depending on patient need, maintenance 50 mg q24h
Available forms include: Tabs 50 mg
Side effects/adverse reactions:
HEMA: ***Thrombocytopenia, agranulocytosis, leukopenia, neutropenia, hemolytic anemia,*** increased pro-time
CNS: Stimulation, drowsiness, dizziness, confusion, convulsion, headache, flushing, hallucinations
GI: Nausea, vomiting, diarrhea, heartburn, anorexia, ***hepatitis***
INTEG: Rash, urticaria, bruising

* Available in Canada only

EENT: Tinnitus, hearing loss
CV: Rapid pulse, pulmonary edema, hypertension
RESP: Wheezing, hyperpnea
Contraindications: Hypersensitivity, opioid dependence, hepatic failure, hepatitis
Precautions: Pregnancy (C)
Pharmacokinetics:
PO: Onset 15-30 min, peak 1-2 hr, duration is dose dependent
Metabolized by liver, excreted by kidneys, crosses placenta, excreted in breast milk, half-life 4 hr, extensive first-pass metabolism

NURSING CONSIDERATIONS

Assess:
- VS q3-5 min
- ABGs including PO_2, PCO_2

Administer:
- Only if resuscitative equipment is nearby

Perform/provide:
- Storage in tight container

Evaluate:
- Therapeutic response: blocking narcotic ingestion
- Signs of withdrawal in drug-dependent individuals
- Cardiac status: tachycardia, hypertension
- Respiratory dysfunction: respiratory depression, character, rate, rhythm; if respirations are <10/min, respiratory stimulant should be administered

nandrolone decanoate/ nandrolone phenpropionate

(nan'droe-lone)
Androlone-50, Androlone-D 50, Deca-Durabolin, Hybolin Decanoate, Anabolin, Anorolone, Durabolin, Hybolin Improved, Nandrobolic, Nandrolin
Func. class.: Androgenic anabolic steroid
Chem. class.: Halogenated testosterone derivative

Action: Increases weight by building body tissue, increases potassium, phosphorus, chloride, nitrogen levels, increases bone development
Uses: Tissue building, severe disease, refractory anemias, metastatic breast cancer
Dosage and routes:
Tissue building (possibly effective)
- *Adult:* IM 50-100 mg q3-4wk (decanoate)
- *Child 2-13 yr:* IM 25-50 mg q3-4wk (decanoate)

Severe disease/refractory anemias
- *Adult:* IM 100-200 mg qwk (decanoate)

Breast cancer
- *Adult:* IM 50-100 mg qwk (phenpropionate)

Available forms include: Phenpropionate inj IM 25, 50 mg/ml; decanoate inj IM 50, 100, 200 mg/ml
Side effects/adverse reactions:
INTEG: Rash, acneiform lesions, oily hair, skin, flushing, sweating, acne vulgaris, alopecia, hirsutism
CNS: Dizziness, headache, fatigue, tremors, paresthesias, flushing, sweating, anxiety, lability, insomnia
MS: Cramps, spasms

N

CV: Increased B/P
GU: ***Hematuria,*** amenorrhea, vaginitis, decreased libido, decreased breast size, clitoral hypertrophy, testicular atrophy
GI: Nausea, vomiting, constipation, weight gain, ***cholestatic jaundice***
EENT: Carpal tunnel syndrome, conjunctional edema, nasal congestion
ENDO: Abnormal GTT

Contraindications: Severe renal disease, severe cardiac disease, severe hepatic disease, hypersensitivity, pregnancy (X), lactation, abnormal genital bleeding, males with CA of breast, prostate

Precautions: Diabetes mellitus, CV disease, MI

Pharmacokinetics:
IM: Metabolized in liver, excreted in urine, crosses placenta, excreted in the breast milk

Interactions/incompatibilities:
- Increased effects of: oral antidiabetics, oxyphenbutazone
- Increased PT: anticoagulants
- Edema: ACTH, adrenal steroids
- Decreased effects of: insulin

NURSING CONSIDERATIONS

Assess:
- Weight daily, notify physician if weekly weight gain is >5 lb
- B/P q4h
- I&O ratio; be alert for decreasing urinary output, increasing edema
- Growth rate in children since growth rate may be uneven (linear/bone growth) when used for extended periods of time
- Electrolytes: K, Na, Cl, Ca; cholesterol
- Liver function studies: ALT, AST, bilirubin

Administer:
- Titrated dose, use lowest effective dose

Perform/provide:
- Diet with increased calories, protein; decrease sodium if edema occurs

Evaluate:
- Therapeutic response: increased appetite, increased stamina
- Edema, hypertension, cardiac symptoms, jaundice
- Mental status: affect, mood, behavioral changes, aggression
- Signs of masculinization in female: increased libido, deepening of voice, breast tissue, enlarged clitoris, menstrual irregularities; male: gynecomastia, impotence, testicular atrophy
- Hypercalcemia: lethargy, polyuria, polydipsia, nausea, vomiting, constipation, drug may need to be decreased
- Hypoglycemia in diabetics; since oral anticoagulant action is decreased

Teach patient/family:
- That drug needs to be combined with complete health plan: diet, rest, exercise
- To notify physician if therapeutic response decreases
- Not to discontinue medication abruptly
- About changes in sex characteristics
- That females should report menstrual irregularities
- That 1-3 mo course is necessary for response in breast cancer
- Procedure for use of buccal tablets: requires 30-60 min to dissolve, change absorption site with each dose; do not eat, drink, chew, or smoke while tablet is in place

Lab test interferences:
Increase: Serum cholesterol, blood glucose, urine glucose
Decrease: Serum calcium, serum potassium, T_4, T_3, thyroid ^{131}I up-

take test, urine 17-OHCS, 17-KS, PBI, BSP

naphazoline HCl

(naf-az'oh-leen)

Privine

Func. class.: Nasal decongestant
Chem. class.: Sympathomimetic amine

Action: Produces vasoconstriction (rapid, long-acting) of arterioles, thereby decreasing fluid exudation, mucosal engorgement

Uses: Nasal congestion

Dosage and routes:

- *Adult:* Instill 2 gtts or sprays to nasal mucosa q3-4h
- *Child 6-12 yr:* Instill 1-2 gtts or sprays, repeat q3-4h prn, not to exceed 5 days

Available forms include: Sol 0.025, 0.05%

Side effects/adverse reactions:

GI: Nausea, vomiting, anorexia
EENT: Irritation, burning, sneezing, stinging, dryness, rebound congestion
INTEG: Contact dermatitis
CNS: Anxiety, restlessness, tremors, weakness, insomnia, dizziness, fever, headache

Contraindications: Hypersensitivity to sympathomimetic amines

Precautions: Child <6 yr, elderly, diabetes, cardiovascular disease, hypertension, hyperthyroidism, increased ICP, prostatic hypertrophy, pregnancy (C), glaucoma

Interactions/incompatibilities:

- Hypertension: MAOIs, β-adrenergic blockers
- Hypotension: methyldopa, mecamylamine, reserpine

NURSING CONSIDERATIONS

Administer:

- No more than q4h
- For <4 consecutive days

Perform/provide:

- Environmental humidification to decrease nasal congestion, dryness
- Storage in light-resistant containers; do not expose to high temperatures

Evaluate:

- Therapeutic response: decreased nasal congestion
- Redness, swelling, pain in nasal passages

Teach patient/family:

- That stinging may occur for several applications; drying of mucosa may be decreased by environmental humidification
- To notify physician if irregular pulse, insomnia, dizziness, or tremors occur
- Proper administration to avoid systemic absorption

naphazoline HCl

(naf-az'oh-leen)

Allerest Eye Drops, AK-Con Ophthalmic, Albalon, Clear Eyes, Muro's Opcon, Nafazair, Naphcon, Vasocon

Func. class.: Ophthalmic vasoconstrictor
Chem. class.: Direct imidazoline derivative

Action: Vasoconstriction of eye arterioles; decreases eye engorgement by stimulation of α-adrenergic receptors

Uses: Relieves hyperemia, irritation in superficial corneal vascularity

Dosage and routes:

- *Adult:* Instill 1-2 gtts q3-4h

Available forms include: Sol 0.1%, 0.02%, 0.025%, 0.05%, 0.03%, 0.012%

Side effects/adverse reactions:

CNS: Headache, dizziness, seda-

N

tion, anxiety, weakness, sweating (systemic absorption)
CV: Hypertension, dysrhythmias, tachycardia, ***CV collapse*** (systemic absorption)
EENT: Pupil dilation, increased intraocular pressure, photophobia
Contraindications: Hypersensitivity, glaucoma (narrow-angle)
Precautions: Hypertension, hyperthyroidism, elderly, severe arteriosclerosis, cardiac disease, pregnancy (C)
Pharmacokinetics:
Instill: Duration 2-3 hr
Interactions/incompatibilities:
• Increased pressor effects: MAOIs, tricyclic antidepressants

NURSING CONSIDERATIONS

Perform/provide:
• Storage in tight, light-resistant container
Evaluate:
• Therapeutic response: vasoconstriction of the eye
Teach patient/family:
• To report change in vision, blurring, or loss of sight; breathing trouble, sweating, flushing, anxiety, weakness
• Method of instillation; tilt head backward, hold dropper over eye, drop medication inside lower lid, using pressure on inside corner of eye hold 1 min, do not touch dropper to eye
• That blurred vision will decrease with repeated use of drug
• To notify physician if headache, spots, redness, pain occur; discontinue use

naproxen/naproxen sodium

(na-prox'en)
Naprosyn/Anaprox
Func. class.: Nonsteroidal antiinflammatory
Chem. class.: Propionic acid derivative

Action: Inhibits prostaglandin synthesis by decreasing an enzyme needed for biosynthesis; possesses analgesic, antiinflammatory, antipyretic properties
Uses: Mild to moderate pain, osteoarthritis, rheumatoid, gouty arthritis
Dosage and routes:
• *Adult:* PO 250-500 mg bid, not to exceed 1 g/day (base); 525 mg, then 275 mg q6-8h prn, not to exceed 1475 mg (sodium)
Available forms include: Tabs 250, 275, 375, 500 mg; susp 125 mg/5 ml
Side effects/adverse reactions:
GI: Nausea, anorexia, vomiting, diarrhea, jaundice, ***cholestatic hepatitis,*** constipation, flatulence, cramps, dry mouth, peptic ulcer
CNS: Dizziness, drowsiness, fatigue, tremors, confusion, insomnia, anxiety, depression
CV: Tachycardia, peripheral edema, palpitations, dysrhythmias
INTEG: Purpura, rash, pruritus, sweating
GU: ***Nephrotoxicity: dysuria, hematuria, oliguria, azotemia***
HEMA: ***Blood dyscrasias***
EENT: Tinnitus, hearing loss, blurred vision
Contraindications: Hypersensitivity, asthma, severe renal disease, severe hepatic disease
Precautions: Pregnancy (B), lac-

tation, children, bleeding disorders, GI disorders, cardiac disorders, hypersensitivity to other antiinflammatory agents, elderly

Pharmacokinetics:

PO: Peak 2-4 hr, half-life 3-3½ hr; metabolized in liver, excreted in urine (metabolites), excreted in breast milk, 99% protein binding

Interactions/incompatibilities:

- May increase action of: heparin
- Increased lithium toxicity: lithium

NURSING CONSIDERATIONS

Assess:

- Renal, liver, blood studies: BUN, creatinine, AST, ALT, Hgb before treatment, periodically thereafter
- Audiometric, ophthalmic exam before, during, after treatment

Administer:

- With food to decrease GI symptoms; best to take on empty stomach to facilitate absorption

Perform/provide:

- Storage at room temperature

Evaluate:

- Therapeutic response: decreased pain, stiffness, swelling in joints, ability to move more easily
- For eye, ear problems: blurred vision, tinnitus (may indicate toxicity)

Teach patient/family:

- To report blurred vision, ringing, roaring in ears (may indicate toxicity)
- To avoid driving or other hazardous activities if dizziness or drowsiness occurs
- To report change in urine pattern, weight increase, edema (face, lower extremities), pain increase in joints, fever, blood in urine (indicates nephrotoxicity)
- That therapeutic effects may take up to 1 mo

Laboratory test interferences:

Increase: BUN, alk phosphatase

False increase: 5-HIAA, 17KGS

---

natamycin (ophthalmic)

(na-ta-mye'sin)

Natacyn

Func. class.: Antiinfective/antifungal

Chem. class.: Tetraene polyene compound

Action: Inhibits transport functions and cell permeability in organism

Uses: Eye infection, fungal blepharitis, conjunctivitis, keratitis

Dosage and routes:

- *Adult and child:* Instill 1 gtt q1-2h × 3-4 days, then decrease to 1 gtt 8×/day, duration of therapy, 14-21 days

Available forms include: Susp 5%

Side effects/adverse reactions:

EENT: Temporary visual haze, overgrowth of nonsusceptible organisms

Contraindications: Hypersensitivity

Precautions: Antibiotic hypersensitivity, pregnancy (C); failure of keratitis to improve after 7-10 days suggests infection not caused by susceptible organism

NURSING CONSIDERATIONS

Administer:

- After washing hands, cleanse crusts or discharge from eye before application

Perform/provide:

- Storage at room temperature

Evaluate:

- Therapeutic response: absence of redness, inflammation, tearing, photophobia
- Allergy: itching, lacrimation, redness, swelling, eye pain

Teach patient/family:

- To use drug exactly as pre-

scribed, shake well before using
• Not to use eye makeup, towels, washcloths, eye medication of others; reinfection may occur
• That drug container tip should not be touched to eye
• To report itching, increased redness, burning, stinging, swelling; drug should be discontinued

neomycin sulfate

(nee-oh-mye'sin)
Mycifradin Sulfate, Neobiotic
Func. class.: Antibiotic
Chem. class.: Aminoglycoside

Action: Inferferes with protein synthesis in bacterial cell by binding to ribosomal subunit causing inaccurate peptide sequence to form in protein chain, causing bacterial death

Uses: Severe systemic infections of CNS, respiratory, GI, urinary tract, eye, bone, skin, soft tissues caused by *P. aeruginosa, E. coli, Enterobacter, K. pneumoniae, P. vulgaris;* also used for hepatic coma, preoperatively to sterilize bowel, infectious diarrhea caused by enteropathogenic *E. coli*

Dosage and routes:

Severe systemic infections
• *Adult:* IM 15 mg/kg/day in 4 divided doses, not to exceed 1 g/day

Hepatic coma
• *Adult:* PO 4-12 g/day in divided doses × 5-6 days
• *Child:* 50-100 mg/kg/day in divided doses

Preoperative bowel sterilization
• *Adult:* PO on 3rd day of a 3 day regimen, give 1 g early PM, repeat in 1 hr, repeat at hs (given with erythromycin); give saline cathartic before giving this drug

Available forms include: Tabs 500 mg; top, inj IM 500 mg; ophthalmic oint, oral sol 125 mg/5 ml

Side effects/adverse reactions:
GU: ***Oliguria, hematuria, renal damage, azotemia, renal failure, nephrotoxicity***
CNS: Confusion, depression, numbness, tremors, ***convulsions,*** muscle twitching, ***neurotoxicity,*** dizziness, vertigo
EENT: ***Ototoxicity,*** deafness, visual disturbances, tinnitus
HEMA: ***Agranulocytosis, thrombocytopenia,*** leukopenia, eosinophilia, anemia
GI: Nausea, vomiting, anorexia, increased ALT, AST, bilirubin, hepatomegaly, ***hepatic necrosis,*** splenomegaly
CV: Hypotension, hypertension, palpitation
INTEG: Rash, burning, urticaria, photosensitivity, dermatitis, alopecia

Contraindications: Bowel obstruction (oral use), severe renal disease, hypersensitivity, infants, children

Precautions: Mild renal disease, pregnancy (C), hearing deficits, lactation, myasthenia gravis, Parkinson's disease

Pharmacokinetics:
PO: Onset rapid, peak 1-2 hr
Plasma half-life 2-3 hr; not metabolized, excreted unchanged in urine, crosses placental barrier

Interactions/incompatibilities:
• Increased ototoxicity, neurotoxicity, nephrotoxicity: other aminoglycosides, amphotericin B, polymyxin, vancomycin, ethacrynic acid, furosemide, mannitol, methoxyflurane, cisplatin, cephalosporins, bacitracin
• Do not mix in solution or syringe: carbenicillin, ticarcillin, amphoter-

icin B, cephalothin, erythromycin, heparin

• Increased effects: nondepolarizing muscle relaxants, succinylcholine, oral anticoagulants when given with oral neomycin

• Decreased effects of: digoxin, penicillin V when given with oral neomycin

NURSING CONSIDERATIONS

Assess:

• Weight before treatment; calculation of dosage is usually done based on ideal body weight, but may be calculated on actual body weight

• I&O ratio, urinalysis daily for proteinuria, cells, casts; report sudden change in urine output

• Urine pH if drug is used for UTI; urine should be kept alkaline

Administer:

• IM injection in large muscle mass, rotate injection sites

• Drug in evenly spaced doses to maintain blood level

• Bicarbonate to alkalinize urine if ordered in treating UTI, as drug is most active in alkaline environment

Perform/provide:

• Adequate fluids of 2-3 L/day unless contraindicated to prevent irritation of tubules

• Supervised ambulation, other safety measures with vestibular dysfunction

Evaluate:

• Therapeutic response: absence of fever, draining wounds, negative C&S after treatment

• Renal impairment by securing urine for CrCl testing, BUN, serum creatinine; lower dosage should be given in renal impairment (CrCl <80 ml/min)

• Deafness by audiometric testing, ringing, roaring in ears, vertigo; assess hearing before, during, after treatment

• Dehydration: high sp gr, decrease in skin turgor, dry mucous membranes, dark urine

• Overgrowth of infection: increased temperature, malaise, redness, pain, swelling, perineal itching, diarrhea, stomatitis, change in cough, sputum

• C&S before starting treatment to identify infecting organism

• Vestibular dysfunction: nausea, vomiting, dizziness, headache; drug should be discontinued if severe

• Injection sites for redness, swelling, abscesses; use warm compresses at site

Teach patient/family:

• To report headache, dizziness, symptoms of overgrowth of infection, renal impairment

• To report loss of hearing, ringing, roaring in ears or a feeling of fullness in head

Treatment of overdose: Hemodialysis, monitor serum levels of drug

neomycin sulfate

(nee-oh-mye'sin)

Drotic, Otocort

Func. class.: Otic, antibiotic
Chem. class.: Aminoglycoside

Action: Inhibits protein synthesis in susceptible microorganisms

Uses: Ear infection (external), short-term use

Dosage and routes:

• *Adult and child:* Instill 2-5 gtt tid-qid

Available forms include: Otic sol in combination with neomycin, hydrocortisone 0.25%, 0.5%

Side effects/adverse reactions:

EENT: Itching, irritation in ear

N

INTEG: Rash, urticaria
Contraindications: Hypersensitivity, perforated eardrum
Precautions: Pregnancy (C)

NURSING CONSIDERATIONS

Administer:

- After removing impacted cerumen by irrigation
- After cleaning stopper with alcohol
- After restraining child if necessary
- Warming solution

Evaluate:

- Therapeutic response: decreased ear pain
- For redness, swelling, fever, pain in ear, which indicates superimposed infection

Teach patient/family:

- Method of instillation using aseptic technique, including not touching dropper to ear
- That dizziness may occur after instillation

neomycin sulfate (topical)

(nee-oh-mye'sin)
Myciguent
Func. class.: Local antibacterial
Chem. class.: Aminoglycoside

Action: Interferes with bacterial protein synthesis
Uses: Skin infections
Dosage and routes:

- *Adult and child:* TOP rub into affected area bid-tid

Available forms include: Oint, cream 0.5%
Side effects/adverse reactions:
INTEG: Rash, urticaria, scaling, redness
Contraindications: Hypersensitivity, large areas, burns, ulcerations
Precautions: Pregnancy (C), lactation, impaired renal function, external ear of perforated eardrum

NURSING CONSIDERATIONS

Administer:

- Enough medication to completely cover lesions
- After cleansing with soap, water before each application, dry well
- To less than 20% of body surface area

Perform/provide:

- Storage at room temperature in dry place

Evaluate:

- Therapeutic response: decrease in size, number of lesions
- Allergic reaction: burning, stinging, swelling, redness
- For signs of nephrotoxicity or ototoxicity

Teach patient/family:

- To use medical asepsis (hand washing) before, after each application
- To apply with glove to prevent further infection
- To avoid use of OTC creams, ointments, lotions unless directed by physician
- To notify physician if condition worsens

neostigmine bromide/neostigmine methylsulfate

(nee-oh-stig'meen)
Prostigmin Bromide/Prostigmin
Func. class.: Cholinergic stimulant
Chem. class.: Quaternary compound

Action: Inhibits destruction of acetylcholine, which increases concentration at sites where acetylcholine is released; this facilitates transmission of impulses across myoneural junction

Uses: Myasthenia gravis, nondepolarizing neuromuscular blocker, antagonist, bladder distention, postoperative ileus

Dosage and routes:

Myasthenia gravis

- *Adult:* PO 15-375 mg/day; IM/IV 0.5-2 mg q1-3h
- *Child:* PO 2 mg/kg/day q3-4h

Tubocurarine antagonist

- *Adult:* IV 0.5-2 mg slowly, may repeat if needed (give 0.6-1.2 mg atropine before this drug)

Abdominal distention/postoperative ileus

- *Adult:* IM/SC 0.25-1 mg q4-6h depending on condition

Available forms include: Tabs 15 mg; inj IM, SC, IV 1:1000, 1:2000, 1:4000

Side effects/adverse reactions:

INTEG: Rash, urticaria, flushing
CNS: Dizziness, headache, sweating, confusion, weakness, ***convulsions,*** incoordination, ***paralysis***
GI: Nausea, diarrhea, vomiting, cramps
CV: Tachycardia, dysrhythmias, bradycardia, hypotension, AV block, ECG changes, ***cardiac arrest***
GU: Frequency, incontinence
RESP: ***Respiratory depression, bronchospasm, constriction, laryngospasm, respiratory arrest***
EENT: Miosis, blurred vision, lacrimation

Contraindications: Obstruction of intestine, renal system, pregnancy (C), bromide sensitivity

Precautions: Bradycardia, hypotension, seizure disorders, bronchial asthma, coronary occlusion, hyperthyroidism, dysrhythmias, peptic ulcer, megacolon, poor GI motility, lactation, children

Pharmacokinetics:

PO: Onset 45-75 min, duration 2½-4 hr
IM/SC: Onset 10-30 min, duration 2½-4 hr
IV onset 4-8 min; duration 2-4 hr; metabolized in liver, excreted in urine

Interactions/incompatibilities:

- Decreased action of: gallamine, metocurine, pancuronium, tubocurarine, atropine
- Increased action of: decamethonium, succinylcholine
- Decreased action of neostigmine: aminoglycosides, anesthetics, procainamide, quinidine, mecamylamine, polymyxin, magnesium

NURSING CONSIDERATIONS

Assess:

- VS, respiration q8h
- I&O ratio; check for urinary retention or incontinence

Administer:

- IV undiluted, give through Y-tube or 3-way stopcock; give 0.5 mg or less over 1 min
- Only with atropine sulfate available for cholinergic crisis
- Only after all other cholinergics have been discontinued
- Increased doses if tolerance occurs
- Larger doses after exercise or fatigue
- With food or milk to decrease GI symptoms
- On empty stomach for better absorption

Perform/provide:

- Storage at room temperature

Evaluate:

- Therapeutic response: increased muscle strength, hand grasp, improved gait, absence of labored breathing (if severe)
- Bradycardia, hypotension, bronchospasm, headache, dizziness, convulsions, respiratory depression; drug should be discontinued if toxicity occurs

N

Teach patient/family:
• That drug is not a cure, it only relieves symptoms
• To wear Medic Alert ID specifying myasthenia gravis, drugs taken

Treatment of overdose: Respiratory support, atropine 1-4 mg (IV)

netilmicin sulfate

(ne-til-mye'sin)
Netromycin
Func. class.: Antibiotic
Chem. class.: Aminoglycoside

Action: Interferes with protein synthesis in bacterial cell by binding to ribosomal subunit, causing inaccurate peptide sequence to form in protein chain, causing bacterial death

Uses: Severe systemic infections of CNS, respiratory, GI, urinary tract, bone, skin, soft tissues caused by *P. aeruginosa, E. coli, Enterobacter, Citrobacter, Staphylococcus, K. pneumoniae, P. mirabilis, Serratia, Shigella, Salmonella, Acinetobacter, Neisseria*

Dosage and routes:
Normal renal function
• *Adult and child >12 yr:* IM/IV 3-6.5 mg/kg/day; may give q8-12h for severe infections
• *Child and infant 6 wk-12 yr:* IM/IV 5.5-8 mg/kg/day in divided doses q8-12h
• *Neonate <6 wk:* IM/IV 4-6.5 mg/kg/day in divided doses q12h

Available forms include: Inj IM, IV 10, 25, 100 mg/ml

Side effects/adverse reactions:
GU: ***Oliguria, hematuria, renal damage, azotemia, renal failure, nephrotoxicity***
CNS: Confusion, depression, numbness, tremors, ***convulsions,*** muscle twitching, ***neurotoxicity,*** dizziness, vertigo
EENT: ***Ototoxicity,*** deafness, visual disturbances, tinnitus
HEMA: ***Agranulocytosis, thrombocytopenia, leukopenia, eosinophilia, anemia***
GI: Nausea, vomiting, anorexia, increased ALT, AST, bilirubin, hepatomegaly, ***hepatic necrosis,*** splenomegaly
CV: Hypotension, hypertension, palpitations
INTEG: Rash, burning, urticaria, dermatitis

Contraindications: Severe renal disease, hypersensitivity

Precautions: Neonates, mild renal disease, pregnancy (D), children <12 yr, lactation, myasthenia gravis, hearing deficit, Parkinson's disease

Pharmacokinetics:
IM: Onset rapid, peak 1-2 hr
IV: Onset immediate, peak 1-2 hr
Plasma half-life 2-3 hr, not metabolized, excreted unchanged in urine, crosses placental barrier

Interactions/incompatibilities:
• Increased ototoxicity, neurotoxicity, nephrotoxicity: other aminoglycosides, amphotericin B, polymyxin, vancomycin, ethacrynic acid, furosemide, mannitol, methoxyflurane, cisplatin, cephalosporins, bacitracin
• Do not mix in solution or syringe: carbenicillin, ticarcillin, amphotericin B, cephalothin, erythromycin, heparin
• Increased effects: nondepolarizing muscle relaxants, succinylcholine

NURSING CONSIDERATIONS

Assess:
• Weight before treatment; calculation of dosage is usually done

based on ideal body weight, but may be calculated on actual body weight
• Daily I&O ratio, urinalysis for proteinuria, cells, casts; report sudden change in urine output
• VS during infusion, watch for hypotension, change in pulse
• IV site for thrombophlebitis including pain, redness, swelling q30 min, change site if needed; apply warm compresses to discontinued site
• Serum peak, drawn at 30-60 min after IV infusion or 60 min after IM injection; trough level drawn just before next dose; blood level should be 2-4 times bacteriostatic level
• Urine pH if drug is used for UTI; urine should be kept alkaline

Administer:
• IM injection in large muscle mass, rotate injection sites
• Drug in evenly spaced doses to maintain blood level
• Bicarbonate to alkalinize urine if ordered in treating UTI, as drug is most active in alkaline environment
• IV diluted in 50-200 ml IV sol, infuse over ½-2 hr

Perform/provide:
• Adequate fluids of 2-3 L/day unless contraindicated to prevent irritation of tubules
• Flush of IV line with NS or D_5W after infusion
• Supervised ambulation, other safety measures with vestibular dysfuncton

Evaluate:
• Therapeutic response: absence of fever, draining wounds, negative C&S after treatment
• Renal impairment by securing urine for CrCl testing, BUN, serum creatinine; a lower dosage should be given in renal impairment (CrCl <80 ml/min)
• Deafness by audiometric testing, ringing, roaring in ears, vertigo; assess hearing before, during, after treatment
• Dehydration: high sp gr, decrease in skin turgor, dry mucous membranes, dark urine
• Overgrowth of infection: increased temperature, malaise, redness, pain, swelling, perineal itching, diarrhea, stomatitis, change in cough or sputum
• C&S before starting treatment to identify infecting organism
• Vestibular dysfunction: nausea, vomiting, dizziness, headache; drug should be discontinued if severe
• Injection sites for redness, swelling, abscesses; use warm compresses at site

Teach patient/family:
• To report headache, dizziness, symptoms of overgrowth of infection, renal impairment
• To report loss of hearing, ringing, roaring in ears or feeling of fullness in head

Treatment of overdose: Hemodialysis, monitor serum levels of drug

---

niacin (vitamin B_3/ nicotinic acid)/niacinamide (nicotinamide)

(nye'a-sin) (nye-a-sin'a-mide)
Niac, Nico-400, Nicobid, Nicolar, Nico-Span, Novoniacin*

Func. class.: Vitamin B_3
Chem. class.: Water-soluble vitamin

Action: Needed for conversion of fats, protein, carbohydrates, by oxidation reduction; acts directly on vascular smooth muscle causing vasodilation; high doses decrease serum lipids

Uses: Pellagra, hyperlipidemias, (niacin) peripheral vascular disease (niacin)

Dosage and routes:

Adjunct in hyperlipidemia

• *Adult:* PO 1.5-3 g qd in 3 divided doses after meals, may be increased to 6 g/day

Pellagra

• *Adult:* IM/SC/PO/IV INF 10-20 mg, not to exceed 500 mg total dose

• *Child:* IM/SC/PO/IV INF 300 mg until desired response

Peripheral vascular disease

• *Adult:* PO 250-800 mg qd in divided doses

Available forms include: Nicotinic acid—tabs 20, 25, 50, 100, 500 mg; caps timed released 125, 250, 300, 400, 500 mg; tabs time released 150 mg; elix 50 mg/5 ml; inj 100 mg/ml; nicotinamide—tabs 50, 100, 500 mg; tabs timed release 1000 mg; inj IV, IM, SC 100 mg/ml

Side effects/adverse reactions:

CNS: Paresthesias, headache, dizziness, anxiety

GI: Nausea, vomiting, anorexia, flatulence, xerostomia, ***jaundice,*** diarrhea, peptic ulcer

GU: Hyperuricemia, ***glycosuria, hypoalbuminemia***

CV: Postural hypotension, vasovagal attacks, dysrhythmias, vasodilation

EENT: Blurred vision, ptosis

INTEG: Flushing, dry skin, rash, pruritus

RESP: Wheezing

Contraindications: Hypersensitivity, peptic ulcer, hepatic disease, lactation, hemorrhage, severe hypotension

Precautions: Glaucoma, cardiovascular disease, CAD, diabetes mellitus, gout, schizophrenia, pregnancy (A)

Pharmacokinetics:

PO: Peak 30-70 min, half-life 45 min, metabolized in liver, 30% excreted unchanged in urine

Interactions/incompatibilities:

• Increased action of: ganglionic blockers

NURSING CONSIDERATIONS

Assess:

• Liver function studies: AST, ALT, bilirubin, alk phosphatase; blood glucose before and during treatment

• Niacin levels while taking this drug

Administer:

• With meals for GI symptoms

Evaluate:

• Therapeutic response: decreased lipids, warm extremities, absence of numbness in extremities

• Cardiac status: rate, rhythm, quality; postural hypotension, dysrhythmias

• Nutritional status: liver, yeast, legumes, organ meat, lean poultry

• Liver dysfunction: clay-colored stools, itching, dark urine, jaundice

• CNS symptoms: headache, paresthesias, blurred vision

Teach patient/family:

• That flushing and increase in feelings of warmth will occur several hours after taking drug (PO) or immediately (IM/IV/SC); time-release product will minimize flushing

• To remain recumbent if postural hypotension occurs

• To abstain from alcohol if drug is prescribed for hyperlipidemia

• To avoid sunlight if skin lesions are present

Lab test interferences:

Increase: Bilirubin, alk phospha-

tase, liver enzymes, LDH, uric acid
Decrease: Cholesterol
False increase: Urinary catecholamines
False positive: Urine glucose

nicardipine HCl

(nye-card'i-peen)
Cardene
Func. class.: Calcium-channel blocker
Chem. class.: Dihydropyridine

Action: Inhibits calcium ion influx across cell membrane during cardiac depolarization; produces relaxation of coronary vascular smooth muscle, peripheral vascular smooth muscle; dilates coronary vascular arteries; increases myocardial oxygen delivery in patients with vasospastic angina
Uses: Chronic stable angina pectoris, hypertension
Dosage and routes:
Angina
Adult: PO 20 mg tid initially, may increase after 3 days (range 20-40 mg tid)
Hypertension
Adult: PO 20 mg tid initially, then increase after 3 days (range 20-40 mg tid)
Available forms include: Caps 20, 30 mg
Side effects/adverse reactions:
CV: Dysrhythmia, edema, CHF, bradycardia, hypotension, palpitations, ***MI, pulmonary edema***
GI: Nausea, vomiting, diarrhea, gastric upset, constipation, ***hepatitis,*** abdominal cramps
GU: Nocturia, polyuria, ***acute renal failure***
INTEG: Rash, pruritus, urticaria, photosensitivity, hair loss
CNS: Headache, fatigue, drowsiness, dizziness, anxiety, depression, weakness, insomnia, confusion, paresthesia, somnolence
OTHER: Blurred vision, flushing, nasal congestion, sweating, shortness of breath, gynecomastia, hyperglycemia, sexual difficulties
Contraindications: Sick sinus syndrome, 2nd or 3rd degree heart block, hypotension less than 90 mm Hg systolic, hypersensitivity
Precautions: CHF, hypotension, hepatic injury, pregnancy (C), lactation, children, renal disease, elderly
Pharmacokinetics:
PO: Onset 10 min, peak 1-2 hr, half-life 2-5 hr; metabolized by liver, excreted in urine (98% as metabolites)
Interactions/incompatibilities:
• Increased effects of: digitalis, neuromuscular blocking agents, theophylline
• Increased effects of: nicardipine, cimetidine

NURSING CONSIDERATIONS

Administer:
• ac, hs
Evaluate:
• Therapeutic response: decreased anginal pain, decreased B/P
• Cardiac status: B/P, pulse, respiration, ECG
Teach patient/family:
• To avoid hazardous activities until stabilized on drug, dizziness is no longer a problem
• To limit caffeine consumption
• To avoid OTC drugs unless directed by physician
• To comply in all areas of medical regimen: diet, exercise, stress reduction, drug therapy
• To notify physician of: irregular heart beat, shortness of breath, swelling of feet and hands, pro-

nounced dizziness, constipation, nausea, hypotension
Treatment of overdose: Defibrillation, β-agonists, IV calcium inotropic agents, diuretics, atropine for AV block, vasopressor for hypotension

---

niclosamide

(ni-kloe'sa-mide)
Niclocide

Func. class.: Anthelmintic
Chem. class.: Salicylanilide derivative

Action: Inhibits synthesis of ATP in mitochondria; leads to destruction in intestine where worm may be digested, removed in feces; not effective for ova or larval stage
Uses: Regular, dwarf tapeworms
Dosage and routes:

- *Adult:* PO 2 g chewed as a single dose for *T saginata* and *D latum*; 2g × 7 days for *Hymenolepis nana*
- *Child >34 kg:* PO 1.5 g chewed as a single dose for *T. saginata* and *D. latum*; 1.5 g as single dose on day 1 followed by 1 g × 6 days for *Hymenolepis nana*
- *Child <34 kg:* PO 1 g chewed as a single dose for *T. saginata* and *D. latum*; 1 g on day 1, then 0.5 g × 6 days for *Hymenolepis nana*

Available forms include: Tabs, chewable 500 mg
Side effects/adverse reactions:
INTEG: Rash, pruritus, pruritus ani, alopecia
CNS: Dizziness, headache, drowsiness, restlessness, sweating, fever
EENT: Bad taste, oral irritation
GI: Nausea, vomiting, anorexia, diarrhea, constipation, rectal bleeding
Contraindications: Hypersensitivity
Precautions: Child <2 yr, pregnancy (B), lactation

NURSING CONSIDERATIONS

Assess:

- Stools during entire treatment, 1, 3 mo after treatment; specimens must be sent to lab while still warm

Administer:

- May be crushed, mixed with water if unable to swallow whole
- Laxatives if constipated; not needed for drug to work
- After breakfast, tab must be chewed, not swallowed

Perform/provide:

- Storage in tight, light-resistant container in cool environment; do not freeze

Evaluate:

- Therapeutic response: expulsion of worms, 3 negative stool cultures after completion of treatment
- For allergic reaction: rash, itching in anal area
- For diarrhea during expulsion of worms
- For infection in other family members since infection from person to person is common

Teach patient/family:

- Proper hygiene after BM including handwashing technique; tell patient to avoid putting fingers in mouth
- That infected person should sleep alone; do not shake bed linen, change bed linen qd, wash in hot water
- To clean toilet qd with disinfectant (green soap solution)
- Need for compliance with dosage schedule, duration of treatment
- To drink fruit juice to remove mucus that intestinal tapeworms burrow in, aids in explusion of worms (dwarf tapeworms only)

Treatment of overdose: Enemas, laxatives; do not induce vomiting

---

* Available in Canada only

nicotine resin complex

(nik'o-teen)

Nicorette, Nicotine Pola Crile

Func. class.: Smoking deterrent
Chem. class.: Ganglionic cholinergic agonist

Action: Agonist at nicotinic receptors in the peripheral and central nervous systems; acts at sympathetic ganglia; on chemoreceptors of the aorta and carotid bodies; also affects adrenal-releasing catecholamines

Uses: Deter cigarette smoking

Dosage and routes:

• *Adult:* Gum 1 piece chewed × ½ hr as needed to abstain from smoking, not to exceed 30/day

Available forms include: Gum 2 mg/piece of gum

Side effects/adverse reactions:

RESP: Breathing difficulty, cough, hoarseness, sneezing, wheezing

EENT: Jaw ache, irritation in buccal cavity

CNS: Dizziness, vertigo, insomnia, headache, confusion, convulsions, depression, euphoria, numbness, tinnitus

GI: Nausea, vomiting, anorexia, indigestion, diarrhea, abdominal pain, constipation, eructation

CV: Dysrhythmias, tachycardia, palpitations

Contraindications: Hypersensitivity, immediate post MI recovery period, severe angina pectoris, pregnancy (X)

Precautions: Vasospastic disease, dysrhythmias, diabetes mellitus, children, hyperthyroidism, pheochromocytoma, coronary disease, esophagitis, peptic ulcer

Pharmacokinetics:

Onset 15-30 min, metabolized in liver, excreted in urine, half-life 2-3 hr, 30-120 hr, (terminal)

Interactions/incompatibilities:

• Smoking cessation increases diuretic effects of; furosemide
• Increased blood levels with cessation of smoking: caffeine, theophylline, petazocine, imipramine

NURSING CONSIDERATIONS

Assess:

• Adverse reaction: irritation of buccal cavity, dislike of taste, jaw ache

Evaluate:

• Therapeutic response: decrease in urge to smoke, decreased need for gum after 3-6 mo

Teach patient/family:

• To chew gum slowly for 30 min to promote buccal absorption of the drug; do not chew over 45 min
• To begin drug withdrawal after 3 mo use; not to exceed 6 mo
• All aspects of drug; give package insert to patient and explain
• That gum will not stick to dentures, dental appliances
• That gum is as toxic as cigarette; it is to be used only to deter smoking
• Not to use during pregnancy; birth defects may occur

nicotine transdermal system

Nicoderm, Habitrol

Func. class.: Smoking deterrent
Chem. class.: Alkaloid

Action: Binds to acetylcholine receptors at autonomic ganglia in the adrenal medulla, at neuromuscular junctions, and in the brain

Uses: Deter cigarette smoking

Dosage and routes:

• *Adult:* Trans 21 mg/day for 6 wk,

then 14 mg/day for 2 wk, then 7 mg/day for 2 wk

Available forms include: Transdermal patch delivering 7, 14, 21 mg/day

Side effects/adverse reactions:

INTEG: Erythema, pruritus, burning at application site, cutaneous hypersensitivity, sweating

GI: Diarrhea, dyspepsia, constipation, nausea, abdominal pain, vomiting

MS: Arthralgia, myalgia

EENT: Dry mouth

CNS: Abnormal dreams, insomnia, nervousness, headache, dizziness, paresthesia

Contraindications: Hypersensitivity, children, pregnancy (D), nonsmokers, during immediate postmyocardial infarction period, life-threatening dysrhythmias, severe or worsening angina pectoris

Precautions: Skin disease, angina pectoris, myocardial infarction, renal or hepatic insufficiency, peptic ulcer, accelerated hypertension, serious cardiac dysrhythmias, hyperthyroidism, pheochromocytoma, insulin-dependent diabetes, elderly

Pharmacokinetics: Half-life 3-4 hr, protein binding <5%, 30% is excreted unchanged in urine

Interactions/incompatibilities:

- Decreased dose at cessation of smoking: acetaminophen, caffeine, imipramine, oxazepam, pentazocine, propranolol, theophylline, insulin, adrenergic antagonists
- Increased dose at cessation of smoking: adrenergic agonists
- Decreased metabolism of: propoxyphene
- Increased diuretic effects of: furosemide

NURSING CONSIDERATIONS

Assess:

- Adverse reactions: irritation, pruritus, burning at patch site

Perform/provide:

- Storage above 86° F

Evaluate:

- Therapeutic response: decrease in urge to smoke, absence of nicotine withdrawal symptoms

Teach patient/family:

- All aspects of drug; give package insert to patient and explain
- That patch is as toxic as cigarettes; it is to be used only to deter smoking
- Not to use during pregnancy; birth defects may occur
- To keep used and unused system out of reach of children and pets
- To apply once a day to a nonhairy, clean, dry area of skin on upper body or upper outer arm
- To stop smoking immediately when beginning treatment with patch
- To apply promptly after removing from protective patch; system may lose strength

nifedipine

(nye-fed'i-peen)

Adalat, Procardia

Func. class.: Calcium-channel blocker

Chem. class.: Dihydropyridine

Action: Inhibits calcium ion influx across cell membrane during cardiac depolarization; produces relaxation of coronary vascular smooth muscle, dilates coronary arteries; increases myocardial oxygen delivery in patients with vasospastic angina; dilates peripheral arteries

Uses: Chronic stable angina pectoris, vasospastic angina, hypertension (sustained release only)

*Available in Canada only

Dosage and routes:
- *Adult:* PO Immediate release: 10 mg tid, increase in 10 mg increments q4-6h, not to exceed 180 mg or single dose of 30 mg
- *Adult:* PO sus rel: 30-60 mg qd, may increase q7-14days, doses >120 mg not recommended

Available forms include: Caps 10, 20 mg, tabs sus rel 30, 60, 90 mg

Side effects/adverse reactions:
CV: Dysrhythmia, edema, ***CHF,*** hypotension, palpitations, ***MI,*** pulmonary edema, tachycardia
GI: Nausea, vomiting, diarrhea, gastric upset, constipation, increased liver function studies, dry mouth
GU: Nocturia, polyuria
INTEG: Rash, pruritus, flushing, photosensitivity, hair loss
MISC: Flushing, sexual difficulties, cough, fever, chills
CNS: Headache, fatigue, drowsiness, dizziness, anxiety, depression, weakness, insomnia, lightheadedness, paresthesia, tinnitus, blurred vision

Contraindications: Hypersensitivity

Precautions: CHF, hypotension, sick sinus syndrome, 2nd or 3rd degree heart block, hypotension less than 90 mm Hg systolic, hepatic injury, pregnancy (C), lactation, children, renal disease

Pharmacokinetics:
PO: Onset 20 min, peak 0.5-6 hr, half-life 2-5 hr; metabolized by liver, excreted in urine (98% as metabolites)

Interactions/incompatibilities:
- Increased effects of: theophylline, β-blockers, antihypertensives, digitalis
- Increased nifedipine level: cimetidine
- Decreased effects: quinidine

NURSING CONSIDERATIONS

Administer:
- Before meals, hs

Evaluate:
- Therapeutic response: decreased anginal pain, B/P
- Cardiac status: B/P, pulse, respiration, ECG

Teach patient/family:
- To avoid hazardous activities until stabilized on drug, dizziness is no longer a problem
- To limit caffeine consumption
- To avoid OTC drugs unless directed by a physician
- To comply to all areas of medical regimen: diet, exercise, stress reduction, drug therapy
- Not to chew, divide, or crush sus rel tabs

Treatment of overdose: Defibrillation, atropine for AV block, vasopressor for hypotension

nitrofurantoin/nitrofurantoin macrocrystals

(nye-troe-fyoor'an-toyn)

Furadantin, Furalan, Furantoin, J-Dantin, Nephronex,* Nitrex, Novofuran,* Sarodant

Func. class.: Urinary tract antiinfective

Chem. class.: Synthetic nitrofuran derivative

Action: Appears to inhibit bacterial enzymes

Uses: Urinary tract infections caused by *E. coli, Klebsiella, Pseudomonas, P. vulgaris, P. morganii, Serratia, Citrobacter, S. aureus*

Dosage and routes:
- *Adult and child >12 yr:* PO 50-100 mg qid pc or 50-100 mg hs for long-term treatment
- *Child 1 mo-3 yr:* PO 5-7 mg/kg/

day in 4 divided doses; 1-3 mg/kg/day for long-term treatment
Available forms include: Caps 25, 50, 100 mg; tabs 50, 100 mg; susp 25 mg/5 ml
Side effects/adverse reactions:
INTEG: Pruritus, rash, urticaria, angioedema, alopecia, tooth staining
CNS: Dizziness, headache, drowsiness, peripheral neuropathy
GI: Nausea, vomiting, abdominal pain, diarrhea, ***cholestatic jaundice***
Contraindications: Hypersensitivity, anuria, severe renal disease
Precautions: Pregnancy (B), lactation
Pharmacokinetics:
PO: Half-life 20-60 min, crosses blood-brain barrier, placenta, enters breast milk, excreted as inactive metabolites in liver
Interactions/incompatibilities:
- Increased levels of nitrofurantoin: probenecid
- Antagonistic effect: nalidixic acid
- Decreased absorption of: magnesium trisilicate antacid

NURSING CONSIDERATIONS
Assess:
- Blood count for patients on chronic therapy
- I&O ratio, urine pH <5.5 is ideal
- Renal and hepatic function

Administer:
- After clean-catch urine is obtained for C&S
- Two daily doses if urine output is high or if patient has diabetes

Evaluate:
- Therapeutic response: decreased dysuria, fever
- CNS symptoms: insomnia, vertigo, headache, drowsiness, convulsions
- Allergy: fever, flushing, rash, urticaria, pruritus

Teach patient/family:
- To take medication with food or milk
- To protect susp from freezing and shake well before taking
- That drug may cause drowsiness; instruct client to seek aid in walking and other activities; advise client not to drive or operate machinery while on medication
- That diabetics to should use ketodiastix, blood glucose level
- That drug may turn urine rust-yellow to brown

nitrofurazone (topical)

(nye-troe-fyoor'a-zone)
Furacin
Func. class.: Local antibacterial
Chem. class.: Synthetic nitrofuran

Action: A broad-spectrum, mostly bactericidal for aerobic, anaeorbic gram-positive organisms, may interfere with enzyme systems needed for carbohydrate metabolism antibacterial action
Uses: Burns (2nd, 3rd degree)
Dosage and routes:
- *Adult and child:* TOP apply to affected area qd or qod

Available forms include: Sol, oint (soluble dressing), cream 0.2%
Side effects/adverse reactions:
INTEG: Rash, urticaria, stinging, burning, superinfections, photosensitivity, local edema
Contraindications: Hypersensitivity, G-6-PD deficiency
Precautions: Pregnancy (C), lactation; superinfection may result in bacterial or fungal overgrowth

NURSING CONSIDERATIONS
Administer:
- Analgesic before application if needed

* Available in Canada only

• Enough medication to completely cover burns
• After cleansing debris from area before each application
• Using sterile technique

Perform/provide:
• Storage at room temperature in dry place

Evaluate:
• Therapeutic response: development of granulation tissue
• Allergic reaction: burning, stinging, swelling, redness

Teach patient/family:
• That drug may be used until grafting is possible
• To avoid sunlight or ultraviolet light
• To stop drug and notify physician if rash or irritation occurs

---

nitroglycerin

(nye-troe-gli'ser-in)

Nitro-Bid, Nitrocap, Nitrodisc, Nitro-Dur, Nitrolingual, Nitrol, Nitrospan, Nitrostat, Tridil, Nitrogard, Nitrone, Nitroglyn, Nitrone, Deponit, Transderm Nitro

Func. class.: Vasodilatory coronary

Chem. class.: Nitrate

Action: Decreases preload, afterload, which is responsible for decreasing left ventricular end-diastolic pressure, systemic vascular resistance

Uses: Chronic stable angina pectoris, prophylaxis of angina pain, CHF associated with acute MI, controlled hypotension in surgical procedures

Dosage and routes:

• *Adult:* SL dissolve tablet under tongue when pain begins; may repeat q5min until relief occurs; take no more than 3 tabs/15 min; use 1 tab prophylactically 5-10 min before activities; Sus cap q6-12h on empty stomach; TOP 1-2 in q8h, increase to 4 in q4h as needed; IV 5 μg/min, then increase by 5 μg/min q3-5min; if no response after 20 μg/min, increase by 10-20 μg/min until desired response; trans apply a pad qd to a site free of hair

Available forms include: Buccal tabs 1, 2, 3 mg; aero 0.4 mg/meter spray; caps 2.5, 6.5, 9 mg; tabs ext rel 2.6, 6.5, 9 mg; inj 0.5, 0.8, 5, 10 mg/ml; SL tabs 0.15, 0.3, 0.4, 0.6 mg; top oint 2%; trans derm syst 2.5, 5, 7.5, 10, 15 mg/24 hr

Side effects/adverse reactions:

CV: Postural hypotension, tachycardia, ***collapse,*** syncope

GI: Nausea, vomiting

INTEG: Pallor, sweating, rash

CNS: Headache, flushing, dizziness

Contraindications: Hypersensitivity to this drug or nitrites, severe anemia, increased intracranial pressure, cerebral hemorrhage

Precautions: Postural hypotension, pregnancy (C), lactation

Pharmacokinetics:

SUS REL: Onset 20-45 min, duration 3-8 hr

SL: Onset 1-3 min, duration 30 min

TRANS DER: Onset ½-1 hr, duration 12-24 hr

IV: Onset immediately, duration variable

TRANSMUC: Onset 3 min, duration 10-30 min

AEROSOL: Onset 2 min, duration 30-60 min

TOP OINT: Onset 30-60 min, duration 2-12 hr

Metabolized by liver, excreted in urine

Interactions/incompatibilities:

• Increased effects: β-blockers, diuretics, antihypertensives, anticoagulants, alcohol

N

• Decreased heparin: IV nitroglycerin

NURSING CONSIDERATIONS

Assess:

• Orthostatic B/P, pulse

Administer:

• IV diluted in amount specified D_5 or NS for infusion; use glass infusion bottles, nonpolyvinyl chloride infusion tubing; titrate to patient response

• With 8 oz of water on empty stomach (oral tablet)

Evaluate:

• Therapeutic response: decrease, prevention of anginal pain

• Pain: duration, time started, activity being performed, character

• Tolerance if taken over long period of time

• Headache, light-headedness, decreased B/P; may indicate a need for decreased dosage

Teach patient/family:

• To place buccal tab between lip and gum above incisors or between cheek and gum; sus rel must be swallowed whole, do not chew; SL should be dissolved under tongue, do not swallow; aerosol should be sprayed under tongue, do not inhale

• To keep tabs in original container

• If 3 SL tabs in 15 min do not relieve pain, activate EMS

• To avoid alcohol

• That drug may cause headache, tolerance usually develops, use nonnarcotic analgesic

• That drug may be taken before stressful activity: exercise, sexual activity

• That SL may sting when drug comes in contact with mucous membranes

• To avoid hazardous activities if dizziness occurs

• To comply with complete medical regimen

• To make position changes slowly to prevent fainting

nitroprusside sodium

(nye-troe-pruss'ide)

Nipride, Nitropress

Func. class.: Antihypertensive

Chem. class.: Peripheral vasodilator

Action: Directly relaxes arteriolar, venous smooth muscle; resulting in reduction in cardiac preload, afterload

Uses: Hypertensive crisis, to decrease bleeding by creating hypotension during surgery

Dosage and routes:

• *Adult:* IV INF dissolve 50 mg in 2-3 ml of D_5W, then dilute in 250-1000 ml of D_5W; run at 0.5-8 μg/kg/min

Available forms include: Inj IV 50 mg

Side effects/adverse reactions:

GI: Nausea, vomiting, abdominal pain

CNS: Dizziness, headache, agitation, twitching, decreased reflexes, ***loss of consciousness,*** restlessness

EENT: Tinnitus, blurred vision

GU: Impotence

INTEG: Pain, irritation at injection site, sweating

Contraindications: Hypersensitivity, hypertension (compensatory)

Precautions: Pregnancy (C), lactation, children, fluid, electrolyte imbalances, hepatic disease, renal disease, hypothyroidism, elderly

Pharmacokinetics:

IV: Onset 1-2 min, duration 1-10 min after IV done, half-life 4 days in patients with abnormal renal function; metabolized in liver, excreted in urine

* Available in Canada only

Interactions/incompatibilities:

• Severe hypotension: ganglionic blockers, volatile liquid anesthetics, halothane, enflurane, circulatory depressants

• Do not mix with any drug in syringe or solution

NURSING CONSIDERATIONS

Assess:

• Electrolytes: K, Na, Cl, CO_2

• Renal function studies: catecholamines, BUN, creatinine

• Hepatic function studies: AST, ALT, alk phosphatase

• B/P by direct means if possible, check ECG continuously

• Weight daily, I&O

• Thiocyanate levels qd if on long-term treatment

Administer:

• Depending on B/P reading q15 min

• IV after diluting 50 mg/2-3 ml of D_5W, further dilute in 250 ml of D_5W; use an infusion pump only, wrap bottle with aluminum foil to protect from light; observe for color change in the infusion, discard if highly discolored (blue, green, dark red), titrate to patient response

Evaluate:

• Therapeutic response: decreased B/P, absence of bleeding

• Nausea, vomiting, diarrhea

• Edema in feet, legs daily

• Skin turgor, dryness of mucous membranes for hydration status

• Rales, dyspnea, orthopnea q30 min

Treatment of overdose: Administer amyl nitrite inhalation until 3% sodium nitrate solution can be prepared for IV administration, then inject sodium thiosulfate IV, correct drop in BP with vasopressor

norepinephrine injection

(nor-ep-i-nef'rin)

Levophed

Func. class.: Adrenergic

Chem. class.: Catecholamine

Action: Causes increased contractility and heart rate by acting on β-receptors in heart; also, acts on α-receptors, causing vasoconstriction in blood vessels; B/P is elevated, coronary blood flow improves, cardiac output increases, B/P elevates

Uses: Acute hypotension

Dosage and routes:

• *Adult:* IV INF 8-12 μg/min titrated to B/P

Available forms include: Inj IV 1 mg/ml

Side effects/adverse reactions:

CNS: Headache, anxiety, dizziness, insomnia, restlessness, tremor

CV: Palpitations, tachycardia, hypertension, ectopic beats, angina

GI: Nausea, vomiting

INTEG: Necrosis, tissue sloughing with extravasation, ***gangrene***

RESP: Dyspnea

GU: Decreased urine output

Contraindications: Hypersensitivity, ventricular fibrillation, tachydysrhythmias, pheochromocytoma, pregnancy (D)

Precautions: Lactation, arterial embolism, peripheral vascular disease, hypertension, hyperthyroidism, elderly, heart disease

Pharmacokinetics:

IV: Onset 1-2 min, metabolized in liver, excreted in urine (inactive metabolites), crosses placenta

Interactions/incompatibilities:

• Do not use within 2 wk of MAOIs, or hypertensive crisis may result

N

• Dysrhythmias: general anesthetics
• Decreased action of norepinephrine: α-blockers
• Increased B/P: oxytocics
• Increased pressor effect: tricyclic antidepressant, MAOIs
• Incompatible with alkaline solutions: Na, HCO_3

NURSING CONSIDERATIONS

Assess:
• I&O ratio; notify MD if output < 30 cc/hr
• ECG during administration continuously, if B/P increases, drug is decreased
• B/P and pulse q5min after parenteral route
• CVP or PWP during infusion if possible

Administer:
• Plasma expanders for hypovolemia
• IV after diluting 500-1000 ml D_5W or NS, give as infusion 2-3 ml/min; titrate to patient response
• Using 2 bottle set up so drug may be discontinued while IV is still running, use infusion pump

Perform/provide:
• Storage of reconstituted solution if refrigerated for no longer than 24 hr
• Do not use discolored solutions

Evaluate:
• Therapeutic response: increased B/P with stabilization
• For paresthesias and coldness of extremities, peripheral blood flow may decrease
• Injection site: tissue sloughing; if this occurs, administer phentolamine mixed with NS

Teach patient/family:
• Reason for drug administration

Treatment of overdose: Administer fluids, electrolyte replacement

norethindrone

(nor-eth-in′drone)
Micronor, Norlutin, Nor-QD
Func. class.: Progestogen
Chem. class.: Progesterone derivative

Action: Inhibits secretion of pituitary gonadotropins, which prevents follicular maturation, ovulation, stimulates growth of mammary tissue, antineoplastic action against endometrial cancer

Uses: Uterine bleeding (abnormal), amenorrhea, endometriosis

Dosage and routes:
• Adult: PO 5-20 mg qd days 5-25 of menstrual cycle

Endometriosis
• Adult: PO 10 mg qd × 2 wk, then increased by 5 mg qd × 2 wk, up to 30 mg qd

Available forms include: Tabs 5 mg

Side effects/adverse reactions:
CNS: Dizziness, headache, migraines, depression, fatigue
CV: Hypotension, thrombophlebitis, edema, ***thromboembolism, stroke, pulmonary embolism, myocardial infarction***
GI: Nausea, vomiting, anorexia, cramps, increased weight, ***cholestatic jaundice***
EENT: Diplopia
GU: Amenorrhea, cervical erosion, breakthrough bleeding, dysmenorrhea, vaginal candidiasis, breast changes, (gynecomastia, testicular atrophy, impotence), endometriosis, ***spontaneous abortion***
INTEG: Rash, urticaria, acne, hirsutism, alopecia, oily skin, seborrhea, purpura, melasma
META: Hyperglycemia

Contraindications: Breast cancer,

*Available in Canada only

hypersensitivity, thromboembolic disorders, reproductive cancer, genital bleeding (abnormal, undiagnosed), pregnancy (X)
Precautions: Lactation, hypertension, asthma, blood dyscrasias, gallbladder disease, CHF, diabetes mellitus, bone disease, depression, migraine headache, convulsive disorders, hepatic disease, renal disease, family history of breast or reproductive tract cancer
Pharmacokinetics:
PO: Duration 24 hr, excreted in urine, feces, metabolized in liver
NURSING CONSIDERATIONS
Assess:
• Weight daily: notify physician of weekly weight gain >5 lb
• B/P at beginning of treatment and periodically
• I&O ratio; be alert for decreasing urinary output, increasing edema
• Liver function studies: ALT, AST, bilirubin, periodically during long-term therapy
Administer:
• Titrated dose, use lowest effective dose
• Oil solution deeply in large muscle mass (IM), rotate sites
• In one dose in AM
• With food or milk to decrease GI symptoms
• After warming to dissolve crystals
Perform/provide:
• Storage in dark area
Evaluate:
• Therapeutic response: decreased abnormal uterine bleeding, absence of amenorrhea
• Edema, hypertension, cardiac symptoms, jaundice
• Mental status: affect, mood, behavioral changes, depression
• Hypercalcemia
Teach patient/family:
• About cushingoid symptoms
• To report breast lumps, vaginal bleeding, edema, jaundice, dark urine, clay-colored stools, dyspnea, headache, blurred vision, abdominal pain, numbness or stiffness in legs, chest pain; male to report impotence or gynecomastia
• To report suspected pregnancy
Lab test interferences:
Increase: Alk phosphatase, nitrogen (urine), pregnanediol, amino acids, factors VII, VIII, IX, X
Decrease: GTT, HDL

norethindrone acetate

(nor-eth-in′drone)
Aygestin, Norlutate
Func. class.: Progestogen
Chem. class.: Progesterone derivative

Action: Inhibits secretion of pituitary gonadotropins, which prevents follicular maturation, ovulation, stimulates growth of mammary tissue, antineoplastic action against endometrial cancer
Uses: Uterine bleeding (abnormal), amenorrhea, endometriosis
Dosage and routes:
• *Adult:* PO 2.5-10 mg qd days 5-25 of menstrual cycle
Endometriosis
• *Adult:* PO 5 mg qd × 2 wk, then increased by 2.5 mg qd × 2 wk, up to 15 mg qd
Available forms include: Tabs 5 mg
Side effects/adverse reactions:
CNS: Dizziness, headache, migraines, depression, fatigue
CV: Hypotension, thrombophlebitis, edema, ***thromboembolism, stroke, pulmonary embolism, myocardial infarction***

N

GI: Nausea, vomiting, anorexia, cramps, increased weight, ***cholestatic jaundice***
EENT: Diplopia
GU: Amenorrhea, cervical erosion, breakthrough bleeding, dysmenorrhea, vaginal candidiasis, breast changes, *gynecomastia, testicular atrophy, impotence,* endometriosis, ***spontaneous abortion***
INTEG: Rash, urticaria, acne, hirsutism, alopecia, oily skin, seborrhea, purpura, melasma
META: Hyperglycemia
Contraindications: Breast cancer, hypersensitivity, thromboembolic disorders, reproductive cancer, genital bleeding (abnormal, undiagnosed), cerebral hemorrhage, pregnancy (X)
Precautions: Lactation, hypertension, asthma, blood dyscrasias, gallbladder disease, CHF, diabetes mellitus, bone disease, depression, migraine headache, convulsive disorders, hepatic disease, renal disease, family history of breast or reproductive tract cancer
Pharmacokinetics:
PO: Duration 24 hr, excreted in urine, feces, metabolized in liver

NURSING CONSIDERATIONS

Assess:
• Weight daily; notify physician of weekly weight gain >5 lb
• B/P at beginning of treatment and periodically
• I&O ratio; be alert for decreasing urinary output, increasing edema
• Liver function studies: ALT, AST, bilirubin, periodically during long-term therapy
Administer:
• Titrated dose, use lowest effective dose
• Oil solution deeply in large muscle mass (IM), rotate sites
• In one dose in AM
• With food or milk to decrease GI symptoms
• After warming to dissolve crystals
Perform/provide:
• Storage in dark area
Evaluate:
• Therapeutic response: decreased abnormal uterine bleeding, absence of amenorrhea
• Edema, hypertension, cardiac symptoms, jaundice
• Mental status: affect, mood, behavioral changes, depression
• Hypercalcemia
Teach patient/family:
• About cushingoid symptoms
• To report breast lumps, vaginal bleeding, edema, jaundice, dark urine, clay-colored stools, dyspnea, headache, blurred vision, abdominal pain, numbness or stiffness in legs, chest pain; male to report impotence or gynecomastia
• To monitor blood sugar, if diabetic
• To report suspected pregnancy
Lab test interferences:
Increase: Alk phosphatase, nitrogen (urine), pregnanediol, amino acids, factors VII, VIII, IX, X
Decrease: GTT, HDL

---

norfloxacin

(nor-flox'-a-sin)
Noroxin
Func. class.: Urinary antiinfective
Chem. class.: Fluoroquinolone antibacterial

Action: Interferes with conversion of intermediate DNA fragments into high-molecular-weight DNA in bacteria
Uses: Adult urinary tract infections (including complicated) caused by *E. coli, E. cloacae, P. mirabilis,*

* Available in Canada only

K. pneumoniae, group D strep, indole-positive *Proteus, C. freundii, S. aureus*

Dosage and routes:

Uncomplicated

• *Adult:* 400 mg bid × 7-10 days 1 hr before or 2 hr after meals

Complicated

• *Adult:* 400 mg bid × 10-21 days; 400 mg qd × 7-10 days in impaired renal function

Available forms include: Tabs 400 mg

Side effects/adverse reactions:

CNS: Headache, dizziness, fatigue, somnolence, depression, insomnia

GI: Nausea, constipation, increased ALT, AST, flatulence, heartburn, vomiting, diarrhea, dry mouth

INTEG: Rash

EENT: Visual disturbances

Contraindications: Hypersensitivity to quinolones

Precautions: Pregnancy (C), lactation, children, renal disease, seizure disorders

Pharmacokinetics:

Peak 1 hr, half-life 3-4 hr; steady state 2 days; excreted in urine as active drug, metabolites

NURSING CONSIDERATIONS

Assess:

• Kidney, liver function studies: BUN, creatinine, AST, ALT

• I&O ratio, urine pH; <5.5 is ideal

Administer:

• After clean-catch urine is obtained for C&S

• Two daily doses if urine output is high or if patient has diabetes

Perform/provide:

• Limited intake of alkaline foods, drugs: milk, dairy products, peanuts, vegetables, alkaline antacids, sodium bicarbonate

Evaluate:

• Therapeutic response: decreased pain, frequency, urgency, C&S, absence of infection

• CNS symptoms: insomnia, vertigo, headache, agitation, confusion

• Allergic reactions: fever, flushing, rash, urticaria, pruritus

Teach patient/family:

• Fluids must be increased to 3 L/day to avoid crystallization in kidneys

• If dizziness occurs, to ambulate, perform activities with assistance

• Complete full course of drug therapy

• To contact physician if adverse reaction occurs

• To take 1 hr before or 2 hr after meals; not to take antacids with or within 2 hr of this drug, use sips of water or hard candy for dry mouth

Lab test interferences:

Increase: AST, ALT, BUN, creatinine, alk phosphatase

---

norgestrel

(nor-jess'trel)

Ovrette, Ovral

Func. class.: Progestogen

Chem. class.: Progesterone derivative

Action: Inhibits secretion of pituitary gonadotropins, which prevents follicular maturation, ovulation, stimulates growth of mammary tissue, antineoplastic action against endometrial cancer

Uses: Female contraception

Dosage and routes:

• *Adult:* PO 1 tablet qd

Available forms include: Tabs 0.35, 0.075 mg

Side effects/adverse reactions:

CNS: Dizziness, headache, migraines, depression, fatigue

CV: Hypotension, thrombophlebi-

tis, edema, ***thromboembolism, stroke, pulmonary embolism, myocardial infarction***
GI: Nausea, vomiting, anorexia, cramps, increased weight, ***cholestatic jaundice***
EENT: Diplopia
GU: Amenorrhea, cervical erosion, breakthrough bleeding, dysmenorrhea, vaginal candidiasis, breast changes, *gynecomastia, testicular atrophy, impotence,* endometriosis, ***spontaneous abortion***
INTEG: Rash, urticaria, acne, hirsutism, alopecia, oily skin, seborrhea, purpura, melasma
META: Hyperglycemia
Contraindications: Breast cancer, hypersensitivity, thromboembolic disorders, reproductive cancer, genital bleeding (abnormal, undiagnosed), cerebral hemorrhage, pregnancy (X)
Precautions: Lactation, hypertension, asthma, blood dyscrasias, gallbladder disease, CHF, diabetes mellitus, bone disease, depression, migraine headache, convulsive disorders, hepatic disease, renal disease, family history of breast or reproductive tract cancer
Pharmacokinetics:
PO: Duration 24 hr, excreted in urine and feces, metabolized in liver

NURSING CONSIDERATIONS

Assess:
- Weight daily; notify physician of weekly weight gain >5 lb
- B/P at beginning of treatment and periodically
- I&O ratio; be alert for decreasing urinary output, increasing edema
- Liver function studies: ALT, AST, bilirubin, periodically during long-term therapy

Administer:
- Titrated dose; use lowest effective dose
- Oil solution deeply in large muscle mass (IM), rotate sites
- In one dose in AM
- With food or milk to decrease GI symptoms
- After warming to dissolve crystals

Perform/provide:
- Storage in dark area

Evaluate:
- Therapeutic response: absence of pregnancy
- Edema, hypertension, cardiac symptoms, jaundice
- Mental status: affect, mood, behavioral changes, depression
- Hypercalcemia

Teach patient/family:
- About cushingoid symptoms
- To report breast lumps, vaginal bleeding, edema, jaundice, dark urine, clay-colored stools, dyspnea, headache, blurred vision, abdominal pain, numbness or stiffness in legs, chest pain
- To report suspected pregnancy
- To monitor blood sugar, if diabetic

Lab test interferences:
Increase: Alk phosphatase, nitrogen (urine), pregnanediol, amino acids, factors VII, VIII, IX, X
Decrease: GTT, HDL

nortriptyline HCl

(nor-trip'ti-leen)
Aventyl, Pamelor
Func. class.: Antidepressant—tricyclic
Chem. class.: Dibenzocycloheptene—secondary amine

Action: Blocks reuptake of norepinephrine, serotonin into nerve endings, increasing action of norepinephrine, serotonin in nerve cells
Uses: Major depression

* Available in Canada only

Dosage and routes:
• *Adult:* PO 25 mg tid or qid, may increase to 150 mg/day; may give daily dose hs
Available forms include: Caps 10, 25, 75 mg; sol 10 mg/5 ml
Side effects/adverse reactions:
HEMA: ***Agranulocytosis, thrombocytopenia, eosinophilia, leukopenia***
CNS: Dizziness, drowsiness, confusion, headache, anxiety, tremors, stimulation, weakness, insomnia, nightmares, EPS (elderly), increased psychiatric symptoms
GI: Constipation, dry mouth, nausea, vomiting, ***paralytic ileus,*** increased appetite, cramps, epigastric distress, jaundice, ***hepatitis,*** stomatitis
GU: Retention, ***acute renal failure***
INTEG: Rash, urticaria, sweating, pruritus, photosensitivity
CV: Orthostatic hypotension, ECG changes, tachycardia, ***hypertension,*** palpitations
EENT: Blurred vision, tinnitus, mydriasis
Contraindications: Hypersensitivity to tricyclic antidepressants, recovery phase of myocardial infarction, convulsive disorders, prostatic hypertrophy
Precautions: Suicidal patients, severe depression, increased intraocular pressure, narrow-angle glaucoma, urinary retention, cardiac disease, hepatic disease, hyperthyroidism, electroshock therapy, elective surgery, pregnancy (C)
Pharmacokinetics:
PO: Steady state 4-19 days; metabolized by liver, excreted by kidneys, crosses placenta, excreted in breast milk, half-life 18-28 hr
Interactions/incompatibilities:
• Decreased effects of: guanethidine, clonidine, indirect-acting sympathomimetics (ephedrine)
• Increased effects of: direct-acting sympathomimetics (epinephrine), alcohol, barbiturates, benzodiazepines, CNS depressants
• Hyperpyretic crisis, convulsions, hypertensive episode: MAOI

NURSING CONSIDERATIONS

Assess:
• B/P (lying, standing), pulse q4h; if systolic B/P drops 20 mm Hg hold drug, notify physician; take vital signs q4h in patients with cardiovascular disease
• Blood studies: CBC, leukocytes, differential, cardiac enzymes if patient is receiving long-term therapy
• Hepatic studies: AST, ALT, bilirubin, creatinine
• Weight qwk, appetite may increase with drug
• ECG for flattening of T wave, bundle branch block, AV block, dysrhythmias in cardiac patients

Administer:
• Increased fluids, bulk in diet if constipation, urinary retention occur
• With food or milk for GI symptoms
• Dosage hs if oversedation occurs during day; may take entire dose hs; elderly may not tolerate once/day dosing
• Gum, hard candy, or frequent sips of water for dry mouth
• Concentrate with fruit juice, water, or milk to disguise taste

Perform/provide:
• Storage in tight, light-resistant container at room temperature
• Assistance with ambulation during beginning therapy since drowsiness/dizziness occurs
• Safety measures including siderails primarily in elderly

• Checking to see PO medication swallowed

Evaluate:

• Therapeutic response: decreased depression

• EPS primarily in elderly: rigidity, dystonia, akathisia

• Mental status: mood, sensorium, affect, suicidal tendencies, increase in psychiatric symptoms: depression, panic

• Urinary retention, constipation; constipation is more likely to occur in children

• Withdrawal symptoms: headache, nausea, vomiting, muscle pain, weakness; do not usually occur unless drug was discontinued abruptly

• Alcohol consumption; if alcohol is consumed, hold dose until morning

Teach patient/family:

• That therapeutic effects may take 2-3 wk

• To use caution in driving or other activities requiring alertness because of drowsiness, dizziness, blurred vision

• To avoid alcohol ingestion, other CNS depressants

• Not to discontinue medication quickly after long-term use, may cause nausea, headache, malaise

• To wear sunscreen or large hat since photosensitivity occurs

Lab test interferences:

Increase: Serum bilirubin, blood glucose, alk phosphatase

False increase: Urinary catecholamines

Decrease: VMA, 5-HIAA

Treatment of overdose: ECG monitoring, induce emesis, lavage, activated charcoal, administer anticonvulsant

nylidrin HCl

(nye'li-drin)

Arlidin, Rolidrin, Adrin

Func. class.: Peripheral vasodilator, β-adrenergic agonist

Chem. class.: β-Adrenergic agonist-phenylisopropylamine

Action: Acts on β-adrenergic receptors to dilate arterioles in skeletal muscles; increases cardiac output, may have direct vasodilatory effect on vascular smooth muscle

Uses: Arteriosclerosis obliterans, thromboangiitis obliterans, diabetic vascular disease, night leg cramps, Raynaud's disease, ischemic ulcer, frostbite, acrocyanosis, acroparesthesia, thrombophlebitis, primary cochlear cell ischemia, cochlear stria ischemia, muscular or ampullar ischemia, other disturbances from labyrinth artery spasm or obstruction

Dosage and routes:

• *Adult:* PO 3-12 mg tid or qid

Available forms include: Tabs 6, 12 mg

Side effects/adverse reactions:

CV: Postural hypotension, palpitations

CNS: Dizziness, anxiety, tremors, weakness, nervousness

GI: Nausea, vomiting

INTEG: Flushing

Contraindications: Hypersensitivity, paroxysmal tachycardia, progressive angina pectoris, thyrotoxicosis, myocardial infarction

Precautions: CHF, pregnancy (C)

Pharmacokinetics:

PO: Onset 10 min, peak 30 min, duration 2 hr; slowly metabolized in liver, excreted in urine, therapeutic effect may take several weeks

Interactions/incompatibilities:
• Increased hypotension: phenothiazines, other vasodilators, antihypertensives

NURSING CONSIDERATIONS

Assess:
• B/P, pulse during treatment until stable; take B/P lying, standing; orthostatic hypotension is common

Administer:
• With meals to reduce GI upset

Perform/provide:
• Storage at room temperature

Evaluate:
• Therapeutic response: ability to walk without pain, increased pulse volume, increased temperature in extremities or orientation, long- and short-term memory

Teach patient/family:
• That medication is not cure, may need to be taken continuously depending on condition; therapeutic response may not be evident for 2-3 mo
• That it is necessary to quit smoking to prevent excessive vasoconstriction
• To avoid hazardous activities until stabilized on medication; dizziness may occur
• That palpitations should subside as therapy continues

---

nystatin

(nye-stat'in)

Mycostatin, Nadostine,* Nilstat, O-V Statin

Func. class.: Antifungal
Chem. class.: Amphoteric polyene

Action: Interferes with fungal DNA replication; binds sterols in fungal cell membrane, which increases permeability, leaking of cell nutrients

Uses: *Candida* species causing oral, vaginal, intestinal infections

Dosage and routes:

Oral infection
• *Adult:* SUSP 400,000-600,000 U qid
• *Child and infants >3 mo:* SUSP 250,000-500,000 U qid
• *Newborn and premature infants:* susp 100,000 U qid

GI infection
• *Adult:* PO 500,000-1,000,000 U tid

Vaginal infection
• *Adult:* VAG TAB 100,000 U inserted high into vagina qd-bid × 2 wk

Available forms include: Tabs 500,000 U; vag tabs 100,000 U; powder 50 mill, 150 mill, 500 mill, 1 bill, 2 bill, 5 bill U; susp 100,000 U; top cream, oint, powder 100,000 U

Side effects/adverse reactions:
INTEG: Rash, urticaria (rare)
GI: Nausea, vomiting, anorexia, diarrhea, cramps

Contraindications: Hypersensitivity

Precautions: Pregnancy (B)

Pharmacokinetics:
PO: Little absorption, excreted in feces

NURSING CONSIDERATIONS

Administer:
• Oral suspension dose by placing ½ in each cheek, then swallow
• Topical dose after cleansing area; mouth may be swabbed

Perform/provide:
• Storage in refrigerator, oral susp, tabs in tight, light-resistant containers at room temperature

Evaluate:
• Therapeutic response: culture negative for *Candida*
• For allergic reaction: rash, urticaria; drug may need to be discontinued

N

• For predisposing factors: antibiotic therapy, pregnancy, diabetes mellitus, sexual partner infection (vaginal infections)

Teach patient/family:

• That long-term therapy may be needed to clear infection; to complete entire course of medication
• Proper hygiene: changing socks if feet are infected, using no commercial mouthwashes for mouth infection
• To avoid getting preparation on hands
• To wear light-day pad for vaginal preparations
• To avoid tight shoes, bandages when using for feet infection
• To avoid sexual contact during treatment to minimize reinfection
• To notify physician if irritation occurs; drug may need to be discontinued
• That relief from itching may occur after 24-72 hr

---

nystatin (topical)

(nye-stat'in)

Mycostatin, Nystex, Nilstat, Mykinac

Func. class.: Local antiinfective
Chem. class.: Antifungal

Action: Interferes with fungal DNA replication; binds sterols in fungal cell membrane, which increases permeability, leaking of cell nutrients

Uses: Cutaneous vulvovaginal candidiasis, mucocutaneous fungal infections

Dosage and routes:

• *Adult and child:* TOP apply to affected area bid-tid × 14 days; vag 1-2 tabs (100,000 U each) inserted into vagina

Available forms include: Cream, oint, powder, spray, vag tabs 100,000 U

Side effects/adverse reactions:

INTEG: Rash, urticaria, stinging, burning

Contraindications: Hypersensitivity

Precautions: Pregnancy (B), lactation

NURSING CONSIDERATIONS

Administer:

• To moist lesions with a swab
• Vaginal tablets by inserting high into vagina with applicator provided
• Enough medication to completely cover lesions
• In gravid client 3-6 wk before term to decrease candidiasis in the newborn
• After cleansing with soap, water before each application, dry well

Perform/provide:

• Storage at room temperature in dry place, protect from light, air, heat

Evaluate:

• Therapeutic response: decrease in size, number of lesions, decreased itching, white patches on vulvae
• Allergic reaction: burning, stinging, swelling, redness

Teach patient/family:

• To discontinue use and notify physician if irritation occurs
• To apply with glove to prevent further infection; drug may stain, pads may protect clothing
• To avoid use of OTC creams, ointments, lotions unless directed by physician
• To use medical asepsis (hand washing) before, after each application

---

ofloxacin

(o-flox'a-sin)

Floxin

Func. class.: Antiinfective
Chem. class.: Fluoroquinolone

Action: Interferes with conversion of intermediate DNA fragments into high-molecular-weight DNA in bacteria

Uses: Treatment of lower respiratory tract infections (pneumonia, bronchitis), genitourinary infections (prostatitis, UTIs) caused by *E. coli, K. pneumoniae, C. trachomatis, N. gonorrhoeae;* skin and skin structure infections

Dosage and routes:

Lower respiratory tract infections/ skin and skin structure infections

• *Adult:* PO 400 mg q12h × 10 days

Cervicitis, urethritis

• *Adult:* PO 300 mg q12h × 7 days

Prostatitis

• *Adult:* PO 300 mg q12h × 6 wk

Acute, uncomplicated gonorrhea

• *Adult:* PO 400 mg as a single dose

Available forms include: Tabs 200, 300, 400 mg

Side effects/adverse reactions:

CNS: Dizziness; headache, fatigue, somnolence, depression, insomnia, lethargy, malaise

GI: Diarrhea, nausea, vomiting, anorexia, flatulence, heartburn, dry mouth, increased AST, ALT, abdominal pain, constipation

INTEG: Rash, pruritus

EENT: Visual disturbances

Contraindications: Hypersensitivity to quinolones

Precautions: Pregnancy (C), lactation, children, elderly, renal disease, seizure disorders, excessive sunlight

Pharmacokinetics:

PO: Peak 1-2 hr, half-life 9 hr, steady state 2 days; excreted in urine as active drug, metabolites, 0.9% bioavailability

Interactions/incompatibilities:

• Decreased effects of ofloxacin: antacids, nitrofurantoin, sucralfate, iron salts, zinc salts

• Increased ofloxacin levels: probenecid

• Increased effects of: warfarin, cyclosporine

NURSING CONSIDERATIONS

Assess:

• Kidney, liver function studies: BUN, creatinine, AST, ALT

• I&O ratio, urine pH; <5.5 is ideal

Administer:

• After clean-catch urine is obtained for C&S

Perform/provide:

• Limited intake of alkaline foods, drugs; milk, dairy products, peanuts, vegetables, alkaline antacids, sodium bicarbonate

Evaluate:

• Therapeutic response: negative C&S

• CNS symptoms: insomnia, vertigo, headache, agitation, confusion

• Allergic reactions: rash, flushing, urticaria, pruritus

Teach patient/family:

• That fluids must be increased to 3L/day to avoid crystallization in kidneys

• That if dizziness or light-headedness occurs, ambulate, perform activities with assistance

• To complete full course of drug therapy

• To contact physician if adverse reactions occur

• To avoid iron- or mineral-containing supplements within 2 hr before or after dose

olsalazine sodium

(ohl-sal'ah-zeen)

Dipentum

Func. class.: Antiinflammatory
Chem. class.: Salicylate derivative

Action: Bioconverted to 5-aminosalicylic acid, which decreases inflammation

Uses: Maintenance of remission of ulcerative colitis in patients intolerant to sulfasalazine

Dosage and routes:

Adult: PO 1 g/day in 2 divided doses

Available forms include: Tabs 250 mg

Side effects/adverse reactions:

SYST: ***Anaphylaxis***

GI: Nausea, vomiting, abdominal pain, stomatitis, hepatitis, pancreatitis, diarrhea, bloating

CNS: Headache, insomnia, hallucinations, depression, vertigo, fatigue, drug fever, chills, dizziness, drowsiness, tremors

HEMA: ***Leukopenia, neutropenia, thrombocytopenia, agranulocytosis, anemia***

INTEG: Rash, dermatitis, urticaria, ***Stevens-Johnson syndrome,*** erythema, photosensitivity, alopecia

GU: Frequency, dysuria, hematuria, impotence

CV: Allergic myocarditis, 2nd degree heart block, hypertension, peripheral edema, chest pain, palpitations

RESP: ***Bronchospasm,*** shortness of breath

Contraindications: Hypersensitivity to salicylates, child <14 yr

Precautions: Pregnancy (C), lactation, impaired hepatic function, severe allergy, bronchial asthma

Pharmacokinetics:

PO: Partially absorbed, peak 1½ hr, half-life 5-10 hr, excreted in urine as 5-aminosalicylic acid and metabolites, crosses placenta

NURSING CONSIDERATIONS

Assess:

- I&O ratio: note color, character, pH of urine if drug is administered for urinary tract infections; output should be 800 ml less than intake; if urine is highly acidic, alkalization may be needed
- Kidney function studies: BUN, creatinine, urinalysis if on long-term therapy

Administer:

- With food in evenly divided doses
- Medication after C&S; repeat C&S after full course of medication completed
- With resuscitative equipment available; severe allergic reactions may occur
- Total daily dose in evenly spaced doses to help minimize GI intolerance

Perform/provide:

- Storage in tight, light-resistant containers at room temperature

Evaluate:

- Therapeutic response: absence of fever, mucus in stools
- Blood dyscrasias: skin rash, fever, sore throat, bruising, bleeding, fatigue, joint pain
- Allergic reaction: rash, dermatitis, urticaria, pruritus, dyspnea, bronchospasm

Lab test interferences:

False positive: Urinary glucose test

* Available in Canada only

omeprazole

(om-ee-pray-zole)

Prilosec

Func. class.: Antisecretory compound

Chem. class.: Benzimidazole

Action: Suppresses gastric secretion by inhibiting hydrogen/potassium ATPase enzyme system in the gastric parietal cell; characterized as a gastric acid pump inhibitor, since it blocks the final step of acid production

Uses: Gastroesophageal reflux disease (GERD), severe erosive esophagitis, poorly responsive systemic GERD, pathologic hypersecretory conditions (Zollinger-Ellison syndrome, systemic mastocytosis, multiple endocrine adenomas); possibly effective for treatment of duodenal ulcers

Dosage and routes:

Severe erosine esophagitis/poorly responsive gastroesophageal reflux disease

• *Adult:* PO 20 mg gd × 4-8 wk

Pathologic hypersecretory conditions

• *Adult:* PO 60 mg/day, may increase to 120 mg tid; daily doses >80 mg should be given in divided doses

Available forms include: Cap, sus rel 20 mg

Side effects/adverse reactions

CNS: Headache, dizziness, asthenia

GI: Diarrhea, abdominal pain, vomiting, nausea, constipation, flatulence, acid regurgitation, abdominal swelling, anorexia, irritable colon, esophageal candidiasis, dry mouth

RESP: Upper respiratory infections, cough, epistaxis

INTEG: Rash, dry skin, urticaria, pruritus, alopecia

META: Hypoglycemia, increased hepatic enzymes, weight gain

EENT: Tinnitus, taste perversion

CV: Chest pain, angina, tachycardia, bradycardia, palpitations, peripheral edema

GU: Urinary tract infection, frequency, increased creatinine, ***proteinuria, hematuria,*** testicular pain, glycosuria

HEMA: ***Pancytopenia, thrombocytopenia, neutropenia, leukocytosis,*** anemia

MISC: Back pain, fever, fatigue, malaise

Contraindications: Hypersensitivity

Precautions: Pregnancy (C), lactation, children

Pharmacokinetics:

Peak: ½-3½ hr, ½ life–½-1 hr, protein binding 95%, eliminated in urine as metabolites and in feces; in the elderly the elimination rate is decreased, bioavailability is increased

Interactions/incompatibilities:

• Increased serum levels: diazepam, phenytoin

• Possible increased bleeding: warfarin

NURSING CONSIDERATIONS

Assess:

• GI system: bowel sounds q8h, abdomen for pain, swelling, anorexia

• Hepatic enzymes: AST, ALT during treatment

Administer:

• Before eating; swallow capsule whole; do not open, chew, or crush

Evaluate:

• Therapeutic response: absence of epigastric pain, swelling, fullness

Teach patient/family:

• To report severe diarrhea; drug may need to be discontinued

• That the diabetic patient should be aware that hypoglycemia may occur

ondansetron HCl

(on-dan-see'tron)

Zofran

Func. class.: Antiemetic

Chem. class.: 5-HT3 receptor antagonist

Action: Prevents nausea, vomiting by blocking serotonin peripherally, centrally, and in the small intestine

Uses: Prevention of nausea, vomiting associated with cancer chemotherapy

Dosage and routes:

• *Adult:* IV 0.15 mg/kg infused over 15 min, 30 min before the start of cancer chemotherapy; 0.15 mg/kg is given 4 hr and 8 hr after first dose; dilute 50 ml of D_5W or 0.9% NaCl before giving

Available forms include: Inj 2 mg/ml

Side effects/adverse reactions:

GI: Diarrhea, constipation, increased AST, ALT

CNS: Headache

MISC: Rash, ***bronchospasm***

Contraindications: Hypersensitivity

Precautions: Pregnancy (B), lactation, children, elderly

Pharmacokinetics:

IV: Mean elimination half-life 3.5-4.7 hr, plasma protein binding 70%-76%; extensively metabolized in the liver

NURSING CONSIDERATIONS

Assess:

• For absence of nausea, vomiting during chemotherapy

• Hypersensitive reaction: rash, bronchospasm

Perform/provide:

• Storage at room temperature for 48 hr after dilution

Evaluate:

• Therapeutic response: absence of nausea, vomiting during cancer chemotherapy

Teach patient/family:

• To report diarrhea, constipation, rash, or changes in respirations

opium tincture/ camphorated opium tincture

(oh'pee-um)

Paregoric, Paregorique*

Func. class.: Antidiarrheal

Chem. class.: Opium/opium and morphine

Controlled Substance Schedule III/II (depending on amount of opium)

Action: Antiperistaltic activity

Uses: Diarrhea (cause undetermined); to treat withdrawal symptoms in infants born to addicted mothers

Dosage and routes:

• *Adult:* PO 0.3-1 ml qid, not to exceed 6 ml/day (tincture) or 5-10 ml qd-qid (camphorated)

• *Child:* PO 0.25-0.5 ml/kg qd-qid (camphorated)

Withdrawal

• *Neonates:* PO 1:25 dilution, 3-6 gtt q3-6hr (tincture), dosage adjustment is made to control symptoms

Available forms include: Liq 2 mg morphine equivalent per 5 ml

Side effects/adverse reactions:

CNS: Dizziness, drowsiness, fainting, flushing, physical dependency ***CNS depression***

GI: Nausea, vomiting, constipation, abdominal pain

* Available in Canada only

Contraindications: Hypersensitivity, severe ulcerative colitis, pseudomembranous colitis
Precautions: Liver disease, addiction-prone individuals, prostatic hypertrophy (severe), pregnancy (B)
Pharmacokinetics:
PO: Duration 4 hr, half-life 2-3 hr; metabolized in liver, excreted in urine
Interactions/incompatibilities:
• Increased action of both drugs: other CNS depressants
• Increased CNS toxicity: cimetidine

NURSING CONSIDERATIONS
Assess:
• Electrolytes (K, Na, Cl) if on long-term therapy
• Skin turgor q8h if dehydration is suspected
Administer:
• Undiluted with water
• For 48 hr only
Evaluate:
• Therapeutic response: decreased diarrhea
• Bowel pattern before; for rebound constipation
• Response after 48 hr; if no response, drug should be discontinued
• Dehydration in children
• Abdominal distention; toxic megacolon may occur in ulcerative colitis
Teach patient/family:
• To avoid OTC products (cough, cold, hay fever preparations) unless directed by physician
• Not to exceed recommended dose
• That drug may be habit-forming
• To avoid hazardous activities, drowsiness may occur

oral contraceptives

Func. class.: Hormone
Chem. class.: Estrogen/progestin combinations

Action: Prevents ovulation by suppressing follicle stimulating, luteinizing hormone
Uses: To prevent pregnancy, endometriosis, hypermenorrhea
Dosage and routes:
• *Adult:* PO 1 qd starting on day 5 of menstrual cycle; day 1 is 1st day of period
20/21 tablet packs
• *Adult:* PO 1 qd starting on day 7 of menstrual cycle; day 1 is 1st day of period, then on 20 or 21 days, off 7 days
28 tablet packs
• *Adult:* PO 1 qd continuously
Biphasic
• *Adult:* 1 qd × 10 days, then next color 1 qd × 11 days
Triphasic
• *Adult:* 1 qd; check package insert for each new brand
Endometriosis
• *Adult:* PO 1 qd × 20 days from day 5 to 24 of cycle
• *Adult:* PO 1 qd; check package insert for specific instructions
Available forms include: Check specific brand
Side effects/adverse reactions:
GI: Nausea, vomiting, cramps, diarrhea, bloating, constipation, change in appetite, ***cholestatic jaundice***
INTEG: Chloasma, melasma, acne, rash, urticaria, erythema, pruritus, hirsutism, alopecia, photosensitivity
CV: Increased B/P, thromboembolic conditions, fluid retention, edema
ENDO: Decreased glucose toler-

ance, increased TBG, PBI, T_4, T_3
GU: Breakthrough bleeding, amenorrhea, spotting, dysmenorrhea, galactorrhea, endocervical hyperplasia, vaginitis, cystitis-like syndrome, breast change
CNS: Depression, fatigue, dizziness, nervousness, anxiety, headache
EENT: Optic neuritis, retinal thrombosis, cataracts
HEMA: Increased fibrinogen, clotting factor

Contraindications: Pregnancy (X), lactation, reproductive cancer, thrombophlebitis, MI, hepatic tumors, hepatic disease, CAD, women 40 and over, CVA

Precautions: Depression, hypertension, renal disease, seizure disorders, lupus erythematosus, rheumatic disease, migraine headache, amenorrhea, irregular menses, breast cancer (fibrocystic), gallbladder disease, diabetes mellitus, heavy smoking, acute mononucleosis, sickle cell disease

Pharmacokinetics: Excreted in breast milk

Interactions/incompatibilities:

- Decreased effectiveness of oral contraceptives: anticonvulsants, rifampin, analgesics, antibiotics, antihistamines, chenodiol, griseofulvin
- Decreased action of: oral anticoagulants
- Increased clotting: aminocaproic acid

NURSING CONSIDERATIONS

Assess:

- Glucose, thyroid function, liver function tests

Evaluate:

- Therapeutic response: absence of pregnancy, endometriosis, hypermenorrhea
- Reproductive changes: change in breasts, tumors, positive Pap smear; drug should be discontinued if changes occur

Teach patient/family:

- About detection of clots using Homan's sign
- To use sunscreen or avoid sunlight; photosensitivity can occur
- To take at same time each day to ensure equal drug level
- To report GI symptoms that occur after 4 mo
- To use another birth control method during 1st week of oral contraceptive use
- To take another tablet as soon as possible if one is missed
- That after drug is discontinued, pregnancy may not occur for several months
- To report abdominal pain, change in vision, shortness of breath, change in menstrual flow, spotting, breakthrough bleeding, breast lumps, swelling, headache, severe leg pain
- That continuing medical care is needed: PAP smear and gynecologic examinations q6mo
- To notify physician and dentist of oral contraceptive use

Lab test interferences:

Increase: Pro-time, clotting factors VII, VIII, IX, X, TBG, PBI, T_4, platelet aggregability, BSP, triglycerides, bilirubin, AST, ALT
Decrease: T_3, antithrombin III, folate, metyrapone test, GTT, 17-OHCS

orphenadrine citrate

(or-fen'a-dreen)

Banflex, Flexon, Myolin, Norflex, Ro-Orphena, X-Otag

Func. class.: Skeletal muscle relaxant, central acting; anticholinergic

Chem. class.: Tertiary amine

Action: Acts centrally on skeletal muscle to relax, inhibit muscle spasm

Uses: Pain in musculoskeletal conditions

Dosage and routes:

- *Adult:* PO 100 mg bid; IM/IV 60 mg q12h

Available forms include: Tabs 100 mg; tabs sus rel 100 mg; inj IM, IV 30 mg/ml

Side effects/adverse reactions:

HEMA: ***Aplastic anemia***

CNS: Dizziness, weakness, fatigue, drowsiness, headache, disorientation, insomnia, stimulation, hallucination, agitation

EENT: Nasal congestion, blurred vision, increased intraocular pressure, mydriasis

CV: Orthostatic hypotension, tachycardia

GI: Nausea, vomiting, constipation, dry mouth

GU: Urinary frequency, hesitancy, retention

INTEG: Rash, pruritus, urticaria

Contraindications: Hypersensitivity, narrow-angle glaucoma, GI obstruction, myasthenia gravis, stenosing peptic ulcer, bladder neck obstruction, cardiospasm

Precautions: Pregnancy (C), children, cardiac disease, tachycardia

Pharmacokinetics:

PO: Peak 2 hr, duration 4-6 hr, half-life 14 hr, metabolized in liver, excreted in urine (unchanged)

Interactions/incompatibilities:

- Increased CNS effects: propoxyphene, other anticholinergics, oral contraceptives

NURSING CONSIDERATIONS

Assess:

- Monitor vital signs q10-15min during administration
- Blood studies: CBC, WBC, differential; blood dyscrasias may occur (rare)
- I&O ratio; check for urinary retention, frequency, hesitancy
- Dosage: even slight overdose can cause toxicity

Administer:

- With meals for GI symptoms
- IV undiluted, or diluted in 5-10 ml sterile H_2O for inj; give 60 mg or less over 5 min
- When giving IV may cause paradoxical initial bradycardia; usually disappears in 2 min

Perform/provide:

- Assistance with ambulation if dizziness, drowsiness occurs

Evaluate:

- Therapeutic response: decreased rigidity, spasms
- Allergic reactions: rash, fever, respiratory distress
- Blood dyscrasias: temperature, bleeding, fatigue (rare)
- CNS symptoms: dizziness, drowsiness, psychiatric symptoms

Teach patient/family:

- Not to discontinue medication quickly; insomnia, nausea, headache will occur
- Not to take with alcohol, other CNS depressants
- To avoid altering activities while taking this drug
- To avoid hazardous activities if drowsiness, dizziness occurs
- To avoid using OTC medication: cough preparations, antihistamines, unless directed by physician

• To use gum, frequent sips of water for dry mouth

---

oxacillin sodium

(ox-a-sill'in)

Bactocill, Prostaphilin

Func. class.: Broad-spectrum antibiotic

Chem. class.: Penicillinase-resistant penicillin

Action: Interferes with cell wall replication of susceptible organisms; osmotically unstable cell wall swells, bursts from osmotic pressure

Uses: Effective for gram-positive cocci *(S. aureus, S. pneumoniae)*, infections caused by penicillinase-producing *Staphylococcus*

Dosage and routes:

• *Adult:* PO 2-6 g/day in divided doses q4-6h; IM/IV 2-12 g/day in divided doses q4-6h

• *Child:* PO 50-100 mg/kg/day in divided doses q6h; IM/IV 50-100 mg/kg/day in divided doses q4-6h

Available forms include: Caps 250, 500 mg; powder for oral susp 250 mg/5 ml; powder for inj IM, IV 250, 500 mg, 1, 2, 4, 10 g; IV INF 1, 2 g

Side effects/adverse reactions:

HEMA: Anemia, increased bleeding time, ***bone marrow depression, granulocytopenia***

GI: Nausea, vomiting, diarrhea, increased AST, ALT, abdominal pain, glossitis, colitis

GU: ***Oliguria, proteinuria, hematuria,*** *vaginitis, moniliasis,* ***glomerulonephritis***

CNS: Lethargy, hallucinations, anxiety, depression, twitching, ***coma, convulsions***

Contraindications: Hypersensitivity to penicillins

Precautions: Pregnancy (B), hypersensitivity to cephalosporins, neonates

Pharmacokinetics:

PO/IM: Peak 30-60 min, duration 4-6 hr

IV: Peak 5 min, duration 4-6 hr, half-life 30-60 min, metabolized in the liver, excreted in urine, bile, breast milk, crosses placenta

Interactions/incompatibilities:

• Decreased antimicrobial effectiveness of oxacillin: tetracyclines, erythromycins

• Increased oxacillin concentrations: aspirin, probenecid

NURSING CONSIDERATIONS

Assess:

• I&O ratio; report hematuria, oliguria since penicillin in high doses is nephrotoxic

• Any patient with compromised renal system since drug is excreted slowly in poor renal system function; toxicity may occur rapidly

• Liver studies: AST, ALT

• Blood studies: WBC, RBC, Hct/Hgb, bleeding time

• Renal studies: urinalysis, protein, blood

• C&S before drug therapy; drug may be taken as soon as culture is taken

Administer:

• IV after diluting 500 mg or less/5 ml sterile H_2O or NaCl for inj; may dilute further in compatible sol and give 1 g/10 min; may be given as infusion over 6 hr

• Drug after C&S has been completed

Perform/provide:

• Adrenalin, suction, tracheostomy set, endotracheal intubation equipment

• Scratch test to assess allergy, after securing order from physician;

---

*Available in Canada only

usually done when penicillin is only drug of choice
• Storage in tight container; refrigerate reconstituted solution up to 2 wk

Evaluate:
• Therapeutic response: absence of fever, draining wounds
• Bowel pattern before and during treatment
• Skin eruptions after administration of penicillin to 1 wk after discontinuing drug
• Respiratory status: rate, character, wheezing, tightness in chest
• Allergies before initiation of treatment, and reaction of each medication; highlight allergies on chart, Kardex

Teach patient/family:
• Aspects of drug therapy including need to complete course of medication to ensure organism death (10-14 days); culture may be taken after completed course
• To report sore throat, fever, fatigue; (could indicate superimposed infection)
• To wear or carry Medic Alert ID if allergic to penicillins
• To take on empty stomach with a full glass of water

Lab test interferences:
False positive: Urine glucose, urine protein

Treatment of overdose: Withdraw drug, maintain airway, administer epinephrine, aminophylline, O_2, IV corticosteroids for anaphylaxis

---

oxamniquine
(ox-am'ni-kwin)
Vansil

Func. class.: Anthelmintic
Chem. class.: Tetrahydroquinonc derivative

Action: Causes paralysis, contraction, leading to dislodgement of suckers; they are carried to liver where phagocytosis takes place

Uses: Schistosomiasis

Dosage and routes:
• *Adult and child >30 kg:* PO 12-15 mg/kg as single dose
• *Child <30 kg:* PO 20 mg/kg in 2 divided doses q2-8h

Available forms include: Caps 250 mg

Side effects/adverse reactions:
INTEG: Rash, pruritus, urticaria
CNS: Dizziness, headache, drowsiness, insomnia, ***convulsions,*** hallucination, personality changes, stimulation
EENT: Bad taste, oral irritation
GI: Nausea, vomiting, anorexia, abdominal pain
HEMA: Increased sed rate, reticulocyte count, increase or decrease in leukocytes

Contraindications: Hypersensitivity

Precautions: Pregnancy (C), lactation, seizure disorders

Pharmacokinetics:
PO: Peak 1-1½ hr, half-life 1-2½ hr, excreted in urine, (unchanged/metabolites)

NURSING CONSIDERATIONS

Assess:
• Stools during entire treatment, 1, 3 mo after treatment; specimens must be sent to lab while still warm

Administer:
• PO after meals to avoid GI symptoms

Perform/provide:
• Storage in tight container, cool environment

Evaluate:
• Therapeutic response: expulsion of worms, 3 negative stool cultures after completion of treatment
• For allergic reaction: rash, itching, urticaria

• For infection in other family members since infection from person to person is common

Teach patient/family:

• Proper hygiene after BM including handwashing technique; tell patient to avoid putting fingers in mouth
• That infected person should sleep alone; do not shake bed linen; change bed linen daily, wash in hot water
• To clean toilet qd with disinfectant (green soap solution)
• Need for compliance with dosage schedule, duration of treatment
• That urine may turn orange or red
• To avoid hazardous activities since drowsiness occurs
• That seizures may recur in patient who is controlled on medication

Lab test interferences:
Interferes: Urinalysis

---

oxandrolone

(ox-an'droe-lone)
Anavar

Func. class.: Androgenic anabolic steroid
Chem. class.: Halogenated testosterone derivative

Action: Increases weight by building body tissue, increases potassium, phosphorus, chloride, nitrogen levels, increases bone development

Uses: Tissue building after steroid therapy, osteoporosis, prolonged immobility

Dosage and routes:

• *Adult:* PO 2.5 mg bid-qid, not to exceed 20 mg qd × 2-3 wk
• *Child:* PO 0.25 mg/kg/day × 2-4 wk, not to exceed 3 mo

Available forms include: Tabs 2.5 mg

Side effects/adverse reactions:
INTEG: Rash, acneiform lesions, oily hair, skin, flushing, sweating, acne vulgaris, alopecia, hirsutism
CNS: Dizziness, headache, fatigue, tremors, paresthesias, flushing, sweating, anxiety, lability, insomnia
MS: Cramps, spasms
CV: Increased B/P
GU: ***Hematuria,*** amenorrhea, vaginitis, decrease libido, decreased breast size, clitoral hypertrophy, testicular atrophy
GI: Nausea, vomiting, constipation, weight gain, ***cholestatic jaundice***
EENT: Carpal tunnel syndrome, conjunctional edema, nasal congestion
ENDO: Abnormal GTT

Contraindications: Severe renal disease, severe cardiac disease, severe hepatic disease, hypersensitivity, pregnancy (X), lactation, genital bleeding (abnormal)

Precautions: Diabetes mellitus, CV disease, MI

Pharmacokinetics:
PO: Metabolized in liver, excreted in urine, crosses placenta, excreted in breast milk

Interactions/incompatibilities:

• Increased effects of: oral antidiabetics, oxyphenbutazone
• Increased PT: anticoagulants
• Edema: ACTH, adrenal steroids
• Decreased effects of: insulin

NURSING CONSIDERATIONS

Assess:

• Weight daily, notify physician if weekly weight gain is >5 lb
• B/P q4h
• I&O ratio; be alert for decreasing urinary output, increasing edema
• Growth rate in children since growth rate may be uneven (linear/

bone growth) when used for extended time
• Electrolytes: K, Na, Cl, Ca; cholesterol
• Liver function studies: ALT, AST, bilirubin
Administer:
• Titrated dose, use lowest effective dose
Perform/provide:
• Diet with increased calories and protein; decrease sodium if edema occurs
• Supportive drug of enemia
Evaluate:
• Therapeutic response: occurs in 4-6 wk in osteoporosis
• Edema, hypertension, cardiac symptoms, jaundice
• Mental status: affect, mood, behavioral changes, aggression
• Signs of masculinization in female: increased libido, deepening of voice, breast tissue, enlarged clitoris, menstrual irregularities; male: gynecomastia, impotence, testicular atrophy
• Hypercalcemia: lethargy, polyuria, polydipsia, nausea, vomiting, constipation; drug may need to be decreased
• Hypoglycemia in diabetics, since oral anticoagulant action is decreased
Teach patient/family:
• That drug needs to be combined with complete health plan: diet, rest, exercise
• To notify physician if therapeutic response decreases
• Not to discontinue this medication abruptly
• About change in sex characteristics
• Women to report menstrual irregularities
• That 1-3 mo course is necessary for response in breast cancer
• Procedure for use of buccal tablets (requires 30-60 min to dissolve, change absorption site with each dose; do not eat, drink, chew, or smoke while tablet is in place)
Lab test interferences:
Increase: Serum cholesterol, blood glucose, urine glucose
Decrease: Serum calcium, serum potassium, T_4, T_3, thyroid ^{131}I uptake test, urine 17-OHCS, 17-KS, PBI, BSP

---

oxazepam

(ox-a'ze-pam)
Apo-Oxazepam,* Novoxapam,* Serax

Func. class.: Antianxiety
Chem. class.: Benzodiazepine

Controlled Substance Schedule IV
Action: Depresses subcortical levels of CNS, including limbic system and reticular formation
Uses: Anxiety, alcohol withdrawal
Dosage and routes:
Anxiety
• *Adult:* PO 10-30 mg tid-qid
Alcohol withdrawal
• *Adult:* PO 15-30 mg tid-qid
Available forms include: Caps 10, 15, 30 mg, tabs 15 mg
Side effects/adverse reactions:
CNS: Dizziness, drowsiness, confusion, headache, anxiety, tremors, fatigue, depression, insomnia, hallucinations, paradoxical excitement, transient amnesia
GI: Nausea, vomiting, anorexia
INTEG: Rash, dermatitis, itching
CV: Orthostatic hypotension, ***ECG changes, tachycardia,*** hypotension
EENT: Blurred vision, tinnitus, mydriasis
Contraindications: Hypersensitiv-

ity to benzodiazepines, narrow-angle glaucoma, psychosis, pregnancy (D), child <12 yr
Precautions: Elderly, debilitated, hepatic disease, renal disease
Pharmacokinetics:
PO: Peak 2-4 hr, metabolized by liver, excreted by kidneys, half-life 5-15 hr
Interactions/incompatibilities:
• Decreased effects of oxazepam: oral contraceptives, valproic acid
• Increased effects of oxazepam: CNS depressants, alcohol, disulfiram, oral contraceptives

NURSING CONSIDERATIONS

Assess:
• B/P (lying, standing), pulse; if systolic B/P drops 20 mm Hg, hold drug, notify physician; respirations q5-15 min if given IV
• Blood studies: CBC during long-term therapy, blood dyscrasias have occurred rarely
• Hepatic studies: AST, ALT, bilirubin, creatinine, LDH, alk phosphatase
Administer:
• With food or milk for GI symptoms
• Sugarless gum, hard candy, frequent sips of water for dry mouth
Perform/provide:
• Assistance with ambulation during beginning therapy; drowsiness/dizziness occurs
• Safety measures, including siderails
• Check to see PO medication has been swallowed
Evaluate:
• Therapeutic response: decreased anxiety, restlessness, insomnia
• Mental status: mood, sensorium, affect, sleeping pattern, drowsiness, dizziness
• Physical dependency, withdrawal symptoms: headache, nausea, vomiting, muscle pain, weakness, tremors, ***convulsions*** after long-term use
• Suicidal tendencies
Teach patient/family:
• That drug may be taken with food
• Not to be used for everyday stress or used longer than 4 mo, unless directed by physician; not to take more than prescribed dose; may be habit forming
• To avoid OTC preparations (cough, cold, hay fever) unless approved by physician
• To avoid driving, activities that require alertness, since drowsiness may ocur
• To avoid alcohol ingestion or other psychotropic medications unless prescribed by physician
• Not to discontinue medication abruptly after long-term use
• To rise slowly or fainting may occur, especially elderly
• That drowsiness might worsen at beginning of treatment
Lab test interferences:
Increase: AST/ALT, serum bilirubin
Decrease: RAIU
False increase: 17-OHCS
Treatment of overdose: Lavage, VS, supportive care

---

oxidized cellulose

Oxycel, Surgicel
Func. class.: Hemostatic
Chem. class.: Cellulose product

Action: Absorbs blood, acts like an artificial clot
Uses: Hemostasis in surgery, oral surgery, exodontia
Dosage and routes:
Adult and child: TOP apply using sterile technique as needed, remove

*Available in Canada only

after bleeding stops, if possible, or leave in place if needed
Available forms include: TOP knitted fabric
Side effects/adverse reactions:
EENT: Sneezing, burning in epistaxis
INTEG: Burning, stinging, encapsulation of fluid, foreign bodies
CNS: Headache in epistaxis
Contraindications: Hypersensitivity, large artery hemorrhage, oozing surfaces, implantation in bone deficit, placement around optic nerve, and chiasm

NURSING CONSIDERATIONS
Administer:
• Dry, use only amount needed to control bleeding
• Loosely, remove excess before closure in surgery; irrigate first, then remove using sterile technique
• Using sterile technique, cannot be resterilized
Evaluate:
• Therapeutic response: decreased bleeding in surgery
• Allergy: fever, rash, itching, burning, stinging

---

oxtriphylline

(ox-trye'fi-lin)
Choledyl, Novotriphyl,* Theophyllinate, Theophylline Choline
Func. class.: Bronchodilator, spasmolytic
Chem. class.: Choline salt of theophylline

Action: Relaxes smooth muscle of respiratory system by blocking phosphodiesterase, which increases cyclic AMP; 64% theophylline
Uses: Acute bronchial asthma, reversible bronchospasm in chronic bronchitis and COPD

Dosage and routes:
• *Adult and child >12 yr:* PO 200 mg qid
• *Child 2-12 yr:* PO 4 mg/kg q6h; may be increased to desired response, therapeutic level
Available forms include: Elix 100 mg/5 ml; syr 50 mg/5 ml; tabs 100, 200, 400, 600 mg
Side effects/adverse reactions:
CNS: Anxiety, restlessness, insomnia, dizziness, ***convulsions,*** headache, light-headedness
CV: Palpitations, sinus tachycardia, hypotension
GI: Nausea, vomiting, anorexia, diarrhea, bitter taste, dyspepsia
RESP: Increased rate
INTEG: Flushing, urticaria
Contraindications: Hypersensitivity to xanthines, tachydysrhythmias
Precautions: Elderly, CHF, cor pulmonale, hepatic disease, active peptic ulcer disease, diabetes mellitus, hyperthyroidism, hypertension, children, pregnancy (C), glaucoma, prostatic hypertrophy
Pharmacokinetics:
SOL: Peak 1 hr, metabolized in liver, excreted in urine, breast milk, crosses placenta
Interactions/incompatibilities:
• Increased action of oxtriphylline: cimetidine, erythromycin, troleandomycin
• May increase effects of: anticoagulants, coffee
• Cardiotoxicity: β-blockers
• Decreased effect of: lithium

NURSING CONSIDERATIONS
Assess:
• Therapeutic blood levels; toxicity may occur with small increase above therapeutic level
• Therapeutic theophylline levels: 11-20
• Smoking reduces effects of theophyllines, requiring larger doses

Administer:
• PO after meals to decrease GI symptoms; absorption may be affected
• After meals, hs

Perform/provide:
• Storage in closed container, away from heat, protect elixir from light

Evaluate:
• Therapeutic response: absence of dyspnea, wheezing
• Respiratory rate, rhythm, depth; auscultate lung fields bilaterally; notify physician of abnormalities
• Allergic reactions: rash, urticaria; if these occur, drug should be discontinued

Teach patient/family:
• To check OTC medications, current prescription medications for ephedrine, which will increase stimulation
• To avoid hazardous activities; dizziness may occur
• If GI upset occurs, to take drug with 8 oz water; avoid food; absorption may be decreased
• To notify physician of toxicity: nausea, vomiting, anxiety, convulsions, insomnia, rapid pulse
• To notify physician of change in smoking habit; may need to change dose

oxybutynin chloride

(ox-i-byoo'ti-nin)
Ditropan
Func. class.: Spasmolytic
Chem. class.: Synthetic tertiary amine

Action: Relaxes smooth muscles in urinary tract
Uses: Antispasmodic for neurogenic bladder
Dosage and routes:
• *Adult:* PO 5 mg bid-tid, not to exceed 5 mg qid
• *Child >5 yr:* PO 5 mg bid, not to exceed 5 mg tid
Available forms include: Sol 5 mg/5 ml; tabs 5 mg
Side effects/adverse reactions:
HEMA: ***Leukopenia, eosinophilia***
CNS: Anxiety, restlessness, dizziness, ***convulsions,*** headache, drowsiness, confusion
CV: Palpitations, sinus tachycardia, hypotension
GI: Nausea, vomiting, anorexia, abdominal pain, constipation
GU: Dysuria, retention, hesitancy
INTEG: Urticaria, dermatitis
EENT: Blurred vision, increased intraocular tension, dry mouth, throat
Contraindications: Hypersensitivity, GI obstruction, GI hemorrhage, GU obstruction, glaucoma, severe colitis, myasthenia gravis, unstable CV status in acute hemorrhage
Precautions: Pregnancy (C), lactation, suspected glaucoma, children <12 yr
Pharmacokinetics: Onset ½-1 hr, peak 3-4 hr, duration 6-10 hr, metabolized by liver, excreted in urine

NURSING CONSIDERATIONS

Evaluate:
• Urinary status: dysuria, frequency, nocturia, incontinence
• Allergic reactions: rash, urticaria; if these occur, drug should be discontinued

Teach patient/family
• To avoid hazardous activities; dizziness may occur

oxycodone HCl

(ox-i-koe'done)
Supeudol*; Combinations—Codoxy, Percocet,* Percocet-Demi, Percodan, Tylox
Func. class.: Narcotic analgesics
Chem. class.: Opiate, semisynthetic derivative

Controlled Substance Schedule II

* Available in Canada only

Action: Inhibits ascending pain pathways in CNS, increases pain threshold, alters pain perception
Uses: Moderate to severe pain
Dosage and routes:
- *Adult:* REC 1-3 supp/day prn (Supeubol)
- *Child:* PO ¼-½ tab q6h prn (Percodan-Demi)
- *Adult:* PO 1-2 tab q6h prn (Combinations)

Available forms include: Tabs 5 mg; sol 5 mg/5ml
Side effects/adverse reactions:
CNS: Drowsiness, dizziness, confusion, headache, sedation, euphoria
GI: Nausea, vomiting, anorexia, constipation, cramps
GU: Increased urinary output, dysuria, urinary retention
INTEG: Rash, urticaria, bruising, flushing, diaphoresis, pruritus
EENT: Tinnitus, blurred vision, miosis, diplopia
CV: Palpitations, bradycardia, change in B/P
RESP: ***Respiratory depression***
Contraindications: Hypersensitivity, addiction (narcotic)
Precautions: Addictive personality, pregnancy (B), lactation, increased intracranial pressure, MI (acute), severe heart disease, respiratory depression, hepatic disease, renal disease, child <18 yr
Pharmacokinetics:
PO: Onset 10-15 min, peak ½-1 hr, duration 4-5 hr; detoxified by liver, excreted in urine, crosses placenta, excreted in breast milk
Interactions/incompatibilities:
- Increased effects with other CNS depressants: alcohol, narcotics, sedative/hypnotics, antipsychotics, skeletal muscle relaxants

NURSING CONSIDERATIONS

Assess:
- I&O ratio; check for decreasing output; may indicate urinary retention

Administer:
- With antiemetic if nausea, vomiting occur
- When pain is beginning to return; determine dosage interval by patient response

Perform/provide:
- Storage in light-resistant area at room temperature
- Assistance with ambulation
- Safety measures: siderails, night light, call bell within easy reach

Evaluate:
- Therapeutic response: decrease in pain
- CNS changes: dizziness, drowsiness, hallucinations, euphoria, LOC, pupil reaction
- Allergic reactions: rash, urticaria
- Respiratory dysfunction: respiratory depression, character, rash, rhythm; notify physician if respirations are <10/min
- Need for pain medication, physical dependence

Teach patient/family:
- To report any symptoms of CNS changes, allergic reactions
- That physical dependency may result when used for extended periods of time
- That withdrawal symptoms may occur: nausea, vomiting, cramps, fever, faintness, anorexia

Lab test interferences:
Increase: Amylase
Treatment of overdose: Narcan 0.2-0.8 IV, O_2, IV fluids, vasopressors

O

oxymetazoline HCl (nasal)

(ox-i-met-az'oh-leen)

Afrin, Afrin Pediatric Nose Drops, Dristan Long-Lasting, Duramist, Duration, Nafrine,* Nostrilla, NTZ Long-Acting, Sinex Long-Lasting, St. Joseph's Decongestant for Children

Func. class.: Nasal decongestant
Chem. class.: Sympathomimetic amine

Action: Produces vasoconstriction (rapid, long-acting) of arterioles, thereby decreasing fluid exudation, mucosal engorgement

Uses: Nasal congestion

Dosage and routes:

- *Adult and child >6 yr:* instill 2-3 gtts or sprays to each nostril bid
- *Child 2-6 yr:* instill 2-3 gtts or sprays .025% sol bid, not to exceed 5 days

Available forms include: Sol 0.025%, 0.05%

Side effects/adverse reactions:

GI: Nausea, vomiting, anorexia

EENT: Irritation, burning, sneezing, stinging, dryness, rebound congestion

INTEG: Contact dermatitis

CNS: Anxiety, restlessness, tremors, weakness, insomnia, dizziness, fever, headache

Contraindications: Hypersensitivity to sympathomimetic amines

Precautions: Child <6 yr, elderly, diabetes, cardiovascular disease, hypertension, hyperthyroidism, increased ICP, prostatic hypertrophy, pregnancy (C), glaucoma

Interactions/incompatibilities:

- Hypertension: MAOIs, β-adrenergic blockers
- Hypotension: methyldopa, mecamylamine, reserpine

NURSING CONSIDERATIONS

Administer:

- No more than q4h
- For <4 consecutive days

Perform/provide:

- Environmental humidification to decrease nasal congestion, dryness
- Storage in light-resistant containers; do not expose to high temperatures

Evaluate:

- Therapeutic response: decreased nasal congestion
- For redness, swelling, pain in nasal passages

Teach patient/family:

- That stinging may occur for a few applications; drying of mucosa may be decreased by environmental humidification
- To notify physician if irregular pulse, insomnia, dizziness, or tremors occur
- Proper administration to avoid systemic absorption

oxymetholone

(ox-i-meth'oh-lone)

Adroyd, Anadrol-50, Anapolon 50*

Func. class.: Androgenic anabolic steroid
Chem. class.: Halogenated testosterone derivative

Action: Increases weight by building body tissue, increases potassium, phosphorus, chloride, and nitrogen levels, increases bone development

Uses: Tissue building after steroid therapy, osteoporosis, aplastic anemia, anemias caused by deficient RBC production

Dosage and routes:

Aplastic anemia

- *Adult and child:* PO 1-5 mg/kg/

*Available in Canada only

day, titrated to patient response, not to exceed 3 months

Osteoporosis/tissue building (possible indication)

• *Adult:* PO 5-15 mg/day, not to exceed 30 mg/day or 3 mo

• *Child >6 yr:* PO up to 10 mg/day, not to exceed 1 mo

• *Child <6 yr:* PO 1.25 mg qd-qid, not to exceed 1 mo

Available forms include: Tabs 50 mg

Side effects/adverse reactions:

INTEG: Rash, acneiform lesions, oily hair, skin, flushing, sweating, acne vulgaris, alopecia, hirsutism

CNS: Dizziness, headache, fatigue, tremors, paresthesias, flushing, sweating, anxiety, lability, insomnia

MS: Cramps, spasms

CV: Increased B/P

GU: ***Hematuria,*** amenorrhea, vaginitis, decreased libido, decreased breast size, clitoral hypertrophy, testicular atrophy

GI: Nausea, vomiting, constipation, weight gain, ***cholestatic jaundice***

EENT: Carpal tunnel syndrome, conjunctional edema, nasal congestion

ENDO: Abnormal GTT

Contraindications: Severe renal disease, severe cardiac disease, severe hepatic disease, hypersensitivity, pregnancy (X), lactation, genital bleeding (abnormal)

Precautions: Diabetes mellitus, CV disease, MI

Pharmacokinetics:

PO: Metabolized in liver, excreted in urine, crosses placenta, excreted in breast milk

Interactions/incompatibilities:

• Increased effects of: oral antidiabetics, oxyphenbutazone

• Increased PT: anticoagulants

• Edema: ACTH, adrenal steroids

• Decreased effects of: insulin

NURSING CONSIDERATIONS

Assess:

• Weight daily, notify physician if weekly weight gain is >5 lb

• B/P q4h

• I&O ratio; be alert for decreasing urinary output, increasing edema

• Growth rate in children since growth rate may be uneven (linear/bone growth) when used for extended period

• Electrolytes: K, Na, Cl, Ca; cholesterol

• Liver function studies: ALT, AST, bilirubin

Administer:

• Titrated dose, use lowest effective dose

Perform/provide:

• Diet with increased calories and protein; decrease sodium if edema occurs

• Supportive drug of anemia

Evaluate:

• Therapeutic response: occurs in 4-6 wk in osteoporosis

• Edema, hypertension, cardiac symptoms, jaundice

• Mental status: affect, mood, behavioral changes, aggression

• Signs of masculinization in female: increased libido, deepening of voice, breast tissue, enlarged clitoris, menstrual irregularities; male: gynecomastia, impotence, testicular atrophy

• Hypercalcemia: lethargy, polyuria, polydipsia, nausea, vomiting, constipation; drug may need to be decreased

• Hypoglycemia in diabetics, since oral anticoagulant action is decreased

Teach patient/family:

• That drug needs to be combined

with complete health plan: diet, rest, exercise
• To notify physician if therapeutic response decreases
• Not to discontinue this medication abruptly
• About changes in sex characteristics
• That women should report menstrual irregularities
• That 1-3 mo course is necessary for response in breast cancer
• Procedure for use of buccal tablets (requires 30-60 min to dissolve, change absorption site with each dose; do not eat, drink, chew, or smoke while tablet is in place)

Lab test interferences:
Increase: Serum cholesterol, blood glucose, urine glucose
Decrease: Serum calcium, serum potassium, T_4, T_3, thyroid ^{131}I uptake test, urine 17-OHCS, 17-KS, PBI, BSP

---

oxymorphone HCl

(ox-i-mor-fone)
Numorphan

Func. class.: Narcotic analgesic
Chem. class.: Opiate, semisynthetic phenanthrene derivative

Controlled Substance Schedule II
Action: Inhibits ascending pain pathways in CNS, increases pain threshold, alters pain perception
Uses: Moderate to severe pain
Dosage and routes:
• *Adult:* IM/SC 1-1.5 mg q4-6h prn; IV 0.5 mg q4-6h prn; REC 2.5-5 mg q4-6h prn
Available forms include: Inj SC, IM, IV 1, 1.5 mg/ml; supp 5 mg
Side effects/adverse reactions:
CNS: Drowsiness, dizziness, confusion, headache, sedation, euphoria
GI: Nausea, vomiting, anorexia, constipation, cramps
GU: Increased urinary output, dysuria, urinary retention
INTEG: Rash, urticaria, bruising, flushing, diaphoresis, pruritus
EENT: Tinnitus, blurred vision, miosis, diplopia
CV: Palpitations, bradycardia, change in B/P
RESP: ***Respiratory depression***
Contraindications: Hypersensitivity, addiction (narcotic)
Precautions: Addictive personality, pregnancy (B), lactation, increased intracranial pressure, MI (acute), severe heart disease, respiratory depression, hepatic disease, renal disease, child $<$18 yr
Pharmacokinetics:
SC/IM: Onset 10-15 min, peak 1-½ hr, duration 2-6 hr
IV: Onset 5-10 min, peak 1-½ hr, duration 3-6 hr
REC: Onset 15-30 min, duration 3-6 hr
Metabolized by liver, excreted in urine, crosses placenta
Interactions/incompatibilities:
• Increased effects with other CNS depressants: alcohol, narcotics, sedative/hypnotics, antipsychotics, skeletal muscle relaxants

NURSING CONSIDERATIONS

Assess:
• I&O ratio; check for decreasing output; may indicate urinary retention
Administer:
• IV after diluting with 5 ml sterile H_2O or NS for inj; give over 5 min through Y-tube or 3-way stopcock
• With antiemetic if nausea, vomiting occur
• When pain is beginning to return; determine dosage interval by patient response

---

* Available in Canada only

Perform/provide:
- Storage in light-resistant area at room temperature
- Assistance with ambulation
- Safety measures: siderails, night light, call bell within easy reach

Evaluate:
- Therapeutic response: decrease in pain
- CNS changes: dizziness, drowsiness, hallucinations, euphoria, LOC, pupil reaction
- Allergic reactions: rash, urticaria
- Respiratory dysfunction: respiratory depression, character, rate, rhythm; notify physician if respirations are <10/min
- Need for pain medication, physical dependence

Teach patient/family:
- To report any symptoms of CNS changes, allergic reactions
- That physical dependency may result when used for extended periods of time
- That withdrawal symptoms may occur: nausea, vomiting, cramps, fever, faintness, anorexia

Lab test interferences:
Increase: Amylase

Treatment of overdose: Narcan 0.2-0.8 IV, O_2, IV fluids, vasopressors

---

oxyphenbutazone

(ox-i-fen-byoo'ta-zone)
Oxalid, Oxybutazone*

Func. class.: Nonsteroidal
Chem. class.: Pyrazolone derivative

Action: Inhibits prostaglandin synthesis by decreasing an enzyme needed for biosynthesis; possesses analgesic, antiinflammatory, antipyretic properties

Uses: Mild to moderate pain, osteoarthritis, rheumatoid arthritis

Dosage and routes:

Pain
- *Adult:* PO 100-200 mg tid-qid

Acute arthritis
- *Adult:* PO 400 mg, then 100 mg q4h × 4 days or until desired response

Available forms include: Tabs 100 mg

Side effects/adverse reactions:
GI: Nausea, anorexia, vomiting, diarrhea, jaundice, ***cholestatic hepatitis,*** constipation, flatulence, cramps, dry mouth, peptic ulcer
CNS: Dizziness, drowsiness, fatigue, tremors, confusion, insomnia, anxiety, depression
CV: Tachycardia, peripheral edema, palpitations, dysrhythmias
INTEG: Purpura, rash, pruritus, sweating
GU: ***Nephrotoxicity: dysuria, hematuria, oliguria, azotemia***
HEMA: ***Blood dyscrasias***
EENT: Tinnitus, hearing loss, blurred vision

Contraindications: Hypersensitivity, asthma, severe renal disease, severe hepatic disease, pregnancy (D)

Precautions: Lactation, children, bleeding disorders, GI disorders, cardiac disorders, hypersensitivity to other antiinflammatory agents

Pharmacokinetics:
PO: Peak 2 hr, half-life 3-3½ hr; metabolized in liver, excreted in urine (metabolites), excreted in breast milk

Interactions/incompatibilities:
- Increased action of: coumarin, phenytoin, sulfonamides

NURSING CONSIDERATIONS

Assess:
- Renal, liver, blood studies: BUN, creatinine, AST, ALT, Hgb before

treatment, periodically thereafter
• Audiometric, ophthalmic exam before, during, after treatment
Administer:
• With food to decrease GI symptoms; best to take on empty stomach to facilitate absorption
Perform/provide:
• Storage at room temperature
Evaluate:
• Therapeutic response: decreased pain, stiffness, swelling in joints, ability to move more easily
• For eye, ear problems: blurred vision, tinnitus (may indicate toxicity)
Teach patient/family:
• To report blurred vision, or ringing, roaring in ears (may indicate toxicity)
• To avoid driving or other hazardous activities if dizziness or drowsiness occurs
• To report change in urine pattern, weight increase, edema, pain increase in joints, fever, blood in urine (indicates nephrotoxicity)
• That therapeutic effects may take up to 1 mo

---

oxytetracycline HCl

(ox-i-tet-ra-sye'kleen)
Dalimycin, Oxlopar, Oxytetraclor, Terramycin, Uri-tet, E.P. Mycin
Func. class.: Broad-spectrum antibiotic/antiinfective
Chem. class.: Tetracycline

Action: Inhibits protein synthesis, phosphorylation in microorganisms by binding to 30S ribosomal subunits, reversibly binding to 50S ribosomal subunits, bacteriostatic
Uses: Syphilis, chlamydia trachomatis, gonorrhea, lymphogranuloma venereum, uncommon gram-positive/negative organisms, rickettsial infections
Dosage and routes:
• *Adult:* PO 250-500 mg q6h; IM 100 mg q8h or 150 mg q12h IV 250-500 mg q12h, 250 mg q24h
• *Child >8 yr:* PO 25-50 mg/kg/day in divided doses q6h; IM 15-25 mg/kg/day in divided doses q8-12h; IV 10-20 mg/kg/day in divided doses q12h
Gonorrhea
• *Adult:* PO 1.5 g, then 500 mg qid for a total of 9 g
Chlamydia trachomatis
• *Adult:* PO 500 mg qid × 7 days
Syphilis
• *Adult:* PO 2-3 g in divided doses × 10-15 days up to 30-40 g total
• Dosage adjustment necessary in renal impairment
Available forms include: Tabs 250 mg; caps 125, 250 mg; powder for inj IV 250, 500 mg; inj IM 50, 125 mg/ml
Side effects/adverse reactions:
CNS: Fever
HEMA: ***Eosinophilia, neutropenia, thrombocytopenia, leukocytosis, hemolytic anemia***
EENT: Dysphagia, glossitis, decreased calcification of deciduous teeth, oral candidiasis
GI: Nausea, abdominal pain, *vomiting, diarrhea,* anorexia, enterocolitis, ***hepatotoxicity,*** flatulence, abdominal cramps, epigastric burning, stomatitis
CV: Pericarditis
GU: Increased BUN
INTEG: Rash, urticaria, photosensitivity, increased pigmentation, ***exfoliative dermatitis,*** pruritus, angioedema, pain at injection site
Contraindications: Hypersensitivity to tetracyclines, children <8 yr, pregnancy (D)

---

* Available in Canada only

Precautions: Renal disease, hepatic disease, lactation

Pharmacokinetics:

PO: Peak 2-4 hr, half-life 6-12 hr; excreted in urine, bile, feces, in active form, crosses placenta 20%-40% protein bound

Interactions/incompatibilities:

• Decreased effect of oxytetracycline: antacids, $NaHCO_3$, dairy products, alkali products, iron, kaolin/pectin, cimetidine

• Increased effect: anticoagulants

• Decreased effect: penicillins, oral contraceptives

• Nephrotoxicity: methoxyflurane

• Do not mix with other drugs

NURSING CONSIDERATIONS

Assess:

• I&O ratio

• Blood studies: PT, CBC, AST, ALT, BUN, creatinine

• Signs of anemia: Hct, Hgb, fatigue

Administer:

• PO with a full glass of water

• IM, deep only

• IV after diluting 250 mg or less/10 ml of sterile H_2O for inj; further dilute with at least 100 ml of D_5W or NS for inj; give 100 mg or less/5 min or more; use within 12 hr, decrease rate or increase volume of diluent if vein irritation occurs; do not give SC

• After C&S obtained

• 2 hr before or after laxative or ferrous products, 3 hr after antacid

Perform/provide:

• Storage in tight, light-resistant container at room temperature

Evaluate:

• Therapeutic response: decreased temperature, absence of lesions, negative C&S

• Allergic reactions: rash, itching, pruritus, angioedema

• Nausea, vomiting, diarrhea; administer antiemetic, antacids as ordered

• Overgrowth of infection: increased temperature, malaise, redness, pain, swelling, drainage, perineal itching, diarrhea, changes in cough or sputum

Teach patient/family:

• To avoid sun exposure since burns may occur; sunscreen does not seem to decrease photosensitivity

• If diabetic to avoid use of Clinistix, Diastix, or Tes-Tape for urine glucose testing

• That all prescribed medication must be taken to prevent superimposed infection

• To avoid milk products, to take with a full glass of water

Lab test interferences:

False negative: Urine glucose with Clinistix or Tes-Tape

False increase: Urinary catecholamines

oxytocin, synthetic injection

(ox-i-toe'sin)

Pitocin, Syntocinon, Uteracon

Func. class.: Oxytocic

Chem. class.: Hormone

Action: Acts directly on myofibrils producing uterine contraction, stimulates milk ejection by the breast

Uses: Stimulation of labor, induction; missed or incomplete abortion; postpartum bleeding

Dosage and routes:

Stimulation of labor

• *Adult:* IV INF 1 ml/1000 ml D_5W or 0.9% NaCl over 1-2 milli U/min; may increase q15-30 min, not to exceed 20 milli U/min

Incomplete abortion

• *Adult:* IV INF 10 U/500 ml D_5W or 0.9% NaCl given at 20-40 milli U/min

Postpartum bleeding

• *Adult:* IV INF 10-40 U/1000 ml D_5W or 0.9% NaCl given at 20-40 milli U/min

Available forms include: Inj IV 10 U/ml

Side effects/adverse reactions:

CNS: Hypertension, convulsions, tetanic contractions

GI: Nausea, vomiting, constipation

CV: Hypotension, dysrhythmias, increased pulse

GU: Abruptio placentae, decreased uterine blood flow

INTEG: Rash

HEMA: Increased hyperbilirubinemia

CV: Bradycardia, tachycardia, PVC

RESP: Anorexia, asphyxia

FETUS: ***Dysrhythmias, jaundice, hypoxia, intracranial hemorrhage***

Contraindications: Hypersensitivity, serum toxemia, cephalopelvic disproportion, fetal distress, hypertonic uterus

Precautions: Cervical/uterine surgery, sepsis (uterine), primipara >35 yr, 1st, 2nd stage of labor

Pharmacokinetics:

IM: Onset 3-7 min, duration 1 hr, half-life 12-17 min

IV: Onset 1 min, duration 30 min, half-life 12-17 min

Interactions/incompatibilities:

• Hypertension: vasopressors

NURSING CONSIDERATIONS

Assess:

• I&O ratio

• Contraction FHT, B/P, pulse, respiration

• B/P, pulse; watch for changes that may indicate hemorrhage

• Respiratory rate, rhythm, depth; notify physician of abnormalities

Administer:

• IV after diluting 10 U/L of 0.9% NS or D_5 NS run at 1-2 mU/min; increase by 1-2 mU/min at 15-30 min intervals to begin normal labor; dilute 10-40 U/L of solution, run 10-20 mU/min, titrate to control pp bleeding; dilute 10 U/500 ml of solution, run 10 U-20 mU/ml, administer by only one route at a time, use infusion pump

• After having crash cart available on unit (Mg^+, SO_4 at bedside)

Evaluate:

• Therapeutic response: stimulation of labor, control of postpartum bleeding

• Length, intensity, duration of contraction; notify physician of contractions lasting over 1 min or absence of contractions, turn patient on her side

• FHTs, fetal distress, watch for acceleration, deceleration, notify physician if problems occur

• For signs and symptoms of water intoxication

Teach patient/family:

• To report increased blood loss, abdominal cramps, increased temperature or foul-smelling lochia

---

oxytocin, synthetic nasal

(ox-i-toe'sin)

Func. class.: Oxytocic hormone

Action: Acts directly on myofibrils producing uterine contraction, stimulates milk ejection by the breast

Uses: Postpartum breast engorgement, initial milk letdown

Dosage and routes:

• *Adult:* Nas spray 1 spray into one or both nostrils q2-3min before breast feeding; nas drops 3 gtts into one or both nostrils q2-3min before breast feeding

Available forms include: Nas spray 40 U/ml; nas drops

Side effects/adverse reactions: None

Pharmacokinetics:

Onset 5-10 min, half-life 1 min

Interactions/incompatibilities:

• Hypertension: vasopressors

NURSING CONSIDERATIONS

Assess:

• I&O ratio

• Environment conducive to let-down reflex

Evaluate

• Therapeutic response: stimulation of milk ejection

Teach patient/family:

• To blow nose before administering

• To rinse dropper with warm water after each use

• Not to over use

---

pamidronate

(pam-i-drone'ate)

Aredia

Func. class.: Bone-resorption inhibitor

Chem. class.: Bisphosphonate

Action: Absorbs calcium phosphate crystals in bone and may directly block dissolution of hydroxyappetite crystals of bone; inhibits bone resorption, apparently without inhibiting bone formation and mineralization

Uses: Moderate to severe hypercalcemia associated with malignancy with or without bone metastases

Dosage and routes:

• *Adult:* IV INF 60-90 mg in moderate hypercalcemia, 90 mg in severe hypercalcemia given over 24 hr

Available forms include: Inj 30 mg pamidronate disodium and 470 mg of mannitol

Side effects/adverse reactions:

INTEG: Redness, swelling, induration, pain on palpitation at site of catheter insertion

GI: Abdominal pain, anorexia, constipation, nausea, vomiting

MS: Bone pain

CV: Hypertension

GU: Urinary tract infection, fluid overload

Contraindications: Hypersensitivity to biphosphonates

Precautions: Children, nursing mothers, pregnancy (C), renal dysfunction

Pharmacokinetics: Rapidly cleared from circulation and taken up mainly by bones, eliminated primarily by kidneys

Interactions/incompatibilities:

• Do not mix with calcium-containing infusion solutions, such as Ringer's solutions

NURSING CONSIDERATIONS

Assess:

• Renal studies and calcium, phosphate, magnesium, potassium

Administer:

• After reconstituting by adding 10 ml of sterile water for inj to each vial, then adding to 1000 ml of sterile 0.45%, 0.9% NaCl, D_5W, run over 24 hr

Perform/provide:

• Storage of infusion solution for up to 24 hr at room temperature

• Reconstituted solution with sterile water may be stored under refrigeration for up to 24 hr

Evaluate:

• Therapeutic response: decrease calcium levels

P

pancreatin

(pan'kree-a-tin)

Elzyme 303 Enseals

Func. class.: Digestant

Chem. class.: Pancreatic enzyme concentrate—bovine/porcine

Action: Pancreatic enzyme needed for proper pancreatic functioning

Uses: Exocrine pancreatic secretion insufficiency, cystic fibrosis (digestive aid)

Dosage and routes:

• *Adult:* PO 8000-24,000 USP U with meals

Available forms include: Tab 650, 2000, 12,000 U

Side effects/adverse reactions:

GI: Anorexia, nausea, vomiting, diarrhea, glossitis, anal soreness

GU: Hyperuricuria, hyperuricemia

INTEG: Rash, hypersensitivity

EENT: Buccal soreness

Contraindications: Hypersensitivity to pork

Precautions: Pregnancy (C), lactation

Interactions/incompatibilities:

• Decreased absorption: cimetidine, antacids, oral iron

NURSING CONSIDERATIONS

Assess:

• I&O ratio, watch for increasing urinary output

• Fecal fat, nitrogen, pro-time, calcium during treatment

Administer:

• After antacid or H_2 blockers; decreased pH inactivates drug

• Whole, not to be crushed, chewed (enteric coated)

• Low fat diet to decrease GI symptoms

Perform/provide:

• Storage in tight container at room temperature

Evaluate:

• For allergy to pork

• For polyuria, polydipsia, polyphagia (may indicate diabetes mellitus)

pancrelipase

(pan-kre-li'pase)

Cotazym, Cotazyme-S, Ilozyme, Ku-Zyme HP, Pancrease, Viokase

Func. class.: Digestant

Chem. class.: Pancreatic enzyme—bovine/porcine

Action: Pancreatic enzyme needed for proper pancreatic functioning

Uses: Exocrine pancreatic secretion insufficiency, cystic fibrosis (digestive aid), steatorrhea, pancreatic enzyme deficiency

Dosage and routes:

• *Adult and child:* PO 1-3 caps/tabs ac or with meals, or 1 caps/tab with snack or 1-2 pdr pkt ac

Available forms include: Tab 8000, 11,000, 30,000 U; caps 8000, 30,000 U; enteric coated caps 4000, 5000, 20,000, 25,000 U; powd 16,800 U

Side effects/adverse reactions:

GI: Anorexia, nausea, vomiting, diarrhea

GU: Hyperuricuria, hyperuricemia

Contraindications: Allergy to pork

Precautions: Pregnancy (C)

Interactions/incompatibilities:

• Decreased absorption: cimetidine, antacids, oral iron

NURSING CONSIDERATIONS

Assess:

• I&O ratio, watch for increasing urinary output

• Fecal fat, nitrogen, pro-time during treatment

Administer:

• After antacid or cimetidine; decreased pH inactivates drug

• Powder mixed in prepared fruit for infants, children
• Whole, not crushed or chewed (enteric coated)
• Low fat diet to decrease GI symptoms
• Powder mixed with pureed fruit, take tabs with or before food

Perform/provide:
• Storage in tight container at room temperature

Evaluate:
• For allergy to pork
• For polyuria, polydipsia, polyphagia (may indicate diabetes mellitus)

pancuronium bromide

(pan-kyoo-roe'nee-um)
Pavulon

Func. class.: Neuromuscular blocker (nondepolarizing)
Chem. class.: Synthetic curariform

Action: Inhibits transmission of nerve impulses by binding with cholinergic receptor sites, antagonizing action of acetylcholine

Uses: Facilitation of endotracheal intubation, skeletal muscle relaxation during mechanical ventilation, surgery, or general anesthesia

Dosage and routes:
• *Adult:* IV 0.04-0.1 mg/kg, then 0.01 mg/kg q½-1hr
• *Child >10 yr:* IV 0.04-0.1 mg/kg, then ⅕ initial dose q½-1hr

Available forms include: Inj IV, IM, 1, 2 mg/ml

Side effects/adverse reactions:
CV: Bradycardia, tachycardia, increased, decreased B/P, ventricular extra systoles
RESP: ***Prolonged apnea, bronchospasm, cyanosis, respiratory depression***
EENT: Increased secretions
MS: Weakness to prolonged skeletal muscle relaxation
INTEG: Rash, flushing, pruritus, urticaria, sweating, salivation

Contraindications: Hypersensitivity to bromide ion

Precautions: Pregnancy (C), renal disease, cardiac disease, lactation, children <2 yr, electrolyte imbalances, dehydration, neuromuscular disease, respiratory disease

Pharmacokinetics:
IV: Onset 30-45 sec, peak 3-5 min; metabolized (small amounts), excreted in urine (unchanged), crosses placenta

Interactions/incompatibilities:
• Increased neuromuscular blockade: aminoglycosides, clindamycin, lincomycin, quinidine, local anesthetics, polymyxin antibiotics, lithium, narcotic analgesics, thiazides, enflurane, isoflurane
• Dysrhythmias: theophylline
• Do not mix with barbiturates in solution or syringe

NURSING CONSIDERATIONS

Assess:
• For electrolyte imbalances (K, Mg), may lead to increased action of this drug
• Vital signs (B/P, pulse, respirations, airway) until fully recovered; rate, depth, pattern of respirations, strength of hand grip
• I&O ratio; check for urinary retention, frequency, hesitancy

Administer:
• With diazepam or morphine when used for therapeutic paralysis; this drug provides no sedation alone
• Using nerve stimulator by anesthesiologist to determine neuromuscular blockade
• Atropine to counteract muscarinic effects

• After succinylcholine effects subside
• Anticholinesterase to reverse neuromuscular blockade
• IV undiluted, give over 1-2 min (only by qualified persons)

Perform/provide:
• Storage in refrigerator; do not store in plastic containers or syringes; use only fresh solutions
• Reassurance if communication is difficult during recovery from neuromuscular blockade
• Frequent (q2h) instillation of artificial tears and covering eyes to prevent drying of cornea

Evaluate:
• Therapeutic response: paralysis of jaw, eyelid, head, neck, rest of body
• Recovery: decreased paralysis of face, diaphragm, leg, arm, rest of body, allow to recover fully before completing a neuro assessment
• Allergic reactions: rash, fever, respiratory distress, pruritus; drug should be discontinued

Treatment of overdose: Edrophonium or neostigmine, atropine, monitor VS; may require mechanical ventilation

Lab test interferences:
Decrease: Cholinesterase

---

papaverine HCl

(pa-pav'er-een)

Cerebid, Cerespan, Lapav, Myobid, Pavabid, Pavacen, Pavadel, Pavasule, Ro-Papav, Vasal, Vasocap, Vasospan, Vazosan

Func. class.: Peripheral vasodilator

Chem. class.: Opium alkaloid (no narcotic activity)

Action: Relaxes all smooth muscle, inhibits cyclic nucleotide phosphodiesterase, which increases intracellular cAMP, causing vasodilation

Uses: Arterial spasm resulting in cerebral and peripheral ischemia; myocardial ischemia, associated with vascular spasm; or dysrhythmias; angina pectoris, peripheral, pulmonary embolism; visceral spasm; as in ureteral, biliary, GI colic PVD

Dosage and routes:
• *Adult:* PO 100-300 mg 3-5 times day; sus rel 150-300 mg q8-12 h; IM/IV 30-120 mg q3h prn

Available forms include: Cap time-release 150, 200, 300 mg; tabs 30, 60, 100, 150, 200, 300 mg; inj IM/IV 30 mg/ml

Side effects/adverse reactions:
CV: ***Tachycardia,*** increased B/P
RESP: Increased depth of respirations
CNS: Headache, dizziness, drowsiness, sedation, vertigo, malaise
GI: Nausea, anorexia, abdominal pain, constipation, diarrhea, jaundice, altered liver enzymes, ***hepatotoxicity***
INTEG: Flushing, sweating, rash

Contraindications: Hypersensitivity, complete AV heart block

Precautions: Cardiac dysrhythmias, glaucoma, pregnancy (C), lactation, drug dependency, children

Pharmacokinetics:
PO: Onset 30 sec, peak 1-2 hr, duration 3-4 hr
SUS REL: Onset erratic
90% bound to plasma proteins, metabolized in liver, excreted in urine (inactive metabolites)

Interactions/incompatibilities:
• Decreased effect of: levodopa
• Increased hypotension: antihypertensives, vasodilators, diazoxide, alcohol

---

* Available in Canada only

• Do not add to LR solution, precipitation will occur

NURSING CONSIDERATIONS

Assess:

• B/P, pulse, respiratory rate, rhythm, character during treatment until stable; take B/P lying, standing; orthostatic hypotension is common

• Hepatic tests: AST, ALT, bilirubin; liver enzymes may increase

Administer:

• With meals to reduce GI upset

• An ordered analgesic if headache develops

• IV undiluted or diluted in equal amount of sterile H_2O, give 30 mg or less/2 min through Y-tube or stopcock

Perform/provide:

• Storage at room temperature

Evaluate:

• Therapeutic response: ability to walk without pain, increased pulse volume, increased temperature in extremities or orientation, long- and short-term memory

• Hepatic hypersensitivity reaction: nausea, vomiting, jaundice; drug should be discontinued if this occurs

Teach patient/family:

• That medication is not cure, may need to be taken continuously depending on condition; therapeutic response may not be evident for 2-3 mo

• That it is necessary to quit smoking to prevent excessive vasoconstriction

• To avoid hazardous activities until stabilized on medication; dizziness may occur

• To notify physician if nausea, flushing, sweating, headache, or jaundice occur

Treatment of overdose: Discontinue medication

paraldehyde

(par-al'de-hyde)

Paral

Func. class.: Anticonvulsant

Chem. class.: Cyclic ether

Controlled Substance Schedule IV

Action: CNS depressant; exact mechanism of action is unknown

Uses: Refractory seizures, status epilepticus, sedation, insomnia, alcohol withdrawal, tetanus, eclampsia

Dosage and routes:

Seizures

• *Adult:* IM 5-10 ml, divide 10 ml into 2 inj; IV 0.2-0.4 ml/kg in NS inj

• *Child:* IM 0.15 ml/kg; REC 0.3 ml/kg q4-6h or 1 ml/yr of age, not to exceed 5 ml, may repeat in 1 hr prn; IV 5 ml/90 ml NS inj, begin infusion at 5 ml/hr, titrate to patient response

Alcohol withdrawal

• *Adult:* PO/REC 5-10 ml, not to exceed 60 ml; IM 5 ml q4-6h × 24 hr, then q6h on following days, not to exceed 30 ml

Sedation

• *Adult:* PO/REC 4-10 ml; IM 5 ml; IV 3-5 ml to be used in emergency only

• *Child:* PO/REC/IM 0.15 ml/kg

Tetanus

• *Adult:* IV 4-5 ml or 12 ml by gastric tube q4h diluted with water; IM 5-10 ml prn

Available forms include: Inj IM, IV; oral and rectal liquid

Side effects/adverse reactions:

HEMA: ***Thrombocytopenia, agranulocytosis, leukopenia, neutropenia, hemolytic anemia,*** increased pro-time

P

CNS: Stimulation, drowsiness, dizziness, confusion, ***convulsion,*** headache, flushing, hallucinations, coma
GI: Foul breath, irritation
GU: Nephrosis
INTEG: Rash, erythema, local pain, sloughing fat necrosis
CV: Pulmonary edema, ***pulmonary hemorrhage, circulatory collapse, respiratory depression***

Contraindications: Hypersensitivity, gastroenteritis with ulceration

Precautions: Asthma, hepatic disease, pulmonary disease, pregnancy (C)

Pharmacokinetics:
PO: Onset 10-15 min, peak 1-2 hr, duration 6-8 hr
REC: Onset slow, duration 4-6 hr; metabolized by liver, excreted by kidneys, lungs, crosses placenta, half-life 7.5 hr

Interactions/incompatibilities:
- Increased blood levels of paraldehyde: alcohol, CNS depressants, general anesthetics, disulfiram
- Increase crystallization in kidneys: sulfonamides

NURSING CONSIDERATIONS

Assess:
- VS q30min after parenteral route
- Blood studies: Hct, Hgb, RBCs, serum folate, vitamin D if on long-term therapy
- Hepatic studies: AST, ALT, bilirubin, creatinine, failure

Administer:
- IM injection in deep large muscle mass, use Z-track method to prevent tissue sloughing, maximum of 5 ml at any one site
- After conservative measures have been tried for insomnia
- Rectal after diluting in cottonseed or olive oil as retention enema or 200 ml NS for enema
- Keep patient's room well ventilated to remove exhaled drug
- Orally with juice or milk to cover taste/smell, decrease GI symptoms
- Using fresh supply; don't expose to air, don't use if brown or odor is vinegary or if container opened >24 h
- Using glass container only, reacts with plastic

Perform/provide:
- Ventilation of room

Evaluate:
- Therapeutic response: increased sedation, decreased seizures
- Mental status: mood, sensorium, affect, memory (long, short)
- Respiratory dysfunction; respiratory depression, character, rate, rhythm; hold drug if respirations are >10/min or if pupils are dilated

Teach patient/family:
- That physical dependency may result when used for extended periods of time
- To avoid driving, other activities that require alertness
- Not to discontinue medication quickly after long-term use, taper over several weeks

Lab test interferences:
False positive: Ketones (serum)(urine), interference, 17-OHCS

---

paramethadione

(par-a-meth-a-dye'one)
Paradione
Func. class.: Anticonvulsant
Chem. class.: Oxazolidinedione

Action: Increases seizure threshold in cortex and basal ganglia; de-

*Available in Canada only

creases synaptic stimulation to low-frequency impulses

Uses: Refractory absence (petit mal) seizures

Dosage and routes:

- *Adult:* PO 300 mg tid, may increase by 300 mg/wk, not to exceed 600 mg qid
- *Child >6 yr:* PO 0.9 g/day in divided doses tid or qid
- *Child 2-6 yr:* PO 0.6 g/day in divided doses tid or qid
- *Child <2 yr:* PO 0.3 g/day in divided doses tid or qid

Available forms include: Caps 150, 300 mg; sol 300 mg/ml

Side effects/adverse reactions:

HEMA: ***Thrombocytopenia, agranulocytosis, leukopenia, neutropenia, hemolytic anemia,*** increased pro-time

CNS: *Drowsiness,* dizziness, fatigue, paresthesia, irritability, headache

GU/GYN: Vaginal bleeding, albuminuria, nephrosis

GI: Nausea, vomiting, abdominal pain, weight loss, bleeding gums, abnormal liver function tests

INTEG: *Exfoliative dermatitis,* rash, alopecia, petechiae, erythema

EENT: Photophobia, diplopia, epistaxis, retinal hemorrhage

CV: Hypertension, hypotension

Contraindications: Hypersensitivity, blood dyscrasias, pregnancy (D)

Precautions: Hepatic disease, renal disease, retinal or optic nerve damage

Pharmacokinetics:

PO: Onset 15-30 min, peak 1-2 hr, duration 4-6 hr

REC: Onset slow, duration 4-6 hr, metabolized by the liver, excreted by the kidneys, crosses placenta, excreted in breast milk, half-life 1-3½ hr

NURSING CONSIDERATIONS

Assess:

- Blood studies: Hct, Hgb, RBCs, serum folate, vitamin D if on long-term therapy; discontinue drug if neutrophil count falls below 2500/mm^3
- Hepatic studies: ALT, AST, bilirubin, creatinine, failure
- Skin: If rash occurs withhold drug

Administer:

- After diluting oral solution with water
- Oral with juice or milk to cover taste-smell, to decrease GI symptoms

Perform/provide:

- Ventilation of room

Evaluate:

- Therapeutic response: decreased seizures
- Mental status: mood, sensorium, affect, memory (long, short)

Teach patient/family:

- To avoid driving, other activities that require alertness
- Not to discontinue medication quickly after long-term use; convulsions may result
- To obtain liver function tests and urinalysis monthly
- To notify physician if sore throat, fever, malaise, bruises, petechiae, or epistaxis occurs
- To wear dark glasses if photosensitivity occurs
- To take drug with food, milk to decrease GI symptoms

---

paramethasone acetate

(par-a-meth'a-sone)

Haldrone

Func. class.: Corticosteroid
Chem. class.: Glucocorticoid, long acting

Action: Decreases inflammation by

suppression of migration of polymorphonuclear leukocytes, fibroblasts, reversal to increase capillary permeability and lysosomal stabilization

Uses: Severe inflammation, collagen disorders, respiratory, dermatologic disorders, adrenal insufficiency

Dosage and routes:

- *Adult:* PO 0.5-6 mg tid-qid
- *Child:* PO 58-800 μg/kg/day in divided doses tid-qid

Available forms include: Tabs 2 mg

Side effects/adverse reactions:

INTEG: Acne, poor wound healing, ecchymosis, petechiae

CNS: Depression, flushing, sweating, headache, mood changes

CV: Hypertension, ***circulatory collapse, thrombophlebitis, embolism,*** tachycardia, edema

HEMA: ***Thrombocytopenia***

MS: Fractures, osteoporosis, weakness

GI: Diarrhea, nausea, abdominal distention, ***GI hemorrhage,*** increased appetite, ***pancreatitis***

EENT: Fungal infections, increased intraocular pressure, blurred vision

Contraindications: Psychosis, hypersensitivity, idiopathic thrombocytopenia, acute glomerulonephritis, amebiasis, fungal infections, nonasthmatic bronchial disease, child <2 yr, AIDS, TB

Precautions: Pregnancy (C), diabetes mellitus, glaucoma, osteoporosis, seizure disorders, ulcerative colitis, CHF, myasthenia gravis, renal disease, esophagitis, peptic ulcer

Pharmacokinetics:

PO: Peak 1-2 hr, duration 2 days

IM: Peak 3-45 hr

Interactions/incompatibilities:

- Decreased action of paramethasone: cholestyramine, colestipol, barbiturates, rifampin, ephedrine, phenytoin, theophylline
- Decreased effects of: anticoagulants, anticonvulsants, antidiabetics, ambenonium, neostigmine, isoniazid, toxoids, vaccines
- Increased side effects: alcohol, salicylates, indomethacin, amphotericin B, digitalis preparations
- Increased action of paramethasone: salicylates, estrogens, indomethacin

NURSING CONSIDERATIONS

Assess:

- Potassium, blood sugar, urine glucose while on long-term therapy; hypokalemia and hyperglycemia
- Weight daily, notify physician of weekly gain >5 lb
- B/P q4h, pulse, notify physician if chest pain occurs
- I&O ratio, be alert for decreasing urinary output and increasing edema
- Plasma cortisol levels during long-term therapy (normal level: 138-635 nmol/L SI units when drawn at 8 AM)

Administer:

- Titrated dose, use lowest effective dose
- In one dose in AM to prevent adrenal suppression, avoid SC administration, damage may be done to tissue
- With food or milk to decrease GI symptoms

Perform/provide:

- Assistance with ambulation in patient with bone tissue disease to prevent fractures

Evaluate:

- Therapeutic response: ease of respirations, decreased inflammation
- Infection: increased temperature,

WBC, even after withdrawal of medication; drug masks symptoms of infection
• Potassium depletion: paresthesias, fatigue, nausea, vomiting, depression, polyuria, dysrhythmias, weakness
• Edema, hypertension, cardiac symptoms
• Mental status: affect, mood, behavioral changes, aggression

Teach patient/family:
• That ID as steroid user should be carried
• To notify physician if therapeutic response decreases; dosage adjustment may be needed
• Not to discontinue this medication abruptly or adrenal crisis can result
• To avoid OTC products: salicylates, alcohol in cough products, cold preparations unless directed by physician
• About cushingoid symptoms
• Symptoms of adrenal insufficiency: nausea, anorexia, fatigue, dizziness, dyspnea, weakness, joint pain

Lab test interferences:
Increase: Cholesterol, sodium, blood glucose, uric acid, calcium, urine glucose
Decrease: Calcium, potassium, T_4, T_3, thyroid ^{131}I uptake test, urine 17-OHCS, 17-KS, PBI
False negative: Skin allergy tests

pargyline HCl

(par'gi-leen)
Eutonyl
Func. class.: Antihypertensive
Chem. class.: MAOI

Action: Inhibits monoamine oxidase, decreasing B/P

Uses: Moderate to severe hypertension

Dosage and routes:
• *Adult:* PO 25 mg daily, increase by 10 mg q7d, not to exceed 200 mg; maintenance dosage: 25-50 mg daily

Available forms include: Tabs 10, 25, 50 mg

Side effects/adverse reactions:
CV: Orthostatic hypotension, tachycardia, chest pain, bradycardia, fluid retention, ***CHF***
CNS: Drowsiness, dizziness, sedation, headache, depression, insomnia, weakness, fatigue, confusion, blurred vision, EPS
GI: Nausea, vomiting, anorexia, constipation, weight gain
EENT: Dry mouth
GU: Impotence
MS: Arthralgia
MISC: Sweating, increased appetite, hypoglycemia

Contraindications: Hypersensitivity, malignant hypertension, paranoid schizophrenia, severe pulmonary failure, pheochromocytoma, hyperthyroidism, advanced renal failure, children $<$12 yr

Precautions: Pregnancy (C), lactation, impaired renal function, liver disease, CAD, parkinsonism, diabetes mellitus

Pharmacokinetics:
Excreted in urine, therapeutic response may take 4 days-3 weeks

Interactions/incompatibilities:
• Hypertensive crisis: amphetamine, cyclopent-amide, ephedrine, pseudoephedrine, metaraminol, methylphenidate, phenylpropanolamine, levodopa, methyldopa, reserpine, tryptamine, tyramine foods
• Hypotension and increased sedation: barbiturates, alcohol, nar-

cotics, CNS depressants, antihypertensive agents

• May potentiate effects: doxapram, narcotics, phenothiazines, other psychotropic agents, tricyclic antidepressants

NURSING CONSIDERATIONS

Assess:

• Electrolytes: K, Na, Cl, CO_2

• Renal function studies: catecholamines, BUN, creatinine

• Hepatic function studies: AST, ALT, alk phosphatase

• Weight daily, I&O

• B/P lying, standing before starting treatment

Administer:

• Gum, frequent rinsing of mouth or hard candy for dry mouth

Evaluate:

• Therapeutic response: decreased B/P

• Nausea, vomiting, diarrhea

• Edema in feet, legs daily

• Skin turgor, dryness of mucous membranes for hydration status

Teach patient/family:

• To report dizziness, palpitations, fainting

• To change position slowly or fainting may occur

• To take drug exactly as prescribed

• Not to eat tyramine-rich foods: beer, wine, pickled products, yeast products, aged cheeses, avocados, chocolate

• May cause drowsiness

• To avoid all OTC products unless directed by physician

Treatment of overdose: Induce emesis or gastric lavage, support respiration, severe hypertension—administer α-blocker, treat CNS stimulation with IV diazepam, maintain fluid or electrolyte balance

paromomycin sulfate

(par-oh-moe-mye'sin)

Humatin

Func. class.: Amebicide

Chem. class.: Aminoglycoside antibiotic

Action: Direct action in intestinal lumen

Uses: Intestinal amebiasis, tapeworms

Dosage and routes:

Intestinal amebiasis

• *Adult and child:* PO 25-35 mg/kg/day in 3 divided doses × 5-10 days pc

Tapeworms

• *Adult:* PO 1 g q15 min × 4 doses

• *Child:* PO 11 mg/kg q15min × 4 doses

Available forms include: Caps 250 mg

Side effects/adverse reactions:

HEMA: ***Eosinophilia***

INTEG: Rash

CNS: Headache, dizziness

EENT: Ototoxicity

GI: Nausea, vomiting, diarrhea, epigastric distress, anorexia, steatorrhea, pruritus ani, hypocholesterolemia

GU: ***Nephrotoxicity, hematuria***

Contraindications: Hypersensitivity, renal disease, GI obstruction

Precautions: GI ulcerations, pregnancy (C)

Pharmacokinetics:

PO: Excreted in feces, urine, slowly

NURSING CONSIDERATIONS

Assess:

• Stools during entire treatment; should be clear at end of therapy, stools should be free of parasite for 1 yr before patient is considered cured

• I&O, stools for number, frequency, character

Administer:

• Cleansing enema if ordered before beginning treatment

• PO after meals to avoid GI symptoms

Perform/provide:

• Storage in tight container

Evaluate:

• Therapeutic response: decreased diarrhea, stools clear on culture

• Allergic reaction: rash, itching; drug should be discontinued if these occur

• Diarrhea for 2-3 days

Teach patient/family:

• Proper hygiene after BM: handwashing technique

• Avoid contact of drug with eyes, mouth, nose, other mucous membranes

• Need for compliance with dosage schedule, duration of treatment

Lab test interferences:

Decrease: Serum cholesterol

---

pemoline

(pem'oh-leen)

Cylert

Func. class.: Cerebral stimulant

Chem. class.: Oxazolidinone derivative

Controlled Substance Schedule IV

Action: Exact mechanism unknown; may act through dopaminergic mechanisms

Uses: Attention deficit disorder with hyperactivity

Dosage and routes:

• *Child >6 yr:* 37.5 mg in AM, increasing by 18.75 mg/wk, not to exceed 112.5 mg/day

Available forms include: Tabs 18.75, 37.5, 75 mg; chewable tabs 37.5 mg

Side effects/adverse reactions:

MISC: Rashes, growth suppression in children

CNS: Hyperactivity, insomnia, restlessness, dizziness, depression, headache, stimulation, irritability, aggressiveness, hallucination seizures, Gilles de la Tourette's disorder, drowsiness, dyskinetic movements

GI: Nausea, anorexia, diarrhea, abdominal pain, increased liver enzymes, hepatitis, jaundice

Contraindications: Hypersensitivity, hepatic insufficiency

Precautions: Renal disease, pregnancy (B), lactation, drug abuse, child <6

Pharmacokinetics:

PO: Peak 2-4 hr, duration 8 hr, metabolized (50%) by liver, excreted (40%) by kidneys, half-life 12 hr

NURSING CONSIDERATIONS

Assess:

• Hepatic function studies: ALT, AST, bilirubin, creatinine

• Child for height, growth rate, since growth retardation occurs

Administer:

• At least 6 hr before hs

• Gum, hard candy, frequent sips of water for dry mouth

Evaluate:

• Therapeutic response: decreased hyperactivity

• Mental status: mood, sensorium, affect, stimulation, insomnia, aggressiveness

Teach patient/family:

• To decrease caffeine consumption (coffee, tea, cola, chocolate), which may increase irritability, stimulation

• To avoid OTC preparations unless approved by physician

- To taper off drug over several weeks
- To avoid alcohol ingestion
- To avoid hazardous activities until patient is stabilized on medication
- That therapeutic effect may take 2-4 wk

penicillin G benzathine

(pen-i-sill'in)

Bicillin L-A, Megacillin,* Permapen

Func. class.: Broad-spectrum antibiotic

Chem. class.: Natural penicillin

Action: Interferes with cell wall replication of susceptible organisms; osmotically unstable cell wall swells, bursts from osmotic pressure

Uses: Respiratory infections, scarlet fever, erysipelas, otitis media, pneumonia, skin and soft tissue infections, gonorrhea; effective for gram-positive cocci *(Staphylococcus, S. pyogenes, S. viridans, S. faecalis, S. bovis, S. pneumoniae)*, gram-negative cocci *(N. gonorrhoeae)*, gram-positive bacilli *(B. anthracis, C. perfringens, C. tetani, C. diphtheriae, L. monocytogenes)*, gram-negative bacilli *(E. coli, P. mirabilis, Salmonella, Shigella, Enterobacter, S. moniliformis)*, spirochetes *(T. pallidum)*, *Actinomyces*

Dosage and routes:

Early syphilis

- *Adult:* IM 2.4 million U in single dose

Congenital syphilis

- *Child <2 yr:* IM 50,000 U/kg in single dose

Prophylaxis of rheumatic fever, glomerulonephritis

- *Adult and child >60 lb:* IM 1.2 million U in single dose qmo or 600,000 U q2wk
- *Child <60 lb:* IM 600,000 U in single dose

Upper respiratory infections (group A streptococcal)

- *Adult:* IM 1.2 million U in single dose, PO 400,000-600,000 U q4-6h
- *Child >27 kg:* IM 900,000 U in single dose
- *Child <27 kg:* IM 50,000 U/kg in single dose

Available forms include: Inj IM 300,000, 600,000 U/ml; tabs 200,000 U

Side effects/adverse reactions:

HEMA: Anemia, increased bleeding time, ***bone marrow depression, granulocytopenia***

GI: Nausea, vomiting, diarrhea, increased AST, ALT, abdominal pain, glossitis, colitis

GU: ***Oliguria, proteinuria, hematuria,*** *vaginitis, moniliasis,* ***glomerulonephritis***

CNS: Lethargy, hallucinations, anxiety, depression, twitching, ***coma, convulsions***

META: Hyperkalemia, hypokalemia, alkalosis, hypernatremia

Contraindications: Hypersensitivity to penicillins; neonates

Precautions: Hypersensitivity to cephalosporins, pregnancy (B)

Pharmacokinetics:

IM: Very slow absorption, duration 21-28 days, half-life 30-60 min, excreted in urine, feces, breast milk, crosses placenta

Interactions/incompatibilities:

- Decreased antimicrobial effect of penicillin: tetracyclines, erythromycins
- Increased penicillin concentrations: aspirin, probenecid

NURSING CONSIDERATIONS

Assess:

- I&O ratio; report hematuria, oli-

* Available in Canada only

guria since penicillin in high doses is nephrotoxic
• Any patient with compromised renal system since drug is excreted slowly in poor renal system function; toxicity may occur rapidly
• Liver studies: AST, ALT
• Blood studies: WBC, RBC, H&H, bleeding time
• Renal studies: urinalysis, protein, blood
• C&S before drug therapy; drug may be taken as soon as culture is taken

Administer:
• Orally on an empty stomach for best absorption
• Drug after C&S has been completed
• After shaking well, deep IM inj in large muscle masses; avoid intravascular inj, aspirate

Perform/provide:
• Adrenalin, suction, tracheostomy set, endotracheal intubation equipment
• Adequate fluid intake (2000 ml) during diarrhea episodes
• Scratch test to assess allergy, after securing order from physician; usually done when penicillin is only drug of choice
• Storage in tight container; refrigerate injection

Evaluate:
• Therapeutic response: absence of fever, purulent drainage, redness, inflammation
• Bowel pattern before and during treatment
• Skin eruptions after administration of penicillin to 1 wk after discontinuing drug
• Respiratory status: rate, character, wheezing, tightness in chest
• Allergies before initiation of treatment, reaction of each medication; highlight allergies on chart, Kardex

Teach patient/family:
• To take oral penicillin on empty stomach with full glass of water
• That culture may be taken after completed course of medication
• To report sore throat, fever, fatigue; (could indicate superimposed infection)
• To wear or carry Medic Alert ID if allergic to penicillins
• To notify nurse of diarrhea

Lab test interferences:
False positive: Urine glucose, urine protein

Treatment of hypersensitivity: Withdraw drug, maintain airway, administer epinephrine, aminophylline, O_2, IV corticosteroids for anaphylaxis

penicillin G potassium

Acrocillin, Burcillin-G, Deltapen, Megacillin,* Novopen G,* Pentids, Pfizerpen

Func. class.: Broad-spectrum antibiotic-penicillin
Chem. class.: Natural penicillin

P

Action: Interferes with cell wall replication of susceptible organisms; osmotically unstable cell wall swells, bursts from osmotic pressure

Uses: Empyema, gangrene, anthrax, gonorrhea, mastoiditis, meningitis, osteomyelitis, pneumonia, tetanus, urinary tract infections, prophylactically in rheumatic fever; effective for gram-positive cocci *(S. aureus, S. pyogenes, S. viridans, S. faecalis, S. bovis, S. pneumoniae)*, gram-negative cocci *(N. gonorrhoeae, N. meningitidis)*, gram-positive bacilli *(B. anthracis, C. perfringens, C. tetani, C. diph-*

theriae, L. monocytogenes), gram-negative bacilli *(Bacteroides, F. nucleatum, P. multocida, S. minor, S. moniliformis),* spirochetes *(T. pallidum, T. pertenue, B. recurrentis, L. icterohaemorrhagiae), Actinomyces*

Dosage and routes:

Pneumococcal/streptococcal infections (mild-moderate)

• *Adult:* PO 400,000-500,000 U q6-8h × 10 days (streptococcal infections) or afebrile × 2 days (pneumococcal infections)

• *Child <12 yr:* PO 25,000-90,000 U/kg/day in 3-6 divided doses

Prevention of recurrence of rheumatic fever

• *Adult:* PO 200,000-250,000 U bid continuously

• *Child <12 yr:* PO 25,000-90,000 U/kg/day in 3-6 divided doses

Vincent's gingivitis/pharyngitis

• *Adult:* PO 400,000-500,000 U q6-8h

Available forms include: Tabs 200,000, 250,000, 400,000, 500,000, 800,000 U; powder for oral sol 200,000, 400,000 U/5 ml

Side effects/adverse reactions:

HEMA: Anemia, increased bleeding time, ***bone marrow depression, granulocytopenia***

GI: Nausea, vomiting, diarrhea, increased AST, ALT, abdominal pain, glossitis, colitis

GU: ***Oliguria, proteinuria, hematuria,*** *vaginitis, moniliasis,* ***glomerulonephritis***

CNS: Lethargy, hallucinations, anxiety, depression, twitching, ***coma, convulsions***

META: Hyperkalemia, hypokalemia, alkalosis, hypernatremia

Contraindications: Hypersensitivity to penicillins; neonates

Precautions: Hypersensitivity to cephalosporins, pregnancy (B)

Pharmacokinetics:

PO: Duration 6 hr, peak 1 hr; excreted in urine unchanged, breast milk, crosses placenta

Interactions/incompatibilities:

• Decreased antimicrobial effectiveness of penicillin: tetracyclines, erythromycins

• Decreased absorption: cholestyramine, colestipol

• Increased penicillin concentrations: aspirin, probenecid

NURSING CONSIDERATIONS

Assess:

• I&O ratio; report hematuria, oliguria since penicillin in high doses is nephrotoxic

• Any patient with compromised renal system since drug is excreted slowly in poor renal system function; toxicity may occur rapidly

• Liver studies: AST, ALT

• Blood studies: WBC, RBC, H&H, bleeding time

• Renal studies: urinalysis, protein, blood

• C&S before drug therapy; drug may be taken as soon as culture is taken

Administer:

• Orally on an empty stomach for best absorption

• Drug after C&S has been completed

Perform/provide:

• Adrenalin, suction, tracheostomy set, endotracheal intubation equipment

• Adequate fluid intake (2000 ml) during diarrhea episodes

• Scratch test to assess allergy, after securing order from physician; usually done when penicillin is only drug of choice

• Storage in dry, tight container; oral susp refrigerated 2 wk, 1 wk at room temperature

* Available in Canada only

Evaluate:
- Therapeutic response: absence of fever, draining wounds
- Bowel pattern before and during treatment
- Skin eruptions after administration of penicillin to 1 wk after discontinuing drug
- Respiratory status: rate, character, wheezing, tightness in chest
- Allergies before initiation of treatment, reaction of each medication; highlight allergies on chart, Kardex

Teach patient/family:
- Aspects of drug therapy, including need to complete course of medication to ensure organism death (10-14 days); culture may be taken after completed course
- To report sore throat, fever, fatigue; (could indicate superimposed infection)
- To wear or carry Medic Alert ID if allergic to penicillins
- To notify nurse of diarrhea

Lab test interferences:
Decrease: Uric acid
False positive: Urine glucose, urine protein

Treatment of overdose: Withdraw drug, maintain airway, administer epinephrine, aminophylline, O_2, IV corticosteroids for anaphylaxis

penicillin G procaine

Crysticillin A.S., Duracillin A.S., Wycillin, Pfizerpen-AS

Func. class.: Broad-spectrum long-acting antibiotic

Chem. class.: Natural penicillin

Action: Interferes with cell wall replication of susceptible organisms; osmotically unstable cell wall swells, bursts from osmotic pressure

Uses: Empyema, gangrene, anthrax, gonorrhea, mastoiditis, meningitis, osteomyelitis, pneumonia, tetanus, urinary tract infections, prophylactically in rheumatic fever; effective for gram-positive cocci *(S. aureus, S. pyogenes, S. viridans, S. faecalis, S. bovis, S. pneumoniae),* gram-negative cocci *(N. gonorrhoeae, N. meningitidis),* gram-positive bacilli *(B. anthracis, C. perfringens, C. tetani, C. diphtheriae, L. monocytogenes),* gram-negative bacilli *(Bacteroides, F. nucleatum, P. multocida, S. minor, S. moniliformis),* spirochetes *(T. pallidum, T. pertenue, B. recurrentis, L. icterohaemorrhagiae), Actinomyces*

Dosage and routes:

Moderate to severe infections
- *Adult and child:* IM 600,000-1.2 million U in one or two doses/day for 10 days to 2 wk
- *Newborn:* 50,000 U/kg IM once daily

Gonorrhea
- *Adult and child >12 yr:* IM 4.8 million units in two injections given 30 min after probenecid 1 g

Pneumonia (pneumococcal)
- *Adult and child >12 yr:* IM 300,000-600,000 U q6-12h

Available forms include: Inj IM 300,000, 500,000, 600,000 U/ml, 600,000 U/1.2 ml, 1,200,000 U/dose, 2,400,000 U/dose

Side effects/adverse reactions:
HEMA: Anemia, increased bleeding time, ***bone marrow depression, granulocytopenia***
GI: Nausea, vomiting, diarrhea, increased AST, ALT, abdominal pain, glossitis, colitis
GU: ***Oliguria, proteinuria, hema-***

P

turia, *vaginitis, moniliasis,* ***glomerulonephritis***

CNS: Lethargy, hallucinations, anxiety, depression, twitching, ***coma, convulsions***

META: Hyperkalemia, hypokalemia, alkalosis, hypernatremia

Contraindications: Hypersensitivity to penicillins, procaine; neonates

Precautions: Hypersensitivity to cephalosporins, pregnancy (B)

Pharmacokinetics:

IM: Peak 1-4 hr, duration 15 hr, excreted in urine

Interactions/incompatibilities:

- Decreased antimicrobial effect of penicillin: tetracyclines, erythromycins
- Increased penicillin concentrations: aspirin, probenecid

NURSING CONSIDERATIONS

Assess:

- I&O ratio; report hematuria, oliguria since penicillin in high doses is nephrotoxic
- Any patient with compromised renal system since drug is excreted slowly in poor renal system function; toxicity may occur rapidly
- Liver studies: AST, ALT
- Blood studies: WBC, RBC, H&H, bleeding time
- Renal studies: urinalysis, protein, blood
- C&S before drug therapy; drug may be taken as soon as culture is taken

Administer:

- Drug after C&S has been completed
- Deep IM, avoid intravascular inj, aspirate

Perform/provide:

- Adrenalin, suction, tracheostomy set, endotracheal intubation equipment
- Adequate fluid intake (2000 ml) during diarrhea episodes
- Scratch test to assess allergy, after securing order from physician; usually done when penicillin is only drug of choice
- Storage in refrigerator

Evaluate:

- Therapeutic response: absence of fever, purulent drainage, redness, inflammation
- Bowel pattern before and during treatment
- Skin eruptions after administration of penicillin to 1 wk after discontinuing drug
- Respiratory status: rate, character, wheezing, tightness in chest
- Allergies before initiation of treatment, reaction of each medication; highlight allergies on chart, Kardex

Teach patient/family:

- That culture may be taken after completed course of medication
- To report sore throat, fever, fatigue (could indicate superimposed infection)
- To wear or carry Medic Alert ID if allergic to penicillins
- To notify nurse of diarrhea

Lab test interferences:

False positive: Urine glucose, urine protein

Treatment of hypersensitivity: Withdraw drug, maintain airway, administer epinephrine, aminophylline, O_2, IV corticosteroids for anaphylaxis

---

penicillin G sodium

Crystapen,* Pfizerpen

Func. class.: Broad-spectrum antibiotic

Chem. class.: Natural penicillin

Action: Acts by interfering with

* Available in Canada only

cell wall replication of susceptible organisms; osmotically unstable cell wall swells and bursts from osmotic pressure

Uses: Empyema, gangrene, anthrax, gonorrhea, mastoiditis, meningitis, osteomyelitis, pneumonia, tetanus, urinary tract infections, prophylactically in rheumatic fever; effective for gram-positive cocci *(S. aureus, S. pyogenes, S. viridans, S. faecalis, S. bovis, S. pneumoniae),* gram-negative cocci *(N. gonorrhoeae, N. meningitidis),* gram-positive bacilli *(B. anthracis, C. perfringens, C. tetani, C. diphtheriae, L. monocytogenes),* gram-negative bacilli *(Bacteroides, E. nucleatum, P. multocida, S. minor, S. moniliformis),* spirochetes *(T. pallidum, T. pertenue, B. recurrentis, L. icterohaemorrhagiae), Actinomyces*

Dosage and routes:

Moderate to severe infections

- *Adult:* IM/IV 12-30 million U/day in divided doses q4h
- *Child:* IM/IV 25,000-300,000 U/day in divided doses q4-12h

Dental surgery prophylaxis for endocarditis

- *Adult:* IM/IV 2 million units ½-1 hr before procedure, then 1 million 6 hr after procedure

Available forms include: Inj IM, IV 1 million, 5 million, 20 million units

Side effects/adverse reactions:

HEMA: Anemia, increased bleeding time, ***bone marrow depression, granulocytopenia***

GI: Nausea, vomiting, diarrhea, increased AST, ALT, abdominal pain, glossitis, colitis

GU: ***Oliguria, proteinuria, hematuria,*** vaginitis, moniliasis, ***glomerulonephritis***

CNS: Lethargy, hallucinations, anxiety, depression, twitching, ***convulsions***

META: Hyperkalemia, hypokalemia, alkalosis, hypernatremia

Contraindications: Hypersensitivity to penicillins; neonates

Precautions: CHF caused by sodium content, pregnancy (B)

Pharmacokinetics:

IM: Peak 1-3 hr, duration 6 hr; excreted in urine

Interactions/incompatibilities:

- Decreased antimicrobial effect of penicillin: tetracyclines, erythromycins
- Increased penicillin concentrations: aspirin, probenecid

NURSING CONSIDERATIONS

Assess:

- I&O ratio; report hematuria, oliguria since penicillin in high doses is nephrotoxic
- Any patient with a compromised renal system since drug is excreted slowly in poor renal system function; toxicity may occur rapidly
- Liver studies: AST, ALT
- Blood studies: WBC, RBC, H&H, bleeding time
- Renal studies: urinalysis, protein, blood
- C&S before drug therapy; drug may be taken as soon as culture is taken

Administer:

- IV after diluting with sterile H_2O, shake, follow manufacturers' instructions for dilution; give by continuous inf, usually over 12 hr
- Drug after C&S has been completed

Perform/provide:

- Adrenalin, suction, tracheostomy set, endotracheal intubation equipment
- Adequate fluid intake (2000 ml) during diarrhea episodes
- Scratch test to assess allergy, af-

P

ter securing order from physician; usually done when penicillin is only drug of choice

• Storage of sterile sol in refrigerator for 1 wk, IV sol at room temperature for 24 hr

Evaluate:

• Therapeutic response: absence of fever, purulent drainage, redness, inflammation

• Bowel pattern before, during treatment

• Skin eruptions after administration of penicillin to 1 wk after discontinuing drug

• Respiratory status: rate, character, wheezing, tightness in chest

• Allergies before initiation of treatment, reaction of each medication; highlight allergies on chart, Kardex

Teach patient family:

• That culture may be taken after completed course of medication

• To report sore throat, fever, fatigue (could indicate superimposed infection)

• To wear or carry Medic Alert ID if allergic to penicillins

• To notify nurse of diarrhea

Lab test interferences:

False positive: Urine glucose, urine protein

Treatment of overdose: Withdraw drug, maintain airway, administer epinephrine, aminophylline, O_2, IV corticosteroids for anaphylaxis

penicillin V potassium

Pen-Vee K*, Deltapen-VK, V-Cillin K, Veetids, PVFK,* Apo-Pen-VK,* Novopen-VK,* Ledercillin-VK, Uticillin-VK, Betapen-VK, Penapar-VK, Robicillin-VK

Func. class.: Broad-spectrum antibiotic

Chem. class.: Natural penicillin

Action: Interferes with cell wall replication of susceptible organisms; osmotically unstable cell wall swells, bursts from osmotic pressure.

Uses: Effective for gram-positive cocci *(S. aureus, S. pyogenes, S. viridans, S. faecalis, S. bovis, S. pneumoniae)*, gram-negative cocci *(N. gonorrhoeae, N. meningitidis)*, gram-positive bacilli *(B. anthracis, C. perfringens, C. tetani, C. diphtheriae, L. monocytogenes)*, gram-negative bacilli *(S. moniliformis)*, spirochetes *(T. pallidum)*, *Actinomyces*

Dosage and routes:

Pneumococcal/staphylococcal infections

• *Adult:* PO 250-500 mg g6h

• *Child <12 yr:* PO 25,000-90,000 U/kg/day in 3-6 divided doses (125 mg = 200,000 U)

Streptococcal infections

• *Adult:* PO 125-250 mg q6-8h × 10 days

Prevention of recurrence of rheumatic fever/chorea

• *Adult:* PO 125-250 mg bid continuously

Vincent's infection of oropharynx

• *Adult:* PO 500 mg q6h

Available forms include: Tabs 125, 250, 500 mg; film-coated tabs 250, 500 mg; powder for oral susp 125, 250 mg/5 ml

* Available in Canada only

Side effects/adverse reactions:
HEMA: Anemia, increased bleeding time, ***bone marrow depression, granulocytopenia***
GI: Nausea, vomiting, diarrhea, increased AST, ALT, abdominal pain, glossitis, colitis
GU: ***Oliguria, proteinuria, hematuria,*** *vaginitis, moniliasis,* ***glomerulonephritis***
CNS: Lethargy, hallucinations, anxiety, ***depression,*** twitching, ***coma, convulsions***
META: Hyperkalemia, hypokalemia, alkalosis
Contraindications: Hypersensitivity to penicillins; neonates
Precautions: Hypersensitivity to cephalosporins, pregnancy (B)
Pharmacokinetics:
PO: Peak 30-60 min, duration 6-8 hr, half-life 30 min, excreted in urine, breast milk
Interactions/incompatibilities:
- Decreased antimicrobial effectiveness of penicillin: tetracyclines, erythromycins
- Increased penicillin concentrations: aspirin, probenecid

NURSING CONSIDERATIONS

Assess:
- I&O ratio; report hematuria, oliguria since penicillin in high doses is nephrotoxic
- Any patient with compromised renal system since drug is excreted slowly in poor renal system function; toxicity may occur rapidly
- Liver studies: AST, ALT
- Blood studies: WBC, RBC, H&H, bleeding time
- Renal studies: urinalysis, protein, blood
- C&S before drug therapy; drug may be taken as soon as culture is taken

Administer:
- Orally on an empty stomach for best absorption
- Drug after C&S has been completed

Perform/provide:
- Adrenalin, suction, tracheostomy set, endotracheal intubation equipment
- Adequate fluid intake (2000 ml) during diarrhea episodes
- Scratch test to assess allergy, after securing order from physician; usually done when penicillin is only drug of choice
- Storage in tight container; after reconstituting, refrigerate for up to 2 wk

Evaluate:
- Therapeutic response: absence of fever, draining wounds
- Bowel pattern before and during treatment
- Skin eruptions after administration of penicillin to 1 wk after discontinuing drug
- Respiratory status: rate, character, wheezing, tightness in chest
- Allergies before initiation of treatment, reaction of each medication; highlight allergies on chart, Kardex

Teach patient/family:
- Aspects of drug therapy, including need to complete entire course of medication to ensure organism death (10-14 days); culture may be taken after completed course
- To report sore throat, fever, fatigue; (could indicate superimposed infection)
- To wear or carry Medic Alert ID if allergic to penicillins
- To notify nurse of diarrhea

Lab test interferences:
False positive: Urine glucose, urine protein
Treatment of overdose: Withdraw drug, maintain airway, administer epinephrine, aminophylline, O_2, IV corticosteroids for anaphylaxis

pentaerythritol tetranitrate

(pen-ta-er-ith'ri-tole)

Desatrate, Duotrate, Nitrin, PETN, Pentraspan, Naptrate, Pentylan, Peritrate, Vasolate

Func. class.: Vasodilatory, coronary

Chem. class.: Nitrate

Action: Decreases preload, afterload; which is responsible for decreasing left ventricular end-diastolic pressure, systemic vascular resistance

Uses: Chronic stable angina pectoris, prophylaxis of angina pain

Dosage and routes:

- *Adult:* PO 10-20 mg tid or qid, max 40 mg qid; sus rel 30-80 mg q12h

Available forms include: Caps ext rel 30, 45, 80 mg; tabs 10, 20, 40, 80 mg; tabs ext rel 80 mg

Side effects/adverse reactions:

CV: Postural hypotension, palpitations, tachycardia, ***collapse,*** syncope

GI: Nausea, vomiting, abdominal pain

INTEG: Pallor, sweating, rash

CNS: Headache, flushing, dizziness, restlessness, weakness, faintness

MISC: Muscle twitching, ***hemolytic anemia, methemoglobinemia***

Contraindications: Hypersensitivity to this drug or nitrites, severe anemia, increased intracranial pressure, cerebral hemorrhage, acute MI

Precautions: Postural hypotension, pregnancy (C), lactation, children

Pharmacokinetics:

PO: Onset 30 min, duration 4-5 hr

SUS REL: Onset 30 min, duration 12 hr

Metabolized by liver, excreted in urine, half-life 10 min

Interactions/incompatibilities:

- Increased effects: β-blockers, diuretics, antihypertensives, alcohol

NURSING CONSIDERATIONS

Assess:

- B/P, pulse, respirations during beginning therapy
- Pain: duration, time started, activity being performed, character

Administer:

- With 8 oz of water on empty stomach

Evaluate:

- Therapeutic response: decrease, prevention of anginal pain
- Tolerance if taken over long period of time
- Headache, light-headedness, decreased B/P; may indicate a need for decreased dosage

Teach patient/family:

- To keep tabs in original container; do not crush or chew sus rel preparations
- To avoid alcohol
- That drug may cause headache, tolerance usually develops
- That drug may be taken before stressful activity: exercise, sexual activity
- To avoid hazardous activities if dizziness occurs
- To comply with complete medical regimen
- To make position changes slowly to prevent fainting

pentamidine isethionate

(pen-tam'i-deen)

Pentam 300, Pentacarinat,* Nebu Pent

Func. class.: Antiprotozoal

Chem. class.: Aromatic diamide derivative

Action: Interferes with DNA/RNA synthesis in protozoa

Uses: *Pneumocystis carinii* infections

Dosage and routes:

- *Adult and child:* IV/IM 4 mg/kg/day × 2 wk: Neb 600 mg/6ml NS via specific nebulizer

Available forms include: Inj IV, IM 300 mg/vial

Side effects/adverse reactions:

CV: Hypotension, ventricular tachycardia, ECG abnormalities

HEMA: Anemia, ***leukopenia, thrombocytopenia***

INTEG: Sterile abscess, pain at injection site, pruritus, urticaria, rash

GU: ***Acute renal failure***

GI: *Nausea, vomiting, anorexia,* increased AST, ALT, ***acute pancreatitis***

CNS: Disorientation, hallucinations, dizziness

META: Hyperkalemia, hypocalcemia, hypoglycemia

Precautions: Blood dyscrasias, hepatic disease, renal disease, diabetes mellitus, cardiac disease, hypocalcemia, pregnancy (C)

Pharmacokinetics: Excreted unchanged in urine (66%)

Interactions/incompatibilities

- Nephrotoxicity: aminoglycosides, amphotercin B, colistin, cisplatin, methoxyflurane, polymyxin B, vancomycin

NURSING CONSIDERATIONS

Assess:

- Blood studies, blood glucose, CBC, platelets
- I&O ratio; report hematuria, oliguria
- ECG for cardiac dysrhythmias, check B/P
- Any patient with compromised renal system; drug is excreted slowly in poor renal system function; toxicity may occur rapidly
- Liver studies: AST, ALT
- Renal studies: urinalysis, BUN, creatinine; nephrotoxicity may occur
- Signs of infection, anemia

Administer:

- IV by intermittent inf over 60 min
- Inhalation through nebulizer over 30-45 min until chamber is empty
- IM diluted in 3 ml sterile H_2O; give deep IM; painful by this route

Perform/provide:

- Storage in refrigerator protected from light

Evaluate:

- Therapeutic response: decreased temperature, ability to breathe
- Bowel pattern before, during treatment
- Sterile abscess, pain at injection site
- Respiratory status: rate, character, wheezing, dyspnea
- Dizziness, confusion, hallucination
- Allergies before treatment, reaction of each medication; place allergies on chart, Kardex in bright red letters; notify all people giving drugs

Teach patient/family:

- To report sore throat, fever, fatigue; could indicate superimposed infection

P

pentazocine HCl/ pentazocine lactate

(pen-taz'oh-seen)

Talwin

Func. class.: Narcotic analgesic, antagonist

Chem. class.: Synthetic benzomorphan

Controlled Substance Schedule IV

Action: Inhibits ascending pain pathways in CNS, increases pain threshold, alters pain perception

Uses: Moderate to severe pain

Dosage and routes:

- *Adult:* PO 50-100 mg q3-4h prn, not to exceed 600 mg/day; IV/IM/SC 30 mg q3-4h prn, not to exceed 360 mg/day

Available forms include: SC, IM, IV 30 mg/ml; tabs 50 mg

Side effects/adverse reactions:

CNS: Drowsiness, dizziness, confusion, headache, sedation, euphoria, hallucinations

GI: Nausea, vomiting, anorexia, constipation, cramps

GU: Increased urinary output, dysuria

INTEG: Rash, urticaria, bruising, flushing, diaphoresis, pruritus

EENT: Tinnitus, blurred vision, miosis, diplopia

CV: Palpitations, bradycardia, change in B/P, tachycardia, increased B/P (high doses)

RESP: ***Respiratory depression***

Contraindications: Hypersensitivity, addiction (narcotic)

Precautions: Addictive personality, pregnancy (B), lactation, increased intracranial pressure, MI (acute), severe heart disease, respiratory depression, hepatic disease, renal disease, child <18 yr

Pharmacokinetics:

SC/IM: Onset 15-30 min, peak 1-2 hr, duration 2-4 hr

IV: Onset 2-3 min, duration 4-6 hr; metabolized by liver, excreted by kidneys, crosses placenta, half-life 2-3 hr, extensive first-pass metabolism with less than 20% entering circulation

Interactions/incompatibilities:

- Increased effects: CNS depressants; alcohol, sedative/hypnotics, antipsychotics, skeletal muscle relaxants
- Decreased effects: narcotics
- Do not mix in solutions or syringe with barbiturates

NURSING CONSIDERATIONS

Assess:

- I&O ratio; check for decreasing output; may indicate urinary retention
- For withdrawal symptoms in narcotic-dependent patients
- Pulmonary embolism, abscesses, ulcerations, vascular occlusion

Administer:

- IV undiluted or diluted 5 mg/ml of sterile H_2O for inj; give 5 mg or less over 1 min
- With antiemetic if nausea, vomiting occur
- When pain is beginning to return; determine dosage interval by patient response

Perform/provide:

- Storage in light-resistant area at room temperature
- Assistance with ambulation
- Safety measures: siderails, night light, call bell within easy reach

Evaluate:

- Therapeutic response: decrease in pain
- CNS changes: dizziness, drowsiness, hallucinations, euphoria, LOC, pupil reaction
- Allergic reactions: rash, urticaria

• Respiratory dysfunction: respiratory depression, character, rate, rhythm; notify physician if respirations are <10/min
• Need for pain medication, physical dependence

Teach patient/family:
• To report any symptoms of CNS changes, allergic reactions
• That physical dependency may result when used for extended periods of time
• That withdrawal symptoms may occur: nausea, vomiting, cramps, fever, faintness, anorexia

Lab test interferences:
Increase: Amylase

Treatment of overdose: Narcan 0.2-0.8 IV, O_2, IV fluids, vasopressors

pentobarbital/pentobarbital sodium

(pen-toe-bar'bi-tal)

Nebralin/Nembutal sodium, Nova-Rectal,* Penital, Pentogen*

Func. class.: Sedative/hypnotic-barbiturate

Chem. class.: Barbitone, short acting

Controlled Substance Schedule II (USA), Schedule G (Canada)

Action: Depresses activity in brain cells primarily in reticular activating system in brain stem; selectively depresses neurons in posterior hypothalamus, limbic structures

Uses: Insomnia, sedation, preoperative medication, increased intracranial pressure, dental anesthetic

Dosage and routes:
• *Adult:* PO 100-200 mg hs; IM 150-200 mg hs; IV 100 mg initially, then up to 500 mg; REC 120-200 mg hs
• *Child:* IM 3-5 mg, not to exceed 100 mg
• *Child 2 mo-1 yr:* REC 30 mg
• *Child 1-4 yr:* REC 30-60 mg
• *Child 5-12 yr:* REC 60 mg
• *Child 12-14 yr:* REC 60-120 mg

Available forms include: Caps 50, 100 mg; elix 18.2 mg/5 ml; powder, rec supp 30, 60, 120, 200 mg; inj IM, IV 50 mg/ml

Side effects/adverse reactions:
CNS: Lethargy, drowsiness, hangover, dizziness, paradoxical stimulation in elderly and children, light-headedness, dependence, ***CNS depression,*** mental depression, slurred speech
GI: Nausea, vomiting, diarrhea, constipation
INTEG: Rash, urticaria, pain, abscesses at injection site, angioedema, thrombophlebitis, ***Stevens-Johnson syndrome***
CV: Hypotension, bradycardia
RESP: ***Depression, apnea, laryngospasm, bronchospasm***
HEMA: ***Agranulocytosis, thrombocytopenia, megaloblastic anemia*** (long-term treatment)

Contraindications: Hypersensitivity to barbiturates, respiratory depression, addiction to barbiturates, severe liver, renal impairment, porphyria, uncontrolled pain

Precautions: Anemia, pregnancy (D), lactation, hepatic disease, renal disease, hypertension, elderly, acute/chronic pain

Pharmacokinetics:
PO: Onset 15-30 min, duration 4-6 hr
REC: Onset slow, duration 4-6 hr
Metabolized by liver, excreted by kidneys (metabolites); half-life 15-48 hr

Interactions/incompatibilities:
• Do not mix with other drugs in solution or syringe

P

• Increased CNS depression: alcohol, MAOIs, sedative, narcotics
• Decreased effect of: oral anticoagulants, corticosteroids, griseofulvin, quinidine
• Increased half-life of: doxycycline

NURSING CONSIDERATIONS

Assess:
• VS q 30min after parenteral route for 2 hr
• Blood studies: Hct, Hgb, RBCs, serum folate, vitamin D (if on long-term therapy); pro-time in patients receiving anticoagulants
• Hepatic studies: AST, ALT, bilirubin; if increased, drug is usually discontinued

Administer:
• After removal of cigarettes, to prevent fires
• IM injection in deep large muscle mass to prevent tissue sloughing and abscesses; do not inject more than 5 ml in one site
• After trying conservative measures for insomnia
• After mixing with sterile water for injection, inject within 30 min of preparation
• IV undiluted or dilute in sterile H_2O, LR, NaCl, give 50 mg or less/min; titrate to patient response; use only clear sol; avoid extravasation
• IV only with resuscitative equipment available, administer at <100 mg/min (only by qualified personnel)
• ½-1 hr before hs for sleeplessness
• On empty stomach for best absorption
• For <14 days since not effective after that; tolerance develops
• Crushed or whole
• Alone, do not mix with other drugs or inject if there is precipitate

Perform/provide:
• Assistance with ambulation after receiving dose
• Safety measure: siderails, nightlight, call bell within easy reach
• Checking to see PO medication has been swallowed
• Storage of suppositories in refrigerator; do not use aqueous solutions that contain precipitate

Evaluate:
• Therapeutic response: ability to sleep at night, decreased amount of early morning awakening if taking drug for insomnia, or decrease in number, severity of seizures if taking drug for seizure disorder
• Mental status: mood, sensorium, affect, memory (long, short)
• Physical dependency: more frequent requests for medication, shakes, anxiety
• Barbiturate toxicity: hypotension; pupillary constriction; cold, clammy skin; cyanosis of lips; insomnia; nausea; vomiting; hallucinations; delirium; weakness; coma; mild symptoms may occur in 8-12 hr without drug
• Respiratory dysfunction: respiratory depression, character, rate, rhythm; hold drug if respirations are <10/min or if pupils are dilated
• Blood dyscrasias: fever, sore throat, bruising, rash, jaundice, epistaxis

Teach patient/family:
• That morning hangover is common
• That drug is indicated only for short-term treatment of insomnia and is probably ineffective after 2 wk
• That physical dependency may result when used for extended periods of time (45-90 days depending on dose)

• To avoid driving or other activities requiring alertness
• To avoid alcohol ingestion or CNS depressants; serious CNS depression may result
• Not to discontinue medication quickly after long-term use; drug should be tapered over 1-2 wk
• To tell all prescribers that a barbiturate is being taken
• That withdrawal insomnia may occur after short-term use; do not start using drug again; insomnia will improve in 1-3 nights
• That effects may take 2 nights for benefits to be noticed
• Alternate measures to improve sleep (reading, exercise several hours before hs, warm bath, warm milk, TV, self-hypnosis, deep breathing)

Lab test interferences:
False increase: Sulfobromophthalein

Treatment of overdose: Lavage, activated charcoal, warming blanket, vital signs, hemodialysis, I&O ratio

pentostatin

(pen-toe-sta'-tin)

Nipent

Func. class.: Antineoplastic-antibiotic

Chem. class.: Streptomyces antibioticus derivative

Action: Inhibits the enzyme adenosine deaminase (ADA), which is able to block DNA synthesis and some RNA synthesis

Uses: Alpha-interferon-refractory hairy cell leukemia

Dosage and routes:
• *Adult:* IV 4 mg/m^2 every other week; may be given IV BOL, or diluted in a larger volume and given over 20-30 min

Available forms include: Powder for inj 10 mg/vial

Side effects/adverse reactions:
CNS: Headache, anxiety, confusion, depression, dizziness, insomnia, nervousness, paresthesia
RESP: Cough, upper respiratory infection, bronchitis, dyspnea, epistaxis, pneumonia, pharyngitis, rhinitis, sinusitis
SYST: Fever, infection, fatigue, pain, allergic reaction, chills, ***death, sepsis,*** chest pain, flu syndrome
HEMA: ***Leukopenia, anemia, thrombocytopenia, ecchymosis, lymphadenopathy,*** petechia
GI: Nausea, vomiting, anorexia, diarrhea, constipation, flatulence, stomatitis, elevated liver function tests
INTEG: Rash, eczema, dry skin, pruritus, sweating, herpes simplex/zoster
GU: ***Hematuria,*** dysuria, increased BUN/creatinine

Contraindications: Hypersensitivity

Precautions: Renal disease, pregnancy (C), lactation, children, bone marrow depression

Pharmacokinetics:
IV: Elimination half-life 5.7 hr, low protein binding, 90% excreted in urine as unchanged drug or metabolites

Interactions/incompatibilities:
• Fatal pulmonary toxicity: fludarabine
• Increased adverse reactions: vidarabine

NURSING CONSIDERATIONS

Assess:
• CBC, differential, platelet count weekly; withhold drug if WBC is 4000/mm^3 or platelet count is

P

<75,000/mm^3; notify physician of these results

- Renal function studies; BUN, serum uric acid, urine CrCl, electrolytes before, during therapy
- I&O ratio; report fall in urine output to <30 ml/hr
- Monitor temperature q4h; fever may indicate beginning infection
- Liver function tests before, during therapy: bilirubin, AST, ALT, alk phosphatase, as needed or monthly

Administer:

- Antiemetic 30-60 min before giving drug to prevent vomiting
- Antibiotics as ordered for prophylaxis of infection
- After diluting, use with 5 ml sterile water for injection and mix thoroughly (2 mg/ml); may be given by bolus or diluted in 25-50 ml of 5% dextrose, or 0.9% NaCl (0.33 or 0.18 mg/ml)

Perform/provide:

- Hydrocortisone, sodium thiosulfate to infiltration area, and ice compress after stopping infusion
- Strict handwashing technique, gloves, protective covering
- Liquid diet: carbonated beverages, gelatin may be added if patient is not nauseated or vomiting
- Rinsing of mouth tid-qid with water, club soda; brushing of teeth bid-qid with soft brush or cotton-tipped applicators for stomatitis; use unwaxed dental floss
- Storage in refrigerator; reconstituted or diluted solution may be stored at room temperature, for no longer than 8 hr

Evaluate:

- Therapeutic response: decrease in tumor size and spread of malignancy
- Bleeding: hematuria, guaiac stools, bruising, petechiae, mucosa or orifices q8h
- Effects of alopecia on body image; discuss feelings about body changes
- Inflammation of mucosa, breaks in skin
- Yellowing of skin, sclera, dark urine, clay-colored stools, itchy skin, abdominal pain, fever, diarrhea
- Buccal cavity q8h for dryness, sores, ulceration, white patches, oral pain, bleeding, dysphagia
- Local irritation, pain, burning at injection site
- Symptoms indicating severe allergic reaction: rash, pruritus, urticaria, purpuric skin lesions, itching, flushing
- GI symptoms: frequency of stools, cramping
- Acidosis, signs of dehydration; rapid respiration, poor skin turgor, decreased urine output, dry skin, restlessness, weakness

Teach patient/family:

- To report any complaints, side effects to nurse or physician
- That hair may be lost during treatment and wig or hairpiece may make patient feel better; tell patient that new hair may be different in color, texture
- To avoid foods with citric acid, hot or rough texture
- To report any bleeding, white spots, ulcerations in mouth to physician; tell patient to examine mouth qd
- To avoid crowds and sources of infection when granulocyte count is low

Lab test interferences:

Increase: Uric acid

pentoxifylline

(pen-tox-i'fi-leen)

Trental

Func. class.: Hemorrheologic agent

Chem. class.: Dimethylxanthine derivative

Action: Decreases blood viscosity, stimulates prostacyclin formation, increases blood flow by increasing flexibility of RBCs; decreases RBC hyperaggregation; reduces platelet aggregation, decreases fibrinogin concentration

Uses: Intermittent claudication related to chronic occlusive vascular disease

Dosage and routes:

• *Adult:* PO 400 mg tid with meals

Available forms include: Tabs, controlled-release 400 mg

Side effects/adverse reactions:

MISC: Epistaxis, flulike symptoms, laryngitis, nasal congestion, leukopenia, malaise, weight changes

EENT: Blurred vision, earache, increased salivation, sore throat, conjunctivitis

CNS: Headache, anxiety, tremors, confusion, dizziness

GI: Nausea, vomiting, anorexia, bloating, belching, constipation, dyspepsia, cholecystitis, dry mouth, thirst, bad taste

INTEG: Rash, pruritus, urticaria, brittle fingernails

CV: Angina, dysrhythmias, palpitation, hypotension, chest pain, dyspnea

Contraindications: Hypersensitivity to this drug or xanthines

Precautions: Pregnancy (C), angina pectoris, cardiac disease, lactation, children, impaired renal function

Pharmacokinetics:

PO: Peak 1 hr, half-life ½-1 hr, degradation in liver, excreted in urine

NURSING CONSIDERATIONS

Assess:

• B/P, respirations of patient taking antihypertensives also

Administer:

• With meals

Evaluate:

• Therapeutic response: decreased pain, cramping, increased ambulation

Teach patient/family:

• That therapeutic response may take 2-4 wk

• That decreased fats, increased cholesterol, increased exercise, decreased smoking are necessary to correct condition

• To observe feet for arterial insufficiency

• To use cotton socks, well-fitted shoes; not to go barefoot

• To watch for bleeding, bruises, petechiae, epistaxis

permethrin

(per-meth'ren)

Nix

Func. class.: Pediculicide

Chem. class.: Synthetic pyrethroid

Action: Acts by disrupting sodium channel current in parasite's nerve cell; delayed repolarization, paralysis of lice

Uses: Lice, nits, ticks, flea nits

Dosage and routes:

• *Adult and child:* Wash hair, towel dry; apply liberally to hair, leave on 10 min, rinse with water

Available forms include: Liq 1%

Side effects/adverse reactions:

INTEG: Pruritus, burning, stinging, rash, tingling, numbness, edema

Contraindications: Hypersensitivity
Precautions: Head rash, children, lactation
Pharmacokinetics:
Metabolized in liver to inactive metabolites, excreted in urine
NURSING CONSIDERATIONS
Administer:
• To body area, scalp only; do not apply to face, lips, mouth, eyes, any mucous membranes, anus, or meatus
• Topical corticosteroids as ordered to decrease contact dermatitis
• Lotions of menthol or phenol to control itching
• Topical antibiotics for infection
Perform/provide:
• Isolation until areas on skin, scalp have cleared and treatment is completed
• Removal of nits by using a fine-tooth comb rinsed in vinegar after treatment
Evaluate:
• Therapeutic response: decreased crusts, nits, itching papules in skin folds
Teach patient/family:
• To wash all inhabitants' clothing, bed-linen using insecticide; preventive treatment may be required of all persons living in same house, using lotion or shampoo to decrease spread of infection
• That itching may continue for 4-6 wk
• That drug must be reapplied if accidently washed off or treatment will be ineffective
• Not to apply to face, apply from neck down for body lice
• To treat sexual contact simultaneously
Treatment of ingestion: Gastric lavage, saline laxatives, IV valium for convulsions

perphenazine
(per-fen'a-zeen)
Trilafon
Func. class.: Antipsychotic/neuroleptic
Chem. class.: Phenothiazine-piperidine

Action: Depresses cerebral cortex, hypothalamus, limbic system, which control activity, aggression; blocks neurotransmission produced by dopamine at synapse; exhibits strong α-adrenergic, anticholinergic blocking action; as antiemetic inhibits medullary chemoreceptor trigger zone; mechanism for antipsychotic effects is unclear
Uses: Psychotic disorders, schizophrenia, alcoholism, nausea, vomiting
Dosage and routes:
Nausea/vomiting/alcoholism
• *Adult and child >12 yr:* IM 5-10 mg prn, max 15 mg in ambulatory patients, 30 mg in hospitalized patients; PO 8-16 mg/day in divided doses, up to 24 mg; IV not to exceed 5 mg, give diluted or slow IV drip
Psychiatric use in hospitalized patients
• *Adults:* PO 8-16 mg bid-qid, gradually increased to desired dose, not to exceed 64 mg/day; IM 5 mg q6h, not to exceed 30 mg/day
• *Child >12 yr:* PO 6-12 mg in divided doses
Nonhospitalized patients
• *Adult:* PO 4-8 mg tid or 8-32 mg repeat-action bid; IM 5 mg q6h
Available forms include: Tabs 2, 4, 8, 16 mg; sol 16 mg/5ml; inj IM 5 mg/ml; sus rel tabs 8 mg
Side effects/adverse reactions:
RESP: ***Laryngospasm,*** dyspnea, ***respiratory depression***

CNS: Extrapyramidal symptoms: pseudoparkinsonism, akathisia, dystonia, tardive dyskinesia, ***seizures,*** *headache*
HEMA: Anemia, ***leukopenia, leukocytosis, agranulocytosis***
INTEG: Rash, photosensitivity, dermatitis
EENT: Blurred vision, glaucoma
GI: Dry mouth, nausea, vomiting, anorexia, constipation, diarrhea, jaundice, weight gain
GU: Urinary retention, urinary frequency, enuresis, impotence, amenorrhea, gynecomastia
CV: Orthostatic hypotension, ***cardiac arrest,*** ECG changes, ***tachycardia***
Contraindications: Hypersensitivity, blood dyscrasias, coma, child <12 yr, brain damage, bone marrow depression
Precautions: Pregnancy (C), lactation, seizure disorders, hypertension, hepatic disease, cardiac disease
Pharmacokinetics:
PO: Onset erratic, peak 2-4 hr
IM: Onset 10 min, peak 1-2 hr, duration 6 hr, occasionally 12-24 hr; metabolized by liver, excreted in urine, crosses placenta, enters breast milk
Interactions/incompatibilities:
- Oversedation: other CNS depressants, alcohol, barbiturate anesthetics
- Toxicity: epinephrine
- Decreased absorption: aluminum hydroxide or magnesium hydroxide antacids
- Decreased effects of: lithium, levodopa
- Increased effects of both drugs: β-adrenergic blockers, alcohol
- Increased anticholinergic effects: anticholinergics

NURSING CONSIDERATIONS

Assess:
- Mental status before initial administration
- Swallowing of PO medication; check for hoarding or giving of medication to other patients
- I&O ratio; palpate bladder if low urinary output occurs
- Bilirubin, CBC, liver function studies monthly
- Urinalysis is recommended before and during prolonged therapy

Administer:
- Antiparkinsonian agent, after securing order from physician to be used if extrapyramidal symptoms occur
- Concentrate mixed in water, orange, pineapple, apricot, prune, tomato, grapefruit juice; do not mix with caffeine beverages (coffee, cola), tannics (tea), or pectinates (apple juice) since incompatibility may result; use 60 ml diluent for each 5 ml of concentrate
- Repeat-action tablets whole; do not crush or chew
- IM injection into a large muscle mass

Perform/provide:
- Decreased noise input by dimming lights, avoiding loud noises
- Supervised ambulation until stabilized on medication; do not involve in strenuous exercise program because fainting is possible; patient should not stand still for long periods of time
- Increased fluids to prevent constipation
- Sips of water, candy, gum for dry mouth
- Storage in tight, light-resistant container

Evaluate:
- Therapeutic response: decrease in emotional excitement, hallucina-

tions, delusions, paranoia, reorganization of patterns of thought, speech
• Affect, orientation, LOC, reflexes, gait, coordination, sleep pattern disturbances
• B/P standing and lying; also include pulse, respirations q4h during initial treatment; establish baseline before starting treatment; report drops of 30 mm Hg
• Dizziness, faintness, palpitations, tachycardia on rising
• Extrapyramidal symptoms including akathisia (inability to sit still, no pattern to movements), tardive dyskinesia (bizarre movements of jaw, mouth, tongue, extremities), pseudoparkinsonism (rigidity, tremors, pill rolling, shuffling gait)
• Skin turgor daily
• For neuroleptic malignant syndrome: hyperthermia, altered mental status, increased CPK, muscle rigidity
• Constipation, urinary retention daily; if these occur, increase bulk, water in diet

Teach patient/family:
• That orthostatic hypotension occurs frequently, and to rise from sitting or lying position gradually, to avoid hazardous activities until stabilized on medication
• To remain lying down after IM injection for at least 30 min
• To avoid hot tubs, hot showers, or tub baths since hypotension may occur
• To avoid abrupt withdrawal of this drug or extrapyramidal symptoms may result; drugs should be withdrawn slowly
• To avoid OTC preparations (cough, hayfever, cold) unless approved by physician since serious drug interactions may occur; avoid use with alcohol or CNS depressants, increased drowsiness may occur
• To use a sunscreen during sun exposure to prevent burns
• Regarding compliance with drug regimen
• About necessity for meticulous oral hygiene since oral candidiasis may occur
• To report sore throat, malaise, fever, bleeding, mouth sores; if these occur, CBC should be drawn and drug discontinued
• In hot weather, that heat stroke may occur; take extra precautions to stay cool

Lab test interferences:
Increase: Liver function tests, cardiac enzymes, cholesterol, blood glucose, prolactin, bilirubin, PBI, cholinesterase, ^{131}I
Decrease: Hormones (blood, urine)
False positive: Pregnancy tests, PKU
False negative: Urinary steroids, 17-OHCS

Treatment of overdose: Lavage if orally injested, provide an airway; *do not induce vomiting*

---

phenacemide

(fe-nass′e-mide)
Phenurone

Func. class.: Anticonvulsant
Chem. class.: Hydantoin

Action: Increases seizure threshold in cortex

Uses: Refractory, generalized tonic-clonic, (grand mal) complex-partial, (psychomotor) absence, (petit mal) atypical seizures

Dosage and routes:
• *Adult:* PO 500 mg tid, may in-

crease by 500 mg/wk, not to exceed 5 g/day
- *Child 5-10 yr:* PO 250 mg tid, may increase by 250 mg/wk, not to exceed 1.5 g/day prn

Available forms include: Tabs 500 mg

Side effects/adverse reactions:

HEMA: ***Agranulocytosis, leukopenia, aplastic anemia***

CNS: Drowsiness, dizziness, insomnia, paresthesias, depression, suicidal tendencies, aggression, headache

GI: Anorexia, weight loss, ***hepatitis,*** jaundice, nausea

GU: Nephritis, ***albuminuria***

INTEG: Rash

Contraindications: Hypersensitivity, psychiatric condition, pregnancy (D)

Precautions: Allergies, hepatic disease, renal disease

Pharmacokinetics:

PO: Duration 5 hr, metabolized by liver, excreted by kidneys

NURSING CONSIDERATIONS

Assess:
- Blood, liver function, renal function studies
- Drug level: drug is extremely toxic

Administer:
- With food to decrease GI symptoms

Evaluate:
- Therapeutic response: decreased seizures
- Mental status: mood, sensorium, affect, memory (long, short); psychosis is common
- Respiratory depression: respirations <10/min, shallow
- Blood dyscrasias: fever, sore throat, bruising, rash, jaundice

Teach patient/family:
- To notify physician if sore throat, fever, rash, fatigue, bleeding, bruising occur (blood dyscrasia)
- To notify physician if dark urine, jaundice, yellow sclerae, itching occur (liver dysfunction)
- To avoid hazardous activities until stabilized on drug
- Never to withdraw abruptly
- To report personality changes

---

phenazopyridine HCl

(fen-az-eh-peer'i-deen)

Baridium, Di-Azo, Diridone, Phenazo,* Phenazodine, Pyridiate, Pyridium, Urodine

Func. class.: Nonnarcotic analgesic

Chem. class.: Azodye

Action: Exerts analgesic, anesthetic action on the urinary tract mucosa; exact mechanism of action unknown

Uses: Urinary tract irritation, infection

Dosage and routes:
- *Adult:* PO 100-200 mg tid
- *Child 6-12 yr:* PO 12 mg/kg/24 hr in divided doses

Available forms include: Tabs 100, 200 mg

Side effects/adverse reactions:

HEMA: ***Thrombocytopenia, agranulocytosis, leukopenia, neutropenia, hemolytic anemia, methemoglobinemia***

CNS: Headache, vertigo

GI: Nausea, vomiting, GI bleeding, diarrhea, heartburn, anorexia, ***hepatic toxicity***

INTEG: Rash, urticaria, skin pigmentation

GU: ***Renal toxicity,*** *orange-red urine*

Contraindications: Hypersensitivity, hepatic disease

Precautions: Pregnancy (B), renal disease

Pharmacokinetics: Metabolized by liver, excreted by kidneys, crosses placenta, duration 6-8 hr

NURSING CONSIDERATIONS

Assess:

- Liver function studies: AST, ALT, bilirubin if patient is on long-term therapy

Administer:

- To patient crushed or whole; chewable tablets may be chewed
- With food or milk to decrease gastric symptoms

Evaluate:

- Therapeutic response: decrease in pain
- Hepatotoxicity: dark urine, clay-colored stools, yellowing of skin, sclera, itching, abdominal pain, fever, diarrhea if patient is on long-term therapy
- Allergic reactions: rash, urticaria; if these occur, drug may need to be discontinued

Teach patient/family:

- To report any symptoms of hepatotoxicity
- Not to exceed recommended dosage, and to take with meals
- To read label on other OTC drugs; many contain aspirin
- Urine may turn red-orange

Lab test interferences:

Interference: Bilirubin, urinary glucose tests, urinalysis, PSP excretion, urinary ketones, steroids, proteins

Treatment of overdose: Methylene blue 1-2 mg/kg IV or 100-200 mg vitamin C PO

phendimetrazine tartrate

(fen-dye-me'tra-zeen)

Adipost, Anorex, Bacarate, Bontril, Delcozine, Di-Ap-Trol, Metra Obalan, Obeval, Obezine, Phenzine, Plegine, SPRX 1, SPRX-105, Statobex, Trimstat, Trimtabs, Melfiat, Weightrol, Weh-less, Trimcaps, Adphen, Dyrexan-OD, Prel-2

Func. class.: Anorexiant

Chem. class.: Morpholine derivative

Controlled Substance Schedule III

Action: Increases release of norepinephrine, dopamine in cerebral cortex to reticular activating system

Uses: Exogenous obesity

Dosage and routes:

Adult: PO 35 mg bid-tid 1 hr ac, not to exceed 70 mg tid, sus rel 105 mg qd ac AM

Available forms include: Tabs 35 mg, caps 35 mg, sus rel cap 105 mg

Side effects/adverse reactions:

CNS: Hyperactivity, insomnia, restlessness, dizziness, tremor headache

INTEG: Urticaria

GI: Nausea, anorexia, dry mouth, diarrhea, constipation, cramps

GU: Dysuria

CV: Palpitations, tachycardia, hypertension

EENT: Blurred vision

Contraindications: Hypersensitivity, hyperthyroidism, hypertension, glaucoma, severe arteriosclerosis, severe cardiovascular disease, children <12 yr, agitated states

Precautions: Drug abuse, anxiety, pregnancy (C), lactation

Pharmacokinetics:
PO: Onset 30 min, peak 1-3 hr, duration 4-20 hr, metabolized by liver, excreted by kidneys, crosses placenta, excreted in breast milk, half-life 2-10 hr
Interactions/incompatibilities:
• Hypertensive crisis: MAOIs or within 14 days of MAOIs
• Increased effect of phendimetrazine: acetazolamide, antacids, sodium bicarbonate
• Decreased effect of phendimetrazine: tricyclics, ascorbic acid, ammonium chloride
• Decreased effect of: guanethidine, other antihypertensives
NURSING CONSIDERATIONS
Assess:
• VS, B/P since this drug may reverse antihypertensives; check patients with cardiac disease more often
• CBC, urinalysis, in diabetes: blood sugar, urine sugar; insulin changes may need to be made since eating will decrease
• Height, growth rate in children; growth rate may decrease
Administer:
• At least 6 hr before hs to avoid sleeplessness
• For obesity only if patient is on weight reduction program, including dietary changes, exercise; patient will develop tolerance, loss of weight won't occur without additional methods, give 1 hr before meals
• Gum, hard candy, frequent sips of water for dry mouth
Teach patient/family:
• Not to crush or chew sus rel preps
• To decrease caffeine consumption (coffee, tea, cola, chocolate), which may increase irritability, stimulation
• To avoid OTC preparations unless approved by physician
• To taper off drug over several weeks, or depression, increased sleeping, lethargy will ensue
• To avoid alcohol ingestion
• To avoid hazardous activities until patient is stabilized on medication
• To get needed rest; patients will feel more tired at end of day
Treatment of overdose: Administer fluids, hemodialysis or peritoneal dialysis; antihypertensive for increased B/P; ammonium Cl for increase excretion

---

phenelzine sulfate

(fen'el-zeen)
Nardil
Func. class.: Antidepressant MAOI
Chem. class.: Hydrazine

Action: Increases concentrations of endogenous epinephrine, norepinephrine, serotonin, dopamine in storage sites in CNS by inhibition of MAO; increased concentration reduces depression
Uses: Depression, when uncontrolled by other means
Dosage and routes:
• *Adult:* PO 45 mg/day in divided doses, may increase to 60 mg/day, dose should be reduced to 15 mg/day, not to exceed 90 mg/day
Available forms include: Tabs 15 mg
Side effects/adverse reactions:
HEMA: Anemia
CNS: Dizziness, drowsiness, confusion, headache, anxiety, tremors, stimulation, weakness, hyperreflexia, mania, insomnia, fatigue, weight gain
GI: Constipation, dry mouth, nau-

P

sea, vomiting, *anorexia,* diarrhea, weight gain
GU: Change in libido, frequency
INTEG: Rash, flushing, increased perspiration
CV: Orthostatic hypotension, hypertension, dysrhythmias, hypertensive crisis
EENT: Blurred vision
ENDO: ***SIADH-like syndrome***

Contraindications: Hypersensitivity to MAOIs, elderly, hypertension, CHF, severe hepatic disease, pheochromocytoma, severe renal disease, severe cardiac disease

Precautions: Suicidal patients, convulsive disorders, severe depression, schizophrenia, hyperactivity, diabetes mellitus, pregnancy (C)

Pharmacokinetics:
Metabolized by liver, excreted by kidneys

Interactions/incompatibilities:
• Increased pressor effects: guanethidine, clonidine, indirect acting sympathomimetics (ephedrine)
• Increased effects of: direct acting sympathomimetics (epinephrine), alcohol, barbiturates, benzodiazepines, CNS depressants, levodopa
• Hyperpyretic crisis, convulsions, hypertensive episode: tricyclic antidepressants, meperidine
• Increased hypoglycemic effect: insulin

NURSING CONSIDERATIONS

Assess:
• B/P (lying, standing), pulse; if systolic B/P drops 20 mm Hg hold drug, notify physician
• Blood studies: CBC, leukocytes, cardiac enzymes if patient is receiving long-term therapy
• Hepatic studies: ALT, AST, bilirubin, creatinine; hepatotoxicity may occur

Administer:
• Increased fluids, bulk in diet if constipation, urinary retention occur
• With food or milk or GI symptoms
• Crushed if patient is unable to swallow medication whole
• Dosage hs if oversedation occurs during day
• Gum, hard candy, or frequent sips of water for dry mouth
• Phentolamine for severe hypertension

Perform/provide:
• Storage in tight container in cool environment
• Assistance with ambulation during beginning therapy since drowsiness/dizziness occurs, especially elderly
• Safety measures including siderails
• Checking to see PO medication swallowed

Evaluate:
• Therapeutic response: decreased depression
• Toxicity: increased headache, palpitation, discontinue drug immediately; prodromal signs of hypertensive crisis
• Mental status: mood, sensorium, affect, memory (long, short); increase in psychiatric symptoms
• Urinary retention, constipation, edema, take weight weekly
• Withdrawal symptoms: headache, nausea, vomiting, muscle pain, weakness

Teach patient/family:
• That therapeutic effects may take 1-4 wk
• To avoid driving or other activities requiring alertness
• To avoid alcohol ingestion, CNS depressants or OTC medications:

---

* Available in Canada only

cold, weight, hay fever, cough syrup
• Not to discontinue medication quickly after long-term use
• To avoid high tyramine foods: cheese (aged), sour cream, beer, wine, pickled products, liver, raisins, bananas, figs, avocados, meat tenderizers, chocolate, yogurt; increase caffeine
• To report headache, palpitation, neck stiffness

Treatment of overdose: Lavage, activated charcoal, monitor electrolytes, vital signs, diazepam IV, $NaHCO_3$

phenmetrazine HCl

(fen-met'ra-zeen)

Preludin

Func. class.: Anorexiant
Chem. class.: Morpholine

Controlled Substance Schedule II

Action: Increases release of norepinephrine, dopamine in cerebral cortex to reticular activating system

Uses: Exogenous obesity

Dosage and routes:
• *Adult:* EXT REL 50-75 mg qd in AM; tab 25 mg bid-tid 1 hr ac not to exceed 75 mg qd

Available forms include: Tabs ext rel 75 mg, tabs 25 mg

Side effects/adverse reactions:
CNS: Hyperactivity, insomnia, restlessness, dizziness, headache
GI: Nausea, anorexia, dry mouth, constipation, abdominal pain
GU: Impotence, change in libido
CV: Palpitations, tachycardia, hypertension
INTEG: Urticaria
EENT: Blurred vision

Contraindications: Hypersensitivity, hyperthyroidism, hypertension, glaucoma, severe arteriosclerosis, angina pectoris, drug abuse, cardiovascular disease, agitation

Precautions: Anxiety, pregnancy (C), lactation

Pharmacokinetics:
EXT REL: Duration 12 hr, metabolized by liver, excreted by kidneys

Interactions/incompatibilities:
• Hypertensive crisis: MAOIs or within 14 days of MAOIs
• Increased effect of phenmetrazine: acetazolamide, antacids, sodium bicarbonate
• Decreased effect of phenmetrazine: tricyclics, ascorbic acid, ammonium chloride
• Decreased effect of: guanethidine, other antihypertensives

NURSING CONSIDERATIONS

Assess:
• VS, B/P since this drug may reverse antihypertensives; check patients with cardiac disease more often
• CBC, urinalysis, in diabetes: blood sugar, urine sugar; insulin changes may need to be made since eating will decrease
• Height, growth rate in children; growth rate may be decreased

Administer:
• At least 6 hr before hs to avoid sleeplessness
• For obesity only if patient is on weight reduction program including dietary changes, exercise; patient will develop tolerance, loss of weight won't occur without additional methods, give 1 hr before meals
• Gum, hard candy, frequent sips of water for dry mouth

Evaluate:
• Therapeutic response: decreased weight
• Mental status: mood, sensorium, affect, stimulation, insomnia, aggressiveness

• Physical dependency: should not be used for extended time; dose should be discontinued gradually, tolerance occurs with long-term use
• Withdrawal symptoms: headache, nausea, vomiting, muscle pain, weakness

Teach patient/family:
• Not to crush or chew sus rel preps
• To decrease caffeine consumption (coffee, tea, cola, chocolate), which may increase irritability, stimulation
• To avoid OTC preparations unless approved by physician
• To taper off drug over several weeks, or depression, increased sleeping, lethargy may ensue
• To avoid alcohol ingestion
• To avoid hazardous activities until patient is stabilized on medication
• To get needed rest; patients will feel more tired at end of day

Treatment of overdose: Administer fluids, hemodialysis or peritoneal dialysis; antihypertensive for increased B/P; ammonium Cl for increased excretion

---

phenobarbital, phenobarbital sodium

(fee-noe-bar'bi-tal)

Bar, Barbita, Eskabarb, Floramine, Luminal, Orpine, SoluBarb, Stental, Luminal sodium

Func. class.: Anticonvulsant
Chem. class.: Barbiturate

Controlled Substance Schedule IV

Action: Decreases impulse transmission, increases seizure threshold at cerebral cortex level

Uses: All forms of epilepsy, status epilepticus, febrile seizures in children, sedation, insomnia, hyperbilirubinemia, chronic cholestasis

Dosage and routes:

Seizures
• *Adult:* PO 100-200 mg/day in divided doses tid or total dose hs
• *Child:* PO 4-6 mg/kg/day in divided doses q12h, may be given as single dose

Status epilepticus
• *Adult:* IV INF 10 mg/kg, run no faster than 50 mg/min, may give up to 20 mg/kg
• *Child:* IV INF 5-10 mg/kg, may repeat q10-15 min, up to 20 mg/kg, run no faster than 50 mg/min

Insomnia
• *Adult:* PO/IM 100-320 mg
• *Child:* PO/IM 3-6 mg/kg

Sedation
• *Adult:* PO 30-120 mg/day in 2-3 divided doses
• *Child:* PO 6 mg/kg/day in 3 divided doses

Preoperative sedation
• *Adult:* IM 100-200 mg 1-1½ hr before surgery
• *Child:* IM 16-100 mg 1-1½ hr before surgery

Hyperbilirubinemia
• *Neonate:* PO 7 mg/kg/day from days 1-5 after birth
IM 5 mg/kg/day on day 1, then PO on days 2-7 after birth

Chronic cholestasis
• *Adult:* PO 90-180 mg/day in 2-3 divided doses
• *Child <12 yr:* PO 3-12 mg/kg/day in 2-3 divided doses

Available forms include: Caps 16 mg; elix 15, 20 mg/5 ml; tabs 8, 15, 16, 30, 32, 60, 65, 100 mg; inj 30, 60, 65, 130 mg/ml

Side effects/adverse reactions:
CNS: Paradoxical excitement (elderly), *drowsiness,* lethargy, hangover headache, flushing, hallucinations, coma

---

* Available in Canada only

GI: Nausea, vomiting
INTEG: Rash, urticaria, ***Stevens-Johnson syndrome, angioedema,*** local pain, swelling, necrosis, thrombophlebitis
Contraindications: Hypersensitivity to barbiturates, porphyria, hepatic disease, respiratory disease, nephritis, hyperthyroidism, diabetes mellitus, elderly, lactation, pregnancy (D)
Precautions: Anemia
Pharmacokinetics:
PO: Onset 20-60 min, peak 8-12 hr, duration 6-10 hr, metabolized by liver, excreted by kidneys, crosses placenta, excreted in breast milk, half-life 53-118 hr
Interactions/incompatibilities:
• Increased effects: CNS depressants, alcohol, chloramphenicol, valproic acid, disulfiram, nondepolarizing skeletal muscle relaxants, sulfonamides
• Increased orthostatic hypotension: furosemide

NURSING CONSIDERATIONS

Assess:
• Blood studies, liver function tests during long-term treatment
• Therapeutic level 15-40 mg/ml
Administer:
• IV after slow dilution with at least 10 ml sterile H_2O for inj; give 65 mg or less/min; titrate to patient response
• Give IM inj deeply into large muscle mass to prevent tissue sloughing
Evaluate:
• Therapeutic response: decreased seizures, increased sedation
• Mental status: mood, sensorium, affect, memory (long, short)
• Respiratory depression
• Blood dyscrasias: fever, sore throat, bruising, rash, jaundice
Teach patient/family:
• To avoid hazardous activities until stabilized on drug
• Never to withdraw drug abruptly
• That therapeutic effects (PO) may not be seen for 2-3 wk
Treatment of overdose: Administer calcium gluconate IV

---

phenolphthalein

(fee-nol-thay'leen)
Alophen, Espotabs, Evac-U-Gen, Evac-U-Lax, Ex-Lax, Feen-A-Mint, Phenolax, Prulet
Func. class.: Laxative, stimulant/irritant
Chem. class.: Diphenylmethane

Action: Directly acts on intestinal smooth muscle by increasing motor activity; thought to irritate colonic intramural plexus
Uses: Constipation, preparation for bowel surgery or examination
Dosage and routes:
• *Adult:* PO 60-270 mg hs
• *Child >6 yr:* 30-60 mg/day
• *Child 2-5 yr:* 15-20 mg/day
Available forms include: Tabs 60 mg; chew tab 60, 64.8, 80, 90, 97.2 mg; chew gum 97.2 mg; susp 22 mg/5 ml
Side effects/adverse reactions:
INTEG: Rash, urticaria, ***Stevens-Johnson syndrome***
GI: Nausea, vomiting, anorexia, diarrhea
META: Hypokalemia, electrolyte, fluid imbalances
Contraindications: Hypersensitivity, GI obstructions, abdominal pain, nausea/vomiting, fecal impaction
Pharmacokinetics:
PO: Onset 6-8 hr; excreted in feces

P

NURSING CONSIDERATIONS

Assess:

- Blood, urine electrolytes if drug is used often by patient
- I&O ratio to identify fluid loss

Administer:

- Alone for better absorption
- In morning or evening (oral dose)

Evaluate:

- Therapeutic response: decrease in constipation
- Cause of constipation; identify whether fluids, bulk, or exercise is missing from lifestyle
- Cramping, rectal bleeding, nausea, vomiting; if these symptoms occur, drug should be discontinued

Teach patient/family:

- To keep out of children's reach, some is fruit or chocolate flavored
- To swallow tabs whole; do not chew
- Not to use laxatives for long-term therapy; bowel tone will be lost
- That normal bowel movements do not always occur daily
- Not to use in presence of abdominal pain, nausea, vomiting
- To notify physician if constipation unrelieved or if symptoms of electrolyte imbalance occur: muscle cramps, pain, weakness, dizziness
- That urine, feces may turn pink to yellow-brown

Lab test interferences:
BSP test

phenoxybenzamine HCl

(fen-ox-ee-ben'za-meen)

Dibenzyline

Func. class.: Antihypertensive
Chem. class.: α-Adrenergic blocker

Action: α-Adrenergic blocker that binds to α-adrenergic receptors, dilating peripheral blood vessels, lowers peripheral resistance, lowers blood pressure

Uses: Pheochromocytoma

Dosage and routes:

- *Adult:* PO 10 mg bid, increase by 10 mg qod, not to exceed 60 mg/day; usual range: 20-40 mg bid-tid

Available forms include: Caps 10 mg

Side effects/adverse reactions:

GI: Dry mouth, nausea, vomiting, diarrhea

CV: Postural hypotension, tachycardia, palpitations

CNS: Dizziness, flushing, drowsiness, sedation, weakness, confusion, headache, malaise

GU: Inhibition of ejaculation

EENT: Nasal congestion, dry mouth, miosis

INTEG: Allergic contact dermatitis

Contraindications: Hypersensitivity, CHF, angina, cerebral vascular insufficiency, coronary arteriosclerosis

Precautions: Severe renal disease, severe pulmonary disease, pregnancy (C)

Pharmacokinetics:

PO: Onset 2 hr, peak 4-6 hr, duration 3-4 days; half-life 24 hr, metabolized in liver, excreted in urine, bile

Interactions/incompatibilities:

- Hypotensive response: epinephrine, antihypertensives

NURSING CONSIDERATIONS

Assess:

- Electrolytes: K, Na, Cl, CO_2
- Weight daily, I&O
- B/P lying, standing before starting treatment, q4h after

Administer:

- Starting with low dose, gradually increasing to prevent side effects
- Gum, frequent rinsing of mouth or hard candy for dry mouth

• With food or milk for GI symptoms

Evaluate:

• Therapeutic response: decreased B/P, increased peripheral pulses

• Nausea, vomiting, diarrhea

• Skin turgor, dryness of mucous membranes for hydration status

Teach patient/family:

• To avoid alcoholic beverages

• To report dizziness, palpitations, fainting

• To change position slowly or fainting may occur

• To take drug exactly as prescribed

• To avoid all OTC products: cough, cold, allergy, unless directed by physician

Treatment of overdose: Administer IV saline, norepinephrine, elevate legs, discontinue drug

phensuximide

(fen-sux'i-mide)

Milontin

Func. class.: Anticonvulsant
Chem. class.: Succinimide

Action: Inhibits spike, wave formation in absence seizures (petit mal), decreases amplitude, frequency, duration

Uses: Absence (petit mal) seizures

Dosage and routes:

• *Adult and child:* PO 500 mg-1 g bid or tid

Available forms include: Caps 500 mg

Side effects/adverse reactions:

HEMA: ***Agranulocytosis, aplastic anemia, thrombocytopenia, leukocytosis, eosinophilia, pancytopenia***

CNS: Drowsiness, dizziness, fatigue, euphoria, lethargy, anxiety, depression, irritability, insomnia, aggressiveness, weakness, headache

GI: Nausea, vomiting, heartburn, anorexia, diarrhea, abdominal pain, cramps, constipation

GU: Vaginal bleeding, ***hematuria, renal damage,*** urinary frequency

INTEG: Urticaria, pruritic erythema, hirsutism, ***Stevens-Johnson syndrome***

EENT: Myopia, gum hypertrophy, tongue swelling, blurred vision

Contraindications: Hypersensitivity to succinimide derivatives

Precautions: Lactation, hepatic disease, pregnancy (D), renal disease

Pharmacokinetics:

PO: Peak 1-4 hr, metabolized by liver, excreted by kidneys, half-life 5-12 hr

Interactions/incompatibilities:

• Antagonist effect: tricyclic antidepressants (imipramine, doxepin)

• Decreased effects of: estrogens, oral contraceptives

NURSING CONSIDERATIONS

Assess:

• Renal studies: urinalysis, BUN, urine creatinine, q6mo

• Blood studies: CBC, Hct, Hgb, reticulocyte counts q3mo

• Hepatic studies: AST, ALT, bilirubin, creatinine q6mo

• Drug levels during initial treatment, therapeutic range (40-80 μg/ml)

Administer:

• With food, milk to decrease GI symptoms

Perform/provide:

• Hard candy, frequent rinsing of mouth, gum for dry mouth

• Assistance with ambulation during early part of treatment; dizziness occurs

Evaluate:

• Therapeutic response: decreased seizures

• Mental status: mood, sensorium, affect, behavioral changes; if mental status changes, notify physician
• Eye problems; need for ophthalmic exam before, during, after treatment (slit lamp, fundoscopy, tonometry)
• Allergic reaction: red raised rash; if this occurs, drug should be discontinued
• Blood dyscrasias: fever, sore throat, bruising, rash, jaundice
• Toxicity: bone marrow depression, nausea, vomiting, ataxia, diplopia

Teach patient/family:
• To carry ID card or Medic-Alert bracelet stating drugs taken, condition, physician's name, phone number
• To avoid driving, other activities that require alertness
• To avoid alcohol ingestion, CNS depressants; increased sedation may occur
• Not to discontinue medication quickly after long-term use
• To call physician if sore throat, fever, malaise, bruises, epistaxis occur
• That drug may color urine pink or red

Lab test interferences:
Increase: Coombs' test

Treatment of overdose: Lavage, activated charcoal, monitor electrolytes, VS

phentermine HCl

(fen'ter-meen)
Anoxine, Fastin, Ionamin, Obe-Nix, Adipex-P, Dapex, Obephen, Obermine, Parmine, Phentrol, Rolaphent, Wilpowr

Func. class.: Cerebral stimulant
Chem. class.: Sympathomimetic amine

Controlled Substance Schedule IV

Action: Stimulates satiety center by action on adrenergic pathways

Uses: Exogenous obesity

Dosage and routes:
• *Adult:* PO 8 mg tid 30 min before meals or 15-37.5 mg qd

Available forms include: Tabs 8, 30, 37.5 mg; caps 15, 18.75, 30, 37.5 mg; caps time rel 30 mg

Side effects/adverse reactions:
CNS: Hyperactivity, insomnia, restlessness, dizziness, tremor, headache
GI: Nausea, anorexia, dry mouth, constipation, unpleasant taste
GU: Impotence, change in libido
CV: *Palpitations, tachycardia,* hypertension
INTEG: Urticaria
EENT: Blurred vision

Contraindications: Hypersensitivity, hyperthyroidism, hypertension, glaucoma, severe arteriosclerosis, angina pectoris, cardiovascular disease, pregnancy (C), child <12 yr

Precautions: Pregnancy (C), lactation, drug abuse, anxiety

Pharmacokinetics:
CON REL: Duration 10-14 hr; metabolized by liver, excreted by kidneys

Interactions/incompatibilities:
• Hypertensive crisis: MAOIs or within 14 days of MAOIs

* Available in Canada only

• Increased effect of phentermine: acetazolamide, antacids, sodium bicarbonate
• Decreased effect of phentermine: tricyclics, ascorbic acid, ammonium chloride
• Decreased effect of: guanethidine, other antihypertensives
• Decreased insulin requirements: diabetes mellitus

NURSING CONSIDERATIONS

Assess:
• VS, B/P since this drug may reverse antihypertensives check patients with cardiac disease more often
• CBC, urinalysis, in diabetes: blood sugar, urine sugar; insulin changes may need to be made since eating will decrease
• Height and growth rate in children; growth rate may be decreased

Administer:
• At least 6 hr before hs to avoid sleeplessness
• For obesity only if patient is on weight reduction program including dietary changes, exercise; patient will develop tolerance, and loss of weight won't occur without additional methods, give 30 min before meals
• Gum, hard candy, frequent sips of water for dry mouth

Perform/provide:
• Check to see PO medication has been swallowed

Evaluate:
• Therapeutic response: decreased weight
• Mental status: mood, sensorium, affect, stimulation, insomnia, aggressiveness
• Physical dependency: should not be used for extended periods of time; dose should be discontinued gradually, tolerance occurs with long-term use
• Withdrawal symptoms: headache, nausea, vomiting, muscle pain, weakness

Teach patient/family:
• To decrease caffeine consumption (coffee, tea, cola, chocolate), which may increase irritability, stimulation
• To avoid OTC preparations unless approved by physician
• To taper off drug over several weeks, or depression, increased sleeping, lethargy may ensue
• To avoid alcohol ingestion
• To avoid hazardous activities until patient is stabilized on medication
• To get needed rest; patients will feel more tired at end of day

Treatment of overdose: Administer fluids, hemodialysis or peritoneal dialysis; antihypertensive for increased B/P; ammonium Cl for increase excretion

---

phentolamine mesylate

(fen-tole'a-meen)

Regitine, Rogitine*

Func. class.: Antihypertensive
Chem. class.: α-Adrenergic blocker

Action: α-Adrenergic blocker, binds to α-adrenergic receptors, dilating peripheral blood vessels, lowering peripheral resistances, lowering blood pressure

Uses: Hypertension, pheochromocytoma, prevention, treatment of dermal necrosis following extravasation of norepinephrine or dopamine

Dosage and routes:

Treatment of hypertensive episodes in pheochromocytoma
• *Adult:* 5 mg IV/IM, repeat if necessary

P

• *Child:* 1 mg IV/IM, repeat if necessary
• *Adult:* 2.5 mg IV, if negative repeat with 5 mg IV
• *Child:* 0.5 mg IV, if negative repeat with 1 mg IV

Prevention, treatment of necrosis
• *Adult:* 5-10 mg/10 ml NS injected into area of norepinephrine extravasation within 12 hr; 10 mg/1000 ml norepinephrine solution is preventive dose

Available forms include: Inj IM, IV 5 mg/ml; tabs 25, 50 mg (only injectable form available in US)

Side effects/adverse reactions:
GI: Dry mouth, nausea, vomiting, diarrhea, abdominal pain
CV: Hypotension, tachycardia, angina, dysrhythmias, ***myocardial infarction***
CNS: Dizziness, flushing, weakness
EENT: Nasal congestion

Contraindications: Hypersensitivity, myocardial infarction, coronary insufficiency, angina

Precautions: Pregnancy (C), lactation

Pharmacokinetics:
IV: Peak 2 min, duration 10-15 min
IM: Peak 15-20 min, duration 3-4 hr; metabolized in liver, excreted in urine

Interactions/incompatibilities:
• Increased effects of: epinephrine, antihypertensives
• Not to be mixed in solution or syringe with any drug except levarterenol

NURSING CONSIDERATIONS

Assess:
• Electrolytes: K, Na, Cl, CO_2
• Weight daily, I&O
• B/P lying, standing before starting treatment, q4h after

Administer:
• IV after diluting 5 mg/1 ml sterile H_2O for inj; may be further diluted with 5-10 ml sterile H_2O for inj; give 5 mg or less/min
• Gum, frequent rinsing of mouth or hard candy for dry mouth
• After having vasopressor nearby
• After discontinuing all medication for 24 hr

Evaluate:
• Therapeutic response: decreased B/P
• Nausea, vomiting, diarrhea, edema in feet, legs daily; skin turgor, dryness of mucous membranes for hydration status, postural hypotension, cardiac system: pulse, ECG

Teach patient/family:
• That bedrest is required during treatment, 1 hr after

Treatment of overdose: Administer norepinephrine, discontinue drug

---

phenylbutazone

(fen-ill-byoo'-ta-zone)

Algoverine, Azolid, Butagesic, Butazolidin, Intrabutazone, Malgesic, Neo-Zoline

Func. class.: Nonsteroidal antiinflammatory

Chem. class.: Pyrazolone derivative

Action: Inhibits prostaglandin synthesis by decreasing an enzyme needed for biosynthesis; possesses analgesic, antiinflammatory, antipyretic properties

Uses: Mild to moderate pain, osteoarthritis, rheumatoid arthritis

Dosage and routes:

Pain
• *Adult:* PO 100-200 mg tid-qid, then after desired response 100 mg tid-qid, not to exceed 600 mg/day

Acute Arthritis
• *Adult:* PO 400 mg, then 100 mg

q4h × 4 days or until desired response
Available forms include: Tabs 100 mg; caps 100 mg
Side effects/adverse reactions:
GI: Nausea, anorexia, vomiting, diarrhea, jaundice, ***cholestatic hepatitis,*** constipation, flatulence, cramps, dry mouth, peptic ulcer
CNS: Dizziness, drowsiness, fatigue, tremors, confusion, insomnia, anxiety, depression
CV: Tachycardia, peripheral edema, palpitations, dysrhythmias
INTEG: Purpura, rash, pruritus, sweating
GU: ***Nephrotoxicity: dysuria, hematuria, oliguria, azotemia***
HEMA: ***Bone marrow suppression***
EENT: Tinnitus, hearing loss, blurred vision
Contraindications: Hypersensitivity, asthma, severe renal disease, severe hepatic disease, pregnancy (D)
Precautions: Lactation, children, bleeding disorders, GI disorders, cardiac disorders, hypersensitivity to other antiinflammatory agents
Pharmacokinetics:
PO: Peak 2 hr, half-life 3-3½ hr; metabolized in liver, excreted in urine (metabolites) excreted in breast milk, 98% protein binding
Interactions/incompatibilities:
- Increased action of: coumarin, phenytoin, sulfonamides when used with this drug

NURSING CONSIDERATIONS

Assess:
- Renal, liver, blood studies: BUN, creatinine, AST, ALT, Hgb, before treatment, periodically thereafter
- Audiometric, ophthalmic exam before, during, after treatment
- For past history of peptic ulcer disease

Administer:
- With food to decrease GI symptoms; best to take on empty stomach to facilitate absorption

Perform/provide:
- Storage at room temperature

Evaluate:
- Therapeutic response: decreased pain, stiffness, swelling in joints, ability to move more easily
- For eye, ear problems: blurred vision, tinnitus (may indicate toxicity)

Teach patient/family:
- To report blurred vision or ringing, roaring in ears (may indicate toxicity)
- To avoid driving or other hazardous activities if dizziness or drowsiness occurs
- To report change in urine pattern, weight increase, edema, pain increase in joints, fever, blood in urine (indicates nephrotoxicity)
- That therapeutic effects may take up to 1 mo
- To report black, tarry stools
- To take with full glass of water

P

phenylephrine HCl

(fen-ill-ef'rin)
Neo-Synephrine
Func. class.: Adrenergic, direct acting
Chem. class.: Substituted phenylethylamine

Action: Powerful and selective (α_1) receptor agonist causing contraction of blood vessels
Uses: Hypotension, paroxysmal supraventricular tachycardia, shock
Dosage and routes:
Hypotension
- *Adult:* SC/IM 2-5 mg, may repeat q10-15min if needed IV 0.1-

0.5 mg, may repeat q10-15min if needed

PVCs

• *Adult:* IV BOL 0.5 mg given rapidly, not to exceed prior dose by >0.1 mg total dose >1 mg

Shock

• *Adult:* IV INF 10 mg/500 ml D_5W given 100-180 gtts/min, then 40-60 gtts/min titrated to B/P

Available forms include: Inj IV, SC, IM, 1% (10 mg/ml)

Side effects/adverse reactions:

CNS: Headache, anxiety, tremor, insomnia, dizziness

CV: Palpitations, tachycardia, hypertension, ectopic beats, angina

GI: Nausea, vomiting

INTEG: Necrosis, tissue sloughing with extravasation, ***gangrene***

Contraindications: Hypersensitivity, ventricular fibrillation, tachydysrhythmias, pheochromocytoma

Precautions: Pregnancy (C), lactation, arterial embolism, peripheral vascular disease

Pharmacokinetics:

IV: Duration 20-30 min

IM/SC: Duration 45-60 min

Interactions/incompatibilities:

• Do not use within 2 wk of MAOIs, or hypertensive crisis may result

• Dysrhythmias: general anesthetics

• Decreased action of phenylephrine: α-blockers

• Increase in B/P: oxytocics

• Increased pressor effect: tricyclic antidepressant, MAOIs

• Incompatible with alkaline solutions: Na HCO_3

NURSING CONSIDERATIONS

Assess:

• I&O ratio, notify MD if output <30 cc/hr

• ECG during administration continuously; if B/P increases, drug is decreased

• B/P and pulse q5min after parenteral route

• CVP or PWP during infusion if possible

Administer:

• Plasma expanders for hypovolemia

• IV after diluting 1 mg/9 ml sterile H_2O for inj; give dose over ½-1 min; may be diluted 10 mg/500 ml of D_5W or NS; titrate to patient response, check for extravastion, check site for infiltration, use infusion pump

Perform/provide:

• Storage of reconstituted solution if refrigerated for no longer than 24 hr

• Elimination of discolored solutions

Evaluate:

• Therapeutic response: increase B/P with stabilization

• For paresthesias and coldness of extremities, peripheral blood flow may decrease

Teach patient/family:

• The reason for drug administration

• To report pain at infusion site immediately

Treatment of overdose: Administer an α-blocker

phenylephrine HCl (nasal)

(fen-ill-ef′rin)

Alconefrin, Coricidin Nasal Mist, Coryzine, Ephrine, Neo-Synephrine, Sinarest Nasal Spray, Sinophen Intranasal, Vacon

Func. class.: Nasal decongestant

Chem. class.: Sympathomimetic amine

Action: Produces vasoconstriction

(rapid, long-acting) of arterioles, thereby decreasing fluid exudation, mucosal engorgement

Uses: Nasal congestion

Dosage and routes:

• *Adult:* INSTILL 2-3 gtts or sprays to nasal mucosa bid (0.25%-1%); TOP apply to nasal mucosa q3-4h prn

• *Child 6-12 yr:* INSTILL 1-2 gtts or sprays (0.25%) q3-4h prn

• *Child <6 yr:* INSTILL 2-3 gtts or sprays (0.125%) q3-4h prn

Available forms include: Sol 0.125%, 0.16%, 0.2%, 0.25%, 0.5%, 1%; jelly 0.5%

Side effects/adverse reactions:

GI: Nausea, vomiting, anorexia

EENT: Irritation, burning, sneezing, stinging, dryness, rebound congestion

INTEG: Contact dermatitis

CNS: Anxiety, restlessness, tremors, weakness, insomnia, dizziness, fever, headache

Contraindications: Hypersensitivity to sympathomimetic amines

Precautions: Child <6 yr, elderly, diabetes, cardiovascular disease, hypertension, hyperthyroidism, increased ICP, prostatic hypertrophy, pregnancy (C), glaucoma

Interactions/incompatibilities:

• Hypertension: MAOIs, β-adrenergic blockers

• Hypotension: methyldopa, mecamylamine, reserpine

NURSING CONSIDERATIONS

Administer:

• No more than q4h

• For <4 consecutive days

Perform/provide:

• Environmental humidification to decrease nasal congestion, dryness

• Storage in light-resistant containers; do not expose to high temperatures

Evaluate:

• Therapeutic response: decreased nasal congestion

• Redness, swelling, pain in nasal passages

Teach patient/family:

• That stinging may occur for a few applications; drying of mucosa may be decreased by environmental humidification

• To notify physician if irregular pulse, insomnia, dizziness, or tremors occur

• Proper administration to avoid systemic absorption

---

phenylephrine HCl (optic)

(fen-ill-ef'rin)

AK-Dilate, Isopto Frin, Neo-Synephrine 10% Plain, Neo-Synephrine Viscous, Prefrin

Func. class.: Ophthalmic vasoconstrictor

Chem. class.: Direct sympathomimetic amine (α-agonist)

Action: Vasoconstriction of eye arterioles; decreases eye engorgement by stimulation of α-adrenergic receptors

Uses: Topical ocular vasoconstrictor

Dosage and routes:

Eye irritation

• *Adult:* INSTILL 2 gtts of a 0.12% sol; may repeat q3-4h

Uveitis/glaucoma/surgery

• *Adult and child:* INSTILL 1 gtt of a 2.5% or 10% sol in upper surface of cornea

Available forms include: Sol 10%, 2.5%, 0.12%

Side effects/adverse reactions:

CNS: Headache, dizziness, weakness

CV: Bradycardia, hypertension,

P

dysrhythmias, ***tachycardia, CV collapse,*** palpitation

EENT: Stinging, lacrimation, blurred vision, conjunctival allergy

Contraindications: Hypersensitivity, glaucoma (narrow-angle)

Precautions: Severe hypertension, diabetes, hyperthyroidism, elderly, severe arteriosclerosis, cardiac disease, infants, pregnancy (C)

Pharmacokinetics:

INSTILL: Peak 1 hr, duration 0.5-7 hr depending on strength

Interactions/incompatibilities:

• Increased pressor effects: MAOIs, tricyclic antidepressants, H_1 antihistamines, guanethedine

NURSING CONSIDERATIONS

Assess:

• B/P, pulse, systemic absorption does occur

Perform/provide:

• Storage in tight, light-resistant container, do not use discolored solutions

Evaluate:

• Therapeutic response: decreased eye irritation

Teach patient/family:

• To report change in vision, blurring, loss of sight; breathing trouble, sweating, flushing

• Method of instillation, tilt head backward, hold dropper over eye, drop medication inside lower lid, using pressure on inside corner of eye hold 1 min, do not touch dropper to eye

• That blurred vision will decrease with repeated use of drug

• To notify physician if headache, spots, redness, pain occurs; discontinue use

• To use sunglasses if photophobia occurs

• To use exactly as prescribed

phenytoin sodium/ phenytoin sodium extended/phenytoin sodium prompt

(fen'i-toy-in)

Dilantin, Dilantin Capsules, Di-Phen, Diphenylan

Func. class.: Anticonvulsant
Chem. class.: Hydantoin

Action: Inhibits spread of seizure activity in motor cortex

Uses: Generalized tonic-clonic seizures, status epilepticus, nonepileptic seizures associated with Reye's syndrome or after head trauma, migraines, trigeminal neuralgia, Bell's palsy, ventricular dysrhythmias uncontrolled by antidysrhythmics

Dosage and routes:

Seizures

• *Adult:* IV loading dose of 900 mg-1.5 g run at 50 mg/min; if patient has received phenytoin, then 100-300 mg run at 50 mg/min; PO loading dose of 900 mg-1.5 g divided tid, then 300 mg/day (extended) or divided tid (extended/prompt)

• *Child:* IV loading dose of 15 mg/kg run at 50 mg/min; if patient has received phenytoin, then 5-7 mg/kg run at 50 mg/min, may repeat in 30 min; PO loading dose of 15 mg/kg divided q8-12h, then 5-7 mg/kg in divided doses q12h

Neuritic pain

• *Adult:* PO 200-400 mg/day

Ventricular dysrhythmias

• *Adult:* PO loading dose 1 g divided over 24 hr, then 500 mg/day × 2 days; IV 250 mg given over 5 min, until dysrhythmias subside or 1 g is given, or 100 mg q15min until dysrhythmias subside or 1 g is given

• *Child:* PO 3-8 mg/kg or 250 mg/m^2/day as single dose or divided in 2 doses; IV 3-8 mg/kg given over several min, or 250 mg/m^2/day as single dose or divided in 2 doses

Available forms include: Susp 30, 125 mg/5 ml; tabs, chewable 50 mg; inj 50 mg/ml; caps ext 30, 100 mg; caps prompt 30, 100 mg

Side effects/adverse reactions:

HEMA: ***Agranulocytosis, leukopenia, aplastic anemia, thrombocytopenia, megloblastic anemia***

CV: Hypotension, ventricular fibrillation

CNS: Drowsiness, dizziness, insomnia, paresthesias, depression, suicidal tendencies, aggression, headache, confusion, slurred speech

GI: Nausea, vomiting, constipation, anorexia, weight loss, ***hepatitis,*** jaundice, ***gingival hyperplasia***

GU: Nephritis, albuminuria

INTEG: Rash, lupus erythematosus, ***Stevens-Johnson syndrome,*** hirsutism

EENT: Nystagmus, diplopia, blurred vision

Contraindications: Hypersensitivity, psychiatric condition, pregnancy (D), bradycardia, SA and AV block, Stokes-Adams syndrome

Precautions: Allergies, hepatic disease, renal disease

Pharmacokinetics:

PO: Duration 5 hr, metabolized by liver, excreted by kidneys

Interactions/incompatibilities:

• Decreased effects of phenytoin: alcohol (chronic use), antihistamines, antacids, antineoplastics, CNS depressants, rifampin, folic acid

NURSING CONSIDERATIONS

Assess:

• Drug level: toxic level 30-50 μg/ml

• Blood studies: CBC, platelets q2wk until stabilized, then qmo × 12, then q3mo; discontinue drug if neutrophils are <1600/mm^3

Administer:

• After diluting with normal saline, never water; inject slowly <50 mg/min, clear IV tubing first with NS sol, use in-line filter, discard 4 hr after preparation; inject into larger veins to prevent purple glove syndrome

Evaluate:

• Therapeutic response: decrease in severity of seizures, or ventricular dysrhythmias

• Mental status: mood, sensorium, affect, memory (long, short)

• Respiratory depression

• Blood dyscrasias: fever, sore throat, bruising, rash, jaundice

Teach patient/family:

• PO doses divided with or after meals to decrease adverse effects

• That urine may turn pink

• Not to discontinue drug abruptly, seizures may occur

• Proper brushing of teeth using a soft toothbrush, flossing to prevent gingival hyperplasia

• To avoid hazardous activities until stabilized on drug

• To carry Medic-Alert ID stating drug use

• That heavy use of alcohol may diminish effect of drug

• Not to change brands or forms once stabilized on therapy

Lab test interferences:

Decrease: Dexamethasone, metyrapone test, PBI, urinary steroids

Increase: Glucose, alk phosphatase, BSP

physostigmine salicylate/physostigmine sulfate

(fi-zoe-stig'meen)

Isopto Eserine Solution/Eserine Sulfate Ointment, Fisostin, Antilirium, Geneserine

Func. class.: Miotic

Chem. class.: Cholinesterase inhibitor

Action: Increases concentration of acetylcholine at cholinergic transmission sites, thus causing prolonged, exaggerated action; produces constriction of ciliary muscles, iris sphincter, causing iris to be pulled away from anterior chamber angle, aiding in aqueous humor drainage

Uses: Used in treatment of wide-angle glaucoma reversal of anticholinergic or antidepressant poisoning

Dosage and routes:

• *Adult and child:* INSTILL OINT ¼ inch strip of 0.25% oint in conjunctival sac; INSTILL SOL 1-2 gtts of a 0.25%-0.5% sol in conjunctival sac qd-qid

Available forms include: Oint 0.25% (sulfate); sol 0.25% (salicylate)

Side effects/adverse reactions:

CNS: ***Convulsions,*** headache

CV: Hypertension, hypotension, bradycardia, irregular pulse

GI: Nausea, vomiting, abdominal cramps

RESP: ***Bronchospasm,*** dyspnea, ***pulmonary edema***

EENT: Blurred vision, conjunctivitis, allergic reactions, rhinorrhea, salivation, eye, brow pain, lacrimation, twitching of eyelids

Contraindications: Asthma, bronchitis, diabetes mellitus, CV disease, inflammatory disease of iris or ciliary body

Precautions: Epilepsy, parkinsonism, bradycardia, pregnancy (C)

Interactions/incompatibilities:

• Benzalkonium chloride in solution or syringe

NURSING CONSIDERATIONS

Administer:

• Topically to conjunctival sac

• Immediately after reconstituting; discard unused portion

Perform/provide:

• Only clear solutions, never pink or brown

Evaluate

• Therapeutic response: decreased intraocular pressure

Teach patient/family:

• To report change in vision, blurring or loss of sight, trouble breathing, sweating, flushing

• Method of instillation, including pressure on lacrimal sac for 1 min, not to touch dropper to eye

• That long-term therapy may be required

• That blurred vision will decrease with repeated use of drug

• That drug is often irritating to eye, rarely tolerated for prolonged periods

• That drug may be prescribed for bedtime use to prevent nocturnal rise in ocular tension

• That maximal effect of topical application is reached in 30 min, may last 12-36 hr

• To observe eyes for irritation, development of cataracts

physostigmine salicylate

(fi-zoe-stig'meen)

Antilirium

Func. class.: Antidote, reversible anticholinesterase

Chem. class.: Tertiary amine

Action: Increases acetylcholine at

cholinergic nerve terminals, reverses central, peripheral anticholinergic effects

Uses: To reverse CNS effects of diazepam; anticholinergic, tricyclic antidepressant, Alzheimer's disease, hereditary ataxia

Dosage and routes:

Overdose of anticholinergics

• *Adult:* IM/IV 2 mg, give no more than 1 mg/min; may repeat

• *Pediatric:* IM/IV inj 0.02 mg/kg, not more than 0.5 mg/min; may repeat at 5-10 min intervals until max dose of 2 mg

Postanesthesia

• *Adult:* IM/IV 0.5-1 mg, give no more than 1 mg/min (IV); can repeat at 10 to 30 min intervals

Available forms include: Inj IM, IV 1 mg/ml

Side effects/adverse reactions:

INTEG: Rash, urticaria

CNS: Dizziness, headache, sweating, confusion, weakness, ***convulsions,*** incoordination, ***paralysis,*** hallucination, delirium

GI: Nausea, diarrhea, vomiting, cramps

CV: Bradycardia, hypotension

GU: Frequency, incontinence

RESP: ***Respiratory depression, bronchospasm, constriction***

EENT: Miosis, blurred vision, lacrimation

Contraindications: Hypotension, obstruction of intestine, renal system, asthma, gangrene, CV disease, choline esters, depolarizing neuromuscular blocking agents

Precautions: Seizure disorders, bronchial asthma, coronary occlusion, hyperthyroidism, dysrhythmias, peptic ulcer, megacolon, poor GI motility, pregnancy (C), Parkinson's disease, bradycardia, lactation

Pharmacokinetics:

IM/IV: Onset 5 min, duration 45-60 min; crosses blood-brain barrier, excreted in urine

Interactions/incompatibilities:

• Decreased action of: gallamine, metocurine, pancuronium, tubocurarine, atropine

• Increased action of: decamethonium, succinylcholine

• Decreased action of physostigmine: aminoglycosides, anesthetics, procainamide, quinidine

NURSING CONSIDERATIONS

Assess:

• VS; respiration q8h

• I&O ratio; check for urinary retention or incontinence

Administer:

• IV undiluted, give through Y-tube or 3-way stopcock; give 1 mg or less/1-3 min

• Only with atropine sulfate available for cholinergic crisis

• Only after all other cholinergics have been discontinued

• Increased doses if tolerance occurs

Perform/provide:

• Storage at room temperature

Evaluate:

• Therapeutic response: LOC—alert

• Drug should be discontinued if toxicity occurs

Treatment of overdose: Can cause cholinergic crisis; atropine is an antagonist

---

phytonadione (vitamin K_1)

(fye-toe-na-dye'one)

AquaMEPHYTON, Konakion, Mephyton

Func. class.: Vitamin K_1, fat-soluble vitamin

Action: Needed for adequate blood

P

clotting (factors II, VII, IX, X)

Uses: Vitamin K malabsorption, hypoprothrombinemia, prevention of hypoprothrombinemia caused by oral anticoagulants

Dosage and routes:

Hypoprothrombinemia caused by vitamin K malabsorption

- *Adult:* PO/IM 2-25 mg may repeat or increase to 50 mg
- *Child:* PO/IM 5-10 mg
- *Infants:* PO/IM 2 mg

Prevention of hemorrhagic disease of the newborn

- *Neonate:* SC/IM 0.5-1 mg after birth, repeat in 6-8 hr if required

Hypoprothrombinemia caused by oral anticoagulants

- *Adult:* PO/SC/IM 2.5-10 mg, may repeat 12-48 hr after PO dose or 6-8 hr after SC/IM dose, based on PT

Available forms include: Tabs 5 mg; inj aqueous colloidal IM, IV; inj aqueous dispersion 2, 10 mg/ml, IM only

Side effects/adverse reactions:

CNS: Headache, ***brain damage*** (large doses)

GI: Nausea, decrease liver function tests

HEMA: ***Hemolytic anemia, hemoglobinuria, hyperbilirubinemia***

INTEG: Rash, urticaria

Contraindications: Hypersensitivity, severe hepatic disease, last few weeks of pregnancy

Precautions: Pregnancy (C), neonates

Pharmacokinetics:

PO/INJ: Metabolized, crosses placenta

Interactions/incompatibilities:

- Decreased action of phytonadione: cholestyramine, mineral oil
- Decreased action of: oral anticoagulants

NURSING CONSIDERATIONS

Assess:

- Pro-time during treatment (2 sec deviation from control time, bleeding time, and clotting time)

Administer:

- IV after diluting with D_5 NS or NS 10 ml or more; give 1 mg/min or more
- IV only when other routes not possible (deaths have occurred)

Perform/provide

- Storage in tight, light-resistant container

Evaluate:

- Therapeutic response: decreased bleeding tendencies, decreased pro-time, decreased clotting time
- Nutritional status: liver (beef), spinach, tomatoes, coffee, asparagus, broccoli, cabbage, lettuce, greens

Teach patient/family

- Not to take other supplements, unless directed by physician
- Necessary foods to be included in diet

---

pilocarpine HCl/pilocarpine nitrate

(pye-loe-kar'peen)

Adsorbocarpine, Akarpine, Almocarpine, Isopto Carpine, Miocarpine,* Ocusert Pilo, Pilocar, Pilocel, Pilomiotin, P.V. Carpine Liquifilm

Func. class.: Miotic, direct-acting

Chem. class.: Cholinergic agonist

Action: Acts directly on cholinergic receptor sites, induces miosis, spasm of accommodation, fall in intraocular pressure, caused by stimulation of ciliary, pupillary sphincter muscles, which leads to pulling away of iris from filtration angle, resulting in increased outflow of aqueous humor

---

* Available in Canada only

Uses: Primary glaucoma, early stages of wide-angle glaucoma (less useful in advanced stages), chronic open-angle glaucoma, acute narrow-angle glaucoma before emergency surgery; also used to neutralize mydriatics used during eye exam; may be used alternately with mydriatics to break adhesions between iris and lens

Dosage and routes:

• *Adult and child:* INSTILL SOL 1-2 gtts of 1% or 2% solution in eye q6-8h; INSTILL 20-40 μg/hr (Ocusert) in cul-de-sac of eye

Available forms include: 0.25% to 10% sol; Ocusert Pilo 20, 40

Side effects/adverse reactions:

CV: Hypotension, tachycardia

RESP: ***Bronchospasm***

GI: Nausea, vomiting, abdominal cramps, diarrhea

EENT: Blurred vision, browache, twitching of eyelids, eye pain with change in focus

Contraindications: Bradycardia, hyperthyroidism, coronary artery disease, obstruction of GI/urinary tracts (or if strength of walls of these structures in question, peptic ulcers), epilepsy, parkinsonism, asthma

Precautions: Bronchial asthma, hypertension, pregnancy (C)

NURSING CONSIDERATIONS

Assess:

• Heart rate, respiratory status, B/P

• Replacement of ocular systems qwk; check system each hs, AM

Administer:

• After shaking vial to mix drug to clear solution, push stopper to mix sterile water with powder

• After cleaning stopper with alcohol

• Excess solution must be wiped away promptly to prevent its flow into lacrimal system, producing systemic symptoms

• Atropine should be readily available as antidote

• Immediately after reconstituting; discard unused portion

Perform/provide:

• Protect solution from light

• Store Ocusert systems between 2° and 8° C

Evaluate:

• Therapeutic response: decreased intraocular pressure

Teach patient/family:

• To report change in vision, blurring or loss of sight, trouble breathing, sweating, flushing

• Method of instillation, including pressure on lacrimal sac for 1 min, not to touch dropper to eye

• That long-term therapy may be required

• That blurred vision will decrease with repeated use of drug

• To discontinue use if local hypersensitivity reaction occurs

• That acuity in dim light will be reduced

• Not to drive while using drug

pinacidil

(pye-na'di-dil)

Pindac

Func. class.: Antihypertensive

Chem. class.: Vasodilator—peripheral

Action: Directly relaxes arteriolar smooth muscle, causing vasodilation

Uses: Severe hypertension not responsive to other therapy; topically to treat alopecia

Dosage and routes:

• *Adult:* PO 12.5-25 mg bid

Available forms include: Tabs 12.5, 25 mg

Side effects/adverse reactions:
CV: Severe rebound hypertension, tachycardia, angina, increased T wave, ***CHF***, pulmonary edema, edema, sodium, water retention
CNS: Drowsiness, dizziness, sedation, headache, depression
GI: Nausea, vomiting, diarrhea, constipation, dry mouth
GU: Gynecomastia, breast tenderness
INTEG: Pruritus, ***Stevens-Johnson syndrome***, rash, hirsutism

Contraindications: Acute myocardial infarction, dissecting aortic aneurysm, hypersensitivity, pheochromocytoma

Precautions: Pregnancy (C), lactation, children, renal disease, CAD, post MI

Pharmacokinetics:
Peak 1 hr, 60% protein bound, metabolized in the liver, excreted in urine/feces (active metabolites), half-life 1½-3 hr

Interactions/incompatibilities:
- Orthostatic hypotension: guanethidine
- Reduced effect of pinacidil: nonsteroidal antiinflammatory drugs

NURSING CONSIDERATIONS

Assess:
- Electrolytes: K, Na, Cl, CO_2
- Renal function studies: AST, ALT, alk phosphatase
- B/P, pulse
- Weight daily, I&O, nausea

Administer:
- With meals for better absorption, to decrease GI symptoms
- With β-blocker and/or diuretic

Evaluate:
- Therapeutic response: decreased B/P or increased hair growth
- Edema in feet, legs daily
- Skin turgor, dryness of mucous membranes for hydration status
- Rales, dyspnea, orthopnea

Teach patient/family:
- That body hair will increase, but is reversible after treatment is discontinued
- Not to discontinue drug abruptly
- To report pitting edema, dizziness, weight gain >5 lb, shortness of breath, bruising or bleeding, heart rate >20 beats/min over normal, severe indigestion, dizziness, light-headedness, panting, new or aggravated symptoms of angina
- To take drug exactly as prescribed or serious side effects may occur

Lab test interferences:
Increase: Renal function studies
Decrease: Hgb/Hct/RBC

Treatment of overdose: Administer normal saline IV, phenylephrine, angiotensin II, vasopressor, dopamine may reverse hypotension

---

pindolol

(pin'doe-lole)
Visken

Func. class.: Antihypertensive
Chem. class.: Nonselective β-blocker

Action: Competitively blocks stimulation of β-adrenergic receptor within vascular smooth muscle; produces chronotropic, inotropic activity (decreases rate of SA node discharge, increases recovery time), slows conduction of AV node, decreases heart rate, which decreases O_2 consumption in myocardium; also, decreases renin-aldosterone-angiotensin system, at high doses inhibits β-2 receptors in bronchial system

Uses: Mild to moderate hypertension

Dosage and routes:
- *Adult:* PO 5 mg bid, usual dose

15 mg/day (5 mg tid), may increase by 10 mg/day q3-4wk to a max of 60 mg/day

Available forms include: Tabs 5, 10 mg

Side effects/adverse reactions:

CV: Hypotension, bradycardia, ***CHF,*** edema, chest pain, palpitation, claudication, tachycardia, ***AV block***

CNS: Insomnia, dizziness, hallucinations, anxiety, fatigue

GI: Nausea, vomiting, ***ischemic colitis,*** diarrhea, *abdominal pain,* ***mesenteric arterial thrombosis***

INTEG: Rash, alopecia, pruritus, fever

HEMA: ***Agranulocytosis, thrombocytopenia, purpura***

EENT: Visual changes, sore throat, *double vision,* dry burning eyes

GU: Impotence, frequency

RESP: ***Bronchospasm,*** *dyspnea,* cough, rales

MISC: Joint pain, muscle pain

Contraindications: Hypersensitivity to β-blockers, cardiogenic shock, heart block (2nd, 3rd degree), sinus bradycardia, CHF, cardiac failure, bronchial asthma

Precautions: Major surgery, pregnancy (B), lactation, diabetes mellitus, renal disease, thyroid disease, COPD, well-compensated heart failure, CAD, nonallergic bronchospasm

Pharmacokinetics:

PO: Peak 2-4 hr; half-life 3-4 hr, excreted 30%-45% unchanged, 60%-65% is metabolized by liver, excreted in breast milk

Interactions/incompatibilities:

- Increased hypotension, bradycardia: reserpine, hydralazine, methyldopa, prazosin, anticholinergics
- Decreased antihypertensive effects: indomethacin, sympathomimetics
- Increased hypoglycemic effect: insulin
- Decreased bronchodilation: theophyllines

NURSING CONSIDERATIONS

Assess:

- I&O, weight daily
- B/P during initial treatment, periodically thereafter; pulse q4h, note rate, rhythm, quality
- Apical/radial pulse before administration; notify physician of any significant changes
- Baselines in renal, liver function tests before therapy begins

Adminster:

- PO ac, hs, tablet may be crushed or swallowed whole
- Reduced dosage in renal dysfunction

Perform/provide:

- Storage in dry area at room temperature, do not freeze

Evaluate:

- Therapeutic response: decreased B/P after 1-2 wk
- Edema in feet, legs daily
- Skin turgor, dryness of mucous membranes for hydration status

Teach patient/family:

- To take with or immediately after meals
- Not to discontinue drug abruptly, taper over 2 wk, may cause precipitate angina
- Not to use OTC products containing α-adrenergic stimulants (nasal decongestants, OTC cold preparations) unless directed by physician
- To report bradycardia, dizziness, confusion, depression, fever, sore throat, shortness of breath to physician
- To take pulse at home, advise when to notify physician
- To avoid alcohol, smoking, sodium intake

• To comply with weight control, dietary adjustments, modified exercise program
• To carry Medic Alert ID to identify drug you are taking, allergies
• To avoid hazardous activities if dizziness if present
• To report symptoms of CHF: difficult breathing, especially on exertion or when lying down, night cough, swelling of extremities
• To take medication at bedtime to prevent orthostatic hypotension
• To wear support hose to minimize effects of orthostatic hypotension

Lab test interferences:
Increase: Liver function tests, renal function tests

Treatment of overdose: Lavage, IV atropine for bradycardia, IV theophylline for bronchospasm, digitalis, O_2, diuretic for cardiac failure, hemodialysis, hypotension; give vasopressor (norepinephrine)

pipecuronium bromide

Arduran

Func. class.: Neuromuscular blocker (nondepolarizing)
Chem. class.: Synthetic curariform

Action: Inhibits transmission of nerve impulses by binding with cholinergic receptor sites, antagonizing action of acetylcholine

Uses: Facilitation of endotracheal intubation, skeletal muscle relaxation during mechanical ventilation, surgery, or general anesthesia

Dosage and routes: Dosage is individualized; in patients with normal renal function who are not obese, initial dose is 70-85 μg/kg; maintenance dose ranges from 10-15 μg/kg

Available forms include: Inj IV 10-mg vials

Side effects/adverse reactions:
CV: Bradycardia, tachycardia, increased or decreased B/P, ventricular extrasystole, ***myocardial ischemia, cardiovascular accident, thrombosis, atrial fibrillation***
RESP: ***Prolonged apnea, bronchospasm, cyanosis, respiratory depression***
GU: ***Anuria***
EENT: Increased secretions
CNS: Hypesthesia, CNS depression
MS: Weakness to prolonged skeletal muscle relaxation
INTEG: Rash, urticaria
METABOLIC: Hypoglycemia, hyperkalemia, increased creatinine

Contraindications: Hypersensitivity to bromide ion

Precautions: Pregnancy (C), renal disease, cardiac disease, lactation, children <3 mo, fluid and electrolyte imbalances, neuromuscular diseases, respiratory disease, obesity

Pharmacokinetics:
IV: Onset 30-45 sec, peak 3-5 min: metabolized (small amounts), excreted in urine (unchanged), crosses placenta

Interactions/incompatibilities:
• Increased neuromuscular blockade: aminoglycosides, quinidine, local anesthetics, polymyxin antibiotics, enflurane, isoflurane, tetracyclines, halothane, magnesium, colistin

NURSING CONSIDERATIONS

Assess:
• For electrolyte imbalances (K, Mg); may lead to increased action of this drug
• Vital signs (B/P, pulse, respirations, airway) until fully recovered: rate, depth, pattern of respirations, strength of hand grip
• I&O ratio; check for urinary retention, frequency, hesitancy

Administer:
- Using nerve stimulator by anesthesiologist to determine neuromuscular blockade
- Atropine to counteract muscarinic effects
- After succinylcholine effects subside
- Anticholinesterase to reverse neuromuscular blockade
- By slow IV over 1-2 min (only by qualified persons, usually an anesthesiologist)
- Only fresh solution

Perform/provide:
- Storage in refrigerator; do not store in plastic containers or syringes
- Reassurance if communication is difficult during recovery from neuromuscular blockade
- Use reconstituted solution within 24 hr
- Frequent (q2h) instillation of artificial tears and covering eyes to prevent drying of cornea

Evaluate:
- Therapeutic response: paralysis of jaw, eyelid, head, neck, rest of body
- Recovery: decreased paralysis of face, diaphragm, leg, arm, rest of body
- Allergic reactions: rash, fever, respiratory distress, pruritus; drug should be discontinued

Treatment of overdose: Neostigmine, atropine, monitor VS; may require mechanical ventilation

---

piperacillin sodium

(pi-per'a-sill-in)

Pipracil

Func. class.: Broad-spectrum antibiotic

Chem. class.: Extended-spectrum penicillin

Action: Interferes with cell wall replication of susceptible organisms; osmotically unstable cell wall swells and bursts from osmotic pressure

Uses: Respiratory, skin, urinary tract, bone infections, gonorrhea, pneumonia; effective for gram-positive cocci *(S. aureus, S. pyogenes, S. viridans, S. faecalis, S. bovis, S. pneumoniae)*, gram-negative cocci *(N. gonorrhoeae, N. meningitidis)*, gram-positive bacilli, *C. perfringens, C. tetani*, gram-negative bacilli *(Bacteroides, F. nucleatum, E. coli, Klebsiella, P. mirabilis, M. morganii, P. vulgaris, P. rehgesii, Enterobacter, Citrobacter, P. aeruginosa, Serratia, Acinetobacter, Peptococcus, Peptostreptococcus, Eubacterium)*

Dosage and routes:

Systemic infections
- *Adult and child >12 yr:* IM/IV 100-300 mg/kg/day in divided doses q4-6h

Prophylaxis of surgical infections
- *Adult:* IV 2g ½-1 hr before procedure, may be repeated during surgery or after surgery

Available forms include: Inj IM, IV 2, 3, 4, 40 g; IV INF 2, 3, 4 g

Side effects/adverse reactions:

HEMA: Anemia, increased bleeding time, ***bone marrow depression***

GI: Nausea, vomiting, diarrhea, increased AST, ALT, abdominal pain, glossitis, colitis

GU: ***Oliguria, proteinuria, hematuria,*** *vaginitis, moniliasis,* ***glomerulonephritis***

CNS: Lethargy, hallucinations, anxiety, depression, twitching, ***coma, convulsions***

META: Hypokalemia, hypernatremia

Contraindications: Hypersensitivity to penicillins; neonates

Precautions: Pregnancy (B),

P

hypersensitivity to cephalosporins, CHF

Pharmacokinetics:

IM: Peak 30-50 min

IV: Peak 20-30 min

Half-life 0.7-1.33 hr, excreted in urine, bile, breast milk, crosses placenta

Interactions/incompatibilities:

• Decreased antimicrobial effect of piperacillin: tetracyclines, erythromycins, aminoglycosides IV

• Increased piperacillin concentrations: aspirin, probenecid

NURSING CONSIDERATIONS

Assess:

• I&O ratio; report hematuria, oliguria since penicillin in high doses is nephrotoxic

• Any patient with compromised renal system since drug is excreted slowly in poor renal system function; toxicity may occur rapidly

• Liver studies: AST, ALT

• Blood studies: WBC, RBC, H&H, bleeding time

• Renal studies: urinalysis, protein, blood

• C&S before drug therapy; drug may be taken as soon as culture is taken

Administer:

• IV after diluting 1 g/5 ml or more sterile H_2O or 0.9% NaCl, shake, give dose over 3-5 min; may further dilute with D_5W, 0.9% NS, and give over ½ hr; discontinue primary IV

• Drug after C&S has been completed

Perform/provide:

• Adrenalin, suction, tracheostomy set, endotracheal intubation equipment on unit

• Adequate intake of fluids (2000 ml) during diarrhea episodes

• Scratch test to assess allergy, after securing order from physician; usually done when penicillin is only drug of choice

• Storage at room temperature, reconstituted solution for 24 hr or 7 days refrigerated

Evaluate:

• Therapeutic response: absence of fever, purulent drainage, redness, inflammation

• Bowel pattern before and during treatment

• Skin eruptions after administration of penicillin to 1 wk after discontinuing drug

• Respiratory status: rate, character, wheezing, tightness in chest

• Allergies before initiation of treatment, reaction of each medication; highlight allergies on chart, Kardex

Teach patient/family:

• That culture may be taken after completed course of medication

• To report sore throat, fever, fatigue; (could indicate superimposed infection)

• To wear or carry Medic Alert ID if allergic to penicillins

• To notify nurse of diarrhea

Lab test interferences:

False positive: Urine glucose, urine protein, Coombs' test

Treatment of overdose: Withdraw drug, maintain airway, administer epinephrine, aminophylline, O_2, IV corticosteroids for anaphylaxis

piperazine adipate/ piperazine citrate

(pi'per-a-zeen)

Antepar, Bryrol, Entacyl,* Pin-Tega Tabs, Ta-Verm, Vermizine

Func. class.: Anthelmintic

Action: Causes paralysis in worm, leading to expulsion

Uses: Pinworm, roundworm

* Available in Canada only

Dosage and routes:

Pinworm

• *Adult and child:* PO 65 mg/kg × 7-8 days, not to exceed 2.5 g/day

Roundworm

• *Adult:* PO 3.5 g in single dose × 2 days

• *Child:* PO 75 mg/kg/day in a single dose × 2 days

Available forms include: Tabs 250, 500 mg; syr 500 mg/5 ml; powder, oral sol 500 mg

Side effects/adverse reactions:

HEMA: ***Hemolytic anemia***

INTEG: Rash, uriticaria, photosensitivity

RESP: ***Bronchospasm***

CNS: Dizziness, headache, paresthesia, convulsions, fever

EENT: Blurred vision, nystagmus, strabismus, cataracts, rhinorrhea

GI: Nausea, vomiting, anorexia, diarrhea, abdominal cramps

Contraindications: Hypersensitivity, renal disease, hepatic disease, seizures

Precautions: Severe malnutrition, seizure disorders, anemia, pregnancy (B)

Pharmacokinetics:

PO: Excreted in urine (unchanged)

Interactions/incompatibilities:

• Increased extrapyramidal symptoms: phenothiazines

NURSING CONSIDERATIONS

Assess:

• Stools during entire treatment, 1, 3 mo after treatment; specimens must be sent to lab while still warm

Administer:

• May be crushed or chewed if unable to swallow whole

• Laxatives if constipated; not needed for drug to work

• Second course after 1 wk off drug, if infection is severe

Perform/provide:

• Storage in tight container at room temperature

Evaluate:

• Therapeutic response: expulsion of worms, 3 negative stool cultures after completion of treatment

• For allergic reaction: rash, itching, urticaria

• For infection in other family members since infection from person to person is common

Teach patient/family:

• Proper hygiene after BM including handwashing technique, tell patient to avoid putting fingers in mouth

• That infected person should sleep alone; do not shake bed linen; change bed linen daily, wash in hot water

• To clean toilet qd with disinfectant (green soap solution)

• Need for compliance with dosage schedule and duration of treatment

• That urine may turn orange or red

• To avoid hazardous activities since drowsiness occurs

• That seizures may recur in patient who is controlled on medication

Lab test interferences:

Decrease: Serum uric acid

P

pirbuterol acetate

(purr-byoo'-ter-ole)

Maxair

Func. class.: Bronchodilator

Chem. class.: β-Adrenergic agonist

Action: Causes bronchodilation with little effect on heart rate by action on β-receptors, causing increased cAMP and relaxation of smooth muscle

Uses: Reversible bronchospasm (prevention, treatment) including asthma; may be given with theophylline or steroids

Dosage and routes:
- *Adult and child >12 yr:* Aerosol 1-2 inh (0.4 mg) q4-6h; do not exceed 12 inh/day

Available forms include: Aerosol delivers 0.2 mg pirbuterol/actuation

Side effects/adverse reactions:
CNS: Tremors, anxiety, insomnia, headache, dizziness, stimulation, restlessness, hallucinations, drowsiness, irritability
EENT: Dry nose, irritation of nose, throat
CV: Palpitations, tachycardia, hypertension, angina, hypotension, dysrhythmias
GI: Heartburn, nausea, vomiting, anorexia
MS: Muscle cramps
RESP: ***Bronchospasm,*** dyspnea, coughing

Contraindications: Hypersensitivity to sympathomimetics, tachycardia

Precautions: Lactation, pregnancy (C), cardiac disorders, hyperthyroidism, diabetes mellitus, prostatic hypertrophy

Pharmacokinetics:
INH: Onset 3 min, peak ½-1 hr, duration 5 hr

Interactions/incompatibilities:
- Increased action of: other aerosol bronchodilators
- Increased action of pirbuterol: tricyclic antidepressants, antihistamines, sodium levothyroxine
- Decreased action of pirbuterol: β-blockers
- Increased dysrhythmias: halogenated hydrocarbon anesthetics

NURSING CONSIDERATIONS

Assess:
- Respiratory function: vital capacity, forced expiratory volume, ABGs, B/P

Administer:
- After shaking, exhale, place mouthpiece in mouth, inhale slowly, hold breath, remove, exhale slowly
- Gum, sips of water for dry mouth

Perform/provide:
- Storage in light-resistant container, do not expose to temperatures over 86° F

Evaluate:
Therapeutic response: absence of dyspnea, wheezing over 1 hr

Teach patient/family:
- Not to use OTC medications; extra stimulation may occur
- Use of inhaler, review package insert with patient
- To avoid getting aerosol in eyes
- To wash inhaler in warm water and dry qd, rinse mouth after use; if used with inhalers containing glucocorticosteroids, wait 5 min before using steroid inhaler
- On all aspects of drug; avoid smoking, smoke-filled rooms, persons with respiratory infections
- To keep fluid intake >2 L/day to liquefy thick secretions

Treatment of overdose: Administer a β-adrenergic blocker

---

piroxicam

(peer-ox'i-kam)
Feldene
Func. class.: Nonsteroidal antiinflammatory
Chem. class.: Oxicam derivative

Action: Inhibits prostaglandin synthesis by decreasing an enzyme needed for biosynthesis; possesses analgesic, antiinflammatory, antipyretic properties

Uses: Mild to moderate pain, osteoarthritis, rheumatoid arthritis

* Available in Canada only

Dosage and routes:

• *Adult:* PO 20 qd or 10 mg bid

Available forms include: Caps 10, 20 mg

Side effects/adverse reactions:

GI: Nausea, anorexia, vomiting, diarrhea, jaundice, ***cholestatic hepatitis,*** constipation, flatulence, cramps, dry mouth, peptic ulcer

CNS: Dizziness, *drowsiness,* fatigue, tremors, confusion, insomnia, anxiety, depression, *headache*

CV: Tachycardia, peripheral edema, palpitations, dysrhythmias

INTEG: Purpura, rash, pruritus, sweating

GU: ***Nephrotoxicity: dysuria, hematuria, oliguria, azotemia***

HEMA: ***Blood dyscrasias***

EENT: Tinnitus, hearing loss, blurred vision

Contraindications: Hypersensitivity, asthma, severe renal disease, severe hepatic disease

Precautions: Pregnancy (C), lactation, children, bleeding disorders, GI disorders, cardiac disorders, hypersensitivity to other antiinflammatory agents

Pharmacokinetics:

PO: Peak 2 hr, half-life 3-3½ hr; metabolized in liver, excreted in urine (metabolites) excreted in breast milk; 99% protein binding

Interactions/incompatibilities:

• Increased action of: coumarin, phenytoin, sulfonamides

NURSING CONSIDERATIONS

Assess:

• Renal, liver, blood studies: BUN, creatinine, AST, ALT, Hgb, before treatment, periodically thereafter

• Audiometric, ophthalmic exam before, during, after treatment

Administer:

• With food to decrease GI symptoms; best to take on empty stomach to facilitate absorption

Perform/provide:

• Storage at room temperature

Evaluate:

• Therapeutic response: decreased pain, stiffness, swelling in joints, ability to move more easily

• For eye, ear problems: blurred vision, tinnitus (may indicate toxicity)

Teach patient/family:

• To report blurred vision or ringing, roaring in ears (may indicate toxicity)

• To avoid driving or other hazardous activities if dizziness or drowsiness occurs

• To report change in urine pattern, weight increase, edema, pain increase in joints, fever, blood in urine (indicates nephrotoxicity)

• That therapeutic effects may take up to 1 mo

plasma protein fraction

Plasmanate, Plasma Plex, Plasmatein, PPF Protenate

Func. class.: Blood derivative

Chem. class.: Human plasma in NaCl

Action: Exerts similar oncotic pressure as human plasma, expands blood volume

Uses: Hypovolemic, shock, hypoproteinemia

Dosage and routes:

Shock

• *Adult:* IV INF 250-500 ml (12.5-25 g protein), not to exceed 10 ml/min

• *Child:* IV INF 22-33 ml/kg at 5-10 ml/min

Hypoproteinemia

• *Adult:* IV INF 1000-1500 ml qd, not to exceed 8 ml/min

Available forms include: Inj IV 50 mg/ml

P

Side effects/adverse reactions:
GI: Nausea, vomiting, increased salivation
INTEG: Rash, urticaria, cyanosis
CNS: Fever, chills, headache, paresthesias, flushing
RESP: Altered respirations, dyspnea, pulmonary edema
CV: Fluid overload, hypotension, erratic pulse
Contraindications: Hypersensitivity, CHF, severe anemia
Precautions: Decreased salt intake, decreased cardiac reserve, lack of albumin deficiency, hepatic disease, renal disease, pregnancy (C)
Pharmacokinetics:
Metabolized as a protein/energy source
Interactions/incompatibilities:
• Incompatible with solution containing alcohol or norepinephrine

NURSING CONSIDERATIONS

Assess:
• Blood studies: Hct, Hgb; if serum protein declines, dyspnea, hypoxemia can result
• B/P (decreased), pulse (erratic), respiration during infusion
• I&O ratio; urinary output may decrease
• CVP, pulmonary wedge pressure (increases if overload occurs)
Administer:
• No dilution required; use infusion pump, use large-gauge needle (20G or >), discard unused portion, infuse slowly
• Within 4 hr of opening
Perform/provide:
• Adequate hydration before administration
• Storage—check type of albumin, date; may need to refrigerate
Evaluate:
• Therapeutic repsonse: increased B/P, decrease edema, increased serum albumin
• Allergy: fever, rash, itching, chills, flushing, urticaria, nausea, vomiting, or hypotension requires discontinuation of infusion; use new lot if therapy reinstituted
• Increased CVP reading: distended neck veins indicate circulatory overload; SOB, anxiety, insomnia, expiratory rales, frothy blood-tinged cough, cyanosis indicate pulmonary overload
Lab test interferences:
False increase: Alk phosphatase

---

plicamycin (mithramycin)

(plik-a-mi'cin)
Mithracin
Func. class.: Antineoplastic, antibiotic
Chem. class.: Crystalline aglycone

Action: Inhibits DNA, RNA, protein synthesis; derived from *Streptomyces plicatus;* replication is decreased by binding to DNA; demonstrates calcium-lowering effect not related to its tumoricidal activity; also acts on osteoclasts and blocks action of parathyroid hormone; a vesicant
Uses: Testicular cancer, hypercalcemia, hypercalciuria, symptomatic treatment of advanced neoplasms
Dosage and routes:
Testicular tumors
• *Adult:* IV 25-30 μg/kg/day × 8-10 days, not to exceed 30 μg/kg/day
Hypercalcemia/hypercalciuria
• *Adult:* IV 25 μg/kg/day × 3-4 days, repeat at intervals of 1 wk
Available forms include: Inj IV 2.5 mg

* Available in Canada only

Side effects/adverse reactions:
META: Decreased serum calcium, phosphorus, potassium
HEMA: ***Hemorrhage, thrombocytopenia,*** decreased pro-time, WBC count
GI: Nausea, vomiting, anorexia, diarrhea, stomatitis, increased liver enzymes
GU: Increased BUN, creatinine, ***proteinuria***
INTEG: Rash, cellulitis, ***extravasation,*** facial flushing
CNS: Drowsiness, weakness, lethargy, headache, flushing, fever, depression
Contraindications: Hypersensitivity, thrombocytopenia, bone marrow depression, bleeding disorders, pregnancy (X)
Precautions: Renal disease, hepatic disease, electrolyte imbalances
Pharmacokinetics: Crosses blood-brain barrier, excreted in urine; little known about pharmacokinetics
Interactions/incompatibilities:
- Increased toxicity: other antineoplastics or radiation

NURSING CONSIDERATIONS

Assess:
- CBC, differential, platelet count weekly; withhold drug if WBC is <4000/mm³ or platelet count is <50,000/mm³; notify physician of results
- Renal function studies: BUN, serum uric acid, urine CrCl, electrolytes before, during therapy
- I&O ratio; report fall in urine output to <30 ml/hr
- Monitor temperature q4h; fever may indicate beginning infection
- Liver function tests before, during therapy: bilirubin, AST, ALT, alk phosphatase prn or monthly

Administer:
- IV dilute 2.5 mg/4.9 ml of sterile H_2O; dilute single dose in 1000 ml of D_5W run over 4-6 hr
- EDTA for extravasation, apply ice compress
- Antiemetic 30-60 min before giving drug and 4-10 hr after treatment to prevent vomiting
- Slow IV infusion using 20-, 21-gauge needle
- Transfusion for anemia
- Antispasmodic for diarrhea, phenothiazine for nausea and vomiting

Perform/provide:
- Liquid diet: carbonated beverages, gelatin may be added if patient is not nauseated or vomiting
- Rinsing of mouth tid-qid with water; brushing of teeth with baking soda bid-tid with soft brush or cotton-tipped applicators for stomatitis; use unwaxed dental floss
- Usage immediately after mixing

Evaluate:
- Therapeutic response: decreased tumor size, spread of malignancy
- Alkalosis if severe vomiting is present
- Toxicity: facial flushing, epistaxis, increased pro-time, thrombocytopenia; drug should be discontinued
- Bleeding: hematuria, guaiac stools, bruising or petechiae, mucosa or orifices q8h
- Food preferences; list likes, dislikes
- Inflammation of mucosa, breaks in skin
- Yellowing of skin, sclera, dark urine, clay-colored stools, itchy skin, abdominal pain, fever, diarrhea
- Buccal cavity q8h for dryness, sores, ulceration, white patches, oral pain, bleeding, dysphagia
- Local irritation, pain, burning at injection site

- Frequency of stools, characteristics, cramping
- Acidosis, signs of dehydration: rapid respirations, poor skin turgor, decreased urine output, dry skin, restlessness, weakness

Teach patient/family:

- To report any complaints or side effects to nurse or physician
- To avoid foods with citric acid, hot or rough texture
- To report to physician any bleeding, white spots, ulcerations in the mouth; tell patient to examine mouth qd
- To avoid driving or activities requiring alertness; drowsiness may occur
- To report leg cramps, tingling of fingertips, weakness; may indicate hypocalcemia
- To avoid crowds or persons with infections when granulocyte count is low

---

podophyllum resin

(poe-doe-fil' um)

Podoben, Podofilm*

Func. class.: Keratolytic

Chem. class.: Podophyllum derivative

Action: Arrests mitosis by binding to tubulin, protein subunit of spindle microtubules; also interferes with movements of chromosomes

Uses: Venereal warts, keratoses, multiple superficial, epitheliomatoses

Dosage and routes:

Warts

- *Adult:* TOP cover wart, cover with wax paper, bandage for 4-6 hr, wash, may repeat qwk if needed

Keratoses/epitheliomatoses

- *Adult:* TOP apply qd with applicator, let dry, remove tissue, may reapply if needed

Available forms include: Sol 11.5%, 25%

Side effects/adverse reactions:

HEMA: ***Thrombocytopenia, leukopenia***

INTEG: Irritation of unaffected areas

CNS: Peripheral neuropathy

Contraindications: Hypersensitivity, pregnancy (X)

Interactions/incompatibilities:

- Necrosis of skin: when used with other keratolytic

NURSING CONSIDERATIONS

Assess:

- Platelets, WBC if systemic absorption occurs

Administer:

- Only to affected area, cover normal skin with petrolatum for protection; do not apply to broken or inflamed skin
- Only to small areas or for short periods of time or absorption (systemic) may occur

Evaluate:

- Therapeutic response: decrease in size and amount of lesions
- Allergic reactions: irritation, redness, itching, stinging, burning; drug should be discontinued
- Blood dyscrasias if systemic absorption is suspected: decrease platelets
- CNS toxicity: peripheral neuropathy; drug should be discontinued

Teach patient/family:

- That discomfort will begin after 24 hr, subside in 2-4 days
- To use soap and water to clean area and remove drug

---

* Available in Canada only

Poliovirus vaccine, live, oral, trivalent

Orimune

Func. class.: Vaccine

Action: Produces specific antibodies for poliomyelitis

Uses: Prevention of polio

Dosage and routes:

• *Adult and child >2 yr:* PO 0.5 ml, given q8wk × 2 doses, then 0.5 ml ½-1 yr after dose 2

• *Infant:* PO 0.5 ml at 2, 4, 18 mo

Available forms include: Oral vaccine

Side effects/adverse reactions:

SYST: ***Paralysis***

Contraindications: Hypersensitivity, active infection, allergy to neomycin/streptomycin, immunosuppression, vomiting or diarrhea

Precautions: Pregnancy

Interactions/incompatibilities:

• Do not use TB skin test or other live virus vaccines within 6 wk of vaccine

• Do not use within 3 mo of transfusion of whole blood, plasma, or use with immune serum globulin

NURSING CONSIDERATIONS

Administer:

• Only PO

• Do not administer within 1 mo of other live virus vaccines

Perform/Provide:

• Storage at 7°F (−13°C)

• Written record of immunization

Evaluate:

• For history of allergies, skin conditions (eczema, psoriasis, dermatitis), reactions to vaccinations

• For anaphylaxis: inability to breathe, bronchospasm

polymyxin B sulfate

(pol-i-mix'in)

Aerosporin

Func. class.: Antibacterial

Chem. class.: Polymyxin

Action: Interferes with phospholipids, penetrates cell wall; changes occur immediately in bacterial membrane causing leakage of essential metabolites

Uses: Serious *P. aeruginosa, E. aerogenes, K. pneumoniae, E. coli, H. influenzae* infections or when other antibiotics cannot be used

Dosage and routes:

• *Adult and child:* IV INF 15,000-25,000 U/kg/day in divided doses q12h, or 25,000 U/kg/day in divided doses q4-8h

P. aeruginosa/H. influenzae

• *Adult and child >2 yr:* INTRATHECAL 50,000 U/day × 3-4 days, then 50,000 U/qod × 2 wk after CSF negative, glucose normal

• *Child <2 yr:* INTRATHECAL 20,000 U/day × 3-4 days, then 25,000 U qod × 2 wk after CSF negative

Available forms include: Inj IV, intrathecal, 500,000 U

Side effects/adverse reactions:

INTEG: Urticaria

CNS: Dizziness, confusion, weakness, drowsiness, paresthesia, slurred speech, ***coma, seizures,*** headache, stiff neck

RESP: ***Paralysis***

GU: ***Proteinuria, hematuria, azotemia, leukocyturia***

Contraindications: Hypersensitivity, severe renal disease

Precautions: Pregnancy (B)

Pharmacokinetics:

IM: Peak 2 hr, half-life 4½-6 hr,

excreted in urine unchanged (60%)
IV: Data not available

Interactions/incompatibilities:

• Increased skeletal muscle relaxation: anesthetics, neuromuscular blockers (tubocurarine decamethonium, succinylcholine, gallamine)

• Increased nephrotoxicity, neurotoxicity: aminoglycosides

• Incompatible with amphotericin B, cephalosporins, penicillins, chloramphenicol, strong acidic/alkalinic agents

NURSING CONSIDERATIONS

Assess:

• I&O ratio; report hematuria, oliguria

• Any patient with compromised renal system; drug is excreted slowly in poor renal system function; toxicity may occur rapidly; monitor BUN, creatinine

• Renal studies: urinalysis, protein, blood

• C&S before drug therapy; drug may be taken as soon as culture is taken; C&S may be done after completion of therapy

Administer:

• IV after diluting 500,000 U/5 ml sterile H_2O or NS for inj; then dilute each dose with 300-500 ml D_5W given over 60-90 min

• Intrathecal after reconstituting with 10 ml NS to yield 50,000 U/ml

Perform/provide:

• Storage in dark area at room temperature

• Do not use procaine HCl in intrathecal injection

• Adrenalin, suction, tracheostomy set, endotracheal intubation equipment on unit

Evaluate:

• Therapeutic response: absence of fever, purulent drainage, C&S negative

• Skin eruptions, itching; drug should be discontinued

• Respiratory status: rate, character, dyspnea, symptoms of neuromuscular blockade, tightness in chest; discontinue drug if these occur

• Allergies before initiation of treatment, reaction of each medication; place allergies on chart, Kardex in bright red letters; notify all people giving drugs

• For flushing of face, dizziness, disorientation, weakness, paresthesia, blurred vision, slurred speech, restlessness, irritability; indicate neurotoxicity

• For headache, fever, stiff neck; after intrathecal administration, indicate meningeal irritation

Teach patient/family:

• To report sore throat, fever, fatigue; could indicate superimposed infection

Treatment of overdose: Withdraw drug, maintain airway, administer epinephrine, aminophylline, O_2, IV corticosteroids

---

polymyxin B sulfate (ophthalmic)

(pol-ee-mix'in)

Func. class.: Antiinfective (ophthalmic)

Action: Inhibits cell wall permeability in susceptible organism

Uses: Superficial external ocular infections

Dosage and routes:

• *Adult and child:* INSTILL 1-2 gtts bid-qid × 7-10 days

Available forms include: Powder for sol; 500,000 U

---

* Available in Canada only

Side effects/adverse reactions:
EENT: Poor corneal wound healing, temporary visual haze, overgrowth of nonsusceptible organisms
Contraindications: Hypersensitivity
Precautions: Antibiotic hypersensitivity, pregnancy (B)

NURSING CONSIDERATIONS

Administer:
- After washing hands, cleanse crusts or discharge from eye before application
- After reconstituting powder to 20-50 ml

Perform/provide:
- Storage in refrigerator

Evaluate:
- Therapeutic response: absence of redness, inflammation, tearing
- Allergy: itching, lacrimation, redness, swelling

Teach patient/family:
- To use drug exactly as prescribed
- Not to use eye makeup, towels, washcloths, eye medication of others; reinfection may occur
- That drug container tip should not be touched to eye
- To report itching, increased redness, burning, stinging, swelling; drug should be discontinued

---

potassium bicarbonate/ potassium acetate/ potassium chloride/ potassium gluconate/ potassium phosphate

Micro-K/K-Lyte, K-Lor, Kaon, Kay Ciel, Slow-K/Klorvess, Kolyum, Kaochlor, Klotrix

Func. class.: Electrolyte
Chem. class.: Potassium

Action: Needed for adequate transmission of nerve impulses and cardiac contraction, renal function intracellular ion maintenance
Uses: Prevention and treatment of hypokalemia
Dosage and routes:
Potassium bicarbonate
- *Adult:* PO dissolve 25-50 mEq in water qd-qid

Potassium acetate—hypokalemia
- *Adult and child:* PO 40-100 mEq/day in divided doses 2-4 days

Hypokalemia (prevention)
- *Adult and child:* PO 20 mEq/day in 2-4 divided doses

Potassium chloride
- *Adult:* PO 40-100 mEq in divided doses tid-qid; IV 20 mEq/hr when diluted as 40 mEq/1000 ml, not to exceed 150 mEq/day

Potassium gluconate
- *Adult:* PO 40-100 mEq in divided doses tid-qid

Potassium phosphate
- *Adult:* IV 1 mEq/hr in sol of 60 mEq/L, not to exceed 150 mEq/day; PO 40-100 mEq/day in divided doses

Available forms include: Tabs for sol 6.5, 25 mEq/inj for prep of IV 2, 4 mEq/caps ext rel 8, 10 mEq; powder for sol 3.3, 5, 6.7, 10, 13.3 mEq/5 ml; tabs 4, 13.4 mEq; tabs ext rel 6.7, 8, 10 mEq; inj for prep of IV 1.5, 2, 2.4, 3, 3.2 mEq/ml; elix 6.7 mEq/5 ml; tabs 2, 5 mEq; oral sol 2.375 mEq/5 ml; inj for prep of IV 4.4, 4.7 mEq/ml
Side effects/adverse reactions:
CNS: Confusion
CV: Bradycardia, ***cardiac depression, dysrhythmias, arrest, peaking T waves, lowered R and depressed RST, prolonged P-R interval, widened QRS complex***
GI: Nausea, vomiting, cramps, pain, diarrhea, ulceration of small bowel
GU: Oliguria

P

INTEG: Cold extremities, rash

Contraindications: Renal disease (severe), severe hemolytic disease, Addison's disease, hyperkalemia, acute dehydration, extensive tissue breakdown

Precautions: Cardiac disease, potassium sparing diuretic therapy, systemic acidosis, pregnancy (A)

Interactions/incompatibilities:

• Hyperkalemia: potassium phosphate IV and products containing calcium or magnesium; potassium sparing, diuretic, or other potassium products

Pharmacokinetics:

PO: Excreted by kidneys and in feces; onset of action ≈ 30 min

IV: Immediate onset of action

NURSING CONSIDERATIONS

Assess:

• ECG for peaking T waves, lowered R, depressed RST, prolonged P-R interval, widening QRS complex, hyperkalemia; drug should be reduced or discontinued

• Potassium level during treatment (3.5-5.0 mg/dl is normal level)

• I&O ratio; watch for decreased urinary output, notify physician immediately

Administer:

• Through large-bore needle, to decrease vein inflammation, check for extravasation

• In large vein, avoiding scalp vein in child (IV)

• Slowly by IV, INF to prevent toxicity, never give IV bolus or IM

• PO, with or pc meal; dissolve effervescent tabs, powder in 8 oz cold water or juice, do not give IM, SC

Perform/provide:

• Storage at room temperature

Evaluate:

• Therapeutic response: absence of fatigue, muscle weakness, and decreased thirst and urinary output, cardiac changes

• Cardiac status: rate, rhythm, CVP, PWP, PAWP, if being monitored directly

Teach patient/family:

• To add potassium-rich foods to diet: bananas, orange juice, avocados; whole grains, broccoli, carrots, prunes, cocoa after this medication is discontinued

• To avoid OTC products: antacids, salt substitutes, analgesics, vitamin preparations, unless specifically directed by physician

• To report hyperkalemia symptoms (lethargy, confusion, diarrhea, nausea, vomiting, fainting, decreased output) or continued hypokalemia symptoms (fatigue, weakness, polyuria, polydipsia, cardiac changes)

• Take capsules with full glass of liquid

• To completely dissolve powder or tablet in at least 120 ml water or juice

• Not to chew time release or extended release preparations

• Emphasize importance of regular follow-up

---

potassium iodide

Iostat, Pima, Potassium Iodide Solution, Strong Iodine Solution, Lugol's Solution, Thyro-Block

Func. class.: Thyroid hormone antagonist

Chem. class.: Iodine product

Action: Inhibits secretion of thyroid hormone, fosters colloid accumulation in thyroid follicles, decreases vascularity of gland

Uses: Preparation for thyroidectomy, thyrotoxic crisis, neonatal

* Available in Canada only

thyrotoxicosis, radiation protectant, thyroid storm

Dosage and routes:

Thyrotoxic crisis

• *Adult and child:* PO 1 ml in water tid after meals (strong iodine solution)

Preparation for thyroidectomy

• *Adult and child:* PO 0.1-0.3 ml tid (Strong Iodine Solution) or 5 gtts in water tid pc × 2-3 wk before surgery (Potassium Iodide Solution)

Available forms include: Solution 5%, 10%, 21 mg/gtt; tabs 130, 300 mg; inj IV 10%, 20%

Side effects/adverse reactions:

ENDO: Hypothyroidism, hyperthyroid adenoma

INTEG: Rash, urticaria, ***angineurotic edema,*** acne, mucosal hemorrhage, fever

CNS: Headache, confusion, paresthesias

GI: Nausea, diarrhea, vomiting, small bowel lesions, upper gastric pain

MS: Myalgia, arthralgia, weakness

EENT: Metallic taste, stomatitis, salivation, periorbital edema, sore teeth and gums, cold symptoms

Contraindications: Hypersensitivity to iodine, pulmonary edema, pulmonary TB, pregnancy (D)

Precautions: Lactation, children

Pharmacokinetics:

PO: Onset 24-48 hr, peak 10-15 days after continuous therapy, uptake by thyroid gland or excreted in urine; crosses placenta

Interactions/incompatibilities:

• Hypothyroidism: lithium, other antithyroid agents

NURSING CONSIDERATIONS

Assess:

• Pulse, B/P, temperature

• I&O ratio; check for edema: puffy hands, feet, periorbit; indicate hypothyroidism

• Weight qd; same clothing, scale, time of day

• T_3, T_4, which is increased; serum TSH, which is decreased; free thyroxine index, which is increased if dosage is too low; discontinue drug 3-4 wk before RAIU

Administer:

• Strong iodine solution after diluting with water or juice to improve taste

• Through straw to prevent tooth discoloration

• With meals to decrease GI upset

• At same time each day, to maintain drug level

• Lowest dose that relieves symptoms, discontinue before RAI

Perform/provide:

• Fluids to 3-4 L/day, unless contraindicated

Evaluate:

• Therapeutic response: weight gain, decreased pulse, T_4, size of thyroid gland

• Overdose: peripheral edema, heat intolerance, diaphoresis, palpitations, dysrhythmias, severe tachycardia, increased temperature delirium, CNS irritability

• Hypersensitivity: rash, enlarged cervical lymph nodes may indicate drug may need to be discontinued

• Hypoprothrombinemia: bleeding, petechiae, ecchymosis

• Clinical response: after 3 wk should include increased weight, pulse; decreased T_4

Teach patient/family:

• To abstain from breast feeding after delivery

• To keep graph of weight, pulse, mood

• To avoid OTC products that contain iodine

• That seafood, other iodine products may be restricted
• Not to discontinue this medication abruptly; thyroid crisis may occur; stress patient response
• That response may take several months if thyroid is large
• To discontinue drug, notify physician if fever, rash, metallic taste, swelling of throat, burning of mouth, throat, sore gums, teeth, severe GI distress, enlargement of thyroid, cold symptoms occur

Lab test interferences:
Interferes: Urinary 17-OHCS

potassium iodide (SSKI)

Pima, Iosat, Thyro-Block
Func. class.: Expectorant

Action: Increases respiratory tract fluid by decreasing surface tension, adhesiveness, which increases removal of mucus

Uses: Bronchial asthma, emphysema, bronchitis, nuclear radiation protection

Dosage and routes:
• *Adult:* PO 0.3-0.6 ml q4-6h
• *Child:* PO 0.25-1 ml saturated sol bid-qid

Radiation protection:
• *Adult:* PO 0.13 ml SSKI before or after initial exposure
• *Infant <1 yr:* Half adult dose

Available forms include: Sol 1 g/ml

Side effects/adverse reactions:
EENT: Burning mouth, throat, eye irritation, swelling of eyelids
GI: Gastric irritation
ENDO: Iodism, goiter, myxedema
RESP: ***Pulmonary edema***
INTEG: ***Angioedema,*** rash
CNS: Frontal headache, ***CNS depression,*** fever, parkinsonism

Contraindications: Hypersensitivity to iodides, pulmonary TB, pregnancy (D), hyperthyroidism, hyperkalemia, acute bronchitis

Precautions: Hypothyroidism, cystic fibrosis, lactation

Pharmacokinetics: Excreted in urine

Interactions/incompatibilities:
• Increased hypothyroid effects: lithium, antithyroid drugs
• Dysrhythmias, hyperkalemia: potassium-sparing diuretics, potassium-containing medication

NURSING CONSIDERATIONS

Administer:
• Decreased dose to elderly patients; their excretion may be slowed
• Diluted water or fruit juice to improve taste, decrease nausea

Perform/provide:
• Storage at room temperature in tight containers
• Increased fluids to liquefy secretions

Evaluate:
• Therapeutic response: absence of cough
• Cough: type, frequency, character including sputum

Teach patient/family:
• Not to use if pregnant
• Symptoms of iodism: eruptions, burning of oral cavity, eye irritation
• Symptoms of hyperthyroidism: CNS depression, fever, glomerulonephritis
• To discontinue, notify physician if fever, rash, metallic taste occur

povidone iodine

(poe'vi-done)
ACU-dyne, Aerodine, Betadine, Efo-dine, Mallisol, Proviodine*
Func. class.: Disinfectant
Chem. class.: Iodophor

Action: Destroys a wide variety of

* Available in Canada only

microorganisms by local irritation, germicidal action

Uses: Cleansing wounds, disinfection, preoperative skin preparation removal

Dosage and routes:

• *Adult and child:* Sol Use as needed, topical only

Available forms include: Top sol 1.5%, 3%

Side effects/adverse reactions:

GU: ***Renal damage***

META: Metabolic acidosis

INTEG: Irritation

Contraindications: Hypersensitivity to iodine, pregnancy (vaginal antiseptic) (D)

Precautions: Extensive burns

Interactions/incompatibilities:

• Do not use with alcohol or hydrogen peroxide

NURSING CONSIDERATIONS

Assess:

• For allergies to seafood, drug should not be used

Perform/provide:

• Storage in tight, light-resistant container

• Bandaging of areas if needed

Evaluate:

• Area of the body involved: irritation, rash, breaks, dryness, scales

Teach patient/family:

• To discontinue use if rash, irritation, or redness occurs

---

pralidoxime chloride

(pra-li-dox'eem)

Protopam chloride, PAM

Func. class.: Cholinesterase reactivator

Chem. class.: Quaternary ammonium oxide

Action: Reactivated enzyme metabolizes and inactivates acetylcholine at both muscarinic and nicotinic sites in the periphery

Uses: Cholinergic crisis in myasthenia gravis, organophosphate poisoning antidote, relief of paralysis of respiratory muscles; used as an adjunct to systemic atropine administration

Dosage and routes:

Anticholinesterase overdosage

• *Adult:* IV 1-2 g, then 250 mg q5min until desired response

Organophosphate poisoning

• *Adult:* IV INF 1-2 g/100 ml NS over 15-30 min, may repeat in 1 hr; PO 1-3 g q5h

• *Child:* IV INF 20-40 mg/kg/dose diluted in 100 ml NS over 15-30 min

Available forms include: Inj IV 600 mg/2 ml; tabs 500 mg; emergency kit 1 g/20-ml vial

Side effects/adverse reactions:

CNS: Dizziness, headache, drowsiness, blurred vision, diplopia, impaired accommodation

GI: Nausea

MS: Weakness, muscle rigidity

CV: Tachycardia

RESP: Hyperventilation, ***laryngospasm***

Contraindications: Hypersensitivity, carbamate insecticide poisoning

Precautions: Myasthenia gravis, pregnancy (C), renal insufficiency, children, lactation

Pharmacokinetics:

PO: Peak 2-3 hr

IV: Peak 5-15 min

IM: Peak 10-20 min

Half-life 1½ hr, metabolized in liver, excreted in urine (unchanged)

Interactions/incompatibilities:

• Avoid use with aminophylline, morphine, phenothiazines, reserpine, succinylcholine, theophylline in organophosphate poisoning

P

NURSING CONSIDERATIONS

Assess:

• For 48-72 hr after poisoning

• B/P, VS, I&O ratio; observe for decreased urinary output for 48-72 hr after poisoning to determine atropine toxicity from poisoning effects

Administer:

• Only with emergency equipment available

• As soon as possible after poisoning; within 4 hr

• IV after diluting 1 g/20 ml sterile H_2O for inj; further dilute/100 ml NS and give 1 g/15-30 min

• Slowly (IV) after dilution with sterile water

• Concurrent atropine 2-4 mg IV or IM if cyanosis is present, to block accumulated acetylcholine in respiratory center; repeat q5-10 min until toxicity occurs: dry mouth, flushing, tachycardia, delirium, hallucinations

• Only with edrophonium (Tensilon) on unit for myasthenia gravis patient

Evaluate:

• Airway, need for assistance with respiration

• Respiratory status: rate, rhythm, characteristics

pramoxine HCl (topical)

(pra-mox'-een)

ProctoFoam, Tronolane, Tronothane

Func. class.: Topical anesthetic

Action: Inhibits nerve impulses from sensory nerves, which produces anesthesia

Uses: Pruritus, sunburn, toothache, sore throat, cold sores, oral pain, rectal pain and irritation

Dosage and routes:

• *Adult and child:* TOP apply q3-4h; REC apply 1 full applicator bid-tid and after each BM

Available forms include: Aero, cream, gel, lotion 1%; rec oint 1%; rec or top aero, cream 1%

Side effects/adverse reactions:

INTEG: Rash, irritation, sensitization

Contraindications: Hypersensitivity, infants <1 yr, application to large areas

Precautions: Child <6 yr, sepsis, pregnancy (C), denuded skin

NURSING CONSIDERATIONS

Administer:

• After cleansing and drying of affected area

• Rectal aerosol using applicator or tissue

• Directly using gauze

Evaluate:

• Therapeutic response: absence of pain, itching of affected area

• Allergy: rash, irritation, reddening, swelling

• Infection: if affected area is infected, do not apply

Teach patient/family:

• To report rash, irritation, redness, swelling

• How to apply

• Not for long-term use, consult physician after 4 wk of use

pravastatin

(prav-i-sta'tin)

Pravachol

Func. class.: Antihyperlipidemic

Action: Inhibits HMG-CoA reductase enzyme, which reduces cholesterol synthesis

Uses: As an adjunct in primary hypercholesterolemia (types IIa, IIb)

Dosage and routes:
• *Adult:* PO 10-20 mg qd at hs (range 10-40 mg qd)
Available forms include: Tabs 10, 20 mg
Side effects/adverse reactions:
INTEG: Rash, pruritus
GI: Nausea, constipation, diarrhea, dyspepsia, flatus, abdominal pain, heartburn, ***liver dysfunction,*** pancreatitis, ***hepatitis***
EENT: Lens opacities, common cold, rhinitis, cough
MS: Muscle cramps, myalgia, ***myositis, rhabdomyolysis***
CNS: Headache, dizziness, psychic disturbances
Contraindications: Hypersensitivity, pregnancy (X), lactation, active liver disease
Precautions: Past liver disease, alcoholics, severe acute infections, trauma, hypotension, uncontrolled seizure disorders, severe metabolic disorders, electrolyte imbalances
Pharmacokinetics: Peak 1-1½ hr, metabolized by the liver, highly protein bound, excreted in urine, feces; crosses placenta, excreted in breast milk
Interactions/incompatibilities:
• Increased effects of: coumadin
• Decreased bioavailability of pravastatin: bile acid sequestrants

NURSING CONSIDERATIONS

Assess:
• Cholesterol levels periodically during treatment
• Liver function studies baseline, q6wk during the first 3 mo, q8wk for remainder of yr, then q6mo; AST, ALT, liver function tests may increase
• Renal studies in patients with compromised renal system: BUN, I&O ratio, creatinine
Administer:
• Without regard to meals, hs
Perform/provide:
• Storage in cool environment in tight container protected from light
Evaluate:
• Therapeutic response: decrease in cholesterol to desired level after 8 wk
Teach patient/family:
• That treatment will be ongoing for several years
• That blood work will be necessary during treatment
• To report blurred vision, severe GI symptoms, dizziness, headache
• That previously prescribed regimen will continue: low-cholesterol diet exercise program
Lab test interferences:
Increase: CPK, liver function tests

---

prazepam

(pra'ze-pam)
Centrax
Func. class.: Antianxiety
Chem. class.: Benzodiazepine

Controlled Substance Schedule IV
Action: Depresses subcortical levels of CNS, including limbic system and reticular formation
Uses: Anxiety
Dosage and routes:
• *Adult:* PO 30 mg in divided doses or at hs
Available forms include: Caps 5, 10, 20 mg; tabs 10 mg
Side effects/adverse reactions:
CNS: Dizziness, drowsiness, confusion, headache, anxiety, tremors, stimulation, fatigue, insomnia, weakness
GI: Constipation, dry mouth, nausea, vomiting, anorexia, diarrhea
INTEG: Rash, dermatitis, itching
CV: Orthostatic hypotension, ***ECG***

P

changes, tachycardia, hypotension, palpitations, syncope
EENT: Blurred vision, tinnitus, mydriasis
Contraindications: Hypersensitivity to benzodiazepines, narrow-angle glaucoma, psychosis, pregnancy (D), child <18 yr
Precautions: Elderly, debilitated, hepatic disease, renal disease
Pharmacokinetics:
PO: Peak 6 hr, duration up to 48 hr, metabolized by liver, excreted by kidneys, crosses placenta, breast milk, half-life 30-100 hr
Interactions/incompatibilities:
• Decreased effects of prazepam: oral contraceptives, valproic acid
• Increased effects of prazepam: CNS depressants, alcohol, disulfiram, oral contraceptives

NURSING CONSIDERATIONS

Assess:
• B/P (lying, standing), pulse; if systolic B/P drops 20 mm Hg, hold drug, notify physician
• Blood studies: CBC
• Hepatic studies: AST, ALT, bilirubin, CrCl
Administer:
• With food or milk for GI symptoms
• Crushed if patient is unable to swallow medication whole
• Gum, hard candy, frequent sips of water for dry mouth
Perform/provide:
• Assistance with ambulation during beginning therapy, since drowsiness/dizziness occurs
• Safety measure including siderails
Evaluate:
• Therapeutic response: decreased anxiety
• Mental status: mood, sensorium, affect
• Physical dependency, withdrawal symptoms: headache, nausea, vomiting, muscle pain, weakness, tremors, ***convulsions*** after long-term use
• Check to see PO medication has been swallowed
Teach patient/family:
• Not to be used for everyday stress or used longer than 4 mo; not to use more than prescribed amount, may be habit forming
• To avoid OTC preparations (cough, cold, hay fever) unless approved by physician
• To avoid driving or other activities that require alertness
• To avoid alcohol ingestion or other psychotropic medications
• Not to discontinue medication quickly after long-term use
• To rise slowly or fainting may occur, especially elderly
Lab test interferences:
Increase: AST, ALT, serum bilirubin, LDH
Decrease: RAIU
False increase: 17-OHCS
Treatment of overdose: Lavage, VS, supportive care

praziquantel

(pray-zi-kwon'tel)
Biltricide
Func. class.: Anthelmintic
Chem. class.: Pyrazinoisoquiolone derivative

Action: Causes contraction, paralysis, leading to dislodgement of suckers; they are carried to liver where phagocytosis takes place
Uses: Schistosomiasis, liver flukes, lung flukes, intestinal flukes, tapeworms
Dosage and routes:
• *Adult and child >4 yr:* PO 20 mg/kg q4-6h × 1 day

* Available in Canada only

Available forms include: Tabs 600 mg

Side effects/adverse reactions:

INTEG: Rash, pruritus, urticaria, internal hypertension

CNS: Dizziness, headache, drowsiness, malaise, increased seizure activity, fever, sweating

GI: Nausea, vomiting, anorexia, diarrhea, abdominal pain, increased liver enzymes

Contraindications: Hypersensitivity, lactation

Precautions: Child <4 yr, seizure disorders, pregnancy (B)

Pharmacokinetics:

PO: Peak 1-3 hr, half-life 48-90 min, metabolized by liver (metabolites), excreted in urine, breast milk, CSF

NURSING CONSIDERATIONS

Assess:

- Liver function test: AST, ALT; watch for increase
- Stools during entire treatment, 1, 3 mo after treatment; specimens must be sent to lab while still warm

Administer:

- Corticosteroids as ordered to reduce CNS effects (cerebral cysticercosis)
- Laxatives before treatment to cleanse bowel
- PO with liquids during meals to avoid GI symptoms, not to be chewed

Perform/provide:

- Storage in tight container in cool environment

Evaluate:

- Therapeutic response: expulsion of worms, 3 negative stool cultures after completion of treatment
- For allergic reaction: rash, urticaria, pruritus
- For diarrhea during expulsion of worms
- For CSF reaction: headache, high fever; if these occur, drug should be discontinued, physician notified

Teach patient/family:

- To avoid driving or hazardous activities on day of, day after treatment
- Proper hygiene after BM including handwashing technique, tell patient to avoid putting fingers in mouth
- Need for compliance with dosage schedule, duration of treatment
- To refrain from breast feeding on day of treatment, 72 hr after

Treatment of overdose: Fast-acting laxative

---

prazosin HCl

(pra'zoe-sin)

Minipress

Func. class.: Antihypertensive

Chem. class.: α-Adrenergic blocker

Action: Peripheral blood vessels are dilated, peripheral resistance lowered, reduction in blood pressure results from α-adrenergic receptors being blocked

Uses: Hypertension, refractory CHF, Raynaud's vasospasm

Dosage and routes:

- *Adult:* PO 1 mg bid or tid, increasing to 20 mg qd in divided doses if required, usual range 6-15 mg/day, not to exceed 1 mg initially

Available forms include: Caps 1, 2, 5 mg

Side effects/adverse reactions:

CV: Palpitations, orthostatic hypotension, tachycardia, edema, rebound hypertension

CNS: Dizziness, headache, drowsiness, anxiety, depression, vertigo, weakness, fatigue

P

GI: Nausea, vomiting, diarrhea, constipation, abdominal pain
GU: Urinary frequency, incontinence, impotence, priapism
EENT: Blurred vision, epistaxis, tinnitus, dry mouth, red sclera
Contraindications: Hypersensitivity
Precautions: Pregnancy (C), children
Pharmacokinetics:
PO: Onset 2 hr, peak 1-3 hr, duration 6-12 hr; half-life 2-3 hr, metabolized in liver, excreted via bile, feces (>90%), in urine (<10%)
Interactions/incompatibilities:
- Increased hypotensive effects: β-blockers, nitroglycerin
- Decreased effect: indomethacin

NURSING CONSIDERATIONS
Assess:
- B/P during initial treatment, periodically thereafter
- Pulse, jugular venous distention q4h
- BUN, uric acid if on long-term therapy
- Weight daily, I&O

Perform/provide:
- Storage in tight containers in cool environment

Evaluate:
- Therapeutic response: decreased B/P
- Edema in feet, legs daily
- Skin turgor, dryness of mucous membranes for hydration status
- Rales, dyspnea, orthopnea q30min

Teach patient/family:
- Fainting occasionally occurs after 1st dose; do not drive or operate machinery for 4 hr after 1st dose or take 1st dose at bedtime

Lab test interferences:
Increased: Urinary norepinephrine, VMA
Treatment of overdose: Administer volume expanders or vasopressors, discontinue drug, place in supine position

---

prednisolone/prednisolone acetate/prednisolone phosphate/prednisolone tebutate

(pred-niss'oh-lone)
Cortalone, Delta-Cortef, Fernisolone-P/Predoxine/Savacort/Hydeltrasol, PSP-IV/Hydeltra-TBA, Metalone-TBA
Func. class.: Corticosteroid
Chem. class.: Glucocorticoid, immediate acting

Action: Decreases inflammation by suppression of migration of polymorphonuclear leukocytes, fibroblasts, reversal to increase capillary permeability and lysosomal stabilization
Uses: Severe inflammation, immunosuppression, neoplasms
Dosage and routes:
- *Adult:* PO 2.5-15 mg bid-qid; IM 2-30 mg (acetate, phosphate) q12h; IV 2-30 mg (phosphate) q12h, 2-30 mg in joint or soft tissue (phosphate), 4-40 mg in joint of lesion (tebutate), 0.25-1 ml qwk in joints (acetate-phosphate)

Available forms include: Tabs 5 mg; inj 25, 50, 100 mg/ml acetate; inj 20 mg/ml terbutate; inj 20 mg/ml phosphate; inj 80 mg/ml acetate/phosphate
Side effects/adverse reactions:
INTEG: Acne, poor wound healing, ecchymosis, petechiae
CNS: ***Depression,*** flushing, sweating, headache, mood changes
CV: Hypertension, ***circulatory collapse, thrombophlebitis, embolism,*** tachycardia

---

* Available in Canada only

HEMA: ***Thrombocytopenia***
MS: Fractures, osteoporosis, weakness
GI: Diarrhea, nausea, abdominal distention, ***GI hemorrhage,*** increased appetite, ***pancreatitis***
EENT: Fungal infections, increased intraocular pressure, blurred vision

Contraindications: Psychosis, hypersensitivity, idiopathic thrombocytopenia, acute glomerulonephritis, amebiasis, fungal infections, nonasthmatic bronchial disease, child <2 yr

Precautions: Pregnancy (C), diabetes mellitus, glaucoma, osteoporosis, seizure disorders, ulcerative colitis, CHF, myasthenia gravis

Pharmacokinetics:
PO: Peak 1-2 hr, duration 2 days
IM: Peak 3-45 hr

Interactions/incompatibilities:
- Decreased action of prednisolone: cholestyramine, colestipol, barbiturates, rifampin, ephedrine, phenytoin, theophylline
- Decreased effects of: anticoagulants, anticonvulsants, antidiabetics, ambenonium, neostigmine, isoniazid, toxoids, vaccines, anticholinesterases, salicylates, somatrem
- Increased side effects: alcohol, salicylates, indomethacin, amphotericin B, digitalis, cyclosporine, diuretics
- Increased action of prednisolone: salicylates, estrogens, indomethacin, oral contraceptives, ketoconazole, macrolide antibiotics

NURSING CONSIDERATIONS

Assess:
- Potassium, blood sugar, urine glucose while on long-term therapy; hypokalemia and hyperglycemia
- Weight daily, notify physician if weekly gain of >5 lb
- B/P q4h, pulse, notify physician if chest pain occurs
- I&O ratio; be alert for decreasing urinary output and increasing edema
- Plasma cortisol levels during long-term therapy (normal level: 138-635 nmol/L SI units when drawn at 8 AM)

Administer:
- IV undiluted or added to NaCl or D_5 and given by IV INF; give 10 mg or less/1 min
- After shaking suspension (parenteral)
- Titrated dose, use lowest effective dose
- IM inj deeply in large mass, rotate sites, avoid deltoid, use 21G needle
- In one dose in AM to prevent adrenal suppression, avoid SC administration, damage may be done to tissue
- With food or milk to decrease GI symptoms

Perform/provide:
- Assistance with ambulation in patient with bone tissue disease to prevent fractures

Evaluate:
- Therapeutic response: ease of respirations, decreased inflammation
- Infection: increased temperature, WBC, even after withdrawal of medication; drug masks symptoms of infection
- Potassium depletion: paresthesias, fatigue, nausea, vomiting, depression, polyuria, dysrhythmias, weakness
- Edema, hypertension, cardiac symptoms
- Mental status: affect, mood, behavioral changes, aggression

Teach patient/family:

- That ID as steroid user should be carried
- To notify physician if therapeutic response decreases; dosage adjustment may be needed
- Not to discontinue this medication abruptly or adrenal crisis can result
- To avoid OTC products: salicylates, alcohol in cough products, cold preparations unless directed by physician
- About cushingoid symptoms
- Symptoms of adrenal insufficiency: nausea, anorexia, fatigue, dizziness, dyspnea, weakness, joint pain

Lab test interferences:

Increase: Cholesterol, sodium, blood glucose, uric acid, calcium, urine glucose

Decrease: Calcium, potassium, T_4, T_3, thyroid ^{131}I uptake test, urine 17-OHCS, 17-KS, PBI

False negative: Skin allergy tests

---

prednisolone acetate (suspension)/prednisolone sodium phosphate (solution)

(pred-niss'oh-lone)

Econopred, Pred-Forte, Pred Mild, Predulose Ophthalmic/Ak-Pred, Hydelthrasol, Inflamase Forte, Inflamase Ophthalmic, Metreton Ophthalmic

Func. class.: Ophthalmic antiinflammatory

Chem. class.: Analog of hydrocortisone

Action: Decreases inflammation, resulting in decreases in pain, photophobia, hyperemia, cellular infiltration

Uses: Inflammation of eye, lids, conjunctiva, cornea, uveitis, iridocyclitis, allergic condition, burns, foreign bodies

Dosage and routes:

- *Adult and child:* Instill 1-2 gtts into conjunctival sac q1h × 2 days, if needed, then bid-qid

Available forms include: Susp 0.12%, 0.125%, 1%; sol 0.125%, 0.5%, 1%

Side effects/adverse reactions:

EENT: ***Increased intraocular pressure,*** poor corneal wound healing, increased possibility of corneal infections, glaucoma exacerbation, ***optic nerve damage,*** decreased acuity, visual field

Contraindications: Hypersensitivity, acute superficial herpes simplex, fungal/viral diseases of eye or conjunctiva, active diabetes mellitus, ocular TB, infections of the eye

Precautions: Corneal abrasions, glaucoma, pregnancy (C)

NURSING CONSIDERATIONS

Evaluate:

- Therapeutic response: absence of swelling, redness, exudate

Administer:

- After shaking

Perform/provide:

- Storage in tight, light-resistant container

Teach patient/family:

- Instillation method: pressure on lacrimal duct for 1 min
- Not to share eye medications with others
- Not to use if purulent drainage is present
- Not to discontinue abruptly, taper over 1-2 wk

---

prednisone

(pred-ni-sone)

Deltasone, Meticorten, Orasone

Func. class.: Corticosteroid

Chem. class.: Glucocorticoid, intermediate acting

Action: Decreases inflammation by suppression of migration of polymorphonuclear leukocytes, fibroblasts, reversal to increase capillary permeability, and lysosomal stabilization

Uses: Severe inflammation, immunosuppression, neoplasms, multiple sclerosis, collagen disorders, dermatologic disorders

Dosage and routes:

• *Adult:* PO 2.5-15 mg bid-qid, then qd or qod maintenance up to 250 mg/day

Nephrosis

• *Child:* 18 mo-4 yr 7.5-10 mg qid initially

• *Child:* 4 yr-10 yr 15 mg qid initially

• *Child:* >10 yr 20 mg qid initially

Multiple sclerosis

• *Adult:* PO 200 mg/day × 1 wk, then 80 mg qod × 1 mo

Available forms include: Tabs 1, 2.5, 5, 10, 20, 25, 50 mg; oral sol 5 mg/5 ml; syr 5 mg/5 ml

Side effects/adverse reactions:

INTEG: Acne, poor wound healing, ecchymosis, petechiae

CNS: Depression, flushing, sweating, headache, mood changes

CV: Hypertension, ***circulatory collapse, thrombophlebitis, embolism,*** tachycardia

HEMA: ***Thrombocytopenia***

MS: Fractures, osteoporosis, weakness

GI: Diarrhea, nausea, abdominal distention, ***GI hemorrhage,*** increased appetite, ***pancreatitis***

EENT: Fungal infections, increased intraocular pressure, blurred vision

Contraindications: Psychosis, hypersensitivity, idiopathic thrombocytopenia, acute glomerulonephritis, amebiasis, fungal infections, nonasthmatic bronchial disease, child <2 yr, AIDS, TB

Precautions: Pregnancy (C), diabetes mellitus, glaucoma, osteoporosis, seizure disorders, ulcerative colitis, CHF, myasthenia gravis, renal disease, esophagitis, peptic ulcer

Pharmacokinetics:

PO: Peak 1-2 hr, duration 1-1½ days, half-life 3½-4 hr

Interactions/incompatibilities:

• Decreased action of prednisone: cholestyramine, colestipol, barbiturates, rifampin, ephedrine, phenytoin, theophylline

• Decreased effects of: anticoagulants, anticonvulsants, antidiabetics, ambenonium, neostigmine, isoniazid, toxoids, vaccines, anticholinesterases, salicylates, somatrem

• Increased side effects: alcohol, salicylates, indomethacin, amphotericin B, digitalis, cyclosporine, diuretics

• Increased action of prednisone: salicylates, estrogens, indomethacin, oral contraceptives, ketoconazole, macrolide antibiotics

NURSING CONSIDERATIONS

Assess:

• Potassium, blood sugar, urine glucose while on long-term therapy; hypokalemia and hyperglycemia

• Weight daily, notify physician of weekly gain >5 lb

• B/P q4h, pulse, notify physician if chest pain occurs

• I&O ratio, be alert for decreasing

urinary output and increasing edema
• Plasma cortisol levels during long-term therapy (normal level: 138-635 nmol/L SI units when drawn at 8 AM)
Administer:
• Titrated dose, use lowest effective dose
• With food or milk to decrease GI symptoms
Perform/provide:
• Assistance with ambulation in patient with bone tissue disease to prevent fractures
Evaluate:
• Therapeutic response: ease of respirations, decreased inflammation
• Infection: increased temperature, WBC, even after withdrawal of medication; drug masks symptoms of infection
• Potassium depletion: paresthesias, fatigue, nausea, vomiting, depression, polyuria, dysrhythmias, weakness
• Edema, hypertension, cardiac symptoms
• Mental status: affect, mood, behavioral changes, aggression
Teach patient/family:
• That ID as steroid user should be carried
• To notify physician if therapeutic response decreases; dosage adjustment may be needed
• Not to discontinue this medication abruptly or adrenal crisis can result
• To avoid OTC products: salicylates, alcohol in cough products, cold preparations unless directed by physician
• About cushingoid symptoms
• Symptoms of adrenal insufficiency: nausea, anorexia, fatigue, dizziness, dyspnea, weakness, joint pain

Lab test interferences:
Increase: Cholesterol, sodium, blood glucose, uric acid, calcium, urine glucose
Decrease: Calcium, potassium, T_4, T_3, thyroid ^{131}I uptake test, urine 17-OHCS, 17-KS, PBI
False negative: Skin allergy tests

primaquine phosphate
(prim'a-kween)

Func. class.: Antimalarial
Chem. class.: Synthetic 8-aminoquinolone

Action: Action is unknown; thought to destroy exoerythrocytic forms by gametocidal action
Uses: Malaria caused by *Plasmodium vivax*
Dosage and routes:
• *Adult:* PO 15 mg (base) qd × 2 wk, 26.3 mg tab is 15 mg base
• *Child:* PO 0.3 mg/kg × 2 wk
Available forms include: Tabs 26.3 mg
Side effects/adverse reactions:
INTEG: Pruritus, skin eruptions
CNS: Headache
EENT: Blurred vision, difficulty focusing
GI: Nausea, vomiting, anorexia, cramps
CV: Hypertension
HEMA: ***Agranulocytosis, granulocytopenia, leukopenia, hemolytic anemia, leukocytosis,*** mild anemia, ***methemoglobinemia***
Contraindications: Hypersensitivity, anemia, lupus erythematosus, methemoglobinemia, porphyria, rheumatoid arthritis, methemoglobin reductase deficiency, G-6-PD deficiency
Precautions: Pregnancy (C)
Pharmacokinetics:
PO: Metabolized by liver (metabolites), half-life 3.7-9.6 hr

*Available in Canada only

Interactions/incompatibilities:
• Toxicity: quinacrine

NURSING CONSIDERATIONS

Assess:
• Ophthalmic test if long-term treatment or drug dosage >150 mg/day
• Liver studies qwk: AST, ALT, bilirubin, if on long-term therapy
• Blood studies: CBC, since blood dyscrasias occur

Administer:
• Before or after meals at same time each day to maintain drug level

Evaluate:
• Therapeutic response: decreased symptoms of malaria
• Allergic reactions: pruritus, rash, urticaria
• Blood dyscrasias: malaise, fever, bruising, bleeding (rare)
• For renal status: dark urine, hematuria, decreased output
• For hemolytic reaction: chills, fever, chest pain, cyanosis; drug should be discontinued immediately

Teach patient/family:
• To report visual problems, fever, fatigue, dark urine, bruising, bleeding; may indicate blood dyscrasias

---

primidone

(pri'mi-done)
Mysoline, Sertan*

Func. class.: Anticonvulsant
Chem. class.: Barbiturate derivative

Action: Raises seizure threshold by conversion of drug to phenobarbital
Uses: Generalized tonic-clonic (grand mal), complex-partial psychomotor seizures
Dosage and routes:
• *Adult and child >8 yr:* PO 250 mg/day, may increase by 250 mg/wk, not to exceed 2 g/day in divided doses qid
• *Child <8 yr:* PO 125 mg/day, may increase by 125 mg/wk, not to exceed 1 g/day in divided doses qid
Available forms include: Tabs 50, 250 mg; susp 250 mg/5 ml
Side effects/adverse reactions:
HEMA: ***Thrombocytopenia, leukopenia, neutropenia, eosinophilia, megaloblastic anemia,*** serum folate level, lymphadenopathy
CNS: Stimulation, drowsiness, dizziness, confusion, sedation, headache, flushing, hallucinations, coma, psychosis, ataxia, vertigo
GI: Nausea, vomiting, anorexia
INTEG: Rash, edema, alopecia, lupuslike syndrome
EENT: Diplopia, nystagmus, edema of eyelids
GU: Impotence, polyuria
Contraindications: Hypersensitivity, porphyria, pregnancy (D)
Precautions: COPD, hepatic disease, renal disease, hyperactive children
Pharmacokinetics:
PO: Peak 4 hr, excreted by kidneys, excreted in breast milk, half-life 3-24 hr
Interactions/incompatibilities:
• Increased blood levels: alcohol, heparin, CNS depressants, isoniazid, phenytoin, phenobarbital

NURSING CONSIDERATIONS

Assess:
• Drug level: therapeutic level 5-10 μg/ml; CBC should be done q6mo

Administer:
• Shake liquid susp well

Evaluate:
• Therapeutic response: decreased seizures
• Mental status: mood, sensorium, affect, memory (long, short)

- Respiratory depression
- Blood dyscrasias: fever, sore throat, bruising, rash, jaundice

Teach patient/family:

- Not to withdraw drug quickly, withdrawal symptoms may occur
- To avoid hazardous activities until stabilized on drug

probenecid

(proe-ben'e-sid)

Benemid, Benn, Benuryl,* Probalan, Probenimead, Robenecid

Func. class.: Uricosuric

Chem. class.: Sulfonamide derivative

Action: Inhibits tubular reabsorption of urates, with increased excretion of uric acids

Uses: Gonorrhea, hyperuricemia in gout, gouty arthritis, adjunct to cephalosporin or penicillin treatment

Dosage and routes:

Gonorrhea

- *Adult:* PO 1 g with 3.5 g ampicillin or 1 g ½ hr before 4.8 mill U of aqueous penicillin G procaine injected into 2 sites IM

Gout/gouty arthritis

- *Adult:* PO 250 mg bid for 1 wk, then 500 mg bid, not to exceed 2 g/day; maintenance: 500 mg/day × 6 mos

Adjunct in penicillin/cephalosporin treatment

- *Adult and child >50 kg:* PO 500 mg qid
- *Child <50 kg:* PO 25 mg/kg, then 40 mg/kg in divided doses qid

Available forms include: Tabs 0.5 g

Side effects/adverse reactions:

CNS: Drowsiness, headache

CV: Bradycardia

GU: Glycosuria, thirst, frequency, ***nephrotic syndrome***

GI: Gastric irritation, nausea, vomiting, anorexia, ***hepatic necrosis***

INTEG: Rash, dermatitis, pruritus, fever

META: Acidosis, hypokalemia, hyperchloremia, hyperglycemia

RESP: ***Apnea,*** irregular respirations

Contraindications: Hypersensitivity, severe hepatic disease, blood dyscrasias, severe renal disease, CrC <50 mg/min, history of uric acid calculus

Precautions: Pregnancy (B), severe respiratory disease, lactation, cardiac edema, child <2 yr

Pharmacokinetics:

PO: Peak 2-4 hr, duration 8 hr, half-life 8-10 hr; metabolized by liver, excreted in urine, crosses placenta

Interactions/incompatibilities:

- Increased activity of: oral anticoagulants
- Increased toxicity: sulfa drugs, dapsone, clofibrate, PAS, indomethacin, rifampin, naproxen, methotrexate, pantothenic acid, oral hypoglycemics
- Decreased action of probenecid: alcohol, salicylates, nitrofurantoin, diazoxides, diuretics
- Decreased action of: oral hypoglycemics

NURSING CONSIDERATIONS

Assess:

- Uric acid levels (3-7 mg/dl)
- Respiratory rate, rhythm, depth; notify physician of abnormalities
- Electrolytes, CO_2 before, during treatment
- Urine pH, output, glucose during beginning treatment

Administer:

- After meals or with milk if GI symptoms occur
- Increase fluid intake 2-3 L/day to prevent urinary calculi

*Available in Canada only

Perform/provide:
• Low purine diet restricting: organ meats, anchovies, sardines, meat gravy, dried beans, meat extracts
Evaluate:
• Therapeutic response: absence of pain, stiffness in joints
• For CNS symptoms: confusion, twitching, hyperreflexia, stimulation, headache; may indicate overdose
Teach patient/family
• To avoid high purine foods, alcohol, urinary calculi may form
• To avoid OTC preparations (aspirin) unless directed by physician
Lab test interferences:
False positive: Urine glucose with copper sulfate test (Clinitest)
False positive: Theophylline levels
Increase: BSP/urinary PSP
Decrease: Urinary 17-KS

---

probucol

(proe'byoo-kole)
Lorelco
Func. class.: Antilipemic

Action: Increases bile acid excretion, catabolism of LDL-cholesterol; increases HDL reverse cholesterol transport and blocks oxidation of LDL-cholesterol
Uses: Severe hypercholesterolemia when other treatment unsuccessful
Dosage and routes:
Adult: PO 500 mg bid with breakfast, supper
Available forms include: Tabs 250, 500 mg
Side effects/adverse reactions:
GI: Nausea, vomiting, diarrhea, flatulence, anorexia
CV: Palpitations, dysrhythmias, ***myocardial infarction,*** prolonged QT interval
EENT: Visual disturbances, ptosis, tinnitus
CNS: Insomnia, dizziness, palpitations, paresthesias, syncope
Contraindications: Hypersensitivity
Precautions: Dysrhythmias, pregnancy (B), lactation, children
Pharmacokinetics:
PO: Excreted in bile/feces
Interactions/incompatibilities:
• Do not use with clofibrate

NURSING CONSIDERATIONS

Assess:
• Hepatic function if patient is on long-term therapy
Administer:
• Drug with meals if GI symptoms occur
Evaluate:
• Therapeutic response: decreased cholesterol levels, (hyperlipidemia), diarrhea, pruritus (excess bile area)
• Bowel pattern daily; increase bulk, water in diet if constipation develops
Teach patient/family:
• That compliance is needed since toxicity may result if doses are missed
• That risk factors should be decreased: high fat diet, smoking, alcohol consumption, absence of exercise
• Birth control should be practiced while on this drug
Lab test interferences:
Increase: Liver function studies, CPK, blood glucose, uric acid, BUN

P

procainamide HCl

(proe-kane-a'mide)

Procan SR, Promine, Pronestyl, Sub-Quin, Rhythmin

Func. class.: Antidysrhythmic (Class IA)

Chem. class.: Procaine HCl amide analog

Action: Depresses excitability of cardiac muscle to electrical stimulation and slows conduction in atrium, bundle of His, and ventricle

Uses: PVCs, atrial fibrillation, PAT, ventricular tachycardia, atrial dysrhythmias, ventricular tachycardia

Dosage and routes:

Atrial fibrillation/PAT

• *Adult:* PO 1-1.25 g, may give another 750 mg if needed, if no response then 500 mg-1g q2h until desired response; maintenance 50 mg/kg in divided doses q6h

Ventricular tachycardia

• *Adult:* PO 1g; maintenance 50 mg/kg/day given in 3 hr intervals; SUS REL TABS 500 mg-1.25 g q6h

Other dysrhythmias

• *Adult:* IV BOL 100 mg q5min, given 25-50 mg/min, not to exceed 500 mg; then IV INF 2-6 mg/min

Available forms include: Caps 250, 375, 500 mg; tabs 250, 375, 500 mg; tabs sus rel 250, 500, 750, 1000 mg; inj IV 100, 500 mg/ml

Side effects/adverse reactions:

CNS: Headache, dizziness, confusion, psychosis, restlessness, irritability, weakness

GI: Nausea, vomiting, anorexia, diarrhea, hepatomegaly

CV: Hypotension, ***heart block, cardiovascular collapse, arrest***

HEMA: SLE syndrome, ***agranulocytosis, thrombocytopenia, neutropenia, hemolytic anemia***

INTEG: Rash, urticaria, edema, swelling (rare), pruritus

Contraindications: Hypersensitivity, myasthenia gravis, severe heart block

Precautions: Pregnancy (C), lactation, children, renal disease, liver disease, CHF, respiratory depression

Pharmacokinetics:

PO: Peak 1-2 hr, duration 3 hr (8 hr extended)

IM: Peak 10-60 min, duration 3 hr; half-life 3 hr, metabolized in liver to active metabolites, excreted unchanged by kidneys (60%)

Interactions/incompatibilities:

• Increased effects of: neuromuscular blockers, anticholinergics, antihypertensives

• Increased procainamide effects: cimetidine

• Decreased effects of procainamide: barbiturates

• Increased toxicity: other antidysrhythmics

NURSING CONSIDERATIONS

Assess:

• ECG continuously to determine increased PR or QRS segments; if these develop, discontinue immediately; watch for increased ventricular ectopic beats, maximum need to rebolus

• Blood levels, 3-10 μg/ml

• B/P continuously for fluctuations

• I&O ratio; electrolytes (K, Na, Cl)

Administer:

• IV after diluting 100 mg/ml of D_5W or sterile H_2O for inject, give 20 mg or less/1 min; may dilute 1 g/250-500 ml D_5W, run at 2-6 mg/min

• IM injection in deltoid; aspirate to avoid intravascular administration; check IV site q8h for infiltration or extravasation

* Available in Canada only

Evaluate:

• Therapeutic response: decreased dysrhythmias

• Malignant hyperthermia: tachypnea, tachycardia, changes in B/P, increased temperature

• Cardiac rate, respiration: rate, rhythm, character

• Respiratory status: rate, rhythm, lung fields, watch for respiratory depression

• CNS effects: dizziness, confusion, psychosis, paresthesias, convulsions; drug should be discontinued

• Lung fields, bilateral rales may occur in CHF patient

• Increased respiration, increased pulse; drug should be discontinued

---

procaine HCl

(proe'-kane)

Novocain, Unicaine

Func. class.: Local anesthetic
Chem. class.: Ester

Action: Competes with calcium for sites in nerve membrane that control sodium transport across cell membrane; decreases rise of depolarization phase of action potential

Uses: Spinal anesthesia, epidural, peripheral nerve block, perineum, lower extremities, infiltration

Dosage and routes:
Varies depending on route of anesthesia

Available forms include: Inj 1%, 2%, 10%

Side effects/adverse reactions:
CNS: Anxiety, restlessness, ***convulsions, loss of consciousness,*** drowsiness, disorientation, tremors, shivering
CV: ***Myocardial depression, cardiac arrest, dysrhythmias,*** bradycardia, hypotension, hypertension, fetal bradycardia
GI: Nausea, vomiting
EENT: Blurred vision, tinnitus, pupil constriction
INTEG: Rash, urticaria, allergic reactions, edema, burning, skin discoloration at injection site, tissue necrosis
RESP: ***Status asthmaticus, respiratory arrest, anaphylaxis***

Contraindications: Hypersensitivity, child <12 yr, elderly, severe liver disease

Precautions: Elderly, severe drug allergies, pregnancy (C)

Pharmacokinetics:
Onset 2-5 min, duration 1 hr; metabolized by liver, excreted in urine (metabolites)

Interactions/incompatibilities:

• Dysrhythmias: epinephrine, halothane, enflurane

• Hypertension: MAOIs, tricyclic antidepressants, phenothiazines

• Decreased action of procaine: chloroprocaine

NURSING CONSIDERATIONS

Assess:

• B/P, pulse, respiration during treatment

• Fetal heart tones if drug is used during labor

Administer:

• Only drugs that are not cloudy, do not contain precipitate

• Only with crash cart, resuscitative equipment nearby

• Only drugs without preservatives for epidural or caudal anesthesia

Perform/provide:

• Use of new solution, discard unused portions

Evaluate:

• Therapeutic response: anesthesia necessary for procedure

• Allergic reactions: rash, urticaria, itching

P

• Cardiac status: ECG for dysrhythmias, pulse, B/P during anesthesia

Treatment of overdose: Airway, O_2, vasopressor, IV fluids, anticonvulsants for seizures

procarbazine HCl

(proe-kar'ba-zeen)

Matulane, Natulan*

Func. class.: Antineoplastic, miscellaneous

Chem. class.: Hydrazine derivative

Action: Inhibits DNA, RNA, protein synthesis; has multiple sites of action; a nonvesicant

Uses: Lymphoma, Hodgkin's disease, cancers resistant to other therapy

Dosage and routes:

• *Adult:* PO 2-4 mg/kg/day for first wk; maintain dosage of 4-6 mg/kg/day until platelets and WBC fall; after recovery, 1-2 mg/kg/day

• *Child:* PO 50 mg/day for 7 days, then 100 mg/m^2 until desired response, leukopenia, or thrombocytopenia occurs; 50 mg/day is maintenance after bone marrow recovery

Available forms include: Caps 50 mg

Side effects/adverse reactions:

HEMA: ***Thrombocytopenia, anemia, leukopenia, myelosuppression, bleeding tendencies,*** purpura, petechiae, epistaxis

GI: Nausea, vomiting, anorexia, diarrhea, constipation, dry mouth, stomatitis

EENT: Retinal hemorrhage, nystagmus, photophobia, diplopia

INTEG: Rash, pruritus, dermatitis, alopecia, herpes, hyperpigmentation

CNS: Headache, dizziness, insomnia, hallucinations, confusion, coma, pain, chills, fever, sweating, paresthesias

RESP: Cough, pneumonitis

MS: Arthralgias, myalgias

GU: Azospermia, cessation of menses

Contraindications: Hypersensitivity, thrombocytopenia, bone marrow depression

Precautions: Renal disease, hepatic disease, pregnancy (D), radiation therapy

Pharmacokinetics: Half-life 1 hr; concentrates in liver, kidney, skin; metabolized in liver, excreted in urine

Interactions/incompatibilities:

• Increased CNS depression: barbiturates, antihistamines, narcotics, hypotensive agents, phenothiazines

• Disulfiram-like reaction: ethyl alcohol, MAOIs, tricyclic antidepressants, tyramine foods, sympathomimetic drugs

• Hypertension: guanethidine, levodopa, methyldopa, reserpine

• Increased hypoglycemia: insulin, oral hypoglycemics

NURSING CONSIDERATIONS

Assess:

• CBC, differential, platelet count weekly; withhold drug if WBC is $<4000/mm^3$ or platelet count is $<100,000/mm^3$; notify physician of these results

• Renal function studies: BUN, serum uric acid, urine CrCl, electrolytes before, during therapy

• I&O ratio, report fall in urine output to <30 ml/hr

• Monitor temperature q4h; fever may indicate beginning infection

• Liver function tests before, during therapy: bilirubin, AST, ALT, alk phosphatase prn or monthly

*Available in Canada only

• CNS changes: confusion, paresthesias, neuropathies, drug should be discontinued
Administer:
• In divided doses and at hs to minimize nausea and vomiting
• Nonphenothiazine antiemetic 30-60 min before giving drug and 4-10 hr after treatment to prevent vomiting
• Transfusion for anemia
• Antispasmodic for GI symptoms
Perform/provide:
• Liquid diet: carbonated beverages, gelatin may be added if patient is not nauseated or vomiting
• Storage in tight, light-resistant container in cool environment
Evaluate:
• Therapeutic response: decreased tumor size, spread of malignancy
• Toxicity: facial flushing, epistaxis, increased pro-time, thrombocytopenia; drug should be discontinued
• Bleeding: hematuria, guaiac stools, bruising or petechiae, mucosa or orifices q8h
• Food preferences; list likes, dislikes
• Effects of alopecia on body image; discuss feelings about body changes
• Inflammation of mucosa, breaks in skin
• Yellowing of skin, sclera, dark urine, clay-colored stools, itchy skin, abdominal pain, fever, diarrhea
• Buccal cavity q8h for dryness, sores or ulceration, white patches, oral pain, bleeding, dysphagia
• Alkalosis if vomiting is severe
• GI symptoms: frequency of stools, cramping
• Acidosis, signs of dehydration: rapid respirations, poor skin turgor, decreased urine output, dry skin, restlessness, weakness
Teach patient/family:
• To report any complaints, side effects to nurse or physician: cough, shortness of breath, fever, chills, sore throat, bleeding, bruising, vomiting blood, black tarry stools
• That hair may be lost during treatment and wig or hairpiece may make patient feel better; tell patient that new hair may be different in color, texture
• To avoid foods with citric acid, hot or rough texture
• To report any bleeding, white spots, ulcerations in mouth to physician; tell patient to examine mouth qd
• To avoid driving or activities requiring alertness; dizziness may occur
• That contraceptive measures are recommended during therapy
• To avoid ingestion of alcohol, tyramine-containing foods; cold, hayfever, or weight-reducing products may cause serious drug interactions
• To avoid crowds or persons with infections if granulocytes are low

P

prochlorperazine edisylate/prochlorperazine maleate

(proe-klor-per'a-zeen)
Chlorazine, Compazine, Stemetil*
Func. class.: Antiemetic
Chem. class.: Phenothiazine, piperazine derivative

Action: Acts centrally by blocking chemoreceptor trigger zone, which in turn acts on vomiting center
Uses: Nausea, vomiting
Dosage and routes:
Postoperative nausea/vomiting

• *Adult:* IM 5-10 mg 1-2 hr before anesthesia; may repeat in 30 min; IV 5-10 mg 15-30 min before anesthesia; IV INF 20 mg/L D_5W or NS 15-30 min before anesthesia, not to exceed 40 mg/day

Severe nausea/vomiting

• Adult: PO 5-10 mg tid-qid; SUS REL 15 mg qd in AM or 10 mg q12h; REC 25 mg/bid; IM 5-10 mg; may repeat q4h, not to exceed 40 mg/day

• *Child 18-39 kg:* PO 2.5 mg tid or 5 mg bid; do not exceed 15 mg/day; IM 0.132 mg/kg

• *Child 14-17 kg:* PO/REC 2.5 mg bid-tid, not to exceed 10 mg/day; IM 0.132 mg/kg

• *Child 9-13 kg:* PO/REC 2.5 mg qd-bid, not to exceed 7.5 mg/day; IM 0.132 mg/kg

Available forms include: Oral sol 5 mg/ml; inj 5 mg/ml; tabs 5, 10, 25 mg; caps ext rel 10, 15, 30 mg

Side effects/adverse reactions:

CNS: Euphoria, ***depression,*** *extrapyramidal symptoms,* restlessness, tremor, dizziness

GI: Nausea, vomiting, anorexia, dry mouth, diarrhea, constipation, weight loss, metallic taste, cramps

CV: ***Circulatory failure, tachycardia***

RESP: ***Respiratory depression***

Contraindications: Hypersensitivity to phenothiazines, coma, seizure, encephalopathy, bone marrow depression

Precautions: Children <2 yr, pregnancy (C), elderly

Pharmacokinetics:

PO: Onset 30-40 min, duration 3-4 hr

EX REL: Onset 30-40 min, duration 10-12 hr

REC: Onset 60 min, duration 3-4 hr

IM: Onset 10-20 min, duration 12 hr, metabolized by liver, excreted by kidneys, crosses placenta, excreted in breast milk

Interactions/incompatibilities:

• Decreased effect of prochlorperazine: barbiturates, antacids

• Increased anticholinergic action: anticholinergics, antiparkinson drugs, antidepressants

• Do not mix with other drug in syringe or solution

NURSING CONSIDERATIONS

Assess:

• VS, B/P; check patients with cardiac disease more often

Administer:

• IM injection in large muscle mass; aspirate to avoid IV administration

• IV after diluting 5 mg/9 ml of NaCl for inj, give 5 mg or less/min; may dilute 10-20 mg/1000 ml NaCl and give as infusion

Evaluate:

• Therapeutic response: absence of nausea, vomiting

• Respiratory status before, during, after administration of emetic; check rate, rhythm, character; respiratory depression can occur rapidly with elderly or debilitated patients

Teach patient/family:

• To avoid hazardous activities, activities requiring alertness; dizziness may occur

---

procyclidine HCl

(proe-sye'kli-deen)

Kemadrin, Procyclid*

Func. class.: Cholinergic blocker
Chem. class.: Tertiary amine

Action: Centrally acting anticholinergic

Uses: Parkinson symptoms

Dosage and routes:

• *Adult:* PO 2.5 mg tid pc, titrated to patient response

*Available in Canada only

Available forms include: Tabs 5 mg

Side effects/adverse reactions:

MS: Weakness, cramping

INTEG: Rash, urticaria, dermatoses

MISC: Increased temperature, flushing, decreased sweating, hyperthermia, heat stroke, numbness of fingers

CNS: Confusion, anxiety, restlessness, irritability, delusions, hallucinations, headache, sedation, depression, incoherence, dizziness, light-headedness, memory loss

EENT: Blurred vision, photophobia, dilated pupils, difficulty swallowing, mydriasis

CV: Palpitations, tachycardia, postural hypotension, bradycardia

GI: Dryness of mouth, constipation, nausea, vomiting, abdominal distress, paralytic ileus, ***epigastric distress***

GU: Hesitancy, retention

Contraindications: Hypersensitivity, narrow-angle glaucoma, myasthenia gravis, GI/GU obstruction, child <3 yr, megacolon, stenosing peptic ulcer

Precautions: Pregnancy (C), elderly, lactation, tachycardia, prostatic hypertrophy, children, kidney, liver disease, drug abuse, hypotension, hypertension, psychiatric patients

Pharmacokinetics:

PO: Onset 30-45 min, duration 4-6 hr

Interactions/incompatibilities:

- Decreased action of: haloperidol, levodopa
- Increased anticholinergic effect: antihistamines, MAOIs, phenothiazines

NURSING CONSIDERATIONS

Assess:

- I&O ratio; retention commonly causes decreased urinary output
- Heart rate, rhythm, B/P

Administer:

- With or after meals for GI upset; may give with fluids other than water
- At hs to avoid daytime drowsiness in patient with parkinsonism

Perform/provide:

- Storage at room temperature in tight container
- Hard candy, frequent drinks, sugarless gum to relieve dry mouth

Evaluate:

- Therapeutic response: decreased involuntary movements
- Parkinsonism: shuffling gait, muscle rigidity, involuntary movements
- Urinary hesitancy, retention; palpate bladder if retention occurs
- Constipation especially elderly; increase fluids, bulk, exercise if this occurs, palpate abdomen
- For tolerance over long-term therapy; dose may need to be increased or changed
- Mental status: affect, mood, CNS depression, worsening of mental symptoms during early therapy

Teach patient/family:

- Not to discontinue this drug abruptly; to taper off over 1 wk
- To avoid driving or other hazardous activities; drowsiness may occur
- To avoid OTC medication: cough, cold preparations with alcohol, antihistamines unless directed by physician
- To avoid alcohol

P

progesterone

(proe-jess'ter-one)

Femotrone, Profac-O, Progelan, Progest-50, Progestaject-50, Progestasert

Func. class.: Progestogen
Chem. class.: Progesterone derivative

Action: Inhibits secretion of pituitary gonadotropins, which prevents follicular maturation, ovulation, stimulates growth of mammary tissue, antineoplastic action against endometrial cancer

Uses: Contraception, amenorrhea, premenstrual syndrome, abnormal uterine bleeding

Dosage and routes:

Amenorrhea/uterine bleeding

• Adult: IM 5-10 mg qd × 6-8 doses

Contraception

• Adult: INSERT 1 placed in uterine cavity, active for 1 yr

PMS

• Adult: REC SUPP/VAG SUPP 200-400 mg

Available forms include: Inj IM 25, 50, 100 mg/ml; IU system 38 mg, rec supp, vag supp

Side effects/adverse reactions:

CNS: Dizziness, headache, migraines, depression, fatigue

CV: Hypotension, thrombophlebitis, edema, ***thromboembolism, stroke, pulmonary embolism, myocardial infarction***

GI: Nausea, vomiting, anorexia, cramps, increased weight, ***cholestatic jaundice***

EENT: Diplopia

GU: Amenorrhea, cervical erosion, breakthrough bleeding, dysmenorrhea, vaginal candidiasis, breast changes, *gynecomastia, testicular atrophy, impotence,* endometriosis, ***spontaneous abortion***

INTEG: Rash, urticaria, acne, hirsutism, alopecia, oily skin, seborrhea, purpura, melasma

META: Hyperglycemia

Contraindications: Breast cancer, hypersensitivity, thromboembolic disorders, reproductive cancer, genital bleeding (abnormal, undiagnosed), cerebral hemorrhage, pregnancy (X)

Precautions: Lactation, hypertension, asthma, blood dyscrasias, gallbladder disease, CHF, diabetes mellitus, bone disease, depression, migraine headache, convulsive disorders, hepatic disease, renal disease, family history of breast or reproductive tract cancer

Pharmacokinetics:

IM: Duration 24 hr

Excreted in urine, feces, metabolized in liver

NURSING CONSIDERATIONS

Assess:

• Weight daily; notify physician of weekly weight gain >5 lb

• B/P at beginning of treatment and periodically

• I&O ratio; be alert for decreasing urinary output, increasing edema

• Liver function studies: ALT, AST, bilirubin periodically during long-term therapy

Administer:

• Titrated dose; use lowest effective dose

• Oil solution deeply in large muscle mass IM, rotate sites

• In one dose in AM

• With food or milk to decrease GI symptoms

• After warming to dissolve crystals

Perform/provide:

• Storage in dark area

* Available in Canada only

Evaluate:
• Therapeutic response: decrease abnormal uterine bleeding, absence of amenorrhea
• Edema, hypertension, cardiac symptoms, jaundice
• Mental status: affect, mood, behavioral changes, depression
• Hypercalcemia

Teach patient/family:
• About cushingoid symptoms
• To report breast lumps, vaginal bleeding, edema, jaundice, dark urine, clay-colored stools, dyspnea, headache, blurred vision, abdominal pain, numbness or stiffness in legs, chest pain
• To report suspected pregnancy
• To monitor blood sugar, if diabetic

Lab test interferences:
Increase: Alk phosphatase, nitrogen (urine), pregnanediol, amino acids, factors VII, VIII, IX, X
Decrease: GTT, HDL

---

promazine HCl

(proe'ma-zeen)
Promanyl,* Prozine, Sparine
Func. class.: Antipsychotic/neuroleptic
Chem. class.: Phenothiazine, aliphatic

Action: Depresses cerebral cortex, hypothalamus, limbic system, which control activity, aggression; blocks neurotransmission produced by dopamine at synapse; exhibits a strong α-adrenergic, anticholinergic blocking action; as antiemetic, inhibits medullary chemoreceptor trigger zone; mechanism for antipsychotic effects is unclear

Uses: Psychotic disorders, schizophrenia, nausea, vomiting, alcohol withdrawal

Dosage and routes:
Psychosis
• *Adult:* PO 10-200 mg q4-6h, max dose 1000 mg/day; IM 50-150 mg, followed in 30 min with additional dose up to a total dose of 300 mg
• *Child >12 yr:* PO 10-25 mg q4-6h

Nausea/vomiting
• *Adult:* PO 25-50 mg q4-6h; IM 50 mg; IV not recommended, but may use in concentrations of <25 mg/ml

Available forms include: Tabs 25, 50, 100 mg; syr 10 mg/5ml; inj IV, IM 25, 50 mg/ml

Side effects/adverse reactions:
RESP: ***Laryngospasm,*** dyspnea, ***respiratory depression***
CNS: Extrapyramidal symptoms: pseudoparkinsonism, akathisia, dystonia, tardive dyskinesia, drowsiness, headache, ***seizures***
HEMA: Anemia, ***leukopenia, leukocytosis, agranulocytosis***
INTEG: Rash, photosensitivity, dermatitis
EENT: Blurred vision, glaucoma, dry eyes
GI: Dry mouth, nausea, vomiting, anorexia, constipation, diarrhea, jaundice, weight gain
GU: Urinary retention, urinary frequency, enuresis, impotence, amenorrhea, gynecomastia
CV: Orthostatic hypotension, ***cardiac arrest,*** ECG changes, ***tachycardia***

Contraindications: Hypersensitivity, blood dyscrasias, coma, child <12 yr, brain damage, bone marrow depression, glaucoma

Precautions: Pregnancy (C), lactation, seizure disorders, hypertension, hepatic disease, cardiac disease

Pharmacokinetics:
PO: Onset erratic, peak 2-4 hr

IM: Onset 15 min, peak 1 hr, duration 4-6 hr; metabolized by liver, excreted in urine, crosses placenta, enters breast milk

Interactions/incompatibilities:

• Oversedation: other CNS depressants, alcohol, barbiturate anesthetics

• Toxicity: epinephrine

• Decreased absorption: aluminum hydroxide or magnesium hydroxide antacids

• Decreased effects of: lithium, levodopa

• Increased effects of both drugs: β-adrenergic blockers, alcohol

• Increased anticholinergic effects: anticholinergics

NURSING CONSIDERATIONS

Assess:

• Mental status before initial administration

• Swallowing of PO medication; check for hoarding or giving of medication to other patients

• I&O ratio; palpate bladder if low urinary output occurs

• Bilirubin, CBC, liver function studies monthly

• Urinalysis is recommended before and during prolonged therapy

Administer:

• Reduced dose in elderly

• IV undiluted, give at 25 mg/min or less over 1 min; may dilute 25-60 mg/9 ml NaCl for inj

• Antiparkinsonian agent, after securing order from physician to be used if EPS occur

• Syrup mixed in citrus- or chocolate-flavored drinks

• IM injection into large muscle mass

Perform/provide:

• Decreased noise input by dimming lights, avoiding loud noises

• Supervised ambulation until stabilized on medication; do not involve in strenuous exercise program because fainting is possible; patient should not stand still for long periods of time

• Increased fluids to prevent constipation

• Sips of water, candy, gum for dry mouth

• Storage in tight, light-resistant container; avoid contact with hands

Evaluate:

• Therapeutic response: decrease in emotional excitement, hallucinations, delusions, paranoia, reorganization of patterns of thought, speech

• Affect, orientation, LOC, reflexes, gait, coordination, sleep pattern disturbances

• B/P standing and lying; also include pulse, respirations, q4h during initial treatment; establish baseline before starting treatment; report drops of 30 mm Hg

• Dizziness, faintness, palpitations, tachycardia on rising

• Extrapyramidal symptoms including akathisia (inability to sit still, no pattern to movements), tardive dyskinesia (bizarre movements of jaw, mouth, tongue, extremities), pseudoparkinsonism (rigidity, tremors, pill rolling, shuffling gait)

• For neuroleptic malignant syndrome: muscle rigidity, altered mental status, hyperthermia, increased CPK

• Skin turgor daily

• Constipation, urinary retention daily, if these occur increase bulk and water in diet

Teach patient/family:

• That orthostatic hypotension occurs frequently, and to rise from sitting or lying position gradually, to avoid hazardous activities until stabilized on medication

---

* Available in Canada only

- To remain lying down after IM injection for at least 30 min
- To avoid hot tubs, hot showers, or tub baths since hypotension may occur
- To avoid abrupt withdrawal of this drug or extrapyramidal symptoms may result; drugs should be withdrawn slowly
- To avoid OTC preparations (cough, hayfever, cold) unless approved by physician since serious drug interactions may occur; avoid use with alcohol or CNS depressants, increased drowsiness may occur
- To use a sunscreen during sun exposure to prevent burns
- Regarding compliance with drug regimen
- About extrapyramidal symptoms and necessity for meticulous oral hygiene since oral candidiasis may occur
- To report sore throat, malaise, fever, bleeding, mouth sores; if these occur, CBC should be drawn and drug discontinued
- In hot weather, heat stroke may occur; take extra precautions to stay cool

Lab test interferences:
Increase: Liver function tests, cardiac enzymes, cholesterol, blood glucose, prolactin, bilirubin, PBI, cholinesterase, ^{131}I
Decrease: Hormones (blood and urine)
False positive: Pregnancy tests, PKU
False negative: Urinary steroids, 17-OHCS, pregnancy tests
Treatment of overdose: Lavage if orally injested, provide an airway; *do not induce vomiting*

promethazine HCl

(proe-meth'a-zeen)
Ganphen, Methazine, Pentazine, Phencen-50, Phenergan, Prorex, Provigan, Remsed, Rolamethazine, Sigazine
Func. class.: Antihistamine, H_1-receptor antagonist
Chem. class.: Phenothiazine derivative

Action: Acts on blood vessels, GI, respiratory system by competing with histamine for H_1-receptor site; decreases allergic response by blocking histamine
Uses: Motion sickness, rhinitis, allergy symptoms, sedation, nausea, preoperative, postoperative sedation
Dosage and routes:
Nausea
- *Adult:* PO/IM 25 mg, may repeat 12.5-25 mg q4-6h
- *Child:* PO/IM 0.5 mg/lb q4-6h

Motion sickness
- *Adult:* PO 25 mg bid
- *Child:* PO/IM/REC 12.5-25 mg bid

Allergy/rhinitis
- *Adult:* PO 12.5 mg qid, or 25 mg hs
- *Child:* PO 6.25-12.5 mg tid or 25 mg hs

Sedation
- *Adult:* PO/IM 25-50 mg hs
- *Child:* PO/IM/REC 12.5-25 mg hs

Sedation (preoperative/postoperative)
- *Adult:* PO/IM/IV 25-50 mg
- *Child:* PO/IM/IV 12.5-25 mg

Available forms include: Tabs 12.5, 25, 50 mg; syr 6.25, 25 mg/5 ml; supp 12.5, 25, 50 mg; inj 25, 50 mg/ml

P

Side effects/adverse reactions:
CNS: Dizziness, drowsiness, poor coordination, fatigue, anxiety, euphoria, confusion, paresthesia, neuritis
CV: Hypotension, palpitations, tachycardia
RESP: Increased thick secretions, wheezing, chest tightness
HEMA: ***Thrombocytopenia, agranulocytosis, hemolytic anemia***
GI: Constipation, dry mouth, nausea, vomiting, anorexia, diarrhea
INTEG: Rash, urticaria, photosensitivity
GU: Retention, dysuria, frequency
EENT: Blurred vision, dilated pupils, tinnitus, nasal stuffiness, dry nose, throat, mouth, photosensitivity

Contraindications: Hypersensitivity to H_1-receptor antagonist, acute asthma attack, lower respiratory tract disease

Precautions: Increased intraocular pressure, renal disease, cardiac disease, hypertension, bronchial asthma, seizure disorder, stenosed peptic ulcers, hyperthyroidism, prostatic hypertrophy, bladder neck obstruction, pregnancy (C)

Pharmacokinetics:
PO: Onset 20 min, duration 4-6 hr, metabolized in liver, excreted by kidneys, GI tract (inactive metabolites)

Interactions/incompatibilities:
- Increased CNS depression: barbiturates, narcotics, hypnotics, tricyclic antidepressants, alcohol
- Decreased effect of: oral anticoagulants, heparin
- Increased effect of promethazine: MAOIs

NURSING CONSIDERATIONS

Assess:
- I&O ratio; be alert for urinary retention, frequency, dysuria; drug should be discontinued if these occur
- CBC during long-term therapy

Administer:
- IV after diluting 25-50 mg/9 ml of NaCl for inj; give 25 mg or less/2 min
- With meals if GI symptoms occur, absorption may slightly decrease
- Deep IM in large muscle; rotate site
- When used for motion sickness, 30 min before travel

Perform/provide:
- Hard candy, gum, frequent rinsing of mouth for dryness
- Storage in tight, light-resistant container

Evaluate:
- Therapeutic response: absence of running, congested nose, rashes, absence of motion sickness, nausea; sedation
- Respiratory status: rate, rhythm, increase in bronchial secretions, wheezing, chest tightness
- Cardiac status: palpitations, increased pulse, hypotension

Teach patient/family:
- That drug may cause photosensitivity; to avoid prolonged sunlight
- To notify physician if confusion, sedation, hypotension occurs
- To avoid driving or other hazardous activity if drowsiness occurs
- To avoid concurrent use of alcohol or other CNS depressants

Lab test interferences:
False negative: Skin allergy tests
False positive: Urine pregnancy test

Treatment of overdose: Administer ipecac syrup or lavage, diazepam, vasopressors, barbiturates (short-acting)

---

propafenone

(proe-pa-fen'one)
Rythmol
Func. class.: Antidysrhythmic, (Class IC)

Action: Able to slow conduction velocity; reduces membrane responsiveness, inhibits automaticity, increases ratio of effective refractory period to action potential duration, β-blocking activity

Uses: Life-threatening dysrhythmias, sustained ventricular tachycardia

Dosage and routes:
- *Adult:* PO 300-900 mg/day in divided doses, 150 mg q8h, allow a 3-4 day interval before increasing dose

Available forms include: Tabs 150, 300 mg

Side effects/adverse reactions:
INTEG: Rash
CV: Dysrhythmias, palpitations, AV block, intraventricular conduction delay, AV dissociation, CHF, ***sudden death,*** atrial flutter
HEMA: ***Leukopenia, agranulocytosis, granulocytopenia, thrombocytopenia,*** anemia
CNS: Headache, dizziness, abnormal dreams, syncope, confusion, ***seizures***
GI: Nausea, vomiting, constipation, dyspepsia, cholestasis, ***hepatitis,*** abnormal liver function studies, dry mouth
RESP: Dyspnea
EENT: Blurred vision, altered taste, tinnitus

Contraindications: 2nd or 3rd degree AV block, right bundle branch block, cardiogenic shock, hypersensitivity, bradycardia, uncontrolled CHF, sick-sinus node syndrome, marked hypotension, bronchospastic disorders

Precautions: CHF, hypokalemia, hyperkalemia, recent MI, nonallergic branchospasm, pregnancy (C), lactation, children, hepatic or renal disease

Pharmacokinetics:
Peak 3-5 hr, half-life 2-10 hr, metabolized in liver, excreted in urine (metabolite)

Interactions/incompatibilities:
- Increased effect of propafenone: cimetidine, quinidine
- Increased anticoagulation: warfarin
- Increased digoxin level: digoxin
- Increased β-blocker effect: propranolol, metoprolol

NURSING CONSIDERATIONS

Assess:
- GI status: bowel pattern, number of stools
- Cardiac status: rate, rhythm, quality
- Chest x-ray, pulmonary function test during treatment
- I&O ratio; check for decreasing output
- B/P for fluctuations
- Lung fields; bilateral rales may occur in CHF patient
- Increased respiration, increased pulse; drug should be discontinued

Evaluate:
- Therapeutic response: absence of dysrhythmias
- Toxicity: fine tremors, dizziness
- Cardiac rate: respiration, rate, rhythm, character continuously

Lab test interferences:
Increase: CPK

Treatment of overdose: O_2, artificial ventilation, ECG, administer dopamine for circulatory depression, administer diazepam or thiopental for convulsions

P

propantheline bromide

(proe-pan'the-leen)

Banlin,* Norpanth, Pro-Banthine, Propanthel*

Func. class.: Gastrointestinal anticholinergic

Chem. class.: Synthetic quarternary ammonium compound

Action: Inhibits muscarinic actions of acetylcholine at postganglionic parasympathetic neuroeffector sites

Uses: Treatment of peptic ulcer disease, irritable bowel syndrome, duodenography, urinary incontinence

Dosage and routes:

- *Adult:* PO 15 mg tid ac, 30 mg hs
- *Elderly:* PO 7.5 mg tid ac

Available forms include: Tabs 7.5, 15 mg

Side effects/adverse reactions:

CNS: Confusion, stimulation in elderly, headache, insomnia, dizziness, drowsiness, anxiety, weakness, hallucinations

GI: Dry mouth, constipation, ***paralytic ileus,*** heartburn, nausea, vomiting, dysphagia, absence of taste

GU: Hesitancy, retention, impotence

CV: Palpitations, tachycardia

EENT: Blurred vision, photophobia, mydriasis, cycloplegia, increased ocular tension

INTEG: Urticaria, rash, pruritus, anhidrosis, fever, allergic reactions

Contraindications: Hypersensitivity to anticholinergics, narrow-angle glaucoma, GI obstruction, myasthenia gravis, paralytic ileus, GI atony, toxic megacolon

Precautions: Hyperthyroidism, coronary artery disease, dysrhythmias, CHF, ulcerative colitis, hypertension, hiatal hernia, hepatic disease, renal disease, pregnancy (C), urinary retention, prostatic hypertrophy

Pharmacokinetics:

PO: Onset 30-45 min, duration 6 hr; metabolized by liver, GI system, excreted in urine, bile

Interactions/incompatibilities:

- Increased anticholinergic effect: amantadine, tricyclic antidepressants, MAOIs, H_1 antihistamines
- Decreased effect of: phenothiazines, levodopa, ketoconazole

NURSING CONSIDERATIONS

Assess:

- VS, cardiac status: checking for dysrhythmias, increased rate, palpitations
- I&O ratio; check for urinary retention or hesitancy

Administer:

- ½-1 hr ac for better absorption
- Decreased dose to elderly patients; their metabolism may be slowed
- Gum, hard candy, frequent rinsing of mouth for dryness of oral cavity

Perform/provide:

- Storage in tight container protected from light
- Increased fluids, bulk, exercise to patient's lifestyle to decrease constipation

Evaluate:

- Therapeutic response: absence of epigastric pain, bleeding, nausea, vomiting
- GI complaints: pain, bleeding (frank or occult), nausea, vomiting, anorexia

Teach patient/family:

- To avoid driving or other hazardous activities until stabilized on medication, may cause blurred vision

* Available in Canada only

• To avoid alcohol or other CNS depressants; will enhance sedating properties of this drug
• To drink plenty of fluids
• To report dysphagia

propofol

(proe-po'foel)

Diprivan

Func. class.: General anesthetic

Controlled Substance Schedule II

Action: Produces dose-dependent CNS depression

Uses: Induction or maintenance of anesthesia, as part of balanced anesthetic technique

Dosage and routes:

Induction

• *Adult:* IV 2-2.5 mg/kg, approximately 40 mg q10sec until inducton onset

• *Elderly:* 1-1.5 mg/kg, approximately 20 mg q10sec until induction onset

Maintenance

• *Adult:* 0.1-0.2 mg/kg/min (6-12 mg/kg/hr)

• *Elderly:* 0.05-0.1 mg/kg/min (3-6 mg/kg/hr)

Intermittent bolus

• *Adult:* Increments of 25-50 mg as needed

Available forms include: Inj 10 mg/ml in 20 ml amp

Side effects/adverse reactions:

CNS: Movement, headache, jerking, fever, dizziness, shivering, tremor, confusion, somnolence, paresthesia, agitation, abnormal dreams, euphoria, fatigue

GI: Nausea, vomiting, abdominal cramping, dry mouth, swallowing, hypersalivation

MS: Myalgia

GU: Urine retention, green urine

EENT: Blurred vision, tinnitus, eye pain, strange taste

CV: Bradycardia, hypotension, hypertension, PVC, PAC, tachycardia, abnormal ECG, ST segment depression

RESP: ***Apnea,*** *cough, hiccups,* dyspnea, hypoventilation, sneezing, wheezing, tachypnea, hypoxia

INTEG: Flushing, phlebitis, hives, burning/stinging at injection site

Contraindications: Hypersensitivity

Precautions: Elderly, respiratory depression, severe respiratory disorders, cardiac dysrhythmias, pregnancy (B), labor and delivery, lactation, children

Pharmacokinetics:

Onset 40 sec, rapid distribution, half-life 1-8 min, terminal elimination half-life 5-10 hr, 70% excreted in urine, metabolized in liver by conjugation to inactivate metabolites

Interactions/incompatibilities:

• Increased CNS depression: alcohol, narcotics, sedative/hypnotics, antipsychotics, skeletal muscle relaxants, inhalational anesthetics

NURSING CONSIDERATIONS

Assess:

• Injection site: phlebitis, burning/stinging

• ECG for changes: PVC, PAC, S-T segment changes

Administer:

• After diluting with D_5W, use only glass containers when mixing, not stable in plastic

• By injection (IV only)

• Alone, do not mix with other agents before using

• Only with resuscitative equipment available

• Only by qualified persons trained in anesthesia

P

Perform/provide:
• Storage in light-resistant area at room temperature
• Coughing, turning, deep breathing for postoperative patients
• Safety measures: siderails, night light, call bell within reach

Evaluate:
• Therapeutic response: induction of anesthesia
• CNS changes: movement, jerking, tremors, dizziness, LOC, pupil reaction
• Allergic reactions: hives
• Respiratory dysfunction: respiratory depression, character, rate, rhythm; notify physician if respirations are <10/min

Treatment of overdose: Discontinue drug, artificial ventilation, administer vasopressor agents or anticholinergics

---

propoxyphene HCl/ propoxyphene napsylate

(proe-pox'i-feen)

Darvon, Dolene, Doraphen, Myospaz, Pargesic-65, Proxagesic, Ropoxy 642*/Darvocet-N, Darvon-N

Func. class.: Narcotic analgesics
Chem. class.: Synthetic opiate

Controlled Substance Schedule IV

Action: Depresses pain impulse transmission at the spinal cord level by interacting with opioid receptors

Uses: Mild to moderate pain

Dosage and routes:
• *Adult:* PO 65 mg q4h prn (HCl)
• *Adult:* PO 100 mg q4h prn (Napsylate)

Available forms include: HCl-tabs 32, 65 mg; napsylate-tabs 100 mg; susp 10 mg/ml

Side effects/adverse reactions:
CNS: Drowsiness, dizziness, confusion, headache, sedation, euphoria, ***convulsions, hyperthermia***
GI: Nausea, vomiting, anorexia, constipation, cramps
GU: Increased urinary output, dysuria
INTEG: Rash, urticaria, bruising, flushing, diaphoresis, pruritus
EENT: Tinnitus, blurred vision, miosis, diplopia
CV: Palpitations, bradycardia, change in B/P, ***dysrhythmias***
RESP: ***Respiratory depression***

Contraindications: Hypersensitivity to ASA products (some preparations), addiction (narcotic)

Precautions: Addictive personality, pregnancy (C), lactation, increased intracranial pressure, MI (acute), severe heart disease, respiratory depression, hepatic disease, renal disease, child <18 yr

Pharmacokinetics:
PO: Onset 15-30 min, peak 2-3 hr, duration 4-6 hr
REC: Onset slow; duration 4-6 hr
Metabolized by liver, excreted by kidneys (as metabolites), crosses placenta, excreted in breast milk, half-life 12 hr (metabolites)

Interactions/incompatibilities:
• Increased effects with other CNS depressants: alcohol, narcotics, sedative/hypnotics, antipsychotics, skeletal muscle relaxants

NURSING CONSIDERATIONS

Assess:
• I&O ratio; check for decreasing output; may indicate urinary retention

Administer:
• With antiemetic if nausea, vomiting occur
• When pain is beginning to return; determine dosage interval by patient response

---

* Available in Canada only

Perform/provide:
• Storage in light-resistant area at room temperature
• Assistance with ambulation
• Safety measures: siderails, night light, call bell within easy reach

Evaluate:
• Therapeutic response: decrease in pain
• CNS changes: dizziness, drowsiness, hallucinations, euphoria, LOC, pupil reaction
• Allergic reactions: rash, urticaria
• Respiratory dysfunction: respiratory depression, character, rate, rhythm; notify physician if respirations are <10/min
• Need for pain medication, physical dependence

Teach patient/family:
• To report any symptoms of CNS changes, allergic reactions
• That physical dependency may result when used for extended periods of time; not to exceed dose
• That withdrawal symptoms may occur: nausea, vomiting, cramps, fever, faintness, anorexia

Lab test interferences:
Increase: Amylase

Treatment of overdose: Narcan 0.2-0.8 IV, O_2, IV fluids, vasopressors

---

propranolol HCl

(proe-pran'oh-lole)
Inderal

Func. class.: Antihypertensive, antianginal
Chem. class.: β-Adrenergic blocker

Action: Nonselective β-blocker with negative inotropic, chronotropic, dromotropic properties

Uses: Chronic stable angina pectoris, hypertension, supraventricular dysrhythmias, migraine, prophylaxis, MI, pheochromocytoma, essential tremor

Dosage and routes:

Dysrythmias
• *Adult:* PO 10-30 mg tid-qid; IV BOL 0.5-3 mg over 1 mg/min; may repeat in 2 min

Hypertension
• *Adult:* PO 40 mg bid or 80 mg qd (sus rel) initially; usual dose 120-240 mg/day bid-tid or 120-160 mg qd (sus rel)

Angina
• *Adult:* PO 80-320 mg in divided doses bid-qid or 80 mg qd (sus rel); usual dose 160 mg qd (sus rel)

MI
• *Adult:* PO 180-240 mg/day tid-qid

Pheochromocytoma
• *Adult:* PO 60 mg/day × 3 days preoperatively in divided doses or 30 mg/day in divided doses (inoperable tumor)

Migraine
• *Adult:* PO 80 mg/day (sus rel) or in divided doses; may increase to 160-240 mg/day in divided doses

Essential tremor
• *Adult:* PO 40 mg bid; usual dose 120 mg/day

Available forms include: Caps ext rel 80, 120, 160 mg; tabs 10, 20, 40, 60, 80, 90 mg; inj 1 mg/ml, oral sol 4 mg, 8 mg/ml, conc oral sol 80 mg/ml, ext rel cap 60 mg

Side effects/adverse reactions:

RESP: Dyspnea, respiratory dysfunction, *bronchospasm*

CV: Bradycardia, hypotension, ***CHF,*** palpitations, AV block, peripheral vascular insufficiency, vasodilation

HEMA: ***Agranulocytosis, thrombocytopenia***

GI: Nausea, vomiting, diarrhea, colitis, constipation, cramps, dry

P

mouth, hepatomegaly, gastric pain, acute pancreatitis
GU: Impotence, decreased libido, urinary tract infections
MS: Joint pain, arthralgia, muscle cramps, pain
MISC: Facial swelling, weight change, Raynaud's phenomenon
INTEG: Rash, pruritus, fever
CNS: Depression, hallucinations, dizziness, fatigue, lethargy, paresthesias, bizarre dreams, disorientation
EENT: Sore throat, ***laryngospasm,*** blurred vision, dry eyes
META: Hyperglycemia, hypoglycemia

Contraindications: Hypersensitivity to this drug, cardiac failure, cardiogenic shock, 2nd or 3rd degree heart block, bronchospastic disease, sinus bradycardia, CHF

Precautions: Diabetes mellitus, pregnancy (C), renal disease, lactation, hyperthyroidism, COPD, hepatic disease, children, myasthenia gravis, peripheral vascular disease, hypotension

Pharmacokinetics:
PO: Onset 30 min, peak 1-1½ hr
IV: Onset 2 min, peak 15 min, duration 3-6 hr; immediate rel half-life 3-5 hr; sus rel half-life 8-11 hr; metabolized by liver, crosses placenta, blood-brain barrier, excreted in breast milk

Interactions/incompatibilities:
- AV block: digitalis, calcium channel blockers
- Increased negative inotropic effects: verapamil, disopyramide
- Increased effects of: reserpine, digitalis, neuromuscular blocking agents
- Decreased β-blocking effects: norepinephrine, isoproterenol, barbiturates, rifampin, dopamine, dobutamine, smoking
- Increased β-blocking effect: cimetidine
- Increased hypotension: quinidine, haloperidol, hydralazine

NURSING CONSIDERATIONS

Assess:
- B/P, pulse, respirations during beginning therapy
- Weight qd, report gain of 5 lb
- I&O ratio, CrCl if kidney damage is diagnosed
- ECG if using as antidysrhythmic
- Hepatic enzymes: AST, ALT, bilirubin

Administer:
- IV undiluted or diluted 10 ml D_5W for inj, give 1 mg or less/min; may be diluted in 50 ml NaCl and run 1 mg over 10-15 min
- With 8 oz of water on empty stomach

Evaluate:
- Therapeutic response: decreased B/P, dysrhythmias
- Pain: duration, time started, activity being performed, character
- Tolerance if taken over long period of time
- Headache, light-headedness, decreased B/P; may indicate a need for decreased dosage

Teach patient/family:
- Not to discontinue abruptly, to take drug at same time each day
- To avoid OTC drugs unless approved by physician
- To avoid hazardous activities if dizziness occurs
- Stress patient compliance with complete medical regimen
- To make position changes slowly to prevent fainting
- To decrease dosage over 2 weeks to prevent cardiac damage

Lab test interferences:
Increase: Serum potassium, serum uric acid, ALT/AST, alk phosphatase, LDH
Decrease: Blood glucose

propylthiouracil (PTU)

(proe-pill-thye-oh-yoor'a-sill)
Propyl-Thyracil*
Func. class.: Thyroid hormone antagonist
Chem. class.: Thioamide

Action: Blocks synthesis of T_3, T_4 (triiodothyronine, thyroxine), inhibits organification of iodine
Uses: Preparation for thyroidectomy, thyrotoxic crisis, hyperthyroidism, thyroid storm
Dosage and routes:
Thyrotoxic crisis
- *Adult and child:* PO same as hyperthyroidism with iodine and propranolol

Preparation for thyroidectomy
- *Adult*: 600-1200 mg/day
- *Child*: 10 mg/kg/day in divided doses

Hyperthyroidism
- *Adult:* PO 100 mg tid increasing to 300 mg q8h, if condition is severe; continue to euthyroid state, then 100 mg qd-tid
- *Child > 10 yr:* PO 100 mg tid, continue to euthyroid state, then 25 mg tid to 100 mg bid
- *Child 6-10 yr:* PO 50-150 mg in divided doses q8h

Available forms include: Tabs 50 mg
Side effects/adverse reactions:
INTEG: Rash, urticaria, pruritus, alopecia, hyperpigmentation, lupuslike syndrome
GU: ***Nephritis***
CNS: Drowsiness, headache, vertigo, fever, paresthesias, neuritis
HEMA: ***Agranulocytosis, leukopenia, thrombocytopenia, hypothrombinemia, lymphadenopathy,*** bleeding, vasculitis, periarteritis
GI: Nausea, diarrhea, vomiting, ***jaundice, hepatits,*** loss of taste
MS: Myalgia, arthralgia, nocturnal muscle cramps
Contraindications: Hypersensitivity, pregnancy (D), lactation
Precautions: Infection, bone marrow depression, hepatic disease
Pharmacokinetics:
PO: Onset 30-40 min, duration 2-4 hr, half-life 1-2 hr, excreted in urine, bile, breast milk, crosses placenta
Interactions/incompatibilities:
- Increased anticoagulant effect: heparin, oral anticoagulants

NURSING CONSIDERATIONS
Assess:
- Pulse, B/P, temperature
- I&O ratio; check for edema: puffy hands, feet, periorbits; indicates hypothyroidism
- Weight qd; same clothing, scale, time of day
- T_3, T_4, which is increased; serum TSH, which is decreased; free thyroxine index, which is increased if dosage is too low; discontinue drug 3-4 wk before RAIU
- Blood work: CBC for blood dyscrasias: leukopenia, thrombocytopenia, agranulocytosis; LFTs

Administer:
- With meals to decrease GI upset
- At same time each day, to maintain drug level
- Lowest dose that relieves symptoms

Perform/provide:
- Storage in light-resistant container
- Fluids to 3-4 L/day, unless contraindicated

Evaluate:
- Therapeutic response: weight gain, decreased pulse, decreased T_4, decreased B/P
- Overdose: peripheral edema, heat intolerance, diaphoresis, palpita-

tions, dysrhythmias, severe tachycardia, increased temperature delirium, CNS irritability
• Hypersensitivity: rash, enlarged cervical lymph nodes, drug may need to be discontinued
• Hypoprothrombinemia: bleeding, petechiae, ecchymosis
• Clinical response: after 3 wk should include increased weight, pulse; decreased T_4
• Bone marrow depression: sore throat, fever, fatigue

Teach patient/family:
• To abstain from breast feeding after delivery
• To take pulse daily
• To report redness, swelling, sore throat, mouth lesions, which indicate blood dyscrasias
• To keep graph of weight, pulse, mood
• To avoid OTC products that contain iodine
• That seafood, other iodine products may be restricted
• Not to discontinue this medication abruptly; thyroid crisis may occur; stress patient response
• That response may take several months if thyroid is large
• Symptoms/signs of overdose: periorbital edema, cold intolerance, mental depression
• Symptoms of inadequate dose: tachycardia, diarrhea, fever, irritability

Lab test interferences:
Increases: Pro-time, AST/ALT, alk phosphatase

protamine sulfate
(proe'ta-meen)

Func. class.: Heparin antagonist
Chem. class.: Low molecular weight protein

Action: Binds heparin making it ineffective
Uses: Heparin overdose
Dosage and routes:
• *Adult:* IV 1 mg of protamine/90-115 U heparin given, administer slowly 1-3 min; give undiluted to 1%, not to exceed 50 mg/10 min
Available forms include: Inj IV 10 mg/ml
Side effects/adverse reactions:
CV: Hypotension, bradycardia
GI: Nausea, vomiting, anorexia
INTEG: *Rash,* dermatitis, urticaria
CNS: Lassitude
HEMA: Bleeding, ***anaphylaxis***
Contraindications: Hypersensitivity
Precautions: Pregnancy (C), lactation, children, allergy to fish
Pharmacokinetics:
IV: Onset 5 min, duration 2 hr

NURSING CONSIDERATIONS

Assess:
• Blood studies (Hct, platelets, occult blood in stools) q3mo
• Coagulation tests (APTT, ACT) 15 min after dose, then in several hours
• VS, B/P, pulse of 30 min; plus 3 hr after dose

Administer:
• IV after diluting 50 mg/5 ml sterile bacteriostatic H_2O for inj; shake, give 20 mg or less over 1-3 min; may further dilute with equal volume of NaCl or D_5W and run over 2-3 hr

Perform/provide:
• Storage at 36°-46° F

Evaluate:
• Therapeutic response: reversal of heparin overdose
• Skin rash, urticaria, dermatitis
• Allergy to fish, use with caution in these patients

*Available in Canada only

protriptyline HCl

(proe-trip'te-leen)

Triptil, Vivactil

Func. class.: Antidepressant—tricyclic

Chem. class.: Dibenzocycloheptene—secondary amine

Action: Blocks reuptake of norepinephrine, serotonin into nerve endings, increasing action of norepinephrine, serotonin in nerve cells

Uses: Depression

Dosage and routes:

• *Adult:* PO 15-40 mg/day in divided doses, may increase to 60 mg/day

Available forms include: Tabs 5, 10 mg

Side effects/adverse reactions:

HEMA: ***Agranulocytosis, thrombocytopenia, eosinophilia, leukopenia***

CNS: Dizziness, drowsiness, confusion, headache, anxiety, tremors, stimulation, weakness, insomnia, nightmares, EPS (elderly), increased psychiatric symptoms, paresthesia

GI: Diarrhea, dry mouth, nausea, vomiting, ***paralytic ileus,*** increased appetite, cramps, epigastric distress, jaundice, ***hepatitis,*** stomatitis

GU: Retention, ***acute renal failure***

INTEG: Rash, urticaria, sweating, pruritus, photosensitivity

CV: Orthostatic hypotension, ECG changes, tachycardia, ***hypertension,*** palpitations

EENT: Blurred vision, tinnitus, mydriasis

Contraindications: Hypersensitivity to tricyclic antidepressants, recovery phase of myocardial infarction, convulsive disorders, prostatic hypertrophy

Precautions: Suicidal patients, severe depression, increased intraocular pressure, narrow-angle glaucoma, urinary retention, cardiac disease, hepatic disease, hyperthyroidism, electroshock therapy, elective surgery, pregnancy (C)

Pharmacokinetics:

PO: Onset 15-30 min, peak 24-30 hr, duration 4-6 hr; therapeutic effect 2-3 wk; metabolized by liver, excreted by kidneys, crosses placenta, half-life 54-98 hr

Interactions/incompatibilities:

• Decreased effects of: guanethidine, clonidine, indirect acting sympathomimetics (ephedrine)

• Increased effects of: direct acting sympathomimetics (epinephrine), alcohol, barbiturates, benzodiazepines, CNS depressants

• Hyperpyretic crisis, convulsions, hypertensive episode: MAOI (pargyline [Eutonyl])

NURSING CONSIDERATIONS

Assess:

• B/P (lying, standing), pulse q4h; if systolic B/P drops 20 mm Hg hold drug, notify physician; take vital signs q4h in patients with cardiovascular disease

• Blood studies: CBC, leukocytes, differential, cardiac enzymes if patient is receiving long-term therapy

• Hepatic studies: AST, ALT, bilirubin, creatinine

• Weight qwk, appetite may increase with drug

• ECG for flattening of T wave, bundle branch block, AV block, dysrhythmias in cardiac patients

Administer:

• Increased fluids, bulk in diet if constipation, urinary retention occur

P

• With food or milk for GI symptoms
• Dosage hs if oversedation occurs during day; may take entire dose hs; elderly may not tolerate once/day dosing
• Gum, hard candy, or frequent sips of water for dry mouth

Perform/provide:
• Storage in tight, light-resistant container at room temperature
• Assistance with ambulation during beginning therapy since drowsiness/dizziness occurs
• Safety measures including siderails, primarily in elderly
• Checking to see PO medication swallowed

Evaluate:
• Therapeutic response: decreased depression
• EPS primarily in elderly: rigidity, dystonia, akathisia
• Mental status: mood, sensorium, affect, suicidal tendencies, increase in psychiatric symptoms: depression, panic
• Urinary retention, constipation; constipation is more likely to occur in children
• Withdrawal symptoms: headache, nausea, vomiting, muscle pain, weakness; do not usually occur unless drug was discontinued abruptly
• Alcohol consumption; if alcohol is consumed, hold dose until morning

Teach patient/family:
• That therapeutic effects may take 2-3 wk
• To use caution in driving or other activities requiring alertness because of drowsiness, dizziness, blurred vision
• To avoid alcohol ingestion, other CNS depressants
• Not to discontinue medication quickly after long-term use; may cause nausea, headache, malaise
• To wear sunscreen or large hat since photosensitivity occurs

Lab test interferences:
Increase: Serum bilirubin, blood glucose, alk phosphatase
False increase: Urinary catecholamines
Decrease: VMA, 5-HIAA

Treatment of overdose: ECG monitoring, induce emesis, lavage, activated charcoal, administer anticonvulsant

---

pseudoephedrine HCl/ pseudoephedrine sulfate

(soo-doe-e-fed'rin)

Besan, Cenafed, Eltor,* First Sign, Novafed, Robidrine, Sudabid, Sudafed/Afrinol Repetabs

Func. class.: Adrenergic
Chem. class.: Substituted phenylethylamine

Action: Causes increased contractility and heart rate by acting on β-receptors in heart; also, acts on α-receptors, causing vasoconstriction in blood vessels

Uses: Decongestant, nasal congestion

Dosage and routes:
• *Adult:* PO 60 mg q6h; EXT REL 60-120 mg q12h
• *Child 6-12 yr:* PO 30 mg q6h, not to exceed 120 mg/day
• *Child 2-6 yr:* PO 15 mg q6h, not to exceed 60 mg/day

Available forms include: Caps ext rel 120 mg; sol 15 mg, 30 mg/5 ml, 7.5 mg/0.8 ml; tabs 30, 60, 120 mg

Side effects/adverse reactions:
CNS: Tremors, anxiety, insomnia,

* Available in Canada only

headache, dizziness, anxiety, hallucinations, ***seizures***
EENT: Dry nose, irritation of nose and throat
CV: Palpitations, tachycardia, hypertension, chest pain, ***dysrhythmias***
GI: Anorexia, nausea, vomiting, dry mouth
GU: Dysuria
Contraindications: Hypersensitivity to sympathomimetics, narrow-angle glaucoma
Precautions: Pregnancy (C), cardiac disorders, hyperthyroidism, diabetes mellitus, prostatic hypertrophy
Pharmacokinetics:
PO: Onset 15-30 min, duration 4-6 hr, 8-12 hr (extended release); metabolized in liver, excreted in feces and breast milk
Interactions/incompatibilities:
• Do not use with MAOIs or tricyclic antidepressants, hypertensive crisis may occur
• Decreased effect of this drug: methyldopa, urinary acidifiers, rauwolfia alkaloids
• Increased effect of this drug: urinary alkalizers
NURSING CONSIDERATIONS
Perform/provide:
• Storage at room temperature
Evaluate:
• Therapeutic response: Decreased nasal congestion
Teach patient/family:
• Reason for drug administration
• Not to use continuously, or more than recommended dose, or rebound congestion may occur
• To check with physician before using other drugs, as drug interactions may occur
• To avoid taking near hs; stimulation can occur
• Not to use if stimulation, restlessness, or tremors occur

psyllium
(sill'i-um)
Effer-Syllium Instant Mix, Hydrocil Instant Powder, Konsyl, L.A. Formula, Metamucil, Metamucil Instant Mix, Metamucil Sugar Free, Modance Bulk, Mucillium, Mucilose, Naturacil, Plain Hydrocil, Prodiem Plain,* Reguloid, Siblin, Syllact, V-Lax
Func. class.: Laxative, bulk
Chem. class.: Psyllium colloid

Action: Bulk-forming laxative
Uses: Chronic constipation, treatment of ulcerative colitis, irritable bowel syndrome
Dosage and routes:
• *Adult:* PO 1-2 tsp in 8 oz of water bid or tid, then 8 oz of water or 1 premeasured packet in 8 oz of water bid or tid, then 8 oz of water
• *Child >6 yr:* 1 tsp in 4 oz of water hs
Available forms include: Chew pieces 1.7 g/piece; pdr 309, 390, 430, 450, 486, 500, 600, 630, 654, 672, 791, 919, 950 mg/g, 1 g/g
Side effects/adverse reactions:
GI: Nausea, vomiting, anorexia, diarrhea, cramps
Contraindications: Hypersensitivity, intestinal obstruction, abdominal pain, nausea/vomiting, fecal impaction
Precautions: Pregnancy (C)
Pharmacokinetics: Excreted in feces
NURSING CONSIDERATIONS
Assess:
• Blood, urine electrolytes if drug is used often by patient
• I&O ratio to identify fluid loss

P

Administer:
- Alone for better absorption
- In morning or evening (oral dose)
- After mixing with water immediately before use

Evaluate:
- Therapeutic response: decrease in constipation or decreased diarrhea in colitis
- Cause of constipation; identify whether fluids, bulk, or exercise is missing from lifestyle
- Cramping, rectal bleeding, nausea, vomiting; if these symptoms occur, drug should be discontinued

Teach patient/family:
- To maintain adequate fluid consumption
- That normal bowel movements do not always occur daily
- Do not use in presence of abdominal pain, nausea, vomiting
- To notify physician if constipation unrelieved or if symptoms of electrolyte imbalance occur: muscle cramps, pain, weakness, dizziness, excessive thirst

pyrantel pamoate

(pi-ran'tel)

Antiminth, Combantrin*

Func. class.: Anthelmintic
Chem. class.: Pyrimidine derivative

Action: Causes paralysis in worm by neuroblockade, caused by stimulation of ganglionic receptors; worms are expelled by normal peristalsis

Uses: Pinworms, roundworms

Dosage and routes:
- *Adult and child >2 yr:* PO 11 mg/kg as single dose, not to exceed 1 g; repeat in 2 wk for pinworms

Available forms include: Oral susp 250 mg/5 ml

Side effects/adverse reactions:
INTEG: Rash
CNS: Dizziness, headache, drowsiness, insomnia, fever, weakness
GI: Nausea, vomiting, anorexia, diarrhea, distention

Contraindications: Hypersensitivity

Precautions: Seizure disorders, hepatic disease, dehydration, anemia, child <2 yr, pregnancy (C)

Pharmacokinetics:
PO: Peak 1-3 hr, metabolized in liver, excreted in feces, urine (unchanged/metabolites)

Interactions/incompatibilities:
- Antagonizes effect of pyrantel: piperazine

NURSING CONSIDERATIONS

Assess:
- Stools during entire treatment; specimens must be sent to lab while still warm

Administer:
- PO after meals to avoid GI symptoms
- After shaking suspension

Perform/provide:
- Storage in tight, light-resistant containers in cool environment

Evaluate:
- Therapeutic response: expulsion of worms, 3 negative stool cultures after completion of treatment
- For allergic reaction: rash
- For diarrhea during expulsion of worms

Teach patient/family:
- Proper hygiene after BM including handwashing technique; tell patient to avoid putting fingers in mouth
- That infected person should sleep alone; do not shake bed linen; change bed linen qd, wash in hot water
- To clean toilet qd with disinfectant (green soap solution)

*Available in Canada only

• Need for compliance with dosage schedule, duration of treatment
• To drink fruit juice to help expel worms
• To wear shoes, wash all fruits, vegetables well before eating

pyrazinamide

(peer-a-zin'a-mide)
Tebrazid*

Func. class.: Antitubercular
Chem. class.: Pyrazinoic acid amine/nicoturimide analog

Action: Bactericidal interference with lipid, nucleic acid biosynthesis
Uses: Tuberculosis, as an adjunct when other drugs are not feasible
Dosage and routes:
• *Adult:* PO 20-35 mg/kg/day in 3-4 divided doses, not to exceed 3 g/day
Available forms include: Tabs 500 mg
Side effects/adverse reactions:
INTEG: Photosensitivity, urticaria
CNS: Headache
GI: ***Hepatotoxicity,*** abnormal liver function tests, peptic ulcer
GU: Urinary difficulty, increased uric acid
HEMA: ***Hemolytic anemia***
Contraindications: Hypersensitivity
Precautions: Pregnancy (C), child <13 yr
Pharmacokinetics:
PO: Peak 2 hr, half-life 9-10 hr; metabolized in liver, excreted in urine (metabolites/unchanged drug)
NURSING CONSIDERATIONS
Assess:
• Signs of anemia: Hct, Hgb, fatigue
• Temperature if <101° F, drug should be reduced
• Liver studies qwk: ALT, AST, bilirubin
• Renal status before, qmo: BUN, creatinine, output, sp gr, urinalysis
Administer:
• With meals to decrease GI symptoms
• After C&S is completed; qmo to detect resistance
Evaluate:
• Therapeutic response: decreased symptoms of TB, culture negative
• Hepatic status: decreased appetite, jaundice, dark urine, fatigue
Teach patient/family:
• That compliance with dosage schedule, length is necessary
• To avoid alcohol while taking this drug
Lab test interferences:
Increase: PBI
Decrease: 17-KS

pyrethrins/piperonyl butoxide

(peer'e-thrins)
A-200 Pyrinate, Barc, Blue, Pyrin-d, Pyrinyl, Rdc, Rid, TISIT, Triple X

Func. class.: Pediculocide
Chem. class.: Pyrethrin/piperonyl butoxide/petroleum distillate

Action: Causes paralysis, death of organism by acting as a contact poison
Uses: Head, body, pubic lice; nits
Dosage and routes:
• *Adult and child:* Apply undiluted to infested area; allow application to remain no longer than 10 min, wash thoroughly with warm water, soap, or shampoo; remove dead lice, eggs with fine-toothed comb; do not exceed 2 consecutive applications within 24 hr
• *Adult and child:* CREAM/LO-

P

TION wash area with soap, water; remove visible crusts, apply to skin surfaces, remove with soap, water in 8-12 hr; may reapply in 1 wk if needed; SHAMPOO using 30 ml, work into lather, rub for 5 min, rinse, dry with towel

Available forms include: Gel, liq, shampoo, cream, lotion

Side effects/adverse reactions:
INTEG: Irritation, pruritus, urticaria, eczema

Contraindications: Hypersensitivity, inflammation of skin, abrasions, or breaks in skin

Precautions: Child/infant, ragweed sensitivity, pregnancy (C)

Pharmacokinetics: Inactivated by GI tract, other data not available

NURSING CONSIDERATIONS

Administer:

- To body areas, scalp only; do not apply to face, lips, mouth, eyes, any mucous membrane, anus, or meatus; apply to neck down for body lice
- Topical corticosteroids as ordered to decrease contact dermatitis
- Lotions of menthol or phenol to control itching
- Topical antibiotics for infection

Perform/provide:

- Storage in tight container
- Isolation until areas on skin, scalp have cleared and treatment is completed
- Removal of nits by using a fine-toothed comb rinsed in vinegar after treatment

Evaluate:

- Therapeutic response: decreased nits, crusts

Teach patient/family:

- To discontinue use and notify physician if irritation or infection occurs
- To flush with water in case of contact with eyes
- To wash all inhabitants' clothing, bed linen using insecticide; preventive treatment may be required of all persons living in same house, using lotion or shampoo to decrease spread of infection
- That itching may continue for 4-6 wk
- That drug must be reapplied if accidently washed off or treatment will be ineffective
- To use externally only
- To treat sexual contacts simultaneously

---

pyridostigmine bromide

(peer-id-oh-stig'meen)

Mestinon, Regonol

Func. class.: Cholinergic
Chem. class.: Tertiary amine carbamate

Action: Inhibits destruction of acetylcholine, which increases concentration at sites where acetylcholine is released; this facilitates transmission of impulses across myoneural junction

Uses: Nondepolarizing muscle relaxant antagonist, myasthenia gravis

Dosage and routes:

Myasthenia gravis

- *Adult:* PO 60-180 mg bid-qid, not to exceed 1.5 g/day; IM/IV 1/30 of PO dose, sus rel 180-540 mg 1-2 × day at intervals of at least 6 hr

Tubocurare antagonist

- *Adult:* 0.6-1.2 mg IV atropine, then 10-30 mg

Available forms include: Tabs 60 mg; tabs sus rel 180 mg; syr 60 mg/5 ml; inj IM/IV 5 mg/ml

Side effects/adverse reactions:
INTEG: Rash, urticaria, flushing
CNS: Dizziness, headache, sweat-

---

* Available in Canada only

ing, confusion, weakness, ***convulsions,*** incoordination, paralysis
GI: Nausea, diarrhea, vomiting, cramps
CV: Tachycardia, dysrhythmias, bradycardia, AV block, hypotension, ECG changes, ***cardiac arrest***
GU: Frequency, incontinence
RESP: ***Respiratory depression, bronchospasm, constriction, laryngospasm, respiratory arrest***
EENT: Miosis, blurred vision, lacrimation

Contraindications: Bradycardia, hypotension, obstruction of intestine, renal system

Precautions: Seizure disorders, bronchial asthma, coronary occlusion, hyperthyroidism, dysrhythmias, peptic ulcer, megacolon, poor GI motility, pregnancy (C)

Pharmacokinetics:
PO: Onset 20-30 min, duration 3-6 hr
IM/IV/SC: Onset 2-15 min, duration 2½-4 hr; metabolized in liver, excreted in urine

Interactions/incompatibilities:
- Decreased action: gallamine, metocurine, pancuronium, tubocurarine, atropine
- Increased action: decamethonium, succinylcholine
- Decreased action of pyridostigmine: aminoglycosides, anesthetics, procainamide, quinidine, mecamylamine, polymyxin, magnesium, corticosteroids, antidysrhythmics

NURSING CONSIDERATIONS

Assess:
- VS, respiration q8h
- I&O ratio; check for urinary retention or incontinence

Administer:
- IV undiluted, give through Y-tube or 3-way stopcock, give 0.5 mg or less/min
- Only with atropine sulfate available for cholinergic crisis
- Only after all other cholinergics have been discontinued
- Increased doses if tolerance occurs
- Larger doses after exercise or fatigue
- With food or milk to decrease GI symptoms
- On empty stomach for better absorption

Perform/provide:
- Storage at room temperature

Evaluate:
- Therapeutic response: increased muscle strength, hand grasp, improved gait, absence of labored breathing (if severe)
- Bradycardia, hypotension, bronchospasm, headache, dizziness, convulsions, respiratory depression; drug should be discontinued if toxicity occurs

Teach patient/family:
- Not to crush or chew sus rel prep
- That drug is not a cure, it only relieves symptoms
- To wear Medic Alert ID specifying myasthenia gravis, drugs taken

Treatment of overdose:
Discontinue drug, atropine 1-4 mg IV

P

pyridoxine HCl (vitamin B_6)

(peer-i-dox-een)

Beesix, HexaBetalin, Hexacrest

Func. class.: Vitamin B_6, water soluble

Action: Needed for fat, protein, carbohydrate metabolism; enhances glycogen release from liver and muscle tissue; needed as coen-

zyme for metabolic transformations of a variety of amino acids
Uses: Vitamin B_6 deficiency associated with inborn errors of metabolism, seizures, isoniazid therapy, oral contraceptives, or alcoholic polyneuritis
Dosage and routes:
Vitamin B_6 deficiency
• *Adult:* PO/IM/IV 10-20 mg qd × 3 wk, then 2-5 mg qd
• *Child:* PO/IM/IV 100 mg until desired response
Inborn errors of metabolism
• *Adult:* IM/IV/PO 600 mg or less qd, then 50 mg qd for life
• *Child:* IM/PO/IV 100 mg, then 2-10 mg IM or 10-100 mg PO qd
Deficiency caused by isoniazid
• *Adult:* PO 100 mg qd × 3 wk, then 50 mg qd
• *Child:* PO dose titrated to patient response
Prevention of deficiency caused by isoniazid
• *Adult:* PO 25-50 mg qd
• *Child:* PO 0.5-1.5 mg qd
• *Infant:* PO 0.1-0.5 mg qd
Available forms include: Tabs 10, 25, 50, 100, 200, 250, 500 mg; tabs time released 500 mg; inj IM-IV 100 mg/ml
Side effects/adverse reactions:
CNS: Paresthesia, flushing, warmth, lethargy (rare with normal renal function)
INTEG: Pain at injection site
Contraindications: Hypersensitivity
Precautions: Pregnancy (A), lactation, children, Parkinson's disease
Pharmacokinetics:
PO/INJ: Half-life 2-3 wk, metabolized in liver, excreted in urine
Interactions/incompatibilities:
• Decreased effects of: levodopa
• Decreased effects of pyridoxine: oral contraceptives, INH, cycloserine, hydralazine, penicillamine

NURSING CONSIDERATIONS
Assess:
• Pyridoxine levels throughout treatment
Administer:
• IV undiluted or added to most IV sol; give 50 mg or less/1 min if undiluted
• Z-tract to minimize pain
Perform/provide:
• Storage in tight, light-resistant container
Evaluate:
• Therapeutic response: absence of nausea, vomiting, anorexia, skin lesions, glossitis, stomatitis, edema, convulsions, restlessness, paresthesia
• Nutritional status: yeast, liver, legumes, bananas, green vegetables, whole grains
Teach patient/family:
• To avoid vitamin supplements unless directed by physician
• To keep out of children's reach
• To increase meat, bananas, potatoes, lima beans, whole grain cereals
• To discuss birth control status with physician

pyrimethamine

(peer-i-meth'a-meen)
Daraprim, Fansidar (with sulfadoxine)
Func. class.: Antimalarial
Chem. class.: Folic acid antagonist

Action: Inhibits folic acid metabolism in parasite, prevents transmission by stopping growth of fertilized gametes
Uses: Malaria, prophylaxis, *Plasmodium vivax*

Dosage and routes:
Prophylaxis of malaria
• *Adult:* PO 1 tab qwk or 2 tabs q2wk (Fansidar)
• *Child 9-14 yr:* PO ¾ tab qwk or 1½ tabs q2wk (Fansidar)
• *Child >10 yr:* PO 25 mg qwk
• *Child 4-10 yr:* PO 12.5 mg qwk
• *Child 4-8 yr:* PO ½ tab qwk or 1 tab q2wk (Fansidar)
• *Child <4 yr:* PO ¼ tab qwk or ½ tab q2wk (Fansidar)
• *Child <4 yr:* PO 6.25 mg qwk
Acute attacks of malaria
• *Adult:* PO 2-3 tabs as a single dose (Fansidar) alone or with quinine or primaquine
• *Child 9-14 yr:* 2 tabs
• *Child 4-8 yr:* 1 tab
• *Child <4 yr:* ½ tab
Toxoplasmosis
• *Adult:* PO 100 mg, then 25 mg qd × 4-5 wk, with 1 g sulfadiazine q6h
• *Child:* PO 1 mg/kg, then 0.25 mg/kg qd × 4-5 wk, with sulfadiazine 100 mg/kg/day in divided doses q6h
Available forms include: Tabs 25 mg; combo tabs 500 mg sulfadoxine/25 mg pyrimethamine
Side effects/adverse reactions:
RESP: ***Respiratory failure***
INTEG: Skin eruptions, photosensitivity
CNS: Stimulation, irritability, ***convulsions,*** tremors, ataxia, fatigue
GI: Nausea, vomiting, cramps, anorexia, diarrhea, atrophic glossitis, gastritis
HEMA: ***Thrombocytopenia, leukopenia, pancytopenia, megaloblastic anemia,*** decreased folic acid, ***agranulocytosis***
Contraindications: Hypersensitivity, chloroquine-resistant malaria, megaloblastic anemia caused by folate deficiency
Precautions: Blood dyscrasias, seizure disorder, pregnancy (C)
Pharmacokinetics:
PO: Peak 2 hr, half-life 111 hr; metabolized in liver, highly protein bound, excreted in urine (metabolites)
Interactions/incompatibilities:
• Synergestic action: para-aminobenzoic acid or folic acid

NURSING CONSIDERATIONS

Assess:
• Folic acid level, megaloblastic anemia occurs
• Blood studies, CBC, platelets, since blood dyscrasias occur; twice weekly if dosage is increased
Administer:
• Leucovorin IM 3-9 mg/day × 3 days if folic acid deficiency occurs
• Before or after meals at same time each day to maintain drug level to decrease GI symptoms
Perform/provide:
• Storage in tight, light-resistant containers
Evaluate:
• Therapeutic response: decreased symptoms of malaria
• For toxicity: vomiting, anorexia, seizure, blood dyscrasia, glossitis; drug should be discontinued immediately
Teach patient/family:
• To report visual problems, fever, fatigue, bruising, bleeding; may indicate blood dyscrasias
Treatment of overdose: Gastric lavage, administer short-acting barbiturate, leucovorin, respiratory support if needed

---

quazepam

Doral

Func. class.: Sedative-hypnotic
Chem. class.: Benzodiazepine derivative

Controlled Substance Schedule IV (USA)

Action: Produces CNS depression at the limbic, thalamic, hypothalamic levels of CNS; may be mediated by neurotransmitter γ-aminobutyric acid (GABA); results are sedation, hypnosis, skeletal muscle relaxation, anticonvulsant activity, anxiolytic action

Uses: Insomnia

Dosage and routes:

Adult: PO 7.5 mg hs, may increase if needed

Available forms include: Tabs 7.5, 15 mg

Side effects/adverse reactions:

HEMA: ***Leukopenia, granulocytopenia*** (rare)

CNS: Lethargy, drowsiness, daytime sedation, dizziness, confusion, light-headedness, headache, anxiety, irritability, weakness, tremor, depression

GI: Nausea, vomiting, diarrhea, heartburn, abdominal pain, constipation, anorexia, taste alteration

CV: Chest pain, pulse changes, palpitations, tachycardia

MISC: Joint pain, congestion, dermatitis, sweating

Contraindications: Hypersensitivity to benzodiazepines, pregnancy, lactation

Precautions: Hepatic disease, renal disease, suicidal individuals, drug abuse, elderly, psychosis, child <18 yr, lactation, depression, pulmonary insufficiency

Pharmacokinetics:

PO: Onset 15-45 min, duration 7-8 hr; metabolized by liver, excreted by kidneys (inactive/active metabolites), crosses placenta, excreted in breast milk

Interactions/incompatibilities:

- Increased effects of quazepam: cimetidine, disulfiram
- Increased CNS depression: alcohol, CNS depressants
- Decreased effect of quazepam: antacids

NURSING CONSIDERATIONS

Assess:

- Blood studies: Hct, Hgb, RBCs (if on long-term therapy)
- Hepatic studies: AST, ALT, bilirubin

Administer:

- After removal of cigarettes, to prevent fires
- After trying conservative measures for insomnia
- ½-1 hr before hs for sleeplessness
- On empty stomach for fast onset, but may be taken with food if GI symptoms occur

Perform/provide:

- Assistance with ambulation after receiving dose
- Safety measure: siderails, night light, call bell within easy reach
- Checking to see PO medication has been swallowed
- Storage in tight container in cool environment

Evaluate:

- Therapeutic response: ability to sleep at night, decreased amount of early morning awakening
- Mental status: mood, sensorium, affect, memory (long, short)
- Blood dyscrasias: fever, sore throat, bruising, rash, jaundice, epistaxis (rare)
- Type of sleep problem: falling asleep, staying asleep

Teach patient/family:

- To avoid driving or other activities requiring alertness until drug is stabilized
- To avoid alcohol ingestion or CNS depressants; serious CNS depression may result
- That effects may take two nights for benefits to be noticed
- Alternate measures to improve sleep: reading, exercise several

* Available in Canada only

hours before hs, warm bath, warm milk, TV, self-hypnosis, deep breathing
• That hangover is common in elderly, but less common than with barbiturates

Lab test interferences:
Increase: AST/ALT, serum bilirubin
Decrease: RAI uptake
Treatment of overdose: Lavage, activated charcoal, monitor electrolytes, vital signs

---

quinacrine HCl

(kwin'a-kreen)
Atabrine

Func. class.: Anthelmintic
Chem. class.: Acridine dye derivative

Action: Causes worm scolex to detach from GI tract
Uses: Giardiasis, tapeworms (cestodiasis), malaria
Dosage and routes:
• *Adult:* PO 100 mg × 5-7 days
• *Child:* PO 7 mg/kg/day in 3 divided doses pc × 5 days, not to exceed 300 mg/day; may repeat in 2 wk if needed; administer 1-3 mo for malaria
Available forms include: Tabs 100 mg
Side effects/adverse reactions:
INTEG: Rash, dermatitis, yellow pigmentation of skin, urticaria
CNS: Dizziness, headache, insomnia, restlessness, confusion, behavioral changes, psychosis, ***convulsions***
EENT: Bad taste, oral irritation, corneal deposits, retinopathy
GI: Nausea, vomiting, anorexia, diarrhea, cramps, hepatitis
HEMA: ***Aplastic anemia, agranulocytosis***
Contraindications: Hypersensitivity, porphyria, psoriasis
Precautions: Seizure disorders, elderly, psychosis, alcoholism, hepatic disease, depression, child <12 yr, G-6-PD deficiency, pregnancy (C)
Pharmacokinetics:
PO: Peak 8 hr, metabolized by the liver (slowly), excreted primarily in urine, crosses placenta, high protein bindings
Interactions/incompatibilities:
• Increased toxicity: primaquine, hepatotoxic drugs
• Disulfiram-like reaction: alcohol

NURSING CONSIDERATIONS

Assess:
• Stools during entire treatment, collect entire stools × 48 hr, pass through sieve, check for scolex (yellow tapeworms)
• CBC, ophthalmic exam if used for long-term treatment
• Stools 2 wk after last dose for giardiasis

Administer:
• By duodenal tube for pork tapeworm; prevents vomiting, transportation of parasites into stomach
• Bland liquid diet, no fat, or no-residue 24-48 hr before beginning therapy; patient should be fasting night before, given saline enemas, cleansing enema before beginning therapy (tapeworms only)
• Laxatives before treatment to cleanse bowel
• After meals with fluids for giardiasis, malaria
• In jam or honey to disguise bitter taste of pulverized tablets (children)

Perform/provide:
• Storage in tight containers

Evaluate:
• Therapeutic response: expulsion

of worms, 3 negative stool cultures after completion of treatment

- For allergic reaction (rash), visual problems (halos, blurring, inability to focus)
- For infection in other family members since infection from person to person is common
- Mental status: affect, mood, behavioral changes

Teach patient/family:

- Proper hygiene after BM including handwashing technique; tell patient to avoid putting fingers in mouth
- To clean toilet qd with disinfectant (green soap solution)
- Need for compliance with dosage schedule, duration of treatment
- That skin, urine may turn deep yellow
- To report any visual changes
- Not to drink alcohol

Lab test interferences:

False positive: Adrenal function tests

Increase: 17-OHCS (Mattingly method)

Treatment of overdose: Induce vomiting

---

quinapril

(kwye'a-preel)

Accupril

Func. class.: Antihypertensive

Chem. class.: Angiotensin converting enzyme (ACE) inhibitor

Action: Selectively suppresses renin-angiotensin-aldosterone system; inhibits ACE, prevents conversion of angiotensin I to angiotensin II; results in dilation of arterial, venous vessels

Uses: Hypertension, alone or in combination with thiazide diuretics

Dosage and routes:

- *Adult:* PO 10 mg qd initially, then 20-80 mg/day divided bid or qd

Available forms: Tabs 5, 10, 20, 40 mg

Side effects/adverse reactions:

CV: Hypotension, postural hypotension, syncope, palpitations, angina pectoris, MI, tachycardia, vasodilation

GU: Increased BUN, creatinine, decreased libido, impotence, urinary tract infection

HEMA: ***Thrombocytopenia, agranulocytosis***

INTEG: ***Angioedema,*** rash, sweating, photosensitivity, pruritus

RESP: Cough, bronchitis

META: Hyperkalemia

GI: Nausea, constipation, vomiting, gastritis, GI hemorrhage, dry mouth

CNS: Headache, dizziness, fatigue, somnolence, depression, malaise, nervousness, vertigo

MISC: Back pain, amblyopia, pharyngitis

MS: Arthralgia, arthritis, myalgia

Contraindications: Hypersensitivity to ACE inhibitors, pregnancy (D), children

Precautions: Impaired renal, liver function, dialysis patients, hypovolemia, blood dyscrasias, CHF, COPD, asthma, elderly, lactation

Pharmacokinetics:

PO: Peak ½-1 hr, serum protein binding, 97%, half-life 2 hr, metabolized by liver (metabolites), metabolities excreted in urine

Interactions/incompatibilities:

- Increased hypotension: diuretics, other antihypertensives, ganglionic blockers, adrenergic blockers, phenothiazines
- Use caution with vasodilators, hydralazine, prazosin, potassium-

sparing diuretics, sympathomimetics
• Decreased absorption of: tetracycline
• Reduced hypotensive effect of quinipril: indomethacin
• Increased toxicity: lithium, digoxin

NURSING CONSIDERATIONS

Assess:
• Blood studies: neutrophils, decreased platelets
• B/P, orthostatic hypotension, syncope
• Renal studies: protein, BUN, creatinine, watch for increased levels that may indicate nephrotic syndrome
• Baselines in renal, liver function tests before therapy begins
• Potassium levels, although hyperkalemia rarely occurs
• Dip-stick of urine for protein qd in first morning specimen; if protein is increased, a 24-hr urinary protein should be collected

Administer:
• IV infusion of 0.9% NaCl (as ordered) to expand fluid volume if severe hypotension occurs

Perform/provide:
• Supine or Trendelenburg position for severe hypotension

Evaluate:
• Therapeutic response: decrease in B/P
• Edema in feet, legs daily
• Allergic reactions: rash, fever, pruritus, urticaria; drugs should be discontinued if antihistamines fail to help
• Renal symptoms: polyuria, oliguria, frequency, dysuria

Teach patient/family:
• Take 1 hr before meals; do not take antacids within 1-2 hr of quinapril
• Not to discontinue drug abruptly
• Not to use OTC products (cough, cold, allergy); not to use salt substitutes containing potassium unless directed by physician
• To comply with dosage schedule, even if feeling better
• To rise slowly to sitting or standing position to minimize orthostatic hypotension
• To notify physician of: mouth sores, sore throat, fever, swelling of hands or feet, irregular heartbeat, chest pain, persistent dry cough
• To report excessive perspiration, dehydration, vomiting, diarrhea; may lead to fall in B/P
• That drug may cause dizziness, fainting, light-headedness; may occur during 1st few days of therapy
• That drug may cause skin rash or impaired taste perception
• How to take B/P, and normal readings for age group

Lab test interferences:
False positive: Urine acetone

Treatment of overdose: 0.9% NaCl IV INF, hemodialysis

---

quinestrol

(kwin-ess'trole)

Estrovis

Func. class.: Estrogen
Chem. class.: Nonsteroidal synthetic estrogen

Action: Needed for adequate functioning of female reproductive system; affects release of pituitary gonadotropins, inhibits ovulation, promotes adequate calcium use in bone structures

Uses: Menopause, atrophic vaginitis, kraurosis vulvae, female castration, female hypogonadism, primary ovarian failure

Dosage and routes:

- *Adult:* PO 100 μg qd × 1 wk, then 100 μg qwk starting 2 wk after beginning treatment; may increase to 200 μg/wk

Available forms include: Tabs 100 μg

Side effects/adverse reactions:

CNS: Dizziness, headache, migraine, depression

CV: Hypotension, thrombophlebitis, edema, ***thromboembolism, stroke, pulmonary embolism, myocardial infarction***

GI: Nausea, vomiting, diarrhea, anorexia, pancreatitis, cramps, constipation, increased appetite, increased weight, ***cholestatic jaundice***

EENT: Contact lens intolerance, increased myopia, astigmatism

GU: Amenorrhea, cervical erosion, breakthrough bleeding, dysmenorrhea, vaginal candidiasis, breast changes, *gynecomastia, testicular atrophy, impotence*

INTEG: Rash, urticaria, acne, hirsutism, alopecia, oily skin, seborrhea, purpura, melasma

META: Folic acid deficiency, hypercalcemia, hyperglycemia

Contraindications: Breast cancer, thromboembolic disorders, reproductive cancer, genital bleeding (abnormal, undiagnosed), pregnancy (X)

Precautions: Hypertension, asthma, blood dyscrasias, gallbladder disease, CHF, diabetes mellitus, bone disease, depression, migraine headache, convulsive disorders, hepatic disease, renal disease, family history of cancer of breast or reproductive tract

Pharmacokinetics:

PO: Degraded in liver, excreted in urine, crosses placenta, excreted in breast milk

Interactions/incompatibilities:

- Decreased action of: anticoagulants, oral hypoglycemics
- Toxicity: tricyclic antidepressants
- Decreased action of quinestrol: anticonvulsants, barbiturates, phenylbutazone, rifampin
- Increased action of: corticosteroids

NURSING CONSIDERATIONS

Assess:

- Urine glucose in patient with diabetes; increased urine glucose may occur
- Weight daily, notify physician of weekly weight gain >5 lb; if increase, diurectic may be ordered
- B/P q4h, watch for increase caused by water and sodium retention
- I&O ratio; be alert for decreasing urinary output and increasing edema
- Liver function studies, including AST, ALT, bilirubin, alk phosphatase

Administer:

- Titrated dose, use lowest effective dose
- With food or milk to decrease GI symptoms

Evaluate:

- Therapeutic response: reversal of menopause or decrease in tumor size in prostatic cancer
- Edema, hypertension, cardiac symptoms, jaundice, calcemia
- Mental status: affect mood, behavioral changes, aggression

Teach patient/family:

- To weigh weekly, report gain >5 lb
- To report breast lumps, vaginal bleeding, edema, jaundice, dark urine, clay-colored stools, dyspnea, headache, blurred vision, abdominal pain, numbness or stiff-

* Available in Canada only

ness in legs, chest pain; male to report impotence or gynecomastia

quinidine gluconate/ quinidine polygalacturonate/quinidine sulfate

(kwin'i-deen)

Biquin Durales,* Duraquin,* Quinaglute Dura-Tabs, Quinate, Quinatime, Quin-Release/Cardioquin, Cin-Quin, Novoquindin, Quine, Quinidex Extentabs, Quinora

Func. class.: Antidysrhythmic (Class IA)

Chem. class.: Quinine dextro isomer

Action: Prolongs action potential duration and effective refractory period, thus decreasing myocardial excitability; anticholinergic properties

Uses: PVCs, atrial fibrillation, PAT, ventricular tachycardia, atrial dysrhythmias

Dosage and routes:

Atrial fibrillation/flutter

• *Adult:* PO 200 mg q2-3h × 5-8 doses, may increase qd until sinus rhythm is restored, max 4 g/day given only after digitalization

Paroxysmal supraventricular tachycardia

• *Adult:* PO 400-600 mg q2-3h

All other dysrhythmias

• *Adult:* PO 50-200 mg as a test dose, then 200-400 mg q4-6h; IM 600 mg, then 400 mg q2h, after test dose (gluconate); IV INF 800 mg in 40 ml D_5W run at 16 mg/min

Available forms include: (Gluconate) tabs sus rel 324, 330 mg; inj IM gluconate 80 mg/ml (sulfate) tabs 100, 200, 300 mg; caps 200, 300 mg; tabs sus rel 300 mg; inj IV (polygalacturonate) tabs 275 mg, sulfate 200 mg/ml

Side effects/adverse reactions:

CNS: Headache, dizziness, involuntary movement, confusion, psychosis, restlessness, irritability, syncope, excitement

EENT: Cinchonism: tinnitus, blurred vision, hearing loss, mydriasis, disturbed color vision

GI: Nausea, vomiting, anorexia, *diarrhea,* ***hepatotoxicity***

CV: Hypotension, bradycardia, PVCs, ***heart block, cardiovascular collapse, arrest***

HEMA: ***Thrombocytopenia,*** hemolytic anemia, agranulocytosis, hypoprothrombinemia

RESP: Dyspnea, ***respiratory depression***

INTEG: Rash, urticaria, angioedema, swelling, photosensitivity

Contraindications: Hypersensitivity, blood dyscrasias, severe heart block, myasthenia gravis

Precautions: Pregnancy (C), lactation, children, renal disease, potassium imbalance, liver disease, CHF, respiratory depression

Pharmacokinetics:

PO: Peak 0.5-6 hr, duration 6-8 hr; half-life 6-7 hr, metabolized in liver, excreted unchanged by kidneys

Interactions/incompatibilities:

• Increased effects of: neuromuscular blockers, digoxin, coumadin

• Increased effects of quinidine: cimetidine, propranolol, thiazides, sodium bicarbonate, carbonic anhydrase inhibitors, antacids, hydroxide suspensions

• May decrease effects of quinidine: barbiturates, phenytoin, rifampin, nifedipine

• Additive vagolytic effect: anticholinergic blockers

• Additive cardiac depression:

other antidysrhythmics, phenothiazines, reserpine

NURSING CONSIDERATIONS

Assess:

• ECG continuously to determine increased PR or QRS segments; if these develop, discontinue or reduce dose

• Blood levels (therapeutic level 2-6 μg/ml)

• B/P continuously for fluctuations

Administer:

• IV after diluting 800 mg/40 ml or more D_5W; give 16 mg or less over 1 min as infusion; use infusion pump

• IM injection in deltoid; aspirate to avoid intravascular administration

• An AV node blocker (digoxin, verapamil) before starting quinidine to avoid increased ventricular rate

Evaluate:

• Therapeutic response: decreased dysrhythmias

• Cinchonism: tinnitus, headache, nausea, dizziness, fever, vertigo, tremor; may lead to hearing loss

• Cardiac rate, respiration: rate, rhythm, character, continuously

• Respiratory status: rate, rhythm, lung fields for rales

• CNS effects: dizziness, confusion, psychosis, paresthesias, convulsions; drug should be discontinued

• Lung fields; bilateral rales may occur in CHF patient

• Increased respiration, increased pulse; drug should be discontinued

Lab test interferences:

Increase: CPK

Treatment of overdose: O_2, artificial ventilation, ECG, administer dopamine for circulatory depression, administer diazepam or thiopental for convulsions

quinine sulfate

(kwye'nine)

Novoquine,* Quinamm, Quine, Quinite, Quiphile, Strema, Quin-260

Func. class.: Antimalarial
Chem. class.: Cinchoma tree alkaloid

Action: Inhibits parasite replications, transcription of DNA to RNA by forming complexes with DNA of parasite

Uses: *Plasmodium falciparum* malaria, nocturnal leg cramps

Dosage and routes:

• *Adult:* PO 650 mg q8h × 10 days, given with pyrimethamine 25 mg q12h × 3 days, with sulfadiazine 500 mg qid × 5 days

Available forms include: Caps 130, 195, 200, 300, 325 mg; tabs 260, 325 mg

Side effects/adverse reactions:

RESP: Dysuria

INTEG: Pruritus, pigmentary changes, skin eruptions, lichen planuslike eruptions, flushing, facial edema, sweating

HEMA: ***Thrombocytopenia, purpura, hypothrombinemia, hemolysis***

CNS: Headache, stimulation, fatigue, irritability, ***convulsion,*** bad dreams, dizziness, fever, confusion, anxiety

EENT: Blurred vision, corneal changes, retinal changes, difficulty focusing, tinnitus, vertigo, deafness, photophobia, diplopia, night blindness

GI: Nausea, vomiting, anorexia, diarrhea, epigastric pain

CV: Angina, dysrhythmias, tachycardia, hypotension, ***acute circulatory failure***

* Available in Canada only

ENDO: Hypoglycemia
Contraindications: Hypersensitivity, G-6-PD deficiency, retinal field changes, pregnancy (X)
Precautions: Blood dyscrasias, severe GI disease, neurologic disease, severe hepatic disease, psoriasis, cardiac dysrhythmias, tinnitus
Pharmacokinetics:
PO: Peak 1-3 hr, metabolized in liver, excreted in urine, half-life 4-5 hr
Interactions/incompatibilities:
- Toxicity: $NaHCO_3$, acetazolamide
- Decreased absorption: magnesium or aluminum salts
- Increase levels of: digoxin, digitoxin, neuromuscular blockers, other anticoagulants

NURSING CONSIDERATIONS
Assess:
- B/P, pulse, if administered IV, watch for hypotension, tachycardia
- Liver studies weekly: ALT, AST, bilirubin
- Blood studies, CBC, since blood dyscrasias occur

Administer:
- By slow IV
- Before or after meals at same time each day to maintain drug level

Perform/provide:
- Storage in tight, light-resistant container

Evaluate:
- Therapeutic response: decreased symptoms of malaria
- For cinchonism: nausea, blurred vision, tinnitus, headache, difficulty focusing

Teach patient/family:
- To avoid OTC preparations: cold preparations, tonic water

Lab test interferences:
Increase: 17-KS
Interference: 17-OHCS

rabies immune globulin, human

Hyperab, Imogam
Func. class.: Immune serum
Chem. class.: IgG

Action: Provides passive immunity; given with HDCV; may be used regardless of time of bite, treatment
Uses: Exposure to rabies
Dosage and routes:
- *Adult and child:* IM 20 IU/kg given at same time as 1st rabies vaccine; infiltrate wound with ½ dose, then administer rest IM, 1 ml dose on each of days 3, 7, 14, 28 after 1st dose

Available forms include: Inj IM 125 IU/ml
Side effects/adverse reactions:
INTEG: Pain at injection site, rash, pruritus
MS: Arthralgia
SYST: Lymphadenopathy, ***anaphylaxis***, fever
CNS: Headache, fatigue, malaise
GI: Abdominal pain
Contraindications: Hypersensitivity to equine products and thimerosal
Interactions/incompatibilities:
- Decreased action of rabies immune globulin: corticosteroids, immunosuppressants

NURSING CONSIDERATIONS
Administer:
- Test dose: dilute drug either with 1:100 or 1:1000 0.9% NaCl for injection, inject 0.1 ml 0.9% NaCl in other arm intradermally, check for wheal 10 mm or > after 10 min; if present, drug should not be used
- Only after epinephrine 1:1000, resuscitative equipment are available

• Only if human immune serum is not available
• As soon as possible after exposure

Perform/provide:
• Storage at 2°-8°C

Evaluate:
• Allergic reactions: dyspnea, rash, pruritus, eruptions

Teach patient/family:
• That pain, swelling, itching may occur at injection site
• To take acetaminophen to alleviate headache, fever, and pain

radioactive iodine (sodium iodide) ^{131}I

Func. class.: Antithyroid
Chem. class.: Radiopharmaceutical

Action: Converted to protein-bound iodine by thyroid gland for use when needed

Uses:
High dose: Thyroid cancer, hyperthyroidism
Low dose: Visualization to determine thyroid cancer, diagnostic aid in thyroid function studies

Dosage and routes:
Thyroid cancer
• *Adult:* PO 50-150 mCi, may repeat depending on clinical status
Hyperthyroidism
• *Adult:* PO 4-10 mCi, depending on serum thyroxine level

Available forms include: Caps 1-50, 0.8-100 mCi; oral sol 7.05 mCi/ml, 3.5-150 mCi/vial

Side effects/adverse reactions:
ENDO: Hypothyroidism, ***hyperthyroid adenoma,*** transient thyroiditis
INTEG: Alopecia
HEMA: ***Eosinophilia, lymphedema, leukemia, bone marrow depression, leukopenia,*** anemia
GI: Nausea, diarrhea, vomiting
EENT: Sore throat, cough

Contraindications: Recent MI, lactation, large nodular goiter, pregnancy (X), <30 yr, vomiting/diarrhea, acute hyperthyroidism, use of thyroid drugs

Pharmacokinetics:
PO: Onset 3-6 days, excreted in urine, sweat, feces, crosses placenta, excreted in breast milk, excreted in 56 days

Interactions/incompatibilities:
• Hypothyroidism: lithium
• Decreased uptake if recent intake of stable iodine, thyroid, antithyroid drugs

NURSING CONSIDERATIONS

Assess:
• Weight qd in same clothing, scale, time of day
• Blood work, including CBC for blood dyscrasias (leukopenia, thrombocytopenia, agranulocytosis)

Administer:
• Only after discontinuing all other antithyroid agents × 5-7 days
• After NPO overnight, food delays action
• After menstruation (10 days) or during

Perform/provide:
• Limited contact with patient ½ hr/day for each person
• Adequate rest after treatment
• Fluids to 3-4 L/day for 48 hr after agent is administered to remove agent from body

Evaluate:
• Therapeutic response: weight gain, decreased pulse, decreased T_4, B/P
• Overdose: peripheral edema, heat intolerance, diaphoresis, palpitations, dysrhythmias, severe tachycardia, increased temperature delirium, CNS irritability

• Hypersensitivity: rash, enlarged cervical lymph nodes; drug may need to be discontinued
• Hypoprothrombinemia: bleeding, petechiae, ecchymosis
• Clinical response: after 3 wk should include increased weight, pulse; decreased T_4
• Bone marrow depression: sore throat, fever, fatigue

Teach patient/family:
• To empty bladder often during treatment, avoids radiation of gonads
• To report redness, swelling, sore throat, mouth lesions; indicate blood dyscrasias
• To avoid extended contact with children or spouse for 1 week
• That bathroom may be used by entire family
• Not to take antithyroid agents but propranolol, which decreases hyperthyroid symptoms, until total effects of ^{131}I has taken effect (about 6 wk)
• Avoid coughing, expectorating for 24 hr (saliva and vomiting are highly radioactive for 6-8 hr)

---

ramipril

(ram-a'prel)
Altace

Func. class.: Antihypertensive
Chem. class.: Angiotensin-converting enzyme (ACE) inhibitor

Action: Selectively suppresses renin-angiotensin-aldosterone system; inhibits ACE, prevents conversion of angiotensin I to angiotensin II; results in dilation of arterial, venous vessels

Uses: Hypertension, alone or in combination with thiazide diuretics

Dosage and routes:
• *Adult:* PO 2.5 mg qd initially, then 2.5-20 mg/day divided bid or qd; renal impairment: 1.25 mg qd with Ccr <40 ml/min/1.73 m^2, increase as needed to maximum or 5 mg/day

Available forms include: Caps 1.25, 2.5, 5, 10 mg

Side effects/adverse reactions:
CV: Hypotension, chest pain, palpitations, angina, syncope, dysrhythmia
GU: ***Proteinuria,*** increased BUN, creatinine, impotence
HEMA: Decreased Hct, Hgb, ***eosinophilia, leukopenia***
INTEG: ***Angioedema,*** rash, sweating, photosensitivity, pruritus
RESP: Cough, dyspnea
META: Hyperkalemia
GI: Nausea, constipation, vomiting, dyspepsia, dysphagia, anorexia, diarrhea, abdominal pain
CNS: Headache, dizziness, anxiety, insomnia, paresthesia, fatigue, depression, malaise, vertigo, ***convulsions,*** hearing loss
MS: Arthralgia, arthritis, myalgia

Contraindications: Hypersensitivity to ACE inhibitors, pregnancy (D), lactation, children

Precautions: Impaired renal, liver function, dialysis patients, hypovolemia, blood dyscrasias, CHF, COPD, asthma, elderly

Pharmacokinetics:
PO: Peak ½-1 hr, serum protein binding 97%, half-life 1-2 hr, metabolized by liver (metabolites excreted in urine, feces)

Interactions/incompatibilities:
• Increased hypotension: diuretics, other antihypertensives, ganglionic blockers, adrenergic blockers
• Increased toxicity: vasodilators, hydralazine, prazosin, potassium-sparing diuretics, sympathomimetics
• Decreased absorption: antacids

• Decreased antihypertensive effect: indomethacin
• Increased serum levels of: digoxin, lithium
• Increased hypersensitivity: allopurinol

NURSING CONSIDERATIONS

Assess:
• Blood studies: neutrophils, decreased platelets
• B/P, orthostatic hypotension, syncope
• Renal studies: protein, BUN, creatinine; watch for increased levels that may indicate nephrotic syndrome
• Baselines in renal, liver function tests before therapy begins
• Potassium levels, although hyperkalemia rarely occurs
• Dipstick of urine for protein qd in first morning specimen; if protein is increased, a 24-hr urinary protein should be collected

Administer:
• IV infusion of 0.9% NaCl (as ordered) to expand fluid volume if severe hypotension occurs

Perform/provide:
• Storage in tight container at 30° C or less
• Supine or Trendelenburg position for severe hypotension

Evaluate:
• Therapeutic response: decrease in B/P
• Edema in feet, legs daily
• Allergic reactions: rash, fever, pruritus, urticaria; drugs should be discontinued if antihistamines fail to help
• Renal symptoms: polyuria, oliguria, frequency, dysuria

Teach patient/family:
• Not to discontinue drug abruptly
• Not to use OTC products (cough, cold, allergy) unless directed by physician; not to use salt substitutes containing potassium without consulting physician
• To comply with dosage schedule, even if feeling better
• To rise slowly to sitting or standing position to minimize orthostatic hypotension
• To notify physician of: mouth sores, sore throat, fever, swelling of hands or feet, irregular heartbeat, chest pain
• To report excessive perspiration, dehydration, vomiting, diarrhea; may lead to fall in B/P
• That drug may cause dizziness, fainting, light-headedness; may occur during 1st few days of therapy
• That drug may cause skin rash or impaired perspiration
• How to take B/P, and normal readings for age group

Lab test interferences:
False positive: Urine acetone

Treatment of overdose: 0.9% NaCl IV INF, hemodialysis

---

ranitidine

(ra-nye' te-deen)
Zantac

Func. class.: H_2 histamine receptor antagonist

Action: Inhibits histamine at H_2 receptor site in parietal cells, which inhibits gastric acid secretion

Uses: Duodenal ulcer, Zollinger-Ellison syndrome, gastric ulcers, hypersecretory conditions, gastroesophageal reflux disease, stress ulcers

Dosage and routes:
• *Adult:* PO 150 mg bid, 300 mg hs; IM 50 mg q6-8h; IV BOL 50 mg diluted to 20 ml over 5 min q6-8h IV int inf 50 mg/100 ml D_5 over 15-20 min, q6-8h

* Available in Canada only

Available forms include: Tabs 150, 300 mg; inj 25 mg/ml IM, IV
Side effects/adverse reactions:
CNS: Headache, sleeplessness, dizziness, confusion, agitation, depression, hallucination
GI: Constipation, abdominal pain, diarrhea, nausea, vomiting, ***hepatotoxicity***
GU: Impotence, gynecomastia
CV: Tachycardia, bradycardia, PVCs
EENT: Blurred vision, increased ocular pressure
INTEG: Urticaria, rash, fever
Contraindications: Hypersensitivity
Precautions: Pregnancy (B), lactation, child <12 yr, hepatic disease, renal disease
Pharmacokinetics:
PO: Peak 2-3 hr, duration 8-12 hr; metabolized by liver, excreted in urine, breast milk, half-life 2-3 hr
Interactions/incompatibilities:
• Increased toxicity; anticoagulants, metoprolol
• Decreased absorption of: ketoconazole
• Decreased absorption of ranitidine: antacids

NURSING CONSIDERATIONS

Assess:
• Gastric pH (>5 should be maintained)
• I&O ratio, BUN, creatinine

Administer:
• With meals for prolonged drug effect
• Antacids 1 hr before or 1 hr after ranitidine
• IV after diluting 50 mg/20 ml of compatible sol and give 50 mg or less/5 min or more; may dilute 50 mg/50-100 ml of compatible sol and give over 15-20 min

Perform/provide:
• Storage at room temperature

Evaluate:
• Therapeutic response: decreased abdominal pain
• Mental status: confusion, dizziness, depression, anxiety, weakness, tremors, psychosis, diarrhea, abdominal discomfort, jaundice; report immediately
• GI complaints: nausea, vomiting, diarrhea, cramps

Teach patient/family:
• That gynecomastia, impotence may occur but are reversible
• To avoid driving or other hazardous activities until patient is stabilized on this medication
• To avoid black pepper, caffeine, alcohol, harsh spices, extremes in temperature of food
• That drug must be continued for prescribed time to be effective

Lab test interferences:
Increase: AST/ALT, alk phosphatase, creatinine, LDH, bilirubin
False positive: Urine protein

---

reserpine

(re-ser'peen)
Broserpine, Elserpine, Hyperine, Rauserpin, Reserfia,* Serpasil, Serpate, Sertina, Tensin, Zepine
Func. class.: Antihypertensive
Chem. class.: Antiadrenergic agent

Action: Inhibits norepinephrine release, depleting norepinephrine stores in adrenergic nerve endings
Uses: Hypertension; relief in agitated psychotic states unable to tolerate phenothiazines or requiring antihypertensive medication
Dosage and routes:
Hypertension
• *Adult:* PO 0.25-0.5 mg qd × 1-2 wk, then 0.1-0.25 mg qd maintenance
• *Child:* PO 0.07 mg/kg or 2 mg/

m² given with hydralzine IM q12-24h

Pyschiatric disorders

• *Adult:* 0.5 mg/day (range 0.1-1 mg)

Available forms include: Tabs 0.2, 0.1, 0.25, 1 mg; caps-time rel 0.5 mg; inj 2.5 mg/ml

Side effects/adverse reactions:

CV: Bradycardia, chest pain, dysrhythmias, prolonged bleeding time, ***thrombocytopenia,*** purpura

CNS: Drowsiness, fatigue, lethargy, dizziness, depression, anxiety, headache, increased dreaming, nightmares, convulsions, Parkinsonism, EPS (high doses)

GI: Nausea, vomiting, cramps, peptic ulcer, dry mouth, increased appetite, anorexia

INTEG: Rash, purpura, alopecia, flushing, warm feeling, pruritus, ecchymosis

EENT: Lacrimation, miosis, blurred vision, ptosis, dry mouth, epistaxis

GU: Impotence, dysuria, nocturia, sodium, water retention, edema, breast engorgement, galactorrhea, gynecomastia

RESP: ***Bronchospasm,*** dyspnea, cough, rales

Contraindications: Hypersensitivity, depression/suicidal patients, active peptic ulcer disease, ulcerative colitis, pregnancy (D)

Precautions: Pregnancy, lactation, seizure disorders, renal disease

Pharmacokinetics:

PO: Peak 4 hr, duration 2-6 wk; half-life 50-100 hr, metabolized by liver, excreted in urine, feces, crosses placenta, blood-brain barrier, excreted in breast milk

Interactions/incompatibilities:

• Increased hypotension: diuretics, hypotension, β-blockers, methotrimeprazine
• Dysrhythmias: cardiac glycosides
• Increased cardiac depression: quinidine, procainamide
• Excitation, hypertension: MAOIs
• Increased CNS depression: barbiturates, alcohol, narcotics
• Increased pressor effects: epinephrine, isoproterenol, norepinephrine
• Decreased pressor effects: ephedrine, amphetamine

NURSING CONSIDERATIONS

Assess:

• Renal function studies in renal impairment (BUN, creatinine)
• Bleeding time, check for ecchymosis, thrombocytopenia, purpura
• I&O in renal disease patient

Evaluate:

• Therapeutic response: decreased hypertension
• Cardiac status: B/P, pulse, watch for hypotension, bradycardia
• Edema in feet, legs daily; take weight daily
• Skin turgor, dryness of mucous membranes for hydration status
• Symptoms of CHF: edema, dyspnea, wet rales

Teach patient/family:

• To avoid driving, hazardous activities if drowsiness occurs
• Not to discontinue drug abruptly
• Not to use OTC products (cough, cold preparations) unless directed by physician
• To report bradycardia, dizziness, confusion, depression, fever, sore throat
• That impotence, gynecomastia may occur but is reversible
• To rise slowly to sitting or standing position to minimize orthostatic hypotension
• That therapeutic effect may take 2-4 wk

Lab test interferences:
Increase: VMA excretion, 5-HIAA excretion
Interferences: 17-OHCS, 17-KS
Treatment of overdose: Lavage, IV atropine for bradycardia, supportive therapy

Rh_o (D) immune globulin, human

Gamulin Rh, HypoRho-D, MICRhoGAM, Mini-Gamulin RH, RHoGAM, Win-Rho*

Func. class.: Immunizing agent
Chem. class.: IgG

Action: Supresses immune response of non-sensitized Rh_o (D or D^u)-negative patients who are exposed to Rh_o (D or D^u)-positive blood
Uses: Prevention of isoimmunization in Rh-negative women exposed to Rh positive blood, given after abortions, miscarriages, amniocentesis
Dosage and routes:
Obstetrical use
• *Adult:* IM 1 vial if fetal packed RBCs <15 ml, or 2 vials if fetal packed RBCs >15 ml; given within 72 hr of delivery or miscarriage
Transfusion error
• *Adult:* IM Give within 72 hr
Available forms include: Inj IM single dose vial
Side effects/adverse reactions:
INTEG: Irritation at injection site, fever
CNS: Lethargy
MS: Myalgia
Contraindications: Previous immunization with this drug, Rh_o (O)-positive/D^u-positive patient
NURSING CONSIDERATIONS
Assess:
• Allergies, reactions to immunizations
Administer:
• After sending newborn's cord blood to lab after delivery for cross match, type, infant must be Rh-positive, with Rh-negative mother
• IM only in deltoid, aspirate
• Only equal lot numbers of drug, cross-match
• Only MICRhoGAM for abortions, or miscarriages < 12 wk unless fetus or father is Rh^-, unless she is Rh_o (D)-positive, D^u-positive, Rh antibodies are present
Evaluate:
• Allergic reaction: rash, urticaria, nausea, fever, wheezing
Perform/provide:
• Storage in refrigerator
Teach patient/family:
• How drug works, that drug does need to be given after subsequent deliveries if baby is Rh positive

riboflavin (vitamin B_2)

(rey'boo-flay-vin)
Riobin-50 and others

Func. class.: Vitamin B_2, water soluble

Action: Needed for respiratory reactions by catalyzing proteins and normal vision
Uses: Vitamin B_2 deficiency or polyneuritis, cheilosis adjunct with thiamine
Dosage and routes:
• *Adult and child >12 yr:* PO 5-50 mg qd
• *Child <12 yr:* PO 2-10 mg qd
Available forms include: Tabs 5, 10, 25, 50, 100 mg
Side effects/adverse reactions:
GU: Yellow discoloration of urine (large doses)
Contraindications: Child <12 yr
Precautions: Pregnancy (A)
Pharmacokinetics:
PO: Half-life 65-85 min, 60% pro-

R

tein-bound, unused amounts excreted in urine (unchanged)

Interactions/incompatibilities:

- Decreased action of: tetracyclines

NURSING CONSIDERATIONS

Administer:

- With food for better absorption

Perform/provide:

- Storage in tight, light-resistant container

Evaluate:

- Therapeutic response: absence of headache, GI problems, cheilosis, skin lesions, depression, burning, itchy eyes, anemia
- Nutritional status: liver, eggs, dairy products, yeast, whole grain, green vegetables

Teach patient/family:

- That urine may turn bright yellow
- About addition of needed foods that are rich in riboflavin

Lab test interferences:

- May cause false elevations of urinary catecholamines

---

rifampin

(rif'am-pin)

Rifadin, Rimactane, Rofact*

Func. class.: Antitubercular

Chem. class.: Rifamycin B derivative

Action: Inhibits DNA-dependent polymerase, decreases tubercle bacilli replication

Uses: Pulmonary tuberculosis, meningococcal carriers (prevention)

Dosage and routes:

- *Adult:* PO 600 mg/day as single dose 1 hr ac or 2 hr pc
- *Child >5 yr:* PO 10-20 mg/kg/day as single dose 1 hr ac or 2 hr pc, not to exceed 600 mg/day, with other antituberculars

Meningococcal carriers

- *Adult:* PO 600 mg bid × 2 days
- *Child >5 yr:* PO 10 mg/kg bid × 2 days, not to exceed 600 mg/dose

Available forms include: Caps 150, 300 mg

Side effects/adverse reactions:

INTEG: Rash, pruritus, urticaria

EENT: Visual disturbances

MS: Atoxia, weakness

MISC: Flulike syndrome, menstrual disturbances, edema, shortness of breath

GI: Nausia, vomiting, anorexia, diarrhea, ***pseudomembranous colitis***, heartburn, sore mouth, tongue, pancreatitis

GU: ***Hematuria, acute renal failure, hemoglobinuria***

CNS: Headache, fatigue, anxiety, drowsiness, confusion

HEMA: ***Hemolytic anemia, eosinophilia, thrombocytopenia, leukopenia***

Contraindications: Hypersensitivity

Precautions: Pregnancy (C), lactation, hepatic disease, blood dyscrasias

Pharmacokinetics:

PO: Peak 2-3 hr, duration >24 hr, half-life 3 hr; metabolized in liver (active/inactive metabolites), excreted in urine as free drug (30% crosses placenta), excreted in breast milk

Interactions/incompatibilities:

- Decreased action: barbiturates, clofibrate, corticosteroids, dapsone, anticoagulants, antidiabetics, hormones, digoxin, PAS, alcohol, oral contraceptives
- Hepatotoxicity: INH

NURSING CONSIDERATIONS

Assess:

- Signs of anemia: Hct, Hgb, fatigue

---

* Available in Canada only

• Liver studies qwk: ALT, AST, bilirubin
• Renal status before, qmo: BUN, creatinine, output, sp gr, urinalysis

Administer:
• On empty stomach, 1 hr ac or 2 hr pc
• Antiemetic if vomiting occurs
• After C&S is completed; qmo to detect resistance

Evaluate:
• Therapeutic response: decreased symptoms of TB, culture negative
• Hepatic status: decreased appetite, jaundice, dark urine, fatigue

Teach patient/family:
• That compliance with dosage schedule, duration is necessary
• That scheduled appointments must be kept; relapse may occur
• To avoid alcohol while taking drug
• That urine, feces, saliva, sputum, sweat, tears may be colored red-orange; soft contact lenses may be permanently stained
• To report flulike symptoms: excessive fatigue, anorexia, vomiting, sore throat; unusual bleeding, yellowish discoloration of skin/eyes

Lab test interferences:
Interference: Folate level, vitamin B_{12}, BSP, gall bladder studies

---

ritodrine HCl

(ri'toe-dreen)

Yutopar

Func. class.: Tocolytic, uterine relaxant

Chem. class.: β_2-adrenergic agonist

Action: Reduces frequency, intensity of uterine contractions by stimulation of the β_2 receptors in uterine smooth muscle

Uses: Preterm labor

Dosage and routes:
• Adult: IV INF 150 mg/500 ml (0.3 mg/ml) given 0.1 mg/min, increased gradually by 0.05 mg/min q10min until desired response; PO 10 mg given ½ hr before termination of IV, then 10 mg q2h × 24 hr, then 10-20 mg q4-6h, not to exceed 120 mg/day

Available forms include: Tabs 10 mg; inj 10 mg/ml

Side effects/adverse reactions:
MISC: Erythema, rash, dyspnea, hyperventilation, glycosuria, lactic acidosis
META: Hyperglycemia
CNS: Headache, restlessness, anxiety, nervousness, sweating, chills, drowsiness, tremor
GI: Nausea, vomiting, anorexia, malaise, bloating, constipation, diarrhea
CV: Altered maternal, fetal heart rate, B/P, dysrhythmias, palpitation, chest pain

Contraindications: Hypersensitivity, eclampsia, hypertension, dysrhythmias, thyrotoxicosis, before 20th wk of pregnancy, antepartum hemorrhage, intrauterine fetal death, maternal cardiac disease, pulmonary hypertension, uncontrolled diabetes, pheochromocytoma

Precautions: Migraine, sulfite sensitivity, pregnancy-induced hypertension, hypertension, diabetes

Pharmacokinetics:
PO: Peak ½-1 hr
IV: Peak 1 hr, distribution half-life 6 min, 1½-2½ hr, >10 hr, metabolized in liver, excreted in urine, crosses placenta

Interactions/incompatibilities:
• Pulmonary edema: corticosteroids
• Increased CV effects of ritodrine: magnesium sulfate, diazoxide, me-

R

peridine, potent general anesthetics
• Increased effects of: sympathomimetic amines
• Systemic hypertension: atropine
• Decreased action of ritodrine: β-blockers

NURSING CONSIDERATIONS

Assess:
• Maternal, fetal heart tones during infusion
• Intensity, length of uterine contractions
• Fluid intake to prevent fluid overload; discontinue if this occurs
• Blood glucose in diabetics

Administer:
• Only clear solutions
• After dilutions: 150 mg/500 ml D_5W or NS, give at 0.3 mg/ml
• After infusion pump, or monitor carefully

Perform/provide:
• Positioning of patient in left lateral recumbent position to decrease hypotension, increase renal blood flow

Evaluate:
• Therapeutic response: decreased intensity, length of contraction, absence of preterm labor, decreased B/P

Teach patient/family:
• To remain in bed during infusion

Lab test interferences:
Increase: Blood glucose, free fatty acids, insulin, GTT
Decrease: Potassium

salicylic acid

Calicylic, Keralyt, Salacid, Salonil
Func. class.: Keratolytic

Action: Corrects abnormal keratinization and causes peeling of skin
Uses: Dandruff, seborrheic dermatitis, psoriasis, multiple superficial epitheliomatoses
Dosage and routes:
• *Adult:* TOP apply as needed, cover at night
Available forms include: Powder, cream 2%, 2.5%, 10%; gel 6%, 17%; oint 25%, 60%; plaster 40%; pledgets 0.5%; shampoo 2%, 4%; solution 0.5%, 13.6%, 17%; stick 2%; susp 2%
Side effects/adverse reactions:
INTEG: Irritation, drying
CNS: ***Salicylism: hearing loss, tinnitus, dizziness, confusion, headache, hyperventilation***
Contraindications: Hypersensitivity
Precautions: Pregnancy (C), diabetes

NURSING CONSIDERATIONS

Assess:
• Platelets, WBC if systemic absorption occurs

Administer:
• Only to intact skin; do not use on inflamed, denuded skin
• After wetting skin, wash thoroughly each AM after treatment
• Using an occlusive dressing to increase absorption, apply more often to areas where occlusion is impossible

Evaluate:
• Therapeutic response: decrease in dandruff, size of lesions
• Salicylism: tinnitus, hearing loss, dizziness, confusion, headache, hyperventilation
• Allergic reactions: irritation, redness

Teach patient/family:
• To avoid contact with eyes, mucous membranes
• To apply lotion if drying occurs
• To avoid applying to large areas, salicylate toxicity may occur

salsalate

(sal-sa'late)

Disalcid, Mono-Gesic

Func. class.: Nonnarcotic analgesic

Chem. class.: Salicylate

Action: Blocks formation of peripheral prostaglandins, which causes pain and inflammation, antipyretic action results from inhibition of hypothalamic heat-regulating center, does not inhibit platelet aggregation

Uses: Mild to moderate pain or fever including arthritis, juvenile rheumatoid arthritis

Dosage and routes:

• *Adult:* PO 3000 mg/day in divided doses

Available forms include: Caps 500 mg; tabs 500, 750 mg

Side effects/adverse reactions:

HEMA: ***Thrombocytopenia, agranulocytosis, leukopenia, neutropenia, hemolytic anemia,*** increased pro-time

CNS: Stimulation, drowsiness, dizziness, confusion, ***convulsions,*** headache, flushing, hallucinations, coma

GI: Nausea, vomiting, GI bleeding, diarrhea, heartburn, anorexia, ***hepatotoxicity***

INTEG: Rash, urticaria, bruising

EENT: Tinnitus, hearing loss

CV: Rapid pulse, ***pulmonary edema***

RESP: Wheezing, hyperpnea

ENDO: Hypoglycemia, hyponatremia, hypokalemia, alteration in acid-base balance

Contraindications: Hypersensitivity to salicylates, NSAIDs, GI bleeding, bleeding disorders, children < 3 yr, vitamin K deficiency

Precautions: Anemia, hepatic disease, renal disease, Hodgkin's disease, pregnancy (C), lactation

Pharmacokinetics: Metabolized by liver, excreted by kidneys, half-life 1 hr, highly protein bound, crosses blood-brain barrier and placenta slowly

Interactions/incompatibilities:

• Decreased effects of salsalate: antacids, steroids, urinary alkalizers

• Increased blood loss: alcohol, heparin, ibuprofen, warfarin

• Increased effects of: anticoagulants, insulin, methotrexate, probenecid

• Decreased effects of: spironolactone, sulfinpyrazone, sulfonylmides, loop diuretics

• Toxic effects: PABA

• Decreased blood sugar levels: salicylates

NURSING CONSIDERATIONS

Assess:

• Liver function studies: AST, ALT, bilirubin, creatinine if patient is on long-term therapy

• Renal function studies: BUN, urine creatinine if patient is on long-term therapy

• Blood studies: CBC, Hct, Hgb, pro-time if patient is on long-term therapy

• I&O ratio; decreasing output may indicate renal failure (long-term therapy)

Administer:

• To patient crushed or whole; chewable tablets may be chewed

• With food or milk to decrease gastric symptoms; give 30 min before or 2 hr after meals

• With full glass of water

Evaluate:

• Therapeutic response: decreased pain, fever

• Hepatotoxicity: dark urine, clay-

colored stools, yellowing of skin, sclera, itching, abdominal pain, fever, diarrhea if patient is on long-term therapy
• Allergic reactions: rash, urticaria; if these occur, drug may need to be discontinued
• Renal dysfunction: decreased urine output
• Ototoxicity: tinnitus, ringing, roaring in ears; audiometric testing is needed before, after long-term therapy
• Visual changes: blurring, halos, corneal and retinal damage
• Edema in feet, ankles, legs
• Prior drug history; there are many drug interactions

Teach patient/family:
• To report any symptoms of hepatotoxicity, renal toxicity, visual changes, ototoxicity, allergic reactions (long-term therapy)
• Not to exceed recommended dosage; acute poisoning may result
• To read label on other OTC drugs; many contain aspirin
• That therapeutic response takes 2 wk (arthritis)
• To avoid alcohol ingestion; GI bleeding may occur

Lab test interferences:
Increase: Coagulation studies, liver function studies, serum uric acid, amylase, CO_2, urinary protein
Decrease: Serum potassium, PBI, cholesterol, blood glucose
Interfere: Urine catecholamines, pregnancy test

Treatment of overdose: Lavage, activated charcoal, monitor electrolytes, VS

---

sargramostim (GM-CSF)
(sare-gram'o-stem)
Leukine, Prokine
Func. class.: Biologic modifier

Action: Stimulates proliferation and differentiation of hematopoietic progenitor cells

Uses: Acceleration of myeloid recovery in patients with non-Hodgkin's lymphoma, acute lymphoblastic leukemia, autologous bone marrow transplantation in Hodgkin's disease; bone marrow transplantation failure or engraftment delay

Dosage and routes:
Myeloid reconstitution after autologous bone marrow transplantation
• *Adult:* IV 250 μg/m²/day × 3 wks, give over 2 hr, given 2-4 hr after autologous bone marrow infusion, and not less than 24 hr after last dose of antineoplastics and 12 hr after last dose of radiotherapy, bone marrow transplantation failure, or engraftment delay
• *Adult:* IV 250 μg/m²/day × 14 days, give over 2 hr, may repeat in 7 days, may repeat 500 μg/m²/day × 14 days after another 7 days if no improvement

Available forms include: Pwd for inj lyophilized 250, 500 μg

Side effects/adverse reactions:
CNS: Fever, malaise, CNS disorder
GI: Nausea, vomiting, diarrhea, anorexia, ***GI hemorrhage,*** stomatitis, ***liver damage***
HEMA: ***Blood dyscrasias, hemorrhage***
INTEG: Alopecia, rash, peripheral edema
GU: Urinary tract disorder, abnormal kidney function

Contraindications: Hypersensitivity to GM-CSF, yeast products, excessive leukemic myeloid blast in the bone marrow or peripheral blood

Precautions: Pregnancy (C), lactation, children, renal, hepatic, lung disease, cardiac disease, pleural, pericardial effusions

Pharmacokinetics: Half-life 2 hr, detected within 5 min after administration, peak 2 hr

Interactions/incompatibilities:

- Do not use this drug concomitantly with antineoplastics
- Increased myeloproliferation: lithium, corticosteroids
- Do not add other medications to infusion solution

NURSING CONSIDERATIONS

Assess:

- Blood studies: CBC, differential count before treatment and twice weekly, leukocytosis may occur (WBC >50,000 cells/mm^3, ANC >20,000 cells/mm^3)
- Renal and hepatic studies before treatment: BUN, creatinine, urinalysis; AST, ALT, alk phosphatase; twice weekly monitoring is needed in renal, hepatic disease
- Hypersensitive reactions, rashes and local injection site reactions may occur and are usually transient
- For increased fluid retention in cardiac disease

Administer:

- After reconstituting with 1 ml sterile water for inj without preservative; do not reenter vial, discard unused portion; direct reconstitution solution at side of vial, rotate contents; do not shake
- Dilute in 0.9% NaCl inj to prepare IV infusion; if final concentration is <10 μg/ml, add human albumin to make a final concentration of 0.1% to the NaCl before adding sargramostim to prevent adsorption; for a final concentration of 0.1% albumin add 1 mg human albumin/1 ml 0.9% NaCl inj; give within 6 hrs after reconstitution

Perform/provide:

- Storage in refrigerator, do not freeze

Evaluate:

- Therapeutic response: WBC and differential recovery

---

scopolamine (transdermal)

(skoe-pol'-a-meen)

Transderm-Scop

Func. class.: Antiemetic, anticholinergic

Chem. class.: Belladonna alkaloid

Action: Competitive antagonism of acetylcholine at receptor site in eye, smooth muscle, cardiac muscle, glandular cells; inhibition of vestibular input to the CNS, resulting in inhibition of vomiting reflex

Uses: Prevention of motion sickness

Dosage and routes:

- *Adult:* PATCH 1 placed behind ear 4-5 hr before travel
- Not recommended for children

Available forms include: Patch, 0.5 mg delivered in 72 hr

Side effects/adverse reactions:

INTEG: Rash, erythema

GU: Difficult urination

CNS: Dizziness, drowsiness, confusion, disorientation, memory disturbances, hallucinations

EENT: Blurred vision, altered depth perception, *dilated pupils,* photophobia, *dry mouth,* dry, itchy, red eyes, acute narrow-angle glaucoma

Contraindications: Hypersensitivity, glaucoma

Precautions: Children, elderly, pregnancy (C), pyloric, urinary, bladder neck, intestinal obstruction, liver, kidney disease

Pharmacokinetics:

PATCH: Onset 4-5 hr, duration 72 hr

S

Interactions/incompatibilities:
• Increased anticholinergic effects: antihistamines, antidepressants

NURSING CONSIDERATIONS

Teach patient/family:
• To avoid hazardous activities, activities requiring alertness; dizziness may occur
• To wash, dry hands before and after applying to surface behind ear
• To change patch q72h
• To apply at least 4 hr before traveling
• If blurred vision, severe dizziness, drowsiness occurs, to discontinue use, use another type of antiemetic
• To read label of all OTC medications; if any scopolamine is found in product, avoid use
• To keep out of children's reach

scopolamine hydrobromide

(skoe-pol'a-meen)

Func. class.: Cholinergic blocker
Chem. class.: Belladonna alkaloid

Action: Inhibits acetylcholine at receptor sites in autonomic nervous system, which controls secretions, free acids in stomach; blocks central muscarinic receptors, which decreases involuntary movements
Uses: Reduction of secretions before surgery, calm delirium, motion sickness
Dosage and routes:
Parkinson symptoms
• *Adult:* IM/SC/IV 0.3-0.6 mg tid-qid diluted using dilution provided
• *Child:* SC 0.006 mg/kg tid-qid or 0.2 mg/m^2
Preoperatively
• *Adult:* SC 0.4-0.6 mg

Available forms include: Inj 0.3, 0.4, 0.86, 1 mg/ml
Side effects/adverse reactions:
CNS: Confusion, anxiety, restlessness, irritability, delusions, hallucinations, headache, sedation, depression, incoherence, dizziness, excitement, delirium, flushing, weakness
INTEG: Urticaria
MISC: Suppression of lactation, nasal congestion, decreased sweating
EENT: Blurred vision, photophobia, dilated pupils, difficulty swallowing, mydriasis, cycloplegia
CV: Palpitations, tachycardia, postural hypotension, paradoxical bradycardia
GI: Dryness of mouth, constipation, nausea, vomiting, abdominal distress, ***paralytic ileus***
GU: Hesitancy, retention
Contraindications: Hypersensitivity, narrow-angle glaucoma, myasthenia gravis, GI/GU obstruction, hypersensitivity to belladonna, barbiturates
Precautions: Pregnancy (C), elderly, lactation, prostatic hypertrophy, CHF, hypertension, dysrhythmia, children, gastric ulcer
Pharmacokinetics:
SC/IM: Peak 30-45 min, duration 7 hr
IV: Peak 10-15 min, duration 4 hr
Excreted in urine, bile, feces (unchanged)
Interactions/incompatibilities:
• Increased anticholinergic effect: alcohol, narcotics, antihistamines, phenothiazines, tricyclics
• Do not mix with diazepam, chloramphenicol, pentobarbital, sodium bicarbonate in syringe or solution

NURSING CONSIDERATIONS

Assess:
• I&O ratio; retention commonly causes decreased urinary output

* Available in Canada only

Administer:
- Parenteral dose with patient recumbent to prevent postural hypotension
- Administer with or after meals for GI upset; may give with fluids other than water
- At hs to avoid daytime drowsiness in patient with parkinsonism
- Parenteral dose slowly; keep in bed for at least 1 hr after dose
- With analgesic to avoid behavioral changes when given as a preop

Perform/provide:
- Storage at room temperature in light-resistant containers
- Hard candy, frequent drinks, sugarless gum to relieve dry mouth

Evaluate:
- Therapeutic response: decreased secretions
- Parkinsonism, extrapyramidal symptoms: shuffling gait, muscle rigidity, involuntary movements
- Urinary hesitancy, retention, palpate bladder if retention occurs
- Constipation; increase fluids, bulk, exercise if this occurs
- For tolerance over long-term therapy; dose may need to be increased or changed
- Mental status: affect, mood, CNS depression, worsening of mental symptoms during early therapy

Teach patient/family:
- Not to discontinue this drug abruptly; to taper off over 1 wk
- To avoid driving or other hazardous activities; drowsiness may occur
- To avoid OTC medication: cough, cold preparations with alcohol, antihistamines unless directed by physician

scopolamine hydrobromide (optic)

(skoe-pol'a-meen)

Isopto-Hyoscine

Func. class.: Mydriatic
Chem. class.: Synthetic alkaloid

Action: Blocks response of iris sphincter muscle, muscle of accommodation of ciliary body to cholinergic stimulation, resulting in dilation, paralysis of accommodation

Uses: Uveitis, iritis

Dosage and routes:
- *Adult:* INSTILL 1-2 gtts before refraction or 1-2 gtts qd-tid for iritis or uveitis
- *Child:* INSTILL 1 gtt bid × 2 days before refraction

Available forms include: Sol 0.25%

Side effects/adverse reactions:
CV: Tachycardia
CNS: Confusion, somnolence, flushing, fever
EENT: Blurred vision, photophobia, increased intraocular pressure, irritation, edema

Contraindications: Hypersensitivity, children <6 yr, narrow-angle glaucoma, increased intraocular pressure, infants

Precautions: Children, elderly, hypertension, hyperthyroidism, diabetes, pregnancy (C)

Pharmacokinetics:
INSTILL: Peak 20-30 min, duration 3-7 days

NURSING CONSIDERATIONS

Evaluate:
- Therapeutic response: decrease in inflammation, cycloplegic refraction
- Eye pain, discontinue use

Teach patient/family:
- To report change in vision, blur-

ring or loss of sight, trouble breathing, inhibition of sweating, flushing
• Method of instillation: pressure on lacrimal sac for 1 min, do not touch dropper to eye
• That blurred vision will decrease with repeated use of drug
• Not to engage in hazardous activities until able to see
• Wait 5 min to use other drops
• Do not blink more than usual

secobarbital/secobarbital sodium

(see-koe-bar'bi-tal)

Seconal/Secogen Sodium,* Seconal Sodium, Seral*

Func. class.: Sedative/hypnotic-barbiturate

Chem. class.: Barbitone (short acting)

Controlled Substance Schedule II (USA), Schedule G (Canada)

Action: Depresses activity in brain cells primarily in reticular activating system in brain stem; selectively depresses neurons in posterior hypothalamus, limbic structures; able to decrease seizure activity by inhibition of epileptic activity in CNS

Uses: Insomnia, sedation, preoperative medication, status epilepticus, acute tetanus convulsions

Dosage and routes:

Insomnia

• *Adult:* PO/IM 100-200 mg hs
• *Child:* IM 3-5 mg/kg, not to exceed 100 mg, not to inject >5 ml in one site; REC 4-5 mg/kg

Sedation/preoperatively

• *Adult:* PO 200-300 mg 1-2 hr preoperatively
• *Child:* PO 50-100 mg 1-2 hr preoperatively; REC 4-5 mg/kg 1-2 hr preoperatively

Status epilepticus

• *Adult and child:* IM/IV 250-350 mg

Acute psychotic agitation

• *Adult and child:* IM/IV 5.5 mg/kg q3-4h

Available forms include: Caps 50, 100 mg; tabs 100 mg, inj IM, IV 50 mg/ml; powder, rec supp 200 mg

Side effects/adverse reactions:

CNS: Lethargy, drowsiness, hangover, dizziness, paradoxical stimulation in the elderly and children, light-headedness, dependence, CNS depression, mental depression, slurred speech

GI: Nausea, vomiting, diarrhea, constipation

INTEG: Rash, urticaria, pain, abscesses at injection site, angioedema, thrombophlebitis, ***Stevens-Johnson syndrome***

CV: Hypotension, bradycardia

RESP: Depression, ***apnea, laryngospasm, bronchospasm***

HEMA: ***Agranulocytosis, thrombocytopenia, megaloblastic anemia*** (long-term treatment)

Contraindications: Hypersensitivity to barbiturates, respiratory depression, addiction to barbiturates, severe liver impairment, porphyria, uncontrolled severe pain

Precautions: Anemia, pregnancy (D), lactation, hepatic disease, renal disease, hypertension, elderly, acute/chronic pain

Pharmacokinetics:

IM: Onset 10-15 min, duration 4-6 hr

REC: Onset slow, duration 3-6 hr; metabolized by liver, excreted by kidneys (metabolites); half-life 15-40 hr

* Available in Canada only

Interactions/incompatibilities:
• Do not mix with other drugs in solution or syringe
• Increased CNS depression: alcohol, MAOIs, sedative, narcotics
• Decreased effect of: oral anticoagulants, corticosteroids, griseofulvin, quinidine
• Decreased half-life of doxycycline

NURSING CONSIDERATIONS

Assess:
• VS q30min after parenteral route for 2 hr
• Blood studies: Hct, Hgb, RBCs, serum folate, vitamin D (if on long-term therapy); pro-time in patients receiving anticoagulants
• Hepatic studies: AST, ALT, bilirubin; if increased, the drug is usually discontinued

Administer:
• After removal of cigarettes, to prevent fires
• IM injection in deep large muscle mass to prevent tissue sloughing and abscesses
• After conservative measures have been tried for insomnia
• Within 30 min of mixing with sterile water for injection, reconstitute after rotating ampule, do not shake, do not use cloudy solution, may be given directly, or indirectly
• IV only with resuscitative equipment available, administer at <100 mg/min (only by qualified personnel)
• ½-1hr before hs for sleeplessness
• On empty stomach for best absorption
• For <14 days since drug is not effective after that; tolerance develops
• Crushed or whole
• Alone, do not mix with other drugs or inject if there is precipitate
• After cleansing enema if given rectally preoperatively in children

Perform/provide:
• Assistance with ambulation after receiving dose
• Safety measure: siderails, nightlight, call bell within easy reach
• Checking to see PO medication has been swallowed
• Storage of suppositories in refrigerator; do not use aqueous solutions containing precipitate

Evaluate:
• Therapeutic response: ability to sleep at night, decreased amount of early morning awakening if taking drug for insomnia, or decrease in number, severity of seizures if taking drug for seizure disorder
• Unresolved pain, as drug may cause severe stimulation if pain is present
• Mental status: mood, sensorium, affect, memory (long, short)
• Physical dependency: more frequent requests for medication, shakes, anxiety
• Barbiturate toxicity: hypotension; pulmonary constriction; cold, clammy skin; cyanosis of lips; insomnia; nausea; vomiting; hallucinations; delirium; weakness; mild symptoms may occur in 8-12 hr without drug
• Respiratory dysfunction: respiratory depression, character, rate, rhythm; hold drug if respirations <10/min or if pupils dilated
• Blood dyscrasias: fever, sore throat, bruising, rash, jaundice, epistaxis
• Perianal irritation if rectal forms used

Teach patient/family:
• That morning hangover is common
• That drug is indicated only for short-term treatment of insomnia

S

and is probably ineffective after 2 wk
• That physical dependency may result when used for extended periods of time (45-90 days depending on dose)
• To avoid driving or other activities requiring alertness
• To avoid alcohol ingestion or CNS depressants; serious CNS depression may result
• Not to discontinue medication quickly after long-term use; drug should be tapered over 1-2 wk
• To tell all prescribers that barbiturate is being taken
• That withdrawal insomnia may occur after short-term use; do not start using drug again, insomnia will improve in 1-3 nights, may experience increased dreaming
• That effects may take 2 nights for benefits to be noticed
• Alternate measures to improve sleep (reading, exercise several hours before hs, warm bath, warm milk, TV, self-hypnosis, deep breathing)

Lab test interferences:
False increase: Sulfobromophthalein

Treatment of overdose: Lavage, activated charcoal, warming blanket, vital signs, hemodialysis, I&O ratio

selegiline HCl (L-Deprenyl)

(sel-ee-gill-ene)
Eldepryl

Func. class.: Antiparkinson agent
Chem. class.: Levorotatory acetylanic derivative of phenethylamine

Action: Increased dopaminergic activity by inhibition of MAO type B activity; not fully understood

Uses: Adjunct management of Parkinson's disease in patients being treated with levodopa/carbidopa who have had a poor response to therapy

Dosage and routes:
• *Adult:* PO 10 mg/day in divided doses 5 mg at breakfast and lunch, after 2-3 days begin to reduce the dose of levodopa/carbidopa 10%-30%

Available forms: Tabs 5 mg

Side effects/adverse reactions:
CNS: Increased tremors, chorea, restlessness, blepharospasm, increased bradykinesia, grimacing, tardive dyskinesia, dystonic symptoms, involuntary movements, increased apraxia, hallucinations, dizziness, mood changes, nightmares, delusions, lethargy, apathy, overstimulation, sleep disturbances, headache, migraine, numbness, muscle cramps, confusion, anxiety, tiredness, vertigo, personality change, back/leg pain
CV: Orthostatic hypotension, hypertension, dysrhythmia, palpitations, angina pectoris, hypotension, tachycardia, edema, sinus bradycardia, syncope
GI: Nausea, vomiting, constipation, weight loss, anorexia, diarrhea, heartburn, rectal bleeding, poor appetite, dysphagia
GU: Slow urination, nocturia, prostatic hypertrophy, hesitation, retention, frequency, sexual dysfunction
INTEG: Increased sweating, alopecia, hematoma, rash, photosensitivity, facial hair
RESP: Asthma, shortness of breath
EENT: Diplopia, dry mouth, blurred vision, tinnitus

Contraindications: Hypersensitivity

Precautions: Pregnancy (C), lactation, children

Pharmacokinetics:
Rapidly absorbed, peak ½-2 hr; rapidly metabolized (active metabolites: N-desmethyldeprenyl, amphetamine, methamphetamine), metabolites excreted in urine
Interactions/incompatibilities:
• **Fatal interaction:** opioids (especially meperidine); do not administer together

NURSING CONSIDERATIONS

Assess:
• B/P, respiration

Administer:
• Drug up until NPO before surgery
• Adjust dosage, depending on patient response
• With meals; limit protein taken with drug
• At doses <10 mg/day because of risks associated with nonselective inhibition of MAO

Perform/provide:
• Assistance with ambulation, during beginning therapy

Evaluate:
• Therapeutic response: decrease in akathisia, increased mood
• Mental status: affect, mood behavioral changes, depression; perform suicide assessment

Teach patient/family:
• To change positions slowly to prevent orthostatic hypotension
• To report side effects: twitching, eye spasms; indicate overdose
• To use drug exactly as prescribed; if drug is discontinued abruptly, parkinsonian crisis may occur

Lab test interferences:
False positive: urine ketones, urine glucose
False negative: urine glucose (glucose oxidase)
False increase: uric acid, urine protein
Decrease: VMA

Treatment of overdose: IV fluids for hypotension, IV dilute pressure agent for B/P titration

selenium sulfide

(cee-leen'ee-um)
Exsel, Selsun, Selsen Blue
Func. class.: Local antiseborrheic, antifungal

Action: Appears to have cytostatic effect on epidural cells and reduces corneocyte production
Uses: Dandruff, seborrhea; dermatitis of the scalp, versicolor
Dosage and routes:
• *Adult and child:* TOP wash hair with 1-2 tsp, leave on 2-3 min; rinse, repeat, use 2 applications/wk × 2 wk, then 3-4 wk or as needed
Available forms include: Shampoo lotion 1%, 2.5%
Side effects/adverse reactions:
INTEG: Oiliness of hair/scalp, alopecia, discoloration of hair
Contraindications: Hypersensitivity to sulfur preparations, inflamed skin
Precautions: Infants, pregnancy (C)

NURSING CONSIDERATIONS

Perform/provide:
• Thorough hair rinsing after use
• Storage at room temperature in tight container

Evaluate:
• Toxicity: tremors, perspiration, pain in abdomen, weakness, anorexia
• Area of body involved, including time involved, what helps or aggravates condition

Teach patient/family:
• To avoid contact with eyes, genital area

• To discontinue use if rash or irritation occurs
• That drug may damage jewelry, remove before application
• That drug is not be taken internally

senna

(sin'na)

Black Draught, Casafru, Senexon, Senokot, X-Prep

Func. class.: Laxative
Chem. class.: Anthraquinone

Action: Stimulates peristalsis by action on Auerbach's plexus
Uses: Constipation, bowel preparation for surgery or examination
Dosage and routes:
• *Adult:* PO 1-8 tabs (Senokot)/day ½ to 4 tsp of granules added to water or juice; REC SUPP 1-2 hs; SYR 1-4 tsp hs, 7.5-15 ml; (Black Draught) ¾ oz dissolved in 2.5 oz liquid given between 2-4 PM the day before procedure (X-Prep)
• *Child >27 kg:* ½ adult dose; do not use Black Draught for children
• *Child 1 mo-1 yr:* SYR 1.25-2.5 ml (Senokot) hs
Available forms include: Supp 625 mg, 30 mg sennosides; powder 662 mg/g, 6, 15 mg sennosides/3g; tabs 8.6 sennosides, 180 mg
Side effects/adverse reactions:
GI: Nausea, vomiting, anorexia, cramps, diarrhea
META: Hypocalcemia, enteropathy, alkalosis, hypokalemia, ***tetany***
Contraindications: Hypersensitivity, GI bleeding, obstruction, CHF, lactation, abdominal pain, nausea/vomiting, appendicitis, acute surgical abdomen
Precautions: Pregnancy (C)
Pharmacokinetics:
PO: Onset 6-24 hr; metabolized by liver, excreted in feces
Interactions/incompatibilities:
• Do not use with antabuse

NURSING CONSIDERATIONS

Assess:
• Blood, urine electrolytes if drug is used often by patient
• I&O ratio to identify fluid loss
Administer:
• In morning or evening (oral dose)
Evaluate:
• Therapeutic response: decrease in constipation
• Cause of constipation; identify whether fluids, bulk, or exercise is missing from lifestyle
• Cramping, rectal bleeding, nausea, vomiting; if these symptoms occur, drug should be discontinued
Teach patient/family:
• That urine, feces may turn yellow-brown to red
• Not to use laxatives for long-term therapy; bowel tone will be lost
• That normal bowel movements do not always occur daily
• Not to use in presence of abdominal pain, nausea, vomiting
• To notify physician if constipation unrelieved or if symptoms of electrolyte imbalance occur: muscle cramps, pain, weakness, dizziness, excessive thirst

sertralline

(sir'trall-en)

Zoloft

Func. class.: Antidepressant

Action: Inhibits serotonin reuptake
Uses: Major depression
Dosage and routes:
• *Adult:* PO 50 mg qd, may increase to a maximum of 200 mg/day; do not change dose at intervals of <1 wk; administer qd in AM, PM
Available forms include: Tabs 50, 100 mg

Side effects/adverse reactions:
CNS: Insomnia, agitation, somnolence, dizziness, headache, tremor, fatigue, paresthesia, twitching, confusion
GU: Male sexual dysfunction, micturition disorder
GI: Diarrhea, nausea, constipation, anorexia, dry mouth, dyspepsia, vomiting, flatulence
CV: Palpitations, chest pain
EENT: Vision abnormalities
Contraindications: Hypersensitivity
Precautions: Pregnancy (B), lactation, elderly, hepatic, renal disease, epilepsy
Pharmacokinetics:
PO: Peak 6-10 hr, plasma protein binding 99%, elimination half-life 25 hr, extensively metabolized, metabolite excreted in urine
Interactions/incompatibilities:
- Increased effects of: alcohol, diazepam, tolbutamide, warfarin
- Fatal reactions: MAOIs
- Altered lithium levels: lithium

NURSING CONSIDERATIONS

Assess:
- Mental status: mood sensorium, affect, suicidal tendencies, increase in psychiatric symptoms, depression, panic
- B/P (lying/standing), pulse q4h; if systolic B/P drops 20 mm Hg, hold drug, notify physician; take vital signs q4h in patients with cardiovascular disease
- Weight weekly; appetite may decrease with drug

Administer:
- Increased fluids, bulk in diet if constipation, urinary retention occur
- With food or milk for GI symptoms
- Crushed if patient is unable to swallow medication whole
- Gum, hard candy, frequent sips of water for dry mouth

Perform/provide:
- Storage at room temperature; do not freeze
- Assistance with ambulation during therapy since drowsiness, dizziness occur
- Safety measures, including side rails, primarily in elderly
- Checking to see that PO medication is swallowed

Evaluate:
- Therapeutic response: significant improvement in depression
- Urinary retention, constipation, especially in elderly
- Withdrawal symptoms: headache, nausea, vomiting, muscle pain, weakness; do not usually occur unless drug is discontinued abruptly
- Alcohol consumption; if alcohol is consumed, hold dose until morning

Teach patient/family:
- That therapeutic effect may take 2-3 wk
- To use caution in driving or other activities requiring alertness because drowsiness, dizziness, blurred vision may occur
- Not to discontinue medication quickly after long-term use; may cause nausea, headache, malaise
- To avoid alcohol ingestion or other CNS depressants
- To notify physician if pregnant or plan to become pregnant or breastfeed

Lab test interferences:
Increase: Serum bilirubin, blood glucose, alk phosphatase
Decreased: VMA, 5-HIAA
False increase: Urinary catecholamines

silver nitrate

Func. class.: Keratolytic

Action: Possesses antiinfective, astringent, caustic properties
Uses: Cauterization of lesions, warts, burns (low concentrations)
Dosage and routes:
• *Adult and child:* TOP apply to area to be treated
Available forms include: Sticks, sol 10%, 25%, 50%
Side effects/adverse reactions:
INTEG: Skin discoloration
Contraindications: Hypersensitivity
Interactions/incompatibilities:
• Not to be used with alkalis, phosphates, thimerosol, benzalkonium chloride, halogenated acids
NURSING CONSIDERATIONS
Administer:
• After moistening stick with water
• To burns using a wet dressing (low concentrations 0.125%)
Evaluate:
• Therapeutic response: absence of lesions, healing of burned areas
Perform/provide:
• Storage in cool area
Teach patient/family:
• To avoid contact with clothing or unaffected areas, discoloration may occur

silver nitrate 1% (ophthalmic)

Func. class.: Antiinfective

Action: Inhibits metabolic actions in susceptible organisms
Uses: Prevention, treatment of gonorrheal ophthalmia neonatorum
Dosage and routes:
• *Neonate:* INSTILL 2 gtts of 1% solution into each eye
Available forms include: Sol
Side effects/adverse reactions:
EENT: Redness, discharge, edema, swelling
Contraindications: Hypersensitivity
Precautions: Antibiotic hypersensitivity, pregnancy (C)
NURSING CONSIDERATIONS
Administer:
• After washing hands
Perform/provide:
• Storage at room temperature, in tight, light-resistant container
Evaluate:
• Allergy: itching, lacrimation, redness, swelling

silver protein, mild

Argyrol S.S., Silvol, Solargentum
Func. class.: Disinfectant
Chem. class.: Silver colloidal compound

Action: Destroys gram-positive, gram-negative organisms
Uses: Eye, nose, throat, swelling, infection
Dosage and routes:
• *Adult and child:* TOP sol use as needed
Available forms include: Top sol 5%, 10%, 25%; eyedrops 20%
Side effects/adverse reactions:
INTEG: Irritation, discoloration of tissue
Contraindications: Hypersensitivity
Precautions: Pregnancy (C)
NURSING CONSIDERATIONS
Administer:
• To area to be treated only; do not apply to healthy skin
Perform/provide:
• Storage in tight container
Evaluate:
• Area of body involved: irritation, rash, breaks, dryness, scales

silver sulfadiazine (topical)

(sul-fa-dye'a-zeen)

Flamazine, Flint SSD, Silvadene

Func. class.: Local antiinfective
Chem. class.: Sulfonamide

Action: Interferes with bacterial cell wall synthesis, broad-spectrum
Uses: Burns (2nd, 3rd degree); prevention of wound sepsis
Dosage and routes:
• *Adult and child:* TOP apply 1/16 in to affected area qd-bid
Available forms include: Cream 10 mg/g
Side effects/adverse reactions:
INTEG: Rash, urticaria, stinging, burning, itching, pain, skin necrosis, erythema
HEMA: Reversible leukopenia
Contraindications: Hypersensitivity, child <2 mo
Precautions: Impaired renal function, pregnancy (C), impaired hepatic function, lactation

NURSING CONSIDERATIONS
Administer:
• Using aseptic technique, use sterile gloves
• Enough medication to completely cover burns, keep covered with medication at all times
• After cleansing debris before each application, bathe daily
• Analgesic before application if needed
Perform/provide:
• Storage at room temperature in dry place
Evaluate:
• Therapeutic response: relief of infection
• Allergic reaction: burning, stinging, swelling, redness
• Renal function studies, check for crystalluria
Teach patient/family:
• That drug may be continued until graft can be done

simethicone

(si-meth'-i-kone)

Gas-X, Mylicon, Ovol,* Phazyme, Silain

Func. class.: Antiflatulent

Action: Disperses, prevents gas pockets in GI system
Uses: Flatulence
Dosage and routes:
• *Adult and child >12 yr:* PO 40-100 mg pc, hs
Available forms include: Chew tabs 40, 80 mg; tabs 50, 60, 95, 125 mg; drops 40 mg/0.6 ml
Side effects/adverse reactions:
GI: Belching, rectal flatus
Contraindications: Hypersensitivity
Precautions: Pregnancy (C)

NURSING CONSIDERATIONS
Evaluate:
• Therapeutic response: absence of flatulence
Teach patient/family:
• That tablets must be chewed
• Shake suspension well before pouring

simvastatin

(sem-va-sta'-tin)

Zocor

Func. class.: Antihyperlipidemic
Chem. class.: Synthetically derived fermentation product

Action: Inhibits HMG-CoA reductase enzyme, which reduces cholesterol synthesis
Uses: As an adjunct in primary hypercholesterolemia (types IIa, IIb)

Dosage and routes:
• *Adult:* PO 5-10 mg qd in PM initially; usually range 5-40 mg/day qd in PM, not to exceed 40 mg/day; dosage adjustments may be made in 4-wk intervals or more
Available forms include: Tabs 5, 10, 20, 40 mg
Side effects/adverse reactions:
INTEG: Rash, pruritus, alopecia
GI: Nausea, constipation, diarrhea, dyspepsia, flatus, abdominal pain, heartburn, ***liver dysfunction,*** pancreatitis
EENT: Lens opacities
MS: Muscle cramps, myalgia, ***myositis, rhabdomyolysis***
CNS: Headache, tremor, vertigo, peripheral neuropathy
Contraindications: Hypersensitivity, pregnancy (X), lactation, active liver disease
Precautions: Past liver disease, alcoholics, severe acute infections, trauma, hypotension, uncontrolled seizure disorders, severe metabolic disorders, electrolyte imbalances
Pharmacokinetics: Peak 1-2 ½ hr, metabolized in liver (active metabolites), highly protein bound, excreted primarily in bile, feces
Interactions/incompatibilities:
• Increased effects of: coumadin
• Increased myalgia, myositis: cyclosporine, gemfibrozil, niacin, erthyromycin
• Increased serum level of: digoxin

NURSING CONSIDERATIONS
Assess:
• Cholesterol levels periodically during treatment
• Liver function studies q1-2mo during the first 1½ yr of treatment; AST, ALT, liver function tests may increase
• Renal studies in patients with compromised renal system: BUN, I&O ratio, creatinine
• Eyes with slit lamp before, 1 mo after treatment begins, annually; lens opacities may occur
Administer:
• Total daily dose in evening
Perform/provide:
• Storage in cool environment in tight container protected from light
Evaluate:
• Therapeutic response: decrease in cholesterol to desired level after 8 wk
Teach patient/family:
• That treatment will be ongoing for several years
• That blood work and eye exam will be necessary during treatment
• To report blurred vision, severe GI symptoms, dizziness, headache
• That previously prescribed regimen will continue: low-cholesterol diet, exercise program
Lab test interferences:
Increase: CPK, liver function tests

sodium bicarbonate

Func. class.: Alkalinizer
Chem. class.: $NaHCO_3$

Action: Orally neutralizes gastric acid, which forms water, NaCl, CO_2; increases plasma bicarbonate, which buffers H^+ ion concentration; reverses acidosis
Uses: Acidosis (metabolic), cardiac arrest, alkalinization (systemic/urinary) antacid
Dosage and routes:
Acidosis
• *Adult and child:* IV INF 2-5 mEq/kg over 4-8 hr depending on CO_2, pH
Cardiac arrest
• *Adult and child:* IV BOL 1 mEq/kg, then 0.5 mEq/kg q10 min, then doses based an ABGs
• *Infant:* IV INF not to exceed 8

* Available in Canada only

mEq/kg/day based on ABGs (4.2% sol)

Alkalinization

- *Adult:* PO 325 mg-2 g qid
- *Child:* PO 12-120 mg/kg/day

Antacid

- *Adult:* PO 300 mg-2 g chewed, taken with water

Available forms include: Tabs 325, 520, 650 mg; powd; inj 4%, 4.2%, 5%, 7.5%, 8.4%

Side effects/adverse reactions:

CNS: Irritability, headache, confusion, stimulation, tremors, *twitching, hyperreflexia, **tetany,*** weakness, ***convulsions*** caused by alkalosis

CV: Irregular pulse, ***cardiac arrest,*** water retention, edema, weight gain

GI: Flatulence, belching, distention, ***paralytic ileus,*** acid rebound

META: Alkalosis

GU: Calculi

RESP: Shallow, slow respirations, cyanosis, ***apnea***

Contraindications: Hypertension, peptic ulcer, renal disease

Precautions: CHF, cirrhosis, toxemia, renal disease, pregnancy (C)

Pharmacokinetics:

PO: Onset 2 min, duration 10 min

IV: Onset 15 min, duration 1-2 hr, excreted in urine

Interactions/incompatibilities:

- Increases effects: amphetamines, mecamylamine, quinine, quinidine, pseudoephedrine
- Decreases effects: lithium, chlorpropamide, barbiturates, salicylates
- Increased sodium and decreased potassium: corticosteroids
- Do not mix solution with other drugs

NURSING CONSIDERATIONS

Assess:

- Respiratory and pulse rate, rhythm, depth, lung sounds, notify physician of abnormalities
- Fluid balance (I&O, weight qd, edema); notify physician of fluid overload
- Electrolytes, blood pH, PO_2, HCO_3, during treatment; ABGs frequently during emergency situations
- Urine pH, urinary output, during beginning treatment
- Extravasation with IV administration (tissue sloughing, ulceration, and necrosis)
- Weight daily with initial therapy

Administer:

- IV diluted in an equal amount of compatible sol

Evaluate:

- Therapeutic response: ABGs, electrolytes, blood pH, HCO_3 WNL
- Alkalosis: irritability, confusion, twitching, hyperreflexia stimulation, slow respirations, cyanosis, irregular pulse
- Milk-alkali syndrome: confusion, headache, nausea, vomiting, anorexia, urinary stones, hypercalcemia

Teach patient/family:

- To chew antacid tablets and drink 8 oz water
- Not to take antacid with milk, or milk-alkali syndrome may result
- Not to use antacid for more than 2 weeks
- To notify physician if indigestion is accompanied by chest pain, dyspnea, diarrhea, dark, tarry stools
- About sodium-restricted diet; to avoid use of baking soda for indigestion

Lab tests interferences:

Increase: Urinary urobilinogen

False positive: Urinary protein, blood lactate

S

sodium biphosphate/ sodium phosphate

Enemeez, Fleet Enema, Phospho-Soda, Saf-tip Phosphate Enema/ Sal-Hepatica

Func. class.: Laxative, saline

Action: Increases water absorption in the small intestine by osmotic action

Uses: Constipation, bowel or rectal preparation for surgery, examination

Dosage and routes:

• *Adult:* PO 5-20 ml with water; powder 4 g dissolved in water; sol 20-46 ml mixed with 4 oz cold water; enema 2-4.5 oz

Available forms include: Powder, sol

Side effects/adverse reactions:

GI: Nausea, cramps, diarrhea

META: Electrolyte, fluid imbalances

Contraindications: Hypersensitivity, rectal fissures, abdominal pain, nausea/vomiting, appendicitis, acute surgical abdomen, ulcerated hemorrhoids, sodium-restricted diets (Sal-Hepatica, PhosphoSoda)

Precautions: Pregnancy (C)

Pharmacokinetics: Excreted in feces

NURSING CONSIDERATIONS

Assess:

• Blood, urine electrolytes if drug is used often by patient

• I&O ratio to identify fluid loss

Administer:

• Alone for better absorption; do not take within 1 hr of other drugs

Evaluate:

• Therapeutic response: decrease in constipation

• Cause of constipation; identify whether fluids, bulk, or exercise is missing from lifestyle

• Cramping, rectal bleeding, nausea, vomiting; if these symptoms occur, drug should be discontinued

Teach patient/family:

• Not to use laxatives for long-term therapy; bowel tone will be lost

• That normal bowel movements do not always occur daily

• Not to use in presence of abdominal pain, nausea, vomiting

• To notify physician if constipation unrelieved or if symptoms of electrolyte imbalance occur: muscle cramps, pain, weakness, dizziness, excessive thirst

• To maintain adequate fluid consumption

sodium chloride, hypertonic

Adsorbonac Ophthalmic Solution, Muro Ointment, Sodium Chloride Ointment

Func. class.: Miscellaneous ophthalmic agent

Chem. class.: Hyperosmolar ophthalmic

Action: Reduces corneal edema by osmosis of water through corneal epithelium, which is semipermeable

Uses: Reduces corneal edema

Dosage and routes:

• *Adult:* INSTILL 1-2 gtts q3-4h or ointment hs

Available forms include: Sol 2%, 5%; oint 5%

Side effects/adverse reactions:

EENT: Stinging

Contraindications: Hypersensitivity

NURSING CONSIDERATIONS

Perform/provide:

• Storage in tight container

Evaluate:

• Therapeutic response: decreased corneal edema

Teach patient/family:

• Method of instillation, including pressure on lacrimal sac for 1 min, and not to touch dropper to eye

• That blurred vision is common with oint

• To report double vision, rapid change in vision, appearance of floating spots, acute redness of eyes

sodium fluoride

Fluor-A-Day,* Fluoritabs, Flura-Drops, Fluotic,* Luride Lozitabs, Karidium, Pediaflor

Func. class.: Trace elements
Chem. class.: Fluorideion

Action: Needed for hard tooth enamel and for resistance to periodontal disease; reduces acid production by dental bacteria

Uses: Prevention of dental caries

Dosage and routes:

• *Adult and child >12 yr:* TOP 10 ml 0.2% sol qd after brushing teeth, rinse mouth for >1 min with sol

• *Child 6-12 yr:* TOP 5 ml 0.2% sol

• *Child >3 yr:* PO 1 mg qd

• *Child <3 yr:* PO 0.5 mg

Available forms include: Tabs chewable 0.25 mg; tabs 0.5, 1 mg, tab effervescent 10 mg; drops 0.125, 0.25, 0.5 mg/ml; rinse supplements 0.2 mg/ml, rinse 0.01%, 0.02%, 0.09%; gel 0.1%, 0.5%, 1.23%

Side effects/adverse reactions:

ACUTE OVERDOSE: ***Black tarry stools, bloody vomit, diarrhea, decreased respiration, increased salivation, watery eyes***

CHRONIC OVERDOSE: ***Hypocalcemia and tetany, respiratory arrest, sores in mouth, constipation, loss of appetite, nausea, vomiting, weight loss, discoloration of teeth*** (white, black, brown)

Contraindications: Hypersensitivity, pregnancy (D)

Precautions: Child < 6 yr

Pharmacokinetics:

PO: Excreted in urine and feces, crosses placenta, breast milk

Interactions/incompatibilities:

• Avoid use with dairy products

NURSING CONSIDERATIONS

Assess:

• Use in children

Administer:

• Drops after meals with fluids or undiluted tablets, may be chewed; do not swallow whole, may be given with water or juice, avoid milk

Evaluate:

• Therapeutic response: absence of dental caries

• Nutritional status: increase fluoride content of water, decrease carbohydrate snacks, increase fish, tea, mineral water

Teach patient/family:

• To monitor children using gel or rinse, not to be swallowed

• Not to drink, eat, or rinse mouth for at least ½ hr

• Not to use during pregnancy

• To apply after brushing and flossing hs

• To store out of children's reach

sodium lactate

Func. class.: Alkalinizer

Action: Removes lactate and hydrogen, which leads to alkalinization; lactate is converted to CO_2 and water

Uses: Acidosis (metabolic), alkalinization (urinary)

Dosage and routes:
Acidosis
• *Adult:* IV 1/6 molar (167 mEq lactate/L)
Alkalinization
• *Adult:* IV 30 ml of 1/6 molar sol/kg in divided doses
Available forms include: Inj IV
Side effects/adverse reactions:
CNS: Irritability, headache, confusion, stimulation, tremors, *twitching, hyperreflexia,* ***tetany,*** weakness, ***convulsions***
CV: Irregular pulse, ***cardiac arrest***
GI: Flatulence, belching, distention, ***paralytic ileus***
META: Alkalosis
RESP: Shallow, slow respirations, cyanosis, ***apnea***
Contraindications: Hypertension, peptic ulcer
Precautions: CHF, cirrhosis, toxemia, renal disease, pregnancy (C)
Pharmacokinetics:
PO: Onset 2 min, duration 10 min
IV: Onset immediate
Interactions/incompatibilities:
• Increased effects: amphetamines, mecamylamine, lithium, barbiturates, salicylates, quinine, quinidine, pseudoephedrine
• Decreased effect: salicylates
• Do not mix solution with other drugs

NURSING CONSIDERATIONS

Assess:
• Respiratory rate, rhythm, depth, notify physician of abnormalities
• Electrolytes, blood pH, PO_2, HCO_3, during treatment
• Urine pH, urinary output, fluid balance during beginning treatment
Administer:
• IV INF; dilute 5 mEq/ml added to IV solutions or TPN; run at 2-5 mEq/kg over 4-8 hr; check for extravasation
Evaluate:
• Therapeutic response: ABGs, blood pH, HCO_3, electrolytes WNL
• Alkalosis: irritability, confusion, twitching, hyperreflexia, stimulation, slow respirations, cyanosis, irregular pulse
Lab tests interferences:
Increase: Urinary urobilinogen
False positive: Urinary protein, blood lactate

sodium polystyrene sulfonate

(pol-ee-stye'-reen)
Kayexalate, SPS Suspension
Func. class.: Potassium-removing resin
Chem. class.: Cation exchange resin

Action: Removes potassium by exchanging sodium for potassium in body; occurs primarily in large intestine
Uses: Hyperkalemia in conjunction with other measures
Dosage and routes:
• *Adult:* PO 15 g qd-qid; rectal enema 30-50 g/100 ml of sorbitol warmer to body temperature q6h
• *Child:* 1 mEq of potassium exchanged/g of resin, approximate dose 1g/kg q6h
Available forms include: Susp, 15 g polystyrene sulfonate, 21.5 ml sorbitol, 1.5 g (65 mEq) sodium/60 ml; powder
Side effects/adverse reactions:
GI: Constipation, anorexia, nausea, vomiting, diarrhea (sorbitol), fecal impaction, gastric irritation
META: Hypocalcemia, hypokalemia, hypomagnesium, sodium retention
Precautions: Pregnancy (C), renal

failure, CHF, severe edema, severe hypertension

Interactions/incompatibilities:

• Decreased effect of sodium polystyrene: antacids, laxatives

NURSING CONSIDERATIONS

Assess:

• Bowel function daily

• Hypotension: confusion, irritability, muscular pain, weakness

Administer:

• Oral dose as susp mixed with water or syrup (20-100 ml)

• Mild laxative as ordered to prevent constipation and fecal impaction

• Sorbitol as ordered to prevent constipation

• Retention enema after mixing with warm water; introduce by gravity, continue stirring, flush with 100 ml of fluid, clamp, and leave in place

Perform/provide:

• Retention of enema for at least ½-1 hr

• Irrigation of colon after enema with 1-2 qt of nonsodium solution, drain

• Storage of freshly prepared solution for 24 hr at room temperature

Evaluate:

• Therapeutic response: Potassium level WNL

• Serum potassium, calcium, magnesium, sodium, acid-base balance

sodium thiosalicylate

Arthrolate, Asproject, Rexolate, Tusal, Thiosal

Func. class.: Nonnarcotic analgesic

Chem. class.: Salicylate

Action: Blocks pain impulses in CNS that occur in response to inhibition of prostaglandin synthesis; antipyretic action results from inhibition of hypothalamic heat-regulating center

Uses: Mild to moderate pain (rheumatic fever, acute gout)

Dosage and routes:

Pain

• *Adult:* IM 50-100 mg qd or qod

Rheumatic fever

• *Adult:* IM 100-150 mg q4-6h for 3 days, then 100 mg bid

Arthritis

• *Adult:* IM 100 mg/day

Available forms include: Inj IM 50 mg/ml

Side effects/adverse reactions:

HEMA: ***Thrombocytopenia, agranulocytosis, leukopenia, neutropenia, hemolytic anemia,*** increased pro-time

CNS: Stimulation, drowsiness, dizziness, confusion, ***convulsions,*** headache, flushing, hallucinations, coma

GI: Nausea, vomiting, GI bleeding, diarrhea, heartburn, anorexia, ***hepatitis***

INTEG: Rash, urticaria, bruising

EENT: Tinnitus, hearing loss

CV: Rapid pulse, ***pulmonary edema***

RESP: Wheezing, hyperpnea

ENDO: Hypoglycemia, hyponatremia, hypokalemia

Contraindications: Hypersensitivity to salicylates, GI bleeding, bleeding disorders, children < 3 yr, vitamin K deficiency, peptic ulcer

Precautions: Anemia, hepatic disease, renal disease, Hodgkin's disease, pregnancy (C), lactation

Pharmacokinetics:

PO: Onset 15-30 min, peak 1-2 hr, duration 4-6 hr

REC: Onset slow, duration 4-6 hr, Metabolized by liver, excreted by kidneys, crosses placenta, excreted in breast milk, half-life 1-3½ hr

Interactions/incompatibilities:
- Decreased effects of sodium thiosalicylate: antacids, steroids, urinary alkalizers
- Increased blood loss: alcohol, heparin
- Increased effects of: anticoagulants, insulin, methotrexate
- Decreased effects of: probenecid, spironolactone, sulfinpyrazone, sulfonylmides
- Toxic effects: PABA

NURSING CONSIDERATIONS

Assess:
- Liver function studies: ALT, AST, bilirubin, creatinine if patient is on long-term therapy
- Renal function studies: BUN, urine creatinine if patient is on long-term therapy
- Blood studies: CBC, Hct, Hgb, pro-time if patient is on long-term therapy
- I&O ratio; decreasing output may indicate renal failure (long-term therapy)

Evaluate:
- Therapeutic response: decreased pain
- Hepatotoxicity: dark urine, clay-colored stools, yellowing of skin, sclera, itching, abdominal pain, fever, diarrhea if patient is on long-term therapy
- Allergic reactions: rash, urticaria; if these occur, drug may need to be discontinued
- Renal dysfunction: decreased urine output
- Ototoxicity: tinnitus, ringing, roaring in ears; audiometric testing is needed before, after long-term therapy
- Visual changes: blurring, halos, corneal, retinal damage
- Edema in feet, ankles, legs
- Prior drug history; there are many drug interactions

Teach patient/family:
- To report any symptoms of hepatotoxicity, renal toxicity, visual changes, ototoxicity, allergic reactions (long-term therapy)
- Not to exceed recommended dosage; acute poisoning may result
- To read label on other OTC drugs; many contain aspirin
- That therapeutic response takes 2 wk (arthritis)
- To avoid alcohol ingestion; GI bleeding may occur

Lab test interferences:
Increase: Coagulation studies, liver function studies, serum uric acid, amylase, CO_2, urinary protein
Decrease: Serum potassium, PBI, cholesterol, blood glucose
Interfere: Urine catecholamines, pregnancy test

Treatment of overdose: Lavage, activated charcoal, monitor electrolytes, VS

---

somatotropin (human growth hormone)

(soe-ma-toe-troe'pin)

Asellacrin, Crescormon, Humatrope*

Func. class.: Pituitary hormone
Chem. class.: Growth hormone

Action: Stimulates growth

Uses: Pituitary growth hormone deficiency (hypopituitary dwarfism)

Dosage and routes:
- *Child:* IM 2 IU 3 ×/wk, less than 48 hr between doses, may give 4 IU if growth is <1 inch/6 mo

Available forms include: Inj IM, IV 2, 4, 10 IU

Side effects/adverse reactions:
GU: Hypercalciuria
INTEG: Rash, urticaria, pain, inflammation at injection site

* Available in Canada only

CNS: Headache, growth of intracranial tumor
ENDO: ***Hyperglycemia, ketosis, hypothyroidism***
SYST: ***Antibodies to growth hormone***
Contraindications: Hypersensitivity to benzyl-alcohol, closed epiphyses, intracranial lesions
Precautions: Diabetes mellitus, hypothyroidism, pregnancy (C)
Pharmacokinetics:
Half-life 15-60 min, duration 7 days; metabolized in liver
Interactions/incompatibilities:
• Decreased growth: glucocorticosteroids
• Epiphyseal closure: androgens, thyroid hormones

NURSING CONSIDERATIONS
Assess:
• Growth hormone antibodies if patient fails to respond to therapy
• Thyroid function tests: T_3, T_4, T_7, TSH to identify hypothyroidism
Administer:
• IM, rotate injection site
• After reconstituting 10 IU/5 ml bacteriostatic water for injection, do not shake
Perform/provide:
• Storage in refrigerator for <1 mo if reconstituted <1 wk; do not use discolored or cloudy solutions
Evaluate:
• Therapeutic response: growth in children
• Allergic reaction: rash, itching, fever, nausea, wheezing
• Hypercalciuria: urinary stones, groin, flank pain, nausea, vomiting, frequency, hematuria, chills
• Growth rate of child at intervals during treatment

spectinomycin hydrochloride
(spek-ti-noe-mye'sin)
Trobicin
Func. class.: Antibiotic
Chem. class.: Aminocyclitol

Action: Inhibits bacterial synthesis by binding to 30S subunit on ribosomes
Uses: Gonorrhea
Dosage and routes:
• *Adult:* IM 2-4 g as single dose
Available forms include: Inj IM 2, 4 g
Side effects/adverse reactions:
CNS: Dizziness, chills, fever, insomnia, headache, anxiety
HEMA: Anemia
GI: *Nausea,* vomiting, increased BUN
GU: Decreased urine output
INTEG: *Pain at injection site,* urticaria, rash, pruritus, fever
Contraindications: Hypersensitivity, syphilis
Precautions: Pregnancy (B), infants, children
Pharmacokinetics:
IM: Peak 1-2 hr, duration >8 hr, half-life 1-3 hr, excreted in urine (active form)

NURSING CONSIDERATIONS
Assess:
• Gonorrhea culture after treatment
• I&O ratio; report decreased output
• Liver studies: AST, ALT, serum alk phosphatase following multiple doses
• Blood studies: Hct, Hgb, BUN if multiple diagnoses given
• Serologic test for syphilis 3 mo after treatment
Administer:
• After shaking vial

• IM in deep muscle mass
• With 20-gauge needle; no more than 5 ml per site

Perform/provide:
• Storage at room temperature; reconstituted solutions should be discarded after 24 hr
• Treatment of partner, report infection

Evaluate:
• Therapeutic response: negative gonorrhea culture after treatment
• Allergies before treatment, reaction of each medication

spironolactone

(speer'on-oh-lak'tone)
Aldactone

Func. class.: Potassium-sparing diuretic
Chem. class.: Aldosterone antagonist

Action: Competes with aldosterone at receptor sites in distal tubule, resulting in excretion of sodium chloride, water, retention of potassium, phosphate

Uses: Edema, hypertension, diuretic-induced hypokalemia, primary hyperaldosteronism (diagnosis, short-term treatment, long-term treatment), nephrotic syndrome, cirrhosis of the liver with ascites

Dosage and routes:
Edema/hypertension
• *Adult:* PO 25-200 mg/qd in single or divided doses
• *Child:* PO 3.3 mg/kg/day in single or divided doses

Hypokalemia
• *Adult:* PO 25-100 mg/day; if PO, K supplements are unable to be used

Primary hyperaldosteronism diagnosis
• *Adult:* PO 400 mg/day × 4 days or 4 wk depending on test, then 100-400 mg/day maintenance

Available forms include: Tab 25, 50, 100 mg

Side effects/adverse reactions:
CNS: Headache, confusion, drowsiness, lethargy, ataxia
GI: Diarrhea, cramps, ***bleeding,*** gastritis, vomiting
INTEG: Rash, pruritus, urticaria
ENDO: Impotence, gynecomastia, irregular menses, amenorrhea, postmenopausal bleeding, hirsutism, deepening voice
HEMA: Decreased WBCs, platelets
ELECT: Hyperchloremic metabolic acidosis, ***hyperkalemia,*** hyponatremia

Contraindications: Hypersensitivity, anuria, severe renal disease, hyperkalemia, pregnancy (D)

Precautions: Dehydration, hepatic disease, lactation

Pharmacokinetics:
PO: Onset 24-48 hr, peak 48-72 hr; metabolized in liver, excreted in urine, crosses placenta

Interactions/incompatibilities:
• Increased action of: antihypertensives, digitalis, lithium
• Increased hyperkalemia: potassium sparing diuretics, potassium products, ACE inhibitors, salt substitutes
• Decreased effect of spironolactone: ASA

NURSING CONSIDERATIONS

Assess:
• Electrolytes: sodium chloride, potassium, BUN, serum creatinine, ABGs, CBC
• Weight, I&O daily to determine fluid loss; effect of drug may be decreased if used qd

Administer:
• In AM to avoid interference with sleep

• With food, if nausea occurs, absorption may be decreased slightly

Evaluate:

• Therapeutic response: improvement in edema of feet, legs, sacral area daily if medication is being used in CHF
• Improvement in CVP q8h
• Signs of metabolic acidosis: drowsiness, restlessness
• Rashes, temperature elevation qd
• Confusion, especially in elderly, take safety precautions if needed
• Hydration: skin turgor, thirst, dry mucous membranes

Teach patient/family:

• That drowsiness, ataxia, mental confusion may occur; observe caution in driving
• To notify physician of cramps, diarrhea, lethargy, thirst, headache, skin rash, menstrual abnormalities, deepening voice, breast enlargement

Lab test interferences:
Interfere: 17-OHCS, 17-KS, radioimmunoassay, digoxin assay

Treatment of overdose: Lavage if taken orally, monitor electrolytes, administer IV fluids, monitor hydration, renal, CV status

---

stanozolol

(stan-oh'zoe'lole)
Winstrol

Func. class.: Androgenic anabolic steroid
Chem. class.: Halogenated testosterone derivative

Action: Increases weight by building body tissue, increases potassium, phosphorus, chloride, and nitrogen levels, increases bone development

Uses: Prevention of hereditary angioedema, aplastic anemia to increase hemoglobin

Dosage and routes:

Aplastic anemia (possibly effective)
• *Adult:* PO 2 mg tid
• *Child 6-12 yr:* PO up to 2 mg tid
• *Child <6 yr:* PO 1 mg bid

Angioedema
• *Adult:* PO 2 mg tid, then decrease q1-3 mo, down to 2 mg qd or q2d

Available forms include: Tabs 2 mg

Side effects/adverse reactions:
INTEG: Rash, acneiform lesions, oily hair, skin, flushing, sweating, acne vulgaris, alopecia, hirsutism
CNS: Dizziness, headache, fatigue, tremors, paresthesias, flushing, sweating, anxiety, lability, insomnia
MS: Cramps, spasms
CV: Increased B/P
GU: ***Hematuria,*** amenorrhea, vaginitis, decreased libido, decreased breast size, clitoral hypertrophy, testicular atrophy
GI: Nausea, vomiting, constipation, weight gain, ***cholestatic jaundice***
EENT: Carpal tunnel syndrome, conjunctional edema, nasal congestion
ENDO: Abnormal GTT

Contraindications: Severe renal disease, severe cardiac disease, severe hepatic disease, hypersensitivity, pregnancy (X), lactation, genital bleeding (abnormal)

Precautions: Diabetes mellitus, CV disease, MI

Pharmacokinetics:
PO: Metabolized in liver, excreted in urine, crosses placenta, excreted in breast milk

Interactions/incompatibilities:
• Increased effects of: oral antidiabetics, oxyphenbutazone

- Increased PT: anticoagulants
- Edema: ACTH, adrenal steroids
- Decreased effects of: insulin

NURSING CONSIDERATIONS

Assess:
- Weight daily, notify physician if weekly weight gain is >5 lb
- B/P q4h
- I&O ratio; be alert for decreasing urinary output, increasing edema
- Growth rate in children since growth rate may be uneven (linear/bone browth) when used for extended period
- Electrolytes: K, Na, Cl, Ca; cholesterol
- Liver function studies: ALT, AST, bilirubin

Administer:
- Titrated dose, use lowest effective dose

Perform/provide:
- Diet with increased calories and protein; decrease sodium if edema occurs
- Supportive drug of anemia

Evaluate:
- Therapeutic response: occurs in 4-6 wk in osteoporosis
- Edema, hypertension, cardiac symptoms, jaundice
- Mental status: affect, mood, behavioral changes, aggression
- Signs of masculinization in female: increased libido, deepening of voice, breast tissue, enlarged clitoris, menstrual irregularities; male: gynecomastia, impotence, testicular atrophy
- Hypercalcemia: lethargy, polyuria, polydipsia, nausea, vomiting, constipation; drug may need to be decreased
- Hypoglycemia in diabetics, since oral anticoagulant action is decreased

Teach patient/family:
- Drug needs to be combined with complete health plan: diet, rest, exercise
- To notify physician if therapeutic response decreases
- Not to discontinue this medication abruptly
- About change in sex characteristics
- Women to report menstrual irregularities
- That 1-3 mo course is necessary for response in breast cancer
- Procedure for use of buccal tablets (requires 30-60 min to dissolve, change absorption site with each dose; do not eat, drink, chew, or smoke while tablet is in place)

Lab test interferences:

Increase: Serum cholesterol, blood glucose, urine glucose

Decrease: Serum calcium, serum potassium, T_4, T_3, thyroid ^{131}I uptake test, urine 17-OHCS

---

streptokinase

(strep-toe-kye'nase)

Kabikinase, Streptase

Func. class.: Thrombolytic enzyme

Chem. class.: β-Hemolytic streptococcus filtrate (purified)

Action: Activates conversion of plasminogen to plasmin (fibrinolysin): plasmin is able to break down clots (fibrin), fibrinogen, factors V, VII, occlusion of venous access lines

Uses: Deep vein thrombosis, pulmonary embolism, arterial thrombosis, arterial embolism, arteriovenous cannula occlusion, lysis of coronary artery thrombi after MI, acute evolving transmural MI

Dosage and routes:

Lysis of coronary artery thrombi

• *Adult:* CC 20,000 IU, then 2000 IU/min over 1 hr as IV INF

Arteriovenous cannula occlusion

• *Adult:* IV INF 250,000 IU/2 ml sol into occluded limb of cannula run over 1/2 hr, clamp for 2 hr, aspirate contents, flush with NaCl sol and reconnect

Thrombosis/embolism

• *Adult:* IV INF 250,000 IU over 1/2 hr, then 100,000 IU/hr for 72 hr for deep thrombosis, 100,000 IU/hr over 24-72 hr for pulmonary embolism

Acute evolving transmural MI:

• *Adult:* IV INF 1,500,000 IU diluted to a volume of 45 ml; give within 1 hr

Available forms include: Inj IV 250,000, 600,000, 750,000 IU

Side effects/adverse reactions:

HEMA: Decreased Hct, ***bleeding***

INTEG: Rash, urticaria, phlebitis at IV inf site, itching, flushing

CNS: Headache, fever

GI: Nausea

RESP: Altered respirations, SOB, ***bronchospasm***

MS: Low back pain

CV: Hypertension, dysrhythmias

EENT: Periorbital edema

SYST: ***GI, GU, intracranial retroperitoneal bleeding,*** surface bleeding, ***anaphylaxis***

Contraindications: Hypersensitivity, active bleeding, intraspinal surgery, neoplasms of the CNS, ulcerative colitis/enteritis, severe hypertension, renal disease, hepatic disease, hypocoagulation, COPD, subacute bacterial endocarditis, rheumatic valvular disease, cerebral embolism/thrombosis/hemorrhage, intraarterial diagnostic procedure or surgery (10 days), recent major surgery

Precautions: Arterial emboli from left side of heart, pregnancy (C)

Pharmacokinetics:

IV: Excreted in bile, urine, half-life <20 min

Interactions/incompatibilities:

• Bleeding potential: aspirin, indomethacin, phenylbutazone, anticoagulants

NURSING CONSIDERATIONS

Assess:

• VS, B/P, pulse, resp, neuro signs, temp at least q4h, temp >104° F are indicators of internal bleeding, cardiac rhythm following intracoronary administration; systolic pressure increase of >25 mm Hg, should be reported to physician

• For neurologic changes that may indicate intracranial bleeding

• Retroperitoneal bleeding: back pain, leg weakness, diminished pulses

Administer:

• As soon as thrombi identified; not useful for thrombi over 1 wk old

• Cryoprecipatate or fresh, frozen plasma if bleeding occurs

• Loading dose at beginning of therapy may require increase loading doses

• Heparin after fibrinogen level is over 100 mg/dl. Heparin infusion to increase PTT to 1.5-2 × baseline for 3-7 days

• After reconstituting with 5 ml of NS or D_5W; do not shake; further dilute to total volume of 45 ml; may be diluted to 500 ml in 45 ml increments; may dilute vial in 15 ml NS, further dilute 750,000 IU/50 ml NS or D_5W; further dilute 1,500,000 IU dose/100 ml or more

• About 10% patients have high streptococcal antibody titers requiring increased loading doses

• IV therapy using 0.8 μm filter

Perform/provide:

• Storage of reconstituted in refrigerator; discard after 24 hr

• Bed rest during entire course of treatment
• Avoidance of venous or arterial puncture, inj, rectal temp
• Treatment of fever with acetaminophen or aspirin
• Pressure for 30 sec to minor bleeding sites; inform physician if this does not attain hemostasis; apply pressure dressing

Evaluate:
• Therapeutic response: resolution of thrombosis, embolism
• Allergy: fever, rash, itching, chills; mild reaction may be treated with antihistamines
• For bleeding during 1st hr of treatment: hematuria, hematemesis, bleeding from mucous membranes, epistaxis, ecchymosis
• Blood studies (Hct, platelets, PTT, PT, TT, APTT) before starting therapy; PT or APTT must be less than × 2 control before starting therapy TT ot PT q3-4h during treatment

Lab test interferences:
Increase: PT, APTT, TT

---

streptomycin sulfate

(strep-toe-mye'sin)

Func. class.: Antibiotic
Chem. class.: Aminoglycoside

Action: Interferes with protein synthesis in bacterial cell by binding to ribosomal subunit, causing inaccurate peptide sequence to form in protein chain, causing bacterial death

Uses: Sensitive strains of *M. tuberculosis,* nontuberculous infections caused by sensitive strains of *Y. pestus, Brucella, H. influenzae, K. pneumoniae, E. coli, E. aerogenes, S. viridans, F. tularensis, Proteus*

Dosage and routes:
Tuberculosis
• *Adult:* IM 1g qd × 2-3 mo, then 1 g 2-3 × /week given with other antitubercular drugs
• *Child:* IM 20-40 mg/kg/day in divided doses given with other antitubercular drugs

Streptococcal endocarditis
• *Adult:* IM 1 g q12h × 1 wk with penicillin, then 500 mg bid for 1 wk

Enterococcal endocarditis
• *Adult:* IM 1 g q12h × 2 wk, then 500 mg q12h × 4 wk with penicillin

Available forms include: Inj IM 1, 5 g: 400 mg/ml

Side effects/adverse reactions:
GU: ***Oliguria, hematuria, renal damage, azotemia, renal failure, nephrotoxicity***
CNS: Confusion, depression, numbness, tremors, ***convulsions,*** muscle twitching, ***neurotoxicity***
EENT: ***Ototoxicity,*** deafness, visual disturbances
HEMA: ***Agranulocytosis, thrombocytopenia, leukopenia, eosinophilia, anemia***
GI: Nausea, vomiting, anorexia, increased ALT, AST, bilirubin, hepatomegaly, ***hepatic necrosis,*** splenomegaly
CV: Hypotension, myocarditis, palpitations
INTEG: Rash, burning urticaria, dermatitis, alopecia

Contraindications: Severe renal disease, hypersensitivity

Precautions: Neonates, mild renal disease, pregnancy (B), myasthenia gravis, lactation, hearing deficits, elderly, Parkinson's disease

Pharmacokinetics:
IM: Onset rapid, peak 1-2 hr; plasma half-life 2-2½ hr, not me-

tabolized, excreted unchanged in urine, crosses placental barrier

Interactions/incompatibilities:

• Increased ototoxicity, neurotoxicity, nephrotoxicity: other aminoglycosides, amphotericin B, polymyxin, vancomycin, ethacrynic acid, furosemide, mannitol, methoxyflurane, cisplatin, cephalosporins, bacitracin

• Do not mix in solution or syringe: carbenicillin, ticarcillin, amphotericin B, cephalothin, erythromycin, heparin

• Increased effects: nondepolarizing muscle relaxants, succinylcholine

NURSING CONSIDERATIONS

Assess:

• Weight before treatment; calculation of dosage is usually done based on ideal body weight, but may be calculated on actual body weight

• I&O ratio, urinalysis daily for proteinuria, cells, casts; report sudden change in urine output

• Serum peak 60 min after IM injection, trough level drawn just before next dose; blood level should be 2-4 times bacteriostatic level

• Urine pH if drug is used for UTI; urine should be kept alkaline

Administer:

• IM injection in large muscle mass, rotate injection sites

• Drug in evenly spaced doses to maintain blood level

Perform/provide:

• Adequate fluids of 2-3 L/day unless contraindicated to prevent irritation of tubules

• Supervised ambulation, other safety measures with vestibular dysfunction

Evaluate:

• Therapeutic effect: absence of fever, draining wounds, negative C&S after treatment

• Renal impairment by securing urine for CrCl testing, BUN, serum creatinine; lower dosage should be given in renal impairment (CrCl <80 ml/min)

• Deafness by audiometric testing, ringing, roaring in ears, vertigo; assess hearing before, during, after treatment

• Dehydration: high sp gr, decrease in skin turgor, dry mucous membranes, dark urine

• Overgrowth of infection: increased temperature, malaise, redness, pain, swelling, perineal itching, diarrhea, stomatitis, change in cough, sputum

• C&S before starting treatment to identify infecting organism

• Vestibular dysfunction: nausea, vomiting, dizziness, headache; drug should be discontinued if severe

• Injection sites for redness, swelling, abscesses; use warm compresses at site

Teach patient/family:

• To report headache, dizziness, symptoms of overgrowth of infection, renal impairment

• To report loss of hearing, ringing, roaring in ears, fullness in head

Treatment of overdose: Hemodialysis, monitor serum levels of drug

S

---

streptozocin

(strep-toe-zoe'sin)

Zanosar

Func. class.: Antineoplastic alkylating agent

Chem. class.: Nitrosourea

Action: Alkylates DNA, RNA; inhibits enzymes that allow synthesis of amino acids in proteins; is also responsible for cross-linking DNA strands

Uses: Metastatic islet cell carcinoma of pancreas

Dosage and routes:

- *Adult:* IV 500 mg/m^2 × 5 days q6wk until desired response, alternate with 1000 mg/m^2 qwk × 2 wk, not to exceed 1500 mg/m^2 in 1 dose

Available forms include: Inj IV 1 g

Side effects/adverse reactions:

HEMA: ***Thrombocytopenia, leukopenia, pancytopenia***

CNS: Confusion, depression, lethargy

GI: Nausea, vomiting, diarrhea, weight loss, ***hepatotoxicity***

GU: ***Azotemia, anuria,*** hypophosphatemia, glycosuria, renal tubular acidosis, ***renal toxicity***

Contraindications: Hypersensitivity

Precautions: Radiation therapy, children, lactation, pregnancy (C), hepatic disease, renal disease

Pharmacokinetics:

IV: Metabolized by liver, excreted in urine, half-life 5 min, terminal 35-40 min

Interactions/incompatibilities:

- Increased toxicity: neurotoxic agents, other antineoplastics
- Increased action of: doxorubicin
- Decreased effect of streptozocin: phenytoin

NURSING CONSIDERATIONS

Assess:

- CBC, differential, platelet count weekly; withhold drug if WBC is <4000 or platelet count is <75,000; notify physician of results
- Renal function studies: BUN, serum uric acid, phosphate urine CrCl before, during therapy
- I&O ratio; report fall in urine output of 30 ml/hr
- Monitor temperature q4h (may indicate beginning infection)
- Liver function tests before, during therapy (bilirubin, AST, ALT, LDH) as needed or monthly

Administer:

- Antiemetic 30-60 min before giving drug to prevent vomiting
- Antibiotics for prophylaxis of infection
- IV after diluting 1 g/9.5 ml 0.9% NaCl or D_5; may be further diluted in 50-250 mg; may be given directly over 5-15 min
- Using 21-, 23-, 25-gauge needle
- Topical or systemic analgesics for pain
- Local or systemic drugs for infection

Perform/provide:

- Storage protected from light; refrigerate reconstituted solution, stable for 48 hr at room temperature
- Strict medical asepsis, protective isolation if WBC levels are low
- Special skin care
- Warm compresses at injection site for inflammation
- Adequate hydration that may reduce renal toxicity

Evaluate:

- Therapeutic response: decreased tumor size, spread of malignancy
- Bleeding: hematuria, guaiac, bruising or petechiae, mucosa or orifices q8h
- Food preferences; list likes, dislikes
- Inflammation of mucosa, breaks in skin
- Yellowing of skin, sclera, dark urine, clay-colored stools, itchy skin, abdominal pain, fever, diarrhea
- Local irritation, pain, burning, discoloration at injection site

• Symptoms indicating severe allergic reaction: rash, urticaria, itching, flushing

Teach patient/family:

• Of protective isolation precautions
• To report signs of infection: increased temperature, sore throat, flu symptoms
• To report signs of anemia: fatigue, headache, faintness, shortness of breath, irritability
• To avoid use of razors or commercial mouthwash
• To avoid use of aspirin products or ibuprofen

---

succimer

(suk-si'mer)

Chemet

Func. class.: Heavy metal antagonist

Chem. class.: Chelating agent

Action: Binds with ions of lead, to form a water-soluble complex excreted by kidneys

Uses: Lead poisoning in children with lead levels above 45 μg/dl; may be beneficial in mercury, arsenic poisoning

Dosage and routes:

• *Child:* PO 10 mg/kg or 350 mg/m² q8h × 5 days, then 10 mg/kg or 350 mg/m² q12h × 2 wk; another course may be required depending on lead levels; 2 wk should be between courses

Available forms include: Caps 100 mg

Side effects/adverse reactions:

SYST: Back, stomach, head, rib flank pain, abdominal cramps, chills, fever, flulike symptoms, head cold, headache

HEMA: ***Increased platelets, intermittent eosinophilia***

GU: ***Proteinuria,*** decreased urination, voiding difficulties

INTEG: Rash, urticaria, pruritus

META: Increased AST, ALT, alk phosphatase, cholesterol

GI: Nausea, vomiting, diarrhea, metallic taste, anorexia

CNS: Drowsiness, dizziness, paresthesia, sensorimotor neuropathy

EENT: Otitis media, watery eyes, film in eyes, plugged ears

RESP: Sore throat, rhinorrhea, nasal congestion, cough

Contraindications: Hypersensitivity

Precautions: Pregnancy (C), lactation, children <1 yr

Pharmacokinetics:

PO: Peak 1-2 hr, 49% excreted as 39% in feces, 9% urine, 1% as CO_2 from the lungs

Interactions/incompatibilities:

• Not recommended to be used concurrently with other chelating agents

NURSING CONSIDERATIONS

Assess:

• Hepatic, renal studies: ALT, AST, alk phosphatase, BUN, creatinine, serum lead level
• I&O
• For lead sources in home, school environment

Administer:

• To children who cannot swallow capsule by separating the capsule and sprinkling content on food or in a spoon followed by a drink

Perform/provide:

• Adequate fluids, check hydration status daily

Evaluate:

• Therapeutic response: decrease in serum lead level
• Allergic reactions: rash, pruritus, urticaria; drugs should be discontinued if antihistamines fail to help

S

Teach patient/family:
- That therapeutic effect may take 1-3 mo
- To report urticaria, rash

succinylcholine chloride

(suk-sin-ill-koe'leen)

Anectine, Anectine Flo-Pack Powder, Quelicin, Brevidil 'm'* (bromide salt), Scaline*, Sucostrin*, Sux-Cert*

Func. class.: Neuromuscular blocker (depolarizing-ultra short)

Action: Inhibits transmission of nerve impulses by binding with cholinergic receptor sites, antagonizing action of acetylcholine

Uses: Facilitation of endotracheal intubation, skeletal muscle relaxation during orthopedic manipulations

Dosage and routes:
- *Adult:* IV 25-75 mg, then 2.5 mg/min as needed; IM 2.5 mg/kg, not to exceed 150 mg
- *Child:* IV/IM 1-2 mg/kg, not to exceed 150 mg IM

Available forms include: Inj IM, IV 20, 50, 100 mg/ml; powder for inj 100, 500 mg/vial, 1 g/vial

Side effects/adverse reactions:

CV: Bradycardia, tachycardia, increased, decreased B/P, ***sinus arrest, dysrhythmias***

RESP: ***Prolonged apnea, bronchospasm, cyanosis, respiratory depression***

EENT: Increased secretions, increased intraocular pressure

MS: Weakness, muscle pain, fasciculations, prolonged relaxation

HEMA: ***Myoglobulinemia***

INTEG: Rash, flushing, pruritus, urticaria

Contraindications: Hypersensitivity, malignant hyperthermia, decreased plasma pseudocholinesterase

Precautions: Pregnancy (C), cardiac disease, severe burns, fractures—fasciculations may increase damage, lactation, children <2 yr, electrolyte imbalances, dehydration, neuromuscular disease, respiratory disease, collagen diseases, glaucoma, eye surgery, penetrating eye wounds, elderly or debilitated patients

Pharmacokinetics:

IV: Onset 1 min, peak 2-3 min, duration 6-10 min

IM: Onset 2-3 min

Hydrolyzed in urine (active/inactive metabolites)

Interactions/incompatibilities:
- Increased neuromuscular blockade: aminoglycosides, clindamycin, lincomycin, quinidine, local anesthetics, polymyxin antibiotics, lithium, narcotic analgesics, thiazides, enflurane, isoflurane
- Dysrhythmias: theophylline
- Do not mix with barbiturates in solution or syringe

NURSING CONSIDERATIONS

Assess:
- For electrolyte imbalances (K, Mg); may lead to increased action of this drug
- Vital signs (B/P, pulse, respirations, airway) until fully recovered; rate, depth, pattern of respirations, strength of hand grip
- I&O ratio; check for urinary retention, frequency, hesitancy

Administer:
- Using nerve stimulator by anesthesiologist to determine neuromuscular blockade
- Anticholinesterase to reverse neuromuscular blockade
- IV INF; dilute 1-2 mg/ml in compatible sol, give 0.5-10 mg/min,

* Available in Canada only

titrate to patient response; may be given directly over 1 min
- Deep IM, preferably high in deltoid muscle

Perform/provide:
- Storage in refrigerator, powder at room temp, close tightly
- Reassurance if communication is difficult during recovery from neuromuscular blockade, postoperative stiffness is normal, soon subsides

Evaluate:
- Therapeutic response: paralysis of jaw, eyelid, head, neck, rest of body
- Recovery: decreased paralysis of face, diaphragm, leg, arm, rest of body
- Allergic reactions: rash, fever, respiratory distress, pruritus; drug should be discontinued

Treatment of overdose: Edrophonium or neostigmine, atropine, monitor VS; may require mechanical ventilation

sucralfate

(soo-kral'fate)

Carafate, Sulcrate*

Func. class.: Protectant

Chem. class.: Aluminum hydroxide/sulfated sucrose

Action: Forms a complex that adheres to ulcer site, adsorbs pepsin

Uses: Duodenal ulcer

Dosage and routes:
- *Adult:* PO 1 g qid 1 hr ac, hs

Available forms include: Tabs 1 g

Side effects/adverse reactions:

CNS: Drowsiness, dizziness

GI: Dry mouth, constipation, nausea, gastric pain, vomiting

INTEG: Urticaria, rash, pruritus

Contraindications: Hypersensitivity

Precautions: Pregnancy (B), lactation, children

Pharmacokinetics:

PO: Duration up to 5 hr

Interactions/incompatibilities:
- Decreased action of: tetracyclines, phenytoin, fat-soluble vitamins

NURSING CONSIDERATIONS

Assess:
- Gastric pH (>5 should be maintained)

Perform/provide:
- Storage at room temperature

Evaluate:
- Therapeutic response: absence of pain, or GI complaints

Teach patient/family:
- To avoid black pepper, caffeine, alcohol, harsh spices, extremes in temperature of food
- To take on empty stomach
- To take full course of therapy
- To avoid antacids within ½ hr of drug

sufentanil citrate

(soo-fen'ta-nil)

Sufenta

Func. class.: Narcotic analgesics

Chem. class.: Opiate, synthetic

Controlled Substance Schedule II

Action: Inhibits ascending pain pathways in CNS, increases pain threshold, alters pain perception

Uses: Primary anesthetic, adjunct to general anesthetic

Dosage and routes:

Primary anesthetic
- *Adult:* IV 8-30 μg/kg given with 100% O_2, a muscle relaxant

Adjunct
- *Adult:* IV 1-8 μg/kg given with nitrous oxide/O_2

Available forms include: Inj IV 50 μg/ml

S

Side effects/adverse reactions:
CNS: Drowsiness, dizziness, confusion, headache, sedation, euphoria
GI: Nausea, vomiting, anorexia, constipation, cramps
GU: Increased urinary output, dysuria, urinary retention
INTEG: Rash, urticaria, bruising, flushing, diaphoresis, pruritus
EENT: Tinnitus, blurred vision, miosis, diplopia
CV: Palpitations, bradycardia, change in B/P
RESP: ***Respiratory depression***
Contraindications: Hypersensitivity, addiction (narcotic)
Precautions: Addictive personality, pregnancy (C), lactation, increased intracranial pressure, MI (acute), severe heart disease, respiratory depression, hepatic disease, renal disease, child <18 yr
Pharmacokinetics:
Half-life 1-2 hr
Interactions/incompatibilities:
- Increased effects with other CNS depressants: alcohol, narcotics, sedative/hypnotics, antipsychotics, skeletal muscle relaxants

NURSING CONSIDERATIONS
Assess:
- I&O ratio; check for decreasing output (may indicate urinary retention)

Administer:
- IV undiluted over 1-2 min or give as INF
- With antiemetic if nausea, vomiting occur

Perform/provide:
- Storage in light-resistant area at room temperature
- Safety measures: siderails, night light, call bell within easy reach

Evaluate:
- Therapeutic response: maintenance of anesthesia
- CNS changes: dizziness, drowsiness, hallucinations, euphoria, LOC, pupil reaction
- Allergic reactions: rash, urticaria
- Respiratory dysfunction: respiratory depression, character, rate, rhythm; notify physician if respirations are <10/min
- Need for pain medication, physical dependence

Teach patient/family:
- To report any symptoms of CNS changes, allergic reactions

Lab test interferences:
Increase: Amylase
Treatment of overdose: Narcan 0.2-0.8 IV, O_2, IV fluids, vasopressors

sulfacetamide sodium (ophthalmic)

(sul-fa-see'ta-mide)
Bleph-10, Cetamide, Isopto Cetamide, Sodium Sulamyd, Sulf-O
Func. class.: Antibacterial

Action: Inhibits folic acid synthesis by preventing PABA use, which is necessary for bacterial growth
Uses: Conjunctivitis, superficial eye infections, corneal ulcers
Dosage and routes:
- *Adult and child:* INSTILL 1-2 gtts q2-3h; TOP apply ½-1 inch oint into conjunctival sac qid-tid and at bedtime

Available forms include: Sterile ophth sol 10%, 15%, 30%; sterile ophth oint 10%
Side effects/adverse reactions:
EENT: Burning, stinging, swelling
Contraindications: Hypersensitivity
Precautions: Antibiotic hypersensitivity, pregnancy (C)

NURSING CONSIDERATIONS
Administer:
- After washing hands, cleanse

crusts or discharge from eye before application

Perform/provide:

• Storage at room temperature

Evaluate:

• Therapeutic response: absence of redness, inflammation, tearing

• Allergy: itching, lacrimation, redness, swelling

Teach patient/family:

• To use drug exactly as prescribed

• Not to use eye makeup, towels, washcloths, eye medication of others; reinfection may occur

• That drug container tip should not be touched to eye

• To report itching, increased redness, burning, stinging; drug should be discontinued

• That drug may cause blurred vision when ointment is applied

---

sulfadiazine

(sul-fa-dye'a-zeen)

Microsulfon

Func. class.: Antibiotic

Chem. class.: Sulfonamide, intermediate acting

Action: Interferes with bacterial biosynthesis of proteins by competitive antagonism of PABA

Uses: Urinary tract infections, rheumatic fever prophylaxis, adjunctive in toxoplasmosis

Dosage and routes:

Urinary tract infections

• *Adult:* PO 2-4 g, then 1-2 g q6h × 10 days

• *Child:* PO 75 mg/kg or 2 g/m^2, then 150 mg/kg/day or 4 g/m^2 in 4-6 divided doses, max. 6 g/day

Rheumatic fever prophylaxis

• *Child >30 kg:* PO 1 g qd

• *Child <30 kg:* PO 500 mg qd

Available forms include: Tabs 500 mg

Side effects/adverse reactions:

SYST: ***Anaphylaxis***

GI: Nausea, vomiting, abdominal pain, stomatitis, ***hepatitis,*** glossitis, pancreatitis, diarrhea, ***enterocolitis,*** anorexia

CNS: Headache, insomnia, hallucinations, depression, vertigo, fatigue, anxiety, ***convulsions,*** drug fever, chills, drowsiness

HEMA: ***Leukopenia, thrombocytopenia, agranulocytosis, hemolytic anemia, aplastic anemia***

INTEG: Rash, dermatitis, urticaria, ***Stevens-Johnson syndrome,*** erythema, photosensitivity, alopecia

GU: ***Renal failure, toxic nephrosis,*** increased BUN, creatinine, crystalluria, hematuria, proteinuria

CV: ***Allergic myocarditis***

Contraindications: Hypersensitivity to sulfonamides, sulfonylureas, thiazide, loop diurectics, salicylates, pregnancy at term

Precautions: Pregnancy (C), lactation, impaired hepatic function, severe allergy, bronchial asthma, renal dysfunction

Pharmacokinetics:

PO: Rapidly absorbed, onset ½ hr, peak 3-6 hr, 30%-50% bound to plasma proteins, half-life 8-10 hr, excreted in urine, breast milk, crosses placenta, metabolized in liver

Interactions/incompatibilities:

• Decreased effectiveness: oral contraceptives

• Increased hypoglycemic response: sulfonylurea agents

• Increased anticoagulant effects: oral anticoagulants

• Decreased renal excretion of: methotrexate

• Decreased hepatic clearance of: phenytoin

NURSING CONSIDERATIONS

Assess:

• I&O ratio; note color, character,

pH of urine if drug administered for urinary tract infections; output should be 800 ml less than intake; if urine is highly acidic, alkalization may be needed
• Kidney function studies: BUN, creatinine, urinalysis if on long-term therapy
Administer:
• With full glass of water to maintain adequate hydration; increase fluids to 2000 ml/day to decrease crystallization in kidneys
• Medication after C&S; repeat C&S after full course of medication completed
• With resuscitative equipment available; severe allergic reactions may occur
Perform/provide:
• Storage in tight, light-resistant containers at room temperature
Evaluate:
• Therapeutic response: absence of pain, fever, C&S negative
• Blood dyscrasias: skin rash, fever, sore throat, bruising, bleeding, fatigue, joint pain
• Allergic reaction: rash, dermatitis, urticaria, pruritus, dyspnea, bronchospasm
Teach patient/family:
• To take each oral dose with full glass of water to prevent crystalluria
• To complete full course of treatment to prevent superimposed infection
• To avoid sunlight or use sunscreen to prevent burns
• To avoid OTC medication (aspirin, vitamin C) unless directed by physician
• To use alternative contraceptive measures; decreased effectiveness of oral contraceptives may result
• To notify physician if skin rash, sore throat, fever, mouth scores, unusual bruising, bleeding occur
Lab test interferences:
False positive: Urinary glucose test (Benedict's method)

sulfamethizole

(sul-fa-meth'i-zole)
Bursul, Microsul, Proklar, Sulfasol, Sulfurine, Thiosulfil, Utrasul
Func. class.: Antibiotic
Chem. class.: Sulfonamide, short acting

Action: Interferes with bacterial biosynthesis of proteins by competitive antagonism of PABA
Uses: Urinary tract infections
Dosage and routes:
• *Adult:* PO 0.5-1 g tid-qid
• Child >2 mo: PO 30-45 mg/kg/day in divided doses q6h
Available forms include: Tabs 250, 500 mg
Side effects/adverse reactions:
SYST: ***Anaphylaxis***
GI: Nausea, vomiting, abdominal pain, stomatitis, ***hepatitis,*** glossitis, pancreatitis, diarrhea, ***enterocolitis***
CNS: Headache, confusion, insomnia, hallucinations, depression, vertigo, fatigue, anxiety, ***convulsions,*** drug fever, chills
HEMA: ***Leukopenia, neutropenia, thrombocytopenia, agranulocytosis, hemolytic anemia***
INTEG: Rash, dermatitis, urticaria, ***Stevens-Johnson syndrome,*** erythema, photosensitivity
GU: ***Renal failure, toxic nephrosis,*** increased BUN, creatinine, crystalluria
CV: ***Allergic myocarditis***
Contraindications: Hypersensitivity to sulfonamides, pregnancy at term
Precautions: Pregnancy (C), lac-

tation, impaired hepatic function, severe allergy, bronchial asthma

Pharmacokinetics:

PO: Rapidly absorbed, peak 2 hr, 90% bound to plasma proteins, excreted in urine, breast milk, crosses placenta

Interactions/incompatibilities:

- Decreased absorption of: digoxin
- Decreased effectiveness: oral contraceptives
- Increased hypoglycemic response: sulfonylurea agents
- Increased anticoagulant effects: oral anticoagulants
- Decreased renal excretion of: methotrexate
- Decreased hepatic clearance of: phenytoin

NURSING CONSIDERATIONS

Assess:

- I&O ratio; note color, character, pH of urine if drug administered for urinary tract infections; output should be 800 ml less than intake; if urine is highly acidic, alkalization may be needed
- Kidney function studies: BUN, creatinine, urinalysis if on long-term therapy

Administer:

- With full glass of water to maintain adequate hydration; increase fluids to 2000 ml/day to decrease crystallization in kidneys
- Medication after C&S; repeat C&S after full course of medication completed
- With resuscitative equipment available; severe allergic reactions may occur

Perform/provide:

- Storage in tight, light-resistant containers at room temperature

Evaluate:

- Therapeutic response: absence of pain, fever, C&S negative
- Blood dyscrasias: skin rash, fever, sore throat, bruising, bleeding, fatigue, joint pain
- Allergic reaction: rash, dermatitis, urticaria, pruritus, dyspnea, bronchospasm

Teach patient/family:

- To take each oral dose with full glass of water to prevent crystalluria
- To complete full course of treatment to prevent superimposed infection
- To avoid sunlight or use sunscreen to prevent burns
- To avoid OTC medication (aspirin, vitamin C) unless directed by physician
- To use alternative contraceptive measures; decreased effectiveness of oral contraceptives may result
- To notify physician if skin rash, sore throat, fever, mouth sores, unusual bruising, bleeding occur

Lab test interferences:

False positive: Urinary glucose test (Benedict's method)

---

sulfamethoxazole

(sul-fa-meth-ox'a-zole)

Gamazole, Gantanol, Urobak

Func. class.: Antibiotic

Chem. class.: Sulfonamide, intermediate acting

Action: Interferes with bacterial biosynthesis of proteins by competitive antagonism of PABA

Uses: Urinary tract infections, lymphogranuloma venereum, systemic infections

Dosage and routes:

- *Adult:* PO 2 g, then 1 g bid or tid for 7-10 days
- Child >2 mo: PO 50-60 mg/kg then 25-30 mg/kg bid, not to exceed 75 mg/kg/day

S

Lymphogranuloma venereum
• Adult: PO 1 g bid × 14 days
Available forms include: Tabs 500 mg; oral susp 500 mg/5ml
Side effects/adverse reactions:
SYST: ***Anaphylaxis***
GI: Nausea, vomiting, abdominal pain, stomatitis, ***hepatitis,*** glossitis, pancreatitis, diarrhea, ***enterocolitis,*** anorexia
CNS: Headache, insomnia, hallucinations, depression, vertigo, fatigue, anxiety, convulsions, drug fever, chills, drowsiness
HEMA: ***Leukopenia, thrombocytopenia, agranulocytosis, hemolytic anemia, aplastic anemia***
INTEG: Rash, dermatitis, urticaria, ***Stevens-Johnson syndrome,*** erythema, photosensitivity, alopecia
GU: ***Renal failure, toxic nephrosis,*** increased BUN, creatinine, crystalluria, hematuria, proteinuria
CV: ***Allergic myocarditis***
Contraindications: Hypersensitivity to sulfonamides, sulfonylureas, thiazide, loop diuretics, salicylates, pregnancy at term
Precautions: Pregnancy (C), lactation, impaired hepatic function, severe allergy, bronchial asthma
Pharmacokinetics:
PO: Poorly absorbed, peak 3-4 hr, 50%-70% bound to plasma proteins, half-life 7-12 hr, excreted in urine (unchanged 90%), breast milk, crosses placenta
Interactions/incompatibilities:
• Decreased effectiveness: oral contraceptives
• Increased hypoglycemic response: sulfonylurea agents
• Increased anticoagulant effects: oral anticoagulants
• Decreased renal excretion of: methotrexate
• Decreased hepatic clearance of: phenytoin

NURSING CONSIDERATIONS
Assess:
• I&O ratio; note color, character, pH of urine if drug administered for urinary tract infections; output should be 800 ml less than intake; if urine is highly acidic, alkalization may be needed
• Kidney function studies: BUN, creatinine, urinalysis if on long-term therapy
Administer:
• With full glass of water to maintain adequate hydration; increase fluids to 2000 ml/day to decrease crystallization in kidneys
• Medication after C&S; repeat C&S after full course of medication completed
• With resuscitative equipment available; severe allergic reactions may occur
Perform/provide:
• Storage in tight, light-resistant containers at room temperature
Evaluate:
• Therapeutic response: absence of pain, fever, C&S negative
• Blood dyscrasias: skin rash, fever, sore throat, bruising, bleeding, fatigue, joint pain
• Allergic reaction: rash, dermatitis, urticaria, pruritus, dyspnea, bronchospasm
Teach patient/family:
• To take each oral dose with full glass of water to prevent crystalluria
• To complete full course of treatment to prevent superimposed infection
• To avoid sunlight or use sunscreen to prevent burns
• To avoid OTC medication (aspirin, vitamin C) unless directed by physician
• To use alternative contraceptive measures; decreased effectiveness

* Available in Canada only

of oral contraceptives may result
• To notify physician if skin rash, sore throat, fever, mouth sores, unusual bruising, bleeding occur
Lab test interferences:
False positive: Urinary glucose test (Benedict's method)

---

sulfasalazine

(sul-fa-sal'a-zeen)

Azulfidine, SAS-500, Salazopyrin*

Func. class.: Antiinflammatory
Chem. class.: Sulfonamide

Action: Drug acts as a prodrug to deliver sulfapyridine and 5-aminosalicylic acid to colon
Uses: Ulcerative colitis
Dosage and routes:
• *Adult:* PO 3-4 g/day in divided doses; maintenance 1.5-2 g/day in divided doses q6h
• *Child >2 yrs.:* PO 40-60 mg/kg/day in 4-6 divided doses, then 20-30 mg/kg/day in 4 doses, max. 2 g/day
Available forms include: Tabs 500 mg; oral susp 250 mg/5ml; enteric-coated tabs 500 mg
Side effects/adverse reactions:
SYST: ***Anaphylaxis***
GI: Nausea, vomiting, abdominal pain, stomatitis, ***hepatitis,*** glossitis, pancreatitis, diarrhea
CNS: Headache, confusion, insomnia, hallucinations, depression, vertigo, fatigue, anxiety, ***convulsions,*** drug fever, chills
HEMA: ***Leukopenia, neutropenia, thrombocytopenia, agranulocytosis, hemolytic anemia***
INTEG: Rash, dermatitis, urticaria, ***Stevens-Johnson syndrome,*** erythema, photosensitivity
GU: ***Renal failure, toxic nephrosis,*** increased BUN, creatinine, crystalluria
CV: ***Allergic myocarditis***
Contraindications: Hypersensitivity to sulfonamides or salicylates, pregnancy at term, child <2 yr intestinal, urinary obstruction
Precautions: Pregnancy (C), lactation, impaired hepatic function, severe allergy, bronchial asthma, impaired renal function
Pharmacokinetics:
PO: Partially absorbed, peak 1½-6 hr, half-life 5-10 hr, excreted in urine as sulfasalazine (15%), sulfapyridine (60%), 5-aminosalicylic acid and metabolites (20%-33%), breast milk, crosses placenta
Interactions/incompatibilities:
• Decreased absorption of: digoxin, folic acid
• Decreased effectiveness: oral contraceptives
• Increased hypoglycemic response: sulfonylurea agents
• Increased anticoagulant effects: oral anticoagulants
• Decreased renal excretion of: methotrexate
• Decreased hepatic clearance of: phenytoin

NURSING CONSIDERATIONS

Assess:
• I&O ratio; note color, character, pH of urine if drug administered for urinary tract infections; output should be 800 ml less than intake; if urine is highly acidic, alkalization may be needed
• Kidney function studies: BUN, creatinine, urinalysis if on long-term therapy
Administer:
• With full glass of water to maintain adequate hydration; increase fluids to 2000 ml/day to decrease crystallization in kidneys
• Medication after C&S; repeat C&S after full course of medication completed

• With resuscitative equipment available; severe allergic reactions may occur
• Total daily dose in evenly spaced doses and after meals to help minimize GI intolerance

Perform/provide:
• Storage in tight, light-resistant containers at room temperature

Evaluate:
• Therapeutic response: absence of fever, mucus in stools
• Blood dyscrasias: skin rash, fever, sore throat, bruising, bleeding, fatigue, joint pain
• Allergic reaction: rash, dermatitis, urticaria, pruritus, dyspnea, bronchospasm

Teach patient family:
• To take each oral dose with full glass of water to prevent crystalluria
• To complete full course of treatment to prevent superimposed infection
• To avoid sunlight or use sunscreen to prevent burns
• To avoid OTC medication (aspirin, vitamin C) unless directed by physician
• To use alternative contraceptive measures; decreased effectiveness of oral contraceptives may result
• To notify physician if skin rash, sore throat, fever, mouth sores, unusual bruising, bleeding occur

Lab test intereferences:
False positive: Urinary glucose test

---

sulfinpyrazone

(sul-fin-peer'a-zone)

Antazone, Anturan,* Anturane, Zynol

Func. class.: Uricosuric
Chem. class.: Pyrazolone

Action: Inhibits tubular reabsorption of urates, with increased excretion of uric acid; inhibits prostaglandin synthesis, which decreases platelet aggregation

Uses: Inhibition of platelet aggregation, gout

Dosage and routes:
Inhibition of platelet aggregation
• *Adult:* PO 200 mg qid

Gout/gouty arthritis
• *Adult:* PO 100-200 mg bid for 1 wk, then 200-400 mg bid, not to exceed 800 mg/day

Available forms include: Tabs 100 mg; caps 200 mg

Side effects/adverse reactions:
CNS: Dizziness, ***convulsions, coma***
EENT: Tinnitus
GU: Renal calculi, hypoglycemia
GI: Gastric irritation, nausea, vomiting, anorexia, ***hepatic necrosis,*** GI bleeding
INTEG: Rash, dermatitis, pruritus, fever, photosensitivity
HEMA: ***Agranulocytosis*** (rare)
RESP: ***Apnea,*** irregular respirations

Contraindications: Hypersensitivity to pyrazolone derivatives, severe hepatic disease, blood dyscrasias, severe renal disease, CrCl <50 mg/min, active peptic ulcer, GI inflammation, renal calculi

Precautions: Pregnancy (C), lactation

Pharmacokinetics:
PO: Peak 1-2 hr, duration 4-6 hr, half-life 3 hr, metabolized by liver, excreted in urine

Interactions/incompatibilities:
• Increased toxicity: sulfa drugs, dapsone, clofibrate, PAS, indomethacin, rifampin, naproxen, methotrexate, pantothenic acid, tolbutamide, warfarin
• Decreased effects of sulfinpyrazone: salicylates, xanthines

NURSING CONSIDERATIONS

Assess:
• Uric acid levels (3-7 mg/dl)

---

* Available in Canada only

• Respiratory rate, rhythm, depth; notify physician of abnormalities
• Renal function
• Bleeding tendencies, RBC and Hct
• I & O
• Electrolytes, CO_2 before, during treatment
• Urine pH, output, glucose during beginning treatment

Administer:

• With glass of milk
• With food for GI symptoms
• Increased fluids to prevent calculi; alkalinization of urine may be required

Evaluate:

• Therapeutic response: absence of pain, stiffness in joints

Lab test interferences:

Increase: PSP, aminohippuric acid

Teach patient/family:

• To avoid aspirin, alcohol, high purine diet

---

sulfisoxazole

(sul-fi-sox'a-zole)

Barazole, Gantrisin, Novosoxazole,* Rosoxol, Soxomide, Urizole

Func. class.: Antibiotic

Chem. class.: Sulfonamide, short acting

Action: Interferes with bacterial biosynthesis of proteins by competitive antagonism of PABA

Uses: Urinary tract, systemic infections; chancroid; trachoma; toxoplasmosis; acute otitis media; lymphogranuloma venereum, eye infections

Dosage and routes:

• *Adult:* PO 2-4 g loading dose, then 1-2 g qid × 7-10 days
• *Child >2 mo:* PO 75 mg/kg or 2 g/m^2 loading dose then 120-150 mg/kg/day or 4 g/m^2/day in divided doses q6h, not to exceed 6 g/day

Available forms include: Tabs 500 mg; syr, pediatric susp 500 mg/5 ml

Side effects/adverse reactions:

SYST: ***Anaphylaxis***

GI: Nausea, vomiting, abdominal pain, stomatitis, ***hepatitis,*** glossitis, pancreatitis, diarrhea, ***enterocolitis,*** anorexia

CNS: Headache, insomnia, hallucinations, depression, vertigo, fatigue, anxiety, ***convulsions,*** drug fever, chills, drowsiness

HEMA: ***Leukopenia, thrombocytopenia, agranulocytosis, hemolytic anemia, aplastic anemia***

INTEG: Rash, dermatitis, urticaria, ***Stevens-Johnson syndrome,*** erythema, photosensitivity, alopecia

GU: ***Renal failure, toxic nephrosis,*** increased BUN, creatinine, crystalluria, hematuria, proteinuria

CV: ***Allergic myocarditis***

Contraindications: Hypersensitivity to sulfonamides, sulfonylureas, thiazide, loop diuretics, salicylates, pregnancy at term

Precautions: Pregnancy (C), lactation, impaired hepatic function, severe allergy, bronchial asthma

Pharmacokinetics:

PO: Rapidly absorbed, peak 2-4 hr, 85% protein bound; half-life 4-7 hr, excreted in urine, crosses placenta

Interactions/incompatibilities:

• Decreased effectiveness: oral contraceptives
• Increased hypoglycemic response: sulfonylurea agents
• Increased anticoagulant effect: oral anticoagulants
• Decreased renal excretion of: methotrexate
• Decreased hepatic clearance of: phenytoin

S

NURSING CONSIDERATIONS

Assess:

• I&O ratio; note color, character, pH of urine if drug administered for urinary tract infections; output should be 800 ml less than intake; if urine is highly acidic, alkalization may be needed

• Kidney function studies: BUN, creatinine, urinalysis if on long-term therapy

Administer:

• With full glass of water to maintain adequate hydration; increase fluids to 2000 ml/day to decrease crystallization in kidneys

• Medication after C&S; repeat C&S after full course of medication completed

• With resuscitative equipment available; severe allergic reactions may occur

Perform/provide:

• Storage in tight, light-resistant containers at room temperature

Evaluate:

• Therapeutic response: absence of pain, fever, C&S negative

• Blood dyscrasias: skin rash, fever, sore throat, bruising, bleeding, fatigue, joint pain

• Allergic reaction: rash, dermatitis, urticaria, pruritus, dyspnea, bronchospasm

Teach patient/family:

• Take each oral dose with full glass of water to prevent crystalluria

• To complete full course of treatment to prevent superimposed infection

• To avoid sunlight or use sunscreen to prevent burns; avoid hazardous activities if dizziness occurs

• To avoid OTC medication (aspirin, vitamin C) unless directed by physician

• To use alternative contraceptive measures; decreased effectiveness of oral contraceptives may result

• To notify physician if skin rash, sore throat, fever, mouth sores, unusual bruising, bleeding occur

Lab test interferences:

False positive: Urinary glucose test

---

sulindac

(sul-in'dak)

Clinoril, Novosudac*

Func. class.: Nonsteroidal antiinflammatory

Chem. class.: Indeneacetic acid derivative

Action: Inhibits prostaglandin synthesis by decreasing an enzyme needed for biosynthesis; possesses analgesic, antiinflammatory, antipyretic properties

Uses: Mild to moderate pain, osteoarthritis, rheumatoid, gouty arthritis

Dosage and routes:

Arthritis

• *Adult:* PO 150 mg bid, may increase to 200 mg bid

Bursitis/acute arthritis

• *Adult:* PO 200 mg bid × 1-2 wk, then reduce dose

Available forms include: Tabs 150, 200 mg

Side effects/adverse reactions:

GI: Nausea, anorexia, vomiting, diarrhea, jaundice, ***cholestatic hepatitis***, constipation, flatulence, cramps, dry mouth, peptic ulcer

CNS: Dizziness, drowsiness, fatigue, tremors, confusion, insomnia, anxiety, depression

CV: Tachycardia, peripheral edema, palpitations, dysrhythmias

INTEG: Purpura, rash, pruritus, sweating

GU: ***Nephrotoxicity: dysuria, hematuria, oliguria, azotemia***

---

* Available in Canada only

HEMA: ***Blood dyscrasias***
EENT: Tinnitus, hearing loss, blurred vision
Contraindications: Hypersensitivity, asthma, severe renal disease, severe hepatic disease
Precautions: Pregnancy (C), lactation, children, bleeding disorders, GI disorders, cardiac disorders, hypersensitivity to other antiinflammatory agents
Pharmacokinetics:
PO: Peak 2 hr, half-life 3-3½ hr; metabolized in liver, excreted in urine (metabolites) excreted in breast milk, 93% protein binding
Interactions/incompatibilities:
- Increased action of: coumarin, phenytoin, sulfonamides when used with this drug

NURSING CONSIDERATIONS

Assess:
- Renal, liver, blood studies: BUN, creatinine, AST, ALT, HgB, before treatment, periodically thereafter
- Audiometric, ophthalmic exam before, during, after treatment

Administer:
- With food to decrease GI symptoms; best to take on empty stomach to facilitate absorption

Perform/provide:
- Storage at room temperature

Evaluate:
- Therapeutic response: decreased pain, stiffness, swelling in joints, ability to move more easily
- For eye, ear problems: blurred vision, tinnitus (may indicate toxicity)

Teach patient/family:
- To report blurred vision or ringing, roaring in ears (may indicate toxicity)
- To avoid driving or other hazardous activities if dizziness or drowsiness occurs
- To report change in urine pattern, weight increase, edema, pain increase in joints, fever, blood in urine (indicates nephrotoxicity)
- That therapeutic effects may take up to 1 mo

---

talbutal

(tal'byoo-tal)
Lotusate

Func. class.: Sedative/hypnotic-barbiturate (intermediate acting)
Chem. class.: Barbitone

Controlled Substance Schedule II (USA), Schedule G (Canada)
Action: Depresses activity in brain cells primarily in reticular activating system in brain stem; selectively depresses neurons in posterior hypothalamus, limbic structures
Uses: Insomnia, short-term treatment only
Dosage and routes:
- *Adult:* PO 120 mg hs

Available forms include: Tabs 120 mg
Side effects/adverse reactions:
CNS: Lethargy, drowsiness, hangover, dizziness, paradoxical stimulation in elderly and children, light-headedness, dependence, CNS depression, mental depression, slurred speech
GI: Nausea, vomiting, diarrhea, constipation
INTEG: Rash, urticaria, pain, abscesses at injection site, angioedema, thrombophlebitis, ***Stevens-Johnson syndrome***
CV: Hypotension, bradycardia
RESP: Depression, apnea, ***laryngospasm, bronchospasm***
HEMA: ***Agranulocytosis, thrombocytopenia, megaloblastic anemia*** (long-term treatment)
Contraindications: Hypersensitiv-

T

ity to barbiturates, respiratory depression, addiction to barbiturates, severe liver impairment, porphyria, pregnancy (D), uncontrolled severe pain

Precautions: Anemia, lactation, hepatic disease, renal disease, hypertension, elderly, acute/chronic pain

Pharmacokinetics:
Onset 30-45 min, duration 4-6 hr; metabolized by liver, excreted by kidneys (metabolites)

Interactions/incompatibilities:
- Increased CNS depression: alcohol, MAOIs, sedative, narcotics
- Decreased effect of: oral anticoagulants, corticosteroids, griseofulvin, quinidine
- Decreased half-life of: doxycycline

NURSING CONSIDERATIONS

Assess:
- Blood studies: Hct, Hgb, RBCs, if blood dyscrasias are suspected
- Hepatic studies: AST, ALT, bilirubin, if hepatic damage has occurred

Administer:
- After removal of cigarettes, to prevent fires
- After trying conservative measures for insomnia
- ½-1 hr before hs for sleeplessness
- On empty stomach for best absorption
- For $<$ 14 days since drug is not effective after that, tolerance develops
- Crushed or whole

Perform/provide:
- Assistance with ambulation after receiving dose
- Safety measure: siderails, nightlight, call bell within easy reach
- Checking to see PO medication has been swallowed
- Storage in tight container in cool environment

Evaluate:
- Therapeutic response: ability to sleep at night, decreased amount of early morning awakening
- Mental status: mood, sensorium, affect, memory (long, short)
- Physical dependency: more frequent requests for medication, shakes, anxiety
- Barbiturate toxicity: hypotension; pupillary constriction; cold, clammy skin; cyanosis of lips; insomnia; nausea; vomiting; hallucinations; delirium; weakness; mild symptoms may occur in 8-12 hr without drug
- Respiratory dysfunction: respiratory depression, character, rate, rhythm; hold drug if respirations are $<$ 10/min or if pupils are dilated (rare)
- Blood dyscrasias: fever, sore throat, bruising, rash, jaundice, epistaxis (rare)

Teach patient/family:
- That morning hangover is common
- That drug is indicated only for short-term treatment of insomnia and is probably ineffective after 2 wk
- That physical dependency may result when used for extended periods of time (45-90 days depending on dose)
- To avoid driving or other activities requiring alertness; sleep occurs within 45-60 min, lasts 6-8 hr
- To avoid alcohol ingestion or CNS depressants; serious CNS depression may result
- To tell all prescribers that barbiturate is being taken
- That withdrawal insomnia may occur after short-term use; do not start using drug again; insomnia

will improve in 1-3 nights; may experience increased dreaming
• That effects may take 2 nights for benefits to be noticed
• Alternate measures to improve sleep (reading, exercise several hours before hs, warm bath, warm milk, TV, self-hypnosis, deep breathing)

Lab test interferences:
False increase: Sulfobromophthalein

Treatment of overdose: Lavage, activated charcoal, warming blanket, vital signs, hemodialysis, I&O ratio

tamoxifen citrate

(ta-mox'i-fen)
Nolvadex, Tamofen,* Tamone*
Func. class.: Antineoplastic
Chem. class.: Hormone, antiestrogen

Action: Inhibits cell division by binding to cytoplasmic receptors (estrogen receptors); resembles normal cell complex but inhibits DNA synthesis

Uses: Advanced breast carcinoma that has not responded to other therapy in estrogen receptor positive patients (usually postmenopausal)

Dosage and routes:
• *Adult:* PO 10-20 mg bid

Available forms include: Tabs 10 mg

Side effects/adverse reactions:
HEMA: ***Thrombocytopenia, leukopenia***
GI: Nausea, vomiting, altered taste (anorexia)
GU: Vaginal bleeding, pruritus vulvae
INTEG: Rash, alopecia
CV: Chest pain
CNS: Hot flashes, headache, lightheadedness, depression
META: Hypercalcemia
EENT: Ocular lesions, retinopathy, corneal opacity, blurred vision (high doses)

Contraindications: Hypersensitivity, pregnancy (D)

Precautions: Leukopenia, thrombocytopenia, lactation, cataracts

Pharmacokinetics:
PO: Peak 4-7 hr, half-life 7 days (1 wk terminal), excreted primarily in feces

NURSING CONSIDERATIONS

Assess:
• CBC, differential, platelet count weekly; withhold drug if WBC is <4000 or platelet count is <75,000; notify physician of results

Administer:
• Antacid before oral agent; give drug after evening meal, before bedtime
• Antiemetic 30-60 min before giving drug to prevent vomiting

Perform/provide:
• Liquid diet, if needed including cola, Jell-O; dry toast or crackers may be added if patient is not nauseated or vomiting
• Increase fluid intake to 2-3 L/day to prevent dehydration
• Nutritious diet with iron, vitamin supplements as ordered
• Storage in light-resistant container at room temperature

Evaluate:
• Therapeutic response: decreased tumor size, spread of malignancy
• Bleeding: hematuria, guaiac, bruising, petechiae, mucosa or orifices q8h
• Food preferences; list likes, dislikes
• Effects of alopecia on body im-

age; discuss feelings about body changes
• Symptoms indicating severe allergic reactions: rash, pruritus, urticaria, purpuric skin lesions, itching, flushing
Teach patient/family:
• To report any complaints, side effects to nurse or physician
• That vaginal bleeding, pruritus, hot flashes, can occur, are reversible after discontinuing treatment
• To immediately report decreased visual acuity, which may be irreversible. Stress need for routine eye exams, who should be told about tamoxifen therapy
• To report vaginal bleeding immediately
• That tumor flare may occur: increase in size of tumor, increased bone pain and will subside rapidly; may take analgesics for pain
• That premenopausal women need to use mechanical birth control because ovulation may be induced
• That hair may be lost during treatment; a wig or hairpiece may make patient feel better; new hair may be different in color, texture
Lab test interferences:
Increase: Serum Ca

temafloxacin HCl

(teh-may′flox-a-sin)
Omniflox

Func. class.: Antiinfective
Chem. class.: Fluoroquinolone

Action: Interferes with conversion of intermediate DNA fragments into high-molecular-weight DNA in bacteria
Uses: Treatment of lower respiratory tract infections (pneumonia, bronchitis), genitourinary infections (prostatitis, UTIs), skin and skin structure infections
Dosage and routes:
Lower respiratory tract infections
• *Adult:* PO 600 mg q12h × 10-14 days
Skin infections
• *Adult:* PO 600 mg q12h × 7-14 days
Uncomplicated UTIs (cystitis)
• *Adult:* PO 400 mg qd × 3 days
Prostatitis
• *Adult:* PO 400 mg q12h × 28-31 days
Complicated UTIs
• *Adult:* PO 400 mg q12h × 10-14 days
Available forms include: Tabs 400, 600 mg
Side effects/adverse reactions:
CNS: Dizziness, headache, nervousness, somnolence, depression, insomnia, confusion, agitation
GI: Diarrhea, nausea, vomiting, anorexia, flatulence, heartburn, dry mouth, increased AST, ALT, constipation, abdominal pain, oral thrush, glossitis, stomatitis
INTEG: Rash, pruritus, urticaria
EENT: Visual disturbances
Contraindications: Hypersensitivity to quinolones
Precautions: Pregnancy (C), lactation, children, elderly, renal disease, seizure disorders
Pharmacokinetics:
PO: Peak 2-3 hr, half-life 8 hr, steady state 2 days; excreted in urine as active drug, metabolites, also excreted in biliary and GI system
Interactions/incompatibilities:
• Decreased effects of temafloxacin: antacids, nitrofurantoin, sucralfate, iron salts, zinc salts
• Increased temafloxacin levels: probenecid, cimetidine

* Available in Canada only

• Increased levels of: caffeine, cyclosporine, warfarin

NURSING CONSIDERATIONS

Assess:

• Kidney, liver function studies: BUN, creatinine, AST, ALT

• I&O ratio, urine pH; <5.5 is ideal

Administer:

• After clean-catch urine is obtained for C&S

Perform/provide:

• Limited intake of alkaline foods, drugs; milk, dairy products, peanuts, vegetables, alkaline antacids, sodium bicarbonate; also limit caffeine intake

Evaluate:

• Therapeutic response: negative C&S

• CNS symptoms: insomnia, vertigo, headache, agitation, confusion

• Allergic reactions: rash, flushing, urticaria, pruritus

Teach patient/family:

• That fluids must be increased to 3 L/day to avoid crystallization in kidneys

• If dizziness, light-headedness occurs, to ambulate, perform activities with assistance

• To take complete full course of drug therapy

• To contact physician if adverse reactions occur

• To avoid iron or mineral-containing supplements within 2 hr before and after administration

---

temazepam

(te-maz'e-pam)

Razepam, Restoril, Temaz

Func. class.: Sedative-hypnotic
Chem. class.: Benzodiazepine

Controlled Substance Schedule IV (USA), Schedule F (Canada)

Action: Produces CNS depression at limbic, thalamic, hypothalamic levels of the CNS; may be mediated by neurotransmitter gamma aminobutyric acid (GABA); results are sedation, hypnosis, skeletal muscle relaxation, anticonvulsant activity, anxiolytic action

Uses: Insomnia

Dosage and routes:

• *Adult:* PO 15-30 mg hs

Available forms include: Caps 15, 30 mg

Side effects/adverse reactions:

HEMA: ***Leukopenia, granulocytopenia*** (rare)

CNS: Lethargy, drowsiness, daytime sedation, dizziness, confusion, light-headedness, headache, anxiety, irritability

GI: Nausea, vomiting, diarrhea, heartburn, abdominal pain, constipation, anorexia

CV: Chest pain, pulse changes

Contraindications: Hypersensitivity to benzodiazepines, pregnancy (X), lactation, intermittent porphyria

Precautions: Anemia, hepatic disease, renal disease, suicidal individuals, drug abuse, elderly, psychosis, child < 15 yr, acute narrow-angle glaucoma, seizure disorders

Pharmacokinetics:

PO: Onset 30-45 min, duration 6-8 hr, half-life 10-20 hr; metabolized by liver, excreted by kidneys, crosses placenta, excreted in breast milk

Interactions/incompatibilities:

• Increased effects of: cimetidine, disulfiram

• Increased action of both drugs: alcohol, CNS depressants

• Decreased effect of: antacids

T

NURSING CONSIDERATIONS

Assess:

• Blood studies: Hct, Hgb, RBCs (if on long-term therapy)

• Hepatic studies: AST, ALT, bilirubin (if on long-term therapy)

Administer:

• After removal of cigarettes, to prevent fires

• After trying conservative measures for insomnia

• ½-1 hr before hs for sleeplessness

• On empty stomach fast onset, but may be taken with food if GI symptoms occur

Perform/provide:

• Assistance with ambulation after receiving dose

• Safety measure: siderails, nightlight, call bell within easy reach

• Checking to see PO medication has been swallowed

• Storage in tight container in cool environment

Evaluate:

• Therapeutic response: ability to sleep at night, decreased amount of early morning awakening if taking drug for insomnia

• Mental status: mood, sensorium, affect, memory (long, short)

• Blood dyscrasias: fever, sore throat, bruising, rash, jaundice, epistaxis (rare)

• Type of sleep problem: falling asleep, staying asleep

Teach patient/family:

• To avoid driving or other activities requiring alertness until drug is stabilized

• To avoid alcohol ingestion or CNS depressants; serious CNS depression may result

• That effects may take 2 nights for benefits to be noticed

• Alternate measures to improve sleep: reading, exercise several hours before hs, warm bath, warm milk, TV, self-hypnosis, deep breathing

• That hangover, memory impairment are common in elderly, but less common than with barbiturates

Lab test interferences:

Increase: ALT/AST, serum bilirubin

Decrease: RAI uptake

False increase: Urinary 17-OHCS

Treatment of overdose: Lavage, activated charcoal, monitor electrolytes, vital signs

---

terazosin HCl

(ter-ay'zoe-sin)

Hytrin

Func. class.: Antihypertensive, anti-adrenergic

Action: Decreases total vascular resistance, which is responsible for a decrease in B/P; this occurs by blockade of α-1 adrenoreceptors

Uses: Hypertension as a single agent or in combination with diuretics or β-blockers

Dosage and routes:

• *Adult:* PO 1 mg hs, may increase dose slowly to desired response; not to exceed 20 mg/day

Available forms include: Tabs 1, 2, 5 mg

Side effects/adverse reactions:

CV: Palpitations, orthostatic hypotension, tachycardia, edema, rebound hypertension

CNS: Dizziness, headache, drowsiness, anxiety, depression, vertigo, weakness, fatigue

GI: Nausea, vomiting, diarrhea, constipation, abdominal pain

GU: Urinary frequency, incontinence, impotence, priapism

EENT: Blurred vision, epistaxis, tinnitus, dry mouth, red sclera, nasal congestion, sinusitis

---

*Available in Canada only

RESP: Dyspnea
Contraindications: Hypersensitivity
Precautions: Pregnancy (C), children, lactation
Pharmacokinetics:
Peak 1 hr, half-life 9-12 hr, highly bound to plasma proteins; metabolized in liver, excreted in urine, feces
Interactions/incompatibilities:
• Increased hypotensive effects: β-blockers, nitroglycerin, verapamil, nifedipine

NURSING CONSIDERATIONS

Assess:
• B/P, pulse, jugular venous distention q4h
• BUN, uric acid if on long-term therapy
• Weight daily, I&O
Perform/provide:
• Storage in tight containers in cool environment
Evaluate:
• Therapeutic response: decreased B/P, edema in feet, legs
• Skin turgor, dryness of mucous membranes for hydration status
• Rales, dyspnea, orthopnea q30min
Teach patient/family:
• That fainting occasionally occurs after first dose; do not drive or operate machinery for 4 hr after first dose or take first dose hs
• To rise slowly from sitting/lying position

---

terbutaline sulfate

(ter-byoo'te-leen)
Brethaire, Brethine, Bricanyl
Func. class.: Selective β_2-agonist
Chem. class.: Catecholamine

Action: Relaxes bronchial smooth muscle by direct action on β_2-adrenergic receptors, through accumulation of cAMP at β-adrenergic receptor sites
Uses: Bronchospasm, premature labor
Dosage and routes:
Bronchospasm
• *Adult and child >12 yr:* INH 2 puffs q1min apart, then q4-6h; PO 2.5-5 mg q8h; SC 0.25 mg q8h
Premature Labor
• *Adult:* IV INF: 0.01 mg/min, increased by 0.005 mg q10min, not to exceed 0.025 mg/min; SC 0.25 mg q1h; PO 5 mg q4h × 48 hr, then 5 mg q6h as maintenance for above doses
Available forms include: Tabs 2.5, 5 mg; aerosol 0.2 mg/actuation
Side effects/adverse reactions:
CNS: Tremors, anxiety, insomnia, headache, dizziness, stimulation
CV: Palpitations, tachycardia, hypertension, ***cardiac arrest***
GI: Nausea, vomiting
Contraindications: Hypersensitivity to sympathomimetics, narrow-angle glaucoma, tachydysrhythmias
Precautions: Pregnancy (B), cardiac disorders, hyperthyroidism, diabetes mellitus, prostatic hypertrophy, lactation, elderly, hypertensive, glaucoma
Pharmacokinetics:
PO: Onset ½ hr, duration 4-8 hr
SC: Onset 6-15 min, duration 1½-4 hr
INH: Onset 5-30 min, duration 3-6 hr
Interactions/incompatibilities:
• Increased effects of both drugs: other sympathomimetics
• Decreased action: β-blockers
• Hypertensive crisis: MAOIs

NURSING CONSIDERATIONS

Assess:
• Respiratory function: vital capac-

ity, forced expiratory volume, ABGs, B/P, pulse

Administer:

- IV, run 10 μg/min; may increase 5 μg q10 min, titrate to response; after ½-1 hr taper dose by 5 μg, switch to PO as soon as possible
- 2 hr before hs to avoid sleeplessness

Perform/provide:

- Storage at room temperature, do not use discolored solutions

Evaluate:

- Therapeutic response: absence of dyspnea, wheezing
- Tolerance over long-term therapy, dose may need to be increased or changed

Teach patient/family:

- Not to use OTC medications; extra stimulation may occur
- Use of inhaler; review package insert with patient
- To avoid getting aerosol in eyes
- To wash inhaler in warm water and dry qd, rinse mouth after use
- On all aspects of drug; avoid smoking, smoke-filled rooms, persons with respiratory infections
- To increase fluids >2 L/day; allow 15 min between inhalation of this drug and inhaler containing steroid

Treatment of overdose: Administer an α-blocker, then norepinephrine for severe hypotension

---

terconazole

(ter-kon′-a-zole)

Terazol 7

Func. class.: Local antiinfective

Chem. class.: Antifungal

Action: Interferes with fungal DNA replication; binds sterols in fungal cell membranes, which increases permeability, leaking of nutrients

Uses: Vaginal, vulvae, vulvovaginal candidiasis (moniliasis)

Dosage and routes:

- *Adult:* Vag 5 g (1 applicator) hs × 7 days

Available forms include: Vag cream 0.4%

Side effects/adverse reactions:

GU: Vulvovaginal burning, itching, pelvic cramps

INTEG: Rash, urticaria, stinging, burning

MISC: Headache, body pain

Contraindications: Hypersensitivity

Precautions: Children <2 yr, pregnancy, lactation

NURSING CONSIDERATIONS

Administer:

- Enough medication to completely cover lesions
- After cleansing with soap, water before each application, dry well

Perform/provide:

- Storage at room temperature in dry place

Evaluate:

- Therapeutic response: decrease in size, number of lesions
- Allergic reactions: burning, stinging, swelling, redness

Teach patient/family:

- To use medical asepsis (hand washing) before, after each application
- To avoid use of OTC creams, ointments, lotions unless directed by physician
- To avoid contact with eyes
- To continue during menses, and even if symptoms subside; refrain from sexual intercourse during treatment

---

* Available in Canada only

terfenadine

(ter-fin'-a-deen)
Seldane
Func. class.: Antihistamine
Chem. class.: Butyrophenone derivative

Action: Acts on blood vessels, GI, respiratory system by competing with histamine for H_1-receptor site; decreases allergic response by blocking histamine
Uses: Rhinitis, allergy symptoms
Dosage and routes:
• *Adult and child >12 yr:* PO 60 mg bid
• *Child <12 yr:* PO 15-30 mg bid
Available forms include: Tabs 60 mg
Side effects/adverse reactions:
CNS: Dizziness, poor coordination
RESP: Increased thick secretions
GI: Anorexia, increased liver function tests, dry mouth
GU: Retention
Contraindications: Hypersensitivity
Precautions: Pregnancy (C)
Pharmacokinetics:
PO: Peak 1-2 hr, 97% bound to plasma proteins, half-life is biphasic 3½ hr, 16-23 hr
NURSING CONSIDERATIONS
Assess:
• I&O ratio; be alert for urinary retention, frequency, dysuria; drug should be discontinued if these occur
• CBC during long-term therapy
Administer:
• With meals if GI symptoms occur; absorption may slightly decrease
Perform/provide:
• Hard candy, gum, frequent rinsing of mouth for dryness
• Storage in tight, light-resistant container
Evaluate:
• Therapeutic response: absence of running or congested nose or rashes
• Respiratory status: rate, rhythm, increase in bronchial secretions, wheezing, chest tightness
Teach patient/family:
• To notify physician if confusion, sedation, hypotension occurs
Lab test interferences:
False negative: Skin allergy tests
Treatment of overdose: Administer ipecac syrup or lavage, diazepam, vasopressors, barbiturates (short-acting)

terpin hydrate

(ter'pin)
Func. class.: Expectorant

Action: Direct action on respiratory tract, which increases fluids, allows for expectoration
Uses: Bronchial secretions
Dosage and routes:
• *Adult:* ELIX 5-10 ml q4-6h
Available forms include: Elix terpin hydrate codeine 10 mg codeine/85 mg terpin hydrate; elix, plain 85 mg/5 ml
Side effects/adverse reactions:
GI: Nausea, vomiting, anorexia
Contraindications: Hypersensitivity, child <12 yr
Precautions: Pregnancy (C)
NURSING CONSIDERATIONS
Administer:
• With glass of water or food to decrease GI irritation
Perform/provide:
• Storage at room temperature
Evaluate:
• Therapeutic response: absence of thick secretions

T

• Cough: type, frequency, character including sputum
Teach patient/family:
• To avoid driving, other hazardous activities until patient is stabilized on this medication (if combined with codeine, drowsiness occurs)
• Not to exceed recommended dosage

testolactone

(tess-toe-lak'tone)
Teslac
Func. class.: Antineoplastic
Chem. class.: Hormone, androgen

Action: Acts on adrenal cortex to suppress activity; reduces estrone synthesis
Uses: Advanced breast carcinoma in postmenopausal women, prostatic cancer
Dosage and routes:
• *Adult:* PO 250 mg qid
Available forms include: Tabs 50 mg
Side effects/adverse reactions:
GI: Nausea, vomiting, anorexia, glossitis
GU: Urinary retention, ***renal failure***
INTEG: Rash, nail changes, facial hair growth
CV: Orthostatic hypertension, edema
CNS: Paresthesias, dizziness
EENT: Deepening voice
META: Hypercalcemia
Contraindications: Hypersensitivity, premenopausal women, carcinoma of male breast
Precautions: Renal disease, hypercalcemia, cardiac disease, pregnancy (C)
Pharmacokinetics: None known
Interactions/incompatibilities:
• Enhanced effects of: oral anticoagulants

NURSING CONSIDERATIONS
Assess:
• CA^+ levels
• B/P q4h, tell patient to rise slowly from sitting or lying down
Administer:
• For at least 3 mo or longer for desired response
Evaluate:
• Therapeutic response: decreased tumor size, spread of malignancy
• Food preferences; list likes, dislikes
• Edema in feet, joint, stomach pain, shaking
• Symptoms indicating severe allergic reaction: rash, pruritus, urticaria, purpuric skin lesions, itching, flushing
• Anorexia, nausea, vomiting, constipation, weakness, loss of muscle tone (indicating hypercalcemia)
Teach patient/family:
• To recognize and report signs of hepatotoxicity, hypercalcemia, virilization, bleeding if on anticoagulants
Lab test interferences:
Increase: Urinary 17-OHCS
Decrease: Estradiol

testosterone

(tess-toss'ter-one)
Histerone, Malogen, Testoject
Func. class.: Androgenic anabolic steroid
Chem. class.: Halogenated testosterone derivative

Action: Increases weight by building body tissue, increases potassium, phosphorus, chloride, nitrogen levels, increases bone development
Uses: Breast engorgement, breast cancer in postmenopausal women,

eunuchoidism, eunuchism, male climacteric

Dosage and routes:

Breast engorgement

• *Adult:* IM 25-50 mg/day × 3-4 days

Breast cancer

• *Adult:* IM 100 mg 3 ×/wk

Male climacteric/eunuchoidism/eunuchism

• *Adult:* IM 10-25 mg 2-5 ×/wk

Available forms include: Inj IM 25, 50, 100 mg/ml

Side effects/adverse reactions:

INTEG: Rash, acneiform lesions, oily hair, skin, flushing, sweating, acne vulgaris, alopecia, hirsutism

CNS: Dizziness, headache, fatigue, tremors, paresthesias, flushing, sweating, anxiety, lability, insomnia

MS: Cramps, spasms

CV: Increased B/P

GU: Hematuria, amenorrhea, vaginitis, decreased libido, decreased breast size, clitoral hypertrophy, testicular atrophy

GI: Nausea, vomiting, constipation, weight gain, ***cholestatic jaundice***

EENT: Carpal tunnel syndrome, conjunctional edema, nasal congestion

ENDO: Abnormal GTT

Contraindications: Severe renal disease, severe cardiac disease, severe hepatic disease, hypersensitivity, pregnancy (X), lactation, genital bleeding (abnormal)

Precautions: Diabetes mellitus, CV disease, MI

Pharmacokinetics:

PO: Metabolized in liver, excreted in urine, crosses placenta, excreted in breast milk

Interactions/incompatibilities:

• Increased effects of: oral antidiabetics, oxyphenbutazone

• Increased PT: anticoagulants

• Edema: ACTH, adrenal steroids

• Decreased effects of: insulin

NURSING CONSIDERATIONS

Assess:

• Weight daily, notify physician if weekly weight gain is >5 lb

• B/P q4h

• I&O ratio; be alert for decreasing urinary output, increasing edema

• Growth rate in children since growth rate may be uneven (linear/bone browth) when used for extended period

• Electrolytes: K, Na, Cl, Ca; cholesterol

• Liver function studies: ALT, AST, bilirubin

Administer:

• Titrated dose, use lowest effective dose

• IM deep into upper outer quadrant of gluteal muscle

Perform/provide:

• Diet with increased calories and protein; decrease sodium if edema occurs

• Supportive drug of anemia

Evaluate:

• Therapeutic response: occurs in 4-6 wk in osteoporosis

• Edema, hypertension, cardiac symptoms, jaundice

• Mental status: affect, mood, behavioral changes, aggression

• Signs of masculinization in female: increased libido, deepening of voice, breast tissue, enlarged clitoris, menstrual irregularities; male: gynecomastia, impotence, testicular atrophy

• Hypercalcemia: lethargy, polyuria, polydipsia, nausea, vomiting, constipation; drug may need to be decreased

• Hypoglycemia in diabetics, since oral anticoagulant action is decreased

Teach patient/family:

• Drug needs to be combined with complete health plan: diet, rest, exercise

• To notify physician if therapeutic response decreases

• Not to discontinue this medication abruptly

• About changes in sex characteristics

• Women to report menstrual irregularities

• That 1-3 mo course is necessary for response in breast cancer

Lab test interferences:

Increase: Serum cholesterol, blood glucose, urine glucose

Decrease: Serum calcium, serum potassium, T_4, T_3, thyroid ^{131}I uptake test, urine 17-OHCS, 17-KS

---

testosterone cypionate/ testosterone enanthate/ testosterone propionate

Andro-Cyp, Andronate, Depotest, Dep-Test, Depo-Testosterone, Duratest/Android-T LA, Andro-LA, Andryl, Delatestryl, Everone, Malogen,* Malogex,* Testostroval-PA/Androlan, Androlin, Testex

Func. class.: Androgenic anabolic steroid

Chem. class.: Halogenated testosterone derivative

Action: Increases weight by building body tissue, increases potassium, phosphorus, chloride, nitrogen levels, increases bone development

Uses: Female breast cancer, eunuchoidism, male climacteric, oligospermia, impotence, osteoporosis

Dosage and routes:

Oligospermia

• *Adult:* IM 100-200 mg q4-6 wk (cypionate or enanthate)

Breast cancer

• *Adult:* IM 50-100 mg 3 ×/wk (propionate) or 200-400 mg q2-4 wk (cypionate or enanthate)

Male climacteric/eunuchoidism/ eunuchism

• *Adult:* IM 10-25 mg 2-4 ×/wk (propionate)

Available forms include: Propionate inj IM 25, 50, 100 mg/ml; enanthate inj IM 100, 200 mg/ml; cypionate inj IM 50, 100, 200 mg/ml

Side effects/adverse reactions:

INTEG: Rash, acneiform lesions, oily hair, skin, flushing, sweating, acne vulgaris, alopecia, hirsutism

CNS: Dizziness, headache, fatigue, tremors, paresthesias, flushing, sweating, anxiety, lability, insomnia

MS: Cramps, spasms

CV: Increased B/P

GU: Hematuria, amenorrhea, vaginitis, decreased libido, decreased breast size, clitoral hypertrophy, testicular atrophy

GI: Nausea, vomiting, constipation, weight gain, ***cholestatic jaundice***

EENT: Carpal tunnel syndrome, conjunctional edema, nasal congestion

ENDO: Abnormal GTT

Contraindications: Severe renal disease, severe cardiac disease, severe hepatic disease, hypersensitivity, pregnancy (X), lactation, genital bleeding (abnormal)

Precautions: Diabetes mellitus, CV disease, MI

Pharmacokinetics:

PO: Metabolized in liver, excreted in urine, breast milk; crosses placenta

Interactions/incompatibilities:

• Increased effects of: oral antidiabetics, oxyphenbutazone

---

* Available in Canada only

• Increased PT: anticoagulants
• Edema: ACTH, adrenal steroids
• Decreased effects of: insulin

NURSING CONSIDERATIONS

Assess:
• Weight daily, notify physician if weekly weight gain is >5 lb
• B/P q4h
• I&O ratio; be alert for decreasing urinary output, increasing edema
• Growth rate in children since growth rate may be uneven (linear/bone growth) used for extended periods of time
• Electrolytes: K, Na, Cl, Ca; cholesterol
• Liver function studies: ALT, AST, bilirubin

Administer:
• Titrated dose; use lowest effective dose
• IM deep into upper outer quadrant of gluteal muscle

Perform/provide:
• Diet with increased calories, protein; decrease sodium if edema occurs
• Supportive drug of anemia

Evaluate:
• Therapeutic response: occurs in 4-6 wk in osteoporosis
• Edema, hypertension, cardiac symptoms, jaundice
• Mental status: affect, mood, behavioral changes, aggression
• Signs of masculinization in female: increased libido, deepening of voice, breast tissue, enlarge clitoris, menstrual irregularities; male: gynecomastia, impotence, testicular atrophy
• Hypercalcemia: lethargy, polyuria, polydipsia, nausea, vomiting, constipation; drug may need to be decreased
• Hypoglycemia in diabetics, since oral anticoagulant action is decreased

Teach patient/family:
• That drug needs to be combined with complete health plan: diet, rest, exercise
• To notify physician if therapeutic response decreases
• Not to discontinue this medication abruptly
• About changes in sex characteristics
• Women to report menstrual irregularities
• That 1-3 mo course is necessary for response in breast cancer
• Procedure for use of buccal tablets (requires 30-60 min to dissolve, change absorption site with each dose; do not eat, drink, chew, or smoke while tablet is in place)

Lab test interferences:
Increase: Serum cholesterol, blood glucose, urine glucose
Decrease: Serum calcium, serum potassium, T_4, T_3, thyroid ^{131}I uptake test, urine 17-OHCS, 17-KS, PBI

---

tetanus toxoid, adsorbed; tetanus toxoid

Func. class.: Toxoid

Action: Produces specific antibodies to tetanus

Uses: Tetanus toxoid: used for prophylactic treatment of wounds

Dosage and routes:
• *Adult and child:* IM 0.5 ml q4-6 wk × 2 doses, then 0.5 ml 1 yr after dose 2 (adsorbed); SC/IM 0.5 ml q4-8wk × 3 doses, then 0.5 ml ½-1 yr after dose 3

Available forms include: Inj adsorbed IM 5, 10 LfU/0.5 ml; inj IM, SC 4, 5 LfU/0.5 ml

Side effects/adverse reactions:
GI: Nausea, vomiting, anorexia

T

INTEG: Skin abscess, urticaria, itching, swelling
CV: Tachycardia, hypotension
SYST: Lymphadenitis, ***anaphylaxis***
CNS: Crying, fretfulness, fever, drowsiness
MS: Osteomyelitis
Contraindications: Hypersensitivity, active infection, poliomyelitis outbreak, immunosuppression
Precautions: Pregnancy

NURSING CONSIDERATIONS

Assess:
• For skin reactions: swelling, rash, urticaria

Administer:
• At least 4 wk apart × 3 doses for children >6 wk old
• Only with epinephrine 1:1000 on unit to treat laryngospasm
• IM only; not to be given SC (vastus lateralis in infants, deltoid in adults)

Perform/provide
• Written record of immunization

Evaluate:
• For history of allergies, skin conditions (eczema, psoriasis, dermatitis), reactions to vaccinations
• For anaphylaxis: inability to breathe, bronchospasm

Teach patient/family:
• That doses are given at least 4 wk apart × 3 doses; booster needed at 10 yr intervals

---

tetracaine/tetracaine HCl (topical)

(tet'-ra-cane)
Cetacaine, Pontocaine
Func. class.: Topical anesthetic

Action: Inhibits nerve impulses from sensory nerves, which produces anesthesia
Uses: Pruritus, sunburn, toothache, sore throat, cold sores, oral pain, rectal pain and irritation, control of gagging
Dosage and routes:
• *Adult and child:* TOP apply to affected area 1 oz for adult ¼ oz for child
Available forms include: Sol 2%; aero spray, liq, oint, gel
Side effects/adverse reactions:
INTEG: Rash, irritation, sensitization
Contraindications: Hypersensitivity, infants <1 yr, application to large areas, PABA allergies
Precautions: Child <6 yr, sepsis, pregnancy (C), denuded skin

NURSING CONSIDERATIONS

Administer:
• After cleansing and drying of affected area

Evaluate:
• Therapeutic response: absence of pain, itching of affected area
• Allergy: rash, irritation, reddening, swelling
• Infection: if affected area is infected, do not apply

Teach patient/family:
• To report rash, irritation, redness, swelling
• How to apply solution

---

tetracaine HCl

(tet'-ra-caine)
Pontocaine
Func. class.: Ophthalmic anesthetic
Chem. class.: Ester

Action: Decreases ion permeability by stabilizing neuronal membrane
Uses: Cataract extraction, tonometry, gonioscopy, removal of foreign objects, corneal suture removal, glaucoma surgery
Dosage and routes:
• *Adult and child:* Instill 1-2 gtts before procedure

Available forms include: Sol 0.5%; oint 0.5%

Side effects/adverse reactions:

EENT: Blurred vision, stinging, burning, lacrimation, photophobia, conjunctival redness

INTEG: Contact dermatitis

Contraindications: Hypersensitivity to paraaminobenzoic acid

Precautions: Abnormal levels of plasma esterases, allergies, hyperthyroidism, hypertension, cardiac disease, pregnancy (C)

Pharmacokinetics:

Instill: Onset 13-30 sec, duration 15-20 min

Interactions/incompatibilities:

- Decreases antibacterial action of: sulfonamides

NURSING CONSIDERATIONS

Assess:

- Previous hypersensitivity to anesthetics

Perform/provide:

- Protective covering for eye
- Storage at room temperature in tight, light resistant container; refrigerate

Teach patient/family:

- To report change in vision, with blurring or loss of sight, trouble breathing, sweating, flushing
- Not to touch or rub eye, which may further damage eye
- That someone must drive the patient home after the appointment

---

tetracaine HCl

(tet-ra'-kane)

Pontocaine

Func. class.: Local anesthetic
Chem. class.: Ester

Action: Competes with calcium for sites in nerve membrane that control sodium transport across cell membrane; decreases rise of depolarization phase of action potential

Uses: Spinal anesthesia, epidural, peripheral nerve block, perineum, lower extremities

Dosage and routes:

Varies depending on route of anesthesia

Available forms include: Inj 0.2%, 0.3%, 1%; powder

Side effects/adverse reactions:

CNS: Anxiety, restlessness, ***convulsions, loss of consciousness,*** drowsiness, disorientation, tremors, shivering

CV: ***Myocardial depression, cardiac arrest, dysrhythmias,*** bradycardia, hypotension, hypertension, fetal bradycardia

GI: Nausea, vomiting

EENT: Blurred vision, tinnitus, pupil constriction

INTEG: Rash, urticaria, allergic reactions, edema, burning, skin discoloration at injection site, tissue necrosis

RESP: ***Status asthmaticus, respiratory arrest, anaphylaxis***

Contraindications: Hypersensitivity, child <12 yr, elderly, severe liver disease

Precautions: Elderly, severe drug allergies, pregnancy (C)

Pharmacokinetics:

Onset 15 min, duration 3 hr; metabolized by liver, excreted in urine (metabolites)

Interactions/incompatibilities:

- Dysrhythmias: epinephrine, halothane, enflurane
- Hypertension: MAOIs, tricyclic antidepressants, phenothiazines
- Decreased action of tetracaine: chloroprocaine

NURSING CONSIDERATIONS

Assess:

- B/P, pulse, respiration during treatment

• Fetal heart tones if drug is used during labor

Administer:

• Only drugs that are not cloudy, do not contain precipitate

• Only with crash cart, resuscitative equipment nearby

• Only drugs without preservatives for epidural or caudal anesthesia

Perform/provide:

• Use of new solution, discard unused portions

Evaluate:

• Therapeutic response: anesthesia necessary for procedure

• Allergic reactions: rash, urticaria, itching

• Cardiac status: ECG for dysrhythmias, pulse, B/P, during anesthesia

Treatment of overdose: Airway, O_2, vasopressor, IV fluids, anticonvulsants for seizures

---

tetracycline HCl

(tet-ra-sye'kleen)

Achromycin, Bicycline, Cefracycline,* Cycline, Cyclopar, Medicycline,* Neo-Tetrine,* Novotetra,* Panmycin, Sarocycline, Sumycin, Tetracyn, Tetralan, Tetralean,* Trexin, Tetracap

Func. class.: Broad-spectrum antibiotic/antiinfective

Chem. class.: Tetracycline

Action: Inhibits protein synthesis and phosphorylation in microorganisms; bacteriostatic

Uses: Syphilis, chlamydia trachomatis, gonorrhea, lymphogranuloma venereum, uncommon gram-positive/negative organisms, rickettsial infections

Dosage and routes:

• *Adult:* PO 250-500 mg q6h; IM 250 mg/day or 150 mg q12h; IV 250-500 mg q8-12h

• *Child >8 yr:* PO 25-50 mg/kg/day in divided doses q6h; IM 15-25 mg/kg/day in divided doses q8-12h; IV 10-20 mg/kg/day in divided doses q12h

Gonorrhea

• *Adult:* PO 1.5 g, then 500 mg qid for a total of 9 g over 7 days

Chlamydia trachomatis

• *Adult:* PO 500 mg qid × 7 days

Syphilis

• *Adult:* PO 2-3 g in divided doses × 10-15 days; if syphilis duration > 1 yr, must treat 30 days

Brucellosis

• *Adult:* PO 500 mg qid × 3 wk with 1 g streptomycin IM 2 ×/day × 1 wk, and 1 ×/day the second wk

Urethral syndrome in women

• *Adult:* PO 500 mg qid × 7 days

Rape Victims

• *Adult:* PO 500 mg qid × 7 days

Acne

• *Adult:* 1 g/day in divided doses, maintenance 125-500 mg per day

Available forms include: Oral susp 125 mg/5 ml, caps 100, 200, 500 mg; tabs 100, 250, 500 mg; powder for inj

Side effects/adverse reactions:

CNS: Fever, headache, paresthesia

HEMA: ***Eosinophilia, neutropenia, thrombocytopenia, leukocytosis, hemolytic anemia***

EENT: Dysphagia, glossitis, decreased calcification of deciduous teeth, oral candidiasis

GI: Nausea, abdominal pain, *vomiting, diarrhea,* anorexia, enterocolitis, ***hepatotoxicity,*** flatulence, abdominal cramps, epigastric burning, stomatitis

CV: Pericarditis

GU: Increased BUN

INTEG: Rash, urticaria, photosen-

---

*Available in Canada only

sitivity, increased pigmentation, ***exfoliative dermatitis,*** pruritus, ***angioedema***
Contraindications: Hypersensitivity to tetracyclines, children <8 yr, pregnancy (D), lactation
Precautions: Renal disease, hepatic disease
Pharmacokinetics:
PO: Peak 2-3 hr, duration 6 hr, half-life 6-10 hr; excreted in urine, crosses placenta, excreted in breast milk, 20%-60% protein bound
Interactions/incompatibilities:
- Decreased effect of tetracycline: antacids, $NaHCO_3$, dairy products, alkali products, iron, kaolin/pectin
- Increased effect: anticoagulants
- Decreased effect: penicillins, oral anticoagulants
- Nephrotoxicity: methoxyflurane
- Do not mix with other drugs

NURSING CONSIDERATIONS
Assess:
- Signs of anemia: Hct, Hgb, fatigue
- I&O ratio
- Blood studies: PT, CBC, AST, ALT, BUN, creatinine

Administer:
- IM: deep; no more than 2 ml/injection site
- IV after diluting 250 mg or less/5 ml of sterile H_2O; may be further diluted with 100 ml or more D_5W or NS; give 100 mg or less over 5 min or more
- After C&S obtained
- 2 hr before or after ferrous products; 3 hr after antacid or kaolin/pectin products

Perform/provide:
- Storage in tight, light-resistant container at room temperature

Evaluate:
- Therapeutic response: decreased temperature, absence of lesions, negative C&S
- Allergic reactions: rash, itching, pruritus, angioedema
- Nausea, vomiting, diarrhea; administer antiemetic, antacids as ordered
- Overgrowth of infection: increased temperature, malaise, redness, pain, swelling, drainage, perineal itching, diarrhea, changes in cough or sputum

Teach patient/family:
- To avoid sun exposure since burns may occur; sunscreen does not seem to decrease photosensitivity
- Of diabetic to avoid use of Clinistix, Diastix, or Tes-Tape for urine glucose testing
- That all prescribed medication must be taken to prevent superimposed infection
- To avoid milk products, take with a full glass of water

Lab test interferences:
False negative: Urine glucose with Clinistix or Tes-Tape
False increase: Urinary catecholamines

tetracycline HCl (ophthalmic)

(tet-ra-sye'kleen)
Achromycin Ophthalmic
Func. class.: Antiinfective

Action: Inhibits bacterial protein synthesis
Uses: Infection of eye, ophthalmia neonatorum
Dosage and routes:
- *Adult and child:* Instill 1-2 gtts bid-qid as needed

Ophthalmia neonatorum
- *Neonate:* TOP 1-2 gtts into each eye immediately after delivery; SOL, 1 gtt q6-12hr more frequently

Available forms include: Oint 1%, Susp drops 1%

Side effects/adverse reactions:
EENT: Poor corneal wound healing, overgrowth of nonsusceptible organisms

Contraindications: Hypersensitivity, pregnancy (D)

Precautions: Antibiotic hypersensitivity

NURSING CONSIDERATIONS

Administer:
• After washing hands, cleanse crusts or discharge from eye before application

Perform/provide:
• Storage at room temperature, in light-resistant container

Evaluate:
• Therapeutic response: absence of redness, inflammation, tearing
• Allergy: itching, lacrimation, redness, swelling

Teach patient/family:
• To use drug exactly as prescribed, shake well before using
• Not to use eye make-up, towels, washcloths, or eye medication of others, or reinfection may occur
• That drug container tip should not be touched to eye
• To report itching, increased redness, burning, stinging, swelling; drug should be discontinued
• That drug may cause blurred vision when ointment is applied

tetracycline HCl (topical)

(tet-ra-sye'kleen)
Achromycin

Func. class.: Local antiinfective
Chem. class.: Tetracycline

Action: Interferes with microorganism protein synthesis

Uses: Acne vulgaris, skin abrasions

Dosage and routes:
• *Adult and child >12 yr:* TOP apply to affected area bid

Available forms include: Oint 3%; sol 0.22%

Side effects/adverse reactions:
INTEG: Rash, urticaria, stinging, burning, redness, swelling, photosensitivity

Contraindications: Hypersensitivity, pregnancy (D)

Precautions: Lactation

NURSING CONSIDERATIONS

Administer:
• Enough medication to completely cover lesions
• After cleansing with soap, water before each application, dry well

Perform/provide:
• Storage at room temperature in dry place, use within 2 mo or discard

Evaluate:
• Therapeutic response: decrease in size, number of lesions
• Allergic reaction: burning, stinging, swelling, redness

Teach patient/family:
• To apply with glove to prevent further infection
• To avoid use of OTC creams, ointments, lotions unless directed by physician
• To use medical asepsis (hand washing) before, after each application, avoid eyes, nose, mouth
• To notify physician if condition worsens
• That some stinging may occur
• To avoid sunlight or ultraviolet light or burning may occur
• That staining of clothing and skin may occur

tetrahydrozoline HCl

(tet-ra-hi-droz-o-leen)

Murine Plus, Optigene, Soothe, Visine

Func. class.: Ophthalmic vasoconstrictor

Chem. class.: Direct sympathomimetic amine

Action: Vasoconstriction of eye arterioles; decreases eye engorgement by stimulation of α-adrenergic receptors

Uses: Ocular congestion, irritation, itching

Dosage and routes:

• *Adult and child >2 yr:* INSTILL 1-2 gtts bid or tid

Available forms include: Sol 0.05%

Side effects/adverse reactions:

CNS: Headache, dizziness, weakness

CV: Bradycardia, hypertension, dysrhythmias, tachycardia, ***CV collapse,*** palpitation

EENT: Stinging, lacrimation, blurred vision, conjunctival allergy

Contraindications: Hypersensitivity, glaucoma (narrow-angle)

Precautions: Severe hypertension, diabetes, hyperthyroidism, elderly, severe arteriosclerosis, cardiac disease, infants, pregnancy (C)

Pharmacokinetics:

INSTILL: Duration 2-3 hr

Interactions/incompatibilities:

• Increased pressor effects: MAOIs, tricyclic antidepressants

NURSING CONSIDERATIONS

Assess:

• B/P, pulse, systemic absorption does occur

Perform/provide:

• Storage in tight, light-resistant container; do not use discolored solutions

Evaluate:

• Therapeutic response: decreased eye irritation, itching

Teach patient/family:

• To report change in vision, blurring, loss of sight; breathing trouble, sweating, flushing

• Method of instillation; tilt head backward, hold dropper over eye, drop medication inside lower lid, using pressure on inside corner of eye hold 1 min, do not touch dropper to eye

• That blurred vision will decrease with repeated use of drug

• To notify physician if headache, spots, redness, pain occurs; discontinue use

• To use sunglasses if photophobia occurs

• To use exactly as prescribed

tetrahydrozoline HCl

(tet-ra-hye-drozz'a-leen)

Tyzine HCl, Tyzine Pediatric

Func. class.: Nasal decongestant

Chem. class.: Sympathomimetic amine

Action: Produces vasoconstriction (rapid, long-acting) of arterioles, thereby decreasing fluid exudation, mucosal engorgement

Uses: Nasal congestion

Dosage and routes:

• *Adult and child >6 yr:* INSTILL 2-4 gtts or sprays q4-6h prn (0.1%)

• *Child 2-6 yr:* INSTILL 2-3 gtts q4-6h prn (0.05%)

Available forms include: Sol 0.05%, 0.1%

Side effects/adverse reactions:

GI: Nausea, vomiting, anorexia

EENT: Irritation, burning, sneezing, stinging, dryness, rebound congestion

INTEG: Contact dermatitis

T

CNS: Anxiety, restlessness, tremors, weakness, insomnia, dizziness, fever, headache
Contraindications: Hypersensitivity to sympathomimetic amines
Precautions: Child <6 yr, elderly, diabetes, cardiovascular disease, hypertension, hyperthyroidism, increased ICP, prostatic hypertrophy, pregnancy (C), glaucoma
Interactions/incompatibilities:
• Hypertension: MAOIs, β-adrenergic blockers
• Hypotension: methyldopa, mecamylamine, reserpine

NURSING CONSIDERATIONS
Administer:
• No more than q4h
• For <4 consecutive days
Perform/provide:
• Environmental humidification to decrease nasal congestion, dryness
• Storage in light-resistant containers; do not expose to high temperatures
Evaluate:
• Therapeutic response: decreased nasal congestion
• Redness, swelling, pain in nasal passages
Teach patient/family:
• That stinging may occur for several applications; drying of mucosa may be decreased by environmental humidification
• To notify physician if irregular pulse, insomnia, dizziness, or tremors occur
• Proper administration to avoid systemic absorption

theophylline, theophylline sodium glycinate

(thee-off'i-lin)

Aquaphyllin, Bronkodyl, Elixophyllin, Slo-Phyllin, Somophyllin-T/Accurbron, Aerolate, Aquaphyllin, Asmalix, Elixicon, Elixomin, Elixophyllin, Lanophyllin, Lixolin, Theo-Dur, Theo-24, Theo-Dur Sprinkle, Theolair, Theolixir, Theon, Theophyl, Lodrane, Slo-bid, Slo-Phyllin, Theovent, Theo-Time

Func. class.: Spasmolytic
Chem. class.: Xanthine, ethylenediamide

Action: Relaxes smooth muscle of respiratory system by blocking phosphodiesterase, which increases cyclic AMP
Uses: Bronchial asthma, bronchospasm of COPD, chronic bronchitis
Dosage and routes:
Bronchospasm, bronchial asthma
• *Adult:* PO 100-200 mg q6h, dosage must be individualized; REC 250-500 mg q8-12h
• *Child:* PO 50-100 mg q6h, not to exceed 12 mg/kg/24 hr
COPD, chronic bronchitis
• *Adult:* PO 330-660 mg q6-8h pc (sodium glycinate)
• *Child >12 yr:* PO 220-330 mg q6-8h pc (sodium glycinate)
• *Child 6-12 yr:* PO 330 mg q6-8h pc (sodium glycinate)
• *Child 3-6 yr:* PO 110-165 mg q6-8h pc (sodium glycinate)
• *Child 1-3 yr:* PO 55-110 mg q6-8h pc (sodium glycinate)
Available forms include: Caps 50, 100, 200, 250 mg; tabs 100, 125, 200, 225, 250, 300 mg; tabs time-release 100, 200, 250, 300, 400, 500 mg; caps time-release 50, 65, 100, 125, 130, 200, 250, 260, 300,

400, 500 mg; elix 80, 11.25 mg/15 ml; sol 80 mg/15 ml; liq 80, 150, 160 mg/15 ml; susp 300 mg/15 ml

Side effects/adverse reactions:

CNS: Anxiety, restlessness, insomnia, dizziness, convulsions, headache, light-headedness, muscle twitching

CV: Palpitations, sinus tachycardia, hypotension, other dysrhythmias

GI: Nausea, vomiting, anorexia, diarrhea, bitter taste, dyspepsia, gastric distress

RESP: Increased rate

INTEG: Flushing, urticaria

Contraindications: Hypersensitivity to xanthines, tachydysrhythmias

Precautions: Elderly, CHF, cor pulmonale, hepatic disease, active peptic ulcer disease, diabetes mellitus, hyperthyroidism, hypertension, children, pregnancy (C)

Pharmacokinetics:

SOL: Peak 1 hr, metabolized in liver, excreted in urine, breast milk, crosses placenta

Interactions/incompatibilities:

• Increased action of theophylline: cimetidine, propranolol, erythromycin, troleandomycin

• May increase effects of: anticoagulants

• Cardiotoxicity: β-blockers

• Decreased effect of: lithium

NURSING CONSIDERATIONS

Assess:

• Theophylline blood levels (therapeutic level is 10-20 μg/ml); toxicity may occur with small increase above 20 μg/ml

• Monitor I&O; diuresis occurs, dehydration may result in elderly or children

• Signs of toxicity: irritability, insomnia, restlessness, tremors, nausea, vomiting

Administer:

• PO after meals to decrease GI symptoms; absorption may be affected

Evaluate:

• Therapeutic response: ability to breathe more easily

• Respiratory rate, rhythm, depth; auscultate lung fields bilaterally; notify physician of abnormalities

• Allergic reactions: rash, urticaria; if these occur, drug should be discontinued

Teach patient/family

• To check OTC medications, current prescription medications for ephedrine, which will increase stimulation, to avoid alcohol or caffeine

• To avoid hazardous activities; dizziness may occur

• That if GI upset occurs, to take drug with 8 oz water; avoid food, absorption may be decreased

• Not to crush, dissolve, or chew slow-release products

• That contents of bead-filled capsule may be sprinkled over food for children's use

• To notify physician of toxicity: nausea, vomiting, anxiety, insomnia, convulsions

• To notify physician of change in smoking habit; dosage may need to be changed

thiabendazole

(thye-a-ben'da-zole)

Mintezol, Minzolum

Func. class.: Anthelmintic

Chem. class.: Benzimadazole derivative

Action: Inhibits anaerobic metabolism, disrupts microtubules

Uses: Pinworm, roundworm, threadworm, whipworm, trichinosis, hookworm, cutaneous larva migrans (creeping eruption)

Dosage and routes:

• *Adult and child:* PO 25 mg/kg in 2 doses qd × 2-5 days, not to exceed 3 g/day

Available forms include: Tabs, chew 500 mg; oral susp 500 mg/5 ml

Side effects/adverse reactions:

SYST: ***Anaphylaxis***

GU: ***Hematuria, nephrotoxicity,*** enuresis, abnormal smell of urine

INTEG: Rash, pruritus

CNS: Dizziness, headache, drowsiness, fever, flushing, ***convulsions,*** behavioral changes

EENT: Tinnitus, blurred vision, xanthopsia

GI: *Nausea, vomiting, anorexia,* diarrhea, jaundice, liver damage, epigastric distress

CV: Hypotension, bradycardia

Contraindications: Hypersensitivity

Precautions: Severe malnutrition, hepatic disease, renal disease, anemia, severe dehydration, child <14 kg, pregnancy (C)

Pharmacokinetics:

PO: Peak 1-2 hr, metabolized completely by liver, excreted in feces, urine

NURSING CONSIDERATIONS

Assess:

• Stools periodically during entire treatment

Administer:

• Suspension after shaking

• PO after meals to avoid GI symptoms

Perform/provide:

• Storage in tight containers

Evaluate:

• Therapeutic response: stools negative for helmintics

Teach patient/family:

• Proper hygiene after BM including handwashing technique; tell patient to avoid putting fingers in mouth

• That infected person should sleep alone; do not shake bed linen; change bed linen qd

• To clean toilet qd with disinfectant (green soap solution)

• Need for compliance with dosage schedule, duration of treatment

• To drink fruit juice to remove mucus that intestinal tapeworms burrow in; aids in expulsion of worms

• To avoid hazardous activities if drowsiness occurs

Treatment of overdose: Induce emesis or gastric lavage

---

thiamine HCl (vitamin B_1)

Apatate Drops, Betaline S, Betaxin,* Revitonus, Thia

Func. class.: Vitamin B_1

Chem. class.: Water soluble

Action: Needed for pyruvate metabolism

Uses: Vitamin B_1 deficiency or polyneuritis, cheilosis adjunct with thiamine beriberi, Wernicke-Korsakoff syndrome, pellagra

Dosage and routes:

Beriberi

• *Adult:* IM 10-500 mg tid × 2 wk, then 5-10 mg qd × 1 mo

• *Child:* IM 10-50 mg qd × 4-6 wk

Anemia/alcoholism/pregnancy/pellagra

• *Adult:* PO 100 mg qd

• *Child:* PO 10-50 mg qd in divided doses

Beriberi with cardiac failure

• *Adult and child:* IV 100-500 mg

Wernicke's encephalopathy

• *Adult:* IV 500 mg or less, then 100 mg bid

Available forms include: Tabs 5,

---

* Available in Canada only

10, 25, 50, 100, 250, 500 mg; inj IM, IV 100, 200 mg/ml
Side effects/adverse reactions:
CNS: Weakness, restlessness
GI: Hemorrhage, ***nausea, diarrhea***
CV: ***Collapse, pulmonary edema,*** hypotension
INTEG: ***Angioneurotic edema,*** cyanosis, sweating, warmth
SYST: ***Anaphylaxis***
EENT: Tightness of throat
Contraindications: None known
Precautions: Pregnancy (A)
Pharmacokinetics:
PO/INJ: Unused amounts excreted in urine (unchanged)

NURSING CONSIDERATIONS

Assess:
- Thiamine levels throughout treatment

Administer:
- By IM injection, rotate sites if pain and inflammation occur; do not mix with alkaline solutions; Z-track to minimize pain
- Application of cold may decrease pain

Perform/provide:
- Storage in tight, light-resistant container

Evaluate:
- Therapeutic response: absence of nausea, vomiting, anorexia, insomnia, tachycardia, paresthesias, depression, muscle weakness
- Nutritional status: yeast, beef, liver, whole or enriched grains, legumes

Teach patient/family:
- Necessary foods to be included in diet: yeast, beef, liver, legumes, whole grain

thiethylperazine maleate

(thye-eth-il-per'-a-zeen)
Torecan
Func. class.: Antiemetic
Chem. class.: Phenothiazine, piperazine derivative

Action: Acts centrally by blocking chemoreceptor trigger zone, which in turn acts on vomiting center
Uses: Nausea, vomiting
Dosage and routes:
- *Adult:* PO/IM/REC 10 mg/qd-tid

Available forms include: Tabs 10 mg; supp 10 mg; inj 5 mg/ml
Side effects/adverse reactions:
GU: Urinary retention, dark urine
CNS: *Euphoria, depression,* restlessness, tremor, extrapyramidal symptoms, ***convulsions,*** drowsiness
GI: Nausea, vomiting, anorexia, dry mouth, diarrhea, constipation, weight loss, metallic taste, cramps
CV: ***Circulatory failure, tachycardia***, postural hypotension, EKG changes
RESP: ***Respiratory depression***
Contraindications: Hypersensitivity to phenothiazines, coma, seizure, encephalopathy, bone marrow depression
Precautions: Children <2 yr, pregnancy (C), elderly
Pharmacokinetics:
PO: Onset 45-60 min
REC: Onset 45-60 min, metabolized by liver, excreted by kidneys, crosses placenta, excreted in breast milk
Interactions/incompatibilities:
- Decreased effect of thiethylperazine: barbiturates, antacids
- Increased anticholinergic action:

anticholinergics, antiparkinson drugs, antidepressants

• Do not mix with other drug in syringe or solution

NURSING CONSIDERATIONS

Assess:

• VS, B/P; check patients with cardiac disease more often

Administer:

• IM injection in large muscle mass; aspirate to avoid IV administration

Evaluate:

• Therapeutic response: absence of nausea, vomiting

• Respiratory status before, during, after administration of emetic; check rate, rhythm, character; respiratory depression can occur rapidly with elderly or debilitated patients

Teach patient/family:

• To avoid hazardous activities, activities requiring alertness; dizziness may occur

---

thioguanine (6-TG)

(thye-oh-gwah'neen)

TG, 6-Thioguanine, Lanvis*

Func. class.: Antineoplastic-antimetabolite

Chem. class.: Purine analog

Action: Interferes with synthesis, utilization of purine nucleotides; effect is related to substitution of ribonucleotides into DNA

Uses: Acute leukemias, chronic granulocytic leukemia, lymphomas, multiple myeloma, solid tumors

Dosage and routes:

• *Adult and child:* PO 2 mg/kg/day, then increase slowly to 3 mg/kg/day after 4 wk

Available forms include: Tabs 40 mg

Side effects/adverse reactions:

HEMA: ***Thrombocytopenia, leukopenia, myelosuppression, anemia***

GI: Nausea, vomiting, anorexia, diarrhea, stomatitis, ***hepatotoxicity,*** gastritis, jaundice

GU: ***Renal failure,*** hyperuricemia, oliguria

INTEG: Rash, dermatitis, dry skin

Contraindications: Prior drug resistance, leukopenia ($<2500/mm^3$), thrombocytopenia ($<100{,}000/mm^3$), anemia, pregnancy (D)

Precautions: Liver disease

Pharmacokinetics: Oral form absorbed only 30%, metabolized in liver, only small amounts excreted in urine (unchanged)

Interactions/incompatibilities:

• Increased toxicity: radiation, other antineoplastics

NURSING CONSIDERATIONS

Assess:

• CBC, differential, platelet count weekly; withhold drug if WBC is $<3500/mm^3$ or platelet count is $<100{,}000/mm^3$; notify physician of these results; drug should be discontinued

• Renal function studies: BUN, serum uric acid, urine CrCl, electrolytes before, during therapy

• I&O ratio; report fall in urine output to <30 ml/hr

• Monitor temperature q4h; fever may indicate beginning infection

• Liver function tests before, during therapy: bilirubin, alk phosphatase, AST, ALT

• Bleeding time, coagulation time during treatment

Administer:

• Antacid before oral agent; give drug after evening meal before bedtime

• Antiemetic 30-60 min before giving drug to prevent vomiting

---

*Available in Canada only

• Allopurinol or sodium bicarbonate to maintain uric acid levels, alkalinization of urine
• Antibiotics for prophylaxis of infection
• Topical or systemic analgesics for pain
• Transfusion for anemia

Perform/provide:
• Strict medical asepsis, protective isolation if WBC levels are low
• Liquid diet: carbonated beverage, Jell-O; dry toast, crackers may be added when patient is not nauseated or vomiting
• Increase fluid intake to 2-3 L/day to prevent urate deposits, calculi formation, unless contraindicated
• Diet low in purines: absence of organ meats (kidney, liver), dried beans, peas to maintain alkaline urine
• Rinsing of mouth tid-qid with water, club soda, brushing of teeth bid-tid with soft brush or cotton-tipped applicators for stomatitis; use unwaxed dental floss
• Nutritious diet with iron, vitamin supplements as ordered
• Storage in tightly closed container in cool environment

Evaluate:
• Therapeutic response: decreased tumor size, spread of malignancy
• Bleeding: hematuria, guaiac, bruising, petechiae, mucosa or orifices q8h
• Food preferences; list likes, dislikes
• Hepatotoxicity: yellowing of skin, sclera, dark urine, clay-colored stools, pruritus, abdominal pain, fever, diarrhea
• Buccal cavity q8h for dryness, sores, ulceration, white patches, oral pain, bleeding, dysphagia
• Symptoms indicating severe allergic reaction: rash, urticaria, itching, flushing

Teach patient/family:
• Why protective isolation precautions are needed
• To report any complaints, side effects to nurse or physician: black tarry stools, chills, fever, sore throat, bleeding, bruising, cough, shortness of breath, dark, bloody urine
• To avoid foods with citric acid, hot or rough texture if stomatitis is present
• To report stomatitis: any bleeding, white spots, ulcerations in mouth; tell patient to examine mouth qd, report symptoms
• That contraceptive measures are recommended during therapy
• To drink 10-12 (8 oz) glasses of fluid/day

Lab test interferences:
Increase: Uric acid (blood, urine)

thiopental sodium

(thye-oh-pen'tal)
Pentothal

Func. class.: General anesthetic
Chem. class.: Barbiturate

Controlled Substance Schedule III

Action: Acts in reticular-activating system to produce anesthesia

Uses: Short general anesthesia, narcoanalysis, induction anesthesia before other anesthetics

Dosage and routes:

Induction
• *Adult:* IV 210-280 mg or 3-5 ml/kg

General anesthetic
• *Adult:* IV 50-75 mg given at 20-40 sec intervals

Narcoanalysis
• *Adult:* IV 200 mg/min, not to exceed 50 ml/min

T

Sedation or narcosis
• *Adult:* Rec 12-20 mg/lb
Available forms include: Inj IV, rectal sus
Side effects/adverse reactions:
RESP: ***Respiratory depression, bronchospasm***
CNS: Retrograde amnesia, prolonged somnolence
CV: Tachycardia, hypotension, ***myocardial depression, dysrhythmias***
EENT: Sneezing, coughing
INTEG: Chills, *shivering,* necrosis, pain at injection site
MS: Muscle irritability
Contraindications: Hypersensitivity, status asthmaticus, hepatic/intermittent porphyrias
Precautions: Severe cardiovascular disease, renal disease, hypotension, liver disease, myxedema, myasthenia gravis, asthma, increased intracranial pressure, pregnancy (C)
Pharmacokinetics:
IV: Onset 30-40 sec; half-life 11½ hr, crosses placenta
Interactions/incompatibilities:
• Increased action: CNS depressants
• Do not mix with atropine or silicone in solution or syringe

NURSING CONSIDERATIONS
Assess:
• VS q3-5min during IV administration, after dose, q4hr postoperatively
Administer:
• IV after diluting 500 mg/20 ml sterile H_2O for inj; give each 25 mg or less/min, titrate to response
• Only with crash cart, resuscitative equipment nearby
Evaluate:
• Therapeutic response: maintenance of anesthesia
• Extravasation, if it occurs use nitroprusside or chloroprocaine to decrease pain, increase circulation
• Dysrhythmias or myocardial depression

thioridazine HCl

(thye-or-rid' a-zeen)
Mellaril, Millazine, Novoridazine,* SK Thioridazine
Func. class.: Antipsychotic/neuroleptic
Chem. class.: Phenothiazine, piperidine

Action: Depresses cerebral cortex, hypothalamus, limbic system, which control activity, aggression; blocks neurotransmission produced by dopamine at synapse; exhibits strong α-adrenergic, anticholinergic blocking action; mechanism for antipsychotic effects is unclear
Uses: Psychotic disorders, schizophrenia, behavioral problems in children, alcohol withdrawal as adjunct, anxiety, major depressive disorders, organic brain syndrome
Dosage and routes:
Psychosis
• *Adult:* PO 25-100 mg tid, max dose 800 mg/day; dose is gradually increased to desired response, then reduced to minimum maintenance
Depression/behavioral problems/organic brain syndrome
• *Adult:* PO 25 tid, range from 10 mg bid-qid to 50 mg tid-qid
• *Child 2-12 yr:* PO 0.5-3 mg/kg/day in divided doses
Available forms include: Tabs 10, 15, 25, 50, 100, 150, 200, 300 mg; conc 30, 100 mg/ml; susp 25, 100 mg/5 ml
Side effects/adverse reactions:
RESP: ***Laryngospasm,*** dyspnea, ***respiratory depression***

*Available in Canada only

CNS: Extrapyramidal symptoms (rare): pseudoparkinsonism, akathisia, dystonia, tardive dyskinesia, ***seizures,*** *headache,* confusion
HEMA: Anemia, ***leukopenia, leukocytosis, agranulocytosis***
INTEG: Rash, photosensitivity, dermatitis
EENT: Blurred vision, glaucoma, dry eyes
GI: Dry mouth, nausea, vomiting, anorexia, constipation, diarrhea, jaundice, weight gain
GU: Urinary retention, urinary frequency, enuresis, impotence, amenorrhea, gynecomastia
CV: Orthostatic hypotension, ***cardiac arrest,*** ECG changes, ***tachycardia***

Contraindications: Hypersensitivity, blood dyscrasias, coma, child <2 yr, brain damage, bone marrow depression

Precautions: Pregnancy (C), lactation, seizure disorders, hypertension, hepatic disease, cardiac disease

Pharmacokinetics:
PO: Onset erratic, peak 2-4 hr; metabolized by liver, excreted in urine, crosses placenta, enters breast milk, half-life 26-36 hr

Interactions/incompatibilities:
- Oversedation: other CNS depressants, alcohol, barbiturate anesthetics
- Toxicity: epinephrine
- Decreased absorption: aluminum hydroxide or magnesium hydroxide antacids
- Decreased effects of: lithium, levodopa
- Increased effects of both drugs: β-adrenergic blockers, alcohol
- Increased anticholinergic effects: anticholinergics

NURSING CONSIDERATIONS

Assess:
- Mental status before initial administration
- Swallowing of PO medication; check for hoarding or giving of medication to other patients
- I&O ratio; palpate bladder if low urinary output occurs
- Bilirubin, CBC, liver function studies monthly
- Urinalysis is recommended before and during prolonged therapy

Administer:
- Antiparkinsonian agent, after securing order from physician to be used if extrapyramidal symptoms occur
- Concentrate mixed in citrus juices or distilled or acidified tap water

Perform/provide:
- Decreased noise input by dimming lights, avoiding loud noises
- Supervised ambulation until stabilized on medication; do not involve in strenuous exercise program because fainting is possible; patient should not stand still for long periods of time
- Increased fluids to prevent constipation
- Sips of water, candy, gum for dry mouth
- Storage in tight, light-resistant container, avoid contact with skin

Evaluate:
- Therapeutic response: decrease in emotional excitement, hallucinations, delusions, paranoia, reorganization of patterns of thought, speech
- Affect, orientation, LOC, reflexes, gait, coordination, sleep pattern disturbances
- B/P standing and lying; also include pulse and respirations q4h during initial treatment; establish

T

baseline before starting treatment; report drops of 30 mm Hg

- Dizziness, faintness, palpitations, tachycardia on rising
- Extrapyramidal symptoms including akathisia (inability to sit still, no pattern to movements), tardive dyskinesia (bizarre movements of jaw, mouth, tongue, extremities), pseudoparkinsonism (rigidity, tremors, pill rolling, shuffling gait)
- For neuroleptic malignant syndrome: altered mental status, muscle rigidity, increased CPK, hyperthermia
- Skin turgor daily
- Constipation, urinary retention daily; if these occur, increase bulk, water in diet

Teach patient/family:

- That orthostatic hypotension occurs frequently, and to rise from sitting or lying position gradually; to avoid hazardous activities until stabilized on medication
- To remain lying down after IM injection for at least 30 min
- To avoid hot tubs, hot showers, or tub baths since hypotension may occur
- To avoid abrupt withdrawal of thioridazine or extrapyramidal symptoms may result; drugs should be withdrawn slowly
- To avoid OTC preparations (cough, hayfever, cold) unless approved by physician since serious drug interactions may occur; avoid use with alcohol or CNS depressants, increased drowsiness may occur
- To use a sunscreen during sun exposure to prevent burns
- Regarding compliance with drug regimen
- About necessity for meticulous oral hygiene since oral candidiasis may occur
- To report sore throat, malaise, fever, bleeding, mouth sores; if these occur, CBC should be drawn and drug discontinued
- In hot weather, heat stroke may occur; take extra precautions to stay cool

Lab test interferences:

Increase: Liver function tests, cardiac enzymes, cholesterol, blood glucose, prolactin, bilirubin, PBI, cholinesterase, ^{131}I

Decrease: Hormones (blood, urine)

False positive: Pregnancy tests, PKU

False negative: Urinary steroids, pregnancy tests

Treatment of overdose: Lavage if orally injested, provide an airway; do not induce vomiting

---

thiotepa

(thye-oh-tep'a)

Thiotepa, TSPA

Func. class.: Antineoplastic

Chem. class.: Alkylating agent

Action: Responsible for cross-linking DNA strands leading to cell death

Uses: Hodgkin's disease, lymphomas; breast, ovarian, lung, bladder, cancer; neoplastic effusions

Dosage and routes:

- *Adult:* IV 50.2 mg/kg × 5 days, then 0.2 mg/kg q1-3 wk

Neoplastic effusions

- *Adult:* Intracavity 10-15 mg

Bladder cancer

- *Adult:* INSTILL 60 mg/60 ml water for inj instilled in bladder for 2 hr once weekly × 4 wk

Available forms include: Inj 15 mg, powder for inj

* Available in Canada only

Side effects/adverse reactions:
CNS: Dizziness, headache
HEMA: ***Thrombocytopenia, leukopenia, pancytopenia***
GI: Nausea, vomiting, anorexia, stomatitis
GU: Hyperuricemia, ***hematuria, amenorrhea, azoospermia***
INTEG: Rash, pruritus

Contraindications: Hypersensitivity, pregnancy (D)

Precautions: Radiation therapy, bone marrow suppression, impaired renal or hepatic function

Pharmacokinetics:
Onset slow, metabolized in liver, excreted in urine

Interactions/incompatibilities:
• Increased apnea: succinylcholine

NURSING CONSIDERATIONS

Assess:
• CBC, differential, platelet count weekly; withhold drug if WBC is <4000 or platelet count is $<75,000$; notify physician of results
• Renal function studies: BUN, serum uric acid, urine CrCl before, during therapy
• I&O ratio, report fall in urine output of 30 ml/hr
• Monitor temperature q4h (may indicate beginning infection)
• Liver function tests before, during therapy (bilirubin, AST, ALT, LDH) as needed or monthly

Administer:
• IV after diluting 15 mg/1.5 ml of sterile H_2O for inj; give over 1-3 min; may be further diluted in 50-100 ml compatible sol
• Antiemetic 30-60 min before giving drug to prevent vomiting
• Allopurinol or sodium bicarbonate to maintain uric acid levels, alkalinization of urine
• Antibiotics for prophylaxis of infection
• Local or systemic drugs for infection

Perform/provide:
• Storage in light-resistant container, refrigerate
• Strict medical asepsis, protective isolation if WBC levels are low
• Special skin care
• Increase fluid intake to 2-3 L/day to prevent urate deposits, calculi formation
• Diet low in purines: organ meats (kidney, liver), dried beans, peas to maintain alkaline urine
• Rinsing of mouth tid-qid with water; brushing of teeth bid-tid with soft brush or cotton-tipped applicators for stomatitis; use unwaxed dental floss
• Warm compresses at injection site for inflammation

Evaluate:
• Therapeutic response: decreased tumor size, spread of malignancy
• Bleeding: hematuria, guaiac, bruising or petechiae, mucosa or orifices q8h
• Food preferences; list likes, dislikes
• Inflammation of mucosa, breaks in skin
• Yellowing of skin, sclera, dark urine, clay-colored stools, itchy skin, abdominal pain, fever, diarrhea
• Buccal cavity q8h for dryness, sores, ulceration, white patches, oral pain, bleeding, dysphagia
• Symptoms indicating severe allergic reaction: rash, pruritus, urticaria, itching, flushing

Teach patient/family:
• Of protective isolation precautions
• That azoospermia or amenorrhea can occur; reversible after discontinuing treatment

- To avoid foods with citric acid, hot or rough texture
- To report any bleeding, white spots or ulcerations in mouth to physician, tell patient to examine mouth qd
- To report signs of infection: increased temperature, sore throat, flu symptoms
- To report signs of anemia: fatigue, headache, faintness, shortness of breath, irritability
- To avoid use of razors or commercial mouthwash
- To avoid use of aspirin products or ibuprofen

---

thiothixene

(thye-oh-thix'een)

Navane

Func. class.: Antipsychotic/neuroleptic

Chem. class.: Thioxanthene

Action: Depresses cerebral cortex, hypothalamus, limbic system, which control activity, aggression; blocks neurotransmission produced by dopamine at synapse; exhibits strong α-adrenergic blocking action; mechanism for antipsychotic effects is unclear

Uses: Psychotic disorders, schizophrenia, acute agitation

Dosage and routes:

- *Adult:* PO 2-5 mg bid-qid depending on severity of condition; dose is gradually increased to 15-30 mg if needed; IM 4 mg bid-qid, max dose is 30 mg qd; administer PO dose as soon as possible

Available forms include: Caps 1, 2, 5, 10, 20 mg; conc 5 mg/ml; inj IM 2 mg/ml; powder for inj 5 mg/ml

Side effects/adverse reactions:

RESP: ***Laryngospasm,*** dyspnea, ***respiratory depression***

CNS: Extrapyramidal symptoms: pseudoparkinsonism, akathisia, dystonia, tardive dyskinesia, seizures, *headache*

HEMA: Anemia, ***leukopenia, leukocytosis, agranulocytosis***

INTEG: Rash, photosensitivity, dermatitis

EENT: Blurred vision, glaucoma

GI: Dry mouth, nausea, vomiting, anorexia, constipation, diarrhea, jaundice, weight gain

GU: Urinary retention, urinary frequency, enuresis, impotence, amenorrhea, gynecomastia

CV: Orthostatic hypotension, hypertension, ***cardiac arrest,*** ECG changes, ***tachycardia***

Contraindications: Hypersensitivity, blood dyscrasias, child <12 yr, bone marrow depression, circulatory collapse, CNS depression, coma, alcoholism, CV disease, hepatic disease, Reye's syndrome, narrow-angle glaucoma

Precautions: Pregnancy (C), lactation, seizure disorders, hypertension, hepatic disease

Pharmacokinetics:

PO: Onset slow, peak 2-8 hr, duration up to 12 hr

IM: Onset 15-30 min, peak 1-6 hr, duration up to 12 hr; metabolized by liver, excreted in urine, crosses placenta, enters breast milk, half-life 34 hr

Interactions/incompatibilities:

- Oversedation: other CNS depressants, alcohol, barbiturate anesthetics
- Toxicity: epinephrine
- Decreased absorption: aluminum hydroxide or magnesium hydroxide antacids
- Decreased effects of thiothixene: lithium, levodopa
- Increased effects of both drugs: β-adrenergic blockers, alcohol

---

* Available in Canada only

• Increased anticholinergic effects: anticholinergics

NURSING CONSIDERATIONS

Assess:

• Mental status before initial administration
• Swallowing of PO medication; check for hoarding or giving of medication to other patients
• I&O ratio, palpate bladder if low urinary output occurs
• Bilirubin, CBC, liver function studies monthly
• Urinalysis is recommended before and during prolonged therapy

Administer:

• Antiparkinsonian agent, after securing order from physician to be used if EPS occur
• Concentrate mixed in citrus juices or distilled or acidified tap water
• IM injection into large muscle mass

Perform/provide:

• Decreased noise input by dimming lights, avoiding loud noises
• Supervised ambulation until stabilized on medication; do not involve in strenuous exercise program because fainting is possible; patient should not stand still for long periods of time
• Increased fluids to prevent constipation
• Sips of water, candy, gum for dry mouth
• Storage in tight, light-resistant container; place reconstituted solutions at room temperature for up to 48 hr, avoid contact with skin

Evaluate:

• Therapeutic response: decrease in emotional excitement, hallucinations, delusions, paranoia, reorganization of patterns of thought, speech
• Affect, orientation, LOC, reflexes, gait, coordination, sleep pattern disturbances
• B/P standing and lying; also include pulse and respirations q4h during initial treatment; establish baseline before starting treatment; report drops of 30 mm Hg
• Dizziness, faintness, palpitations, tachycardia on rising
• EPS including akathisia (inability to sit still, no pattern to movements), tardive dyskinesia (bizarre movements of jaw, mouth, tongue, extremities), pseudoparkinsonism (rigidity, tremors, pill rolling, shuffling gait)
• For neuroleptic malignant syndrome: muscle rigidity, altered mental status, increased CPK, hyperthermia
• Constipation, urinary retention daily; if these occur, increase bulk, water in diet

Teach patient/family:

• That orthostatic hypotension occurs frequently, and to rise from sitting or lying position gradually; to avoid hazardous activities until stabilized on medication
• To remain lying down after IM inj for at least 30 min
• To avoid hot tubs, hot showers, or tub baths since hypotension may occur
• To avoid abrupt withdrawal of this drug or EPS may result; drugs should be withdrawn slowly
• To avoid OTC preparations (cough, hayfever, cold) unless approved by physician since serious drug interactions may occur; avoid use with alcohol or CNS depressants, increased drowsiness may occur
• To use a sunscreen during sun exposure to prevent burns
• Regarding compliance with drug regimen

• About EPS and necessity for meticulous oral hygiene since oral candidiasis may occur
• To report sore throat, malaise, fever, bleeding, mouth sores; if these occur, CBC should be drawn and drug discontinued
• In hot weather, heat stroke may occur; take extra precautions to stay cool

Lab test interferences:
Increase: Liver function tests, cardiac enzymes, cholesterol, blood glucose, prolactin, bilirubin, PBI, cholinesterase, ^{131}I
Decrease: Uric acid

Treatment of overdose: Lavage if orally injested, provide an airway; *do not induce vomiting*

thrombin

Thrombinar, Thrombostat

Func. class.: Hemostatic
Chem. class.: Bovine thrombin

Action: Converts fibrinogen to fibrin, promotes clotting

Uses: GI hemorrhage, bleeding in dental, plastic, nasal, laryngeal surgery, skin grafting

Dosage and routes:
• *Adult:* TOP apply 100 U/1 ml sterile isotonic NaCl or distilled water in light to moderate bleeding, or 1000-2000 U/ml sterile isotonic NaCl in severe bleeding; dry area before applying

Available forms include: Powder 1000, 5000, 10,000, 20,000, 50,000 U

Side effects/adverse reactions:
INTEG: Rash, allergic reactions
HEMA: ***Intravascular clotting when entering large blood vessels***

Contraindications: Hypersensitivity to bovine products

Precautions: Pregnancy (C)

NURSING CONSIDERATIONS

Administer:
• Only to area sponged free of blood
• After preparing with NS, isotonic saline
• After having blood available for transfusion

Perform/provide:
• Storage in refrigerator, use reconstituted solution within 3 hr, discard unused portion

Evaluate:
• Therapeutic response: control of bleeding
• For allergic reactions: fever, rash, itching, changes in VS; thrombosis formation

thyroglobulin

(thye-roe-glob'yoo-lin)
Proloid

Func. class.: Thyroid hormone
Chem. class.: Combination of natural T_4/T_3; ratio 2.5 to 1

Action: Increases metabolic rates, increases cardiac output, O_2 consumption, body temperature, blood volume, growth, development at cellular level

Uses: Hypothyroidism

Dosage and routes:
Hypothyroidism
Adult: 32 mg/day increasing q2-3wk to desired response; maintenance 65-200 mg/day

Available forms include: Tabs 32, 65, 100, 130, 200 mg

Side effects/adverse reactions:
INTEG: Sweating, alopecia
CNS: Anxiety, insomnia, tremors, headache, heat intolerance, fever, coma, thyroid storm
CV: Tachycardia, palpitations, angina, dysrhythmias, hypertension, CHF

GI: Nausea, diarrhea, increased or decreased appetite, cramps
GU: Menstrual irregularities
Contraindications: Adrenal insufficiency, myocardial infarction, thyrotoxicosis
Precautions: Elderly, angina pectoris, hypertension, ischemia, cardiac disease, pregnancy (A), lactation
Pharmacokinetics:
PO: Peak 12-48 hr, half-life 6-7 days
Interactions/incompatibilities:
• Decreased absorption of thyroglobulin: cholestyramine
• Increased effects of: anticoagulants, sympathomimetics, tricyclic antidepressants, catecholamines
• Decreased effects of: digitalis drugs, insulin, hypoglycemics
• Decreased effects of liothyronine: estrogens

NURSING CONSIDERATIONS

Assess:
• B/P, pulse before each dose
• I&O ratio
• Weight qd in same clothing, using same scale, at same time of day
• Height, growth rate if given to a child
• T_3, T_4, which are decreased, radioimmunoassay of TSH, which is increased, radio uptake, which is decreased if patient is on too low a dose of medication
• Pro-time may require decreased anticoagulant, check for bleeding, bruising
Administer:
• In AM if possible as a single dose to decrease sleeplessness
• At same time each day to maintain drug level
• Only for hormone imbalances, not to be used for obesity, male infertility, menstrual conditions, lethargy
• Lowest dose that relieves symptoms
Perform/provide:
• Removal of medication 4 wk before RAIU test
Evaluate:
• Therapeutic response: absence of depression, increased weight loss, diuresis, pulse, appetite, absence of constipation, peripheral edema, cold intolerance, pale, cool dry skin, brittle nails, alopecia, coarse hair, menorrhagia, night blindness, paresthesias, syncope, stupor, coma, rosy cheeks
• Increased nervousness, excitability, irritability, which may indicate too high dose of medication usually after 1-3 wk of treatment
• Cardiac status: angina, palpitation, chest pain, change in VS
Teach patient/family:
• To report excitability, irritability, anxiety, which indicate overdose
• Not to switch brands unless approved by physician
• That hypothyroid child will show almost immediate behavior/personality change
• That drug is not to be taken to reduce weight
• To avoid OTC preparations with iodine, read labels
• To avoid iodine food, salt iodinized, soy beans, tofu, turnips, some seafood, some bread
Lab test interferences:
Increase: CPK, LDH, AST, PBI, blood glucose
Decrease: TSH, ^{131}I uptake test, uric acid, triglycerides

thyroid USP (desiccated)

(thye-roid)

Armour Thyroid, Cholaxin,* S-P-T, Thyrar, Thyro-Teric, Thyroid Serone, Thyroid USP Enseals

Func. class.: Thyroid hormone
Chem. class.: Active thyroid hormone in natural state and ratio

Action: Increases metabolic rates, increases cardiac output, O_2 consumption, body temperature, blood volume, growth, development at cellular level

Uses: Hypothyroidism, cretinism, myxedema

Dosage and routes:

Hypothyroidism

• *Adult:* PO 65 mg qd, increased by 65 mg q30d until desired response, maintenance dose 65-195 mg qd

• *Geriatric:* PO 7.5-15 mg qd, double dose q6-8wk until desired response

Cretinism/juvenile hypothyroidism

• *Child over 1 yr:* PO up to 180 mg qd titrated to response

• *Child 4-12 mo:* PO 30-60 mg qd

• *Child 1-4 mo:* PO 15-30 mg qd, may increase q2wk, titrated to response, maintenance dose 30-45 mg qd

Myxedema

• *Adult:* PO 16 mg qd, double dose q2wk, maintenance 65-195 mg/day

Available forms include: Tabs 16, 32, 65, 98, 130, 195, 260, 325 mg; tabs enteric coated 32, 65, 130 mg; sugar-coated tabs 32, 65, 130, 195 mg; caps 65, 130, 195, 325 mg

Side effects/adverse reactions:

CNS: Insomnia, tremors, headache, thyroid storm

CV: Tachycardia, palpitations, angina, dysrhythmias, hypertension, ***cardiac arrest***

GI: Nausea, diarrhea, increased or decreased appetite, cramps

MISC: Menstrual irregularities, weight loss, sweating, heat intolerance, fever

Contraindications: Adrenal insufficiency, myocardial infarction, thyrotoxicosis

Precautions: Elderly, angina pectoris, hypertension, ischemia, cardiac disease, pregnancy (A), lactation

Pharmacokinetics:

PO: Peak 12-48 hr, half-life 6-7 days

Interactions/incompatibilities:

• Decreased absorption of thyroid: cholestyramine

• Increased effects of: anticoagulants, sympathomimetics, tricyclic antidepressants, catecholamines

• Decreased effects of: digitalis drugs, insulin, hypoglycemics

• Decreased effects of thyroid: estrogens

NURSING CONSIDERATIONS

Assess:

• B/P, pulse before each dose

• I&O ratio

• Weight qd in same clothing, using same scale, at same time of day

• Height, growth rate if given to a child

• T_3, T_4, which are decreased; radioimmunoassay of TSH, which is increased; radio uptake, which is decreased if patient is on too low a dose of medication

• Pro-time may require decreased anticoagulant, check for bleeding, bruising

Administer:

• In AM if possible as a single dose to decrease sleeplessness

• At same time each day to maintain drug level

* Available in Canada only

• Only for hormone imbalances; not to be used for obesity, male infertility, menstrual conditions, lethargy
• Lowest dose that relieves symptoms

Perform/provide:
• Removal of medication 4 wk before RAIU test

Evaluate:
• Therapeutic response: absence of depression, increased weight loss, diuresis, pulse, appetite, absence of constipation, peripheral edema, cold intolerance, pale, cool dry skin, brittle nails, alopecia, coarse hair, menorrhagia, night blindness, paresthesias, syncope, stupor, coma, rosy cheeks
• Increased nervousness, excitability, irritability, may indicate too high dose of medication usually after 1-3 wk of treatment
• Cardiac status: angina, palpitation, chest pain, change in VS

Teach patient/family:
• That hair loss will occur in child, is temporary
• To report excitability, irritability, anxiety; indicates overdose
• Not to switch brands unless directed by physician
• That hypothyroid child will show almost immediate behavior/personality change
• That treatment drug is not to be taken to reduce weight
• To avoid OTC preparations with iodine; read labels
• To avoid iodine food, salt-iodinized, soy beans, tofu, turnips, some seafood, some bread

Lab test interferences:
Increase: CPK, LDH, AST, PBI, blood glucose
Decrease: TSH, ^{131}I uptake test, uric acid, triglycerides

thyrotropin (thyroid-stimulating hormone, or TSH)

(thye-roe-troe'pin)
Thytropar
Func. class.: Thyroid hormone
Chem. class.: TSH

Action: Increases uptake of iodine by thyroid gland, increases production of thyroid hormone, increases release of thyroid hormone
Uses: Diagnosis of thyroid cancer, diagnosis of primary/secondary hypothyroidism
Dosage and routes:
Diagnosis of hypothyroidism
• *Adult:* IM/SC 10 Units qd × 1-3 days
Diagnosis of thyroid cancer
• *Adult:* IM/SC 10 IU qd × 3-7 days
Treatment of thyroid cancer
• *Adult:* IM/SC 10 Units qd × 3-8 days
Available forms include: Powder for inj 10 IU/vial
Side effects/adverse reactions:
INTEG: Urticaria
CNS: Headache, fever
CV: Tachycardia, angina, ***atrial fibrillation, CHF,*** hypotension
GI: Nausea, vomiting
SYST: ***Anaphylactic reactions***
Contraindications: Hypersensitivity, coronary thrombosis, untreated Addison's disease
Precautions: Angina pectoris, adrenal insufficiency, pregnancy (C), lactation, children
Pharmacokinetics:
IM/SC: Onset 8 hr, peak 24-48 hr

NURSING CONSIDERATIONS

Administer:
• After dilution with 2 ml sterile saline solution

- Three-day dose schedule for myxedema (pituitary)
- In combination with ^{131}I to treat thyroid cancer

Treatment of overdose: Discontinue drug, administer supportive care

---

ticarcillin disodium

(tye-kar-sill'in)

Ticaripen,* Ticar

Func. class.: Broad-spectrum antibiotic

Chem. class.: Extended-spectrum penicillin

Action: Interferes with cell wall replication of susceptible organisms; osmotically unstable cell wall swells, bursts from osmotic pressure.

Uses: Respiratory, soft tissue, urinary tract infections, bacterial septicemia; effective for gram-positive cocci *(S. aureus, S. faecalis, S. pneumoniae)*, gram-negative cocci *(N. gonorrhoeae)*, gram-positive bacilli *(C. perfringens, C. tetani)*, gram-negative bacilli *(Bacteroides, F. nucleatum, E. coli, P. mirabilis, Salmonella, M. morganii, P. rettgeri, Enterobacter, P. aeruginosa, Serratia, Peptococcus, Peptostreptococcus, Eubacterium)*

Dosage and routes:

- *Adult:* IV/IM 12-24 g/day in divided doses q3-6h, infuse over ½-2 hr
- *Child:* IV/IM 50-300 mg/kg/day in divided doses q4-8h
- *Neonates:* IV INF 75-100 mg/kg/8-12 hr

Available forms include: Inj IM, IV 1, 3, 6, 20, 30 g, IV INF 3 g

Side effects/adverse reactions:

HEMA: Anemia, increased bleeding time, ***bone marrow depression, granulocytopenia***

GI: Nausea, vomiting, diarrhea, increased AST, ALT, abdominal pain, glossitis, colitis

GU: Oliguria, proteinuria, hematuria, *vaginitis, moniliasis,* ***glomerulonephritis***

CNS: Lethargy, hallucinations, anxiety, depression, twitching, ***coma, convulsions***

META: Hypokalemia

Contraindications: Hypersensitivity to penicillins

Precautions: Hypersensitivity to cephalosporins, pregnancy (B)

Pharmacokinetics:

IM: Peak 1 hr, duration 4-6 hr

IV: Peak 30-45 min, duration 4 hr, Half-life 70 min, small amount metabolized in liver, excreted in urine, breast milk

Interactions/incompatibilities:

- Decreased antimicrobial effect of ticarcillin: tetracyclines, erythromycins, aminoglycosides IV
- Increased ticarcillin concentrations: aspirin, probenecid

NURSING CONSIDERATIONS

Assess:

- I&O ratio; report hematuria, oliguria since penicillin in high doses is nephrotoxic
- Any patient with compromised renal system since drug is excreted slowly in poor renal system function; toxicity may occur rapidly
- Liver studies: AST, ALT
- Blood studies: WBC, RBC, H&H, bleeding time
- Renal studies: urinalysis, protein, blood
- C&S before drug therapy; drug may be taken as soon as culture is taken

Administer:

- IV after diluting 1 g or less/4 ml

---

* Available in Canada only

sterile H_2O for inj; dilute further with 10-20 ml or more compatible sol; give 1 g or less/5 min or more or by intermittent INF over ½-2 hr or by continuous INF
• Drug after C&S has been completed

Perform/provide:
• Adrenalin, suction, tracheostomy set, endotracheal intubation equipment
• Adequate fluid intake (2000 ml) during diarrhea episodes
• Scratch test to assess allergy, after securing order from physician; usually done when penicillin is only drug of choice
• Storage at room temperature, reconstituted solution for 72 hr at room temperature

Evaluate:
• Therapeutic response: absence of fever, purulent drainage, redness, inflammation
• Bowel pattern before, during treatment
• Skin eruptions after administration of penicillin to 1 wk after discontinuing drug
• Respiratory status: rate, character, wheezing, tightness in chest
• Allergies before initiation of treatment, reaction of each medication; highlight allergies on chart, Kardex

Teach patient/family:
• That culture may be taken after completed course of medication
• To report sore throat, fever, fatigue (could indicate superimposed infection)
• To wear or carry Medic Alert ID if allergic to penicillins
• To notify nurse of diarrhea

Lab test interferences:
False positive: Urine glucose, urine protein

Treatment of overdose: Withdraw drug, maintain airway, administer epinephrine, aminophylline, O_2, IV corticosteroids for anaphylaxis

---

ticarcillin disodium/ clavulanate potassium

Timentin

Func. class.: Broad-spectrum antibiotic

Chem. class.: Extended-spectrum penicillin

Action: Interferes with cell wall replication of susceptible organisms; osmotically unstable cell wall swells, bursts from osmotic pressure

Uses: Respiratory, soft tissue, and urinary tract infections, bacterial septicemia; effective for gram-positive cocci *(S. aureus, S. faecalis, S. pneumoniae),* gram-negative cocci *(N. gonorrhoeae),* gram-positive bacilli *(C. perfringens, C. tetani),* gram-negative bacilli *(Bacteroides, F. nucleatum, E. coli, P. mirabilis, Salmonella, M. morganii, P. rettgeri, Enterobacter, P. aeruginosa, Serratia, Peptococcus, Peptostreptococcus, Eubacterium)*

Dosage and routes:
• *Adult:* IV INF 1 vial containing ticarcillin 3 g, clavulanate potassium 0.1 g q4-6h, infuse over 30 min
• *Child <60 kg:* 200-300 mg ticarcillin/kg/day in divided doses q4-6h

Available forms include: Inj IM, IV 3 g ticarcillin and 0.1g clavulanate; IV INF 3 g ticarcillin and 0.1 g clavulanate

Side effects/adverse reactions:
HEMA: Anemia, increased bleeding

time, ***bone marrow depression, granulocytopenia***
GI: Nausea, vomiting, diarrhea, increased AST, ALT, abdominal pain, glossitis, colitis
GU: Oliguria, proteinuria, hematuria, *vaginitis, moniliasis,* ***glomerulonephritis***
CNS: Lethargy, hallucinations, anxiety, depression, twitching, ***coma, convulsions***
META: Hyperkalemia, hypokalemia, alkalosis, hypernatremia
Contraindications: Hypersensitivity to penicillins; neonates
Precautions: Hypersensitivity to cephalosporins, pregnancy (B)
Pharmacokinetics:
IV: Peak 30-45 min, duration 4 hr, half-life 64-68 min
Interactions/incompatibilities:
• Decreased antimicrobial effect of ticarcillin: tetracyclines, erythromycins, aminoglycosides IV
• Increased ticarcillin concentrations: aspirin, probenecid

NURSING CONSIDERATIONS

Assess:
• I&O ratio; report hematuria, oliguria since penicillin in high doses is nephrotoxic
• Any patient with compromised renal system, since drug is excreted slowly in poor renal system function; toxicity may occur rapidly
• Liver studies: AST, ALT
• Blood studies: WBC, RBC, H&H, bleeding time
• Renal studies: urinalysis, protein, blood
• C&S before drug therapy; drug may be taken as soon as culture is taken
Administer:
• IV after diluting 3.1 g or less/13 ml of sterile H_2O or NaCl, shake; may further dilute in 50-100 ml or more compatible sol and run over ½ hr
• Drug after C&S has been completed
Perform/provide:
• Adrenalin, suction, tracheostomy set, endotracheal intubation equipment
• Adequate fluid intake (2000 ml) during diarrhea episodes
• Scratch test to assess allergy, after securing order from physician; usually done when penicillin is only drug of choice
• Storage at room temperature, reconstituted solution for 12-24 hr or 3-7 days refrigerated
Evaluate:
• Therapeutic response: absence of fever, purulent drainage, redness, inflammation
• Bowel pattern before, during treatment
• Skin eruptions after administration of penicillin to 1 wk after discontinuing drug
• Respiratory status: rate, character, wheezing, and tightness in chest
• Allergies before initiation of treatment, reaction of each medication; highlight allergies on chart, Kardex
Teach patient/family:
• That culture may be taken after completed course of medication
• To report sore throat, fever, fatigue (could indicate superimposed infection)
• To wear or carry Medic Alert ID if allergic to penicillins
Lab test interferences:
False positive: Urine glucose, urine protein
Treatment of overdose: Withdraw drug, maintain airway, administer epinephrine, aminophylline,

O_2, IV corticosteroids for anaphylaxis

ticlopidine

(tye-klo'-pa-deen)

Ticlid

Func. class.: Platelet aggregation inhibitor

Action: Inhibits first and second phases of ADP-induced effects in platelet aggregation

Uses: Reducing the risk of stroke in high-risk patients

Dosage and routes:

• *Adult:* PO 250 mg bid with food

Available forms include: Tabs 250 mg

Side effects/adverse reactions:

INTEG: Rash, pruritus

GI: Nausea, vomiting, diarrhea, GI discomfort, ***cholestatic jaundice, hepatitis,*** increased cholesterol, LDL, VLDL

HEMA: ***Bleeding (epistaxis, hematuria, conjunctival hemorrhage, GI bleeding), agranulocytosis, neutropenia, thrombocytopenia, erythroleukemia***

Contraindications: Hypersensitivity, active liver disease, blood dyscrasias

Precautions: Past liver disease, renal disease, elderly, pregnancy (B), lactation, children, increased bleeding risk

Pharmacokinetics: Peak 1-3 hr, metabolized by the liver, excreted in urine, feces; half-life increases with repeated dosing

Interactions/incompatibilities:

• Increased bleeding tendencies: anticoagulants, aspirin

• Decreased plasma levels of ticlopidine: antacids

• Decreased plasma levels of: digoxin

• Increased effects of ticlopidine: cimetidine

• Increased effects of: theophylline

NURSING CONSIDERATIONS

Assess:

• Liver function studies: AST, ALT, bilirubin, creatinine if patient is on long-term therapy

• Blood studies: CBC, HCt, Hgb, pro-time if patient is on long-term therapy

Administer:

• With food to decrease gastric symptoms

Evaluate:

• Therapeutic response: absence of stroke

Teach patient/family:

• That blood work will be necessary during treatment

• To report any unusual bleeding to physician

• To take with food or just after eating to minimize GI discomfort

• To report side effects such as diarrhea, skin rashes, subcutaneous bleeding, signs of cholestasis (yellow skin, sclera, dark urine, light-colored stools)

timolol maleate

(tye'moe-lole)

Blocadren

Func. class.: Antihypertensive

Chem. class.: Nonselective β-blocker

Action: Competitively blocks stimulation of β-adrenergic receptor within vascular smooth muscle; produces chronotropic, inotropic activity (decreases rate of SA node discharge, increases recovery time), slows conduction of AV node, decreases heart rate, which decreases O_2 consumption in myocardium; also, decreases renin-al-

T

dosterone-angiotensin system, at high doses inhibits β-2 receptors in bronchial system

Uses: Mild to moderate hypertension, sinus tachycardia, persistent atrial extrasystoles, tachydysrhythmias, prophylaxis of angina pectoris, reduction of mortality after MI

Dosage and routes:

Hypertension

• *Adult:* PO 10 mg bid, or 100 mg qd, may increase by 10 mg q2-3d, not to exceed 60 mg/day

Myocardial infarction

• *Adult:* 10 mg bid

Available forms include: Tabs 5, 10, 20 mg

Side effects/adverse reactions:

CV: Hypotension, bradycardia, ***CHF,*** edema, chest pain, bradycardia, claudication

CNS: Insomnia, dizziness, hallucinations, anxiety

GI: Nausea, vomiting, ***ischemic colitis,*** diarrhea, *abdominal pain,* ***mesenteric arterial thrombosis***

INTEG: Rash, alopecia, pruritus, fever

HEMA: ***Agranulocytosis, thrombocytopenia, purpura***

EENT: Visual changes, sore throat, *double vision,* dry burning eyes

GU: Impotence, frequency

RESP: ***Bronchospasm,*** *dyspnea,* cough, rales

META: Hypoglycemia

MUSC: Joint pain, muscle pain

Contraindications: Hypersensitivity to β-blockers, cardiogenic shock, heart block (2nd, 3rd degree), sinus bradycardia, CHF, cardiac failure

Precautions: Major surgery, pregnancy (C), lactation, diabetes mellitus, renal disease, thyroid disease, COPD, well compensated heart failure, CAD, nonallergic bronchospasm

Pharmacokinetics:

PO: Peak 2-4 hr; half-life 3-4 hr, excreted 30%-45% unchanged, 60%-65% is metabolized by liver, excreted in breast milk

Interactions/incompatibilities:

• Increased hypotension, bradycardia: reserpine, hydralazine, methyldopa, prazosin, anticholinergics

• Decreased antihypertensive effects: idomethacin

• Increased hypoglycemic effects: insulin

• Decreased bronchodilation: theophyllines

NURSING CONSIDERATIONS

Assess:

• I&O, weight daily

• B/P during initial treatment, periodically thereafter, pulse q4h; note rate, rhythm, quality

• Apical/radial pulse before administration; notify physician of any significant changes

• Baselines in renal, liver function tests before therapy begins

Administer:

• PO ac, hs, tablet may be crushed or swallowed whole

• Reduced dosage in renal dysfunction

Perform/provide:

• Storage in dry area at room temperature, do not freeze

Evaluate:

• Therapeutic response: decreased B/P after 1-2 wk

• Edema in feet, legs daily

• Skin turgor, dryness of mucous membranes for hydration status

Teach patient/family:

• To take with or immediately after meals

• Not to discontinue drug abruptly,

taper over 2 wk; may cause precipitate angina
- Not to use OTC products containing α-adrenergic stimulants (nasal decongestants, cold preparations) unless directed by physician
- To report bradycardia, dizziness, confusion, depression, fever, sore throat, shortness of breath to physician
- To take pulse at home, advise when to notify physician
- To avoid alcohol, smoking, sodium intake
- To comply with weight control, dietary adjustments, modified exercise program
- To carry Medic Alert ID to identify drug you are taking, allergies
- To avoid hazardous activities if dizziness is present
- To report symptoms of CHF: difficult breathing, especially on exertion or when lying down, night cough, swelling of extremities
- To take medication hs to maintain effect of orthostatic hypotension
- To wear support hose to minimize effects of orthostatic hypotension

Lab test interferences:
Increase: Liver function tests, renal function tests, K, uric acid
Decrease: Hct, Hgb, HDL

Treatment of overdose: Lavage, IV atropine for bradycardia, IV theophylline for bronchospasm, digitalis, O_2, diuretic for cardiac failure, hemodialysis, administer vasopressor (norepinephrine)

timolol maleate (optic)

(tye'moe-lole)
Timoptic Solution

Func. class.: β-Adrenergic blocker
Chem. class.: l-isomer

Action: Reduces production of aqueous humor by unknown mechanism

Uses: Ocular hypertension, chronic open-angle glaucoma, secondary glaucoma, aphakic glaucoma

Dosage and routes:
- *Adult:* INSTILL 1 gtt of 0.25% sol in affected eye(s) bid, then 1 gtt for maintenance, may increase to 1 gtt of 0.5% sol bid if needed

Available forms include: Sol 0.25%, 0.5%

Side effects/adverse reactions:
CNS: Weakness, fatigue, depression, anxiety, headache, confusion
GI: Nausea, anorexia, dyspepsia
EENT: Eye irritation, conjunctivitis, keratitis
INTEG: Rash, urticaria
CV: Bradycardia, hypotension, dysrhythmias
RESP: ***Bronchospasm***

Contraindications: Hypersensitivity, asthma, 2nd or 3rd degree heart block, right ventricular failure, congenital glaucoma (infants), COPD

Pharmacokinetics:
INSTILL: Onset 15-30 min, peak 1-2 hr, duration 24 hr

Interactions/incompatibilities:
- Toxicity: β-adrenergic blockers
- Increased effect: propranolol, metoprolol

NURSING CONSIDERATIONS

Evaluate:
- Therapeutic response: decreased intraocular pressure

Teach patient/family:
- To report change in vision, with

T

blurring or loss of sight, trouble breathing, sweating, flushing, since systemic absorption may occur
• Method of instillation, including pressure on lacrimal sac for 1 min, and not to touch dropper to eye
• That long-term therapy may be required
• That blurred vision will decrease with continued use of drug

tiopronin

(tye-o-pro'-nen)
Thiola
Func. class.: Orphan drug
Chem. class.: Active reducing, complexing thiol compound

Action: Prevents cystine (kidney) stone formation by increasing amount of water-soluble cystine
Uses: Prevention of kidney stone formation in patients with severe homozygous cystinuria with urinary cystine greater than 500 mg/day, who are resistant to conservative treatment
Dosage and routes:
• *Adult:* PO 800-1000 mg/day, given in divided doses tid at least 1 hr before or 2 hr after meals
• *Child:* PO 15 mg/kg/day, given in divided doses tid at least 1 hr before or 2 hr after meals
Available forms include: Tabs 100 mg
Side effects/adverse reactions:
MISC: Blunting of taste
INTEG: Erythema, maculopapular rash, wrinkling skin, lupuslike syndrome (fever, arthralgia, lymphadenopathy), pruritus
CNS: Drug fever
META: Vitamin B_6 deficiency
Contraindications: History of agranulocytosis, thrombocytopenia, aplastic anemia
Precautions: Pregnancy (C), lactation, myasthenia gravis, Goodpasture's syndrome, children <9 yr
Pharmacokinetics:
Reduction of urinary cystine of 250-500 mg on 1-2 g/day may be expected; excreted in urine 78% in 3 days

NURSING CONSIDERATIONS

Assess:
• I&O during treatment, check urine for stones, strain all urine, keep output at 2 L/day
• Diet for alkaline foods: dairy products, prevent overindulgence of sodium alkali foods since hypercalcinuria results
• Urine pH, notify physician of pH over 7
• Urinary cystine 1 mo after treatment, q3mo thereafter
Administer:
• After adequate hydration, conservative treatment: 3 L/day of fluid, 16 oz of fluid at meals and hs
Perform/provide:
• Storage at room temperature
Evaluate:
• Therapeutic response: decrease in urinary cystine to <250 mg/L, absence of pain or hematuria
Teach patient/family:
• To watch for lupuslike syndrome: fever, joint pain, swollen lymph glands; drug may need to be discontinued

tobramycin (ophthalmic)

(toe-bra-mye'sin)
Nebcin, Tobrex
Func. class.: Antiinfective
Chem. class.: Aminoglycoside

Action: Inhibits bacterial protein synthesis
Uses: Infection of eye

* Available in Canada only

Dosage and routes:
• *Adult and child:* INSTILL 1-2 gtts q1-4h depending on infection; OINT: 1 cm bid-tid
Available forms include: Oint 0.3%; sol 0.3%
Side effects/adverse reactions:
EENT: Poor corneal wound healing, visual haze, (temporary), overgrowth of nonsusceptible organisms
Contraindications: Hypersensitivity
Precautions: Antibiotic hypersensitivity, pregnancy (D)

NURSING CONSIDERATIONS
Administer:
• After washing hands, cleanse crusts or discharge from eye before application
• Apply pressure on lacrimal sac for 1 min
Perform/provide:
• Storage at room temperature
Evaluate:
• Therapeutic response: absence of redness, inflammation, tearing
• Allergy: itching, lacrimation, redness, swelling
Teach patient/family:
• To use drug exactly as prescribed
• Not to use eye make-up, towels, washcloths, or eye medication of others, or reinfection may occur
• That drug container tip should not be touched to eye
• To report itching, increased redness, burning, stinging; drug should be discontinued
• That drug may cause blurred vision when ointment is applied

---

tobramycin sulfate
(toe-bra-mye'sin)
Nebcin
Func. class.: Antibiotic
Chem. class.: Aminoglycoside

Action: Interferes with protein synthesis in bacterial cell by binding to ribosomal subunit, causing inaccurate peptide sequence to form in protein chain, causing bacterial death
Uses: Severe systemic infections of CNS, respiratory, GI, urinary tract, bone, skin, soft tissues caused by *P. aeruginosa, E. coli, Enterobacter, Providencia, Citrobacter, Staphylococcus, Proteus, Klebsiella, Serratia*
Dosage and routes:
• *Adult:* IM/IV 3 mg/kg/day in divided doses q8h; may give up to 5 mg/kg/day in divided doses q6-8h
• *Child:* IM/IV 6-7.5 mg/kg/day in 3-4 equally divided doses
• *Neonates <1 wk:* IM up to 4 mg/kg/day in divided doses q12h; IV up to 4 mg/kg/day in divided doses q12h diluted in 50-100 mg NS or D_5W; give over 30-60 min
Available forms include: Inj IM, IV 10, 40 mg/ml; powder for inj 1.2 g; inj 20 mg/2 ml
Side effects/adverse reactions:
GU: ***Oliguria, hematuria, renal damage, azotemia, renal failure, nephrotoxicity***
CNS: Confusion, depression, numbness, tremors, ***convulsions,*** muscle twitching, ***neurotoxicity,*** dizziness, vertigo
EENT: ***Ototoxicity,*** deafness, visual disturbances, tinnitus
HEMA: ***Agranulocytosis, thrombocytopenia, leukopenia, eosinophilia,*** anemia
GI: Nausea, vomiting, anorexia, increased ALT, AST, bilirubin, hepatomegaly, ***hepatic necrosis,*** splenomegaly
CV: Hypotension, hypertension, palpitation
INTEG: Rash, burning, urticaria, dermatitis, alopecia
Contraindications: Severe renal

T

disease, hypersensitivity to aminoglycosides

Precautions: Neonates, mild renal disease, pregnancy (D), myasthenia gravis, lactation, hearing deficits, Parkinson's disease

Pharmacokinetics:

IM: Onset rapid, peak 1-2 hr

IV: Onset immediate, peak 1-2 hr

Plasma half-life 1-3 hr, not metabolized, excreted unchanged in urine, crosses placental barrier

Interactions/incompatibilities:

- Increased ototoxicity, neurotoxicity, nephrotoxicity: other aminoglycosides, amphotericin B, polymyxin, vancomycin, ethacrynic acid, furosemide, mannitol, methoxyflurane, cisplatin, cephalosporins, bacitracin
- Do not mix in solution or syringe: carbenicillin, ticarcillin, amphotericin B, cephalothin, erythromycin, heparin
- Increased effects: nondepolarizing muscle relaxants, succinylcholine

NURSING CONSIDERATIONS

Assess:

- Weight before treatment; calculation of dosage is usually done based on ideal body weight, but may be calculated on actual body weight
- I&O ratio, urinalysis daily for proteinuria, cells, casts; report sudden change in urine output
- VS during infusion, watch for hypotension, change in pulse
- IV site for thrombophlebitis including pain, redness, swelling q30min, change site if needed; apply warm compresses to discontinued site
- Serum peak, drawn at 30-60 min after IV infusion or 60 min after IM injection, trough level drawn just before next dose; blood level should be 2-4 times bacteriostatic level
- Urine pH if drug is used for UTI; urine should be kept alkaline

Administer:

- IV diluted in 50-100 ml NS or D_5W (adult), infuse over 20-60 min
- IM injection in large muscle mass, rotate injection sites
- Drug in evenly spaced doses to maintain blood level
- Bicarbonate to alkalinize urine if ordered in treating UTI, as drug is most active in an alkaline environment

Perform/provide:

- Adequate fluids of 2-3 L/day unless contraindicated to prevent irritation of tubules
- Flush of IV line with NS or D_5W after infusion
- Supervised ambulation, other safety measures with vestibular dysfunction

Evaluate:

- Therapeutic response: absence of fever, draining wounds, negative C&S after treatment
- Renal impairment by securing urine for CrCl testing, BUN, serum creatinine; lower dosage should be given in renal impairment (CrCl <80 ml/min)
- Deafness by audiometric testing, ringing, roaring in ears, vertigo; assess hearing before, during, after treatment
- Dehydration: high sp gr, decrease in skin turgor, dry mucous membranes, dark urine
- Overgrowth of infection: increased temperature, malaise, redness, pain, swelling, perineal itching, diarrhea, stomatitis, change in cough, sputum
- C&S before starting treatment to identify infecting organism
- Vestibular dysfunction: nausea,

vomiting, dizziness, headache, drug should be discontinued if severe

• Injection sites for redness, swelling, abscesses; use warm compresses at site

Teach patient/family:

• To report headache, dizziness, symptoms of overgrowth of infection, renal impairment

• To report loss of hearing, ringing, roaring in ears, feeling of fullness in head

Treatment of overdose: Hemodialysis, monitor serum levels of drug

---

tocainide HCl

(toe-kay'nide)

Tonocard

Func. class.: Antidysrhythmic (Class IB)

Chem. class.: Lidocaine analog

Action: Decreases sodium and potassium, resulting in decreased excitability of myocardial cells

Uses: PVCs, ventricular tachycardia

Dosage and routes:

• *Adult:* PO 600 mg loading dose, then 400 mg q8h

Available forms include: Tabs 400, 600 mg

Side effects/adverse reactions:

CNS: Headache, dizziness, involuntary movement, confusion, psychosis, restlessness, irritability, paresthesias, tremors, ***seizures***

EENT: Tinnitus, blurred vision, hearing loss

GI: Nausea, vomiting, anorexia, diarrhea, hepatitis

CV: Hypotension, bradycardia, angina, PVCs, ***heart block, cardiovascular collapse, arrest, CHF,*** chest pain, tachycardia

RESP: Dyspnea, ***respiratory depression, pulmonary fibrosis***

INTEG: Rash, urticaria, edema, swelling

HEMA: ***Blood dyscrasias: leukopenia, agranulocytosis, hypoplastic anemia, thrombocytopenia***

Contraindications: Hypersensitivity to amides, severe heart block

Precautions: Pregnancy (C), lactation, children, renal disease, liver disease, CHF, respiratory depression, myasthenia gravis, blood dyscrasias

Pharmacokinetics:

PO: Peak 0.5-3 hr; half-life 10-17 hr, metabolized by liver, excreted in urine

Interactions/incompatibilities:

• Increased effects: propranolol, quinidine and all other antidysrhythmics

NURSING CONSIDERATIONS

Assess:

• Chest x-ray, pulmonary function tests, liver enzymes during treatments

• CBC during beginning treatment

• I&O ratio; check for decreasing output

• Blood levels (therapeutic level 4-10 μg/ml)

• B/P continuously for fluctuations

• Lung fields, bilateral rales may occur in CHF patient

• Increased respiration, increased pulse; drug should be discontinued

Evaluate:

• Therapeutic response: decreased dysrhythmia

• Toxicity: fine tremors, dizziness

• Blood dyscrasias: fatigue, sore throat, fever, bruising, increased temperature

• Cardiac rate, respiration: rate, rhythm, character

Lab test interferences:

Increase: CPK

Positive: ANA titer

T

Treatment of overdose: O_2, artificial ventilation, ECG, administer dopamine for circulatory depression, administer diazepam or thiopental for convulsions

---

tolazamide

(tole-az'a-mide)

Ronase, Tolamide, Tolinase

Func. class.: Antidiabetic

Chem. class.: Sulfonylurea (1st generation)

Action: Causes functioning β-cells in pancreas to release insulin, leading to drop in blood glucose levels; may improve binding to insulin receptors or increase the number of insulin receptors; this drug not effective if patient lacks functioning β-cells

Uses: Type II (NIDDM) diabetes mellitus

Dosage and routes:

• *Adult:* PO 100 mg/day for FBS <200 mg/dl or 250 mg/day for FBS >200 mg/dl; dose should be titrated to patient response (1 g or less/day)

Available forms include: Tabs 100, 250, 500 mg

Side effects/adverse reactions:

CNS: Headache, weakness, fatigue, lethargy, dizziness, vertigo, tinnitus

GI: Nausea, vomiting, diarrhea, constipation, gas, ***hepatotoxicity, jaundice,*** heartburn

HEMA: ***Leukopenia, thrombocytopenia, agranulocytosis, aplastic anemia, pancytopenia, hemolytic anemia***

INTEG: Rash, (rare) allergic reactions, pruritus, urticaria, eczema, photosensitivity, erythema

ENDO: ***Hypoglycemia***

Contraindications: Hypersensitivity to sulfonylureas, juvenile or brittle diabetes

Precautions: Pregnancy (C), elderly, cardiac disease, thyroid disease, severe hypoglycemic reactions, renal disease, hepatic disease

Pharmacokinetics:

PO: Completely absorbed by GI route; onset 4-6 hr, peak 4-8 hr, duration 12-24 hr; half-life 7 hr; metabolized in liver, excreted in urine (metabolites), breast milk, highly protein bound

Interactions/incompatibilities:

• Increased hypoglycemic reaction: oral anticoagulants, chloramphenicol, cimetidine, MAOIs, insulin, guanethidine, methyldopa, nonsteroidal antiinflammatories, salicylates, probenecid, sulfonamides, ranitidine

• Mask symptoms of hypoglycemia: β-blockers

• Decreased effects of both drugs: diazoxide

• Decreased action of tolazamide: calcium-channel blockers, corticosteroids, oral contraceptives, thiazide diuretics, thyroid preparations, estrogens, phenothiazines, phenytoin, rifampin, isoniazide, phenobarbital, sympathomimetics

• Disulfiram-like reaction: alcohol

NURSING CONSIDERATIONS

Administer:

• Drug 30 min before meal

Perform/provide:

• Storage in tight container in cool environment

Evaluate:

• Therapeutic response: decrease in polyuria, polydipsia, polyphagia, clear sensorium, absence of dizziness, stable gait

• Hypoglycemic / hyperglycemic reaction that can occur soon after meals

---

*Available in Canada only

Teach patient/family:

- To check for symptoms of cholestatic jaundice (dark urine, pruritus, yellow sclera); if these occur a physician should be notified
- To use a capillary blood glucose test while on this drug
- To test urine glucose levels with Chemstrip 3 × /day
- The symptoms of hypo/hyperglycemia, what to do about each
- That this drug must be continued on a daily basis; explain consequence of discontinuing drug abruptly
- To take drug in morning to prevent hypoglycemic reactions at night
- To avoid OTC medications and alcohol unless prescribed by a physician
- That diabetes is a lifelong illness, drug will not cure disease
- That all food included in diet plan must be eaten to prevent hypoglycemia
- To carry a Medic-Alert ID for emergency purposes

Treatment of overdose: 10%-50% glucose solution IV or 1 mg glucagon

tolazoline HCl

(toe-laz'a-leen)

Priscoline

Func. class.: Peripheral vasodilator

Chem. class.: Imidazoline derivative

Action: Peripheral vasodilation occurs by direct relaxation on vascular smooth muscle; also has weak α- and β-adrenergic properties

Uses: Persistent pulmonary hypertension of newborn

Dosage and routes:

- *Newborn:* IV 1-2 mg/kg via scalp vein; IV INF 1-2 mg/kg/hr

Available forms include: Inj SC, IM, IV 25 mg/ml

Side effects/adverse reactions:

CV: Orthostatic hypotension, ***tachycardia,*** dysrhythmias, hypertension, ***cardiovascular collapse***

RESP: ***Pulmonary hemorrhage***

GU: Edema, oliguria, hematuria

GI: Nausea, vomiting, diarrhea, peptic ulcer, ***GI hemorrhage, hepatitis***

INTEG: Flushing, tingling, rash, chills, sweating, increased pilomotor activity

HEMA: ***Thrombocytopenia, leukopenia***

Contraindications: Hypersensitivity, CVA, CAD

Precautions: Pregnancy (C), active peptic ulcer, lactation, mitral stenosis

Pharmacokinetics:

IM/SC: Peak 30-60 min, duration 3-4 hr, excreted in urine, half-life 3-10 hr

Interactions/incompatibilities:

- Increased effects with alcohol, β-blockers, antihypertensive
- Decrease B/P, rebound hypertension: epinephrine
- Do not mix in syringe or solution with any other drugs

NURSING CONSIDERATIONS

Assess:

- ABGs, electrolytes, VS in newborn
- B/P, pulse during treatment until stable; take B/P lying, standing; orthostatic hypotension is common
- Hepatic tests: AST, ALT, bilirubin; liver enzymes may increase
- Blood studies: CBC, platelets; watch for thrombocytopenia, agranulocytosis

Administer:

• IV undiluted, give 10 mg or less over 1 min; may be diluted in compatible sol, run over 1 hr

• Ordered analgesic if headache develops

• Intraarterially to patient in supine position

• To patient who is sitting or lying down during treatment

Perform/provide:

• Storage at room temperature, protect from light

Evaluate:

• Therapeutic response: decrease in pulmonary hypertension or pulse volume, increased temperature in extremities, ability to walk without pain

• Hepatic involvement: nausea, vomiting, jaundice; drug should be discontinued if this occurs

• For bleeding from GI tract: coffee grounds vomitus, increased pulse, pain in upper gastric area

• Affected areas for changes in temperature, color

Teach patient/family:

• To report jaundice, dark urine, joint pain, fatigue, malaise, bruising, easy bleeding, which may indicate blood dyscrasias

• That it is necessary to quit smoking to prevent excessive vasoconstriction if prescribed for PVD

• To avoid hazardous activities until stabilized on medication; dizziness may occur

Treatment of overdose: Administer IV fluids, head-low position

---

tolbutamide

(tole-byoo'ta-mide)

Mobenol,* Novobutamide,* Orinase, Oramide, Tolbutone*

Func. class.: Antidiabetic

Chem. class.: Sulfonylurea (1st generation)

Action: Causes functioning β-cells in pancreas to release insulin, leading to drop in blood glucose levels; may improve binding to insulin receptors or increase the number of insulin receptors; this drug is not effective if patient lacks functioning β-cells

Uses: Type II (NIDDM) diabetes mellitus

Dosage and routes:

• *Adult:* PO 1-2 g/day in divided doses, titrated to patient response

Available forms include: Tabs 250, 500 mg

Side effects/adverse reactions:

CNS: Headache, weakness, paresthesia, tinnitus, dizziness, vertigo

GI: Nausea, fullness, heartburn, ***hepatotoxicity, cholestatic jaundice,*** taste alteration, diarrhea

HEMA: ***Leukopenia, thrombocytopenia, agranulocytosis, aplastic anemia,*** increased AST, ALT, alk phosphatase

INTEG: Rash, allergic reactions, pruritus, urticaria, eczema, photosensitivity, erythema

ENDO: ***Hypoglycemia***

MS: Joint pains

Contraindications: Hypersensitivity to sulfonylureas, juvenile or brittle diabetes

Precautions: Pregnancy (C), elderly, cardiac disease, thyroid disease, severe hypoglycemic reactions, renal disease, hepatic disease

Pharmacokinetics:

PO: Completely absorbed by GI route; onset 30-60 min, peak 3-5 hr, duration 6-12 hr; half-life 4-5 hr; metabolized in liver, excreted in urine (metabolites), breast milk, 90%-95% is plasma protein bound

Interactions/incompatibilities:

• Increased hypoglycemic reaction: oral anticoagulants, chloramphenicol, cimetidine, MAOIs, insulin, guanethidine, methyldopa, nonste-

---

*Available in Canada only

roidal antiinflammatories, salicylates, probenecid, sulfonamides, ranitidine
• Mask symptoms of hypoglycemia: β-blockers
• Decreased effects of both drugs: diazoxide
• Increased effects of tolbutamide: insulin, MAOIs
• Decreased action of tolbutamide: calcium-channel blockers, corticosteroids, oral contraceptives, thiazide diuretics, thyroid preparations, estrogens, phenobarbital, phenytoin, rifampin, phenothiazines, sympathomimetics

NURSING CONSIDERATIONS

Administer:
• Drug 30 min before meals

Perform/provide:
• Storage in tight container in cool environment

Evaluate:
• Therapeutic response: decrease in polyuria, polydipsia, polyphagia, clear sensorium, absence of dizziness, stable gait
• Hypo/hyperglycemic reaction that can occur soon after meals

Teach patient/family:
• To check for symptoms of cholestatic jaundice (dark urine, pruritus, yellow sclera); if these occur a physician should be notified
• To use a capillary blood glucose test while on this drug
• To test urine glucose levels with Chemstrip 3 × /day
• The symptoms of hypo/hyperglycemia, what to do about each
• That this drug must be continued on a daily basis; explain consequence of discontinuing drug abruptly
• To take drug in morning to prevent hypoglycemic reactions at night
• To avoid OTC medications and alcohol unless prescribed by a physician
• That diabetes is a lifelong illness, drug will not cure disease
• That all food included in diet plan must be eaten to prevent hypoglycemia
• To carry a Medic-Alert ID for emergency purposes

Lab test interferences:
Decrease: RAIU test
Interfere: Urinary albumin

Treatment of overdose: 10%-50% glucose solution IV or 1 mg glucagon

---

tolmetin sodium

(tole'met-in)

Tolectin, Tolectin DS

Func. class.: Nonsteroidal antiinflammatory
Chem. class.: Pyrrole acetic acid derivative

Action: Inhibits prostaglandin synthesis by decreasing an enzyme needed for biosynthesis; possesses analgesic, antiinflammatory, antipyretic properties

Uses: Mild to moderate pain, osteoarthritis, rheumatoid arthritis

Dosage and routes:
• *Adult:* PO 400 mg tid-qid, not to exceed 2 g/day
• *Child >2 yr:* PO 15-30 mg/kg/day in 3 or 4 divided doses

Available forms include: Caps 400 mg; tabs 200 mg

Side effects/adverse reactions:
GI: Nausea, anorexia, vomiting, diarrhea, jaundice, ***cholestatic hepatitis,*** constipation, flatulence, cramps, dry mouth, peptic ulcer
CNS: Dizziness, drowsiness, fatigue, tremors, confusion, insomnia, anxiety, depression

T

CV: Tachycardia, peripheral edema, palpitations, dysrhythmias
INTEG: Purpura, rash, pruritus, sweating
GU: ***Nephrotoxicity: dysuria, hematuria, oliguria, azotemia***
HEMA: ***Blood dyscrasias***
EENT: Tinnitus, hearing loss, blurred vision
Contraindications: Hypersensitivity, asthma, severe renal disease, severe hepatic disease
Precautions: Pregnancy (B), lactation, children, bleeding disorders, GI disorders, cardiac disorders, hypersensitivity to other antiinflammatory agents, peptic ulcer disease
Pharmacokinetics:
PO: Peak 2 hr, half-life 3-3½ hr; metabolized in liver, excreted in urine (metabolites), excreted in breast milk, 99% protein binding
Interactions/incompatibilities:
• Increased action of: coumarin, phenytoin, sulfonamides when used with this drug

NURSING CONSIDERATIONS
Assess:
• Renal, liver, blood studies: BUN, creatinine, AST, ALT, Hgb before treatment, periodically thereafter
• Audiometric, ophthalmic exam before, during, after treatment
Administer:
• With food to decrease GI symptoms; best to take on empty stomach to facilitate absorption
Perform/provide:
• Storage at room temperature
Evaluate:
• Therapeutic response: decreased pain, stiffness, swelling in joints, ability to move more easily
• For eye, ear problems: blurred vision, tinnitus (may indicate toxicity)
Teach patient/family:
• To report blurred vision or ringing, roaring in ears (may indicate toxicity)
• To avoid driving or other hazardous activities if dizziness or drowsiness occurs
• To report change in urine pattern, weight increase, edema, pain increase in joints, fever, blood in urine (indicates nephrotoxicity)
• That therapeutic effects may take up to 1 mo

tolnaftate (topical)

(tole-naf'tate)
Aftate, Footwork, Fungatin, Genaspor, NP-27, Pitrex, Tinactin, Zeasorb-AF

Func. class.: Local antiinfective
Chem. class.: Antifungal

Action: Interferes with fungal cell membrane, which increases permeability, leaking of cell nutrients
Uses: Tinea pedis, tinea cruris, tinea corporis, tinea capitis, tinea unguium, versicolor
Dosage and routes:
• *Adult and child:* TOP apply to affected area bid for 2-6 wk, rub in
Available forms include: Cream, powder, aerosol powder, aerosol liq, gel, pump spray liquid 1%
Side effects/adverse reactions:
INTEG: Rash, urticaria, stinging
Contraindications: Hypersensitivity, nail infections
Precautions: Pregnancy (C), lactation

NURSING CONSIDERATIONS
Administer:
• Aerosol powder after shaking
• Enough medication to completely cover lesions
• After cleansing with soap, water before each application, dry well

Perform/provide:
- Storage at room temperature in dry place; do not puncture or incinerate aerosol container

Evaluate:
- Therapeutic response: decrease in size, number of lesions
- Allergic reaction: burning, stinging, swelling, redness

Teach patient/family:
- To use medical asepsis (hand washing) before, after each application
- To apply with glove to prevent further infection
- To avoid use of OTC creams, ointments, lotions unless directed by physician
- To avoid contact with eyes
- To notify physician if condition worsens or does not improve in 10 days; continue even if symptoms improve

trace elements (chromium, copper, iodide, manganese, selenium, zinc)

Func. class.: Minerals

Action: Needed for adequate absorption and synthesis of amino acids

Uses: Prevention of trace element deficiency

Dosage and routes:

Chromium
- *Adult:* IV 10-15 μg qd
- *Child:* IV 0.14-0.20 μg/kg/day

Copper
- *Adult:* IV 0.5-1.5 mg/day
- *Child:* IV .05-0.2 mg/kg/day

Iodine
- *Adult:* IV 1 μg/kg/day

Manganese
- *Adult:* IV 1-3 mg/day

Selenium
- *Adult:* 40-120 μg/day
- *Child:* 3 μg/kg/day

Zinc
- *Adult:* IV 2-4 mg/day
- *Child:* IV 0.05 mg/kg/day

Available forms include: Many forms available—see particular elements

Side effects/adverse reactions: None known

Precautions: Liver, biliary disease

NURSING CONSIDERATIONS

Assess:
- Trace element levels, notify physician if low copper 0.07-0.15 mg/ml, zinc 0.05-0.15 mg/100 ml, manganese 4-20 μg/100 ml, selenium 0.1-0.19 μg/ml

Administer:
- By IV infusion, often mixed with TPN solution

Evaluate:
- Therapeutic response: absence of element deficiency
- Trace element deficiency if patient is receiving TPN for extended periods of time

tranylcypromine sulfate

(tran-ill-sip'roe-meen)

Parnate

Func. class.: Antidepressant-MAOI

Chem. class.: Nonhydrazine

Action: Increases concentrations of endogenous epinephrine, norepinephrine, serotonin, dopamine in storage sites in CNS by inhibition of MAO; increased concentration reduces depression

Uses: Depression, when uncontrolled by other means

Dosage and routes:
- *Adult:* PO 10 mg bid, may increase to 30 mg/day after 2 wk

T

Available forms include: Tabs 10 mg

Side effects/adverse reactions:

HEMA: Anemia

CNS: Dizziness, drowsiness, confusion, headache, anxiety, tremors, stimulation, weakness, hyperreflexia, mania, insomnia, fatigue, weight gain

GI: Constipation, dry mouth, nausea, vomiting, *anorexia,* diarrhea, weight gain

GU: Change in libido, frequency

INTEG: Rash, flushing, increased perspiration

CV: Orthostatic hypotension, hypertension, dysrhythmias, hypertensive crisis

EENT: Blurred vision

ENDO: ***SIADH-like syndrome***

Contraindications: Hypersensitivity to MAOIs, elderly, hypertension, CHF, severe hepatic disease, pheochromocytoma, severe renal disease, severe cardiac disease

Precautions: Suicidal patients, convulsive disorders, severe depression, schizophrenia, hyperactivity, diabetes mellitus, pregnancy (C)

Pharmacokinetics:

Metabolized by liver, excreted by kidneys, crosses placenta, excreted in breast milk

Interactions/incompatibilities:

• Increased pressor effects: guanethidine, clonidine, indirect acting sympathomimetics (ephedrine)

• Increased effects of: direct acting sympathomimetics (epinephrine), alcohol, barbiturates, benzodiazepines, CNS depressants, levodopa

• Hyperpyretic crisis, convulsions, hypertensive episode: tricyclic antidepressants, meperidine

• Hypoglycemic effect increased: insulin

NURSING CONSIDERATIONS

Assess:

• B/P (lying, standing), pulse; if systolic B/P drops 20 mm Hg, stop drug, notify physician

• Blood studies: CBC, leukocytes, cardiac enzymes if patient is receiving long-term therapy

• Hepatic studies: ALT, AST, bilirubin, creatinine; hepatotoxicity may occur

Administer:

• Increased fluids, bulk in diet if constipation, urinary retention occur

• With food or milk for GI symptoms

• Crushed if patient is unable to swallow medication whole

• Dosage hs if oversedation occurs during day

• Gum, hard candy, or frequent sips of water for dry mouth

• Phentolamine for severe hypertension

Perform/provide:

• Storage in tight container in cool environment

• Assistance with ambulation during beginning therapy since drowsiness/dizziness occurs

• Safety measures including siderails

• Checking to see PO medication swallowed

Evaluate:

• Therapeutic response: decreased depression

• Toxicity: increased headache, palpitation, discontinue drug immediately; prodromal signs of hypertensive crisis

• Mental status: mood, sensorium, affect, memory (long, short), increase in psychiatric symptoms

• Urinary retention, constipation, edema, take weight weekly

• Withdrawal symptoms: head-

* Available in Canada only

ache, nausea, vomiting, muscle pain, weakness

Teach patient/family:

- That therapeutic effects may take 1-4 wk
- To avoid driving or other activities requiring alertness
- To avoid alcohol ingestion, CNS depressants or OTC medications: cold, weight, hay fever, cough syrup
- Not to discontinue medication quickly after long-term use
- To avoid high tyramine foods: cheese (aged), sour cream, beer, wine, pickled products, liver, raisins, bananas, figs, avocados, meat tenderizers, chocolate, yogurt; increase caffeine
- To report headache, palpitation, neck stiffness

Treatment of overdose: Lavage, activated charcoal, monitor electrolytes, vital signs, diazepam IV, $NaHCO_3$

---

trazodone HCl

(tray'zoe-done)

Desyrel

Func. class.: Antidepressant, miscellaneous

Chem. class.: Triazolopyridine

Action: Selectively inhibits serotonin uptake by brain, potentiates behavorial changes

Uses: Depression

Dosage and routes:

- *Adult:* PO 150 mg/day in divided doses, may be increase by 50 mg/day q3-4d, not to exceed 600 mg/day

Available forms include: Tabs 50, 100, 150, 300 mg

Side effects/adverse reactions:

HEMA: ***Agranulocytosis, thrombocytopenia, eosinophilia, leukopenia***

CNS: *Dizziness, drowsiness,* confusion, headache, anxiety, tremors, stimulation, weakness, insomnia, nightmares, EPS (elderly), increase in psychiatric symptoms

GI: *Diarrhea, dry mouth,* nausea, vomiting, ***paralytic ileus,*** increased appetite, cramps, epigastric distress, jaundice, ***hepatitis,*** stomatitis

GU: *Retention,* ***acute renal failure, priapism***

INTEG: Rash, urticaria, sweating, pruritus, photosensitivity

CV: *Orthostatic hypotension, ECG changes, tachycardia,* ***hypertension,*** palpitations

EENT: *Blurred vision,* tinnitus, mydriasis

Contraindications: Hypersensitivity to tricyclic antidepressants, recovery phase of myocardial infarction, convulsive disorders, prostatic hypertrophy

Precautions: Suicidal patients, severe depression, increased intraocular pressure, narrow-angle glaucoma, urinary retention, cardiac disease, hepatic disease, hyperthyroidism, electroshock therapy, elective surgery, pregnancy (C)

Pharmacokinetics:

Metabolized by liver, excreted by kidneys, feces; half-life 4.4-7.5 hr

Interactions/incompatibilities:

- Decreased effects of: guanethidine, clonidine, indirect acting sympathomimetics (ephedrine)
- Increased effects of: direct acting sympathomimetics (epinephrine), alcohol, barbiturates, benzodiazepines, CNS depressants
- Hyperpyretic crisis, convulsions, hypertensive episode: MAOI (pargyline [Eutonyl])

NURSING CONSIDERATIONS

Assess:

• B/P (lying, standing), pulse q4h; if systolic B/P drops 20 mm Hg hold drug, notify physician; take vital signs q4h in patients with cardiovascular disease

• Blood studies: CBC, leukocytes, differential, cardiac enzymes if patient is receiving long-term therapy

• Hepatic studies: AST, ALT, bilirubin, creatinine

• Weight qwk, appetite may increase with drug

• ECG for flattening of T wave, bundle branch block, AV block, dysrhythmias in cardiac patients

Administer:

• Increased fluids, bulk in diet if constipation, urinary retention occur, especially in elderly

• With food or milk for GI symptoms

• Dosage hs if oversedation occurs during day; may take entire dose hs; elderly may not tolerate once/day dosing

• Gum, hard candy, or frequent sips of water for dry mouth

Perform/provide:

• Storage in tight, light-resistant container at room temperature

• Assistance with ambulation during beginning therapy since drowsiness/dizziness occurs

• Safety measures including siderails, primarily in elderly

• Checking to see PO medication swallowed

Evaluate:

• Therapeutic response: decreased depression

• EPS primarily in elderly: rigidity, dystonia, akathisia

• Mental status: mood, sensorium, affect, suicidal tendencies, increase in psychiatric symptoms: depression, panic

• Urinary retention, constipation; constipation is more likely to occur in children

• Withdrawal symptoms: headache, nausea, vomiting, muscle pain, weakness; do not usually occur unless drug was discontinued abruptly

• Alcohol consumption; if alcohol is consumed, hold dose until morning

Teach patient/family:

• That therapeutic effects may take 2-3 wk

• To use caution in driving or other activities requiring alertness because of drowsiness, dizziness, blurred vision

• To avoid alcohol ingestion, other CNS depressants

• Not to discontinue medication quickly after long-term use; may cause nausea, headache, malaise

• To wear sunscreen or large hat since photosensitivity occurs

Lab test interferences:

Increase: Serum bilirubin, blood glucose, alk phosphatase

False increase: Urinary catecholamines

Decrease: VMA, 5-HIAA

Treatment of overdose: ECG monitoring, induce emesis, lavage, activated charcoal, administer anticonvulsant

tretinoin (vitamin A acid, retinoic acid)

(tret'i-noyn)

Retin-A, Stievaa*

Func. class.: Vitamin A acid/acne product

Chem. class.: Tretinoin derivative

Action: Decreases cohesiveness of follicular epithelium, decreases microcomedone formation

* Available in Canada only

Uses: Acne vulgaris (grades 1-3); unlabeled use: skin cancer

Dosage and routes:

• *Adult and child:* TOP cleanse area, apply hs; cover lightly

Available forms include: Top cream 0.1%, 0.05%; top gel 0.025%, 0.01%; top liq 0.05%

Side effects/adverse reactions:

INTEG: Rash, stinging, warmth, redness, erythema, blistering, crusting, peeling, contact dermatitis, hypo/hyperpigmentation

Contraindications: Hypersensitivity

Precautions: Pregnancy (B), lactation, eczema, sunburn

Pharmacokinetics:

TOP: Poor absorption, excreted in urine

Interactions/incompatibilities:

• Increase peeling: medication containing agents such as sulfur, benzoyl peroxide, resorcinol, salicylic acid

• Use with caution medicated or abrasive soaps or cleansers that have drying effect, products with high concentrations of alcohol astringents

NURSING CONSIDERATIONS

Administer:

• Once daily before hs; cover area lightly using gauze

Perform/provide:

• Storage at room temperature

• Washing of hands after application

Evaluate:

• Therapeutic response: decrease in size and number of lesions

• Area of body involved, including time involved, what helps or aggravates condition

Teach patient/family:

• To avoid application on normal skin or getting cream in eyes, nose, or other mucous membranes

• To avoid sunlight or sunlamps

• That treatment may cause warmth, stinging; dryness, peeling will occur

• That cosmetics may be used over drug, do not use shaving lotions

• That rash may occur during first 1-3 wk of therapy

• That drug does not cure condition, only relieves symptoms

---

triamcinolone/triamcinolone acetonide/triamcinolone diacetate/triamcinolone hexacetonide

(trye-am-sin'oh-lone)

Aristocort, Kenacort, Azmacort, Kenalog/Amcort/Cenocort Forte, Triam-Forte, Trisoject/Aristospan

Func. class.: Corticosteroid

Chem. class.: Glucocorticoid, intermediate-acting

Action: Decreases inflammation by suppression of migration of polymorphonuclear leukocytes, fibroblasts, reversal to increase capillary permeability and lysosomal stabilization

Uses: Severe inflammation, immunosuppression, neoplasms, asthma (steroid dependent), collagen, respiratory, dermatologic disorders

Dosage and routes:

• *Adult:* PO 4-48 mg/day in divided doses qd-qid; IM 40 mg qwk (acetonide, or diacetate), 5-48 mg into neoplasms (diacetate, acetonide), 2-40 mg into joint or soft tissue (diacetate, acetonide), 0.5 mg/sq in of affected intralesional skin (hexacetonide), 2-20 mg into joint or soft tissue (hexacetonide)

Asthma

• *Adult:* INH 2 tid-qid, not to exceed 16 INH/day

T

• *Child 6-12 yr:* INH 1-2 tid-qid, not to exceed 12 INH/day

Available forms include: Tabs 1, 2, 4, 8, 16 mg; syr 2 mg/5 ml, 4.85 mg/5 ml; inj 25, 40 mg/ml diacetate; inj 3, 10, 40 mg/ml acetonide; inj 20, 5 mg/ml hexacetonide

Side effects/adverse reactions:
INTEG: Acne, poor wound healing, ecchymosis, petechiae
CNS: Depression, flushing, sweating, headache, mood changes
CV: Hypertension, ***circulatory collapse, thrombophlebitis, embolism,*** tachycardia, edema
HEMA: ***Thrombocytopenia***
MS: Fractures, osteoporosis, weakness
GI: Diarrhea, nausea, abdominal distention, ***GI hemorrhage,*** *increased appetite,* ***pancreatitis***
EENT: Fungal infections, increased intraocular pressure, blurred vision

Contraindications: Psychosis, hypersensitivity, idiopathic thrombocytopenia, acute glomerulonephritis, amebiasis, fungal infections, nonasthmatic bronchial disease, child <2 yr, AIDS, TB

Precautions: Pregnancy (C), diabetes mellitus, glaucoma, osteoporosis, seizure disorders, ulcerative colitis, CHF, myasthenia gravis, renal disease, esophagitis, peptic ulcer

Pharmacokinetics:
PO/IM: Peak 1-2 hr, 2 days, 1-6 wk (IM), half-life 2-5 hr

Interactions/incompatibilities:
• Decreased action of triamcinolone: cholestyramine, colestipol, barbiturates, rifampin, ephedrine, phenytoin, theophylline
• Decreased effects of: anticoagulants, anticonvulsants, antidiabetics, ambenonium, neostigmine, isoniazid, toxoids, vaccines, anticholinesterases, salicylates, somatrem
• Increased side effects: alcohol, salicylates, indomethacin, amphotericin B, digitalis, cyclosporine, diuretics
• Increased action of triamcinolone: salicylates, estrogens, indomethacin, oral contraceptives, ketoconazole, macrolide antibiotics

NURSING CONSIDERATIONS

Assess:
• Potassium, blood sugar, urine glucose while on long-term therapy; hypokalemia and hyperglycemia
• Weight daily; notify physician if weekly gain >5 lb
• B/P q4h, pulse; notify physician if chest pain occurs
• I&O ratio; be alert for decreasing urinary output and increasing edema
• Plasma cortisol levels during long-term therapy (normal level: 138-635 nmol/L SI units when drawn at 8 AM)

Administer:
• After shaking suspension (parenteral)
• Titrated dose, use lowest effective dose
• IM injection deeply in large mass, rotate sites, avoid deltoid, use 21G needle
• In one dose in AM to prevent adrenal suppression, avoid SC administration, damage may be done to tissue
• With food or milk to decrease GI symptoms

Perform/provide:
• Assistance with ambulation in patient with bone tissue disease to prevent fractures

Evaluate:
• Therapeutic response: ease of respirations, decreased inflammation

---

• Infection: increased temperature, WBC, even after withdrawal of medication. Drug masks infections symptoms
• Potassium depletion: paresthesias, fatigue, nausea, vomiting, depression, polyuria, dysrhythmias, weakness
• Edema, hypertension, cardiac symptoms
• Mental status: affect, mood, behavioral changes, aggression

Teach patient/family:
• That ID as steroid user should be carried
• To notify physician if therapeutic response decreases; dosage adjustment may be needed
• Not to discontinue this medication abruptly or adrenal crisis can result
• To avoid OTC products: salicylates, alcohol in cough products, cold preparations unless directed by physician
• About cushingoid symptoms
• Symptoms of adrenal insufficiency: nausea, anorexia, fatigue, dizziness, dyspnea, weakness, joint pain

Lab test interferences:
Increase: Cholesterol, sodium, blood glucose, uric acid, calcium, urine glucose
Decrease: Calcium, potassium, T_4, T_3, thyroid ^{131}I uptake test, urine 17-OHCS, 17-KS, PBI
False negative: Skin allergy tests

triamcinolone acetonide

(trye-am-sin'oh-lone)
Acetospan, Azmacort, Aristocort, Cenocort A_2, Kenalog, Tramacort, Triami-A, Triamonide, Tri-kort, Trilog

Func. class.: Topical corticosteroid
Chem. class.: Synthetic fluorinated agent, group II potency (0.5%), group III potency (0.1%), group IV potency (0.025%)

Action: Possesses antipruritic, antiinflammatory actions
Uses: Psoriasis, eczema, contact dermatitis, pruritus
Dosage and routes:
• *Adult and child:* Apply to affected area bid-qid
Available forms include: Oint 0.025%, 0.1%, 0.5%; cream 0.025%, 0.1%, 0.5%; lotion 0.025%, 0.1%; aerosol 0.2 mg/2 sec; paste 0.1%
Side effects/adverse reactions:
INTEG: Burning, dryness, itching, irritation, acne, folliculitis, hypertrichosis, perioral dermatitis, hypopigmentation, atrophy, striae, miliaria, allergic contact dermatitis, secondary infection
Contraindications: Hypersensitivity to corticosteroids, fungal infections
Precautions: Pregnancy (C), lactation, viral infections, bacterial infections

NURSING CONSIDERATIONS

Assess:
• Temperature; if fever develops, drug should be discontinued

Administer:
• Only to affected areas; do not get in eyes
• Medication, then cover with occlusive dressing (only if prescribed), seal to normal skin,

T

change q12h; use occlusive dressing with extreme caution (group II potency), systemic absorption may occur
• Only to dermatoses; do not use on weeping, denuded, or infected area

Perform/provide:
• Cleansing before application of drug; apply to slightly moist skin; use gloves and a cotton-tipped applicator
• Treatment for a few days after area has cleared
• Storage at room temperature

Evaluate:
• Therapeutic response: absence of severe itching, patches on skin, flaking
• For systemic absorption: increased temperature, inflammation, irritation

Teach patient/family:
• To avoid sunlight on affected area; burns may occur

---

triamcinolone acetonide (topical-oral)

(trye-am-sin'oh-lone)
Kenalog in Orabase

Func. class.: Topical anesthetic
Chem. class.: Synthetic fluorinated adrenal corticosteroid

Action: Inhibits nerve impulses from sensory nerves
Uses: Oral pain
Dosage and routes:
• *Adult and child:* TOP press ¼ inch into affected area until film appears, repeat bid-tid
Available forms include: Paste 0.1%
Side effects/adverse reactions:
INTEG: Rash, irritation, sensitization
Contraindications: Hypersensitivity, infants <1 yr, application to large areas, presence of fungal, viral, or bacterial infections of mouth or throat
Precautions: Child <6 yr, sepsis, pregnancy (C), denuded skin

NURSING CONSIDERATIONS

Administer:
• After cleansing oral cavity

Evaluate:
• Therapeutic response: absence of pain in affected area
• Allergy: rash, irritation, reddening, swelling
• Infection: if affected area is infected, do not apply

Teach patient/family:
• To report rash, irritation, redness, swelling
• How to apply paste

---

triamterene

(trye-am'ter-een)
Dyrenium

Func. class.: Potassium-sparing diuretic
Chem. class.: Pteridine derivative

Action: Acts on distal tubule to inhibit reabsorption of sodium, chloride; increase potassium retention
Uses: Edema; may be used with other diuretics, hypertension
Dosage and routes:
• *Adults:* PO 100 mg bid pc, not to exceed 300 mg
Available forms include: Cap 50, 100 mg
Side effects/adverse reactions:
GI: Nausea, diarrhea, vomiting, dry mouth, jaundice, liver disease
ELECT: Hyperkalemia, hyponatremia, hypochloremia
CNS: Weakness, headache, dizziness
INTEG: Photosensitivity, rash
HEMA: ***Thrombocytopenia, mega-***

* Available in Canada only

loblastic anemia, low folic acid levels
GU: ***Azotemia, interstitial nephritis,*** increased BUN, creatinine, renal stones
Contraindications: Hypersensitivity, anuria, severe renal disease, severe hepatic disease, hyperkalemia, pregnancy (D)
Precautions: Dehydration, hepatic disease, lactation, CHF, renal disease, cirrhosis
Pharmacokinetics:
PO: Onset 2 hr, peak 6-8 hr, duration 12-16 hr; half-life 3 hr; metabolized in liver, excreted in bile and urine
Interactions/incompatibilities:
• Nephrotoxicity: indomethacin
• Enhanced action of: antihypertensives, lithium, amantadine
• Increased hyperkalemia: other potassium sparing diuretics, potassium products, ACE inhibitors, salt substitutes
NURSING CONSIDERATIONS
Assess:
• Weight, I&O daily to determine fluid loss; effect of drug may be decreased if used qd
• Electrolytes: potassium, sodium, chloride; include BUN, blood sugar, CBC, serum creatinine, blood pH, ABGs, liver function tests
Administer:
• In AM to avoid interference with sleep
• With food if nausea occurs; absorption may be decreased slightly
Evaluate:
• Therapeutic response: improvement in edema of feet, legs, sacral area daily if medication is being used in CHF
• Improvement in CVP q8h
• Signs of metabolic acidosis: drowsiness, restlessness
• Rashes, temperature elevation qd
• Confusion, especially in elderly; take safety precautions if needed
• Hydration: skin turgor, thirst, dry mucous membranes
Teach patient/family:
• To take medication after meals for GI upset
• To avoid prolonged exposure to sunlight since photosensitivity may occur
• To notify physician if weakness, headache, nausea, vomiting, dry mouth, fever, sore throat, mouth sores, unusual bleeding or bruising occurs
Lab test interferences:
Interfere: quinidine serum levels, LDH
Treatment of overdose: Lavage if taken orally, monitor electrolytes, administer IV fluids, dialysis, monitor hydration, CV, renal status

---

triazolam

(trye-ay'zoe-lam)
Halcion
Func. class.: Sedative-hypnotic
Chem. class.: Benzodiazepine

Controlled Substance Schedule IV (USA), Schedule F (Canada)
Action: Produces CNS depression at limbic, thalamic, hypothalamic levels of CNS; may be mediated by neurotransmitter γ-aminobutyric acid (GABA); results are sedation, hypnosis, skeletal muscle relaxation, anticonvulsant activity, anxiolytic action
Uses: Insomnia
Dosage and routes:
• *Adult:* PO 0.125-0.5 mg hs
• *Elderly:* PO 0.125-0.25 mg hs
Available forms include: Tabs 0.125, 0.25, 0.5 mg

T

Side effects/adverse reactions:
HEMA: ***Leukopenia, granulocytopenia*** (rare)
CNS: Headache, lethargy, drowsiness, daytime sedation, dizziness, confusion, light-headedness, anxiety, irritability, amnesia, poor coordination
GI: Nausea, vomiting, diarrhea, heartburn, abdominal pain, constipation
CV: Chest pain, pulse changes

Contraindications: Hypersensitivity to benzodiazepines, pregnancy (X), lactation, intermittent porphyria

Precautions: Anemia, hepatic disease, renal disease, suicidal individuals, drug abuse, elderly, psychosis, child < 15 yr, acute narrow-angle glaucoma, seizure disorders

Pharmacokinetics:
PO: Onset 30-45 min, duration 6-8 hr; metabolized by liver, excreted by kidneys (inactive metabolites), crosses placenta, excreted in breast milk; half-life 2-3 hr

Interactions/incompatibilities:
- Increased effects of: cimetidine, disulfiram, erythromycin
- Increased action of both drugs: alcohol, CNS depressants
- Decreased effect of: antacids

NURSING CONSIDERATIONS

Assess:
- Blood studies: Hct, Hgb, RBCs, if blood dyscrasias are suspected (rare)
- Hepatic studies: AST, ALT, bilirubin if liver damage has occurred

Administer:
- After removal of cigarettes, to prevent fires
- After trying conservative measures for insomnia
- ½-1 hr before hs for sleeplessness
- On empty stomach fast onset, but may be taken with food if GI symptoms occur

Perform/provide:
- Assistance with ambulation after receiving dose
- Safety measure: siderails, nightlight, call bell within easy reach
- Checking to see PO medication has been swallowed
- Storage in tight container in cool environment

Evaluate:
- Therapeutic response: ability to sleep at night, decreased amount of early morning awakening if taking drug for insomnia
- Mental status: mood, sensorium, affect, memory (long, short)
- Blood dyscrasias: fever, sore throat, bruising, rash, jaundice, epistaxis (rare)
- Type of sleep problem: falling asleep, staying asleep

Teach patient/family:
- That dependence is possible after long-term use
- To avoid driving or other activities requiring alertness until drug is stabilized
- To avoid alcohol ingestion or CNS depressants; serious CNS depression may result
- That effects may take 2 nights for benefits to be noticed
- Alternate measures to improve sleep: reading, exercise several hours before hs, warm bath, warm milk, TV, self-hypnosis, deep breathing
- That hangover is common in elderly, but less common than with barbiturates; rebound insomnia may occur for 1-2 nights after discontinuing drug

Lab test interferences:
Increase: ALT, AST, serum bilirubin
Decrease: RAI uptake

False increase: Urinary 17-OHCS
Treatment of overdose: Lavage, activated charcoal, monitor electrolytes, vital signs

trientine HCl

(trye-in'-teen)

Cuprid

Func. class.: Heavy metal antagonist

Chem. class.: Chelating agent (thiol compound)

Action: Binds with ions of lead, mercury, copper, iron, zinc to form a water-soluble complex excreted by kidneys
Uses: Wilson's disease
Dosage and routes:
• *Adult:* PO 750-2000 mg in divided doses bid-qid
• *Child:* PO 500-1500 mg in divided doses bid-qid
Available forms include: Caps 125, 250 mg; tabs 250 mg
Side effects/adverse reactions:
HEMA: Anemia, *iron deficiency*
INTEG: Urticaria, fever
SYST: Hypersensitivity
GI: Epigastric distress, anorexia, heartburn
Contraindications: Hypersensitivity
Precautions: Pregnancy (C)
Pharmacokinetics:
PO: Peak 1 hr, metabolized in liver, excreted in urine
Interactions/incompatibilities:
• Decreased action: mineral supplements

NURSING CONSIDERATIONS

Assess:
• Monitor hepatic, renal studies: ALT/AST, alk phosphatase, BUN, creatinine, serum copper level
• Monitor I&O
• For anemia: fatigue, Hct, Hgb
Administer:
• On an empty stomach, ½-1 hr before meals or 2 hr after meals
• B_6 daily; depleted when this drug is used
Evaluate:
• Therapeutic response: improvement in neurologic, psychiatric symptoms
• Allergic reactions (rash, urticaria); if these occur, drug should be discontinued
Teach patient/family:
• That therapeutic effect may take 1-3 mo or longer
• To report urticaria, fever, fatigue

trifluoperazine HCl

(trye-floo-oh-per'a-zeen)

Novoflurazine,* Solazine,* Suprazine, Stelazine, Terfluzine,* Triflurin*

Func. class.: Antipsychotic/neuroleptic

Chem. class.: Phenothiazine, piperazine

Action: Depresses cerebral cortex, hypothalamus, limbic system, which control activity, aggression; blocks neurotransmission produced by dopamine at synapse; exhibits strong α-adrenergic, anticholinergic blocking action; mechanism for antipsychotic effects is unclear
Uses: Psychotic disorders, nonpsychotic anxiety, schizophrenia
Dosage and routes:
Psychotic disorders
• *Adult:* PO 2-5 mg bid, usual range 15-20 mg/day, may require 40 mg/day or more; IM 1-2 mg q4-6h
• *Child >6 yr:* PO 1 mg qd or bid; IM *not recommended for children,* but 1 mg may be given qd or bid

T

Nonpsychotic anxiety

• *Adult:* PO 1-2 mg bid, not to exceed 5 mg/day; do not give longer than 12 wk

Available forms include: Tabs 1, 2, 5, 10, 20 mg; conc 10 mg/ml; inj IM 2 mg/ml

Side effects/adverse reactions:

RESP: ***Laryngospasm,*** dyspnea, ***respiratory depression***

CNS: Extrapyramidal symptoms: pseudoparkinsonism, akathisia, dystonia, tardive dyskinesia, seizures, *headache*

HEMA: Anemia, ***leukopenia, leukocytosis, agranulocytosis***

INTEG: Rash, photosensitivity, dermatitis

EENT: Blurred vision, glaucoma, dry eyes

GI: Dry mouth, nausea, vomiting, anorexia, constipation, diarrhea, jaundice, weight gain

GU: Urinary retention, urinary frequency, enuresis, impotence, amenorrhea, gynecomastia

CV: Orthostatic hypotension, hypertension, ***cardiac arrest,*** ECG changes, ***tachycardia***

Contraindications: Hypersensitivity, cardiovascular disease, coma, blood dyscrasias, severe hepatic disease, child <6 yr, glaucoma

Precautions: Breast cancer, seizure disorders, pregnancy (C), lactation, diabetes mellitus, respiratory conditions, prostatic hypertrophy

Pharmacokinetics:

PO: Onset rapid, peak 2-3 hr, duration 12 hr

IM: Onset immediate, peak 1 hr, duration 12 hr

Metabolized by liver, excreted in urine, crosses placenta, enters breast milk

Interactions/incompatibilities:

• Oversedation: other CNS depressants, alcohol, barbiturate anesthetics

• Toxicity: epinephrine

• Decreased absorption: aluminum hydroxide or magnesium hydroxide antacids

• Decreased effects of: lithium, levodopa

• Increased effects of both drugs: β-adrenergic blockers, alcohol

• Increased anticholinergic effects: anticholinergics

NURSING CONSIDERATIONS

Assess:

• Mental status before initial administration

• Swallowing of PO medication; check for hoarding or giving of medication to other patients

• I&O ratio; palpate bladder if low urinary output occurs

• Bilirubin, CBC, liver function studies monthly

• Urinalysis is recommended before and during prolonged therapy

Administer:

• Antiparkinsonian agent, after securing order from physician to be used if EPS occur

• Conc in 120 ml of tomato or fruit juice, milk, orange, carbonated beverage, coffee, tea, water, or semisolid foods (soup, pudding)

Perform/provide:

• Decreased noise input by dimming lights, avoiding loud noises

• Supervised ambulation until stabilized on medication; do not involve in strenuous exercise program because fainting is possible; patient should not stand still for long periods of time

• Increased fluids to prevent constipation

• Sips of water, candy, gum for dry mouth

• Storage in tight, light-resistant container, oral solutions in amber bottles; slight yellowing of inj or conc is common, does not affect potency.

Evaluate:

• Therapeutic response: decrease in emotional excitement, hallucinations, delusions, paranoia, reorganization of patterns of thought, speech

• Affect, orientation, LOC, reflexes, gait, coordination, sleep pattern disturbances

• B/P standing and lying; also include pulse, respirations q4h during initial treatment; establish baseline before starting treatment; report drops of 30 mm Hg

• Dizziness, faintness, palpitations, tachycardia on rising

• EPS including akathisia (inability to sit still, no pattern to movements), tardive dyskinesia (bizarre movements of jaw, mouth, tongue, extremities), pseudoparkinsonism (rigidity, tremors, pill rolling, shuffling gait)

• Skin turgor daily

• Constipation, urinary retention daily; if these occur increase bulk, water in diet

Teach patient/family:

• That orthostatic hypotension occurs frequently, and to rise from sitting or lying position gradually; avoid hazardous activities until stabilized on medication

• To remain lying down after IM injection for at least 30 min

• To avoid hot tubs, hot showers, or tub baths since hypotension may occur

• To avoid abrupt withdrawal of this drug or EPS may result; drugs should be withdrawn slowly

• To avoid OTC preparations (cough, hayfever, cold) unless approved by physician since serious drug interactions may occur; avoid use with alcohol or CNS depressants, increased drowsiness may occur

• To use a sunscreen during sun exposure to prevent burns

• Regarding compliance with drug regimen

• About necessity for meticulous oral hygiene since oral candidiasis may occur

• To report sore throat, malaise, fever, bleeding, mouth sores; if these occur, CBC should be drawn and drug discontinued

• In hot weather, that heat stroke may occur; take extra precautions to stay cool

Lab test interferences:

Increase: Liver function tests, cardiac enzymes, cholesterol, blood glucose, prolactin, bilirubin, PBI, cholinesterase, ^{131}I

Decrease: Hormones (blood and urine)

False positive: Pregnancy tests, PKU

False negative: Urinary steroids, 17-OHCS, pregnancy tests

Treatment of overdose: Lavage if orally ingested, provide an airway; *do not induce vomiting*

---

trifluproMAZINE HCl

(trye-floo-proe'ma-zeen)

Vesprin

Func. class.: Antipsychotic/neuroleptic

Chem. class.: Phenothiazine, aliphatic

Action: Depresses cerebral cortex, hypothalamus, limbic system, which control activity, aggression; blocks neurotransmission produced by dopamine at synapse; exhibits strong α-adrenergic, anticholiner-

T

gic blocking action; mechanism for antipsychotic effects is unclear

Uses: Psychotic disorders, schizophrenia, acute agitation, nausea, vomiting

Dosage and routes:

Psychosis

• *Adult:* PO 10-50 mg bid-tid depending on severity of condition; dose is gradually increased to desired dose; IM 60 mg; not to exceed 150 mg/day

• *Child >2 yr:* PO 0.5-2 mg/kg/day in 3 divided doses; may increase to 10 mg if needed; IM 0.2 to 0.25 mg/kg to a maximum total dose of 10 mg/day

Nausea/vomiting

• *Adult:* PO 20-30 mg qd; IV 1-3 mg; IM 5-15 mg, q4h, max 60 mg qd

• *Child >2 yr:* PO/IM 0.2 mg/kg, max 10 mg qd

Acute agitation

• *Adult:* IM 60-150 mg/qd in 3 divided doses

• *Child >2 yr:* IM 0.2-0.25 mg/kg/day in divided doses, max 10 mg/qd

Available forms include: Tabs 10, 25, 50 mg (Canada only); inj IM, IV 10, 20 mg/ml

Side effects/adverse reactions:

RESP: ***Laryngospasm,*** dyspnea, ***respiratory depression***

CNS: Extrapyramidal symptoms: pseudoparkinsonism, akathisia, dystonia, tardive dyskinesia, drowsiness, headache, ***seizures***

HEMA: Anemia, ***leukopenia, leukocytosis, agranulocytosis***

INTEG: Rash, photosensitivity, dermatitis

EENT: Blurred vision, glaucoma

GI: Dry mouth, nausea, vomiting, anorexia, constipation, diarrhea, jaundice, weight gain

GU: Urinary retention, urinary frequency, enuresis, impotence, amenorrhea, gynecomastia

CV: Orthostatic hypotension, hypertension, ***cardiac arrest,*** ECG changes, ***tachycardia***

Contraindications: Hypersensitivity, blood dyscrasias, coma, child <2½ yr, brain damage, bone marrow depression

Precautions: Pregnancy (C), lactation, seizure disorders, hepatic disease, cardiac disease

Pharmacokinetics:

PO: Onset erratic, peak 2-4 hr, duration 4-6 hr

IM: Onset 15-30 min, peak 15-20 min, duration 4-6 hr; metabolized by liver, excreted in urine and feces, crosses placenta, enters breast milk

Interactions/incompatibilities:

• Oversedation: other CNS depressants, alcohol, barbiturate anesthetics

• Toxicity: epinephrine

• Decreased absorption: aluminum hydroxide or magnesium hydroxide antacids

• Decreased effects of: lithium, levodopa

• Increased effects of both drugs: β-adrenergic blockers, alcohol

• Increased anticholinergic effects: anticholinergics

NURSING CONSIDERATIONS

Assess:

• Swallowing of PO medication; check for hoarding or giving of medication to other patients

• I&O ratio; palpate bladder if low urinary output occurs

• Bilirubin, CBC, liver function studies monthly

• Urinalysis is recommended before and during prolonged therapy

Administer:

• Reduced dose to elderly

• IV after diluting 10 mg/9 ml of NS; give 1 mg or less/2 min
• Antiparkinsonian agent, after securing order from physician to be used if extrapyramidal symptoms occur
• IM injection into large muscle mass, avoid contact with skin

Perform/provide:
• Decreased noise input by dimming lights, avoiding loud noises
• Supervised ambulation until stabilized on medication; do not involve in strenuous exercise program because fainting is possible; patient should not stand still for long periods of time
• Increased fluids to prevent constipation
• Sips of water, candy, gum for dry mouth
• Storage in tight, light-resistant container

Evaluate:
• Therapeutic response: decrease in emotional excitement, hallucinations, delusions, paranoia, reorganization of patterns of thought, speech
• Affect, orientation, LOC, reflexes, gait, coordination, sleep pattern disturbances
• B/P standing and lying; also include pulse, respirations q4h during initial treatment; establish baseline before starting treatment; report drops of 30 mm Hg
• For neuroleptic malignant syndrome: altered mental status, muscle rigidity, increased CPK, hyperthermia
• Dizziness, faintness, palpitations, tachycardia on rising
• Extrapypramidal symptoms including akathisia (inability to sit still, no pattern to movements), tardive dyskinesia (bizarre movements of jaw, mouth, tongue, extremities), pseudoparkinsonism (rigidity, tremors, pill rolling, shuffling gait)
• Constipation, urinary retention daily; if these occur increase bulk, water in the diet

Teach patient/family:
• That orthostatic hypotension occurs frequently, and to rise from sitting or lying position gradually; to avoid hazardous activities until stabilized on medication
• To remain lying down after IM injection for at least 30 min
• To avoid hot tubs, hot showers, or tub baths since hypotension may occur
• To avoid abrupt withdrawal of this drug or extrapyramidal symptoms may result; drugs should be withdrawn slowly
• To avoid OTC preparations (cough, hayfever, cold) unless approved by physician since serious drug interactions may occur; avoid use with alcohol or CNS depressants, increased drowsiness may occur
• To use sunscreen during sun exposure to prevent burns
• Regarding compliance with drug regimen
• About necessity for meticulous oral hygiene since oral candidiasis may occur
• To report sore throat, malaise, fever, bleeding, mouth sores; if these occur, CBC should be drawn and drug discontinued
• That in hot weather, heat stroke may occur; take extra precautions to stay cool

Lab test interferences:
Increase: Liver function tests, cardiac enzymes, cholesterol, blood glucose, prolactin, bilirubin, PBI, cholinesterase, ^{131}I

Decrease: Hormones (blood and urine)
False positive: Pregnancy tests, PKU
False negative: Urinary steroids, pregnancy tests
Treatment of overdose: Lavage if orally ingested, provide an airway; *do not induce vomiting*

---

trifluridine (ophthalmic)

(trye-flure'i-deen)
Viroptic Ophthalmic Solution
Func. class.: Antiviral
Chem. class.: Pyrimidine nucleoside

Action: Inhibits viral DNA synthesis and replication
Uses: Primary keratoconjunctivitis, recurring epithelial keratitis
Dosage and routes:
• *Adult and child:* INSTILL 1 gtt q2h, not to exceed 9 gtts/day, until corneal epithelium is regrown, then 1 gtt q4h × 1 wk
Available forms include: Sol 1%
Side effects/adverse reactions:
EENT: Burning, stinging, swelling, photophobia
Contraindications: Hypersensitivity
Precautions: Antibiotic hypersensitivity, pregnancy (C)
NURSING CONSIDERATIONS
Administer:
• After washing hands, cleanse crusts or discharge from eye before application
Perform/provide:
• Storage in refrigerator
Evaluate:
• Therapeutic response: absence of redness, inflammation, tearing
• Allergy: itching, lacrimation, redness, swelling
Teach patient/family:
• To use drug exactly as prescribed
• Not to use eye make-up, towels, washcloths, or eye medication of others, or reinfection may occur
• That drug container tip should not be touched to eye
• To report itching, increased redness, burning, stinging; drug should be discontinued

---

trihexyphenidyl HCl

(trye-hex-ee-fen'i-dill)
Aparkane,* Aphen, Artane, Hexaphen, Novohexidyl,* T.H.P., Trihexane, Trihexidyl, Trihexy
Func. class.: Cholinergic blocker
Chem. class.: Synthetic tertiary amine

Action: Blocks central muscarinic receptors, which decreases involuntary movements
Uses: Parkinson symptoms
Dosage and routes:
Parkinson symptoms
• *Adult:* PO 1 mg, increased by 2 mg q3-5d to a total of 6-10 mg/day
Drug-induced extrapyramidal symptoms
• *Adult:* PO 1 mg/day; usual dose 5-15 mg/day
Available forms include: Tabs 2, 5 mg; caps sus-rel 5 mg; elix 2 mg/5 ml
Side effects/adverse reactions:
CNS: Confusion, anxiety, restlessness, irritability, delusions, hallucinations, headache, sedation, depression, incoherence, dizziness, flushing, weakness
EENT: Blurred vision, photophobia, dilated pupils, difficulty swallowing
CV: Palpitations, tachycardia, postural hypotension
INTEG: Urticaria, rash

* Available in Canada only

MISC: Suppression of lactation, nasal congestion, decreased sweating, increased temperature
MS: Weakness, cramping
GI: Dryness of mouth, constipation, nausea, vomiting, abdominal distress, ***paralytic ileus***
GU: Hesitancy, retention
Contraindications: Hypersensitivity, narrow-angle glaucoma, myasthenia gravis, GI/GU obstruction, tachycardia, myocardial ischemia, unstable CV disease
Precautions: Pregnancy (C), elderly, lactation, tachycardia, prostatic hypertrophy, abdominal obstruction, infection, children, gastric ulcer
Pharmacokinetics:
PO: Onset 1 hr, peak 2-3 hr, duration 6-12 hr, excreted in urine
Interactions/incompatibilities:
- Increased anticholinergic effects: antihistamines, phenothiazines, amantadine

NURSING CONSIDERATIONS
Assess:
- I&O ratio; retention commonly causes decreased urinary output
- B/P, pulse frequently while dose is being determined

Administer:
- With or after meals for GI upset; may give with fluids other than water
- At hs to avoid daytime drowsiness in patient with parkinsonism

Perform/provide:
- Storage at room temperature in light resistant containers
- Hard candy, frequent drinks, sugarless gum to relieve dry mouth

Evaluate:
- Therapeutic response: parkinsonism: shuffling gait, muscle rigidity, involuntary movements
- Urinary hesitancy, retention; palpate bladder if retention occurs
- Constipation; increase fluids, bulk, exercise if this occurs
- For tolerance over long-term therapy; dose may need to be increased or changed
- Mental status: affect, mood, CNS depression, worsening of mental symptoms during early therapy

Teach patient/family:
- Not to discontinue this drug abruptly; to taper off over 1 wk
- To avoid driving or other hazardous activities; drowsiness may occur
- To avoid OTC medications: cough, cold preparations with alcohol, antihistamines unless directed by physician
- To avoid sudden position changes
- To avoid hot climates, overheating may occur

trilostane

(trye-loss-tane)
Modrastane

Func. class.: Antineoplastic
Chem. class.: Hormone, adrenal steroid inhibitor

Action: Inhibits DNA, RNA, protein synthesis; derived from *Streptomyces verticillus;* replication is decreased by binding to DNA, which causes strand splitting; drug is phase specific in G_2, M phases
Uses: Metastatic breast cancer, adrenal cancer, suppression of adrenal function in Cushing's syndrome
Dosage and routes:
- *Adult:* PO 30 mg qid, may increase q3-4d up to 480 mg/day

Available forms include: Caps 30, 60 mg
Side effects/adverse reactions:
HEMA: ***Thrombocytopenia, leukopenia, myelosuppression, anemia***

T

GI: Nausea, vomiting, anorexia, ***hepatotoxicity***
GU: Hirsutism
INTEG: Rash, pruritus
CV: Hypotension, tachycardia
CNS: Dizziness, headache
Contraindications: Hypersensitivity, hypothyroidism, pregnancy (X)
Precautions: Renal disease, hepatic disease, respiratory disease
Pharmacokinetics: Half-life 13 hr, metabolized in liver, excreted in urine, crosses placenta

NURSING CONSIDERATIONS

Assess:

- CBC, differential, platelet count weekly; withhold drug if WBC is <4000 or platelet count is <75,000; notify physician of results
- Renal function studies: BUN, serum uric acid, urine CrCl, electrolytes before, during therapy
- I&O ratio; report fall in urine output of 30 ml/hr
- Monitor temperature q4h (may indicate beginning infection)
- Liver function tests before, during therapy (bilirubin, AST, ALT, LDH) as needed or monthly
- RBC, Hct, Hgb since these may be decreased

Administer:

- Medications by oral route; if possible avoid IM, SC, IV routes to prevent infections
- Antacid before oral agent, give last dose of drug after evening meal, before bedtime
- Antiemetic 30-60 min before giving drug to prevent vomiting
- Local or systemic drugs for infection

Perform/provide:

- Nutritious diet with iron, vitamin supplements as ordered

Evaluate:

- Therapeutic response: decreased tumor size, spread of malignancy
- Bleeding: hematuria, guaiac, bruising, petechiae, mucosa or orifices q8h
- Food preferences; list likes, dislikes
- Inflammation of mucosa, breaks in skin
- Yellowing of skin, sclera, dark urine, clay-colored stools, itchy skin, abdominal pain, fever, diarrhea
- Symptoms indicating severe allergic reactions: rash, pruritus, urticaria, purpuric skin lesions, itching, flushing

Teach patient/family:

- To report any complaints, side effects to nurse or physician
- That masculinization can occur, is reversible after discontinuing treatment

---

trimeprazine tartrate

(trye-mep'ra-zeen)
Panectyl,* Temaril
Func. class.: Antihistamine
Chem. class.: Phenothiazine analog, H_1-receptor antagonist

Action: Acts on blood vessels, GI, respiratory system by competing with histamine for H_1-receptor site; decreases allergic response by blocking histamine
Uses: Pruritus
Dosage and routes:

- *Adult:* PO 2.5 mg qid; TIME-REL 5 mg bid
- *Child 3-12 yr:* PO 2.5 mg tid or hs
- *Child 6 mo-1 yr:* PO 1.25 mg tid or hs

Available forms include: Tabs 2.5 mg; spans 5 mg; syr 2.5 mg/5 ml
Side effects/adverse reactions:
CNS: Dizziness, drowsiness, poor

* Available in Canada only

condition, fatigue, anxiety, euphoria, confusion, paresthesia, neuritis
CV: Hypotension, palpitations, tachycardia
RESP: Increased thick secretions, wheezing, chest tightness
HEMA: ***Thrombocytopenia, agranulocytosis, hemolytic anemia***
GI: Dry mouth, nausea, vomiting, anorexia, constipation, diarrhea
INTEG: Rash, urticaria, photosensitivity
GU: Retention, dysuria, frequency
EENT: Blurred vision, dilated pupils, tinnitus, nasal stuffiness, dry nose, throat, mouth

Contraindications: Hypersensitivity to H_1-receptor antagonist, acute asthma attack, lower respiratory tract disease

Precautions: Increased intraocular pressure, renal disease, cardiac disease, hypertension, bronchial asthma, seizure disorder, stenosed peptic ulcers, hyperthyroidism, prostatic hypertrophy, bladder neck obstruction, pregnancy (C)

Interactions/incompatibilities:
- Increased CNS depression: barbiturates, narcotics, hypnotics, tricyclic antidepressants, alcohol
- Decreased effect of: oral anticoagulants, heparin
- Increased effect of trimeprazine: MAOIs

NURSING CONSIDERATIONS

Assess:
- I&O ratio; be alert for urinary retention, frequency, dysuria; drug should be discontinued if these occur
- CBC during long-term therapy

Administer:
- Coffee, tea, cola (caffeine) to decrease drowsiness
- With meals if GI symptoms occur; absorption may slightly decrease
- Sustained-release formulation only to adults

Perform/provide:
- Hard candy, gum, frequent rinsing of mouth for dryness
- Storage in tight container at room temperature

Evaluate:
- Therapeutic response: decreased itching associated with pruritus
- Respiratory status: rate, rhythm, increase in bronchial secretions, wheezing, chest tightness
- Cardiac status: palpitations, increased pulse, hypotension

Teach patient/family:
- To notify physician if confusion, sedation, hypotension occurs
- To avoid driving or other hazardous activity if drowsiness occurs
- To avoid concurrent use of alcohol or other CNS depressants

Lab test interferences:
False negative: Skin allergy tests

Treatment of overdose: Administer ipecac syrup or lavage, diazepam, vasopressors, barbiturates (short-acting)

trimethadione

(trye-meth-a-dye'one)
Tridione
Func. class.: Anticonvulsant
Chem. class.: Oxazolidinedione

Action: Decreases seizures in cortex, basal ganglia; decreases synaptic stimulation to low-frequency impulses

Uses: Refractory absence (petit mal) seizures

Dosage and routes:
- *Adult:* PO 300 mg tid, may increase by 300 mg/wk, not to exceed 600 mg qid

• *Child:* PO 20-50 mg/kg/day, may increase by 150-300 mg/wk
Available forms include: Caps 300 mg; chew tabs 150 mg; sol 200 mg/5 ml; oral sol 40 mg/ml
Side effects/adverse reactions:
HEMA: ***Thrombocytopenia, agranulocytosis, leukopenia, neutropenia, hemolytic anemia,*** increased pro-time, ***eosinophilia, aplastic anemia***
CNS: Drowsiness, dizziness, fatigue, paresthesia, irritability, headache, insomnia
GU: Vaginal bleeding, albuminuria, nephrosis, abdominal pain, weight loss
GI: Nausea, vomiting, bleeding gums, abnormal liver function tests
INTEG: ***Exfoliative dermatitis,*** rash, alopecia, petechiae, erythema
EENT: Photophobia, diplopia, epistaxis, retinal hemorrhage
CV: Hypertension, hypotension
Contraindications: Hypersensitivity, blood dyscrasias, pregnancy (D)
Precautions: Hepatic disease, renal disease
Pharmacokinetics:
PO: Peak 30 min-2 hr, excreted by kidneys, half-life 6-13 days

NURSING CONSIDERATIONS

Assess:
• Blood studies: Hct, Hgb, RBCs, serum folate, vitamin D; hepatic studies: AST, ALT, bilirubin, creatinine; drug should be stopped if neutrophil count falls below 2500/mm^3 if on long-term therapy
Administer:
• After diluting oral solution with water, give slowly through lavage needle
• Oral with juice or milk to cover taste/smell; decreases GI symptoms
Perform/provide:
• Ventilation of room
Evaluate:
• Therapeutic response: decreased seizures
• Mental status: mood, sensorium, affect, memory (long, short)
• Rash, alopecia, convulsions; discontinue drug if these occur
Teach patient/family:
• To notify physician if skin rash, alopecia, sore throat, fever, bruising, epistaxis occur
• That physical dependency may result when used for extended periods
• To avoid driving, other activities that require alertness
• Not to discontinue medication quickly after long-term use; convulsions may result

trimethaphan camsylate

(trye-meth'a-fan)
Arfonad

Func. class.: Antihypertensive
Chem. class.: Ganglionic blocker

Action: Occupies receptor site, prevents acetylcholine from attaching to postsynaptic nerve endings in sympathetic, parasympathetic ganglia
Uses: Hypertensive emergencies, production of controlled hypotension during surgery
Dosage and routes:
• *Adult:* IV INF dilute 500 mg in 500 ml of 5% dextrose injection, run at 3-4 mg/min, adjust to maintain B/P at desired rate; range 0.3-6.0 mg/min
• *Child:* 50-150 μg/kg/min
Available forms include: Inj IV 50 mg/ml
Side effects/adverse reactions:
CV: Orthostatic hypotension, angina, tachycardia, edema

GI: Nausea, vomiting, anorexia, dry mouth, diarrhea, constipation
CNS: Headache, agitation, weakness, restlessness
INTEG: Rash, urticaria, pruritus
RESP: ***Respiratory arrest***
EENT: Blurred vision, diplopia, pupillary dilation
GU: Urinary retention

Contraindications: Uncorrected respiratory insufficiency, hypersensitivity, pregnancy (C), hypovolemic shock, glaucoma, uncorrected anemia

Precautions: Elderly, debilitated, allergic individuals, cardiac disease, degenerative CNS disease, hepatic disease, renal disease, diabetes mellitus, Addison's disease, children

Pharmacokinetics:
IV: Onset 1-2 min, duration up to 30 min; excreted in urine, crosses placenta

Interactions/incompatibilities:
- Increased effects of diuretics, antihypertensives, anesthetics
- Do not mix with any drug in syringe or solution

NURSING CONSIDERATIONS

Assess:
- Electrolytes: K, Na, Cl, CO_2
- Renal function studies: BUN, creatinine
- B/P during initial treatment, periodically thereafter
- Weight daily, I&O
- ECG throughout treatment if there is a history of cardiac problems

Administer:
- IV infusion by microdrip regulator
- Diluted solution only (500 mg of drug/500 ml or more of D_5W)

Perform/provide:
- Artificial ventilation equipment nearby
- Use of only freshly prepared solution
- Elevate patient's head to control B/P

Evaluate:
- Therapeutic response: decreased B/P, primarily systolic B/P
- Nausea, vomiting, diarrhea
- Edema in feet, legs daily
- Skin turgor, dryness of mucous membranes for hydration status
- Constipation: number of stools, consistency, give stool softener as ordered or increase bulk in diet if constipation occurs, or antidiarrheal for diarrhea
- Respiratory dysfunction: bronchospasm, wheezing, tachypnea, respiratory arrest
- Signs of peripheral vascular collapse

Teach patient/family:
- That lying in bed is needed during infusion

Treatment of overdose: Administer vasopressors, phenylephrine, mephentermine

trimethobenzamide

(trye-meth-oh-ben'za-mide)
Spengan, Ticon, Tigan
Func. class.: Antiemetic, anticholinergic
Chem. class.: Ethanolamine derivative

Action: Acts centrally by blocking chemoreceptor trigger zone, which in turn acts on vomiting center

Uses: Nausea, vomiting, prevention of postoperative vomiting

Dosage and routes:
Postoperative vomiting
- *Adult:* IM/REC 200 mg before or during surgery; may repeat 3 hr after

Discontinuing anesthesia
- *Child 13-40 kg:* PO/REC 100-200 mg tid-qid
- *Child <13 kg:* PO/REC 100 mg tid-qid

Nausea/vomiting
- *Adult:* PO 250 mg tid-qid; IM/REC 200 mg tid-qid

Available forms include: Caps 100, 250 mg; supp 100, 200 mg; inj IM 100 mg/ml

Side effects/adverse reactions:
CNS: Drowsiness, restlessness, headache, dizziness, insomnia, confusion, nervousness, tingling, *vertigo,* extrapyramidal symptoms
GI: Nausea, anorexia, diarrhea, vomiting, constipation
CV: Hypertension, hypotension, palpitation
INTEG: Rash, urticaria, fever, chills, flushing
EENT: Dry mouth, blurred vision, diplopia, nasal congestion, photosensitivity

Contraindications: Hypersensitivity to narcotics, shock, children (parenterally)

Precautions: Children, cardiac dysrhythmias, elderly, asthma, pregnancy (C), prostatic hypertrophy, bladder-neck obstruction, narrow-angle glaucoma, stenosing peptic ulcer, pyloroduodenal obstruction

Pharmacokinetics:
PO: Onset 20-40 min, duration 3-4 hr
IM: Onset 15 min, duration 2-3 hr; metabolized by liver, excreted by kidneys

Interactions/incompatibilities:
- Increased effect: CNS depressants
- May mask ototoxic symptoms associated with antibiotics

NURSING CONSIDERATIONS

Assess:
- VS, B/P; check patients with cardiac disease more often

Administer:
- IM injection in large muscle mass; aspirate to avoid IV administration
- Tablets may be swallowed whole, chewed, allowed to dissolve

Evaluate:
- Therapeutic response: decreased nausea, vomiting
- Signs of toxicity of other drugs or masking of symptoms of disease: brain tumor, intestinal obstruction
- Observe for drowsiness, dizziness

Teach patient/family:
- To avoid hazardous activities, activities requiring alertness; dizziness may occur; instruct patient to request assistance with ambulation
- To avoid alcohol, other depressants
- To keep out of children's reach

---

trimethoprim

(trye-meth'oh-prim)
Proloprim, Trimpex

Func. class.: Urinary antiinfective
Chem. class.: Folate antagonist

Action: Prevents bacterial synthesis by blocking enzyme reduction of dihyodrofolic acid

Uses: *E.coli, P. mirabilis, Klebsiella, Enterobacter* urinary tract infections

Dosage and routes:
- *Adult:* PO 100 mg q12h

Available forms include: Tabs 100, 200 mg

Side effects/adverse reactions:
*INTEG: **Exfoliative dermatitis,*** pruritus, rash
*HEMA: **Thrombocytopenia, leukopenia, neutropenia, megaloblastic anemia*** (rare)
GI: Nausea, vomiting, abdominal pain, abnormal taste, increased

AST, ALT, bilirubin, creatinine
CNS: Fever
Contraindications: Hypersensitivity, CrCl <15 ml/min, renal disease, hepatic disease, megaloblastic anemia
Precautions: Folate deficiency, pregnancy (C), lactation, fragile X chromosome, children <12-yr-old
Pharmacokinetics:
PO: Peak 1-4 hr, half-life 8-11 hr; metabolized in liver, excreted in urine (unchanged 60%), breast milk, crosses placenta
Interactions/incompatabilities:
• Increased action of: phenytoin

NURSING CONSIDERATIONS
Assess:
• Nocturia; may indicate drug resistance
• Signs of infection, anemia
• AST/ALT, BUN, bilirubin, creatinine, urine cultures
• C&S before drug therapy; drug may be taken as soon as culture is obtained
Administer:
• With full glass of water
Perform/provide:
• Storage in tight, light-resistant container
• Adequate intake of fluids (2000 ml) to decrease bacteria in bladder
Evaluate:
• Therapeutic response: absence of pain in bladder area, negative C&S
• Skin eruptions
Teach patient/family:
• Aspects of drug therapy: need to complete entire course of medication to ensure organism death (10-14 days); culture may be taken after completed course of medication
• That drug must be taken in equal intervals around clock to maintain blood levels
• To notify nurse of nausea, vomiting

trimipramine maleate
(tri-mip'ra-meen)
Surmontil
Func. class.: Antidepressant—tricyclic
Chem. class.: Tertiary amine

Action: Selectively inhibits serotonin uptake by brain; potentiates behavioral changes
Uses: Depression, enuresis in children
Dosage and routes:
• *Adult:* PO 75 mg/day in divided doses, may be increased to 200 mg/day
• *Child >6 yr:* 25 mg hs, may increase to 50 mg in children <12 yr or 75 mg in children >12 yr
Available forms include: Caps 25, 50, 100 mg
Side effects/adverse reactions:
HEMA: ***Agranulocytosis, thrombocytopenia, eosinophilia, leukopenia***
CNS: Dizziness, drowsiness, confusion, headache, anxiety, tremors, stimulation, weakness, insomnia, nightmares, EPS (elderly), increase in psychiatric symptoms
GI: Diarrhea, dry mouth, nausea, vomiting, ***paralytic ileus,*** increased appetite, cramps, epigastric distress, jaundice, ***hepatitis,*** stomatitis
GU: Retention, ***acute renal failure***
INTEG: Rash, urticaria, sweating, pruritus, photosensitivity
CV: Orthostatic hypotension, ECG changes, tachycardia, ***hypertension,*** palpitations
EENT: Blurred vision, tinnitus, mydriasis
Contraindications: Hypersensitivity to tricyclic antidepressants, recovery phase of myocardial infarc-

tion, convulsive disorders, prostatic hypertrophy
Precautions: Suicidal patients, severe depression, increased intraocular pressure, narrow-angle glaucoma, urinary retention, cardiac disease, hepatic disease, hyperthyroidism, electroshock therapy, elective surgery, pregnancy (C)
Pharmacokinetics:
Metabolized by liver, excreted by kidneys, steady state 2-6 days; half-life 7-30 hr
Interactions/incompatibilities:
• Decreased effects of: guanethidine, clonidine, indirect acting sympathomimetics (ephedrine)
• Increased effects of: direct acting sympathomimetics (epinephrine), alcohol, barbiturates, benzodiazepines, CNS depressants
• Hyperpyretic crisis, convulsions, hypertensive episode: MAOI (pargyline [Eutonyl])

NURSING CONSIDERATIONS

Assess:
• B/P (lying, standing), pulse q4h; if systolic B/P drops 20 mm Hg hold drug, notify physician; take vital signs q4h in patients with cardiovascular disease
• Blood studies: CBC, leukocytes, differential, cardiac enzymes if patient is receiving long-term therapy
• Hepatic studies: AST, ALT, bilirubin, creatinine
• Weight qwk, appetite may increase with drug
• ECG for flattening of T wave, bundle branch block, AV block, dysrhythmias in cardiac patients
Administer:
• Increased fluids, bulk in diet if constipation, urinary retention occur
• With food or milk for GI symptoms
• Dosage hs if oversedation occurs during day; may take entire dose hs; elderly may not tolerate once/day dosing
• Gum, hard candy, or frequent sips of water for dry mouth
Perform/provide:
• Storage in tight, light-resistant container at room temperature
• Assistance with ambulation during beginning therapy since drowsiness/dizziness occurs
• Safety measures, including siderails primarily in elderly
• Checking to see PO medication swallowed
Evaluate:
• Therapeutic response: decreased depression or enuresis
• EPS primarily in elderly: rigidity, dystonia, akathisia
• Mental status: mood, sensorium, affect, suicidal tendencies, increase in psychiatric symptoms: depression, panic
• Urinary retention, constipation; constipation is more likely to occur in children, elderly
• Withdrawal symptoms: headache, nausea, vomiting, muscle pain, weakness; do not usually occur unless drug is discontinued abruptly
• Alcohol consumption; if alcohol is consumed, hold dose until morning
Teach patient/family:
• That therapeutic effects may take 2-3 wk
• To use caution in driving or other activities requiring alertness because of drowsiness, dizziness, blurred vision
• To avoid alcohol ingestion, other CNS depressants
• Not to discontinue medication quickly after long-term use, may cause nausea, headache, malaise

• To wear sunscreen or large hat since photosensitivity occurs

Lab test interferences:
Increase: Serum bilirubin, blood glucose, alk phosphatase
False increase: Urinary catecholamines
Decrease: VMA, 5-HIAA

Treatment of overdose: ECG monitoring, induce emesis, lavage, activated charcoal, administer anticonvulsant

---

tripelennamine HCl

(tri-pel-een'a-meen)

PBZ-SR, Pelamine, Pyribenzamine, Ro-Hist

Func. class.: Antihistamine
Chem. class.: Ethylenediamine derivative

Action: Acts on blood vessels, GI, respiratory system, by competing with histamine for H_1-receptor site; decreases allergic response by blocking histamine

Uses: Rhinitis, allergy symptoms

Dosage and routes:
• *Adult:* PO 25-50 mg q4-6h, not to exceed 600 mg/day; TIME-REL 100 mg bid-tid, not to exceed 600 mg/day
• *Child >5 yr:* TIME-REL 50 mg q8-12hr, not to exceed 300 mg/day
• *Child <5 yr:* PO 5 mg/kg/day in 4-6 divided doses, not to exceed 300 mg/day

Available forms include: Tab 25, 50 mg; time-rel tab 100 mg; elix 37.5 mg/5 ml

Side effects/adverse reactions:
CNS: Dizziness, drowsiness, poor coordination, fatigue, anxiety, euphoria, confusion, paresthesia, neuritis
CV: Hypotension, palpitations, tachycardia
RESP: Increased thick secretions, wheezing, chest tightness
HEMA: ***Thrombocytopenia, agranulocytosis, hemolytic anemia***
GI: Constipation, dry mouth, nausea, vomiting, anorexia, diarrhea
INTEG: Rash, urticaria, photosensitivity
GU: Retention, dysuria, frequency
EENT: Blurred vision, dilated pupils, tinnitus, nasal stuffiness, dry nose, throat, mouth

Contraindications: Hypersensitivity to H_1-receptor antagonist, acute asthma attack, lower respiratory tract disease

Precautions: Increased intraocular pressure, renal disease, cardiac disease, hypertension, bronchial asthma, seizure disorder, stenosed peptic ulcers, hyperthyroidism, prostatic hypertrophy, bladder neck obstruction, pregnancy (C)

Pharmacokinetics:
PO: Onset 15-30 min, duration 4-6 hr, detoxified in liver, excreted by kidneys

Interactions/incompatibilities:
• Increased CNS depressants: barbiturates, narcotics, hypnotics, tricyclic antidepressants, alcohol
• Decreased effect of: oral anticoagulants, heparin
• Increased effect of tripelennamine: MAOIs

NURSING CONSIDERATIONS

Assess:
• I&O ratio; be alert for urinary retention, frequency, dysuria; drug should be discontinued if these occur
• CBC during long-term therapy

Administer:
• With meals if GI symptoms occur; absorption may slightly decrease
• Time-release tab to adults only

T

Perform/provide:
• Hard candy, gum, frequent rinsing of mouth for dryness
• Storage in tight container at room temperature

Evaluate:
• Therapeutic response: decrease itching associated with pruritus
• Respiratory status: rate, rhythm, increase in bronchial secretions, wheezing, chest tightness
• Cardiac status: palpitations, increased pulse, hypotension

Teach patient/family:
• All aspects of drug use; to notify physician if confusion, sedation, hypotension occurs
• To avoid driving or other hazardous activity if drowsiness occurs
• To avoid concurrent use of alcohol or other CNS depressants

Lab test interferences:
False negative: Skin allergy test
False positive: Urine pregnancy tests

Treatment of overdose: Administer ipecac syrup or lavage, diazepam, vasopressors, barbiturates (short-acting)

---

triprolidine HCl

(trye-proe'li-deen)
Actifed,* Actidil, Bayidyl
Func. class.: Antihistamine
Chem. class.: Alkylamine, H_1-receptor antagonist

Action: Acts on blood vessels, GI, respiratory system, by competing with histamine for H_1-receptor site; decreases allergic response by blocking histamine

Uses: Rhinitis, allergy symptoms

Dosage and routes:
• *Adult:* PO 2.5 mg tid-qid
• *Child >6 yr:* PO 1.25 mg tid-qid
• *Child 4-6 yr:* PO 0.9 mg tid-qid
• *Child 2-4 yr:* PO 0.6 mg tid-qid
• *Child 4 mo-2 yr:* 0.3 mg tid-qid

Available forms include: Tab 2.5 mg; syr 1.25 mg/5 ml

Side effects/adverse reactions:
CNS: Dizziness, drowsiness, poor coordination, fatigue, anxiety, euphoria, confusion, paresthesia, neuritis
CV: Hypotension, palpitations, tachycardia
RESP: Increased thick secretions, wheezing, chest tightness
HEMA: ***Thrombocytopenia, agranulocytosis, hemolytic anemia***
GI: Constipation, dry mouth, nausea, vomiting, anorexia, diarrhea
INTEG: Rash, urticaria, photosensitivity
GU: Retention, dysuria, frequency
EENT: Blurred vision, dilated pupils, tinnitus, nasal stuffiness, dry nose, throat, mouth

Contraindications: Hypersensitivity to H_1-receptor antagonist, acute asthma attack, lower respiratory tract disease

Precautions: Increased intraocular pressure, renal disease, cardiac disease, hypertension, bronchial asthma, seizure disorder, stenosed peptic ulcers, hyperthyroidism, prostatic hypertrophy, bladder neck obstruction, pregnancy (C)

Pharmacokinetics:
PO: Onset 20-60 min, duration 8-12 hr, detoxified in liver, excreted by kidneys (metabolites/free drug), half-life 20-24 hr

Interactions/incompatibilities:
• Increased CNS depressants: barbiturates, narcotics, hypnotics, tricyclic antidepressants, alcohol
• Decreased effect of: oral anticoagulants, heparin
• Increased effect of triprolidine: MAOIs

---

* Available in Canada only

NURSING CONSIDERATIONS

Assess:

• I&O ratio; be alert for urinary retention, frequency, dysuria; drug should be discontinued if these occur

• CBC during long-term therapy

Administer:

• With meals if GI symptoms occur; absorption may slightly decrease

• Time-release formulation to adults only

Perform/provide:

• Hard candy, gum, frequent rinsing of mouth for dryness

• Storage in tight container at room temperature

Evaluate:

• Therapeutic response: decreased itching associated with pruritus

• Respiratory status: rate, rhythm, increase in bronchial secretions, wheezing, chest tightness

• Cardiac status: palpitations, increased pulse, hypotension

Teach patient/family:

• All aspects of drug use; to notify physician if confusion, sedation, hypotension occurs

• To avoid driving or other hazardous activity if drowsiness occurs

• To avoid concurrent use of alcohol or other CNS depressants while taking this drug

Lab test interferences:

False negative: Skin allergy tests

Treatment of overdose: Administer ipecac syrup or lavage, diazepam, vasopressors, barbiturates (short-acting)

---

tromethamine

(troe-meth'a-meen)

Tham, Tham-E

Func. class.: Alkalinizer
Chem. class.: Amine

Action: Proton acceptor that corrects acidosis by combining with hydrogen ions to form bicarbonate and buffer; acts as diuretic (osmotic)

Uses: Acidosis (metabolic) associated with cardiac disease or COPD

Dosage and routes:

• *Adult:* 0.3 M required = kg of weight × HCO_3 deficit (mEq/L)

• *Child:* Same as above given over 3-6 hr, not to exceed 40 ml/kg

Available forms include: Inj IV 36 mg/ml, powd for inj IV 36 g

Side effects/adverse reactions:

CV: Irregular pulse, ***cardiac arrest***
META: *Alkalosis*, hypoglycemia
RESP: Shallow, slow respirations, cyanosis, ***apnea***
GI: ***Hepatic necrosis***
INTEG: Infection at injection site, extravasation, phlebitis

Contraindications: Hypersensitivity, anuria, uremia

Precautions: Severe respiratory disease/respiratory depression, pregnancy (C), cardiac edema, renal disease, infants

Pharmacokinetics:

IV: Excreted in urine

NURSING CONSIDERATIONS

Assess:

• Respiratory rate, rhythm, depth, notify physician of abnormalities that may indicate acidosis

• Electrolytes, blood glucose, chloride CO_2, before, during treatment

• Urine pH, urinary output, urine glucose during beginning treatment

• I&O ratio, report large increase or decrease

• IV site for extravasation, phlebitis, thrombosis

• For signs of K^+ depletion

Administer:

• IV slowly to avoid pain at infusion site and toxicity

T

• IV undiluted as INF or added to priming fluid or ACD blood; give 5 ml or less/min

Evaluate:

• Therapeutic response: decreased metabolic acidosis

Teach patient/family:

• To increase K+ in diet: bananas, oranges, cantaloupe, honeydew, spinach, potatoes, dried fruit

tropicamide (optic)

(troe-pik'a-mide)

Mydriacyl

Func. class.: Mydriatic, cycloplegia, anticholingeric

Chem. class.: Belladonna alkaloid

Action: Blocks response of sphincter muscle of iris and ciliary body dilation and paralysis of accommodation

Uses: Fundus exam, cycloplegic refraction

Dosage and routes:

• *Adult and child:* INSTILL 1-2 gtts of 1% sol, repeat in 5 min (refraction) or 1-2 gtts of 0.5% sol 15-20 min before fundus examination

Available forms include: Sol 0.5%, 1%

Side effects/adverse reactions:

SYST: Tachycardia, confusion, hallucinations, emotional changes in children, fever, flushing, dry skin, dry mouth, abdominal discomfort (infants: bladder distention, irregular pulse, ***respiratory depression***)

Contraindications: Hypersensitivity, infants <3 mo, glaucoma, conjunctivitis

Precautions: Pregnancy (C)

Pharmacokinetics:

INSTILL: Peak 20-40 min, (mydriasis), 20-35 min, (cycloplegia)

NURSING CONSIDERATIONS

Evaluate:

• Eye pain, discontinue use

Teach patient/family:

• To report change in vision, with blurring or loss of sight, trouble breathing, flushing

• Method of instillation, including pressure on lacrimal sac for 1 min, and not to touch dropper to eye

• That blurred vision will decrease with repeated use of drug

• Not to engage in hazardous activities until able to see

• To wait 5 min to use other drops

• Not to blink more than usual

• That dark glasses may be worn if photophobia occurs

tubocurarine chloride

(too-boe-kyoo-ar'een)

Tubarine*

Func. class.: Neuromuscular blockers

Chem. class.: Curare alkaloid

Action: Inhibits transmission of nerve impulses by binding with cholinergic receptor sites, antagonizing action of acetylcholine

Uses: Facilitation of endotracheal intubation, skeletal muscle relaxation during mechanical ventilation, surgery, or general anesthesia

Dosage and routes:

• *Adult:* IV BOL 0.4-0.5 mg/kg, then 0.08-0.10 mg/kg 20-45 min after 1st dose if needed for prolonged procedures

Available forms include: Inj IV 3 mg/ml, 20 U/ml

Side effects/adverse reactions:

CV: Bradycardia, tachycardia, increased, decreased B/P

RESP: ***Prolonged apnea, bronchospasm, cyanosis, respiratory depression***

* Available in Canada only

EENT: Increased secretions
INTEG: Rash, flushing, pruritus, urticaria
Contraindications: Hypersensitivity
Precautions: Pregnancy (C), cardiac disease, lactation, children <2 yr, electrolyte imbalances, dehydration, neuromuscular disease, respiratory disease
Pharmacokinetics:
IV: Onset 15 sec, peak 2-3 min, duration ½-1½ hr; half-life 1-3 hr, degraded in liver, kidney (minimally), excreted in urine (unchanged) crosses placenta
Interactions/incompatibilities:
• Increased neuromuscular blockade: aminoglycosides, clindamycin, lincomycin, quinidine, local anesthetics, polymyxin antibiotics, lithium, narcotic analgesics, thiazides, enflurane, isoflurane
• Dysrhythmias: theophylline
• Do not mix with barbiturates in solution or syringe

NURSING CONSIDERATIONS
Assess:
• For electrolyte imbalances (K, Mg); may lead to increased action of this drug
• Vital signs (B/P, pulse, respirations, airway) q15min until fully recovered; rate, depth, pattern of respirations, strength of hand grip
• I&O ratio; check for urinary retention, frequency, hesitancy
Administer:
• With diazepam, or morphine when used for therapeutic paralysis; this drug provides no sedation alone
• Using nerve stimulator by anesthesiologist to determine neuromuscular blockade
• Anticholinesterase to reverse neuromuscular blockade
• IV undiluted 3 mg/ml; give single dose over 1-1½ sec by qualified person
Perform/provide:
• Storage in light-resistant area; use only fresh solution
• Reassurance if communication is difficult during recovery from neuromuscular blockade
Evaluate:
• Therapeutic response: paralysis of jaw, eyelid, head, neck, rest of body
• Recovery: decreased paralysis of face, diaphragm, leg, arm, rest of body; allow to fully recover before completing a neurologic assessment
• Allergic reactions: rash, fever, respiratory distress, pruritus; drug should be discontinued
Treatment of overdose: Edrophonium or neostigmine, atropine, monitor VS; may require mechanical ventilation

---

undecylenic acid (topical)

(un-dek'-sye-lin-ik)
Cruex, Desenex, NP-27, Ting, Unde-Jen
Func. class.: Local antiinfective
Chem. class.: Antifungal, antibacterial

Action: Interferes with fungal cell membrane permeability
Uses: Tinea cruris, tinea pedis, diaper rash, minor skin irritations
Dosage and routes:
• *Adult and child:* TOP apply to affected areas bid
Available forms include: Powder, oint, cream, liq, foam, soap
Side effects/adverse reactions:
INTEG: Rash, urticaria, stinging, burning

U

Contraindications: Hypersensitivity

Precautions: Pregnancy (C), lactation; impaired circulation; diabetes mellitus; broken, pustular skin; puncture wounds

NURSING CONSIDERATIONS

Administer:

- Enough medication to completely cover lesions
- After cleansing with soap, water before each application, dry well

Perform/provide:

- Storage at room temperature in dry place

Evaluate for:

- Therapeutic response: decrease in size, number of lesions
- Allergic reaction: burning, stinging, swelling, redness

Teach patient/family:

- To use medical asepsis (hand washing) before, after each application
- To apply with glove to prevent further infection
- To avoid use of OTC creams, ointments, lotions unless directed by physician
- To avoid inhaling and contact with eyes or other mucous membranes; to seek medical attention if symptoms persist

uracil mustard

(yoor'a-sill)

Func. class.: Antineoplastic alkylating agent

Chem. class.: Nitrogen mustard

Action: Responsible for cross-linking DNA strands leading to cell death

Uses: Hodgkin's disease, lymphomas; cervix, ovarian, lung cancer; chronic lymphocytic, myelocytic leukemia; reticulum cell sarcoma, mycosis fungoides; polycythemia vera

Dosage and routes:

- *Adult:* PO 1-2 mg/day × 3 mo or desired response, then 1 mg/day for 3 out of 4 wk until desired response or 3-5 mg × 7 days, not to exceed total dose of 0.5 mg/kg then 1 mg/day until desired response, then 1 mg/day 3 out of 4 wk

Available forms include: Caps 1 mg

Side effects/adverse reactions:

HEMA: ***Thrombocytopenia, leukopenia,*** anemia

GI: Nausea, vomiting, diarrhea, ***hepatotoxicity***

GU: Amenorrhea, azoospermia

INTEG: Alopecia, dermatitis, pruritus, rash

Contraindications: Severe thrombocytopenia/leukopenia, hypersensitivity, pregnancy (X)

Precautions: Radiation therapy

Pharmacokinetics:

Excreted unchanged in urine

Interactions/incompatibilities:

- Increased toxicity: antineoplastics, radiation

NURSING CONSIDERATIONS

Assess:

- CBC, differential, platelet count weekly; withhold drug if WBC is <4000 or platelet count is <75,000; notify physician of results
- Renal function studies: BUN, serum uric acid, urine CrCl before, during therapy
- I&O ratio; report fall in urine output of 30 ml/hr
- Monitor temperature q4h (may indicate beginning infection)
- Liver function tests before, during therapy (bilirubin, AST, ALT, LDH) as needed or monthly

* Available in Canada only

Administer:

• Medications by oral route if possible; avoid IM, SC, IV routes to prevent infections

• Antacid before oral agent; give drug after evening meal, before bedtime

• Antiemetic 30-60 min before giving drug to prevent vomiting

• Antibiotics for prophylaxis of infection

• Topical or systemic analgesics for pain

• Local or systemic drugs for infection

Perform/provide:

• Storage in tight container at room temperature

• Strict medical asepsis, protective isolation if WBC levels are low

• Special skin care

• Liquid diet, including cola, Jell-O; dry toast or crackers may be added if patient is not nauseated or vomiting

• Increase fluid intake to 2-3 L/day to prevent urate deposits, calculi formation

Evaluate:

• Therapeutic response: decreased tumor size, spread of malignancy

• Bleeding: hematuria, guaiac, bruising or petechiae, mucosa or orifices q8h

• Food preferences; list likes, dislikes

• Yellowing of skin, sclera, dark urine, clay-colored stools, itchy skin, abdominal pain, fever, diarrhea

• Effects of alopecia on body image; discuss feelings about body changes

• Inflammation of mucosa, breaks in skin

• Symptoms indicating severe allergic reaction: rash, pruritus, urticaria, itching

• Check for tartrazine dye allergy

Teach patient/family:

• Of protective isolation precautions

• To report signs of infection: increased temperature, sore throat, flu symptoms

• To report signs of anemia: fatigue, headache, faintness, shortness of breath, irritability

• To avoid use of razors or commercial mouthwash

• To avoid use of aspirin products or ibuprofen

• That azoospermia, amenorrhea can occur; are reversible after discontinuing treatment

• That hair may be lost during treatment; a wig or hairpiece may make patient feel better; new hair may be different in color, texture

• To avoid foods with citric acid, hot or rough texture

urea

(yoor-ee'a)

Ureaphil, Carbamex*

Func. class.: Diuretic, osmotic
Chem. class.: Carbonic acid diamide salt

Action: Elevates plasma osmolality increasing flow of water into the extracellular compartment

Uses: To decrease intracranial pressure, intraocular pressure

Dosage and routes:

• *Adult:* IV 1-1.5 g/kg of a 30% sol over 1-3 hr; do not exceed 120 g/day

• *Child >2 yr:* IV 0.5-1.5 g/kg, not to exceed 4 ml/min

• *Child <2 yr:* IV 0.1 g/kg, not to exceed 4 ml/min

Available forms include: Inj IV 40 g/150 ml

Side effects/adverse reactions:

CNS: Dizziness, headache, disori-

U

entation, fever, syncope, headache
GI: Nausea, vomiting
INTEG: Venous thrombosis, phlebitis, extravasation
CV: Postural hypotension
Contraindications: Severe renal disease, active intracranial bleeding, marked dehydration, liver failure
Precautions: Hepatic disease, renal disease, pregnancy (C), electrolyte imbalances, lactation
Pharmacokinetics:
IV: Onset ½-1 hr, peak 1 hr, duration 3-10 hr, (diuresis) 5-6 hr (intraocular pressure); half-life 1 hr, excreted in urine, crosses placenta, excreted in breast milk
Interactions/incompatibilities:
• Incompatible with whole blood, in solution or syringe with any other drug or solution
• Increased renal excretion of: lithium

NURSING CONSIDERATIONS
Assess:
• Weight, I&O daily to determine fluid loss; effect of drug may be decreased if used qd
• Rate, depth, rhythm of respiration, effect of exertion
• B/P lying, standing, postural hypotension may occur
• Electrolytes: potassium, sodium, chloride; include BUN, blood sugar, CBC, serum creatinine, blood pH, ABGs, liver function tests
Administer:
• IV after diluting 30 g/100 ml diluent with D_5, D_{10}; run 30% sol over 1-2 hr; check for extravasation; do not exceed 4 ml/min, may cause bleeding; use IV filter
• Within minutes of reconstitution; solution becomes ammonia on standing
Evaluate:
• Therapeutic response: improvement in edema of feet, legs, sacral area daily if medication is being used in CHF
• Improvement in CVP q8h
• Signs of metabolic acidosis: drowsiness, restlessness
• Signs of hypokalemia: postural hypotension, malaise, fatigue, tachycardia, leg cramps, weakness
• Temperature elevation, signs of extravasation qd
• Confusion, especially in elderly, take safety precautions if needed
• Hydration: skin turgor, thirst, dry mucous membranes
Teach patient/family:
• That drug will cause diuresis in ½ hr
Treatment of overdose: Lavage if taken orally, monitor electrolytes, administer IV fluids, monitor BUN, hydration, CV status

---

urofollitropin
(yoor-oo-foll'aa-tropin)
Metrodin
Func. class.: Ovulation stimulant
Chem. class.: Gonadotropin

Action: Stimulates ovarian follicular growth in primary ovarian failure
Uses: Induction of ovulation in polycystic ovarian disease in those who have elevated LH/FSH ratios and have failed to respond to other treatment
Dosage and routes:
• *Adult:* IM 75 IU/day × 7-12 days, then 5000-10,000 U HCG 1 day after last urofollitropin, if pregnancy does not occur; may repeat for 2 courses before increasing dose to 150 IU/day 7-12 days then 5000-10,000 U HCG 1 day after last uro-

* Available in Canada only

follitropin; may repeat for 2 more courses

Available forms include: Powder for injection 0.83 mg (76 IU FSH)/amp

Side effects/adverse reactions:

CNS: Malaise

GI: Nausea, vomiting, constipation, increased appetite, abdominal pain

INTEG: Rash, dermatitis, urticaria, alopecia

GU: Polyuria, frequency, birth defects, spontaneous abortions, multiple ovulation, breast pain

Contraindications: Hypersensitivity, pregnancy, undiagnosed vaginal bleeding, intracranial lesion, ovarian cyst not caused by polycystic ovarian disease

Precautions: Lactation, arterial thromboembolism

Pharmacokinetics:

Detoxified in liver, excreted in feces, stored in fat

NURSING CONSIDERATIONS

Assess:

- At same time qd to maintain drug level

Evaluate:

- Therapeutic response: ovulation, pregnancy

Teach patient/family:

- That multiple births are common after taking this drug
- To notify physician if low abdominal pain occurs; may indicate ovarian cyst, cyst rupture
- Method of taking, recording basal body temperature to determine whether ovulation has occurred
- That if ovulation can be determined (there is a slight decrease then a sharp increase for ovulation), to attempt coitus 3 days before and qod until after ovulation
- If pregnancy is suspected, physician must be notified immediately

urokinase

(yoor-oh-kin'ase)

Abbokinase, Win-Kinase

Func. class.: Thrombolytic enzyme

Chem. class.: β-Hemolytic streptococcus filtrate (purified)

Action: Promotes thrombolysis by enhancing the change of plasminogen to plasmin

Uses: Venous thrombosis, pulmonary embolism, arterial thrombosis, arterial embolism, arteriovenous cannula occlusion, lysis of coronary artery thrombi after myocardial infarction

Dosage and routes:

Lysis of pulmonary emboli

- *Adult:* IV 4400 IU/kg/hr × 12-24 hr not to exceed 200 ml; then IV heparin, then anticoagulants

Coronary artery thrombosis

- *Adult:* INSTILL 6000 IU/min into occluded artery for 1-2 hr after giving IV bol of heparin 2500-10,000 U

Venous catheter occlusion

- *Adult:* INSTILL 5000 IU into line, wait 5 min, then aspirate, repeat aspiration attempts q5min × ½ hr; if occlusion has not been removed, then cap line and wait ½-1 hr then aspirate; may need 2nd dose if still occluded

Available forms include: Inj

Side effects/adverse reactions:

HEMA: Decreased Hct, ***bleeding***

INTEG: Rash, urticaria, phlebitis at IV infusion site, itching, flushing

CNS: Headache, fever,

GI: Nausea

RESP: Altered respirations, SOB, ***bronchospasm***

MS: Low back pain

CV: Hypertension, dysrhythmias

U

EENT: Periorbital edema
SYST: ***GI, GU, intracranial, retroperitoneal bleeding,*** surface bleeding, ***anaphylaxis***

Contraindications: Hypersensitivity, active bleeding, intraspinal surgery, neoplasms of CNS, ulcerative colitis/enteritis, severe hypertension, renal disease, hepatic disease, hypocoagulation, COPD, subacute bacterial endocarditis, rheumatic valvular disease, cerebral embolism/thrombosis/hemorrhage, intraarterial diagnostic procedure or surgery (10 days), recent major surgery

Precautions: Arterial emboli from left side of heart, pregnancy (B)

Pharmacokinetics:
IV: Half-life 10-20 min, small amounts excreted in urine

Interactions/incompatibilities:
- Bleeding potential: aspirin, indomethacin, phenylbutazone, anticoagulants

NURSING CONSIDERATIONS

Assess:
- VS, B/P, pulse, resp, neurologic signs, temp at least q4h, temp >104° F or indicators of internal bleeding, cardiac rhythm following intracoronary administration
- For neurologic changes that may indicate intracranial bleeding
- Retroperitoneal bleeding: back pain, leg weakness, diminished pulses
- Peripheral pulses, lung sounds, respiratory function

Administer:
- Using infusion pump, terminal filter (0.45 μm or smaller)
- IV reconstitute only with 5.2 ml sterile water for injection (not bacteriostatic water), and roll (not shake) to enhance reconstitution; further dilute with 190 ml; give as intermittent inf or give to clear cannula by using 1 ml of diluted drug; inject into cannula slowly, clamp 5 min, aspirate clot
- As soon as thrombi identified; not useful for thrombi over 1 wk old
- Cryoprecipitate or fresh, frozen plasma if bleeding occurs
- Loading dose at beginning of therapy may require increased loading doses
- Heparin therapy after thrombolytic therapy is discontinued, TT or APTT less than 2 times control (about 3-4 hr)
- About 10% patients have high streptococcal antibody titres, requiring increased loading doses

Perform/provide:
- Storage in refrigerator; use immediately after reconstitution
- Bed rest during entire course of treatment, use caution in handling patients
- Avoidance of venous or arterial puncture procedures: inj, rectal temp
- Treatment of fever with acetaminophen or aspirin
- Placement of sign above patient's bed stating urokinase therapy
- Pressure for 30 sec to minor bleeding sites; inform physician if hemostasis not attained, apply pressure dressing

Evaluate:
- Therapeutic response: decreased clotting, thrombosis, embolism
- Allergy: fever, rash, itching, chills; mild reaction may be treated with antihistamines
- Bleeding during 1st hr of treatment (hematuria, hematemesis, bleeding from mucous membranes, epistaxis, ecchymosis)
- Blood studies (Hct, platelets, PTT, PT, TT, APTT) before starting therapy; PT or APTT must be less than 2 × control before starting

therapy TT ot PT q3-4h during treatment
Lab test interferences:
Increase: PT, APTT, TT

ursodiol

(your-soo′-dee-ol)
Actigall
Func. class.: Gallstone solubilizing agent
Chem. class.: Ursodeoxycholic acid

Action: Suppresses hepatic synthesis, secretion of cholesterol; inhibits intestinal absorption of cholesterol
Uses: Dissolution of radiolucent, noncalcified gallbladder stones (less than 20 mm in diameter) in which surgery is not indicated
Dosage and routes:
• *Adult:* PO 8-10 mg/kg/day in 2-3 divided doses using gallbladder ultrasound q6mo; determine if stones have dissolved, if so continue therapy, repeat ultrasound within 1-3 mo
Available forms include: Caps 300 mg
Side effects/adverse reactions:
GI: Diarrhea, nausea, vomiting, abdominal pain, constipation, stomatitis, flatulence, dyspepsia, biliary pain
INTEG: Pruritus, rash, urticaria, dry skin, sweating, alopecia
CNS: Headache, anxiety, depression, insomnia, fatigue
MS: Arthralgia, myalgia, back pain
OTHER: Cough, rhinitis
Contraindications: Calcified cholesterol stones, radiopaque stones, radiolucent bile pigment stones, chronic liver disease, hypersensitivity
Precautions: Pregnancy (B), lactation, children
Pharmacokinetics: 80% excreted in feces, 20% metabolized, excreted into bile, lost in feces
Interactions/incompatibilities:
• Reduced action of ursodiol: cholestyramine, colestipol, aluminum-based antacids

NURSING CONSIDERATIONS

Assess:
• GI status: diarrhea, abdominal pain, nausea, vomiting; drug may have to be discontinued if side effects are severe
• Skin for pruritus, rash, urticaria, dry skin; provide soothing lotion to lesions
• Muscular/skeletal status: aches or stiffness in joints
Administer:
• For up to 9-12 mo; if no improvement is seen, discontinue drug
Evaluate:
• Therapeutic response: decreasing size of stones on ultrasound
Teach patient/family:
• That anxiety, depression, insomnia are side effects and are reversible after discontinuing drug

valproate sodium/valproate sodium–valproic acid/valproic acid

(val-proe′ate)
Depakene Syrup, Myproic Acid Syrup/Depakote/Depakene, Myproic Acid
Func. class.: Anticonvulsant
Chem. class.: Carboxylic acid derivative

Action: Increases levels of γ-aminobutyric acid (GABA) in brain
Uses: Simple, complex (petit mal) absence, mixed, tonic-clonic (grand mal) seizures

Dosage and routes:

• *Adult and child:* PO 15 mg/kg/day divided in 2-3 doses, may increase by 5-10 mg/kg/day qwk, not to exceed 30 mg/kg/day in 2-3 divided doses

Available forms include: Caps 250 mg; tabs 125, 250, 500 mg; syr 250 mg/5 ml

Side effects/adverse reactions:

HEMA: ***Thrombocytopenia, leukopenia, lymphocytosis,*** increased pro-time

CNS: Sedation, drowsiness, dizziness, headache, incoordination, paresthesia, depression, hallucinations, behavioral changes, tremors, aggression, weakness

GI: Nausea, vomiting, constipation, diarrhea, heartburn, anorexia, cramps, ***hepatic failure, pancreatitis, toxic hepatitis,*** stomatitis

INTEG: Rash, alopecia, bruising

GU: Enuresis, irregular menses

Contraindications: Hypersensitivity

Precautions: MI (recovery phase), hepatic disease, renal disease, Addison's disease, pregnancy (D), lactation

Pharmacokinetics:

PO: Onset 15-30 min, peak 1-4 hr, duration 4-6 hr

REC: Onset slow, duration 4-6 hr

Metabolized by liver, excreted by kidneys, feces, crosses placenta, excreted in breast milk, half-life 6-16 hr

Interactions/incompatibilities:

• Increased effects: CNS depressants

• Increased toxicity: salicylates, warfarin, sulfinpyrazone

NURSING CONSIDERATIONS

Assess:

• Blood studies: Hct, Hgb, RBCs, serum folate, pro-time vitamin D if on long-term therapy

• Hepatic studies: AST, ALT, bilirubin, creatinine, failure

• Blood levels: therapeutic level 50-100 μg/ml

Administer:

• Tablets or capsules whole

• Elixir alone; do not dilute with carbonated beverage; do not give syrup to patients on sodium restriction

• Give with food or milk to decrease GI symptoms

Evaluate:

• Therapeutic response: decreased seizures

• Mental status: mood, sensorium, affect, memory (long, short)

• Respiratory dysfunction: respiratory depression, character, rate, rhythm; hold drug if respirations are <12/min or if pupils are dilated

Teach patient/family:

• That physical dependency may result when used for extended periods

• To avoid driving, other activities that require alertness

• Not to discontinue medication quickly after long-term use; convulsions may result

Lab test interferences:

False-positive: Ketones

vancomycin HCl

(van-koe-mye'sin)

Vancocin

Func. class.: Antibacterial

Chem. class.: Tricyclic glycopeptide

Action: Inhibits bacterial cell wall synthesis

Uses: Resistant staphylococcal infections, pseudomembranous colitis, staphylococcal enterocolitis, endocarditis prophylaxis for dental procedures

Dosage and routes:

Serious staphylococcal infections

• *Adult:* IV 500 mg q6h or 1 g q12h

• *Child:* IV 40 mg/kg/day divided q6h

• *Neonates:* IV 15 mg/kg initially followed by 10 mg/kg q8-12h

Pseudomembranous/staphylococcal enterocolitis

• *Adult:* PO 500 mg -2 g/day in 3-4 divided doses for 7-10 days

• *Child:* PO 40 mg/kg/day divided q6h, not to exceed 2 g/day

Endocarditis prophylaxis

• *Adult:* IV 1 g over 1 hr, 1 hr before dental procedure

Available forms include: Pulvules 125, 250 mg; powder for oral sol 1, 10 g; powder for inj IV 500 mg, 1 g

Side effects/adverse reactions:

CV: ***Cardiac arrest, vascular collapse***

EENT: ***Ototoxicity, permanent deafness,*** tinnitus

HEMA: ***Leukopenia, eosinophilia, neutropenia***

GI: ***Nausea***

RESP: Wheezing, dyspnea

SYST: ***Anaphylaxis***

GU: ***Nephrotoxicity,*** *increased BUN, creatinine, albumin,* ***fatal uremia***

INTEG: Chills, fever, rash, thrombophlebitis at injection site, urticaria, pruritus, necrosis

Contradindications: Hypersensitivity, decreased hearing

Precautions: Renal disease, pregnancy (C), lactation, elderly, neonates

Pharmacokinetics:

Peak 5 min IV trough 12 hr, half-life 4-8 hr, excreted in urine (active form), crosses placenta

Interactions/incompatibilities:

• Ototoxicity or nephrotoxicity: aminoglycosides, cephalosporins, colistin, polymyxin, bacitracin, cisplatin, amphotericin B

• Do not mix in solution or syringe with alkaline solutions; check product information

NURSING CONSIDERATIONS

Assess:

• I&O ratio; report hematuria, oliguria since nephrotoxicity may occur

• Any patient with compromised renal system; drug is excreted slowly in poor renal system function; toxicity may occur rapidly

• Blood studies: WBC

• C&S before drug therapy; drug may be taken as soon as culture is taken

• Auditory function during, after treatment

• B/P during administration; sudden drop may indicate Redman's syndrome

• Signs of infection

Administer:

• After reconstitution with 10 ml sterile water for injection 500 mg/10 ml; further dilution is needed for IV

• Infuse over >60 min; avoid extravasation

• Antihistamine if Redman's syndrome occurs: decreased B/P, flushing of neck, face

• Dose based on serum concentration

Perform/provide:

• Storage at room temperature for up to 2 wk after reconstitution

• Adrenalin, suction, tracheostomy set, endotracheal intubation equipment on unit; anaphylaxis may occur

• Adequate intake of fluids (2000 ml) to prevent nephrotoxicity

Evaluate:

• Therapeutic response: absence of fever, sore throat

• Hearing loss, ringing, roaring in ears; drug should be discontinued

• Skin eruptions

• Respiratory status: rate, character, wheezing, tightness in chest

• Allergies before treatment, reaction of each medication; place allergies on chart, Kardex in bright red letters; notify all people giving drugs

Teach patient/family:

• Aspects of drug therapy: need to complete entire course of medication to ensure organism death (7-10 days); culture may be taken after completed course of medication

• To report sore throat, fever, fatigue; could indicate superimposed infection

• That drug must be taken in equal intervals around clock to maintain blood levels

vasopressin (antidiuretic hormone)/vasopressin tannate

(vay-soe-press'in)

Pitressin Synthetic/Pitressin Tannate

Func. class.: Pituitary hormone
Chem. class.: Lysine vasopressin

Action: Promotes reabsorption of water by action on renal tubular epithelium; causes vasoconstriction

Uses: Diabetes insipidus (nonnephrogenic/nonpsychogenic), abdominal distention postoperatively, bleeding esophageal varices

Dosage and routes:

Diabetes insipidus

• *Adult:* IM/SC 5-10 units bid-qid as needed; IM/SC 2.5-5 units q2-3 days (Pitressin Tannate) for chronic therapy

• *Child:* IM/SC 2.5-10 units bid-qid as needed; IM/SC 1.25-2.5 units q2-3 days (Pitressin Tannate) for chronic therapy

Abdominal distention

• *Adult:* IM 5 units, then q3-4h, increasing to 10 units if needed (aqueous)

Available forms include: Inj IM, SC 20, 5 U/ml (tannate), spray, cotton pledgets

Side effects/adverse reactions:

EENT: Nasal irritation, congestion, rhinitis

CNS: Drowsiness, headache, lethargy, flushing

GU: Vulval pain

GI: Nausea, heartburn, cramps

CV: Increased B/P

MISC: Tremor, sweating, vertigo, urticaria, bronchial constriction

Contraindications: Hypersensitivity, chronic nephritis

Precautions: CAD, pregnancy (C)

Pharmacokinetics:

NASAL: Onset 1 hr, duration 3-8 hr, half-life 15 min; metabolized in liver, kidneys, excreted in urine

NURSING CONSIDERATIONS

Assess:

• Pulse, B/P, when giving drug IV or IM

• I&O ratio, weight daily, check for edema in extremities, if water retention is severe, diuretic may be prescribed

Evaluate:

• Therapeutic response: absence of severe thirst, decreased urine output, osmolality

• Water intoxication: lethargy, behavioral changes, disorientation, neuromuscular excitability

vecuronium bromide

(vek-yoo-roe'nee-um)
Norcuron
Func. class.: Neuromuscular blocker

Action: Inhibits transmission of nerve impulses by binding with cholinergic receptor sites, antagonizing action of acetylcholine
Uses: Facilitation of endotracheal intubation, skeletal muscle relaxation during mechanical ventilation, surgery, or general anesthesia
Dosage and routes:
• *Adult and child >9 yr:* IV BOL 0.08-0.10 mg/kg, then 0.010-0.015 mg/kg for prolonged procedures
Available forms include: IV 10 mg/5 ml
Side effects/adverse reactions:
CNS: Skeletal muscle weakness or paralysis, rarely
RESP: ***Prolonged apnea, possible respiratory paralysis***
Contraindications: Hypersensitivity
Precautions: Pregnancy (C), cardiac disease, lactation, children <2 yr, electrolyte imbalances, dehydration, neuromuscular disease, respiratory disease
Pharmacokinetics:
IV: Onset 15 min, peak 3-5 min, duration 45-60 min; half-life 65-75 min, not metabolized, excreted in feces, crosses placenta
Interactions/incompatibilities:
• Increased neuromuscular blockade: aminoglycosides, clindamycin, lincomycin, quinidine, local anesthetics, polymyxin antibiotics, lithium, narcotic analgesics, thiazides, enflurane, isoflurane
• Dysrhythmias: theophylline
• Do not mix with barbiturates in solution or syringe

NURSING CONSIDERATIONS

• For electrolyte imbalances (K, Mg); may lead to increased action of this drug
• Vital signs (B/P, pulse, respirations, airway) q15min until fully recovered; rate, depth, pattern of respirations, strength of hand grip
• I&O ratio; check for urinary retention, frequency, hesitancy
Administer:
• With diazepam or morphine when used for therapeutic paralysis; this drug provides no sedation alone
• Using nerve stimulator by anesthesiologist to determine neuromuscular blockade
• Anticholinesterase to reverse neuromuscular blockade
• IV after diluting with diluent provided; further dilute each dose/5-10 ml; may give as continuous inf 10-20 mg/100 ml, titrate to patient response (only by qualified person)
Perform/provide:
• Storage in refrigerator, discard in 24 hr
• Reassurance if communication is difficult during recovery from neuromuscular blockade
Evaluate:
• Therapeutic response: paralysis of jaw, eyelid, head, neck, rest of body
• Recovery: decreased paralysis of face, diaphragm, leg, arm, rest of body; allow to recover fully before completing a neurologic assessment
• Allergic reactions: rash, fever, respiratory distress, pruritus; drug should be discontinued
Treatment of overdose: Edrophonium or neostigmine, atropine, monitor VS; may require mechanical ventilation

V

verapamil HCl

(ver-ap'-a-mill)

Calan, Isoptin

Func. class.: Calcium-channel blocker

Chem. class.: Phenylalkylamine

Action: Inhibits calcium ion influx across cell membrane during cardiac depolarization; produces relaxation of coronary vascular smooth muscle, dilates coronary arteries, decreases SA/AV node conduction, dilates peripheral arteries

Uses: Chronic stable angina pectoris, vasospastic angina, dysrhythmias, hypertension

Dosage and routes:

• *Adult:* PO 80 mg tid or qid, increase qwk; IV BOL 5-10 mg > 2 min, repeat if necessary in 30 min

• *Child 0-1 yr:* IV BOL 0.1-0.2 mg/kg > 2 min with ECG monitoring, repeat if necessary in 30 min

• *Child 1-15 yr:* IV BOL 0.1-0.3 mg/kg over > 2 min, repeat in 30 min, not to exceed 10 mg in a single dose

Available forms include: Tabs 40, 80, 120; sus rel tabs, 240 mg; inj 2.5 mg/ml

Side effects/adverse reactions:

*CV: Edema, **CHF,*** bradycardia, hypotension, palpitations, AV block

GI: Nausea, diarrhea, gastric upset, constipation, increased liver function studies

GU: Nocturia, polyuria

CNS: Headache, drowsiness, dizziness, anxiety, depression, weakness, insomnia, confusion, lightheadedness

Contraindications: Sick sinus syndrome, 2nd or 3rd degree heart block, hypotension less than 90 mm Hg systolic, cardiogenic shock, severe CHF

Precautions: CHF, hypotension, hepatic injury, pregnancy (C), lactation, children, renal disease, concomitant β-blocker therapy

Pharmacokinetics:

IV: Onset 3 min, peak 3-5 min, duration 10-20 min

PO: Onset variable, peak 3-4 hr, duration 17-24 hr, half-life (biphasic) 4 min, 3-7 hr (terminal); metabolized by liver, excreted in urine (96% as metabolites)

Interactions/incompatibilities:

• Increased hypotension: prazosin, quinidine

• Increased effects: β-blockers, antihypertensives, cimetidine

• Decreased effects of: lithium

• Increased levels of: digoxin, theophylline, cyclosporine, carbamazepine, nondepolarizing muscle relaxants

NURSING CONSIDERATIONS

Administer:

• IV undiluted through Y-tube or 3-way stopcock of compatible sol; give over 2 min, or 3 min elderly

• Before meals, hs, sus rel give with food

Evaluate:

• Therapeutic response: decreased anginal pain, decreased B/P, dysrhythmias

• Cardiac status: B/P, pulse, respiration, ECG intervals (PR, QRS, QT)

Teach patient/family:

• How to take pulse before taking drug; record or graph should be kept

• To avoid hazardous activities until stabilized on drug, dizziness is no longer a problem

• To limit caffeine consumption

• To avoid OTC drugs unless directed by a physician

• To comply with all areas of med-

ical regimen: diet, exercise, stress reduction, drug therapy
Lab test interferences:
Increase: Liver function tests
Treatment of overdose: Defibrillation, atropine for AV block, vasopressor for hypotension

---

vidarabine (ophthalmic)

(vye-dare'a-been)
Vira-A Ophthalmic
Func. class.: Antiviral
Chem. class.: Purine nucleoside

Action: Inhibits viral DNA synthesis by blocking DNA polymerase
Uses: Herpes simplex, cytomegalovirus, varicella zoster
Dosage and routes:
• *Adult and child:* TOP ½ inch oint into conjunctival sac q3h, 5 times daily
Available forms include: Oint 3%
Side effects/adverse reactions:
EENT: Burning, stinging, photophobia, pain, temporary visual haze
Contraindications: Hypersensitivity
Precautions: Antibiotic hypersensitivity, pregnancy (C)

NURSING CONSIDERATIONS
Administer:
• After washing hands, cleanse crusts or discharge from eye before application
Perform/provide:
• Storage at room temperature
Evaluate:
• Therapeutic response: absence of redness, inflammation, tearing
• Allergy: itching, lacrimation, redness, swelling
Teach patient/family:
• To use drug exactly as prescribed
• Not to use eye makeup, towels, washcloths, or eye medication of others, or reinfection may occur
• That drug container tip should not be touched to eye
• To report itching, increased redness, burning, stinging, photophobia, drug should be discontinued
• That drug may cause blurred vision when ointment is applied
• To use sunglasses to prevent photophobia

---

vidarabine

(vye-dare'a-been)
Vira-A
Func. class.: Antibacterial, antiviral
Chem. class.: Purine nucleoside

Action: Inhibits bacterial/viral replication by preventing DNA synthesis
Uses: Herpes simplex virus encephalitis, varicella-zoster encephalomyelitis
Dosage and routes:
• *Adult and child:* IV INF 15 mg/kg/day × 10 days; infuse over 12-24 hr
Available forms include: Inj IV 200 mg/ml
Side effects/adverse reactions:
CNS: Psychosis, hallucinations, dizziness, weakness, tremors, ***fatal metabolic encephalopathy,*** confusion, malaise
GU: SIADH
HEMA: ***Anemia, thrombocytopenia, neutropenia***
GI: Nausea, vomiting, anorexia, diarrhea, weight loss
INTEG: Pain, thrombophlebitis at injection site
Contraindications: Hypersensitivity
Precautions: Renal disease, liver disease, lactation, pregnancy (C)
Pharmacokinetics: Crosses blood-

V

brain barrier, excreted by kidneys (metabolites), crosses placenta, half-life 1½-3 hr

Interactions/incompatibilities:

• Increased neurologic side effects: allopurinol

NURSING CONSIDERATIONS

Assess:

• Liver studies: AST, ALT

• Blood studies: WBC, diff, RBC, Hct, Hgb, platelets

• Renal studies: urinalysis, protein, blood

• C&S before drug therapy; drug may be taken as soon as culture is taken; C&S may be taken after therapy

Administer:

• Shake solution; dilute to 450 mg/L IV; give fluid at constant rate over 12-24 hr, using in-line filter with mean pore diameter of 0.45 mm or less

Evaluate:

• Therapeutic response: decreased amount of lesion, itching

• Bowel pattern before, during treatment

• Fluid overload; drug requires large volume to stay in solutions

• Weakness, tremors, confusion, dizziness, psychosis; if these occur, drug might need to be decreased or discontinued

---

vinblastine sulfate (VLB)

(vin-blast'een)

Velban, Velbe*

Func. class.: Antineoplastic

Chem. class.: Vinca rosea alkaloid

Action: Inhibits mitotic activity, arrests cell cycle at metaphase; inhibits RNA synthesis, blocks cellular use of glutamic acid needed for purine synthesis; a vesicant

Uses: Breast, testicular cancer, lymphomas, neuroblastoma, Hodgkin's non-Hodgkin's lymphomas, mycosis fungoides, histiocytosis, Kaposi's sarcoma

Dosage and routes:

• *Adult and child:* IV 0.1 mg/kg or 3.7 mg/m² qwk or q2wk, not to exceed 0.5 mg/kg or 18.5 mg/m² qwk in adults

Available forms include: Inj IV, powder 10 mg for 10 ml IV inj

Side effects/adverse reactions:

HEMA: ***Thrombocytopenia, leukopenia, myelosupppression***

GI: Nausea, vomiting, ileus, *anorexia, stomatitis,* constipation, abdominal pain, GI, rectal bleeding, ***hepatotoxicity,*** pharyngitis, stomatitis

GU: Urinary retention, ***renal failure***

INTEG: Rash, alopecia, photosensitivity

RESP: ***Fibrosis, pulmonary infiltrate***

CV: Tachycardia, orthostatic hypotension

CNS: Paresthesias, peripheral neuropathy, depression, headache, ***convulsions***

META: SIADH

Contraindications: Hypersensitivity, infants, pregnancy (D)

Precautions: Renal disease, hepatic disease

Pharmacokinetics: Half-life (triphasic) 35 min, 53 min, 19 hr, metabolized in liver, excreted in urine, feces, crosses blood-brain barrier

Interactions/incompatibilities:

• Increased action of: methotrexate

• Do not use with radiation

• Synergism: bleomycin

• Decreased phenytoin level: phenytoin

• Bronchospasm: mitomycin

NURSING CONSIDERATIONS

Assess:

• CBC, differential, platelet count

---

* Available in Canada only

weekly, withhold drug if WBC is <4000 or platelet count is <75,000; notify physician of results
• Pulmonary function tests, chest x-ray studies before, during therapy; chest x-ray film should be obtained q2wk during treatment
• Neurologic status: sensory-vibratory evaluation if side effects occur
• Renal function studies: BUN, serum uric acid, urine CrCl, electrolytes before, during therapy
• I&O ratio; report fall in urine output of 30 ml/hr
• Monitor temperature q4h; may indicate beginning infection
• Liver function tests before, during therapy (bilirubin, AST, ALT, LDH) as needed or monthly
• RBC, Hct, Hgb since these may be decreased

Administer:
• IV after diluting 10 mg/10 ml NaCl; give through Y-tube or 3-way stopcock or directly over 1 min
• Hyaluronidase 150 U/ml in 1 ml NaCl, warm compress for extravasation
• Antacid before oral agent; give drug after evening meal before bedtime
• Antiemetic 30-60 min before giving drug and prn to prevent vomiting
• Local or systemic drugs for infection
• Transfusion for anemia
• Antispasmodic for GI symptoms

Perform/provide:
• Deep-breathing exercises with patient 3-4 × day; place in semi-Fowler's position
• Liquid diet: cola, Jell-O; dry toast or crackers may be added if patient is not nauseated or vomiting
• Increase fluid intake to 2-3 L/day to prevent urate deposits, calculi formation
• Rinsing of mouth 3-4 × day with water
• Brushing of teeth 2-3 × day with soft brush or cotton-tipped applicators for stomatitis; use unwaxed dental floss
• Nutritious diet with iron, vitamin supplements
• HOB raised to facilitate breathing

Evaluate:
• Therapeutic response: decreased tumor size, spread of malignancy
• Bleeding: hematuria, guaiac, bruising or petechiae, mucosa of orifices q8h
• Dyspnea, rales, unproductive cough, chest pain, tachypnea, fatigue, increased pulse, pallor, lethargy
• Food preferences; list likes, dislikes
• Effects of alopecia on body image; discuss feelings about body changes
• Sensitivity of feet/hands, which precedes neuropathy
• Inflammation of mucosa, breaks in skin
• Yellowing of skin and sclera, dark urine, clay-colored stools, itchy skin, abdominal pain, fever, diarrhea
• Buccal cavity q8h for dryness, sores or ulceration, white patches, oral pain, bleeding, dysphagia
• Local irritation, pain, burning, discoloration at injection site
• Symptoms indicating severe allergic reaction: rash, pruritus, urticaria, purpuric skin lesions, itching, flushing
• Frequency of stools and characteristics: cramping, acidosis; signs of dehydration: rapid respirations, poor skin turgor, decreased urine

output, dry skin, restlessness, weakness

Teach patient/family:

• To report any complaints or side effects to the nurse or physician

• To report any changes in breathing or coughing

• That hair may be lost during treatment, a wig or hairpiece may make patient feel better; tell patient that new hair may be different in color, texture

• To report change in gait or numbness in extremities; may indicate neuropathy

• To avoid foods with citric acid, hot or rough texture

• To report any bleeding, white spots or ulcerations in mouth to physician; tell patient to examine mouth qd

vincristine sulfate (VCR)

(vin-kris'teen)

Oncovin

Func. class.: Antineoplastic

Chem. class.: Vinca alkaloid

Action: Inhibits mitotic activity, arrests cell cycle at metaphase; inhibits RNA synthesis, blocks cellular use of glutamic acid needed for purine synthesis; a vesicant

Uses: Breast, lung cancer, lymphomas, neuroblastoma, Hodgkin's disease, acute lymphoblastic and other leukemias, rhabdomyosarcoma, Wilms' tumor, osteogenic and other sarcomas

Dosage and routes:

• *Adult:* IV 1-2 mg/m^2/wk, not to exceed 2 mg

• *Child:* IV 1.5-2 mg/m^2/wk, not to exceed 2 mg

Available forms include: Inj IV 1 mg/ml

Side effects/adverse reactions:

INTEG: Alopecia

HEMA: ***Thrombocytopenia, leukopenia, myelosuppression, anemia***

GI: Nausea, vomiting, anorexia, stomatitis, constipation, ***paralytic ileus,*** *abdominal pain,* ***hepatotoxicity***

CV: Orthostatic hypotension

CNS: Decreased reflexes, numbness, weakness, motor difficulties, CNS depression, cranial nerve paralysis, ***seizures***

Contraindications: Hypersensitivity, infants, pregnancy (D)

Precautions: Renal disease, hepatic disease, hypertension, neuromuscular disease

Pharmacokinetics: Half-life (triphasic) 0.85 min, 7.4 min, 164 min, metabolized in liver, excreted in bile, feces, crosses placental barrier, crosses blood-brain barrier

Interactions/incompatibilities:

• Increased action of: methotrexate

• Do not use with radiation

• Neurotoxicity: peripheral nervous system drugs

• Decreased digoxin level: digoxin

• Decreased action of vincristine: L-asparaginase

• Acute pulmonary reactions: Mitomycin-c

NURSING CONSIDERATIONS

Assess:

• CBC, differential, platelet count weekly; withhold drug if WBC is <4000 or platelet count is <75,000; notify physician of results

• Renal function studies: BUN, serum uric acid, urine CrCl, electrolytes before, during therapy

• I&O ratio, report fall in urine output of 30 ml/hr

• Monitor temperature q4h; may indicate beginning infection

• Liver function tests before, dur-

ing therapy (bilirubin, AST, ALT, LDH) as needed or monthly
• RBC, Hct, Hgb since these may be decreased
• Deep tendon reflexes; drug is neurotoxic

Administer:
• Agents to prevent constipation
• Antiemetic 30-60 min before giving drug and prn to prevent vomiting
• IV after diluting with diluent provided or 1 mg/10 ml of sterile H_2O or NaCl; give through Y-tube or 3-way stopcock or directly over 1 min
• Hyaluronidase 150 U/ml in 1 ml NaCl, apply warm compress for extravasation
• Transfusion for anemia
• Antispasmodic for GI symptoms

Perform/provide:
• Liquid diet: cola, Jell-O; dry toast or crackers may be added if patient is not nauseated or vomiting
• Rinsing of mouth 3-4 × day with water
• Brushing of teeth 2-3 × day with soft brush or cotton-tipped applicators for stomatitis; use unwaxed dental floss
• Nutritious diet with iron, vitamin supplements

Evaluate:
• Therapeutic response: decreased tumor size, spread of malignancy
• Sensitivity of feet/hands, which precedes neuropathy
• Bleeding: hematuria, guaiac, bruising or petechiae, mucosa of orifices q8h
• Food preferences; list likes, dislikes
• Effects of alopecia on body image, discuss feelings about body changes
• Inflammation of mucosa, breaks in skin
• Yellowing of skin and sclera, dark urine, clay-colored stools, itchy skin, abdominal pain, fever, diarrhea
• Buccal cavity q8h for dryness, sores or ulceration, white patches, oral pain, bleeding, dysphagia
• Symptoms indicating severe allergic reaction: rash, pruritus, urticaria, purpuric skin lesions, itching, flushing
• Frequency of stools, characteristics: cramping, acidosis; signs of dehydration: rapid respirations, poor skin turgor, decreased urine output, dry skin, restlessness, weakness

Teach patient/family:
• To report change in gait or numbness in extremities; may indicate neuropathy
• To report any complaints or side effects to nurse or physician
• To report any bleeding, white spots or ulcerations in mouth to physician; tell patient to examine mouth qd

vitamin A

Acon, Afaxin, Aquasol A, Natola
Func. class.: Vitamin, fat soluble
Chem. class.: Retinol

Action: Needed for normal bone and teeth development, visual dark adaptation, skin disease, mucosa tissue repair, assists in production of adrenal steroids, cholesterol, RNA

Uses: Vitamin A deficiency

Dosage and routes:
• *Adult and child >8 yr:* PO 100,000-500,000 IU qd 3 days, then 50,000 qd × 2 wk; dose based on severity of deficiency; maintenance 10,000-20,000 IU for 2 mo

• *Child 1-8 yr:* IM 17,500-35,000 IU qd × 10 days
• *Infants <1 yr:* IM 7500-15,000 IU × 10 days
Maintenance
• Child 4-8 yr: IM 15,000 IU qd × 2 mo
• Child <4 yr: IM 10,000 IU qd × 2 mo
Available forms include: Caps 10,000, 25,000, 50,000 IU; drops 5,000 IU; inj 50,000 IU/ml
Side effects/adverse reactions:
GI: Nausea, vomiting, anorexia, abdominal pain, ***jaundice***
CNS: Headache, increased intracranial pressure, intracranial hypertension, lethargy, malaise
EENT: Gingivitis, papilledema, exophthalmos, inflammation of tongue and lips
INTEG: Drying of skin, pruritus, increased pigmentation, night sweats, alopecia
MS: Arthraglia, retarded growth, hard areas on bone
META: Hypomenorrhea, hypercalcemia
Contraindications: Hypersensitivity to vitamin A, malabsorption syndrome (PO)
Precautions: Lactation, impaired renal function, pregnancy (A)
Pharmacokinetics:
PO/INJ: Stored in liver, kidneys, fat; excreted (metabolites) in urine, feces
Interactions/incompatibilities:
• Decreased absorption of vitamin A: mineral oil
• Increased levels of vitamin A: corticosteroids

NURSING CONSIDERATIONS
Administer:
• With food (PO) for better absorption
Perform/provide:
• Storage in tight, light-resistant container
Evaluate:
• Therapeutic response: increased growth rate, weight; absence of dry skin and mucous membranes, night blindness
• Nutritional status: yellow and dark green vegetables, yellow/orange fruits, vitamin A fortified foods, liver, egg yolks
• Vitamin A deficiency: decreased growth, night blindness, dry, brittle nails, hair loss, urinary stones, increased infection, hyperkeratosis of skin, drying of cornea
Teach patient/family:
• Not to use mineral oil while taking this drug
• To notify a physician of nausea, vomiting, lip cracking, loss of hair, headache
• Not to take more than the prescribed amount
Lab test interferences:
False increase: Bilirubin, serum cholesterol
Treatment of overdose: Discontinue drug

---

vitamin D (cholecalciferol, vitamin D_3 or ergocalciferol, vitamin D_2)

Calciferol, Deltalin, Drisdol, Hytakerol, Radiostol,* Radiostol Forte*
Func. class.: Vitamin D
Chem. class.: Fat soluble

Action: Needed for regulation of calcium, phosphate levels, normal bone development, parathyroid activity, neuromuscular functioning
Uses: Vitamin D deficiency, rickets, renal osteodystrophy, hypoparathyroidism, hypophosphatemia, psoriasis, rheumatoid arthritis
Dosage and routes:
• *Adult:* PO/IM 12,000 IU qd,

*Available in Canada only

then increased to 500,000 IU/day
• *Child:* PO/IM 1500/5000 IU qd × 2-4 wk, may repeat after 2 wk or 600,000 IU as single dose
Hypoparathyroidism
• *Adult and child:* PO/IM 200,000 IU given with 4 g calcium tab
Available forms include: Tabs 400, 1000, 50,000 IU; caps 25,000, 50,000; liq 8000 IU/ml; inj 500,000 IU/ml, 500,000 IU/5 ml IM
Side effects/adverse reactions:
GI: Nausea, vomiting, anorexia, cramps, diarrhea, constipation, metallic taste, dry mouth, decreased libido
CNS: Fatigue, weakness, drowsiness, ***convulsions,*** headache, psychosis
GU: Polyuria, nocturia, ***hematuria, albuminuria, renal failure***
CV: Hypertension, dysrhythmias
MS: Decreased bone growth, early joint pain, early muscle pain
INTEG: Pruritus, photophobia
Contraindications: Hypersensitivity, hypercalcemia, renal dysfunction, hyperphosphatemia
Precautions: Cardiovascular disease, renal calculi, pregnancy (A)
Pharmacokinetics:
PO/INJ: Half-life 7-12 hr, stored in liver, duration 2 mo, excreted in bile (metabolites) and urine
Interactions/incompatibilities:
• Decreased effects of vitamin D: cholestyramine, colestipol, phenobarbital, phenytoin
• Increased toxicity: diuretics (thiazides), antacids, verapamil

NURSING CONSIDERATIONS

Assess:
• Vitamin D levels q2 wk during treatment
• Ca, PO_4, Mg, BUN, alk phosphatase, urine Ca, creatinine
Administer:
• IM injection in deep muscle mass, administer slowly
Evaluate:
• Therapeutic response: absence of rickets/osteomalacia, adequate calcium/phosphate levels, decrease in bone pain
• Nutritional status: egg yolk, fortified dairy products, cod, halibut, salmon, sardines
Teach patient/family:
• Necessary foods to be included in diet
• To avoid vitamin supplements unless directed by physician
• To keep doctor's appointments since line between therapeutic and toxic doses is narrow
• To report weakness, lethargy, headache, anorexia, loss of weight
• Nausea, vomiting, abdominal cramps, diarrhea, constipation, excessive thirst, polyuria, muscle and bone pain
• To decrease intake of antacids containing magnesium

vitamin E

Alfacol, Aquasol E, Daltose,* E-Ferol, Eprolin, Hy-E-Plex, Kell-E, Lethopherol, Maxi-E, Pertropin, Tocopher-Caps, Tocopherol
Func. class.: Vitamin E
Chem. class.: Fat soluble

Action: Needed for digestion and metabolism of polyunsaturated fats, decreased platelet aggregation, decreases blood clot formation, promotes normal growth, and development of muscle tissue, prostaglandin synthesis
Uses: Vitamin E deficiency, impaired fat absorption, hemolytic anemia in premature neonates, prevention of retrolental fibroplasia,

V

sickle cell anemia, supplement in malabsorption syndrome

Dosage and routes:

• *Adult:* PO/IM 60-75 IU qd, not to exceed 300 IU/day

• *Child:* PO/IM 1 mg/0.6 g of dietary fat

Available forms include: Caps 50, 100, 200, 400, 500, 600, 1000 IU; 74, 165, 294, 331 mg; tabs 200, 400 IU; 331 mg; drops 50 mg/ml

Side effects/adverse reactions:

META: Altered metabolism of hormones, thyroid, pituitary, adrenal, altered immunity

MS: Weakness

CNS: Headache, fatigue

GI: Nausea, cramps, diarrhea

GU: Gonadal dysfunction

CV: Increased risk thrombophlebitis

EENT: Blurred vision

INTEG: Sterile abscess, contact dermatitis

Contraindications: None significant

Precautions: Pregnancy (A)

Pharmacokinetics:

PO: Metabolized in liver, excreted in bile

Interactions/incompatibilities:

• Increased action of: oral anticoagulants

NURSING CONSIDERATIONS

Assess:

• BUN, creatinine

• Vitamin E levels during treatment

• CBC; hemolytic anemia may occur

Administer:

• Topically to moisturize dry skin

Perform/provide:

• Storage in tight, light-resistant container

Evaluate:

• Therapeutic response: absence of hemolytic anemia, adequate vitamin E levels, improvement in skin lesions, decreased edema

• Nutritional status: wheat germ, dark green leafy vegetables, nuts, eggs, liver, vegetable oils, dairy products, cereals

Teach patient/family:

• Necessary foods to be included in diet

• To avoid vitamin supplements unless directed by physician

---

warfarin sodium

(war'far-in)

Coumadin, Panwarfin, Sofarin, Carfin, Warfilone Sodium,* Warnerin*

Func. class.: Anticoagulant

Action: Interferes with blood clotting by indirect means; depresses hepatic synthesis of vitamin K-dependent coagulation factors (II, VII, IX, X)

Uses: Pulmonary emboli, deep vein thrombosis, myocardial infarction, atrial dysrhythmias

Dosage and routes:

• *Adult:* PO 10-15 mg × 3 days, then titrated to PT qd or 40-60 mg for 1 day, then 2-10 mg qd titrated to PT level

Available forms include: Tabs 1 mg, 2, 2.5, 5, 7.5, 10 mg; inj 50 mg/2 ml

Side effects/adverse reactions:

GI: Diarrhea, nausea, vomiting, anorexia, stomatitis, cramps, ***hepatitis***

GU: ***Hematuria***

INTEG: Rash, dermatitis, urticaria, alopecia, pruritus

CNS: Fever

HEMA: ***Hemorrhage, agranulocytosis, leukopenia, eosinophilia***

Contraindications: Hypersensitivity, hemophilia, leukemia with bleeding, peptic ulcer disease, thrombocytopenic purpura, hepatic

---

*Available in Canada only

disease (severe), severe hypertension, subacute bacterial endocarditis, acute nephritis, blood dyscrasias, pregnancy (D), eclampsia, preeclampsia, lactation

Precautions: Alcoholism, elderly

Pharmacokinetics:

PO: Onset 12-24 hr, peak 1½-3 days, duration 3-5 days, half-life 1½-2½ days; metabolized in liver, excreted in urine/feces (active/inactive metabolites), crosses placenta 99% bound to plasma proteins

Interactions/incompatibilities:

• Increased action of warfarin: allopurinol, chloramphenicol, amiodarone, diflunisal, heparin, steroids, cimetidine, disulfiram, thyroid, glucagon, metronidazole, quinidine, sulindac, sulfinpyrazone, sulfonamides, clofibrate, salicylates, ethacrynic acids, indomethacin, mefenamic acid, oxyphenbutazones, phenylbutazone

• Decreased action of warfarin: barbiturates, griseofulvin, ethchlorvynol, carbamazepine, rifampin, oral contraceptives, phenytoin, estrogens, vitamin K, cholestyramine

• Increased toxicity: oral sulfonylureas, phenytoin

NURSING CONSIDERATIONS

Assess:

• Blood studies (Hct, platelets, occult blood in stools) q3mo

• Prothrombin time, which should be 1½-2 × control, PT; often done qd initially

Administer:

• At same time each day to maintain steady blood levels

• Tabs whole or crushed

• Avoiding all IM injections that may cause bleeding

Perform/provide:

• Storage in tight container

Evaluate:

• Therapeutic response: decrease of deep vein thrombosis

• Bleeding gums, petecchiae, ecchymosis, black tarry stools, hematuria

• Fever, skin rash, urticaria

• Needed dosage change q1-2wk; when stable, PT q3wk

Teach patient/family:

• To avoid OTC preparations that may cause serious drug interactions unless directed by physician

• To use soft-bristle toothbrush to avoid bleeding gums, electric razor

• To carry a Medic-Alert ID identifying drug taken

• Importance of compliance

• To report any signs of bleeding: gums, under skin, urine, stools

• To avoid hazardous activities (football, hockey, skiing) or dangerous work

• Importance of avoiding unusual changes in vitamin intake, diet or lifestyle

• To inform dentists and other physicians of anticoagulant intake

• That smoking increases dose requirements

Lab test interferences:

Increase: T_3 uptake

Decrease: Uric acid

Treatment of overdose: Administer vitamin K

xylometazoline HCl (nasal)

(xye-loe-met-az'oh-leen)

Neo-Synephrine II, Otrivin, Sine-Off Nasal Spray, Sinex-LA

Func. class.: Nasal decongestant

Chem. class.: Sympathomimetic amine

Action: Dilates arterioles of nasal

membrane, which decreases congestion

Uses: Nasal congestion

Dosage and routes:

• *Adult and child >12 yr:* INSTILL 2-3 gtts or 2 sprays q8-10h (0.1%)

• *Child <12 yr:* INSTILL 2-3 gtts or 1% spray q8-10h (0.05%)

Available forms include: Sol 0.05%, 0.1%

Side effects/adverse reactions:

EENT: Irritation, burning, sneezing, stinging, dryness, rebound congestion

INTEG: Contact dermatitis

Contraindications: Hypersensitivity to sympathomimetic amines

Precautions: Pregnancy (C), glaucoma

Pharmacokinetics:

INSTILL: Onset 5-10 min, duration 5-6 hr

NURSING CONSIDERATIONS

Administer:

• No more than q4h

• For <4 consecutive days

Perform/provide:

• Environmental humidification to decrease nasal congestion, dryness

• Storage in light-resistant containers; do not expose to high temperatures

Evaluate:

• Therapeutic response: decreased nasal congestion

• Redness, swelling, pain in nasal passages

Teach patient/family:

• To avoid contamination of container

• That stinging may occur for a few applications; drying of mucosa may be decreased by environmental humidification

• To notify physician if irregular pulse, insomnia, dizziness, or tremors occur

• Proper administration to avoid systemic absorption

zidovudine (formerly azidothymidine or AZT)

(zid-oo'-vue-dine)

Retrovir

Func. class.: Antiviral

Chem. class.: Thymidine analog

Action: Inhibits replication of HIV virus by interfering with transcription of RNA and DNA

Uses: Symptomatic HIV infections (AIDS, ARC), confirmed *P. carinii* pneumonia, or absolute CD4 lymphocytes of <200/mm^3

Dosage and routes:

• *Adult:* PO 200 mg q4h; may need to stop treatment if severe bone marrow depression occurs, and restart after bone marrow recovery

Available forms include: Caps 100 mg

Side effects/adverse reactions:

HEMA: ***Granulocytopenia, anemia***

CNS: Fever, headache, malaise, diaphoresis, dizziness, insomnia, paresthesia, somnolence, chills, tremor, twitching, anxiety, confusion, depression, lability, vertigo, loss of mental acuity

GI: Nausea, vomiting, diarrhea, anorexia, cramps, dyspepsia, constipation, dysphagia, flatulence, rectal bleeding, mouth ulcer

RESP: Dyspnea

EENT: Taste change, hearing loss, photophobia

INTEG: Rash, acne, pruritus, urticaria

MS: Myalgia, arthralgia, muscle spasm

GU: Dysuria, polyuria, frequency, hesitancy

Contraindications: Hypersensitivity

*Available in Canada only

Precautions: Granulocyte count <1000/mm_3 or Hgb <9.5 g/dl, pregnancy (C), lactation, children, severe renal disease, severe hepatic function

Pharmacokinetics:

PO: Rapidly absorbed from GI tract, peak ½-1½ hr, metabolized in liver (inactive metabolites), excreted by kidneys

Interactions/incompatibilities:

• Toxicity: amphotericin B, dapsone, flucytosine, adriamycin, interferon vincristine, vinblastine, pentamidine, probenecid, experimental nucleoside analogs, benzodiazepines, cimetidine, morphine, sulfonamides

• Granulocytopenia: acetaminophen, aspirin, indomethacin

NURSING CONSIDERATIONS

Assess:

• Blood counts q2wk, watch for decreasing granulocytes, Hgb; if low, therapy may need to be discontinued and restarted after hematologic recovery; blood transfusions may be required

Administer:

• By mouth, capsules should be swallowed whole

• Trimethoprim-sulfamethoxazole, pyrimethamine, or acyclovir as ordered to prevent opportunistic infections; if these drugs are given, watch for neurotoxicity

Perform/provide:

• Storage in cool environment, protect from light

Evaluate:

• Blood dyscrasias (anemia, granulocytopenia): bruising, fatigue, bleeding, poor healing

Teach patient/family:

• That drug is not cure for AIDS, but will control symptoms

• To call physician if sore throat, swollen lymph nodes, malaise, fever occur since other infections may occur

• That even with drug administration, patient is still infective and may pass AIDS virus on to others

• That follow-up visits must be continued since serious toxicity may occur, blood counts must be done q2wk

• That drug must be taken q4h around clock even during night

• That serious drug interactions may occur if OTC products are ingested, check with physician first if taking aspirin, acetaminophen, indomethacin

• That other drugs may be necessary to prevent other infections

• That drug may cause fainting or dizziness

---

zinc sulfate

Eye-Sed Ophthalmic, Op-Thal-Zin

Func. class.: Ophthalmic vasoconstrictor

Chem. class.: Zinc product

Action: Vasoconstriction occurs by action on conjunctiva

Uses: Ocular congestion, irritation, itching

Dosage and routes:

• *Adult and child >2 yr:* INSTILL 1-2 gtts bid or tid

Available forms include: Sol 0.217%, 0.25%

Side effects/adverse reactions:

EENT: Eye irritation, burning

Contraindications: Hypersensitivity

Precautions: Narrow-angle glaucoma, pregnancy (C)

NURSING CONSIDERATIONS

Perform/provide:

• Storage in tight container

Evaluate:

• Therapeutic response: decreased

ocular irritation, itching, congestion

Teach patient/family:
• To report change in vision, or irritation
• Method of instillation; tilt head backward, hold dropper over eye, drop medication inside lower lid, using pressure on inside corner of eye hold 1 min, do not touch dropper to eye

---

zinc sulfate

Orazinc

Func. class.: Trace element

Action: Needed for adequate healing, bone and joint development (23% zinc)

Uses: Prevention of zinc deficiency, adjunct to vitamin A therapy

Dosage and routes:
• *Adult:* PO 200-220 mg tid
• *Child:* PO 0.3 mg/kg/day

Available forms include: Tabs 110, 200, 220 mg; caps 110, 220 mg

Side effects/adverse reactions:
GI: Nausea, vomiting, cramps, heartburn, ulcer formation
OVERDOSE: Diarrhea, rash, dehydration, restlessness

Precautions: Pregnancy (A)

Interactions/incompatibilities:
• Decreased absorption of: other covalent cations

NURSING CONSIDERATIONS

Assess:
• Zinc levels during treatment

Administer:
• With meals to decrease gastric upset; avoid dairy products

Evaluate:
• Therapeutic response: absence of zinc deficiency

Teach patient/family:
• That element will need to be taken for 2 mo to be effective
• To immediately report nausea, diarrhea, rash, severe vomiting, restlessness

Appendix a

Abbreviations

ā before
aa of each
AB abortion
abd abdomen
ABGs arterial blood gases
ac before meals
ACE angiotensin-converting enzyme
ad lib as desired
ADA American Diabetes Association
ADH antidiuretic hormone
AKA also known as
ALT alanine aminotransferase, serum
AMA against medical advice
amb ambulation
ANA antinuclear antibodies
ant anterior
AP anteroposterior
APTT activated partial thromboplastin time
AROM active range of motion
ASA acetylsalicylic acid, aspirin
ASAP as soon as possible
AST aspartate aminotransferase, serum
ASHD arteriosclerotic heart disease
AV atrioventricular
BAL blood alcohol level
bid twice a day
BM bowel movement
BMR basal metabolism rate
B/P blood pressure
BPH benign prostatic hypertrophy
bpm beats per minute
BS blood sugar
BSP bromsulphalein
BUN blood urea nitrogen
Bx biopsy
c̄ with
cap capsules
C Celsius (centigrade)
Ca cancer
CAD coronary artery disease
cath catheterization or catheterize
CC chief complaint
cc cubic centimeter
CBC complete blood count
CHF congestive heart failure

cm centimeter
CNS central nervous system
CO_2 carbon dioxide
c/o complains of
COPD chronic obstructive pulmonary disease
CPAP continuous positive airway pressure
CPK creatinine phosphokinase
CPR cardiopulmonary resuscitation
CrCl creatinine clearance
C section cesarean section
C&S culture and sensitivity
CSF cerebrospinal fluid
CV cardiovascular
CVA cerebrovascular accident
CVP central venous pressure
D&C dilatation and curettage
DM diabetes mellitus
DOA dead on arrival
DOB date of birth
dr dram
dsg dressing
D_5W 5% glucose in distilled water
dx diagnosis
ECG electrocardiogram (EKG)
EDTA ethylenediaminetetraacetic acid
EEG electroencephalogram
EENT ear, eye, nose, and throat
elix elixir
EPS extrapyramidal symptoms
ESR erythrocyte sedimentation rate
F Farenheit
FBS fasting blood sugar
FHT fetal heart tones
FIo_2 inspired oxygen concentration
FSH follicle-stimulating hormone
fx fracture
g gram
gal gallon
gr grain
GTT glucose tolerance test
gtt drop
GI gastrointestinal
GU genitourinary
Gyn gynecology
H hypodermically
H & H hematocrit and hemoglobin
Hct hematocrit
HCG human chorionic gonadotropin
HDCV human diploid cell rabies vaccine
Hgb hemoglobin
5-HIAA 5-hydroxyindoleacetic acid
H_2O water
HOB head of bed
HR heart rate
hr hour
hs at bedtime
Hx history
IgG immunoglobulin G

IM intramuscular
INH inhalation
inj injection
IPPB intermittent positive pressure breathing
I&O intake and output
ITP idiopathic thrombocytopenic purpura
IUD intrauterine contraceptive device
IV intravenous
IVAC intravenous controller
IVP intravenous pyelogram
IVPB intravenous piggyback
K potassium
kg kilogram
L or l left
L liter
lat lateral
lb pound
LDH lactic dehydrogenase
LE lupus erythematosus
LH luteinizing hormone
liq liquid
LLQ left lower quadrant
LMP last menstrual period
LOC loss of consciousness
LR lactated Ringer's solution
LUQ left upper quadrant
M meter
m minim
m^2 square meter
MAOI monoamine oxidase inhibitor
MCA motorcycle accident
mEq milliequivalent
mg milligram
μg microgram
MI myocardial infarction
min minute
mixt mixture
ml milliliter
mm millimeter
mo month
MRC medical research council
MVA motor vehicle accident
Na sodium
NC nasal cannula
neg negative
NKA no known allergies
noc night
NPO nothing by mouth (Lat. *nulla per os*)
NS normal saline
NV neurovascular
O_2 oxygen
OBS organic brain syndrome
OD right eye
OOB out of bed
OR operating room
ORIF open reduction, internal fixation
OS left eye
os mouth
OTC over the counter
OU each eye
oz ounce
p̄ after
p pulse

P56 plasma-lyte 56
Pa_{CO_2} arterial carbon dioxide tension (pressure)
Pa_{O_2} arterial oxygen tension (pressure)
PBI protein-bound iodine
PAT paroxysmal atrial tachycardia
PCN penicillin
PCWP pulmonary capillary wedge pressure
PE physical examination
PEEP positive end expiratory pressure
PERRLA pupils equal, round, react to light and accommodation
pH hydrogen ion concentration
PO by mouth
postop postoperatively
PP postprandial
PPD purified protein derivative
preop preoperatively
prep preparation
prn as needed
pro-time, PT prothrombin time
PTT partial thromboplastin time
PVC premature ventricular contraction
q every
qAM every morning
qd every day
qh every hour
qid four times a day
qod every other day
qPM every night
qs quantity sufficient
qt quart
q2h every 2 hours
q3h every 3 hours
q4h every 4 hours
q6h every 6 hours
q12h every 12 hours
R respirations, rectal
r right
RAIU radioactive iodine uptake
RBC(s) red blood count or cell(s)
REM rapid eye movement
RLQ right lower quadrant
R/O rule out
ROM range of motion
RUQ right upper quadrant
Rx therapy, treatment, or prescription
s̄ without
SAN sinoatrial node
SC subcutaneous
sig label
SIMV synchronous intermittent mandatory ventilation
SL sublingual
SOB short of breath
sol solution
ss one half
stat at once
surg surgical
Sx symptoms
supp suppository
syr syrup
T temperature

T&A tonsillectomy and adenoidectomy
tab tablet
TAH total abdominal hysterectomy
tbsp tablespoon
temp temperature
tid three times daily
tinc tincture
TPN total parenteral nutrition
TPR temperature, pulse, respirations
top topical
TSH thyroid-stimulating hormone
tsp teaspoon
TT thrombin time
U unit
UA urinalysis
UV ultraviolet
vag vaginal
VD veneral disease
VMA vanillylmandelic acid
VO verbal order
vol volume
VS vital signs
WBC white blood count
wk week
WNL within normal limits
wt weight
yr year
$>$ greater than
$<$ less than
$=$ equal
$\neq$ not equal
$\uparrow$ increase
$\downarrow$ decrease
2° secondary
° degree
% percent
@ at

Appendix b

Commonly used antibiotics in adults and children

amoxicillin
Adult: PO 750 mg-1.5 g qd in divided doses q8h
Child: PO 20-40 mg/kg/day in divided doses q8h

ampicillin
Adult: PO 1-2 g qd in divided doses q6h
IM/IV 2-8 g qd in divided doses q4-6h
Child: PO 50-100 mg/kg/day in divided doses q6h
IM/IV 100-200 mg/kg/day in divided doses q6h

cefaclor
Adult: PO 250-500 mg q8h
Child: PO 24-40 mg/kg/day in divided doses q8h

cephalexin
Adult: PO 250-500 mg q6h
Child: PO 25-50 mg/kg/day in 4 equal doses

chloramphenicol
Adult and child >3 mo: 50-100 mg/kg/day in divided doses q6h

clindamycin
Adult: PO 150-450 mg q6h
IM/IV 300 mg q6-12h
Child >1 mo: PO 8-25 mg/kg/day in divided doses q6-8h
IM/IV 15-40 mg/kg/day in divided doses q6-8h

erythromycin
Adult: 250 mg-500 mg q6h
Child: 30-50 mg/kg/day in divided doses q6h

gentamicin
Adult: IV INF 3-5 mg/kg/day in divided doses q8h
Child: IV/IM 2-2.5 mg/kg q8h
Neonates and infants: IV/IM 2.5 mg/kg q8h

kanamycin
Adult and child: IV INF/IM 15 mg/kg/day in divided doses q8-12h

methicillin
Adult: IM/IV 4-12 g/day in divided doses q4-6h
Child: IM/IV 50-300 mg/kg/day in divided doses q4-12h
PO 25-50 mg/kg/day in divided doses q6h
Neonates: IM 10 mg/kg q12h

nafcillin

Adult: PO/IM/IV 2-6 g/day in divided doses q4-6h
Child: IM 25 mg/kg q12h

oxacillin

Adult: PO 2-6 g/day in divided doses q4-6h
IM/IV 2-12 g/day in divided doses q4-6h
Child: PO/IM/IV 50-100 mg/kg/day in divided doses q6h

penicillin G benzathine

Adult: IM 1.2 million U

penicillin G potassium

Adult: PO 400,000-500,000 U q6-8h
Child <12 yr: PO 25,000-90,000 U/kg/day in 3-6 divided doses

penicillin G procaine

Adult and child: IM 600,000-1.2 million U in 1-2 doses/day
Newborn: IM 50,000 U/kg qd

nitrofurantoin

Adult and child >12 yr: PO 50-100 mg qid pc

sulfisoxazole

Adult: PO 2-4 g loading dose, then 1-2 g qid
Child >2 mo: PO 75 mg/kg or 2 g/m^2 loading dose then 150 mg/kg/day or 4 g/m^2 day in divided doses q6h

ticarcillin

Adult: IV/IM 12-24 g/day in divided doses q3-6h
Child: IV/IM 50-300 mg/kg/day in divided doses q4-8h
Neonates: IV INF 75-100 mg/kg q8-12h

Appendix c

Nomogram for calculation of body surface area

Place a straight edge from the patient's height in the left column to his weight in the right column. The point of intersection on the body surface area column indicates the body surface area (BSA). Reproduced from Behrman, R.E., and Vaughn, V.C. (editors): Nelson's textbook of pediatrics, ed. 12, Philadelphia, 1983, W.B. Saunders Co.

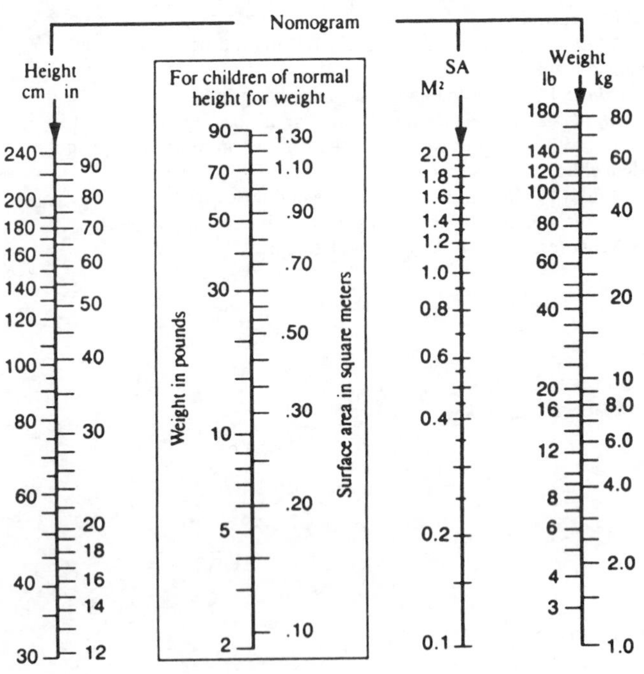

Appendix d

How to prepare a medication card

Medication cards are easy to develop from Mosby–Year Book's Nursing Drug Reference because all the information can be easily found in each individual drug monograph. The key is to use only the most essential information in the monograph since space on the medication card is more limited.

First, locate the generic drug (1) and trade name (2) in the drug monograph and place them, as well as the functional classification (3), on the card. If you are unfamiliar with how to pronounce the generic name, you should also include the pronunciation (4) in the upper right-hand corner of the card. The action (5) should be simplified so you will be able to explain the basic physiologic response of the drug. Identify the reason your patient is receiving this particular drug and place that use (6) first, with all other uses listed afterward.

Next, dosage and routes (7) should be copied exactly as given in the drug monograph; identify the dosage and route your patient is receiving. Side effects/adverse reactions (8) should be listed by body system. Only include the most common *(italicized)* and life-threatening ***(bold italic);*** you can refer to the others in the drug handbook, if needed. Contraindications and precautions (9) can be grouped together and checked before giving the medication. Also, copy the pharmacokinetics (10) so you can refer to this information after you administer the drug. Important drug interactions and incompatibilities (11) should be listed on the card and carefully checked before administering the drug.

Nursing considerations (12), which are grouped under the headings of assess, administer, perform/provide, evaluate, and teach patient/family, can be placed on the back of the card for easy reference. These nursing considerations can be simplified to save space. For example, the following assessment criteria from the drug monograph can be abbreviated as shown below:

Assess:

- I&O, report hematuria, oliguria since penicillin in high doses is neurotoxic
- Culture, sensitivity before drug therapy; drug may be taken as soon as culture is taken

Assess:

- I&O, report hematuria, oliguria
- C&S—begin drug after culture is taken

Example of medication card

FRONT

<table>
<tr><td>(1) Generic drug:
(2) Trade name:
(3) Classification:</td><td>(4) Pronunciation:</td></tr>
<tr><td colspan="2">(5) Action:
(6) Uses:
(7) Dosage and routes:
(8) Side effects/adverse reactions:
(9) Contraindications/precautions:
(10) Pharmacokinetics:
(11) Interactions/incompatibilities:</td></tr>
</table>

BACK

<table>
<tr><td>(12) Nursing considerations
Assess:
Administer:
Perform/provide:
Evaluate:
Teach patient/family:</td></tr>
</table>

Appendix e

Controlled substance chart

Drugs	United States	Canada
Heroin, LSD, peyote, marijuana, mescaline	Schedule I	Schedule H
Opium (morphine), meperidine, amphetamines, cocaine, short-acting barbiturates (secobarbital)	Schedule II	Schedule F
Glutethimide, paregoric, phendimetrazine	Schedule III	Schedule F
Chloral hydrate, chlordiazepoxide, diazepam, mazindol, meprobamate, phenobarbital	Schedule IV	Schedule F
Antidiarrheals with opium, antitussives	Schedule V	

Appendix f

FDA pregnancy categories

A No risk demonstrated to the fetus in any trimester

B No adverse effects in animals, no human studies available

C Only given after risks to the fetus are considered; animal studies have shown adverse reactions, no human studies available

D Definite fetal risks, may be given in spite of risks if needed in life-threatening conditions

X Absolute fetal abnormalities; not to be used anytime during pregnancy

Appendix g

Bibliography

Clark JB, Queener SF, Karb VB: *Pharmacological basis of nursing practice,* ed 3, St Louis, 1990, Mosby–Year Book.

Drug Information 92: Bethesda, 1992, American Hospital Formulary Service.

Facts and Comparisons: Philadelphia, updated monthly, JB Lippincott.

Gahart BL: *Intravenous medications,* ed 8, St Louis, 1992, Mosby–Year Book.

Goodman A, and others: *Goodman and Gilman's The pharmacological basis of therapeutics,* ed 8, New York, 1990, Pergamon Press.

McKenry LM and Salerno E: Mosby's pharmacology in nursing, ed 18, St Louis, 1992, Mosby–Year Book.

Mediphor Editorial Group: *Drug interaction facts,* Philadelphia, updated quarterly, JB Lippincott.

Appendix h

Combination products

Aceta with Codeine, Empracet with Codeine No. 3, Tylenol with Codeine No. 3: acetaminophen 300 mg with codeine phosphate 30 mg
Alazide, Altexide: spironolactone 25 mg with hydrochlorothiazide 25 mg
Aldactazide 25/25: spironolactone 25 mg with hydrochlorothiazide 25 mg
Aldactazide 50/50: spironolactone 50 mg with hydrochlorothiazide 50 mg
Aldoclor-15: methyldopa 250 mg with chlorothiazide 15 mg
Aldoclor-150: methyldopa 250 mg with chlorothiazide 150 mg
Aldoclor-250: methyldopa 250 mg with chlorothiazide 250 mg
Aldoril-15: methyldopa 250 mg with hydrochlorothiazide 15 mg
Aldoril-25: methyldopa 250 mg with hydrochlorothiazide 25 mg
Aldoril D30: methyldopa 500 mg with hydrochlorothiazide 30 mg
Aldoril D50: methyldopa 500 mg with hydrochlorothiazide 50 mg
Amaphen with Codeine No. 3: acetaminophen 325 mg with butalbital 50 mg, caffeine 40 mg, codeine phosphate 30 mg
Ambenyl: diphenhydramine HCl 12.5 mg/5 ml with codeine phosphate 10 mg/5 ml
Anexsia: hydrocodone bitartrate 7.5 mg with acetaminophen 325 mg
Anexsia with Codeine, Empirin with Codeine 30 mg No. 3: codeine 30 mg with acetaminophen 325 mg
Anguen No. 1: pentaerythritol tetranitrate 20 mg, phenobarbital 15 mg
Anodynos-DHC, DIA-Gesic: acetaminophen 150 mg with aspirin 230 mg, caffeine 30 mg, hydrocodone bitartrate 5 mg
Antrocol: atropine sulfate 0.195 mg with phenobarbital 16 mg
Antrocol Elixir: atropine sulfate 0.039 mg/ml with phenobarbital 3 mg/ml
Apresazide 25/25: hydralazine HCl 25 mg with hydrochlorothiazide 25 mg
Apresazide 50/50: hydralazine HCl 50 mg with hydrochlorothiazide 50 mg
Apresazide 100/50: hydralazine HCl 100 mg with hydrochlorothiazide 50 mg
Apresodex, Apresoline-Esidrix: hydralazine HCl 25 mg with hydrochlorothiazide 15 mg
Aralen Phosphate with Primaquine Phosphate: chloroquine phosphate 300 mg (of chloroquine) with primaquine phosphate 45 mg (of primaquine)
Arcotrate No. 3: pentaerythritol tetranitrate 20 mg, phenobarbital 8 mg

A.S.A. and Codeine Compound No. 3 Pulvules: codeine 30 mg with aspirin 380 mg, caffeine 30 mg

Ascriptin with Codeine No. 2: aspirin 325 mg with codeine phosphate 15 mg, buffers

Ascriptin with Codeine No. 3: aspirin 325 mg with codeine phosphate 30 mg, buffers

Atropine, Demerol Injection: meperidine HCl 50 mg/ml with atropine sulfate 0.4 mg/ml

Atropine, Demerol Injection: meperidine HCl 75 mg/ml with atropine sulfate 0.4 mg/ml

Augmentin, clavulin: amoxicillin 250 mg with clavulanate potassium 125 mg; amoxicillin 500 mg with clavulanate potassium 125 mg; amoxicillin 125 mg with potassium clavulanate 31.5 mg/5 ml; amoxicillin 250 mg with potassium clavulanate 31.5 mg/5 ml

Axotal: aspirin 650 mg with butalbital 50 mg

Azo Gantanol, Azo Sulfamethoxazole, UroGantanol: sulfamethoxazole 500 mg with phenazopyridine HCl 100 mg

Azo-Gantrisin, Azo-Suldiazo, Azo-Sulfamethoxazole: sulfisoxazole 500 mg with phenazopyridine HCl 50 mg

B-A-C: aspirin 650 mg with butalbital 50 mg, caffeine 40 mg, buffers

B-A-C No. 3: aspirin 325 mg with butalbital 50 mg, caffeine 40 mg, codeine phosphate 30 mg, buffers

Bancap: acetaminophen 325 mg with butalbital 50 mg

Bancap HC, Dolacet, Hydrocet, Zydone: hydrocodone bitartrate 5 mg with acetaminophen 500 mg

Barbidonna: belladonna alkaloids, atropine sulfate 0.025 mg, hyoscyamine sulfate 0.1286 mg, phenobarbital 16 mg, scopolamine hydrobromide 0.0074 mg

Barbidonna Elixir: belladonna alkaloids, atropine sulfate 0.034 mg/5 ml, hyoscyamine sulfate 0.0174 mg/5 ml, phenobarbital 21.6 mg/ml, scopolamine hydrobromide 0.01 mg/5 ml

Barbidonna No. 2: belladonna alkaloids, atropine sulfate 0.025 mg, hyoscyamine sulfate 0.1286 mg, phenobarbital 32 mg, scopolamine hydrobromide 0.0074 mg

BC Powder: aspirin 650 mg with caffeine 32 mg, salicylamide 195 mg

Belap, Pheno-Bella: belladonna extract 10.8 mg (0.135 mg of alkaloids of belladonna leaf) with phenobarbital
16.2 mg

Belladenal-S: levorotatory belladonna alkaloids malates 0.25 mg (of levorotatory belladonna alkaloids) with phenobarbital 50 mg

Bellalphen, Donnatal, Hyosophen: belladonna alkaloids atropine sulfate 0.0194 mg, hyoscyamine sulfate 0.1037 mg, phenobarbital 16.2 mg, scopolamine hydrobromide 0.0065 mg

Bellergal-S: ergotamine tartrate 0.6 mg with levorotatory belladonna alkaloids malates 0.2 mg (of lavorotatory belladonna alkaloids 40 mg)

Benadryl: diphenhydramine HCl 25 mg with pseudoephedrine HCl 60 mg

Benylin: diphenhydramine HCl 12.5 mg/5 ml with pseudoephedrine HCl 30 mg/5 ml

Benylin DM: dextromethorphan hydrobromide 5 mg/5 ml with guaifenesin 100 mg/5 ml

Bexophene, Darvon Compound-

65, Dolene Compound-65, Doxaphene Compound, Propoxyphene-AC, Propoxyphene Compound-65: propoxyphene HCl 65 mg with aspirin 389 mg, caffeine 32.4 mg
Bicillin C-R: 150,000 units (of penicillin G) per ml with penicillin G benzathine 150,000 units (of penicillin G) per ml
Bicillin C-R: penicillin G procaine 300,000 units (of penicillin G) per ml with penicillin G benzathine 300,000 units (of penicillin G) per ml
Bicillin C-R 900/300: penicillin G procaine 150,000 units (of penicillin G) per ml with penicillin G benzathine 450,000 units (of penicillin G) per ml
Biphetamine 12½: dextroamphetamine 6.25 mg, amphetamine 6.25 mg
Biphetamine 20: dextroamphetamine 10 mg, amphetamine 10 mg
Bitrate: pentaerythritol tetranitrate 15 mg, phenobarbital 20 mg
Blanex: chlorzoxazone 250 mg, acetaminophen 300 mg
Bromo-seltzer: acetaminophen 325 mg/capful measure with citric acid 2.224 g/capful measure, sodium bicarbonate 2.871 g/capful measure
Butibel: belladonna extract 15 mg (0.187 mg of alkaloids of belladonna leaf) with butabarbital sodium 15 mg
Butibel Elixir: belladonna extract 15 mg (0.187 mg of alkaloids of belladonna leaf) with butabarbital sodium 15 mg
Cafergot: ergotamine tartrate 1 mg with caffeine 100 mg
Cafergot suppositories: ergotamine tartrate 2 mg, caffeine 100 mg
Caladryl: diphenhydramine HCl 1% with calamine 8%, camphor 0.1%
Calcidrine: codeine 8.4 mg/5 ml with calcium iodide anhydrous 152 mg/5 ml
CAM-AP-ES: hydrochlorothiazide 15 mg, hydralazine 25 mg, reserpine 0.1 mg
Cantri, Vagilia: sulfisoxazole 10% with allantoin 2%, aminacrine HCl 0.2%
Capital and Codeine: codeine 30 mg with acetaminophen 325 mg
Capital with Codeine: acetaminophen 120 mg/5 ml with codeine 12 mg/5 ml
Capozide 25/15: captopril 25 mg with hydrochlorothiazide 15 mg
Capozide 25/25: captopril 25 mg with hydrochlorothiazide 25 mg
Capozide 50/15: captopril 50 mg with hydrochlorothiazide 15 mg
Capozide 50/25: captopril 50 mg with hydrochlorothiazide 25 mg
Carisoprodol Compound, Soprodol Compound, Soma Compound, Soprodol Compound: risoprodol 200 mg with aspirin 325 mg
Clindex, Clinoxide, Clipoxide, Librax, Lidox, Lidoxide: clidinium bromide 2.5 mg with chlordiazepoxide HCl 5 mg
Chardonna-2: belladonna extract 15 mg (0.187 mg of alkaloids of belladonna leaf) with phenobarbital 15 mg
Cherapas, Ser-A-Gen, Ser-Ap-Es, Serathide, Serpazide, Tri-Hydroserpine, Unipres: reserpine 0.1 mg with hydralazine HCl 25 mg, hydrochlothiazide 15 mg
Children's Hold 4 Hour: dextro-

methorphan hydrobromide 3.75 mg with phenylpropanolamine HCl 6.25 mg
Chlorofon-F, Chlorzone Forte, Paracet Forte, Parafon Forte, Zoxaphen: chlorzoxazone 250 mg with acetaminophen 300 mg
Chloroserp-250, Chloroserpine-250, Diupres-250: reserpine 0.125 mg with chlorothiazide 250 mg
Chloroserp-500, Chloropserpine-500, Diupres-500: reserpine 0.125 mg with chlorothiazide 500 mg
Clindex, Clinoxide, Clipoxide, Librax, Lidox: chlordiazepoxide HCl 5 mg with clidinium bromide 2.5 mg
Co-Gesic, Damacet-P, Duradyne, Hy-Phen, Norcet, Vicodin: hydrocodone bitartrate 5 mg with acetaminophen 500 mg
Codalan No. 1: acetaminophen 500 mg with caffeine 30 mg, codeine phosphate 8 mg
Codalan No. 2: acetaminophen 500 mg with caffeine 30 mg, codeine phosphate 15 mg
Codalan No. 3: acetaminophen 500 mg with caffeine 30 mg, codeine phosphate 30 mg
Codoxy, Percodan, Roxiprin: oxycodone HCl 4.5 mg, oxycodone terephthalate 0.38 mg with aspirin 325 mg
Combipres 0.1 mg: clonidine HCl 0.1 mg with chlorthalidone 15 mg
Combipres 0.2 mg: clonidine HCl 0.2 mg with chlorthalidone 15 mg
Comtrex: dextromethorphan hydrobromide 10 mg with acetaminophen 325 mg, chlorpheniramine maleate 2 mg, phenylpropanolamine hydrochloride 12.5 mg
Comtrex: dextromethorphan hydrobromide 3.3 mg/5 ml with acetaminophen 108.3 mg/5 ml, chlorpheniramine maleate 0.67 mg/5 ml, phenylpropanolamine HCl 4.2 mg/5 ml
Conar: dextromethorphan hydrobromide 15 mg with acetaminophen 300 mg, guaifenesin 100 mg, phenylephrine HCl 10 mg
Conar Expectorant: dextromethorphan hydrobromide 15 mg/5 ml with guaifenesin 100 mg/5 ml, phenylephrine HCl 10 mg/5 ml
Conar Syrup: dextromethorphan hydrobromide 15 mg/5 ml with phenylephrine HCl 10 mg/5 ml
Congespirin: phenylpropanolamine HCl 6.25 mg/5 ml with acetaminophen 130 mg/5 ml
Congespirin, Aspirin-Free: acetaminophen 81 mg with phenylephrine HCl 81 mg
Contac Jr.: dextromethorphan hydrobromide 5 mg/5 ml with acetaminophen 160 mg/5 ml, pseudoephedrine HCl 15 mg/5 ml
Contac Severe Cold Formula, Nyquil Nighttime Cold Medicine, Nytime Cold Medicine, Quiet Nite: dextromethorphan hydrobromide 5 mg/5 ml with acetaminophen 167 mg/5 ml, doxylamine succinate 1.25 mg/5 ml, pseudoephedrine HCl 10 mg/5 ml
Copavin Pulvules: codeine sulfate 15 mg with papaverine HCl 15 mg
Corzide 40/5: bendroflumethiazide 5 mg with nadolol 40 mg
Corzide 80/5: bendroflumethiazide 5 mg with nadolol 80 mg
CoTylenol: dextromethorphan hydrobromide 5 mg/5 ml with acetaminophen 108.3 mg/5 ml, chlorpheniramine maleate 0.67

mg/5 ml, pseudoephedrine HCl 10 mg/5 ml

CoTylenol Cold Medication Tablets: dextromethorphan hydrobromide 15 mg with acetaminophen 325 mg, chlorpheniramine maleate 2 mg, pseudoephedrine HCl 30 mg

Cremacoat 3: dextromethorphan hydrobromide 6.7 mg/5 ml with guaifenesin 66.7 mg/5 ml, phenylpropanolamine HCl 12.5 mg/5 ml

Cremacoat 4: dextromethorphan hydrobromide 6.7 mg/5 ml with doxylamine succinate 2.5 mg/5 ml, phenylpropanolamine HCl 12.5 mg/5 ml

Cyclomydril Ophthalmic: cyclopentolate HCl 0.2%, phenylephrine HCl 1%

Cystex: methenamine 165 mg, salicylamide 65 mg, sodium salicylate 97 mg, benzoic acid 32 mg

Damason-P: hydrocodone bitartrate 5 mg with aspirin 224 mg, caffeine 32 mg

Darvocet-N 50, Propoxyphene Napsylate with Acetaminophen Tablets: acetaminophen 325 mg with propoxyphene napsylate 50 mg

Darvocet-N 100, Doxapap-N, Propacet 100: propoxyphene napsylate 100 mg with acetaminophen 650 mg

Darvon Compound Pulvules: aspirin 389 mg with caffeine 32.4 mg propoxyphene HCl 32 mg

Darvon Compound-65 Pulvules, Dolene Compound-65, SK-65-Compound: aspirin 389 mg with caffeine 32.4 mg, propoxyphene HCl 65 mg

Darvon with A.S.A. Pulvules: aspirin 325 mg with propoxyphene HCl 65 mg

Darvon-N and A.S.A.: aspirin 325 mg with propoxyphene napsylate 100 mg

Decadron with Xylocaine: dexamethasone PO_4 4 mg, lidocaine HCl 10 mg/ml

Demerol APAP: acetaminophen 300 mg with meperidine HCl 50 mg

Demi-Regroton: chlorthalidone 25 mg with reserpine 0.125 mg

Deprol: meprobamate 400 mg with benactyzine HCl 1 mg

Dihydrocodeine Compound Modified, Synalgos: aspirin 356.4 mg with caffeine 30 mg and dihydrocodeine bitartrate 16 mg

Dilantin with Phenobarbital: phenytoin sodium 100 mg, phenobarbital 32 mg

Dilantin with Phenobarbital: phenobarbital 16 mg, phenytoin sodium 100 mg

Dimetane-DX Cough Syrup: dextromethorphan hydrobromide 10 mg/5 ml with brompheniramine maleate 2 mg/5 ml, pseudoephedrine HCl 30 mg/5 ml

Dimycor: pentaerythritol tetranitrate 10 mg, phenobarbital 15 mg

Diupres-250: chlorothiazide 250 mg, reserpine 0.125 mg

Diupres-500: chlorothiazide 500 mg, reserpine 0.125 mg

Diurese, Matatensin No. 4, Trichlormethiazide with Reserpine Tablets, Trichlortensin: trichlormethiazide 4 mg with reserpine 0.1 mg

Diutensen: methyclothiazide 2.5 mg with cryptenamine tannates 2 mg (of cryptenamine)

Diutensen: reserpine 0.1 mg with methyclothiazide 2.5 mg

Diutensin-R: methyclothiazide 25 mg with reserpine 0.1 mg

Dolene AP-65: acetaminophen 650 mg with propoxyphene HCl 65 mg
Donnagel-PG: powdered opium 24 mg, Kaolin 6 g, pectin 142.8 mg, hyoscyamine SO_4 0.1037 mg, atropine SO_4 0.0194 mg, scopolamine hydrobromide 0.0065 mg, alcohol 5%/30 ml susp
Donnagel Suspension: Kaolin 6 g, pectin 142.8 mg, hyoscyamine SO_4 0.1037 mg, atropine SO_4 0.0194 mg, scopolamine hydrobromide 0.0065 mg, alcohol 3.8%/30 ml susp
Donnatal: belladonna alkaloids atropine sulfate 0.0194 mg, hyoscyamine sulfate 0.1037 mg, phenobarbital 32.4 mg, scopolamine hydrobromide 0.0065 mg
Donnatal Elixir, Hyosophen Elixir: belladonna alkaloids atropine sulfate 0.0194 mg/5 ml, hyoscyamine sulfate 0.1037 mg/5 ml, phenobarbital 16.2 mg/5 ml, descopolamine hydrobromide 0.0065/5 ml
Donnatal Extentabs: belladonna alkaloids atropine sulfate 0.0582 mg, hyoscyamine sulfate 0.3111 mg, phenobarbital 48.6 mg, scopolamine hydrobromide 0.0195 mg
Donnatal, Hyosophen: belladonna alkaloids atropine sulfate 0.0194 mg, hyoscyamine sulfate 0.1037 mg, phenobarbital 16.2 mg, scopolamine hydrobromide 0.0065 mg
Dorcol Children's Cough Syrup: dextromethorphan hydrobromide 5 mg/5 ml with guaifenesin 50 mg/5 ml, pseudoephedrine HCl 15 mg/5 ml
DUO-Medihaler: isoproterenol HCl 160 μg/metered spray with phenylephrine bitartrate 240 μg/metered spray
Dyazide: hydrochlorothiazide 25 mg with triamterene 50 mg
E-Pilo: epinephrine bitartrate 1%, pilocarpine HCl 1%, 2%, 3%, 4%, 6%
Empirin with Codeine 15 mg No. 2: codeine 15 mg with aspirin 325 mg
Empirin with Codeine 60 mg No. 4: aspirin 325 mg with codeine phosphate 60 mg
Empracet with Codeine Phosphate 60 mg No. 4, Tylenol with Codeine No. 4: acetaminophen 300 mg with codeine phosphate 60 mg
Endecon, Phenapap No. 2: phenylpropanolamine HCl 25 mg with acetaminophen 325 mg
Enduronyl-Forte, Eserdine Forte, Methyclothiazide and Deserpidine Tablets 5 mg/0.5 mg, Methy-Deserpidine Forte, Methy-Deserpidine Strong: methyclothiazide 5 mg with deserpidine 0.5 mg
Enduronyl, Eserdine, Methychlothiazide, Deserpidine Tablets 5 mg/0.25 mg: deserpidine 0.25 mg with methychlothiazide 5 mg
Entex: guaifenesin 200 mg with phenylephrine HCl 5 mg with phenylpropanolamine HCl 45 mg
Entex LA: guaifenesin 400 mg with phenylpropanolamine HCl 75 mg
Epromate, Equagesic, Equazine-M, Hepto-M, Mepro Compound, Meprogesic, Micranin: meprobamate 200 mg with aspirin 325 mg
Equagesic, Equazine-M, Mepro-Analgesic, Mepor Compound, Micrainin: aspirin 325 mg with meprobamate 200 mg

Ergocaff: ergotamine tartrate 1 mg, caffeine 100 mg
Esgic, Fioricet: acetaminophen 325 mg with butalbital 50 mg, caffeine 40 mg
Esimil: guanethidine monosulfate 10 mg (equivalent to guanethidine sulfate 8.4 mg) with hydrochlorothiazide 25 mg
Estratest: esterified estrogens 1.25 mg, methyltestosterone 2.5 mg
Estratest HS: esterified estrogens 0.625 mg, methyltestosterone 1.25 mg
Etrafon 2-10: perphenazine 2 mg, amitriptyline HCl 10 mg
Etrafon: perphenazine 2 mg, amitriptyline HCl 10 mg
Etrafon-A: perphenazine 4 mg, amitriptyline HCl 10 mg
Etrafon-Forte: perphenazine 4 mg, amitriptyline HCl 25 mg
Euthroid-½: levothyroxine sodium 30 μg, liothyronine sodium 7.5 μg
Euthroid-1: levothyroxine sodium 60 μg, liothyronine sodium 15 μg
Euthroid-2: levothyroxine sodium 120 μg, liothyronine sodium 30 μg
Euthroid-3: levothyroxine sodium 180 μg, liothyronine sodium 45 μg
Eutron Filmtab: pargyline HCl 25 mg with methyclothiazide 5 mg
Excedrin: acetaminophen 194 mg with aspirin 227 mg, caffeine 33 mg, buffers
Excedrin: aspirin 250 mg with acetaminophen 250 mg, caffeine 65 mg
Excedrin P.M.: acetaminophen 500 mg with diphenhydramine citrate 38 mg
Exna-R Tablets: benzthiazide 50 mg, reserpine 0.125 mg
Femguard, Sulfa-Gyn, Sultrin, Sulfa, Trysul: miscellaneous sulfonamide-sulfonamide sulfabenzamide 3.7%, sulfacetamide 2.85%, sulfiazole 3.42%, and urea 0.64%
Fermalox: ferrous SO_4 200 mg, magnesium hydroxide, dried aluminum hydroxide gel 200 mg
Ferocyl: iron (fumarate) 50 mg, docusate sodium 100 mg
Ferro-Sequels: iron (fumarate) 50 mg, docusate sodium 100 mg
Fiorinal: aspirin 325 mg with butalbital 50 mg, caffeine 40 mg
Fiorinal with Codeine No. 1: aspirin 325 mg with butalbital 50 mg, caffeine 40 mg, codeine phosphate 7.5 mg
Fiorinal with Codeine No. 2: aspirin 325 mg with butalbital 50 mg, caffeine 40 mg, and codeine phosphate 15 mg
Fiorinal with Codeine No. 3: aspirin 325 mg with butalbital 50 mg, caffeine 40 mg, codeine phosphate 30 mg
Gemnisyn: acetaminophen 325 mg with aspirin 325 mg
Hexalol: methenamine 40.8 mg, phenyl salicylate 18.1 mg, atropine SO_4 0.03, hyoscyamine 0.03 mg, benzoic acid 4.5 mg, methylene blue 5.4 mg
Hybephen: belladonna alkaloids atropine sulfate 0.0233 mg, hyoscyamine sulfate 0.1277 mg, phenobarbital 15 mg, scopolamine hydrobromide 0.0094 mg
Hydergine: dihydroergocorine mesylate 0.167 mg
Hydrogesic: hydrocodone bitartrate 7.5 mg with acetaminophen 650 mg
Hydromox R: quinethazone 50 mg with reserpine 0.125 mg
Hydropres-25, Hydro-Reserpine-

25, Hydroserp, Hydroserpine No. 1, Hydrosine 25 mg, Mallopress: reserpine 0.125 mg with hydrochlorothiazide 25 mg
Hydropres-50, Hydro-Reserpine-50, Hydroserp, Hydroserpine No. 2, Hydrosine 50 mg, Hydrotensin, Hydroserpalan: reserpine 0.125 mg with hydrochlorothiazide 50 mg
Inderide 40/25, Propranolol HCl, Hydrochlorothiazide Tablets 40/25: propranolol HCl 40 mg with hydrochlorothiazide 25 mg
Inderide 80/25, Propranolol HCl, Hydrochlorothiazide Tablets 80/25: propranolol HCl 80 mg with hydrochlorothiazide 25 mg
Inderide LA 80/50: propranolol HCl 80 mg with hydrochlorothiazide 50 mg
INH: isoniazid 1 tablet, isoniazid 300 mg
Iophen DM, Tussi-Organidin DM: dextromethorphan hydrobromide 10 mg/5 ml with iodinated glycerol 30 mg/5 ml
Isoptop-ES: pilocarpine HCl 2%, physostigmine salicylate 0.25%
Kinesed: belladonna alkaloids atropine sulfate 0.02 mg, hyoscyamine sulfate 0.12 mg, phenobarbital 16 mg, scopolamine hydrobromide 0.007 mg
Levsin with Phenobarbital Tablets, Anaspaz: hyoscyamine sulfate 0.125 mg with phenobarbital
Levsinex with Phenobarbital Elixir: hyoscyamine sulfate 0.125 mg/5 ml with phenobarbital 15 mg/5 ml
Levsinex with Phenobarbital Time-caps: hyoscyamine sulfate 0.375 mg with phenobarbital 45 mg
Levsin-PB: hyoscyamine sulfate 0.125 mg/ml with phenobarbital 15 mg/ml
Librax: chlordiazepoxide HCl 5 mg, clidinium bromide 2.5 mg
Limbitrol 5-12.5: chlordiazepoxide 5 mg, amitriptyline HCl 12.5 mg
Limbitrol 10-25: chlordiazepoxide 10 mg, amitriptyline HCl 25 mg
Lobac: chlorzoxazone 250 mg, acetaminophen 300 mg
Lopressor HCT 50/25: metoprolol tartrate 50 mg with hydrochlorothiazide 25 mg
Lopressor HCT 100/25: metoprolol tartrate 100 mg with hydrochlorothiazide 25 mg
M-KYA, Q-VEL: quinine SO_4 64.8 mg, vit. E. 400 U, lecithin
Maxzide: hydrochlorothiazide 50 mg with triamterene 75 mg
Mediqueall: dextromethorphan hydrobromide 15 mg with pseudoephedrine HCl 30 mg
Menrium 5-2: chlordiazepoxide 5 mg with esterified estrogens 0.2 mg
Menrium 5-4: chlordiazepoxide 5 mg with esterified estrogens 0.4 mg
Menrium 10-4: chlordiazepoxide 10 mg with esterified estrogens 0.4 mg
Mepergan: meperidine HCl 25 mg/ml with promethazine HCl 25 mg/ml
Mepergan Fortis: meperidine HCl 50 mg with promethazine HCl 25 mg
Metatensin No. 2: reserpine 0.1 mg with trichlormethiazide 2 mg
Midol Caplets: aspirin 454 mg with caffeine 32.4 mg, cinnamedrine HCl 14.9 mg
Midol PMS Caplets: acetamino-

phen 500 mg with pamabrom 25 mg, pyrilamine maleate 15 mg
Migral: ergotamine tartrate 1 mg, caffeine 50 mg, cyclizine HCl 25 mg
Milprem-200, PMB 200: meprobamate 200 mg with conjugated estrogens 0.45 mg
Milprem-400, PMB 400: meprobamate 400 mg with conjugated estrogens 0.45 mg
Minizide 1: prazosin HCl 1 mg (of prazosin) with polythiazide 0.5 mg
Minizide 2: prazosin HCl 2 mg (of prazosin) with polythiazide 0.5 mg
Minizide 5: prazosin HCl 5 mg (of prazosin) with polythiazide 0.5 mg
Mixtard injection: 100 mg/ml isophane purified pork insulin susp, purified pork insulin inj
Moduretic: amiloride HCl 5 mg, hydrochlorothiazide 50 mg
Morphine, Atropine Sulfate Injection: morphine sulfate 16 mg/ml with atropine sulfate 0.4 mg/ml
Murocoll-2: scopolamine hydrobromide 0.3%, phenylephrine hydrochloride 10%
Mus-Lax: chlorzoxazone 250 mg, acetaminophen 300 mg
Myapap with Codeine, Tylenol with Codeine: acetaminophen 120 mg/5 ml with codeine phosphate 12 mg/5 ml
Mysteclin F: amphotericin B 25 mg/5 ml with tetracycline equivalent to tetracycline HCl 25 mg/5 ml
Mysteclin-F: amphotericin B 50 mg with tetracycline equivalent to tetracycline HCl 250 mg
Mysteclin-F: tetracycline equivalent to 125 mg tetracycline HCl per 5 ml with amphotericin B 25 mg/5 ml
Mysteclin-F: tetracycline equivalent to 350 mg tetracycline HCl with amphotericin B 50 mg/5 ml
Mysteclin-F Syrup: tetracycline equivalent to 125 mg tetracycline HCl per 5 ml with amphotericin B 25 mg/5 ml
Naldecon-DX Adult: dextromethorphan hydrobromide 15 mg/5 ml with guaifenesin 200 mg/5 ml, phenylpropanolamine HCl 18 mg/5 ml
Naldecon-DX Children's Syrup: dextromethorphan hydrobromide 7.5 mg/5 ml with guaifenesin 100 mg/5 ml, phenylpropanolamine HCl 9 mg/5 ml
Naldegisic: acetaminophen 325 mg with pseudoephedrine HCl 15 mg
Naquival: trichlormethiazide 4 mg, reserpine 0.1 mg
Naturetin with K 2.5, mg: bendroflumethiazide 2.5, potassium chloride 500 mg
Naturetin with K 5 mg: bendroflumethiazide 5 mg with potassium chloride 500 mg
Neosporin G.U. Irrigant: polymyxin B sulfate 200,000 units (of polymyxin B)
Nitrotym-Plus: nitroglycerin 2.5 mg, butabarbital 48 mg
Norgesic: orphenadrine citrate 25 mg, aspirin 385 mg, caffeine 30 mg
Norgesic Forte: orphenadrine citrate 50 mg, aspirin 770 mg, caffeine 60 mg
Normozide 100/25: labetalol hydrochloride 100 mg, hydrochlorothiazide 25 mg
Normozide 200/25: labetalol hydrochloride 200 mg, hydrochlorothiazide 25 mg
Normozide 300/25: labetalol hy-

drochloride 300 mg, hydrochlorothiazide 25 mg
Novahistine Cough and Cold Formula: dextromethorphan hydrobromide 10 mg/5 ml with chlorpheniramine maleate 2 mg/5 ml, pseudoephedrine HCl 30 mg/5 ml
Opium and Belladonna: powdered opium 60 mg with belladonna extract 15 mg (equivalent to belladonna alkaloids 0.2 mg)
Oreticyl 25: deserpidine 0.125 mg with hydrochlorothiazide 25 mg
Oreticyl 50: deserpidine 0.125 mg with hydrochlorothiazide 50 mg
Oreticyl Forte: deserpidine 0.25 mg with hydrochlorothiazide 50 mg
Ornex: phenylpropanolamine HCl 12.5 mg with acetaminophen 325 mg
Orthoxicol Cough Syrup: dextromethorphan hydrobromide 10 mg/5 ml with methoxyphenamine HCl 17 mg/5 ml
Oxymycin, Terramycin Intramuscular Solution: oxytetracycline 50 mg/ml with lidocaine 2%
Pamprin: acetaminophen 325 mg with pamabrom 25 mg, pyrilamine maleate 12.5 mg
Pamprin Maximum Cramp Relief: acetaminophen 500 mg with pamabrom 25 mg, pyrilamine maleate 15 mg
Paracet Forte: chlorzoxazone 250 mg, acetaminophen 300 mg
Parepectolin: opium 15 mg, kaolin 5.85 g, pectin 162 mg, alcohol 0.69%/30 ml susp
Pathibamate-200: meprobamate 200 mg with tridihexethyl chloride 25 mg
Pathibamate-400: meprobamate 400 mg with tridihexethyl chloride 25 mg
Pediazole: erythromycin ethlysuccinate 200 mg (of erythromycin) per 5 ml with sulfisoxazole acetyl 600 mg (of sulfisoxazole) per 5 ml
Penntuss: codeine polistirex equivalent to codeine 10 mg/5 ml with chlorpheniramine polistirex equivalent to chlorpheniramine maleate 4 mg/5 ml
Perbuzem: pentaerythritol tetranitrate 10 mg, butabarbital 15 mg
Percodan-Demi: aspirin 325 mg with oxycodone HCl 2.25 mg, oxycodone terephthalate 0.19 mg
Percogesic: acetaminophen 325 mg with phenyltoloxamine citrate 30 mg
Peri-Colace: docusate sodium 100 mg with cusanthranol 30 mg
Persistin: salsalate 487.5 mg with aspirin 162.5 mg
Phenaphen with Codeine No. 2: acetaminophen 325 mg with codeine phosphate 15 mg
Phenaphen with Codeine No. 2, Proval No. 3: codeine 30 mg with acetaminophen 325 mg
Phenaphen with Codeine No. 3, Proval No. 2: acetaminophen 325 mg with codeine phosphate 30 mg
Phenaphen with Codeine No. 4: acetaminophen 325 mg with codeine phosphate 60 mg
Phenaphen-650 with Codeine: acetaminophen 650 mg with codeine phosphate 30 mg
Phenergan: promethazine HCl 6.25 mg/5 ml with phenylephrine HCl 5 mg/5 ml
Phenergan-D: promethazine HCl 6.25 mg with pseudoephedrine HCl 60 mg
Phenergan VC Syrup, Promethazine HCl VC: promethazine

HCl 6.25 mg/5 ml with phenylephrine HCl 5 mg/5 ml
Phenergan with Dextromethorphan: dextromethorphan hydrobromide 15 mg/5 ml with promethazine HCl 6.35 mg/5 ml
Phrenilin: acetaminophen 325 mg with butalbital 50 mg, caffeine 40 mg
Phrenilin Forte: acetaminophen 650 mg, butalbital 50 mg
Phrenilin with Codeine No. 3: acetaminophen 325 mg, butalbital 50 mg, codeine phosphate 30 mg
Polycillin-PRB: ampicillin trihydrate 3.5 g with probenecid 1 g
Polyflex: chlorzoxazone 250 mg, acetaminophen 300 mg
Propoxyphene HCl/65, Wygesic: acetaminophen 650 mg, propoxyphene HCl 65 mg
Principen with Probenecid: ampicillin trihydrate 3.5 g with probenecid 1 g
Prunicodeine: terpin hydrate 29 mg/5 ml, codeine sulfate 10 mg/5 ml
Rautrax: rauwolfia 50 mg, flumethiazide 400 mg, potassium chloride 400 mg
Rautrax-N: bendroflumethiazide 4 mg, rauwolfia serpentina 50 mg, potassium chloride 400 mg
Rauzide: bendroflumethiazide 4 mg, rauwolfia serpentina 50 mg
Regroton: reserpine 0.25 mg, chlorthalidone 50 mg
Renese-R: reserpine 0.25 mg, polythiazide 2 mg
Rifamate: isoniazid 150 mg with rifampin 300 mg
Rimactane: isoniazid 2 capsules, rifampin 300 mg
Rimactane: rifampin 1 tablet, isoniazid 300 mg
Rimactane: rifampin 2 capsules, rifampin 300 mg
Robaxisal, Robomol/ASA: methocarbamol 400 mg, aspirin 325 mg
Robitussin-DM: dextromethorphan hydrobromide 15 mg/5 ml, guaifenesin 100 mg/5 ml
Roxicet: oxycodone HCl 5 mg/5 ml, acetaminophen 325 mg/5 ml
S-A-C: salicylamide 230 mg, acetaminophen 150 mg, caffeine 30 mg
Salimeth Forte: salicylamide 600 mg, acetaminophen 250 mg
S.B.P.: secobarbital sodium 50 mg, butabarbital sodium 30 mg, phenobarbital 15 mg
Ser-a-Gen: hydrochlorothiazide 15 mg, hydralazine hydrochloride 25 mg, resepine 0.1 mg
Serpasil-Apresoline HCl No. 1: hydralazine HCl 25 mg, reserpine 0.1 mg
Serpasil-Apresoline HCl No. 2: hydralazine HCl 25 mg, reserpine 0.2 mg
Serpasil-Esidrix No. 1: reserpine 0.1 mg, hydrochlorothiazide 25 mg
Serpasil-Esidrix No. 2: reserpine 0.1 mg, hydrochlorothiazide 50 mg
Simron: iron (gluconate) 10 mg, polysorbate 20, 400 mg
Sine-Aid: acetaminophen 325 mg, pseudoephedrine HCl 30 mg
Sine-Aid Extra Strength Caplets, Tylenol Sinus Maximum Strength Caplets: acetaminophen 500 mg, pseudoephedrine HCl 30 mg
Sine-Off Extra Strength, Sinutab: acetaminophen 500 mg, pseudoephedrine HCl 30 mg
Sinubid: acetaminophen 600 mg, phenylpropanolamine HCl 100 mg, phenyltoloxamine citrate 66 mg
Sinutab Maximum Nighttime:

acetaminophen 167 mg/5 ml, diphenhydramine HCl
8.3 mg/5 ml, pseudoephedrine HCl 10 mg/5 ml
Sinutab II Maximum, Tylenol maximum strength sinus: acetaminophen 500 mg, pseudoephedrine HCl 30 mg
SK-APAP with Codeine, Tylenol with Codeine No. 2: codeine 5 mg with acetaminophen 300 mg
Skelez: chlorzoxazone 250 mg, acetaminophen 300 mg
Soma Compound: carisoprodol 200 mg, aspirin 325 mg
Soma Compound with Codeine: codeine 16 mg, aspirin 325 mg, carisoprodol 200 mg
Spec-T: Phenylpropanolamine 10.5 mg with Benzocaine 10 mg, Phenylephrine HCl 5 mg
Spec-T Sore Throat Cough Suppressant: dextromethorphan hydrobromide 10 mg with benzocaine 10 mg
Spironazide: spironolactone 25 mg, hydrochlorothiazide 25 mg
Spirozide: spironolactone 25 mg, hydrochlorothiazide 25 mg
Sudafed Cough Syrup: dextromethorphan hydrobromide 5 mg/5 ml with guaifenesin 100 mg/5 ml, pseudoephedrine HCl 15 mg/5 ml
Sultrin: miscellaneous sulfonamide-sulfonamide sulfabenzamide 184 mg, sulfacetamide 143.75 mg, sulfathiazole 172.5 mg, urea 31.83 mg
Talacen: pentazocine HCl 25 mg (of pentazocine) with acetaminophen 650 mg
Talwin Compound Caplets: aspirin 325 mg with pentazocine HCl 12.5 mg (of pentazocine)
Tenoretic 50: atenolol 50 mg with chlorthalidone 25 mg
Tenoretic 100: atenolol 100 mg with chlorthalidone 25 mg
Terpin Hydrate and Codeine: terpin hydrate 85 mg/5 ml with dextromethorphan hydrobromide 10 mg/5 ml (with alcohol 39%-44%)
Terramycin Intramuscular Solution: oxytetracycline 125 mg/ml with lidocaine 2%
T-Gesic: hydrocodone bitartrate 5 mg with acetaminophen 325 mg, butalbital 30 mg, caffeine 40 mg
Thiacide: methenamine mandelate 500 mg, potassium acid phosphate 250 mg
Thyrolar-¼: levothyroxine sodium 12.5 mg, liothyronine sodium 3.1 μg
Thyrolar-½: levothyroxine sodium 25 μg, liothyronine sodium 6.25 μg
Thyrolar-1: levothyroxine sodium 50 μg, liothyronine sodium 12.5 μg
Thyrolar-2: levothyroxine sodium 100 μg, liothyronine sodium 25 μg
Thyrolar-3: levothyroxine sodium 150 μg, liothyronine sodium 37.5 μg
Timentin Inj: ticarcillin disodium 3 g with clavulanate potassium 100 mg
Timolide 10/25: timolol maleate 10 mg with hydrochlorothiazide 25 mg
TracTabs 2X: methenamine 120 mg, methylene blue 6 mg, phenyl salicylate 30 mg, atropine 0.06, hyoscyamine SO_4 0.03 mg, benzoic acid 7.5 mg
Trendar: acetaminophen 325 mg with pamabrom 25 mg
Triaminic-DM Cough Formula: dextromethorphan hydrobromide 10 mg/5 ml with phenylpropanolamine HCl 12.5 mg/5 ml

Triaminicol: dextromethorphan hydrobromide 10 mg/5 ml with chlorpheniramine maleate 2 mg/5 ml, phenylpropanolamine HCl 12.5 mg/5 ml
Triavil 2-10, Triavil 4-10, Triavil 2-25, Triavil 4-25 (see Etrafon—same products)
Triavil 4-50: perphenazine 4 mg, amitriptyline HCl 50 mg
Tri-Barb Capsules: phenobarbital 32 mg, butabarbital sodium 32 mg, secobarbital sodium 32 mg
Trigesic: aspirin 230 mg with acetaminophen 125 mg, caffeine 30 mg
Triple Sulfa: sulfadiazine 167 mg, sulfamerazine 167 mg, sulfamethazine 167 mg
Tuinal 200 mg Pulvules: secobarbital sodium 100 mg with amobarbital sodium 100 mg
Tylenol with Codeine No. 1: acetaminophen 300 mg with codeine phosphate 7.5 mg
Tylenol with Codeine No. 2: acetaminophen 300 mg with codeine phosphate 15 mg
Tylenol with Codeine No. 3: acetaminophen 300 mg with codeine phosphate 30 mg
Tylenol with Codeine No. 4: acetaminophen 300 mg with codeine phosphate 60 mg
Tylox: acetaminophen 500 mg with oxycodone HCl 5 mg
Unasyn Inj: ampicillin sodium 1 g with sulbactam sodium 500 mg; ampicillin sodium 2 g with sulbactam sodium 1 g
Unipres: hydrochlorothiazide 15 mg, reserpine 0.1 mg, hydralazine hydrochloride 25 mg
Urisedamine: methenamine mandelate 500 mg, hyoscyamine 0.15 mg
Urobiotic-250: oxytetracycline HCl 250 mg (of oxytetracycline) with phenazopyridine HCl 50 mg, sulfamethizole 250 mg
Uroquid-Acid No. 2: methenamine mandelate 500 mg, sodium acid phosphate 500 mg
Vanquish Caplets: aspirin 227 mg with acetaminophen 194 mg, caffeine 30 mg, buffers
Vaseretic: enalapril maleate 10 mg with hydrochlorothiazide 25 mg
Vicks Childrens Cough Syrup: dextromethorphan hydrobromide 3.5 mg/5 ml with guaifenesin 25 mg/5 ml
Vicks Cough Silencers: dextromethorphan hydrobromide 2.5 mg with benzocaine 1 mg
Vicks Daycare: dextromethorphan hydrobromide 10 mg with acetaminophen 325 mg, guaifenesin 100 mg, pseudoephedrine HCl 30 mg
Vicks Daycare: dextromethorphan hydrobromide 3.3 mg/5 ml with acetaminophen 108.3 mg/5 ml, guaifenesin 33.3 mg/5 ml, pseudoephedrine HCl 10 mg/5 ml
Vicks Formula 44 Cough Control Discs: dextromethorphan hydrobromide 5 mg with benzocaine 1.25 mg
Vicks Formula 44 Cough Mixture: dextromethorphan hydrobromide 15 mg/ 5 ml with doxylamine succinate 3.75 mg/5 ml
Vicks Formula 44D: dextromethorphan hydrobromide 10 mg/5 ml with guaifenesin 66.7 mg/5 ml, pseudoephedrine HCl 20 mg/5 ml
Vicks Formula 44M: dextromethorphan hydrobromide 7.4 mg/5 ml with acetaminophen 125 mg/5 ml, guaifenesin 50 mg/5

ml, pseudoephedrine HCl 15 mg/5 ml

Wigraine: ergotamine tartrate 1 mg, caffeine 100 mg, levorotatory belladonna alkaloids 0.1 mg, phenacetin 130 mg

Wigraine Suppositories: ergotamine tartrate 2 mg, caffeine 100 mg, tartaric acid 21.5 mg

Wyanoids: belladonna extract 15 mg (0.19 mg of alkaloids of belladonna leaf) with ephedrine 3 mg

Zoxaphen: chlorzoxazone 250 mg, acetaminophen 300 mg

Ziradyl: diphenhydramine HCl 2% with zinc oxide 2%

Index

Entries can be identified as follows: generic name, Trade Name, DRUG CATEGORY, *Combination Product*.

Entries can be identified as follows: generic name, Trade Name, DRUG CATEGORY, *Combination Product*.

Entries can be identified as follows: generic name, Trade Name, DRUG CATEGORY, *Combination Product*.

Entries can be identified as follows: generic name, Trade Name, DRUG CATEGORY, *Combination Product*.

Entries can be identified as follows: generic name, Trade Name, DRUG CATEGORY, *Combination Product*.

C

Entries can be identified as follows: generic name, Trade Name, DRUG CATEGORY, *Combination Product*.

INDEX

Entries can be identified as follows: generic name, Trade Name, DRUG CATEGORY, *Combination Product*.

Entries can be identified as follows: generic name, Trade Name, DRUG CATEGORY, *Combination Product*.

Entries can be identified as follows: generic name, Trade Name, DRUG CATEGORY, *Combination Product*.

Entries can be identified as follows: generic name, Trade Name, DRUG CATEGORY, *Combination Product*.

Entries can be identified as follows: generic name, Trade Name, DRUG CATEGORY, *Combination Product*.

Entries can be identified as follows: generic name, Trade Name, DRUG CATEGORY, *Combination Product*.

Entries can be identified as follows: generic name, Trade Name, DRUG CATEGORY, *Combination Product*.

Entries can be identified as follows: generic name, Trade Name, DRUG CATEGORY, *Combination Product*.

Entries can be identified as follows: generic name, Trade Name, DRUG CATEGORY, *Combination Product*.

Entries can be identified as follows: generic name, Trade Name, DRUG CATEGORY, *Combination Product*.

INDEX

Entries can be identified as follows: generic name, Trade Name, DRUG CATEGORY, *Combination Product*.

J

K

L

Entries can be identified as follows: generic name, Trade Name, DRUG CATEGORY. *Combination Product*.

INDEX

Entries can be identified as follows: generic name, Trade Name, DRUG CATEGORY, *Combination Product*.

Entries can be identified as follows: generic name, Trade Name, DRUG CATEGORY, *Combination Product*.

Entries can be identified as follows: generic name, Trade Name, DRUG CATEGORY, *Combination Product*.

Entries can be identified as follows: generic name, Trade Name, DRUG CATEGORY, *Combination Product*.

Entries can be identified as follows: generic name, Trade Name, DRUG CATEGORY, *Combination Product*.

O

P

Entries can be identified as follows: generic name, Trade Name, DRUG CATEGORY, *Combination Product*.

Entries can be identified as follows: generic name, Trade Name, DRUG CATEGORY, *Combination Product*.

INDEX

Entries can be identified as follows: generic name, Trade Name, DRUG CATEGORY, *Combination Product*.

Entries can be identified as follows: generic name, Trade Name, DRUG CATEGORY, *Combination Product*.

Q

R

Entries can be identified as follows: generic name, Trade Name, DRUG CATEGORY, *Combination Product*.

S

Entries can be identified as follows: generic name, Trade Name, DRUG CATEGORY, *Combination Product*.

Entries can be identified as follows: generic name, Trade Name, DRUG CATEGORY, *Combination Product*.

T

Entries can be identified as follows: generic name, Trade Name, DRUG CATEGORY, *Combination Product*.

Entries can be identified as follows: generic name, Trade Name, DRUG CATEGORY, *Combination Product*.

Entries can be identified as follows: generic name, Trade Name, DRUG CATEGORY, *Combination Product*.

U

Entries can be identified as follows: generic name, Trade Name, DRUG CATEGORY, *Combination Product*.

Entries can be identified as follows: generic name, Trade Name, DRUG CATEGORY, *Combination Product*.

NOTES

NOTES

NOTES

NOTES

NOTES

NOTES

NOTES

NOTES

NOTES

NOTES

NOTES